FIRST AID
Q&A FOR THE
USMLE
STEP 2 CK

FOUNDING SENIOR EDITORS

TAO LE, MD, MHS
Assistant Clinical Professor of Medicine and Pediatrics
Chief, Section of Allergy and Immunology
Department of Medicine
University of Louisville

ANIL SHIVARAM, MD
Resident
Department of Ophthalmology
Boston University

JOSHUA KLEIN, MD, PhD
Resident
Department of Neurology
Massachusetts General Hospital
Brigham and Women's Hospital

FOUNDING EDITORS

POURYA M. GHAZI, MD
Intern
Department of Internal Medicine
San Joaquin General Hospital

JESSICA MERLIN, MD, MBA
Resident
Department of Internal Medicine
Hospital of the University of Pennsylvania

RUSSELL J. H. RYAN, MD
Resident
Department of Anatomy and Clinical Pathology
Massachusetts General Hospital

ESTEBAN SCHABELMAN, MD, MBA
Resident
Department of Emergency Medicine
University of Maryland Medical System

FLORA WAPLES, MD
Resident
Department of Emergency Medicine
University of Chicago

OMEED ZARDKOOHI, MD
Resident
Department of Internal Medicine
Massachusetts General Hospital

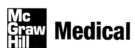 **Medical**

New York / Chicago / San Francisco / Lisbon / London / Madrid / Mexico City
Milan / New Delhi / San Juan / Seoul / Singapore / Sydney / Toronto

First Aid™ Q&A for the USMLE Step 2 CK

1 2 3 4 5 6 7 8 9 0   QPD/QPD   0 9 8 7

ISBN 978-0-07-148173-1
MHID 0-07-148173-7
ISSN 1937-3309

NOTICE

Medicine is an ever-changing science. As new research and clinical experience broaden our knowledge, changes in treatment and drug therapy are required. The authors and the publisher of this work have checked with sources believed to be reliable in their efforts to provide information that is complete and generally in accord with the standards accepted at the time of publication. However, in view of the possibility of human error or changes in medical sciences, neither the authors nor the publisher nor any other party who has been involved in the preparation or publication of this work warrants that the information contained herein is in every respect accurate or complete, and they disclaim all responsibility for any errors or omissions or for the results obtained from use of the information contained in this work. Readers are encouraged to confirm the information contained herein with other sources. For example and in particular, readers are advised to check the product information sheet included in the package of each drug they plan to administer to be certain that the information contained in this work is accurate and that changes have not been made in the recommended dose or in the contraindications for administration. This recommendation is of particular importance in connection with new or infrequently used drugs.

This book was set in Electra LH by Rainbow Graphics.
The editors were Catherine A. Johnson and Penny Linskey.
The production supervisor was Phil Galea.
Project management was provided by Rainbow Graphics.
Quebecor Dubuque was printer and binder.

This book is printed on acid-free paper.

To the contributors to this and future editions, who took time to share their knowledge, insight, and humor for the benefit of residents and clinicians.

and

To our families, friends, and loved ones, who supported us in the task of assembling this guide.

CONTENTS

FOUNDING AUTHORS

J. GEOFF ALLEN, MD
Resident
Department of Surgery
Johns Hopkins University School of Medicine

NEETI BATHIA, MD
Resident
Physical Medicine and Rehabilitation
Kessler Institute for Rehabilitation
University of Medicine and Dentistry of New Jersey

DONALD LEE BOYER, MD
Resident Physician
The Children's Hospital of Philadelphia

ARIANNE BOYLAN
Yale School of Medicine
Class of 2007

BENJAMIN BRUCKER, MD
Resident
Department of Urology
University of Pennsylvania School of Medicine

JESSICA BUCKLEY, MD
Resident
Department of Pediatrics
University of California, San Francisco

KERRY CASE, MD
Resident
Department of Family Medicine
Medical College of Wisconsin

CONNIE YOUHUA CHANG, MD
Resident
Preliminary Medicine
Lenox Hill Hospital in New York City

KIMBERLLY S. CHHOR, MD
Resident
Department of Orthopedic Surgery
Johns Hopkins School of Medicine

ALANA COHEN, MD
Resident
Department of Medicine
Columbia Presbyterian Medical Center

MELINDA COSTA, MD
Resident
Department of Plastic and Reconstructive Surgery
University of Southern California

MONYA DE, MD
University of California-Berkeley School of Public Health

STEVEN DONG, MD
Resident
Department of Urology
Thomas Jefferson University Hospital

DANIEL J. DURAND, MD
Resident
Department of Radiology
Johns Hopkins Hospital

TREVOR ELLISON, MD
Resident
Department of General Surgery
Johns Hopkins Hospital

DOUGLAS ELWOOD, MD, MBA
Resident Clinical Instructor
Department of Physical Medicine and Rehabilitation
New York University Medical Center

VICTOR IKECHUKWU ESENWA, MD
Resident
Department of Radiology
New York University Presbyterian Hospital

PAYAM FARJOODI, MD
Resident
Department of Orthopedic Surgery
Johns Hopkins Hospital

JORGE GALVEZ, MD
Resident
Department of Anesthesiology
Yale Primary Care Program
Yale University School of Medicine

JESSE A. GOLDSTEIN, MD
House Officer
Department of Plastic and Reconstructive Surgery
Georgetown University Hospital

RENU GUPTA, MD
Resident
Department of Psychiatry
University of Illinois-Chicago

ALIA HBEIB, MD
Intern
Department of General Surgery
Department of Neurological Surgery
Case Western Reserve School of Medicine

PETER W. HENDERSON, MD

Resident
Department of General Surgery
New York University Presbyterian Hospital

CHRISTINE ELIZABETH HILL, MD

University of Pennsylvania School of Medicine

STEVEN Y. HUANG, MD

University of Pennsylvania School of Medicine

DANIEL JAMIESON, MD

Resident
Department of Internal Medicine
University of Colorado

PHOEBE ESTE KOCH, MD

Resident
Department of Dermatology
Yale University School of Medicine

CINDY MAN-YAN KU, MD

Resident
Department of Anesthesiology
New York Hospital Medical Center of Queens

ERICA LEE, MD

Transitional Intern
Albert Einstein College of Medicine

JASON DAVID LEE, MD

Resident
Department of Pediatrics
Harbor-UCLA Medical Center

DAVID M. LIEBERMAN, MD

Resident
Department of Otolaryngology
Stanford University

EMILY NELSON MAHER, MD

Resident
Department of Anesthesiology, Perioperative, and Pain Medicine
Brigham and Women's Hospital

NICHOLAS MAHONEY, MD

Resident
Scheie Eye Institute

TZIVIA MOREEN, MD

Resident
Department of Internal Medicine
Weill Medical College of Cornell University

IKECHI JOHN NWANKWO, MD

Resident
Department of Radiology
St. Vincent's Hospital in New York

STEPHAN G. PILL, MD

University of Pennsylvania School of Medicine

ELEANOR PITT, MD

Resident
Department of Internal Medicine
Vanderbilt University Medical Center

HINDI E. STOHL POSY, MD

Resident
Department of Obstetrics & Gynecology
Johns Hopkins University

SIVA P. RAMAN, MD

Resident
Department of Radiology
University of Washington

AMY JOSEPHINE REED, MD

University of Pennsylvania School of Medicine

REBECCA L. RUEBNER, MD

University of Pennsylvania School of Medicine

SARAH SCHELLHORN, MD

Resident
Beth Israel Deaconess Medical Center

LINDSEY SUKAY, MD

Pediatric Resident
The Children's Hospital Denver

MATHEW A. THOMAS, MD

Resident
Department of Surgery
Massachusetts General Hospital

ASSOCIATE AUTHORS

ANNA AWDANKIEWICZ, MD

Resident
Department of Internal Medicine
Vanderbilt Medical Center

RAVI KANT BASHYAL, MD

Resident
Department of Orthopedic Surgery
Barnes-Jewish Hospital
Washington University School of Medicine

LISA McDONALD, MD

Yale University School of Medicine

PREFACE

With *First Aid Q&A for the USMLE Step 2 CK*, we continue our commitment to providing students with the most useful and up-to-date preparation guides for the USMLE Step 2 CK. This new addition to the *First Aid* series represents an outstanding effort by a talented group of authors and includes the following:

- 1,000 high-yield USMLE-style questions from the *USMLERx Qmax Step 2 CK Test Bank* (www.usmlerx.com)
- Concise yet complete explanations to correct and incorrect questions
- Organized as a perfect complement to *First Aid for the USMLE Step 2 CK*
- Eight full-length test blocks simulate the actual exam experience
- High-yield images, diagrams, and tables complement the questions and answers
- Timely updates and corrections at **www.firstaidteam.com.**

We invite you to share your thoughts and ideas to help us improve *First Aid Q&A for the USMLE Step 2 CK*. See How to Contribute, p. xv.

Louisville	Tao Le
Boston	Anil Shivaram
Boston	Joshua Klein

ACKNOWLEDGMENTS

This has been a collaborative project from the start. We gratefully acknowledge the thoughtful comments and advice of the medical students, residents, international medical graduates, and faculty who have supported the authors in the development of *First Aid Q&A for the USMLE Step 2 CK*.

We also want to thank Tawia A. Apenteng, Melissa DeJesus, Christine Dillon, William Joseph Grande, Elizabeth Sarah Hart, Tamar Mirensky, David Beck Schatz, and Alejandro Marin Spiotta for their author-level contributions to the manuscript.

Additional thanks to the following for their review of the manuscript: Andy Armstrong, Douglas Barber, Minoo Battiwalla, Charles Bergstrom, Brian Bosworth, Michael Brucculeri, Dickson Cheung, Mary Dahling, Diana Feldman, Colin Gillespie, Rachel Glaser, Shama Jari, Kenneth Katz, Amy Kelley, Kristina Kudelko, Bruce Leuchter, Sameer Nagda, Geoffrey Nguyen, Gal Omry, Jordan Orange, Alan Pao, Karen Rosenbaum, Lisa Roy, Dr. Schless, Dhwani Shah, Veronique Tache, Meredith Turetz, Karen Warburton, Christopher Warlick, Matthew Weissler, Theo Zaoutis, and April Zhu.

For support and encouragement throughout the process, we are grateful to Thao Pham, Selina Franklin, Louise Petersen, Jonathan Kirsch, and Vikas Bhushan. Thanks to our publisher, McGraw-Hill, for the valuable assistance of their staff. For enthusiasm, support, and commitment to this challenging project, thanks to our editor, Catherine Johnson. For outstanding editorial work, we thank Emma D. Underdown. A special thanks to Rainbow Graphics for remarkable production work.

Louisville	Tao Le
Boston	Anil Shivaram
Boston	Joshua Klein

SECTION I

Organ Systems

CHAPTER 1

Cardiovascular

1. A 66-year-old retired carpenter presents with chronic shortness of breath upon exertion. He has smoked a pack of cigarettes per day for the past 5 years and drinks alcohol regularly. On physical examination, a displaced point of maximal impulse and hepatosplenomegaly are noted. His medications include pantoprazole for gastroesophageal reflux and sertraline for depression. Echocardiogram reveals an ejection fraction of 30% and dilated left and right ventricles. Laboratory test results are:

Na⁻	129 mEq/L
K⁺	5.2 mEq/L
Cl⁻	101 mEq/L
Blood urea nitrogen	45 mg/dL
Creatinine	1.3 mg/dL
Glucose	134 mg/dL
Aspartate aminotransferase	220 U/L
Alanine aminotransferase	140 U/L
Alkaline phosphatase	280 U/L

Which of the following is the most likely etiology of his cardiac findings?

(A) *Borrelia burgdorferi*
(B) Cigarette smoking
(C) Coxsackie B virus
(D) Ethanol
(E) Pantoprazole toxicity
(F) *Trypanosoma cruzi*

2. A 52-year-old man presents to his primary care physician's office for routine care. He has hypertension, hypercholesterolemia, and diabetes mellitus type 2, and has smoked one pack of cigarettes per day for the past 30 years. Medications include hydrochlorothiazide, atorvastatin, and glipizide. There is a family history of myocardial infarction in the maternal grandfather at age 60. The patient has undergone screening for colon and prostate cancer. Physical examination reveals a pleasant, obese man who is 1.5 m, 22.9 cm (5 ft, 9 in) tall and weights 108 kg (238 lb). His blood pressure is 155/81 mm Hg, heart rate is 78/min, respiratory rate is 14/min, and temperature is 36.8°C (98.3°F). What one action would most reduce the patient's stroke risk?

(A) Blood glucose reduction
(B) Blood pressure reduction
(C) Serum cholesterol reduction
(D) Smoking cessation
(E) Weight loss

3. A newborn girl is evaluated in the nursery by a pediatrician. She was born 6 hours ago at 37 weeks' gestation via spontaneous vaginal delivery after an uncomplicated pregnancy to a 35-year-old woman who had good prenatal care. On physical examination, her skin is pink with no rashes or lesions. Her eyes appear regularly shaped and spaced, and she has a red reflex present in both eyes. Her lips and nose are normal, and her palate has a high arch. She has a webbed neck that is flexible. Her chest is shield shaped with widely spaced nipples. Her lungs are clear to auscultation bilaterally, and her breathing is unlabored with a respiratory rate of 50/min. Her femoral pulses are delayed compared to her radial pulses. She is able to move all extremities equally but has edematous hands and feet. She is alert and has normal Moro and rooting reflexes. Which of the following cardiac examination findings is most likely?

(A) Continuous machinery murmur at the left upper sternal border
(B) Harsh holosystolic murmur at the left lower sternal border
(C) Single loud S2
(D) Systolic murmur loudest below the left scapula
(E) Widely split fixed S2 and systolic ejection murmur at the left upper sternal border

4. An 81-year-old man is hospitalized for acute onset of shortness of breath and lower extremity edema. Although he lives by himself, it is very difficult for him to move around his apartment without experiencing fatigue. He has not seen his physician in years but was told in the past that he had high blood pressure. On physical examination, his jugular venous pulse is seen 9 cm above his sternal notch, inspiratory crackles are heard at his lung bases, and there

is 3+ lower extremity edema. Which of the following is most likely to confirm the diagnosis?

(A) Cardiac angiography
(B) Echocardiography
(C) Electrocardiogram
(D) Endomyocardial biopsy
(E) Pulmonary function tests
(F) X-ray of the chest

5. A 42-year-old man presents to clinic for routine evaluation. His medical history is significant only for gallstones. The patient denies smoking and drinks alcohol occasionally. His mother had a heart attack at the age of 63. His vital signs are significant for a blood pressure of 134/77 mm Hg and on physical examination, he is overweight with well-healed laparoscopic cholecystectomy scars. His fasting lipid panel and other laboratory values are:

Aspartate aminotransferase	37 U/L
Alanine aminotransferase	28 U/L
Alkaline phosphatase	88 U/L
Total cholesterol	268 mg/dL
LDL cholesterol	183 mg/dL
HDL cholesterol	46 mg/dL
Triglycerides	166 mg/dL

What is the most appropriate next step in the patient's management?

(A) A trial of lifestyle modification alone (diet, exercise, and weight loss)
(B) A trial of lifestyle modification combined with statin and niacin therapy
(C) A trial of lifestyle modification combined with statin therapy
(D) Niacin therapy
(E) Statin therapy

6. A 72-year-old man with a history of coronary artery disease and hypertension is hospitalized after suffering a myocardial infarction 5 days ago. He suddenly complains of severe chest pain. His blood pressure is 90/60 mm Hg and his heart rate is 65/min. Auscultation reveals no murmurs or rubs. An ECG reveals sinus rhythm with an acute ST segment elevation in the anteroseptal area. Urgent bedside echocardiography showed anteroseptal, lateral, and apical akinesis, mild left ventricular systolic dysfunction, and severe pericardial effusion. Within 20 minutes he is unconscious with undetectable pulses and blood pressure. What is the most likely cause of the patient's sudden decompensation?

(A) Free wall rupture
(B) Left ventricular thrombus
(C) Mitral regurgitation
(D) Pericarditis
(E) Ventricular septal rupture

7. A 56-year-old woman was recently started on medication for high blood pressure. At her next office visit her hypertension is under good control, but she now complains of "feeling strange" since she started the medication. On further questioning, she reports feeling chest tightness several times over the past 2 weeks, and has also noticed pain in her elbows and knees. Her blood pressure is 124/78 mm Hg (146/82 mm Hg on last visit), heart rate is 102/min, and respiratory rate is 14/min. Her examination is notable for several erythematous plaques on the malar distribution of the face, arms, and upper torso. What medication was she likely started on during her last visit?

(A) Captopril
(B) Furosemide
(C) Hydralazine
(D) Metoprolol
(E) Verapamil

8. A 42-year-old stockbroker with a known history of coronary artery disease presents to the emergency department with complaints of worsening chest pain which he began to experience during his walk earlier that morning. His wife insisted that he see a physician because he has been experiencing palpitations, dyspnea, and angina over the past 3 days. His vital signs are blood pressure 70/50 mm Hg, heart rate 140/min and irregular, respiratory rate 22/min, and oxygen saturation 94% on room air. On physical examination he is fully oriented but slightly confused and distressed. An ECG was taken and is shown in the image. What is the next best step in management?

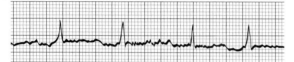

Reproduced, with permission, from USMLERx.com.

(A) Anticoagulation with warfarin
(B) Close clinical observation
(C) Echocardiogram
(D) Electrocardioversion
(E) Rate control with a β-blocker

9. A 19-year-old woman was attacked while coming home from a party and brought to the emergency department (ED). She recalls being punched in the side of the head and stabbed in the left flank. Her speech is slow, and she complains of a bad headache. Her pulse is 110/min, blood pressure is 90/50 mm Hg, and respiratory rate is 25/min. On examination, she has a stab wound at the left costal margin in the midaxillary line. Two large-bore intravenous lines are inserted, and after infusion of 2 L of lactated Ringer's solution, her blood pressure rises to 95/55 mm Hg. What is the most appropriate next step in management?

(A) Abdominal ultrasound
(B) Diagnostic peritoneal lavage
(C) Exploratory laparotomy
(D) Noncontrast CT of the head
(E) Peritoneal laparoscopy

10. A 48-year-old man presents to the ED complaining of crushing substernal chest pain. He is diaphoretic, anxious, and dyspneic. His pulse is 110/min, blood pressure is 175/112 mm Hg, and respiratory rate is 30/min. His oxygen saturation is 94%. Aspirin, oxygen, sublingual nitroglycerin, and morphine are given, but they do not relieve his pain. ECG shows ST segment elevation in V_2 to V_4. The duration of symptoms is now approximately 30 minutes. What is the most appropriate treatment for this patient at this time?

(A) Calcium channel blocker
(B) Intravenous angiotensin-converting enzyme inhibitor
(C) Intravenous β-blocker
(D) Magnesium sulfate
(E) Tissue plasminogen activator

11. A 70-year-old woman presents to the ED complaining of dizziness. She is disoriented to the date and her location and it is difficult to gather an accurate history. Her vital signs are pulse 48/min, blood pressure 84/60 mm Hg, and respiratory rate 12/min. On examination her extremities are cool and clammy. Her capillary refill time is 5 seconds. What is the most appropriate therapy for this patient?

(A) Adenosine
(B) Amiodarone
(C) Atropine
(D) Isoproterenol
(E) Metoprolol

12. A 77-year-old man, complaining of abdominal pain, anorexia, and nausea and vomiting over the past 24 hours, presents to the clinic with his son. The son reveals that his father has also complained of blurred vision. On physical examination, the patient's vital signs are stable and his abdomen is soft, but he appears to be somewhat confused. He is currently maintained on metoprolol, digoxin, and hydrochlorothiazide for ischemic congestive heart failure. His son says that sometimes his father confuses his medications. The patient also has renal insufficiency with a baseline serum creatinine of 2.6 mg/dL. The ECG reveals a widened QRS complex and a new first-degree heart block. Which of the following is the most likely cause of this patient's symptoms?

(A) Digoxin toxicity
(B) Gastroenteritis
(C) Hypocalcemia
(D) Hypovolemia secondary to thiazide diuretic overuse
(E) Myocardial infarction

13. An 89-year-old man presents to the ED with 2 days of painful lower extremity swelling and shortness of breath. His blood pressure is 176/88 mm Hg with significant peripheral edema, elevated jugular venous pulsations, and rales on pulmonary examination. Laboratory values are:

Na^+	34 mEq/L
K^+	5.3 mEq/L
Cl^-	101 mEq/L
Blood urea nitrogen	54 mg/dL
Creatinine	1.7 mg/dL
Glucose	189 mg/dL
WBC count	6400/mm³
Hematocrit	37%
Platelet count	226,000/mm³
Troponin I	0.09 ng/dL
Creatine kinase, myocardial bound	6 ng/mL

The physician suggests x-ray of the chest and echocardiography to investigate further. The patient's ejection fraction is 70%. Which of the following features is most consistent with the diagnosis of diastolic dysfunction?

(A) Decreased end-diastolic pressure
(B) Decreased end-diastolic volume
(C) Decreased ejection fraction
(D) Decreased ratio of ventricular wall thickness to ventricular cavity size
(E) Normal exercise capacity
(F) Normal x-ray of the chest

14. A 49-year-old man presents to the clinic for a health maintenance visit. He has no complaints, but he requests a prescription for his "pressure pills," as he lost his original prescription. On physical examination, his blood pressure is 220/130 mm Hg. A full physical examination otherwise is within normal limits. Laboratory tests show:

Na^+	142 mEq/L
K^+	3.8 mEq/L
Cl^-	105 mEq/L
Carbon dioxide	25 mEq/L
Blood urea nitrogen	20 mg/dL
Creatinine	1.0 mg/dL
Glucose	33 mg/dL

His urinalysis is within normal limits, and his ECG is normal. Which of the following is the most effective management?

(A) Administer intravenous nitroprusside for management of hypertensive emergency
(B) Administer intravenous nitroprusside for management of hypertensive urgency
(C) Administer oral furosemide for management of hypertensive emergency
(D) Administer oral metoprolol for management of hypertensive urgency
(E) Administer sublingual nifedipine for management of hypertensive emergency

15. A 60-year-old man with a history of coronary artery disease, peptic ulcer disease, and gout presents to the ED with a 24-hour history of abdominal pain. The pain, which is most intense in the upper abdomen, was sudden in onset and has become progressively more severe. Free air in the abdomen is detected on x-ray. The patient is in an agitated state. His extremities are cool and capillary refill time is 3 seconds. His blood pressure is 80/40 mm Hg and his heart rate is 130/min. The neck veins are flat, and the lungs are clear to auscultation. His hemoglobin is 13.8 g/dL. A urinary catheter is inserted and only 10 mL of urine is drained. What is the most appropriate treatment for this patient at this time?

(A) Broad-spectrum antibiotics for presumed sepsis
(B) Infusion of isotonic fluid
(C) Infusion of norepinephrine
(D) Inotropic support with dopamine, vasopressin, or dobutamine
(E) Transfuse with 1 unit packed red blood cells

16. A 29-year-old woman presents to the ED with a 3-week history of being awakened by a dull, prolonged chest pain that occurs about three or four times a week. She is a smoker but has never suffered a myocardial infarction (MI) or had chest pain before and has no family history of early MI. A 12-lead ECG is normal. Her first set of cardiac enzymes (creatine kinase, creatine kinase Mb, troponin I) is negative. If coronary angiography were taken at the time of her chest pain, which would be the most likely finding in her condition?

    (A) Coronary artery spasm
    (B) Greater than 80% stenosis in at least two coronary arteries
    (C) No findings
    (D) Plaque rupture and thrombosis

17. A 42-year-old man presents to the ED with a complaint of increasing shortness of breath when walking to get his newspaper, difficulty breathing while lying flat, and a 4.5-kg (10-lb) weight gain over the last month. He is afebrile, his pulse is 75/min, and his blood pressure is 98/50 mm Hg. On examination he smells of alcohol and has 2+ pitting edema in the lower extremities and a third heart sound. X-ray of the chest reveals cardiomegaly. What findings, other than those listed above, must be present in order to confirm this man's underlying diagnosis?

    (A) Hepatojugular reflux and pulmonary congestion
    (B) Left ventricular dilation and aortic insufficiency
    (C) Left ventricular dilation and systolic dysfunction
    (D) Myocardial thickening and diastolic dysfunction
    (E) Pulmonary congestion and diastolic dysfunction

18. A 69-year-old man with a history of rheumatic heart disease presents to the ED complaining of a fever and weakness on his left side. On physical examination, the patient is weak in his left upper extremity and he draws only the right half of a clock. Shortly after his presentation, however, he expires, and an autopsy is performed. A gross photograph of the patient's heart is shown in the image. Which of the following is a risk factor for the type of lesion pictured?

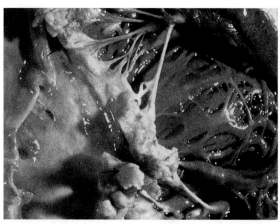

Reproduced, with permission, from Kasper DL, Braunwald E, Fauci AS, Hauser SL, Longo DL, Jameson LJ, Isselbacher KJ, eds. *Harrison's Online*. New York: McGraw-Hill, 2005: Figure 109-1.

    (A) Coronary artery disease
    (B) Hypertension
    (C) Mitral valve prolapse
    (D) Prolonged bed rest
    (E) Prosthetic valve replacement

19. A 28-year-old man with a history of intravenous drug abuse presents to the ED with a 2-day history of fever, chills, and shortness of breath. On physical examination, the patient has a new heart murmur, small retinal hemorrhages, and subungual petechiae. What is the most likely causative organism?

    (A) Group A streptococcus
    (B) *Mycobacterium tuberculosis*
    (C) *Staphylococcus aureus*
    (D) *Staphylococcus epidermidis*
    (E) Streptococcus viridans

20. A boy is delivered at 37 weeks' gestation via spontaneous vaginal delivery. He is the product of a normal pregnancy and was delivered without complications. Maternal prenatal laboratory test results are rubella immune, blood type B, Rh antibody negative, group B streptococci negative, rapid plasma reagin negative, hepatitis B surface antigen negative, and gonorrhea and chlamydia negative. The patient

appears cyanotic. He is breathing at a rate of 60/min and his heart rate is 130/min. He has a normal S1 and S2. There is a harsh holosystolic murmur that is loudest at the left lower sternal border. His examination reveals palpable nonbounding peripheral pulses bilaterally. Which of the following is the most likely diagnosis?

(A) Coarctation of the aorta
(B) Dextraposed transposition of the great arteries
(C) Patent ductus arteriosus
(D) Tetralogy of Fallot
(E) Truncus arteriosus

21. A 32-year-old man is stabbed in the left chest and presents to the ED in distress. His vital signs are pulse 130/min, blood pressure 70/50 mm Hg, and respiratory rate 39/min. The stab wound is found to be located in the left fifth intercostal space in the midaxillary line. On examination his trachea is deviated to the right, jugular veins are distended bilaterally, and he has absent breath sounds and hyperresonance to percussion on the left side. Subcutaneous emphysema is palpated on the left thoracic wall. What is the next best step in management?

(A) Chest tube thoracostomy
(B) Diagnostic peritoneal lavage
(C) Immediate decompression by needle thoracotomy
(D) Pericardiocentesis
(E) Surgical exploration

22. A 75-year-old man comes into the ED with a 10-minute history of crushing substernal chest pain radiating to his left arm. This man is well known to the ED staff due to his long history of chest pain. An ECG is done and his cardiac enzyme levels are drawn. His creatine kinase–myocardial bound fraction percentage of total creatine phosphokinase is 6% with a troponin T level of 0.4 ng/mL. What is the correct diagnosis of this patient?

(A) Acute myocardial infarction
(B) Hypochondriasis
(C) Prinzmetal's angina

(D) Stable angina
(E) Unstable angina

23. A 91-year-old woman presents to the ED with a chief complaint of shortness of breath over the past 2 days. She has a history of hypertension and coronary artery bypass surgery 25 years earlier. Her blood pressure is 178/92 mm Hg and she has jugular venous distention, hepatomegaly, and 3+ lower extremity edema. ECG is remarkable for left ventricular hypertrophy, no ST-segment elevations or depressions, no Q waves, and no T-wave abnormalities. Echocardiogram reveals an ejection fraction of 60% and left atrial dilatation. There is universal left ventricular thickening. No valvular regurgitation or stenosis was noted. Which of the following underlying conditions is the **most** likely cause of this patient's symptoms?

(A) Hypertensive heart disease
(B) Hypertrophic obstructive cardiomyopathy
(C) Ischemic heart disease
(D) Mitral valve prolapse
(E) Myocarditis

24. A 39-year-old white man with a past medical history significant for essential hypertension presents for a routine health maintenance visit. He has no complaints and reports compliance with his hydrochlorothiazide. His pulse is 70/min, blood pressure is 145/92 mm Hg, and respiratory rate is 16/min. His body mass index is 24 kg/m^2. His physical examination is within normal limits. For which condition is the patient at increased risk?

(A) End-stage renal disease
(B) Hypercholesterolemia
(C) Hypertrophic cardiomyopathy
(D) Second-degree Mobitz I atrioventricular block
(E) Type 2 diabetes mellitus

25. An 83-year-old woman is being evaluated for confusion. She was admitted 3 days ago after having an acute myocardial infarction (MI). Her hospital course has been complicated by narrow-complex ventricular tachycardia, which has finally been stabilized on an antiarrhythmic medication. She was also started on a post-MI protocol and an antidepressant. One day after beginning these medications, she begins to develop confusion and slurred speech. Her temperature is 36.7°C (98.1°F), blood pressure is 138/60 mm Hg, pulse is 88/min, and respiratory rate is 14/min. She is alert and oriented to person, but she does not realize she is in the hospital. Additionally, she exhibits difficulty with word articulation, although she speaks fluently, and she demonstrates a mild resting tremor. The remainder of her examination is normal. Which of the following medications is most likely to cause these central nervous system effects?

    (A) Aspirin
    (B) Enalapril
    (C) Fluoxetine
    (D) Lidocaine
    (E) Metoprolol

26. A 43-year-old woman presents to the ED with a chief complaint of chest pain, shortness of breath, and worsening fatigue for the past day. The chest pain initially worsened with lying down and improved with leaning forward, but now it seems equal in intensity over all positions. On physical examination, she has labored, fast breathing and appears to be in pain. She has jugular venous distention. She is tachycardic, has a regular rhythm, and has distant heart sounds with a friction rub. Her lungs are clear to auscultation bilaterally, her abdominal examination is benign, and she has no peripheral edema. Her vital signs in triage are: temperature 39.0°C (102.2°F), pulse 126/min, blood pressure 89/66 mm Hg, respiratory rate 32/min, and oxygen saturation 98%. X-ray of the chest is shown in the image. Which of the following is the most likely diagnosis?

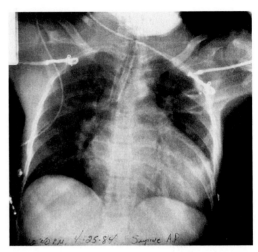

Reproduced, with permission, from Hall JB, Schmidt GA, Wood LDH. *Principles of Critical Care*, 3rd ed. New York: McGraw-Hill, 2005: Figure 28.8.

    (A) Cardiac tamponade
    (B) Decompensated congestive heart failure
    (C) Panic attack
    (D) Pericarditis
    (E) Tension pneumothorax

27. An elderly man presents to the ED with chest pain. He has a history of stable angina and recent-onset diabetes mellitus, but now the chest pain comes on with less exertion and takes longer to go away. An ECG and cardiac enzymes are ordered. If this man has unstable angina, what are the expected findings on ECG and cardiac enzymes?

    (A) Delta waves on the ECG and positive cardiac enzymes
    (B) Low-voltage ECG and positive cardiac enzymes
    (C) No changes on ECG and positive cardiac enzymes
    (D) ST depressions on ECG and normal cardiac enzymes
    (E) ST elevations with Q waves and normal cardiac enzymes

28. A 71-year-old retired banker is hospitalized for shortness of breath of unknown origin. The symptoms have included decreased exercise tolerance and fatigue worsening over the past

month. He has a past history of an acute myocardial infarction at the age of 63 and hypertension. The physician suspects diastolic dysfunction as the cause of his symptoms. Which of the following statements about diastolic dysfunction is true?

(A) Diastolic dysfunction carries a worse prognosis than systolic dysfunction
(B) Ejection fraction is most often normal
(C) Ischemic heart disease causes only systolic dysfunction
(D) Pulmonary congestion is not seen in the setting of diastolic dysfunction
(E) The condition shows a decreased incidence with age

29. A 47-year-old woman who is 2 weeks post triple bypass surgery presents to the ED with a chief complaint of sudden-onset, sharp chest pain for several hours. She is fatigued and short of breath. On physical examination, she has distended neck veins that grow more distended on inspiration. Muffled heart sounds are heard. Her temperature is 37.0°C (101.8°F), pulse is 133/min, blood pressure is 70/50 mm Hg, and respiratory rate is 30/min. Her O_2 saturation is 100%. An echocardiogram shows a large pericardial effusion and chamber collapse; therefore, pericardiocentesis is performed. Although a large amount of blood is aspirated, the patient's clinical picture acutely worsens. Her pain level increases substantially, with pulse 150/min, blood pressure 60/41 mm Hg, and respiratory rate 30/min. Her O_2 saturation is 100%. Repeat echocardiogram shows an even larger pericardial effusion with chamber collapse. Which complication of pericardiocentesis is most likely in this patient?

(A) Acute left ventricular failure with pulmonary edema
(B) Aspiration of 10 mL air into the pericardium
(C) Laceration of a coronary vessel
(D) Pneumothorax
(E) Puncture of the left ventricle

30. A 57-year-old man presents to the ED with worsening substernal chest pain occurring over the past 20 minutes. He has a medical history significant for a 2-pack-per-day smoking history, gout, obesity, hypercholesterolemia, hypertension, osteoarthritis of both knees, inflammatory bowel disease, and recently diagnosed type 2 diabetes that is well controlled on oral antiglycemics (hemoglobin A_{1c} of 7.8%). On physical examination, he is in moderate distress, diaphoretic, and nauseous, and has a temperature of 37.5°C (99.5°F), a pulse of 112/min, blood pressure of 142/85 mm Hg, and a respiratory rate of 22/min. He tests positive for myocardial infarction (MI) by serial cardiac enzymes. He is started on the appropriate therapy and is ready for discharge the following evening. What is the number one preventive measure the patient can take that will decrease his immediate risk for a second MI?

(A) Decrease the amount of cholesterol in his diet
(B) Exercise three times a week
(C) Lower his blood pressure to the 120/80 mm Hg range
(D) Lower his blood sugar levels to achieve a hemoglobin A_{1c} level < 7%
(E) Quit smoking

31. A 64-year-old man in the surgical intensive care unit goes into rapid atrial fibrillation on postoperative day one after a decortication for a loculated pulmonary empyema. He is given an appropriate loading dose of digoxin, but 4 hours after his second dose, the patient complains of increased palpitations and dizziness. The patient is conscious and hemodynamically stable. Stat serum electrolytes show a potassium level of 5.0 mEq/dL, and all others, including divalents, are also in the normal range. The digitalis level is above the therapeutic range at 4 ng/mL (therapeutic range = 0.5–2 ng/mL). Cardiac telemetry is shown below. Which of the following should be administered immediately?

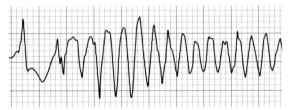

Reproduced, with permission, from USMLERx.com.

(A) Calcium
(B) Furosemide
(C) Magnesium
(D) Potassium
(E) Sodium polystyrene sulfonate

32. A 37-year-old woman with a history of sarcoidosis presents to her primary care physician complaining of progressive fatigue and shortness of breath over the past 3 months. She also reports that her socks and shoes do not fit the way they used to and that she fainted a few weeks ago for the first time in many years. She denies any recent illness and only takes medications to control her sarcoid. She states that she is more comfortable sitting than lying down. On physical examination, she has jugular venous distention, which increases with inspiration. Her blood pressure is 134/87 mm Hg, respiratory rate is 17/min, pulse is 96/min, and temperature is 37.2°C (98.9°F). She also has decreased breath sounds bilaterally at the bases. An ECG shows decreased QRS voltage. An echocardiogram shows a thick left ventricle. What is the most likely diagnosis?

(A) Aortic stenosis
(B) Cardiac tamponade
(C) Hypertensive heart disease
(D) Pericarditis
(E) Restrictive cardiomyopathy

33. A 1-week-old infant presents to her general pediatrician's office for a well-child visit. She was born at 37 weeks' gestation without complications. Her temperature is 37.0°C (98.6°F), pulse is 130/min, blood pressure is 72/54 mm Hg, and respiratory rate is 28/min. She is currently at the 50th percentile for weight and 75th percentile for height. She is acyanotic and has a wide, fixed split S2 with a 2/6 systolic ejection murmur at the left upper sternal border. The remainder of the examination is unremarkable. What is the most likely diagnosis?

(A) Atrial septal defect
(B) Coarctation of the aorta
(C) Dextraposed transposition of the great arteries
(D) Tetralogy of Fallot
(E) Ventricular septal defect

34. A 26-year-old white nonsmoking woman returns for a follow-up appointment with her primary care provider. At a routine health maintenance visit 8 months earlier, her blood pressure was 179/97 mm Hg. Since then, she has adhered to a low-fat diet and exercises regularly. On repeat measurement 1 month later, her blood pressure was still elevated, despite her compliance with the prescribed hydrochlorothiazide and lisinopril. She has no complaints and denies headaches, chest pain, or mental status changes. On physical examination, she is a slender woman in no apparent distress. An abdominal bruit that lateralizes to the left is heard. Her blood pressure is 178/99 mm Hg in her left arm and 181/95 mm Hg in her right arm. A basic metabolic panel and complete blood count are within normal range. Which is the most appropriate next step in patient care?

(A) Add a statin to the patient's current drug regimen to decrease fatty arterial plaques
(B) Admit patient to the hospital and start intravenous nitroprusside

(C) Increase the dosage of her antihypertensive regimen

(D) Order duplex imaging of the renal arteries and proceed to percutaneous transluminal angioplasty if renal artery stenosis is found

(E) Order duplex imaging of the renal arteries and proceed to surgical revascularization if renal artery stenosis is found

35. A college sophomore is found by his roommate to be poorly responsive and brought to the ED. After resuscitation, the man complains of a severe headache and photophobia that is accompanied by dizziness, nausea, vomiting, and neck pain. Physical examination was noteworthy for positive Kernig's and Brudzinski's signs as well as petechiae on the trunk and mucocutaneous bleeding. A lumbar puncture was obtained in which *Neisseria meningitidis* was isolated from the cerebrospinal fluid. A complete blood cell count revealed a WBC count of 17,000/mm^3, hemoglobin of 11 g/dL, and platelet count of 70,000/mm^3. Coagulation studies revealed a bleeding time of 10 minutes, prothrombin time of 17 seconds, activated partial thromboplastin time of 47 seconds, and thrombin time of 18 seconds. A peripheral blood smear was obtained and is shown in the image. What is the most likely diagnosis?

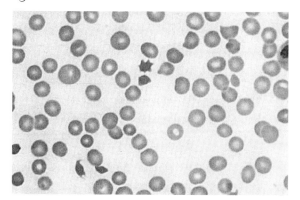

Reproduced, with permission, from Lichtman MA, Beutler E, Kipps TJ, Seligsohn U, Kaushansky K, Prchal JT. *Williams Hematology*, 7th ed. New York: McGraw-Hill, 2006: Plate III-2.

(A) Disseminated intravascular coagulation

(B) Factor V Leiden

(C) Immune thrombocytopenic purpura

(D) Protein C deficiency

(E) Thrombotic thrombocytopenic purpura

36. A 58-year-old man is admitted to the coronary care unit for telemetric monitoring after an episode of bradycardia. While in the unit, he suddenly loses consciousness. His pulse is undetectable, and his blood pressure drops to 40 mm Hg. His airway is clear and patent, and he is still breathing on his own. An ECG shows electrical activity. Chest compressions are started, and he is quickly given a bolus of intravenous sodium bicarbonate and atropine. When his tracing does not improve, the boluses are repeated twice, and finally his tracing returns to normal sinus rhythm. Moments later, when he regains consciousness, he complains of a dry mouth, blurred vision, and feeling flushed. What is the most appropriate next step in the management of this patient?

(A) This patient has atropine toxicity and requires urgent administration of a cholinergic agonist

(B) This patient has atropine toxicity and requires urgent administration of a muscarinic agonist

(C) This patient has bicarbonate toxicity and requires urgent administration of calcium citrate

(D) This patient is experiencing transient adverse effects of atropine and requires only supportive measures

(E) This patient is experiencing transient adverse effects of bicarbonate and requires only supportive measures

37. A 62-year-old man with a history of benign prostatic hypertrophy and hypertension presents to his primary care provider for a routine health maintenance visit. He reports that he feels "better than ever" and explains that his daughter made him come in for his annual visit. He takes prazosin daily and occasionally some acetaminophen. He has no drug allergies and denies smoking, drinking, or the use of illicit drugs. His physical examination is within normal range except for his rectal examination, which revealed an enlarged prostate. His temperature is 36.8°C (98.2°F), respiratory rate is 13/min, pulse is 82/min, and blood pressure is 138/86 mm Hg. Which of the following is one of the common possible effects of α_1-adrenergic blockade in this patient?

    (A) Decreased urine flow
    (B) Increased blood pressure
    (C) Increased sexual drive
    (D) Irritability
    (E) Orthostatic hypotension

38. A 2-year-old girl is referred to the hospital for evaluation of her inability to gain weight. She is well fed by her parents, but appears to tire during feedings and has been losing weight despite frequent high-calorie meals. There is no family history of developmental delay or short stature. She is well dressed, her hair is brushed, and she's playful but tires quickly. Her vital signs are temperature 36.5°C (97.7°F), pulse 110/min, blood pressure 90/50 mm Hg, and respiratory rate 24/min. She has a harsh 2/6 holosystolic murmur that is best heard at the left sternal border, which is unchanged and has been present since birth. Which of the following is the most appropriate next step in management?

    (A) Continue to monitor the patient for increased weight loss and increased shunting
    (B) pH probe for gastroesophageal reflux disease
    (C) Refer for evaluation and possible closure of her ventricular septal defect
    (D) Skeletal survey
    (E) Stool culture

39. A 72-year-old man presents with shortness of breath and increased home oxygen requirement. The patient has a history of coronary artery disease, status post two previous myocardial infarctions, and a history of chronic obstructive pulmonary disease requiring 2 L of continuous home oxygen. The patient has a 45-pack-year history of smoking. He is unable to walk more than a block and the swelling in his legs has worsened. The physician suggests measuring a brain natriuretic peptide (BNP) level to distinguish a cardiac from a pulmonary cause of his symptoms. Which of the following statements regarding BNP is true?

    (A) Brain natriuretic peptide acts to decrease venous capacitance and increase preload
    (B) Brain natriuretic peptide is decreased in the setting of left ventricular dysfunction
    (C) Brain natriuretic peptide is secreted by the cardiac atria
    (D) Brain natriuretic peptide is secreted in response to hypovolemia
    (E) Brain natriuretic peptide levels cannot differentiate systolic and diastolic dysfunction
    (F) Brain natriuretic peptide secretion results in pressure overload

40. A 77-year-old man with a history of hypertension, hypercholesterolemia, an abdominal aortic aneurysm, chronic obstructive pulmonary disease, and a 90-pack-year smoking history presents to the ED with lethargy and abdominal pain. At presentation, his temperature was 36.9°C (98.5°F), blood pressure was 82/54 mm Hg, pulse was 125/min, and respiratory rate was 16/min. On physical examination, there is a pulsatile abdominal mass that is palpable just superior to the umbilicus. There is also diffuse abdominal tenderness, though rebound tenderness and guarding are absent. There is also slight skin discoloration noted in the left lower back. Which of the following is the most likely diagnosis?

    (A) Aortic dissection
    (B) Mesenteric ischemia
    (C) Perforated gastric ulcer
    (D) Ruptured abdominal aortic aneurysm
    (E) Stroke

41. A 52-year-old African-American man with a history of smoking and asthma presents to the ED complaining of shortness of breath. He has

alcohol on his breath and admits to drinking 3–4 beers each night plus an occasional "mixed drink." He denies drug use and states that he has been feeling well until recently, when he began to sleep with more pillows and to become out of breath when walking. His blood pressure is 143/89 mm Hg, respiratory rate is 21/min, pulse is 112/min, and he is afebrile. On physical examination, he has a laterally displaced point of maximal impulse and an S3 gallop, as well as rales over his right lung base. An x-ray of the chest is completed, which shows cardiomegaly and a pleural effusion. Echocardiogram reveals an ejection fraction of 25%. What is the most likely diagnosis?

(A) Asthma exacerbation
(B) Delirium tremens
(C) Dilated cardiomyopathy
(D) Endocarditis
(E) Hypothyroidism

42. A cardiologist is called to consult on the care of a 2-day-old girl delivered at 33 weeks' gestation. The infant is lying supine in her isolette. She is acyanotic, but has a heart rate of 192/min and a respiratory rate of 60/min. She has a nonradiating continuous machinery murmur at the left upper sternal border that remains the same with compression of the ipsilateral, then contralateral jugular veins. Her first and second heart sounds are normal. Her peripheral pulses are bounding. What is the most likely diagnosis?

(A) Aortic stenosis with aortic regurgitation
(B) Patent ductus arteriosus
(C) Systemic arteriovenous fistula
(D) Venous hum
(E) Ventricular septal defect

43. A 23-year-old Chinese-American man with a history of bronchitis at age 15 and influenza at age 19 presents to the ED with shortness of breath and chest pain. He was at home "playing video games" when he started to feel lightheaded. He says that over the next few hours it got worse. On admission, his blood pressure is 136/90 mm Hg, respiratory rate is 22/min, pulse is 108/min, and temperature is 37.2°C (98.9°F). His laboratory values are normal, and his examination reveals a murmur that is very

faint and difficult to classify. However, his ECG shows mild left ventricular hypertrophy, and an echocardiogram shows some outflow tract obstruction and a septum:posterior wall ratio > 1.3. What is the most likely diagnosis?

(A) Cor pulmonale
(B) Hypertrophic cardiomyopathy
(C) Mitral valve prolapse
(D) Pericarditis
(E) Restrictive cardiomyopathy

44. A 56-year-old woman with a history of chronic renal disease presents to the ED with a chief complaint of severe, sharp, retrosternal chest pain which radiates to her jaw. The pain worsens when the patient lies down, and she is most comfortable leaning forward and hugging her knees. She takes erythropoietin, furosemide, calcitriol, and sodium polystyrene sulfonate. She is scheduled for dialysis three times per week, but she admits to sometimes missing sessions. She stopped drinking and smoking 20 years ago, and she has no family history of heart or renal problems. Upon auscultation of the heart, a friction rub is heard. Laboratory values from the ED are:

WBC count	12,000/mm^3
Hemoglobin	10.0 g/dL
Hematocrit	30.0%
Platelet count	150,000/mm^3
Na$^+$	141 mEq/L
K$^+$	4.8 mEq/L
Cl$^-$	101 mEq/L
HCO$_3^-$	22 mEq/L
Blood urea nitrogen	63 mg/dL
Creatinine	3.2 mg/dL
Glucose	111 mg/dL

The emergency medicine physician urges the patient to be more compliant with her dialysis, but the patient complains that she is too tired to go to dialysis all of the time and that it is ruining her life. Which of the following is the most likely complication if the patient's condition remains untreated?

(A) Cardiac tamponade
(B) Decreased jugular venous pressure
(C) Mitral regurgitation
(D) Restrictive cardiomyopathy
(E) Septic shock

45. A 60-year-old man with a history of congestive heart failure presents to his physician. He has a 5-year history of excessive daytime sleepiness and snoring. He also admits to three drinks of alcohol per day. His temperature is 36.6°C (98.0°F), pulse is 85/min, blood pressure is 138/82 mm Hg, respiratory rate is 14/min, and oxygen saturation is 99% on room air. His body mass index is 31 kg/m². Physical examination is significant for macroglossia and a short neck. Polysomnography is obtained and is significant for multiple nocturnal episodes of airflow cessation at the nose and mouth, despite evidence of continuing respiratory effort. Which one of the following is the most effective management for this patient?

(A) Avoidance of alcohol
(B) Avoidance of supine posture
(C) Nasal continuous positive airway pressure
(D) Uvulopalatopharyngoplasty
(E) Weight reduction

46. A 14-year-old girl is found to have a late apical systolic murmur preceded by a click during a screening physical examination for participation in high school sports. The rest of the examination is unremarkable. Echocardiography show superior displacement of the mitral leaflets of > 2 mm during systole into the left atrium, with a thickness of 8 mm. In addition, she states that her father also has some type of heart "murmur," but she knows nothing else about it. Which of the following would be appropriate for management at this time?

(A) Digoxin
(B) Instruct the patient to avoid all forms of strenuous activity
(C) Metoprolol
(D) Mitral valve replacement
(E) Prophylactic antibiotics for dental procedures

47. A 20-year-old woman college student arrives at the ED actively seizing with QRS prolongation on ECG per paramedics. The patient's roommate called emergency medical services after the patient collapsed, was not responsive to questioning, and began having clonic jerks bilaterally in her upper extremities. The patient's roommate denies any knowledge of the patient consuming alcohol or illicit drugs. She does not believe the patient had any plan of harming herself, but does acknowledge that the patient has seemed "down" lately and was recently prescribed medication for generalized anhedonia. What is the correct first-line treatment?

(A) Activated charcoal
(B) Diazepam
(C) Flumazenil
(D) Physostigmine
(E) Sodium bicarbonate and diazepam

48. A 78-year-old woman presents to a nursing home physician complaining of palpitations over the last several months. Her episodes are not associated with any chest pain, dizziness, or loss of consciousness. The patient reports that she spent several weeks in the hospital as a child with rheumatic fever. Her ECG appears in the image. Which is the patient's most likely diagnosis?

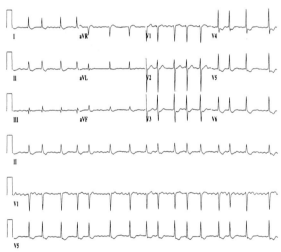

Reprinted, with permission, from Crawford MH. *Current Diagnosis & Treatment in Cardiology*, 2nd ed. New York: McGraw-Hill, 2003: Figure 20-1.

(A) Atrial fibrillation
(B) Atrial flutter
(C) Multifocal atrial tachycardia
(D) Paroxysmal atrial tachycardia
(E) Paroxysmal supraventricular tachycardia

49. A 65-year-old man with a history of chronic atrial fibrillation presented to the ED with a cold, pulseless right lower extremity. Furthermore, he complained of right leg paresthesias and extreme pain, as well as the inability to plantarflex his foot. An emergent popliteal em-

bolectomy was performed that resulted in bilateral palpable pedal pulses. However, the patient was still unable to plantarflex his foot, and continued to experience intense pain and paresthesia. Which of the following is the most appropriate next step in management?

(A) CT of the right leg
(B) Electromyography
(C) Measurement of posterior compartment pressure
(D) Right lower extremity elevation
(E) Right lower extremity fasciotomy

50. A 32-year-old man is brought to the ED by paramedics after being found wandering downtown, apparently delirious and agitated. During transport to the hospital the patient becomes diaphoretic and tremulous and is found to be hypertensive to 163/100 mm Hg, tachycardic with a pulse of 102/min, and febrile to 39°C (102.2°F). On examination, the patient is found to have dilated pupils and ulcerations of his nasal septum mucosa with the residue of a white powder along the nasal alae in addition to his tachycardia, hypertension, hyperthermia, and agitation. What is the reasoning behind avoiding β-blockers in this patient?

(A) Increased risk of late vasospasm
(B) Risk of acutely worsening hypertension through vasoconstriction
(C) Risk of causing acute hypotension
(D) Risk of causing dyspnea
(E) Risk of ventricular arrhythmia

51. A 59-year-old man presents to his internist for a routine visit. He has no complaints, and review of symptoms is negative. His past medical history is significant for poorly controlled hypertension for 15 years due to noncompliance with antihypertensive medications. He takes hydrochlorothiazide 25 mg orally four times a day. His family history is significant for hypertension, heart failure, and stroke. He has a 30

pack-year smoking history and drinks two beers a day. On physical examination, he is a mildly obese man in no acute distress. He has a normal jugular venous pressure. He has a prominent point of maximum impulse, regular rate and rhythm, normal S1, loud S2, and audible S4 with no murmurs. His lungs are clear to auscultation bilaterally, and he has no signs of edema. His abdominal and neurologic examinations are within normal limits. His temperature is 37.0°C (98.6°F), pulse is 81/min, respiratory rate is 12/min, and blood pressure is 165/96 mm Hg. His O_2 saturation is 100%. His ECG shows normal sinus rhythm with large amplitude of the S wave in V_1 and V_2 and of the R wave in V_5 and V_6. Also present are diffuse ST/T wave changes, widened bifid P waves, and prolonged QRS waveforms. Which of the following is the most likely diagnosis?

(A) Acute myocardial infarction
(B) Cerebrovascular accident
(C) Dilated cardiomyopathy
(D) Left ventricular hypertrophy
(E) Pericarditis

52. A 60-year-old woman is transferred to a physician from an outside hospital following a motor vehicle collision. Her medical history is notable for Osler-Weber-Rendu syndrome. She is otherwise healthy. Which of the following triads is most likely to characterize her medical history prior to the collision?

(A) Hypertension, bradycardia, and irregular respirations
(B) Jaundice, fever, and right upper quadrant pain
(C) Symptoms of hypoglycemia, low blood sugar, and relief with increase in blood sugar
(D) Telangiectasia, recurrent epistaxis, and positive family history
(E) Venous stasis, hypercoagulability, and endothelial damage

53. A girl is delivered at 34 weeks' gestation via spontaneous vaginal delivery. She is the product of a pregnancy that was complicated by preterm labor. Maternal prenatal laboratory values are rubella immune, blood type A, Rh antibody negative, group B streptococci negative, rapid plasma reagin negative, hepatitis B surface antigen negative, and gonorrhea and chlamydia negative. There is no meconium. Her birth weight is 2 kg (4 lb, 8 oz). She is pale and cyanotic. She has grunting, nasal flaring, and intercostal retractions. Her respiratory rate is 70/min, and she does not respond to administration of blow-by oxygen. Cardiac auscultation reveals a continuous machinery murmur heard at the left upper sternal border. A prominent apical impulse is also palpable. Pulmonary auscultation reveals decreased breath sounds and crackles at her lung bases bilaterally, bounding peripheral pulses bilaterally, and rooting reflexes. What is the most appropriate next step in management of this patient's heart defect?

    (A) Balloon atrial septostomy
    (B) Coil embolization
    (C) Indomethacin
    (D) Prostaglandin E
    (E) Surgical ligation

EXTENDED MATCHING

Questions 54 and 55

For each patient with chest pain, select the most likely diagnosis.

    (A) Acute aortic dissection
    (B) Acute myocardial infarction
    (C) Angina pectoris
    (D) Cardiac tamponade
    (E) Compression fracture of the spine
    (F) Coronary vasospasm
    (G) Esophageal spasm
    (H) Myocarditis
    (I) Panic disorder
    (J) Pericarditis
    (K) Pneumonia
    (L) Pulmonary embolus
    (M) Rib fracture
    (N) Tension pneumothorax

54. A 47-year-old man presents to the ED via emergency medical services. He was found unconscious and bleeding from a 4-cm wound over his lateral left chest. On admission, he is in respiratory distress and vital signs are significant for tachycardia and hypotension with a blood pressure of 68/43 mm Hg. On physical examination, the patient has an elevated jugular venous pulse and heart sounds are difficult to auscultate.

55. A 66-year-old woman presents to the ED with a chief complaint of nausea, vague abdominal pain, and epigastric discomfort. The pain began while she was climbing stairs in the morning and increased gradually. It was relieved after 10 minutes of sitting down, but she remains concerned. Her pulse is 105/min and her blood pressure is 146/82 mm Hg.

Questions 56 and 57

For each of the following patients with fatigue, select the most appropriate pharmacologic intervention.

    (A) Candesartan
    (B) Digoxin
    (C) Erythropoietin
    (D) Folate
    (E) Heparin
    (F) Isoniazid
    (G) Lisinopril
    (H) Metoprolol
    (I) Warfarin

56. A 36-year-old woman presents 18 weeks pregnant with a chief complaint of fatigue. Her history is significant for leukemia 7 years prior treated successfully with a course of doxorubicin chemotherapy. On physical examination, she has bilateral rales throughout her lung fields and 3+ pitting edema. Echocardiogram reveals a dilated left ventricular chamber and an ejection fraction of 40%.

57. A 75-year-old retired anesthesiologist with a history of two previous myocardial infarctions presents with extreme fatigue upon exertion. He is unable to walk more than two blocks and

requires three pillows to sleep comfortably at night. On physical examination there is jugular venous distention noted. He had previously been unable to tolerate enalapril due to excessive coughing.

Questions 58–60

Select the most effective management for each patient with pericardial disease.

(A) Antibiotics
(B) Chest tube placement
(C) Colchicine
(D) Corticosteroids
(E) Emergency cardiac catheterization
(F) Emergent pericardiocentesis
(G) Intravenous fluids
(H) Loop diuretics
(I) Morphine
(J) Multidrug antituberculous therapy
(K) Nitroglycerin
(L) Nonsteroidal anti-inflammatory drugs
(M) Renal dialysis

58. A 45-year-old man with chronic renal disease on dialysis presents with a chief complaint of sharp chest pain for several days that has not improved with acetaminophen. In addition, he has had increasing fatigue and dyspnea over the past few days with a bothersome cough. On physical examination, he appears in mild distress. He has slightly distended neck veins. His heart sounds are muffled, and a pericardial friction rub is heard. His vital signs at triage are temperature 37.5°C (99.5°F), pulse 85/min, blood pressure 100/72 mm Hg, and respiratory rate 20/min. His O_2 saturation is 99%. An echocardiogram shows a large pericardial effusion.

59. A 37-year-old man with a history of angina and a positive stress test presents for cardiac catheterization. During the procedure, one of his coronary arteries is lacerated. The patient develops tachycardia and becomes hypotensive. The anesthesiologist notices that his systolic pressure falls even further on inspiration. A bedside echocardiogram is performed and shows a small pericardial effusion.

60. An otherwise healthy 17-year-old girl presents to the ED after 2 weeks of chest pain. She describes the pain as sharp, localized to the left side of her chest, and radiating to her jaw and neck. The pain worsens when she lies down and improves on leaning forward. Her physical examination is significant for a soft pericardial friction rub. Her vital signs are temperature 37.5°C (99.5°F), pulse 81/min, blood pressure 139/81 mm Hg, and respiratory rate 15/min. Her O_2 saturation is 100%. An x-ray of the chest shows cardiomegaly, and echocardiography shows a moderate pericardial effusion.

1. **The correct answer is D.** Dilated cardiomyopathy is a common cause of congestive heart failure. It is usually due to causes such as ischemic heart disease or hypertension, but in this case, it is likely due to the toxic effects of chronic alcohol consumption. The liver function tests and physical examination results are consistent with chronic alcoholism and alcoholic cirrhosis.

Answer A is incorrect. Lyme disease, caused by *Borrelia burgdorferi*, can induce a dilated cardiomyopathy, but there is nothing in the question stem to indicate this is the most likely etiology.

Answer B is incorrect. Cigarette smoking is a risk factor for coronary artery disease that can lead to ischemic cardiomyopathy. However, his smoking history is not likely significant enough to lead to this series of events.

Answer C is incorrect. Coxsackie B virus is a common cause of myocarditis, which can also lead to diastolic cardiomyopathy and congestive heart failure. This should be suspected in younger individuals without underlying medical problems.

Answer E is incorrect. Pantoprazole is not associated with toxicity to the heart.

Answer F is incorrect. Chagas disease, caused by *Trypanosoma cruzi*, can also be responsible for heart failure and dysrhythmias, but this is highly unlikely given that the distribution of the pathogen is mostly in Latin America.

2. **The correct answer is B.** Hypertension is the most important controllable risk factor for stroke, and the stroke risk attributable to this patient's high blood pressure is larger than any other factor. The other answers, although important for improving the patient's health and longevity, are less tightly correlated to reducing stroke risk.

Answer A is incorrect. Blood glucose reduction would lessen the patient's risk for diabetic complications, including retinopathy, neuropathy, and nephropathy, but is not as significant a risk reduction for cerebrovascular accident as reducing hypertension.

Answer C is incorrect. Reducing serum cholesterol does impact stroke risk but does not have a greater impact on stroke risk than reducing hypertension. Stroke prevention studies have implicated hypertension as the greatest contributing risk factor to stroke.

Answer D is incorrect. Smoking cessation would improve the patient's overall health and longevity and should be encouraged. Cerebrovascular accident can be multifactorial, but because hypertension is believed to have the largest effect on stroke risk, any stroke reduction program in this patient must effectively control his hypertension.

Answer E is incorrect. Weight loss would improve this patient's glycemic control, as well as overall cardiovascular health, but would not have a larger impact on stroke risk than reducing hypertension.

3. **The correct answer is D.** This female infant most likely has Turner's syndrome with the high-arched palate, webbed neck, widely spaced nipples, and edematous hands and feet. Turner's syndrome, or gonadal dysgenesis, is due to the absence of part or all of an X chromosome. It is the most common abnormality of the X chromosome, with an incidence of 1:2000 to 5000 liveborn girls. In the neonate, other possible findings include dysplastic nails and a short fourth metacarpal. Twenty percent or more of patients with Turner's syndrome also have a congenital heart defect. Bicuspid aortic valve and coarctation of the aorta are the most common cardiovascular malformations in Turner's syndrome patients. This patient's delayed femoral pulses suggest coarctation of the aorta, which is associated with a systolic murmur loudest below the left scapula. If tested, those with coarctation of the aorta will also have decreased blood pressures in the lower extremities versus the upper. If the ductus arteriosus is patent, patients may be asymptomatic. If it is closed, neonates may present

with heart failure and be pale, irritable, diaphoretic, and dyspneic.

Answer A is incorrect. A continuous machinery murmur at the left upper sternal border is associated with a patent ductus arteriosus (PDA), which is a possible finding in a neonate but is not the most common congenital heart defect associated with Turner's syndrome. A small PDA would be asymptomatic, whereas a large PDA would present in infancy with signs of heart failure, including failure to thrive, poor feeding, and respiratory distress.

Answer B is incorrect. A harsh holosystolic murmur at the left lower sternal border is associated with a ventricular septal defect (VSD). Neonates with isolated small VSDs are usually asymptomatic, whereas those with large VSDs present with signs of heart failure by 3–4 weeks of age. In fact, murmurs may not present until several weeks postnatally because the pulmonary vascular resistance decreases more slowly in these infants.

Answer C is incorrect. A single, loud S2 is a common finding in transposition of the great arteries or in tetralogy of Fallot. Children with tetralogy of Fallot present with cyanotic spells. The survival of infants with transposition of the great arteries depends on the presence of other defects that allow for the mixing of the circulations (patent ductus arteriosus, ventricular septal defect, or atrial septal defect).

Answer E is incorrect. A widely split, fixed S2 and systolic ejection murmur at the left upper sternal border is associated with an atrial septal defect (ASD). Small ASDs do not cause symptoms in infancy and childhood. Those with large ASDs may develop heart failure, or present later in life with dyspnea, fatigue, and atrial arrhythmias.

4. The correct answer is B. The patient most likely has an acute congestive heart failure exacerbation with the underlying etiology being hypertension. Echocardiography is an essential test in all patients with newly diagnosed heart failure and is an excellent, noninvasive method of assessing chamber size, function, and ejection fraction.

Answer A is incorrect. Cardiac angiography can determine cardiac pressures, but given the invasive nature of the procedure, it is best reserved for congestive heart failure patients in whom coronary artery disease is suspected as the underlying cause.

Answer C is incorrect. ECG in heart failure may show left ventricular hypertrophy in this patient, but is unlikely to be helpful if acute ischemia is not suspected.

Answer D is incorrect. Biopsy does play a role in the evaluation of heart failure, but is generally reserved for cases of unknown origin or acute cases in young patients. Certain causes of heart failure such as infiltrative disease can be confirmed by biopsy, but it is not likely to be useful here.

Answer E is incorrect. Pulmonary function tests have a role in the evaluation of dyspnea. However, they are not necessary if a cardiac cause is strongly suspected.

Answer F is incorrect. X-ray of the chest in heart failure may show pulmonary congestion or cardiomegaly, but these findings are relatively nonspecific.

5. The correct answer is A. You should be familiar with the goals of cholesterol-adjusting therapies. This patient has only one risk factor (family history) and his goal of LDL cholesterol is 160 mg/dL. Therapeutic lifestyle changes in the form of a 12-week trial of diet, exercise, and weight loss should be attempted given his current LDL level.

Answer B is incorrect. Combination therapies may prove necessary for management of his cholesterol at some later point. As this is his first presentation, therapeutic lifestyle changes should be instituted as first-line therapy.

Answer C is incorrect. Combination therapies may prove necessary for management of his cholesterol at some later point. As this is his first presentation, therapeutic lifestyle changes should be instituted as first-line therapy.

Answer D is incorrect. Niacin is a cheap and effective cholesterol-adjusting medication, particularly in raising levels of HDL cholesterol. Adverse effects include flushing and pruritus and this drug is often poorly tolerated. As with the statins, drug therapy is not necessary given his lipid profile and risk factors.

Answer E is incorrect. While statin therapy is effective in lowering LDL cholesterol, current guidelines suggest that first priority should be given to a trial of therapeutic lifestyle changes. Drug therapy should be initiated at an LDL cholesterol level ≤ 190 mg/dL. Hepatic dysfunction occurs in a small percentage of patients on statins, mostly within the first few months of treatment. The normal liver function tests presented here are reassuring if statin therapy is instituted at a later time.

6. **The correct answer is A.** Myocardial rupture is a sudden postinfarction complication that typically occurs 5–10 days post–myocardial infarction (peak at 7 days). During this time, the integrity of the cardiac wall is compromised by macrophage and mononuclear infiltration, fibrovascular response, and other inflammatory mediators, as they replace necrotic tissue with scar tissue. Old age, first infarction, and a history of hypertension are risk factors. The clinical manifestations, as depicted here, are a sudden loss of heart rate, blood pressure, and consciousness, while the ECG continues to show a sinus rhythm. Measures to prevent cardiac rupture include the administration of β-blockers, angiotensin-converting enzyme inhibitors, and the avoidance of steroidal and nonsteroidal anti-inflammatory agents such as ibuprofen and indomethacin.

Answer B is incorrect. A left ventricular thrombus can occur as a post–myocardial infarction complication. Although an embolus could result in stroke and subsequent mental status change, this would not cause a sudden loss of pulses and blood pressure.

Answer C is incorrect. Papillary muscle rupture will lead to sudden pulmonary edema, shortness of breath, effusions and crackles, and a new mitral regurgitation murmur on chest examination.

Answer D is incorrect. Pericarditis would likely result in a pericardial rub on physical examination and it usually causes ECG changes. The acute nature of this decompensation does not suggest pericarditis.

Answer E is incorrect. Although septal rupture could result in acute decompensation, a new harsh murmur could likely be picked up on physical examination. The electromechanical dissociation is more consistent with free wall rupture.

7. **The correct answer is C.** This patient displays symptoms of angina, tachycardia, rash, and joint pains. This lupus-like syndrome is a well-described adverse effect of hydralazine therapy. The vasodilatory action of hydralazine can result in reflex tachycardia and decreased oxygen delivery to the myocardium in patients with existing coronary artery disease. Other agents known to cause a systemic lupus erythematosus–like syndrome include isoniazid, procainamide, and phenytoin.

Answer A is incorrect. Angiotensin-converting enzyme inhibitors are most commonly associated with a dry cough (10–20% of people). Other important adverse effects include hyperkalemia (due to the blockade of aldosterone secretion), angioedema, and renal failure, especially in patients with known kidney disease.

Answer B is incorrect. In addition to the more common adverse effects of hypotension and hypokalemia, furosemide can lead to ototoxicity. It is not a known cause of tachycardia or a lupus-like syndrome.

Answer D is incorrect. β-Blockers are associated with depression and erectile dysfunction. They can also facilitate hypoglycemia through their adrenergic blockade and lead to hyperkalemia by similar mechanisms. Another important adverse effect of β-blockers is an increase in pulmonary reactivity; as a result, they are contraindicated in patients with asthma and chronic obstructive pulmonary disease. Furthermore, β-blockers lead to bradycardia, not tachycardia.

Answer E is incorrect. Calcium channel blockers such as verapamil act as reverse chronotropes, and thus can lead to bradycardia and even atrioventricular block. Other common adverse effects include gingival hyperplasia and constipation. There is no known association with lupus.

8. **The correct answer is D.** The ECG reveals atrial fibrillation, which was likely caused by cardiac ischemia in this patient. Since the patient is presenting with worsening symptoms, the atrial fibrillation can be considered unstable and therefore requires electrocardioversion.

Answer A is incorrect. Anticoagulation will not convert the patient out of an unstable rhythm, which should be the top priority at this point. Once the patient is stable, anticoagulation is an important intervention to prevent the risk of thromboembolism.

Answer B is incorrect. Although close clinical observation is important, it does not provide the definitive intervention required to convert the unstable cardiac rhythm.

Answer C is incorrect. An echocardiogram can be helpful to rule out a thrombus prior to electrical or chemical conversion if the atrial fibrillation has lasted at least 48 hours. However, the unstable nature of this patient's atrial fibrillation requires immediate electrocardioversion per the advanced cardiac life support protocol.

Answer E is incorrect. Rate control is very important in stable atrial fibrillation to maintain adequate cardiac output. However, this patient needs more urgent intervention.

9. **The correct answer is C.** A stab wound in a patient who is hemodynamically unstable requires immediate exploratory laparotomy. This patient is in shock, and the source of bleeding should be found.

Answer A is incorrect. If this patient were hemodynamically stable, this would have been a viable option. However, there should be no delay in getting this patient to the operating room.

Answer B is incorrect. This would have been another viable option if the patient was hemodynamically stable. However, shock is a contraindication to diagnostic peritoneal lavage, and no time should be spared getting the patient to the operating room.

Answer D is incorrect. Although a head injury is likely, the proper flow in management

should entail the **ABCD's** (**A**irway, **B**reathing, **C**irculation, and **D**isability). Controlling hemorrhage that is manifesting as shock takes priority over dealing with a concomitant head injury.

Answer E is incorrect. Hemorrhage control cannot be adequately achieved with laparoscopy. An expeditious laparotomy is indicated in the setting of hypovolemic shock.

10. **The correct answer is E.** This patient is presenting with a classic acute myocardial infarction, and he has fulfilled all indications for fibrinolytic therapy: acute chest pain suggesting myocardial infarction, time to therapy less than 12 hours, and ST segment elevation > 2–3 mm in the chest leads and 1 mm in the limb leads. Contraindications to fibrinolytic therapy must still be ruled out.

Answer A is incorrect. Calcium channel blockers have not been shown to affect mortality after myocardial infarction and may even be harmful in some patients.

Answer B is incorrect. Angiotensin-converting enzyme inhibitors are important once the patient is stable. They limit infarct expansion and improve structural remodeling in the days following an acute myocardial infarction.

Answer C is incorrect. β-Blockers are recommended to all patients with an ST elevation after myocardial infarction to decrease myocardial oxygen consumption and mortality.

Answer D is incorrect. Magnesium is not routinely used in acute myocardial infarction.

11. **The correct answer is C.** This patient has symptomatic bradycardia as evidenced by her altered mental status and hypoperfusion. In an elderly patient, it is most likely caused by an inferior wall myocardial infarction or sick sinus syndrome, but certain medications like nitroglycerin, β-blockers, angiotensin-converting enzyme inhibitors, or barbiturates can mimic a shock-like state. Atropine is the drug of choice for symptomatic bradycardia.

Answer A is incorrect. Adenosine is not part of the bradycardia algorithm. It is used for atrioventricular nodal reentrant tachycardia such as Wolff-Parkinson-White syndrome.

Answer B is incorrect. Amiodarone is not part of the bradycardia algorithm. It is a class III antiarrhythmic used for wide-complex tachycardia such as atrial fibrillation.

Answer D is incorrect. While isoproterenol is a part of the advance cardiac life support bradycardia algorithm, it is not a first-line agent. The mnemonic for the algorithm is "All Trained Dogs Eat Iams": Atropine, Transcutaneous pacing, Dopamine, Epinephrine, and Isoproterenol, given in that order.

Answer E is incorrect. Metoprolol is not part of the bradycardia algorithm. It is a β-blocker and would therefore slow the heart rate, exacerbating the problem.

12. **The correct answer is A.** Digoxin toxicity often presents with vague abdominal complaints, accompanied by neurologic (headache, delirium) complaints; visual (altered color perception, scotomata) complaints; and, most notably, cardiac arrhythmias. This patient may have taken too many digoxin pills. Plasma digoxin will help confirm the diagnosis (therapeutic range is 0.5–2 ng/mL). However, toxicity can also exist at normal levels, particularly in persons who are elderly. Because digoxin is renally excreted, the patient may have acute renal failure precipitating his toxicity; this must be investigated. Note that digoxin levels taken within 6–8 hours of ingestion do not reflect the steady state and are not reliable predictors of prognosis. Antidigoxigenin antibody Fab fragments are first-line therapy in the setting of life-threatening arrhythmia.

Answer B is incorrect. Although gastroenteritis can present with abdominal pain and nausea, the most likely diagnosis is digoxin toxicity because of the ECG changes.

Answer C is incorrect. Although hypercalcemia may present with abdominal pains, hypocalcemia does not present in this fashion.

Answer D is incorrect. Hypovolemia would not explain the clinical symptoms or the ECG findings.

Answer E is incorrect. Although patients who are elderly have atypical presentations of myocardial infarction (MI), the ECG changes are not suggestive of an acute MI.

13. **The correct answer is B.** Diastolic heart failure refers to the clinical evidence of heart failure (dyspnea and increased venous pressure) in the setting of a normal ejection fraction and normal valvular function. Diastolic failure is due to the inability of the ventricle to relax and properly fill during diastole. This results in a normal or decreased end-diastolic volume.

Answer A is incorrect. Elevated end-diastolic pressure can be found in both systolic and diastolic dysfunction.

Answer C is incorrect. Because contractile strength is usually maintained in the setting of a reduced end-diastolic volume, the ejection fraction can actually be elevated in diastolic heart failure.

Answer D is incorrect. One of the hallmarks of diastolic dysfunction is a large, stiff ventricle with an increased, not decreased, ratio of wall thickness to cavity size. This can be the result of hypertrophy or infiltrative disease.

Answer E is incorrect. Both systolic and diastolic dysfunction are associated with similar clinical symptoms, including a reduced exercise capacity.

Answer F is incorrect. Both systolic and diastolic dysfunction are associated with the typical findings of pulmonary venous congestion on x-ray of the chest, including cephalization of pulmonary vessels.

14. **The correct answer is D.** This patient is in hypertensive urgency: he has a diastolic blood pressure > 130 mm Hg but has no signs of end-organ damage. His ECG, laboratory values, and physical examination results are all normal. Initial management of hypertensive urgency involves administration of an oral antihypertensive. β-Blockers, loop diuretics, angiotensin-converting enzyme inhibitors, or calcium channel blockers are recommended, and two agents should be started if initial treatment fails to lower pressures to a safe level in 3–6 hours. Therefore, oral metoprolol would be appropriate management for our patient in hypertensive urgency.

Answer A is incorrect. The patient is not in hypertensive emergency because he does not have end-organ damage. Intravenous nitroprusside is first-line treatment in hypertensive emergency, but not hypertensive urgency. There is no proven benefit from rapid reduction in blood pressure in asymptomatic patients who have no evidence of end-organ damage.

Answer B is incorrect. Although this patient does meet requirements for hypertensive urgency, intravenous nitroprusside is a poor choice, as a rapid reduction in blood pressure may lead to end-organ damage.

Answer C is incorrect. While diuretics may lower the circulating blood volume and therefore the blood pressure, β-blockers, calcium channel blockers, and angiotensin-converting enzyme inhibitors tend to be more effective. Loop diuretics may be used as an adjunct if initial treatment fails.

Answer E is incorrect. The patient does not have signs or symptoms of end-organ damage, such as headaches, confusion, visual changes, chest pain, papilledema, retinal hemorrhages, or hematuria; therefore he is not in hypertensive emergency. In addition, sublingual nifedipine works quickly and may decrease the blood pressure into a range in which hypoperfusion and ischemia may occur. Therefore, it should generally be avoided in hypertensive emergency or urgency.

15. **The correct answer is B.** This patient is most likely suffering from hypovolemic shock secondary to perforation of a peptic ulcer, which is confirmed by the finding of free air in the abdomen. Initial resuscitation requires rapid re-expansion of the effective blood volume along with interventions to control ongoing losses. This is best accomplished with a rapid infusion of isotonic saline or lactated Ringer's solution through two large-bore intravenous lines.

Answer A is incorrect. Antibiotics are indicated in the setting of septic shock. Given the patient's age, it is possible that a perforated diverticulum could cause septic shock and have a similar presentation. However, a perforated ulcer is more likely because his pain was epigastric, whereas diverticular pain tends to localize to the lower abdomen. Furthermore, even if this patient were in septic shock, volume resuscitation would still be the initial step in treatment.

Answer C is incorrect. Infusing norepinephrine can increase arterial pressure by raising peripheral resistance. However, this is inappropriate other than as a temporizing measure in severe shock while the effective blood volume is being reexpanded with fluid resuscitation.

Answer D is incorrect. Inotropic support is particularly important in cardiogenic shock. The flat jugular veins suggest hypovolemic shock in this case. In the presence of severe or prolonged hypovolemia, inotropic support may be needed to maintain adequate cardiac output, but this should occur after effective blood volume has been restored.

Answer E is incorrect. Resuscitation should begin with crystalloid solutions. Banked blood products are hyperkalemic and acidotic, which can worsen reperfusion injury as the peripheral reperfusion flushes products of anaerobic metabolism back to the heart. This can lead to transient myocardial depression. It should be noted that although the patient's hemoglobin is normal, it takes time to equilibrate, even during an acute bleed. He may require red blood cells in the future.

16. **The correct answer is A.** This patient most likely suffers from Prinzmetal's angina, which is caused by coronary artery spasm. This type of angina usually occurs in smokers younger than those with unstable angina due to atherosclerotic disease. The pain is intermittent and can wake them up in the morning. During chest pain, an ECG will show multilead ST elevations that can resolve with the administration of nitroglycerin.

Answer B is incorrect. Stenosis of this type would result in persistent stable angina for the patient, while she describes more intermittent chest pain. Therefore, it is unlikely that she has such an extent of arterial stenosis, and the picture does not demonstrate any blockages.

Answer C is incorrect. The patient may have normal coronary arteries in between episodes, but the chest pain is brought on by coronary artery spasm so that is what should be seen on angiography. Spasm can be provoked by intracoronary acetylcholine or hyperventilation.

Answer D is incorrect. Plaque rupture and thrombosis leads to acute myocardial infarction, which would not present as chronic anginal pain of 3–4 weeks' duration.

17. **The correct answer is C.** The patient has dilated cardiomyopathy, a diagnosis that requires evidence of left ventricular dilation and systolic dysfunction with left ventricular ejection fraction < 40% on echocardiography. Dilation of the left ventricle (LV) results in decreased ability to contract and eject blood from the chamber, resulting in decreased LV ejection fraction. Patients usually present with symptoms of heart failure, arrhythmias, or even sudden death. Fifty percent of cases are of idiopathic etiology but the most common known causes are ischemic cardiomyopathy due to coronary artery disease, myocarditis, and infiltrative disease. Alcohol is a poorly understood but significant risk factor for dilated cardiomyopathy, and abstinence can result in remarkable recovery of cardiac function.

Answer A is incorrect. Although hepatojugular reflux and pulmonary congestion are both often seen in heart failure due to dilated cardiomyopathy, neither specifically is required for a diagnosis of dilated cardiomyopathy.

Answer B is incorrect. Ventricular dilation is a key component of dilated cardiomyopathy. However, aortic insufficiency is not usually found. Furthermore, this patient does not have any physical examination findings suggestive of aortic insufficiency, such as a diastolic murmur, Corrigan's pulse (water-hammer pulse), de Musset's sign (head bobbing), Traube's sign (pistol-shot sound over the femoral artery), Duroziez's sign (to-and-fro murmur over the femoral artery), Quincke's pulse (capillary pulsation in the nail beds), or Hill's sign (popliteal artery pressure greatly increased over brachial pressure).

Answer D is incorrect. Dilation of the ventricle(s) leads to impaired contraction of the myocardium and eventually to hypotrophy of the myocardium. Again, diastolic dysfunction is not a defining feature of dilated cardiomyopathy.

Answer E is incorrect. Pulmonary congestion is a result of heart failure and a common occurrence in dilated cardiomyopathy patients. However, the pathogenesis of dilated cardiomyopathy lies in systolic dysfunction, not diastolic dysfunction. Diastolic heart failure is characterized by symptoms of heart failure in the context of normal left ventricular (LV) systolic function (normal LV ejection fraction) and diastolic dysfunction (abnormal or elevated LV filling pressures). Common causes of diastolic heart failure include restrictive cardiomyopathy that results in decreased ability for LV filling, chronic hypertension with LV hypertrophy, hypertrophic cardiomyopathy, and ischemic heart disease.

18. **The correct answer is C.** The arrow in the photograph points to a vegetative growth on a native mitral valve. Mitral valve prolapse, particularly as a complication of rheumatic heart disease, is a risk factor for native valve infective endocarditis. This is because altered blood flow around a damaged valve provides the opportunity for a clot to develop and harbor bacteria, which gain access to the blood through a wound, dental work, surgery, or intravenous drug use. It can be prevented by replacing the valve with a prosthetic valve.

Answer A is incorrect. Coronary artery disease (CAD) could lead to valvular disease that would increase the risk of infective endocarditis, but CAD does not directly increase the risk of developing infective endocarditis.

Answer B is incorrect. Hypertension can lead to strain on the heart and its valves if poorly controlled, but it does not directly increase the risk of developing infective endocarditis.

Answer D is incorrect. Prolonged bedrest can lead to the development of deep venous blood clots. This could lead to pulmonary embolism as the clot travels in the venous return and through the right side of the heart. It would be extremely rare for the clot to find a path from the right side of the heart to the left-sided mitral valve. Even if this occurred, the concerning complication would be embolus to the brain, not lodging of the clot in the valve to serve as a site for bacterial growth.

Answer E is incorrect. While an artificial valve is a risk factor for infective endocarditis, it does not contribute to native valve endocarditis.

19. The correct answer is C. In patients with infective endocarditis and a history of intravenous drug abuse, *Staphylococcus aureus* is the causative agent in the vast majority of cases and is more likely to cause acute rather than subacute endocarditis. If the patient has a prosthetic valve, then coagulase-negative staphylococcus is the predominant organism. Bacterial endocarditis is an infectious process of the endothelial surface of the heart. Symptoms include fever, fatigue, malaise, vascular phenomena such as Janeway lesions, and immunologic phenomena such as Osler nodes. Diagnosis is usually based on the Duke criteria, and laboratory studies include blood culture and echocardiography. Treatment is through intravenous antibiotics and surgery for valve repair or replacement, if necessary.

Answer A is incorrect. Group A streptococcus, if untreated, can lead to rheumatic fever, damaging heart valves and muscle. Rheumatic fever can predispose the patient to subsequent development of infective endocarditis, but it does not cause the disease initially.

Answer B is incorrect. Tuberculosis can cause cardiac disease, but in this patient, especially with the history of intravenous drug abuse, *Staphylococcus aureus* is the most likely organism.

Answer D is incorrect. If the patient has a prosthetic valve, coagulase-negative staphylococcus is the predominant organism. Within 2 months of surgery, the most common organisms are nosocomial: coagulase-negative staphylococcus, *Staphylococcus aureus*, facultative gram-negative bacilli, diphtheroids, and fungi. Twelve months after surgery, the organisms are similar to those that cause community-acquired endocarditis.

Answer E is incorrect. *Streptococcus viridans* is the most common pathogen for left-sided subacute bacterial endocarditis.

20. The correct answer is B. Dextraposed transposition of the great arteries (D-TGA) is the most common cause of cyanotic heart disease in neonates. It accounts for 5% of congenital heart defects. With this defect, the aorta arises from the right ventricle and the pulmonary artery arises from the left ventricle. This leads to pulmonary and systemic circuits that are in parallel as opposed to in series. The deoxygenated blood is therefore recirculated through the body in the systemic circulation, while the oxygenated blood only flows through the pulmonary circulation. A lesion, such as an ASD, VSD, or PDA, is therefore required for mixing of the systemic and pulmonary circulations for survival. D-TGA usually presents at birth with cyanosis and tachypnea. Plain-film radiographs demonstrate an egg-shaped silhouette due to the absent main pulmonary artery stem and small heart base. Prostaglandin E$_1$ is used to keep the PDA open and increase mixing of deoxygenated and oxygenated blood. Balloon atrial septostomy can also be used if necessary. An arterial switch surgical procedure is used to repair the defect.

Answer A is incorrect. Coarctation of the aorta is a cause of acyanotic heart disease. It accounts for 8% of congenital heart defects, with a 2:1 male-to-female predominance. Coarctation of the aorta may be associated with a bicuspid aortic valve in 80% of cases. Congestive heart failure may develop in infancy in approximately 10% of patients. It manifests as a systolic ejection murmur at the left upper sternal border, radiating to the interscapular region. Physical examination is also remarkable for weak and delayed femoral pulses relative to the upper extremity pulses, and hypertension in the upper extremities. A "reverse 3" sign may be seen on x-ray of the chest due to constriction of the aorta at the coarctation and dilation of the aorta pre- and postcoarctation. Notching of the ribs may also be seen due to collateral circulation through the intercostal arteries, and erosion of the ribs by the collaterals. The defect may be repaired via angioplasty or surgery.

Answer C is incorrect. PDA causes acyanotic congenital heart disease. PDAs account for 10% of congenital heart disease, occurring with a high incidence in preterm infants and a 2:1 female-to-male predominance. Small PDAs are asymptomatic, while large ones may cause congestive heart failure, failure to thrive, and recurrent lower respiratory tract infections. On physical examination, a continuous machinery murmur heard best at the left upper sternal border, and bounding peripheral pulses may be present. There may also be a prominent apical impulse and a thrill. X-ray of the chest may show cardiomegaly and increased pulmonary vascular markings. PDAs usually close within the first month of life. In preterm infants, indomethacin may be administered to close the PDA. PDAs may also be surgically ligated or coil embolized if necessary.

Answer D is incorrect. Tetralogy of Fallot (TOF) is the third most common cause of cyanotic heart disease in neonates, after dextra-posed transposition of the great arteries and hypoplastic left heart syndrome. It is composed of four defects: right ventricular outflow tract obstruction, ventricular septal defect, right ventricular hypertrophy, and an overriding aorta. TOF usually presents in infancy with cyanotic spells and agitation. The spells either resolve spontaneously or can lead to hypoxia, metabolic acidosis, and death. On physical examination, these infants have a normal S1, single S2, and a harsh systolic crescendo-decrescendo ejection murmur (due to right ventricular outflow tract obstruction), which is loudest over the left upper sternal border and radiates to the back. A boot-shaped heart may be seen on x-ray of the chest and there are increased pulmonary vascular markings. Tetralogy of Fallot is corrected surgically.

Answer E is incorrect. Truncus arteriosus is a rare congenital heart defect that causes cyanotic and congestive heart disease. It is characterized by a single great arterial trunk arising from the ventricles, branching into the pulmonary arteries distal to the coronary arteries and proximal to the first brachiocephalic branch of the aortic arch. There is always an associated VSD for complete mixing of pulmonary and systemic blood, resulting in identical oxygen saturation in the pulmonary arteries and aorta. Thirty percent of these infants have a right-sided aortic arch. A harsh holosystolic murmur is present at the left lower sternal border due to the VSD, and there is a prominent single S2. Arterial pulses are bounding and there is a widened pulse pressure. Cardiomegaly and increased pulmonary vascular markings are present on chest x-ray. Digoxin and diuretics may be used in the initial management, and the defect may then be repaired with surgery.

21. **The correct answer is C.** This patient presented with a tension pneumothorax, which results from a parenchymal wound that acts as a one-way valve that allows free air into the pleural space but prevents its escape, causing collapse of the lung on the affected side. It is a medical emergency, as the building pressure in the pleural space causes shifting or displacement of the mediastinum to the contralateral side and subsequently compromises cardiopulmonary function. Compression of the opposite lung impairs proper gas exchange while impingement on the heart impairs proper cardiac function. The most common mechanisms of this type of injury are blunt or penetrating injuries, or secondary to medical procedures. A large-bore needle should be inserted in the second intercostal space in the midclavicular line to facilitate decompression and reestablish cardiopulmonary function. The needle is left in place until a thoracostomy tube can be inserted.

Answer A is incorrect. Although tube thoracotomy is also needed, tension pneumothorax is a medical emergency and demands urgent decompression. A large release of air after needle insertion confirms the diagnosis, and can then be followed by a thoracotomy. The chest tube is then attached to a vacuum to continuously remove air from the pleural cavity until healing of the parenchyma occurs.

Answer B is incorrect. The location of the wound in the fifth intercostal space implies that abdominal injury is possible. However, in following the ABCs as part of advanced trauma life support protocol, breathing must be adequately treated before evaluating circulation and proceeding to a diagnostic peritoneal lavage.

Answer D is incorrect. Pericardiocentesis is the treatment of choice for cardiac tamponade, which can also present with tachycardia, jugular venous distention, and decreased blood pressure. However, the location of the wound, the tracheal deviation, absent breath sounds, hyperresonance to percussion, and severity of dyspnea suggest tension pneumothorax.

Answer E is incorrect. Exploratory thoracotomy is the treatment for massive hemothorax. However, tension pneumothorax is best managed with needle thoracostomy followed by tube thoracotomy.

22. **The correct answer is A.** This man has a cardiac enzyme leak of specific myocardial markers that suggests acute myocardial infarction. Unstable angina (UA) is defined as either rest angina more than 20 minutes in duration, new-onset angina, or increasing angina that is more frequent, longer in duration, or occurs with less exertion than previous angina. Unstable angina and non-ST elevation myocardial infarction (NSTEMI) are part of the continuum of acute coronary syndromes, in which plaque rupture and coronary thrombosis compromise blood flow to a region of viable myocardium. In UA and NSTEMI, ST elevation and pathologic Q waves are absent. They are treated with medical management (antiplatelet therapy, nitroglycerin, β-blockade, and morphine), and considered for revascularization.

Answer B is incorrect. This man has the signs, symptoms, and laboratory test results of somebody undergoing a myocardial infarction, so hypochondriasis can be ruled out.

Answer C is incorrect. Prinzmetal's angina does not produce positive cardiac enzymes. It is due to coronary vasospasm, and can be treated with medical therapy (calcium channel blockers).

Answer D is incorrect. Stable angina does not produce positive cardiac enzymes. It is defined as chest pain that is reproducible with a certain degree of exertion. These patients may be treated with medical management if low-risk, or with revascularization if high-risk (i.e., left

main artery disease or three-vessel disease), or if they have refractory symptoms.

Answer E is incorrect. Unstable angina (UA) does not produce positive cardiac enzymes. However, the initial management of UA and non-ST segment myocardial infarction are similar (medical management with nitroglycerin, β-blockade, antiplatelet/anticoagulation, and consideration of angiography and revascularization).

23. **The correct answer is A.** You should be able to recognize diastolic dysfunction as a cause of heart failure. In diastolic heart failure, left ventricular ejection fraction is normal (> 50%). Heart failure results from an inability of the left ventricle to fill during diastole rather than an inability of the left ventricle to eject blood into systemic flow. Hypertensive heart disease is one of the most common causes of diastolic heart failure. This patient's medical history of hypertension, in-office measurement indicating high blood pressure, and the ECG showing left ventricular hypertrophy is consistent with this diagnosis.

Answer B is incorrect. Hypertrophic obstructive cardiomyopathy (HOCM) may manifest with hypertension and an ECG showing left ventricular hypertrophy. However, echocardiography of patients with HOCM typically shows asymmetric septal wall thickening (septum-to-ventricular wall thickness ratio > 1.3). Subaortic stenosis oftentimes results from septal wall thickening, causing obstruction across the aortic outflow tract. HOCM is oftentimes familial and is manifest earlier in life (childhood through young adulthood). Patients rarely present in the ninth decade of life.

Answer C is incorrect. Ischemic heart disease is one of the most common causes of diastolic dysfunction and must always be included on the differential. However, an ECG showing lack of ST elevation (indicating acute infarct) or depression (indicating ischemia), Q waves, or T-wave inversions (indicating previous infarct) makes this diagnosis less likely.

Answer D is incorrect. This patient's normal left ventricular ejection fraction (LVEF) is more consistent with diastolic heart failure.

Mitral valve prolapse results in systolic heart failure instead of diastolic heart failure. Increased regurgitation over the mitral valve results in an increased preload and inability of the ventricle to eject this increased volume (decreased LVEF). Furthermore, no regurgitation was noted on Doppler flow on echocardiography, making this answer choice unlikely.

Answer E is incorrect. Myocarditis can be associated with diastolic heart failure, but is less likely in this case given no recent viral illness. This patient's age, past medical history, and ECG are all consistent with hypertensive heart disease.

24. **The correct answer is A.** Hypertension is a risk factor for both chronic renal insufficiency and end-stage renal disease. Hypertension can directly cause renal disease and accelerate the progression of underlying renal pathology. In addition, hypertension increases a patient's risk of premature cardiovascular disease, heart failure, stroke, and intracerebral hemorrhage.

Answer B is incorrect. Hypertension does not increase a patient's risk of hypercholesterolemia; however, both hypertension and hypercholesterolemia increase a patient's risk of cardiovascular disease.

Answer C is incorrect. Hypertension does not increase a patient's risk of hypertrophic cardiomyopathy. Hypertrophic cardiomyopathy is a disease in which the heart muscle thickens and therefore has impaired functioning. Hypertrophic cardiomyopathy is an inherited disorder due to autosomal dominant gene mutations. This disease may cause angina and dyspnea, but often the first symptom of the disease is sudden cardiac death.

Answer D is incorrect. Hypertension does not increase a patient's risk of atrioventricular (AV) block. The most common etiologies of second-degree Mobitz I AV block are drugs, acute inferior myocardial infarction, and enhanced vagal tone.

Answer E is incorrect. Hypertension does not increase a patient's risk of type 2 diabetes; however, both hypertension and diabetes increase a patient's risk of cardiovascular disease.

25. **The correct answer is D.** Lidocaine is an important agent used for the acute treatment of ventricular arrhythmias, especially those following acute MI. It is a class IB antiarrhythmic and thus acts on the ventricular myocardium by mildly blocking sodium channels, slowing repolarization in Purkinje cells, and increasing the firing threshold in pacemaker cells. It has relatively few serious adverse effects; however, patients on lidocaine may experience significant neurologic complications. This patient is displaying the classic neurologic adverse effects of lidocaine, including slurred speech and confusion. Other common adverse effects include tremor, personality and mood changes, and hallucinations. These effects are entirely reversible with the removal of therapy.

Answer A is incorrect. Salicylates are not associated with central nervous system adverse effects with normal dosing. With normal dosing, they may cause renal disease, bleeding, and gastrointestinal upset. In toxic quantities, however, they can lead to an altered mental status and tinnitus.

Answer B is incorrect. Angiotensin-converting enzyme inhibitors are commonly associated with hyperkalemia, renal failure, and dry cough. More rarely, they cause angioedema. They do not commonly cause central nervous system disturbances.

Answer C is incorrect. Selective serotonin reuptake inhibitors are commonly associated with sexual dysfunction and anxiety. Even in overdose, they have few adverse effects, which are mostly limited to the gastrointestinal tract.

Answer E is incorrect. β-Blockers are mainly associated with depression and sexual adverse effects. They can also produce sleep disturbances but are not associated with more severe central nervous system effects.

26. **The correct answer is A.** This patient has the characteristic symptoms and signs of cardiac tamponade. She complains of chest pain, fatigue, and dyspnea, all characteristic of tamponade. On physical examination, she has Beck's triad, a group of signs characterized by hypotension, distant heart sounds, and distended neck veins. The fluid accumulation

around the heart decreases the ventricular filling pressure, which decreases cardiac output. She also has tachycardia and tachypnea, both found in patients with cardiac tamponade. X-ray of the chest showing cardiomegaly is due to a large pericardial effusion, and the echocardiogram would show a large pleural effusion with chamber collapse, a characteristic echocardiographic sign of tamponade.

Answer B is incorrect. Although the patient's x-ray of the chest showed cardiomegaly, this was secondary to a large pericardial effusion leading to tamponade, not an enlarged heart as seen in heart failure. It would be unlikely to see such an acute onset of decompensated heart failure in this otherwise healthy, young woman. In addition, the patient has the classic physical findings of cardiac tamponade.

Answer C is incorrect. Although panic attacks can present as chest pain, tachypnea, and tachycardia, this patient has several findings on physical examination and diagnostic studies that support the diagnosis of cardiac tamponade.

Answer D is incorrect. Although this patient most likely has pericarditis, this diagnosis alone cannot explain her clinical picture. Her pericardial effusion has progressed to cause cardiac tamponade. Her distended neck veins, muffled heart sounds, and hypotension are all signs of cardiac tamponade and do not occur with simple pericarditis.

Answer E is incorrect. Although a tension pneumothorax can lead to tachypnea, tachycardia, and hypotension, the patient's x-ray of the chest would have shown a pneumothorax had one existed.

27. **The correct answer is D.** Unstable angina is acute myocardial ischemia without evidence of myocardial necrosis, manifesting as angina that is new-onset, crescendos, or occurs at rest. It can present with or without ECG changes, including ST depressions, but by definition cardiac enzymes are normal. Treatment involves relief of ischemic pain, assessment of hemodynamic status, and antithrombotic therapy if necessary. If this patient was having an acute myocardial infarction, you would expect to see ST elevations and positive cardiac enzymes.

Answer A is incorrect. Delta waves are associated with Wolff-Parkinson-White syndrome and would only be an incidental finding in this patient as opposed to a finding produced by his angina. Also, unstable angina should not produce positive cardiac enzymes.

Answer B is incorrect. Low-voltage ECG can be caused by poorly placed leads, hemopericardium, emphysema, or massive obesity. Unstable angina would not cause a low-voltage ECG and would not cause positive cardiac enzymes.

Answer C is incorrect. Positive enzymes with no ECG changes can occur but are not indicative of unstable angina. This scenario can be seen days after a cardiac event, as enzymes can remain positive for many days, or as a result of an enzyme leak secondary to a cardiac insult.

Answer E is incorrect. The presence of Q waves (in addition to ST elevations) indicates previous insult to the myocardium, as Q waves do not appear until days after the insult. Therefore it is unlikely that we would see Q waves associated with this patient's unstable angina.

28. **The correct answer is B.** Diastolic dysfunction should be expected in the setting of an elderly patient with heart failure but a normal ejection fraction. Heart failure due to systolic dysfunction is more common, and is usually due to a weak heart that cannot contract normally. The heart can still fill with blood but cannot pump out as much blood as it used to; therefore, the ejection fraction decreases. Heart failure due to diastolic dysfunction is a result of stiff and thick heart walls that do not allow the ventricles to fill normally with blood. Consequently, blood backs up in the left atrium and lung (pulmonary) blood vessels, resulting in congestion. Nonetheless, the heart may be able to pump out a normal percentage of the blood it receives, which is why the ejection fraction can be unchanged.

Answer A is incorrect. Systolic dysfunction is more often due to ischemic heart disease and coronary artery disease and carries with it a worse prognosis than diastolic dysfunction.

Answer C is incorrect. While ischemic heart disease is more often seen in the setting of systolic dysfunction, it is one of the important causes of diastolic dysfunction as well. Other causes of diastolic dysfunction include restrictive cardiomyopathies, constrictive pericarditis, and hypertrophic heart disease.

Answer D is incorrect. All the clinical manifestations of systolic dysfunction (including pulmonary congestion) can be seen in diastolic dysfunction.

Answer E is incorrect. Diastolic dysfunction increases with age and is most often seen in patients older than 70.

29. **The correct answer is C.** Laceration of a coronary vessel is the most dangerous complication of pericardiocentesis. It can lead to worsened cardiac tamponade, myocardial infarction, and even death. This patient has worsening chest pain and hemodynamics during pericardiocentesis, the most likely cause of which is laceration of a coronary vessel.

Answer A is incorrect. Acute left ventricular failure with pulmonary edema is a rare complication of pericardiocentesis. This patient's lungs are clear to auscultation bilaterally after the procedure, which makes this complication unlikely.

Answer B is incorrect. Aspiration of air into the pericardium typically does not cause clinical signs or symptoms, unless the amount of air aspirated into the pericardium exceeds the amount of fluid withdrawn.

Answer D is incorrect. Pneumothorax is a rare complication of pericardiocentesis. This patient's lung examination and x-ray of the chest are not consistent with the diagnosis of pneumothorax.

Answer E is incorrect. Puncture of the left ventricle during pericardiocentesis rarely causes significant bleeding. Although a small pericardial bleed may be painful, it typically resolves on its own and does not lead to hemodynamic compromise.

30. **The correct answer is E.** The patient can best decrease his risk of a second myocardial infarc-

tion by quitting smoking. In some studies, patients who already had an initial coronary event and subsequently quit smoking decreased their risk of a second coronary event by 50%. Those who quit smoking, even those with known coronary vascular disease (CVD), reduced their risk of CVD development to nearly that of a nonsmoker within 3 years.

Answer A is incorrect. Secondary prevention of CVD by treating hyperlipidemia has shown reductions in CVD in the 20–35% range in 5-year follow-up.

Answer B is incorrect. Exercise has only been shown to offer mild to moderate reduction in risk for coronary vascular disease. In this case, the patient should undergo a symptom-limited stress test within 4–12 weeks and start an exercise program monitored by a physician.

Answer C is incorrect. This patient is barely in the hypertensive range (> 140/90 mm Hg) and so better control of his hypertension will not bring as dramatic an effect as modification of his smoking habit.

Answer D is incorrect. Tight glycemic control has not been shown to dramatically decrease the risk of coronary vascular disease.

31. **The correct answer is C.** Nearly any dysrhythmia may be precipitated by acute digitalis toxicity, but atrial tachycardia with 2:1 block, accelerated junctional rhythm, and bidirectional ventricular tachycardia (Torsades de pointes) are frequently seen, due to the combination of decreased atrioventricular node conduction and increased automaticity. Magnesium sulfate is the drug of choice for treating Torsades de pointes, including in the setting of digitalis toxicity, since it decreases calcium influx and thus reduces the early afterdepolarizations that perpetuate this dysrhythmia. A therapeutic level is 4–5 mEq/L. Additional treatment for torsades in the setting of digoxin overdose include anti-digitalis Fab fragments, lidocaine, and direct current cardioversion.

Answer A is incorrect. Calcium gluconate is used for prophylaxis against dysrhythmia in the setting of hyperkalemia. However, it is not recommended in the setting of digitalis toxicity, since intracellular calcium levels are already high. Also, the patient's potassium is high-normal.

Answer B is incorrect. A loop diuretic would not be indicated in this setting, since it could exacerbate electrolyte abnormalities and contribute to hypotension.

Answer D is incorrect. Potassium administration is important in the setting of digitalis toxicity if serum potassium is low, since hypokalemia slows repolarization of the myocyte and may perpetuate dysrhythmias such as Torsades de pointes. The patient's potassium is currently high-normal so potassium administration would not be indicated; however, this should be carefully monitored, as the extracellular potassium shift caused by digitalis may mask low intracellular potassium levels.

Answer E is incorrect. Sodium polystyrene sulfonate (Kayexalate) is a potassium-binding resin used in the treatment of hyperkalemia in renal failure and other settings. It should not be used in the setting of digitalis toxicity, since hyperkalemia in that case is generally due to an extracellular shift, not increased whole-body potassium.

32. **The correct answer is E.** This is a classic description of restrictive cardiomyopathy (RCM). RCM is almost always associated with infiltrative diseases such as amyloidosis, sarcoidosis, or hemochromatosis. These conditions restrict left ventricle filling, causing decreased output and compliance, and increased filling pressure. Consequently, patients begin to experience congestive heart failure symptoms. Here, this patient complains of dyspnea (positional and with exertion), syncope, and peripheral edema. She also has the classic Kussmaul's sign (increased jugular venous distension with inspiration) that, although it is not specific for this condition, contributes to making the diagnosis. The combination of the echocardiogram and ECG signs listed are also classic for making the diagnosis. Treatment of this condition is to control the underlying cause (e.g., iron chelation for hemochromatosis), diuretics, angiotensin-converting enzyme inhibitors, and nitrates.

Answer A is incorrect. Aortic stenosis (AS) is important because it is currently the leading indication for valve replacement. AS usually presents in older individuals (age $\geq$ 60 years) and features the classic triad of angina, syncope, and heart failure. Physical examination reveals pulsus parvus et tardus (small and slowly rising carotid pulse).

Answer B is incorrect. Cardiac tamponade usually presents as subacute dyspnea, fatigue, or anxiety that waxes and wanes. It is often associated with end-stage renal disease or other conditions that may involve the pericardium. Physical examination is characterized by Beck's triad (jugular venous distention, hypotension, and muffled heart sounds). It can be caused by pericarditis.

Answer C is incorrect. This patient's blood pressure is within normal limits, and there is low suspicion for hypertensive heart disease. However, hypertensive heart disease can manifest as concentric and eventually dilated heart failure. On echocardiography, a dilated heart with an elevated end-diastolic volume and low ejection fraction would be detected. Arrhythmias and angina may accompany a hypertensive crisis.

Answer D is incorrect. Pericarditis is most often confused with restrictive cardiomyopathy (RCM). To differentiate these two conditions, first look at the history. Pericarditis patients will likely have had a viral infection 1–2 weeks preceding the complaints. Physical examination is also helpful because pericarditis patients will often have a pericardial knock or rub and a prominent S4 heart sound. On biopsy, pericarditis samples will be normal, and RCM will be abnormal.

33. **The correct answer is A.** Atrial septal defects are often asymptomatic and cause acyanotic heart disease. As described in this patient, physical examination may be remarkable for a wide, fixed, split S2 with a systolic ejection murmur at the left upper sternal border. Some patients also have a mid-diastolic rumble at the left lower sternal border. Both murmurs represent increased blood flow across the pulmonic and tricuspid valves.

Answer B is incorrect. Coarctation of the aorta may produce a systolic ejection murmur at the left upper sternal border, radiating to the interscapular region. Physical examination is also remarkable for weak and delayed femoral pulses relative to upper extremity pulses, and hypertension in the upper extremities.

Answer C is incorrect. Transposition of the great arteries (TGA) occurs when the aorta arises from the right ventricle (RV) and the pulmonary artery (PA) rises from the left ventricle. Dextraposed TGA (D-TGA) describes the form in which the aorta is anterior and to the right of the PA. It usually presents with cyanosis and tachypnea within hours of birth because the systemic and pulmonary circulations are parallel rather than serial. Oxygenated blood circulates through the lungs repeatedly, while deoxygenated blood is pumped to the body. D-TGA is incompatible with life unless there are other defects present, such as atrial or ventricular septal defects or a PDA, that allow for mixing between the two parallel circulations and delivery of oxygen to the body.

Answer D is incorrect. Tetralogy of Fallot (TOF) is composed of four defects: right ventricular outflow tract obstruction, VSD, right ventricular hypertrophy, and an overriding aorta. TOF usually presents in infancy, with cyanotic spells, a normal S1, single S2, and a harsh systolic crescendo–decrescendo ejection murmur (due to right ventricular outflow tract obstruction). This murmur is heard best over the left upper sternal border and radiates to the back. It is also possible to have a holosystolic murmur at the left lower sternal border from the VSD and a continuous machinery murmur if a PDA is present.

Answer E is incorrect. VSDs are the most common congenital heart defect. They are usually associated with a holosystolic murmur that is loudest at the left lower sternal border.

34. **The correct answer is D.** This patient most likely has fibromuscular dysplasia leading to renal artery stenosis. She has early-onset hypertension that is refractory to pharmacotherapy. In addition, she has an abdominal bruit, suggestive of renal artery stenosis. Young women with early onset of hypertension refractory to pharmacotherapy are the most common patient population for fibromuscular dysplasia.

Fibromuscular dysplasia can be diagnosed by duplex imaging of the renal arteries, and percutaneous transluminal angioplasty is the treatment of choice in young patients with this disease and refractory hypertension.

Answer A is incorrect. This patient's renal artery stenosis is most likely due to fibromuscular dysplasia, not atherosclerosis. Adding a statin may decrease her cholesterol, but there is no reason to suspect that her cholesterol is elevated or that decreasing her cholesterol will affect her blood pressure.

Answer B is incorrect. Nitroprusside is the treatment of choice in a hypertensive emergency. Although this patient has stage 2 hypertension, she has no signs of end-organ damage; therefore, she is not in a hypertensive emergency, and nitroprusside is not indicated.

Answer C is incorrect. Although therapy with a thiazide diuretic and an angiotensin-converting enzyme (ACE) inhibitor may be sufficient to control hypertension from renal artery stenosis in some individuals, these medications are not achieving goal pressures in this young woman. In addition, it is important to establish a diagnosis in this patient, rather than treating her hypertension without knowing its etiology. ACE inhibitors can cause an elevation in creatinine in patients with bilateral renal artery stenosis because the glomerular filtration depends largely on angiotensin II in the setting of decreased renal blood flow.

Answer E is incorrect. Although duplex imaging of the renal arteries is an appropriate diagnostic step, percutaneous transluminal angioplasty is the treatment of choice for fibromuscular dysplasia. It has a high success rate, a low restenosis rate, and minimal risk; therefore, angioplasty would be preferred over more invasive surgical revascularization in this setting.

35. **The correct answer is A.** Disseminated intravascular coagulation (DIC) is a consumptive coagulopathy that has been associated with a number of clinical conditions, including bacterial infections such as meningococcemia. DIC involves activation of the coagulation pathways, excessive fibrin formation, and

platelet activation. Subsequent bleeding results because of the depletion of coagulation factors and platelets in the circulation. Because of the consumption of coagulation factors and activation of platelets, patients present with prolonged bleeding time, prothrombin time, activated partial thromboplastin time, and thrombin time, and thrombocytopenia and schistocytes on peripheral blood smear. Although not specific, the presence of D-dimer and fibrinogen degradation products supports a diagnosis of DIC.

Answer B is incorrect. Factor V Leiden involves a genetic mutation that renders factor V of the coagulation pathway resistant to degradation by activated protein C. Factor Va therefore does not get cleaved, but rather remains active, leading to a hypercoagulable state. Thrombocytopenia and bleeding are not manifestations of factor V Leiden and therefore are not supported by the clinical history, laboratory findings, or peripheral smear.

Answer C is incorrect. Immune thrombocytopenic purpura refers to immune-mediated platelet destruction by autoantibodies. Although ITP may present with petechiae and thrombocytopenia, the peripheral smear often shows larger, younger platelets that are produced to compensate for the increased platelet destruction. ITP may present with spontaneous bleeding if the platelet count is below 10,000/mm^3. Like DIC, ITP may present with increased bleeding time due to a decrease in the number of platelets available. ITP, however, is not associated with a prolonged prothrombin time, activated partial thromboplastin time, or thrombin time as seen in DIC.

Answer D is incorrect. Protein C deficiency causes a procoagulant-anticoagulant imbalance. Without protein C, there is increased propensity to form clots and decreased anticoagulation. Thrombocytopenia and increased bleeding are not manifestations of protein C deficiency and therefore are not supported by the clinical history, laboratory findings, or peripheral smear.

Answer E is incorrect. Thrombotic thrombocytopenic purpura (TTP) involves vascular aggregation of platelets that leads to thrombocytopenia and mechanical injury to red blood cells. TTP may be caused by drugs, HIV, pregnancy, autoimmune disease, familial causes, or can be idiopathic; TTP has not been associated directly with meningococcemia. Although one may see thrombocytopenia with prolonged bleeding time in the presence of schistocytes, the prothrombin time, activated partial thromboplastin time, and thrombin time would not be prolonged in the case of TTP.

36. **The correct answer is D.** Pulseless electrical activity (PEA) is an important reversible bradyarrhythmia. It often represents an underlying disorder such as pulmonary embolism, tamponade, or severe acidosis. Advanced cardiac life support recommends initial basic life support stabilization of a patient with demonstrated PEA. Once airway and breathing have been secured, several medications can be administered to address the PEA. These include several doses each of empiric bicarbonate, epinephrine, and atropine. After the administration of each medication, reassessment of the ECG is important. Atropine works on the heart by antagonizing muscarinic receptors and releasing the vagal stimulus on the heart. As an anticholinergic agent, it has several characteristic and uncomfortable adverse effects. Although they are rarely life threatening, they can be quite concerning to a patient experiencing them. They include blurry vision (blind as a bat), cutaneous flushing (red as a beet, hot as a hare), confusion (mad as a hatter), and dry mucous membranes (dry as a bone). Because these adverse effects are uncomfortable, they should be treated supportively.

Answer A is incorrect. This patient does not need to be treated. Therefore, a cholinergic agonist is not needed.

Answer B is incorrect. A muscarinic agonist is incorrect because no medication is needed to treat these adverse effects of atropine.

Answer C is incorrect. This patient is not experiencing bicarbonate toxicity. Symptoms of bicarbonate toxicity include respiratory depression, hypernatremia, hypokalemia, and edema.

Answer E is incorrect. The patient is not experiencing transient adverse effects of bicarbonate.

37. The correct answer is E. When patients stand, baroreceptors in the carotids and aorta typically sense decreased blood flow as blood pools in the venous system due to gravity. This leads to a sympathetic response which stimulates α_1-adrenergic receptors, causing a reflexive vasoconstriction and increased resistance in order to maintain blood pressure. If a patient is taking an α_1-adrenergic blocking agent, this reflexive vasoconstriction and increased resistance is blocked, and patients often experience orthostatic hypotension.

Answer A is incorrect. Prazosin is used to treat benign prostatic hypertrophy (BPH). α_1-adrenergic blockade leads to decreased tone in the smooth muscle of the prostate and urethra, thereby improving urine flow in patients with BPH.

Answer B is incorrect. Prazosin decreases blood pressure by α_1-adrenergic blockade. Stimulation of α_1-adrenergic receptors causes vasoconstriction and increased resistance, which leads to an increase in blood pressure. If stimulation of these receptors is blocked with prazosin, then there is vasodilation, decreased resistance, and a decrease in blood pressure.

Answer C is incorrect. α_1-Adrenergic blockade is not known to change sexual drive.

Answer D is incorrect. α_1-Adrenergic blockade is not known to cause irritability.

38. The correct answer is C. Feeding is a strenuous activity for many infants and can lead to failure to thrive in children with congenital heart disease. Most small ventricular septal defects (VSDs) close spontaneously during the first few years of life; however, this child's VSD is still present given the unchanged murmur, and is leading to weight loss. A high-calorie intake has not led to resolution of the failure to thrive. Therefore, referral for possible closure of the VSD is the correct choice.

Answer A is incorrect. The child is currently below the fifth percentile for weight with an identifiable etiology. As delayed head growth may also prevent normal brain development, this child should be referred for possible closure of her ventricular septal defect.

Answer B is incorrect. Though a pH probe could be placed, there are no signs of gastro-esophageal reflux disease (GERD) to support this decision. The child has an uncorrected VSD, which is the more likely cause of failure to thrive in this case. Frequent spitting up or vomiting and crying or irritability after feedings would be typical presenting symptoms of GERD.

Answer D is incorrect. Given the appropriate interaction between the child and her parents, her well-kept appearance, and no physical evidence of abuse such as bruises or other scars, it is less likely that abuse is the cause of her weight loss. A skeletal survey is not necessary.

Answer E is incorrect. This patient does not have a fever or elevated WBC count. Furthermore, the child's symptoms and history are more consistent with failure to thrive from her VSD, not an infection.

39. The correct answer is E. Brain natriuretic peptide (BNP) levels are increasingly utilized in the management of heart failure. It is often used in the setting of shortness of breath when differentiating between a pulmonary and a cardiac etiology. Levels can predict heart failure from a systolic and diastolic cause with approximately equal accuracy; however, BNP cannot differentiate between the two. Note that N-pro-BNP (a peptide cleaved in BNP release) is often tested because levels rise higher in patients with left ventricular dysfunction.

Answer A is incorrect. The cardiac natriuretic peptides have numerous effects and act as counterregulatory hormones in heart failure. The main physiologic effects are diuresis, hypotension, and antagonism of the renin-angiotensin system. This results in increased venous capacitance and decreased preload.

Answer B is incorrect. One of the main uses of the plasma BNP is in the diagnosis and prognosis of congestive heart failure. Numerous studies have shown an increase (not decrease) in levels in the setting of left ventricular dysfunction.

Answer C is incorrect. As the name suggests, brain natriuretic peptide was initially discovered in the brain but is mainly secreted by stretch of the cardiac ventricles, not the atria. Atrial natriuretic peptide is secreted by the cardiac atria.

Answer D is incorrect. BNP is secreted in response to volume overload (not hypovolemia), which has a similar stretch effect on the ventricles as pressure overload.

Answer F is incorrect. BNP does not cause an increase in pressure, but rather is secreted in response to pressure overload, which manifests as stretch of the cardiac ventricles.

40. **The correct answer is D.** This patient presents with the classic triad of symptoms for the diagnosis of a ruptured abdominal aortic aneurysm (AAA): abdominal pain, pulsatile abdominal mass, and hypotension. In addition, this patient has several risk factors for an AAA rupture, including hypertension and chronic obstructive pulmonary disease. The skin discoloration along the left lower back may be due to a retroperitoneal hematoma that is associated with a ruptured AAA. Patients with AAA diameters between 5 and 7 cm have a 5-year risk of rupture of about 33%. The diagnosis of a ruptured AAA is lethal and demands immediate surgical attention. When ruptured AAA is highly suspicious, the patient should be taken immediately to the operating room for surgical repair without further diagnostic tests.

Answer A is incorrect. Aortic dissections may present with acute-onset abdominal pain and/or back pain and are associated with many of the same risk factors as AAA, including hypertension and hypercholesterolemia. Patients with aortic dissections do not typically present with a pulsatile abdominal mass. This patient's presentation and history supports a diagnosis of ruptured AAA rather than aortic dissection.

Answer B is incorrect. Although patients with mesenteric ischemia may present with acute-onset severe abdominal pain with negative abdominal physical examination findings, this patient is more likely to have a diagnosis of ruptured AAA due to the presence of hypotension and a pulsatile abdominal mass that are not explained by mesenteric ischemia.

Answer C is incorrect. Patients with a perforated gastric ulcer often present with severe abdominal pain and distension with free intraperitoneal air that can be seen on an upright chest x-ray. A diagnosis of a perforated gastric ulcer would not explain the hypotension or pulsatile abdominal mass that this patient presents with. This patient's presentation and history supports a diagnosis of ruptured AAA rather than perforated gastric ulcer.

Answer E is incorrect. This patient's presentation and history supports a diagnosis of ruptured AAA rather than stroke. The patient complains of some lightheadedness, which may be seen in stroke victims; however, there appear to be no neurologic abnormalities noted.

41. **The correct answer is C.** Dilated cardiomyopathy may be caused by a number of factors, one of the most important of which is alcohol. Other causes include chronic coronary artery disease, myocarditis, doxorubicin toxicity, and viral infection. The dilated pericardium leads to decreased contractility and the symptoms of congestive heart failure. The physical examination and diagnostic test findings are classic for this malady.

Answer A is incorrect. Although this patient has a history of asthma, this episode involves his cardiovascular system. He also lacks most of the significant signs and symptoms typically associated with asthma (such as wheezing and change in breath sounds).

Answer B is incorrect. Delirium tremens (DT) is important to consider whenever a patient has a history of excessive alcohol use. In this case, however, the patient still has alcohol on his breath, indicating recent use. DT is caused by withdrawal of alcohol and should be especially suspected if a patient has been admitted to the hospital for a number of days and then begins to undergo changes associated with DT.

Answer D is incorrect. There are three types of endocarditis: native valve, prosthetic valve, and that related to intravenous drug use. There is no mention here of a replacement valve. The other two etiologies are possible in this case, but the patient is not suffering from fever or chills, two prominent symptoms in endocarditis. Anorexia, weight loss, and malaise are other clues that would point to this condition as the cause, and they are absent in this case.

Answer E is incorrect. Hypothyroidism may masquerade in a variety of ways. However, there are many prominent signs and symptoms that are classic for this condition that are not mentioned here, including weakness, menstrual irregularities, lethargy, cold intolerance, constipation, loss of hair, skin changes, and hypothermia.

42. **The correct answer is B.** PDA is a vascular connection that exists between the aorta and main pulmonary artery. It causes acyanotic congenital heart disease. PDAs account for 10% of congenital heart disease, occurring with a high incidence in preterm infants and a 2:1 female-to-male predominance. Small PDAs are asymptomatic, while large ones may cause congestive heart failure, failure to thrive, and recurrent lower respiratory tract infections. On physical examination, a continuous machinery murmur heard best at the left upper sternal border, and bounding peripheral pulses may be present. There may also be a prominent apical impulse and a thrill. X-ray of the chest may show cardiomegaly and increased pulmonary vascular markings. PDAs usually close within the first month of life. In preterm infants, indomethacin may be administered to close the PDA. PDAs also may be surgically ligated or coil embolized if necessary.

Answer A is incorrect. The murmur of aortic stenosis with aortic regurgitation is loudest over the right sternal border and radiates to the neck and apex. The murmur is usually preceded by an ejection click heard best at the left lower sternal border.

Answer C is incorrect. Systemic arteriovenous fistulas are usually extracardiac in location and can produce continuous murmurs. However, the murmur would not be expected to occur in the location described. The rest of the physical examination findings are also most consistent with a PDA.

Answer D is incorrect. The continuous murmur of venous hum is usually loudest on the right (but can also be present on the left)

supra- and infraclavicular areas. It usually is inaudible with the patient in the supine position, but intensifies when the patient is sitting. It also disappears with compression of the ipsilateral jugular vein. It is an innocent murmur that is produced by alteration in blood flow through veins.

Answer E is incorrect. VSDs are the most common congenital heart defects. They usually are associated with a holosystolic murmur that is loudest at the left lower sternal border.

43. **The correct answer is B.** Hypertrophic cardiomyopathy (HCM) is an autosomal dominant disease that is caused by a disordered growth of sarcomeres, leading to outflow tract obstruction and arrhythmias. Because this patient's ECG and echocardiogram both establish clear signs of ventricular hypertrophy, the physician must consider this diagnosis. If the physician is still unsure, a biopsy may be performed, which would show characteristic myofibrillar disarray as the myofibrils cross each other in a disorganized manner. However, the appearance is more normal adjacent to these areas, with parallel arrays of myofibrils.

Answer A is incorrect. Cor pulmonale is more often an adult disease and may be precipitated by chronic obstructive pulmonary disease. Echocardiogram would show right ventricular overload. A physical examination would exhibit signs of underlying lung disease (e.g., an increase in chest diameter or hyperresonance to percussion).

Answer C is incorrect. Mitral valve prolapse may present with these symptoms but would not show outflow tract obstruction on echocardiogram.

Answer D is incorrect. Pericarditis is most often confused with restrictive cardiomyopathy, not HCM, and is usually preceded by a viral infection 1–2 weeks before the patient begins to report symptoms. On biopsy, pericarditis samples will be normal.

Answer E is incorrect. Restrictive cardiomyopathy (RCM) is characterized by normal contractility, little hypertrophy, and a small ventricular cavity. The ECG and echocardiogram results would point to a different etiology. Additionally, RCM is nearly always caused by another underlying condition, such as amyloidosis or sarcoidosis, so the biopsy would show evidence of these diseases.

44. **The correct answer is A.** This patient has symptoms consistent with pericarditis, or inflammation of the pericardial sac. The condition is most often idiopathic (84% of cases), with other major causes being neoplasia, tuberculosis, infection, and collagen vascular diseases. Uremia in patients with chronic renal failure can cause pericarditis, and uremic pericarditis is an indication for emergent dialysis. Pericarditis can be complicated by cardiac tamponade, recurrent pericarditis, or pericardial constriction if left untreated. In patients with cardiac tamponade, ventricular filling is limited, which leads to decreased cardiac output and can lead to shock. Pericarditis is diagnosed by the presence of two of the following three factors: pleuritic chest pain, pericardial friction rub, or widespread ST-segment elevation on ECG. Ten to thirty percent of patients with acute pericarditis may go on to develop recurrent or incessant disease, termed chronic autoreactive pericarditis.

Answer B is incorrect. If the patient's pericarditis were complicated by cardiac tamponade, jugular venous pressure would be increased, not decreased, due to elevated right heart filling pressures.

Answer C is incorrect. Mitral regurgitation is not a common complication of pericarditis, although it could possibly occur in the setting of myocardial ischemia, leading to acute papillary muscle rupture.

Answer D is incorrect. Pericardial constriction and RCM can have similar signs and symptoms. RCM is defined as impaired ventricular filling due to decreased compliance, and is caused in some cases by infiltrative diseases, such as amyloidosis. Pericardial constriction also impairs ventricular filling, but it is caused by scarring from pericarditis with loss of elasticity of the pericardial sac. Although pericardial constriction is a possible complication of pericarditis, RCM is not. Therefore, RCM is an incorrect answer choice.

Answer E is incorrect. Shock can occur secondary to cardiac tamponade, but an infectious etiology would be unlikely. Furthermore, the hemodynamics of septic shock and shock secondary to tamponade are different. In septic shock, cardiac filling pressures are low, while there are elevated filling pressures in tamponade.

45. **The correct answer is C.** The definitive event in obstructive sleep apnea (OSA) is closure of the patient's upper airway, usually at the level of the oropharynx. OSA can occur at any age but is more common in men 30–60 years old. The definitive investigation is polysomnography, and the key diagnostic finding is episodes of airflow cessation at the nose and/or mouth, despite evidence of continuing respiratory effort. Several approaches to the management of OSA have been outlined. For patients with ischemic heart disease or congestive heart failure who also have OSA, treatment should begin with nasal continuous positive airway pressure (CPAP). This is the only treatment modality that has been tested and proved efficacious for patients with ischemic heart disease or congestive heart failure and OSA. Nasal CPAP prevents upper airway occlusion by propping the airway open with positive pressure delivered via face mask, with the air acting as a pneumatic stent.

Answer A is incorrect. Alcohol is a frequent contributor to the pathogenesis of OSA because alcohol has a depressant effect on the muscles of the upper airway. The structural integrity of the airway is compromised, and thus the airway is predisposed to occlusion. Avoidance of alcohol should be advocated in patients with mild to moderate OSA and a history of alcohol consumption. However, in patients with congestive heart failure, nasal CPAP is the only treatment that has been efficacious and is therefore the treatment of choice.

Answer B is incorrect. Avoidance of supine posture should be attempted in patients with mild to moderate OSA. Although it would be reasonable to attempt weight reduction and avoidance of alcohol and supine posture in our patient, the best management is nasal CPAP, given his history of congestive heart failure.

Answer D is incorrect. Uvulopalatopharyngoplasty is a last-resort surgical procedure that increases the airway lumen by reducing the quantity of redundant soft tissue. This procedure results in a long-term cure in less than 50% of patients with OSA.

Answer E is incorrect. Mild to moderate OSA can often be managed by moderate weight reduction. However, in patients with congestive heart failure, nasal CPAP is the only treatment that has been efficacious and is therefore the treatment of choice.

46. **The correct answer is E.** Mitral valve prolapse (MVP) occurs when the leaflets of the mitral valve bulge backward into the left atrium during systole, resulting in a characteristic mid- to late-systolic murmur, often associated with a preceding click. It is caused by an underlying structural abnormality of the mitral valve, and seems to be more common in adolescent girls. Antibiotic prophylaxis shoud be considered in patients with a mid-systolic click and late-systolic mitral regurgitation murmur, including those with increased leaflet thickening or redundancy, left atrial enlargement, and left ventricular dilatation, even in the absence of correlated clinical findings. Due to the transient bacteremia following dental procedures, prophylactic antibiotics are recommended since the prolapsed valve can serve as a nidus for colonization.

Answer A is incorrect. Digoxin does not play a role in the management of MVP.

Answer B is incorrect. MVP, unlike HCM, does not have an increased risk of sudden death and therefore does not require restriction of activity.

Answer C is incorrect. β-Blockers are not indicated since the patient is asymptomatic and without a history of known cardiac disease.

Answer D is incorrect. Surgical valvular replacement is reserved for more advanced cases of valvular disease in which the patient has refractory symptoms. Various symptoms (including atypical chest pain, exertional dyspnea, palpitations, syncope, and anxiety) and clinical findings (including low blood pressure and electrocardiographic repolarization abnormali-

ties) have been associated with MVP and have been termed mitral valve prolapse syndrome. Valve surgery is clearly warranted for patients with symptomatic severe mitral regurgitation, mitral regurgitation accompanied by atrial fibrillation or pulmonary hypertension, and those who are asymptomatic but have left ventricular enlargement or even mildly reduced systolic function.

47. **The correct answer is E.** Tricyclic antidepressant (TCA) overdose presents with sedation, coma, anticholinergic effects, seizures, and arrhythmias. First-line treatment includes sodium bicarbonate for QRS prolongation, diazepam or lorazepam for seizures, and careful cardiac monitoring for arrhythmias. Sodium bicarbonate is indicated for QRS widening > 100 msec, ventricular arrhythmias, and/or hypotension. The benefit of sodium bicarbonate is due both to an increase in serum pH and extracellular sodium. Elevated serum pH lowers free drug concentrations and favors the neutral form of the drug, making less available to bind to sodium channels. Increasing extracellular sodium increases the electrochemical gradient across cardiac cell membranes, thus attenuating TCA-induced blockade of rapid sodium channels.

Answer A is incorrect. Activated charcoal is important for patients who do not have neurologic or cardiovascular components to their presentation. For patients who are neurologically depressed, an endotracheal airway must first be established prior to giving charcoal. Activated charcoal shows the greatest benefit when administered within 1 hour of ingestion. Some agents that are not absorbed well by activated charcoal include heavy metals such as lead and mercury, inorganic ions such as calcium or potassium, acids or alkali, hydrocarbons, and alcohols such as acetone or ethylene glycol.

Answer B is incorrect. Diazepam will control the seizure activity but not the cardiac or anticholinergic components. TCAs are thought to induce seizure by decreasing central GABAergic tone. Benzodiazepines are the preferred antiseizure agents due to the resulting increase in GABAergic tone. Antiseizure medications that block sodium channels, such as phenytoin, should be avoided, as they promote ventricular arrhythmias by potentiating the sodium channel blockade already present from the TCA toxicity.

Answer C is incorrect. Flumazenil is used for benzodiazepine sedation reversal but has been associated with onset of ventricular arrhythmias and seizures.

Answer D is incorrect. Physostigmine is the antidote for anticholinergic overdose and should be avoided in patients with a TCA overdose secondary to association with seizures and cardiac arrest.

48. **The correct answer is A.** This patient has persistent atrial fibrillation. Her risk for the disorder is greatly increased by her history of rheumatic fever and presumed rheumatic heart disease and is varied depending on the severity of valvular disease. The ECG shown is characteristic of atrial fibrillation, showing an irregular baseline, no clear P waves, and irregular and varied QRS complexes. Rheumatic heart disease can cause deformity of the valve cusps, fusion of the commissures, and shortening and fusion of the chordae tendineae. Stenosis of the mitral valve is present in 50–60% of the cases, and combined aortic/mitral valve lesions occur about 20% of the time. Therefore, an astute clinician should auscultate for a mitral stenosis murmur (a diastolic opening snap followed by a late rumbling diastolic murmur). The increased pressure in the left atrium from the mitral stenosis can cause atrial fibrillation (which will need to be anticoagulated). This patient should also receive prophylactic antibiotics for dental, urologic, and surgical procedures to prevent endocarditis.

Answer B is incorrect. The ECG of a patient with atrial flutter would reveal a regular rhythm and P waves in a sawtooth pattern.

Answer C is incorrect. The presence of multiple pacemakers or reentrant pathways in multifocal atrial tachycardia leads to multiple (> 3), varied P-wave morphologies.

Answer D is incorrect. An unusual P wave before each normal QRS complex would be seen in paroxysmal atrial tachycardia, in which an

ectopic atrial pacemaker overrides the native rhythm of the heart.

Answer E is incorrect. An atrioventricular nodal reentry circuit in paroxysmal supraventricular tachycardia leads to P waves hidden within normal QRS complexes on ECG.

49. **The correct answer is E.** The treatment of a compartment syndrome is generally based on the physical examination and clinical judgment. A compartment syndrome is a common finding postoperatively after an embolectomy, so one must have a low threshold for diagnosis. It develops in part due to the absence of collateral flow while the blockage is in place, causing local ischemia that leads to profound edema during the brisk reperfusion of tissue that occurs after removal of the embolus. Treatment requires immediate recognition and open fasciotomy.

Answer A is incorrect. A CT of the extremity would not result in a timely diagnosis, nor would it measure the pressure in the posterior compartment. Although it may aid in detecting damage to structures through direct visualization, it would not be indicated acutely.

Answer B is incorrect. Electromyography would play little role in the acute management of a compartment syndrome and would delay treatment.

Answer C is incorrect. Given the high pretest probability of a compartment syndrome in this patient, it is likely that the pressure in the posterior compartment would be abnormal. Therefore, taking time to measure the compartmental pressure would further delay treatment.

Answer D is incorrect. Although elevation of the extremity would aid in recovery postoperatively, it would be an inadequate measure to relieve the pressure acutely.

50. **The correct answer is B.** Cocaine toxicity produces a hyperadrenergic state which is identified by hypertension, tachycardia, tonic-clonic seizures, dyspnea, and ventricular arrhythmias. Cocaine produces vasoconstriction in coronary arteries, resulting in hypertension and bradycardia. β-Adrenergic blockade may worsen this

effect, suggesting that this vasoconstriction may be mediated by α-adrenergic receptors and antagonized by β-adrenergic receptor–mediated vasodilatation.

Answer A is incorrect. Cocaine withdrawal produces a late, dopamine-related vasospasm. However, β-blockers do not worsen this effect.

Answer C is incorrect. Hypertension is a hyperadrenergic effect of cocaine toxicity. Using a β-blocker will cause vasoconstriction, which may exacerbate hypertension and bradycardia but will not cause hypotension.

Answer D is incorrect. Dyspnea is not directly related to cocaine toxicity. Pulmonary complications associated with cocaine ingestion include pulmonary hemorrhage, barotrauma, asthma exacerbation, pneumonitis, and pulmonary edema. β-Blocker toxicity can be associated with pulmonary complications such as bronchospasm and wheezing.

Answer E is incorrect. Ventricular arrhythmias are associated with cocaine toxicity but not specifically a result of β-blocker treatment of cocaine induced hypertension. Cocaine can cause dysrhythmias, myocarditis, myocardial ischemia, infarction and cardiomyopathy.

51. **The correct answer is D.** Left ventricular hypertrophy (LVH) occurs as a consequence of uncontrolled hypertension. Increased pressures lead to increased workload for the heart and cardiac muscle hypertrophy. Patients with LVH may have a prominent point of maximum impulse, loud S2, and audible S4 from an atrial kick. In addition, there may be signs of LVH on ECG; however, LVH can often be detected with echocardiography far earlier than it can be detected on an ECG. On this patient's ECG, the large amplitude of the S in V_1 and V_2 and of the R in V_5 and V_6, the diffuse ST/T wave changes, the widened bifid P waves (indicating left atrial enlargement), and the prolonged QRS all suggest LVH.

Answer A is incorrect. Acute MI is unlikely in this patient because he is asymptomatic. This patient has ST/T changes on his ECG, but these changes are displacements in the opposite direction to the major deflection of the QRS complex, which is more suggestive of left ventricular hypertrophy, not acute MI.

Answer B is incorrect. Although hypertension increases a patient's risk of cerebrovascular accident (CVA), this patient has no signs or symptoms that would suggest a CVA, which makes this diagnosis unlikely.

Answer C is incorrect. Hypertension can lead to left ventricular hypertrophy and then eventually to dilated cardiomyopathy if allowed to progress. After the ventricle hypertrophies from excess workload, it can later dilate and its ejection fraction can decrease. However, this patient has no signs or symptoms that would suggest dilated cardiomyopathy, which makes this diagnosis unlikely.

Answer E is incorrect. This patient has no signs (pericardial friction rub) or symptoms (pleuritic chest pain, dyspnea, cough, and fever) that would suggest pericarditis. In addition, if the patient had pericarditis, one would expect to see diffuse ST-segment elevation on ECG. Although this patient's ECG shows ST/T changes, it does not show diffuse ST-segment elevation.

52. **The correct answer is D.** Osler-Weber-Rendu syndrome, also known as hereditary hemorrhagic telangiectasia, is an autosomal dominant fibrovascular dysplasia in which vascular lesions (telangiectasias, arteriovenous malformations, and aneurysms) are found throughout the body, particularly in the lungs, brain, and gastrointestinal tract.

Answer A is incorrect. Hypertension, bradycardia, and irregular respirations constitute Cushing's triad, which is suggestive of increased intracranial pressure. Although the patient may have suffered a head injury in the motor vehicle collision, there is no reason to suspect that she had increased cranial pressure prior to the collision.

Answer B is incorrect. Jaundice, fever, and right upper quadrant (RUQ) pain constitute Charcot's triad, which is suggestive of ascending cholangitis. Osler-Weber-Rendu syndrome can result in hepatomegaly and RUQ pain secondary to hepatic atrial ventricular fistulas, but fever would not be present in such patients.

Answer C is incorrect. Symptoms of hypoglycemia, documented low blood sugar and relief of symptoms with increase in blood sugar constitute Whipple's triad, the gold standard for diagnosing hypoglycemia.

Answer E is incorrect. Venous stasis, hypercoagulability, and endothelial damage constitute Virchow's triad, which lists possible etiologies for thrombosis.

53. **The correct answer is C.** PDA is a vascular connection that exists between the aorta and the main pulmonary artery. It is more common in preterm infants, particularly those who have respiratory distress syndrome as described in this patient. PDAs account for 10% of congenital heart disease. Small PDAs are asymptomatic, while large ones may cause congestive heart failure, failure to thrive, and recurrent lower respiratory tract infections. On physical examination, a continuous machinery murmur heard best at the left upper sternal border and left infraclavicular region is present. There may also be a prominent apical impulse and a thrill. X-ray of the chest may show cardiomegaly and increased pulmonary vascular markings. PDAs are kept open by prostaglandin E_2 and nitric oxide; however, they usually close within the first month of life. In preterm infants, indomethacin is the initial treatment used to close clinically significant PDAs.

Answer A is incorrect. Balloon atrial septostomy is used to create a connection between the atria in transposition of the great arteries, to allow mixing of deoxygenated and oxygenated blood for patient survival.

Answer B is incorrect. Coil embolization may also be used if the PDA fails to close with indomethacin.

Answer D is incorrect. Prostaglandin E would actually keep the ductus arteriosus patent and is used in congenital heart defects when a PDA contributes to patient survival, such as in transposition of the great arteries.

Answer E is incorrect. Surgical ligation is used if the PDA fails to close with indomethacin.

Questions 54 and 55

54. **The correct answer is D.** The patient presents with the classic triad of hypotension, jugular venous distention, and distant heart sounds (Beck's triad), indicative of cardiac tamponade. There is also a plausible mechanism given the traumatic left chest wound.

55. **The correct answer is C.** Symptoms of cardiac ischemia are often atypical in the setting of female patients, the elderly, and diabetics. Note that the usual duration of angina is a few minutes to half an hour, with pain gradually increasing and improved with rest.

Answer A is incorrect. Acute aortic dissection can be catastrophic and often presents as "tearing" chest pain radiating to the back.

Answer B is incorrect. An acute myocardial infarction can present atypically in the elderly and women. The transient nature of the symptoms in the second vignette suggests that angina is a more likely cause

Answer E is incorrect. A compression fracture of the spine can often be diagnosed by palpation of the spinal column. This is common in elderly patients.

Answer F is incorrect. Coronary vasospasm can often occur idiopathically in young women or is often seen in the setting of cocaine use. ECG may reveal transient ST-segment changes.

Answer G is incorrect. Be aware that esophageal spasm can be very similar to cardiac chest pain. In both cases, there is another more likely etiology.

Answer H is incorrect. Myocarditis has a wide range of presentations from chest pain to sudden death, depending on the etiology. It often manifests as fatigue, decreased exercise tolerance, or heart failure in a previously healthy individual.

Answer I is incorrect. Panic disorder is a frequent cause of chest pain. However, in both cases, there is another likely etiology.

Answer J is incorrect. Pericarditis is often manifest by severe chest pain, a rub on cardiac examination, and diffuse ST-segment changes on ECG.

Answer K is incorrect. Pneumonia can present as chest pain, but look for other signs of infection.

Answer L is incorrect. Pulmonary embolus can often present as chest pain associated with shortness of breath and hemoptysis. Look for risk factors of deep venous thrombosis (hypercoagulability, malignancy, elderly, nonambulatory, and recent surgery).

Answer M is incorrect. A rib fracture can obviously result in chest pain but usually in the setting of trauma. Nothing in either vignette suggests a rib fracture.

Answer N is incorrect. A tension pneumothorax occurs when there is a one-way valve created by an abnormal connection between the lungs and the pleural space. It manifests as respiratory distress, deviated trachea, hypoxemia, jugular venous distension, and distant breath sounds on the affected side. Treat with immediate decompression.

Questions 56 and 57

56. **The correct answer is H.** This patient likely suffered dilated cardiomyopathy as a result of doxorubicin toxicity, which is now being exacerbated by the cardiopulmonary stress of pregnancy. Any medical intervention should take into account the possible teratogenic effects on the child. A β-blocker such as metoprolol would be an appropriate treatment for heart failure in this case.

57. **The correct answer is A.** Angiotensin-converting enzyme (ACE) inhibitors and angiotensin receptor blockers (ARBs) are the most effective treatments for congestive heart failure. Since many patients suffer from cough as an idiopathic side effect of ACE inhibitors, you should be familiar with ARBs as a possible alternative. ARBs can have serious potential side effects on the fetus.

Answer B is incorrect. Digoxin is an effective symptomatic treatment for heart failure, but has no proven effect on mortality or disease progression.

Answer C is incorrect. Erythropoietin would be useful in treating certain types of anemia, which can cause fatigue. However, since the fatigue described in the question is most likely due to congestive heart failure, this medication would be inappropriate.

Answer D is incorrect. Folate would be indicated in patients with signs and symptoms of folate deficiency as a cause of fatigue.

Answer E is incorrect. Heparin is safe and effective during pregnancy but requires intravenous access. However, neither patient is in need of anticoagulation.

Answer F is incorrect. Isoniazid is a treatment for tuberculosis, another possible cause of fatigue, but it is not suggested in either question stem.

Answer G is incorrect. Lisinopril and other angiotensin-converting enzyme (ACE) inhibitors are considered teratogenic because they cause renal failure in neonates, renal tubular dysgenesis, and decreased skull ossification, and should be avoided in pregnancy. An ACE inhibitor would be considered one of the first-line treatments for congestive heart failure, as it has been shown to decrease mortality. But, as mentioned in one of the question stems, the ACE inhibitor is making the patient cough, so an angiotensin receptor blocker is preferred.

Answer I is incorrect. Warfarin is also a teratogen causing skeletal and central nervous system defects, and should be avoided in pregnancy. Warfarin is not a treatment for congestive heart failure.

Questions 58–60

58. **The correct answer is M.** The patient has cardiac tamponade secondary to uremic pericarditis. The usual treatment for cardiac tamponade is pericardiocentesis. However, in relatively stable patients with cardiac tamponade secondary to uremic pericarditis, the treatment of choice is to initiate or intensify dialysis.

59. **The correct answer is F.** The patient has cardiac tamponade secondary to a hemopericardium. If fluid is rapidly introduced into the

pericardium, it cannot stretch to accommodate the additional volume; therefore, the intrapericardial pressure rises quickly. A very small volume of fluid in the pericardium can lead to tamponade if introduced rapidly enough, as seen in this patient. Emergent pericardiocentesis is recommended in the case of cardiac tamponade in a hemodynamically unstable patient.

60. **The correct answer is L.** The patient has signs and symptoms that would suggest viral pericarditis. Although she has a moderate pericardial effusion seen on x-ray of the chest and echocardiogram, her pericardium has stretched to accommodate the excess fluid, so she is not experiencing cardiac tamponade. High-dose nonsteroidal anti-inflammatory drugs are first-line therapy in viral or idiopathic pericarditis. Her effusion should resolve over time without pericardiocentesis.

Answer A is incorrect. Antibiotics are useful in the treatment of bacterial pericarditis.

Answer B is incorrect. Chest tubes are not indicated in pericarditis, pericardial effusion, or cardiac tamponade.

Answer C is incorrect. Colchicine is often used in combination with nonsteroidal anti-inflammatory drugs (NSAIDs) to treat pericarditis, but NSAIDs are first-line treatment for pericarditis.

Answer D is incorrect. Corticosteroids can be used to treat pericarditis but are only recommended in recurrent pericarditis refractory to nonsteroidal anti-inflammatory drugs and colchicine- or immune-mediated pericarditis.

Answer E is incorrect. Emergency cardiac catheterization is not indicated in the treatment of pericarditis or cardiac tamponade.

Answer G is incorrect. Intravenous (IV) fluids are often given in cardiac tamponade. IV resuscitation can be helpful in cardiac tamponade if the patient is hypovolemic at baseline, but aggressive IV fluid administration can worsen or precipitate cardiac tamponade in patients who are euvolemic or hypervolemic at baseline.

Answer H is incorrect. Loop diuretics are used in the treatment of congestive heart failure, among other disease states, but are not indicated in the treatment of pericarditis or cardiac tamponade.

Answer I is incorrect. Morphine is used in the treatment of myocardial ischemia or infarction.

Answer J is incorrect. Multidrug antituberculous therapy is used to treat tuberculous pericarditis. Pericardial involvement can occur with any bacterial infection; however, the most frequent pathogens are *Staphylococcus*, *Pneumococcus*, *Streptococcus* (rheumatic pancarditis), *Haemophilus*, and *Mycobacterium tuberculosis*.

Answer K is incorrect. Nitroglycerin is used in the treatment of myocardial ischemia or infarction. Pericarditis and effusion are common events following acute myocardial infarction. Acute inflammation associated with the infarct can cause early post-MI pericardial disease. Pericardial disease that occurs weeks to months after the MI is related to immunologic mechanisms.

CHAPTER 2

Dermatology

1. A 17-year-old boy presents to the physician's office complaining of a rash. He first noticed a dry, red patch on his back. Then smaller patches started to appear on his shoulders, and over the past week the rash has spread to his trunk. The rash itches, but he otherwise feels well. He had a slightly sore throat 2 weeks ago but denies fever, cough, or other symptoms of upper respiratory infection. He is sexually active with his girlfriend and they use condoms. He denies travel or exposure to tick bites. On examination there are erythematous scaly papules and plaques as shown in the image. The lesions are erythematous with slight central clearing. There are no other significant findings on examination. Rapid plasma reagin (RPR) test is negative. Which of the following is the most likely diagnosis?

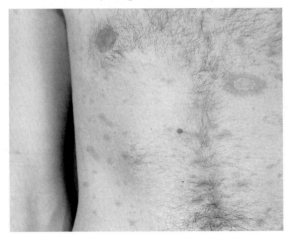

Reproduced, with permission, from Wolff K, Johnson RA, Surmond D. *Fitzpatrick's Color Atlas & Synopsis of Clinical Dermatology*, 5th ed. New York: McGraw-Hill, 2005: Figure 7-1.

(A) Guttate psoriasis
(B) Lyme disease
(C) Pityriasis rosea
(D) Secondary syphilis
(E) Tinea corporis

2. A 14-year-old girl has just returned from a camping vacation and presents to her physician with a pruritic rash on both hands and on her right cheek. The rash consists of vesicles on erythematous plaques arranged linearly with slight crusting. She denies fever or sore throat and otherwise feels well. She does not have a history of eczema or sick contacts. Which of the following is the most likely diagnosis?

(A) Atopic dermatitis
(B) Contact dermatitis
(C) Erythema infectiosum
(D) Impetigo
(E) Seborrheic dermatitis

3. A 42-year-old man presents for evaluation of a mole on his back that his wife noticed has changed in size. She is not present but told him that it used to be smaller. He is fair skinned and admits to never using sunscreen. He has always had numerous freckles and moles but has no personal or family history of skin cancer. Examination shows the lesion seen in the image. He also has > 30 other small, round nevi on his arms and back. Which of the following features is most predictive of poor outcome in this case?

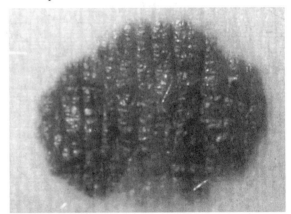

Reprinted, with permission, from PEIR Digital Library (http://peir.net).

(A) Asymmetric shape
(B) Diameter > 6 mm
(C) Irregular borders
(D) Tumor thickness
(E) Variation in color

4. A 26-year-old man presents to the emergency department with burns on his chest. He had a fight with his girlfriend and she threw boiling water at him, splashing his chest and arms.

The burns occurred about an hour ago, and are distributed on the upper third of his left anterior trunk and cover most of his left proximal arm. The patient's temperature is 37.4°C (99.4°F), blood pressure is 127/74 mm Hg, pulse is 80/min, respiratory rate is 18/min, and oxygen saturation is 99% on room air. Physical examination reveals that the burns are quite painful, swollen, and erythematous, with blister formation. The application of pressure produces blanching and is quite painful. What is the most appropriate management of this patient?

(A) Admission to hospital and intravenous antibiotic administration
(B) Cleaning and dressing of the burns, and analgesics as needed
(C) Lubricant application and analgesics as needed
(D) Referral to a burn center
(E) Surgical evaluation for debridement and grafting

5. A 28-year-old man presents with a rash that developed 3 weeks ago that is not resolving. He feels well, and denies pain or pruritus. He is not sexually active and has no history of sexually transmitted diseases. The rash is located on his right axilla, as shown in the image. There is slight, fine scaling. Which of the following will most likely lead to the correct diagnosis?

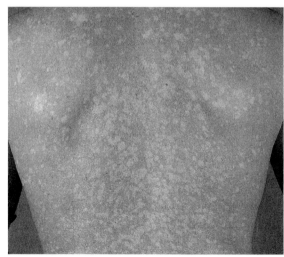

Reproduced, with permission, from Wolff K, Johnson RA, Surmond D. *Fitzpatrick's Color Atlas & Synopsis of Clinical Dermatology*, 5th ed. New York: McGraw-Hill, 2005: Figure 23-37.

(A) Allergy and pulmonary function testing
(B) Further information will not be helpful
(C) Human leukocyte antigen typing
(D) Microscopic examination of scale prepared with 10% potassium hydrochloride
(E) RPR and Venereal Disease Research Laboratory serologies

6. A 47-year-old man with a history of recent subclinical hepatitis C infection presents complaining of rash and mouth pain for the past week. The rash is pruritic. Examination reveals lesions on his wrists, ankles, and scalp; the lesions are shiny, violaceous, sharply demarcated, confluent papules containing fine white lines in a lacy pattern on their surfaces. Examination of his oropharynx reveals an erosion on the left buccal mucosa with the same fine white reticulation. Which of the following is the most likely diagnosis?

(A) Erythema multiforme
(B) Hypersensitivity vasculitis
(C) Lichen planus
(D) Secondary syphilis
(E) Viral exanthema

7. A 19-year-old woman presents to her primary care physician complaining of excessive bruising on her legs for the past 3 days. She denies injury. She was treated for streptococcal throat infection 10 days ago and recently completed antibiotic therapy. She has had some cramping abdominal pain, but she is premenstrual and says the pain is similar to her usual cramps. She took ibuprofen for the pain, with good relief. She has a boyfriend but is not sexually active. She denies previous history of bruising or bleeding easily. Inspection of her legs reveals diffuse tender, erythematous, indurated patches and nodules over the anterior aspects of her tibias bilaterally. Which of the following is the most likely cause of her symptoms?

(A) Delayed hypersensitivity reaction following streptococcal infection
(B) Domestic violence
(C) Henoch-Schönlein purpura
(D) Idiopathic thrombocytopenic purpura
(E) Secondary syphilis

8. A 25-year-old HIV-positive man presents to his primary physician because he has been exposed to herpes. He is concerned because he had a friend with AIDS who developed a fatal disseminated herpes infection and is afraid the same thing might happen to him. The exposure occurred 2 days ago when he shared a ice cream bar with his niece, who had an oral lesion. To his knowledge, he has never had an oral lesion. Neither he nor his partner has ever had "cold sores." Which of the following is the most appropriate approach to this patient?

(A) Admit to hospital for initiation of intravenous anti–herpes simplex virus immunoglobulin therapy
(B) Admit to hospital for intravenous acyclovir therapy
(C) Follow patient closely for development of complications, but it is too late to initiate acyclovir therapy
(D) Prescribe oral acyclovir, five times daily for 7 days and follow closely for clinical disease
(E) Reassure him that he is unlikely to develop severe disease and that he will probably contract herpes simplex virus-1 sooner or later

9. A 68-year-old man presents to his primary care physician for evaluation of "scabs" on his face that have failed to resolve over the past year. He is a retired vineyard manager and has worked outside for most of his career. He does not have any family or personal history of skin cancer. On examination he has two macular, scaling lesions on his right cheek. They are hyperkeratotic with surrounding erythema (see image). This lesion should be biopsied and observed carefully to prevent which of the following?

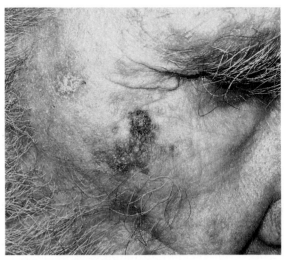

Reproduced, with permission, from Wolff K, Johnson RA, Surmond D. *Fitzpatrick's Color Atlas & Synopsis of Clinical Dermatology*, 5th ed. New York: McGraw-Hill, 2005: Figure 10-21.

(A) Local extension and tissue destruction
(B) Progression to basal cell carcinoma
(C) Progression to malignant melanoma
(D) Progression to squamous cell carcinoma
(E) This lesion does not have malignant potential and further evaluation is not necessary

10. A 55-year-old woman presents to her gynecologist complaining of vaginal discomfort. It first started approximately 6 months ago and has fluctuated in intensity, most recently causing itching and some slight pain when she has intercourse with her husband. She otherwise has been well. She has been postmenopausal for 3 years. Her older sister recommended an estrogen cream, which she has used consistently for > 3 months without any change in symptoms. On examination the introital mucosa and labia minora are whitish-pink, with abnormal wrinkling and a small fissure on the right labia minora. Which of the following is the most likely diagnosis?

(A) Candidiasis
(B) Estrogen deficiency
(C) Lichen sclerosus
(D) Sexual abuse
(E) Vitiligo

1. **The correct answer is C.** Pityriasis rosea may be preceded by a prodrome of headache, malaise, and/or sore throat, but is most often asymptomatic. The diagnosis is made based on history and physical examination. The rash is pruritic and begins with a herald patch. It then classically spreads downward or centrifugally on the trunk and proximal extremities. The herald patch is erythematous, round, and clears centrally with a peripheral scale. The following lesions are oval or oblong, with the long axes aligned with skin cleavage lines. The rash resolves spontaneously within 2–3 months. The etiology of pityriasis rosea is not well understood but is thought to be virally mediated, possibly secondary to a reactivation of human herpesvirus-7.

Answer A is incorrect. Guttate psoriasis usually occurs as an acute eruption of small (1–10 mm) salmon pink papules without central clearing, primarily involving the trunk. Eruption may occur after a streptococcal infection (usually pharyngitis) in a child or young adult. Though this patient describes a recent sore throat, the rash described is not typical for guttate psoriasis.

Answer B is incorrect. Erythema migrans secondary to Lyme disease is an erythematous oval lesion with central clearing that may be confused with the herald patch of pityriasis rosea. The classic "bull's-eye" occurs in only a minority of cases. Erythema migrans may even itch. However, this lesion typically occurs near the tick bite, in warm areas of the body. The location of the herald patch in this case and the subsequent appearance of multiple lesions are very atypical for erythema migrans.

Answer D is incorrect. The rash of secondary syphilis is typically symmetric and characteristically involves the palms and soles. The lesions are red and often scaled. While sore throat may occur as part of secondary syphilis, other symptoms including headache, fever, anorexia, myalgias, and diffuse lymphadenopathy are not present in this case. A negative rapid plasma reagin test effectively rules out secondary syphilis as a possible etiology.

Answer E is incorrect. While tinea corporis may be confused with the herald patch of pityriasis rosea, tinea corporis does not typically result in the numerous lesions seen in this patient. Extensive eruptions of tinea corporis may occur in immunocompromised patients such as those with diabetes mellitus or HIV infection, but there is no history to suggest that this is the case here.

2. **The correct answer is B.** Contact dermatitis causes an acute eczematous rash and results from a type IV hypersensitivity reaction to an allergen. In this case, the allergen was likely poison ivy resin because she presents with a characteristic rash. In addition, the lesions are arranged perfectly linearly, suggesting that the cause is external to the patient (i.e., a plant), rather than an internal dermatologic disease.

Answer A is incorrect. Patients with eczema typically manifest symptoms by ages 5–7 years. Lesions in atopic dermatitis are not characterized by linear distributions. In adolescents and adults, the most common sites of involvement are flexural surfaces, wrists/forearms, and face.

Answer C is incorrect. Erythema infectiosum, or fifth disease, typically causes the "slapped cheek" rash (edematous, erythematous plaques) in a febrile patient. Parvovirus B19 is the infectious agent.

Answer D is incorrect. Impetigo is an epidermal infection with staphylococci or streptococci, which typically occurs on the face, neck, or extremities. The rash is vesicular with honey-colored crusting and can be intensely pruritic, but it is not typically described as linear.

Answer E is incorrect. Seborrheic dermatitis can resemble the rash described but occurs in a distribution consistent with the locations of sebaceous glands. Thus, although the eyebrows, nasolabial folds, and scalp are common locations, the hands are not.

3. **The correct answer is D.** The lesion pictured is a malignant melanoma. Melanomas are recognizable by the **ABCDE's** (Asymmetric

shape, **B**orders irregular, **C**olor variation, **D**iameter > 6 mm, and **E**nlargement or Evolution of the lesion). This mnemonic is a useful way for both patients and physicians to recognize when a previously ordinary mole should be evaluated for melanoma. However, this mnemonic is not useful for determining the prognosis for survival of a patient with primary melanoma. Tumor thickness (or Breslow depth) determined on biopsy has been shown to be the most powerful prognostic factor in primary melanomas.

Answer A is incorrect. Asymmetry can be a worrisome feature in nevi, but this is not a useful prognostic feature once the lesion is identified as malignant.

Answer B is incorrect. A lesion > 6 mm in diameter should be considered malignant until proven otherwise (by biopsy), but it is the depth of the lesion that will best predict survival.

Answer C is incorrect. Absence of a round, clear-cut border (whether raised or flat) raises suspicion for the presence of a malignant lesion but is not useful for predicting survival.

Answer E is incorrect. Variation of color within the lesion is suspicious for malignancy but does not correlate with prognosis.

4. **The correct answer is B.** The burns described here are superficial partial-thickness burns (also called second-degree burns, affecting the epidermis and portions of the dermis), involving approximately 10% of his body surface area (BSA) according to the "rule of nines" (anterior trunk represents 18% BSA total, so one-third = 6%, and each arm represents 9%, so one-half = 4.5%). Pain, swelling, and blistering helps distinguish partial-thickness burns. These burns can be managed in the ambulatory setting, with appropriate cleansing, debridement if necessary, dressing, and appropriate pain management. These burns should heal in 1–3 weeks with minimal scarring, but may potentially result in pigmentation changes. First-degree burns, such as the typical sunburn, affect the epidermis only. Tissue is erythematous and blanches to pressure, and damage is minimal. Healing occurs sponta-

neously. Third-degree burns, or full-thickness burns, affect the entire epidermis and dermis. The area of the burn itself is painless, though surrounding tissue is usually tender due to adjacent areas of partial-thickness burn. The skin may be charred or white in color, with visible blood vessels. Healing is slower than with less severe burns, because sweat glands and hair follicles (the source of skin stem cells) are destroyed. Fourth-degree burns involve underlying muscle and/or bone.

Answer A is incorrect. Intravenous antibiotics are only indicated for treatment of infected burns. There is no proven benefit associated with prophylactic intravenous or oral antibiotic treatment of burn patients.

Answer C is incorrect. Analgesics (and antihistamines for pruritus) are used to symptomatically treat superficial or first-degree burns. These burns can be distinguished from superficial partial-thickness or second-degree burns by the absence of blister formation. Lubricants and moisturizers (including aloe vera) may also provide symptomatic relief; however, they are recommended only for first-degree burns and second-degree burns smaller than 2–3 inches in diameter.

Answer D is incorrect. Criteria for referral to a burn center include: partial-thickness burn covering > 20% total body surface area (BSA) in an adult or > 10% in a child < 10 years old or an adult > 50 years old, or full-thickness burn of > 5% BSA at any age. Special circumstances indicating referral to a burn center include inhalational injury; suspicion of abuse; significant burns to face, genitalia, or joints; and significant associated injuries (i.e., fractures). This patient does not meet these criteria.

Answer E is incorrect. Surgical evaluation for debridement and grafting is indicated if burns become infected, or if necrotic tissue is present.

5. **The correct answer is D.** With this preparation, both spores and hyphae of the yeast *Malassezia furfur* (*Pityrosporum ovale*) should be visible in the typical "spaghetti and meatballs" pattern. This infection causes abnormal

pigmentation of the skin and can be hypo- or hyperpigmented or salmon pink, as in this case. The saprophytic yeast is part of the normal skin flora but may convert to the symptomatic hyphal form if triggered by hot and humid weather or oils.

Answer A is incorrect. Atopic history combined with dry, erythematous rash is suggestive of eczema. However, eczematous lesions are more pruritic and often have more prominent scaling than is seen with tinea versicolor.

Answer B is incorrect. Although the diagnosis of tinea versicolor is suggested by the history and examination, the diagnosis can be made definitively with a potassium hydrochloride preparation, biopsy, or Wood's lamp examination.

Answer C is incorrect. Psoriasis has been associated with various human leukocyte antigen haplotypes and may be confused with the lesion pictured. An erythematous, scaling rash and other examination findings such as nail pitting point to the diagnosis of psoriasis. However, psoriatic lesions have thicker, silvery scales and more pronounced erythema than the lesions described.

Answer E is incorrect. These are tests for syphilis that appear negative during primary infection but become positive by the time secondary symptoms are evident. Secondary syphilis usually gives rise to a symmetric, papular rash that typically involves the palms and soles. Systemic symptoms may also be present.

6. **The correct answer is C.** This is a classic description of lichen planus; remember the "5 P's": Purple, Polygonal, Pruritic, Papules, and Planar) and Wickham's striae. Lichen planus is an uncommon disease of unclear though possibly autoimmune etiology. It affects middle-aged adults and may be associated with hepatitis C infection and/or drug exposure (including β-blockers, penicillamines, angiotensin-converting enzyme inhibitors, and sulfonylureas). Lichen planus is often self-limited, resolving within 8–12 months. Antihistamines and topical corticosteroids are recommended for milder cases. Systemic steroids (e.g., intramuscular triamcinolone every 3 months) or

oral psoralen with ultraviolet-A light therapy may be effective for managing severe symptoms; however, the patient should be made aware of the increased side effects.

Answer A is incorrect. The rash of erythema multiforme typically involves the extremities, palms, and soles, and may consist of erythematous or purpuric plaques and bullae with central clearing. Painful lesions are typical, though pruritus can be present as well. Mucous membrane involvement is common.

Answer B is incorrect. Hypersensitivity vasculitis is typically drug-induced but may also result from hepatitis B or C infection. It manifests as palpable purpura and skin biopsy shows a leukocytoclastic vasculitis.

Answer D is incorrect. The rash of secondary syphilis may consist of mucous membrane and genital lesions with a more diffuse rash (usually erythematous and macular) affecting the palms and soles. Wickham's striae are absent.

Answer E is incorrect. Though recent viral infection can result in rashes of widely varying morphology, these most commonly occur in children and are typically more erythematous and macular, as opposed to the violaceous and papular lesions described here.

7. **The correct answer is A.** Pretibial erythematous, tender nodules in a young woman is a classic presentation of erythema nodosum (EN), which is caused by inflammation of subcutaneous fat. Most cases of EN are idiopathic. The second most common cause of EN is strep pharyngitis, and other known causes include hypersensitivity reaction secondary to drugs (e.g., oral contraceptives and nonsteroidal anti-inflammatory drugs), sarcoidosis, tuberculosis, and inflammatory bowel disease.

Answer B is incorrect. This is a very atypical distribution for bruises or injury secondary to violence. Domestic violence may present with unusual bruising, lacerations, or fractures, but more often is seen in the context of vague somatic complaints, anxiety, and depression. Furthermore, there is a more likely explanation for this patient's skin findings and no reason to suspect domestic violence.

Answer C is incorrect. The combination of abdominal pain and lower-extremity rash is concerning for Henoch-Schönlein purpura (HSP), a small-vessel vasculitis. HSP classically occurs on the buttocks and/or lower extremities. The tetrad of HSP includes arthralgias, abdominal pain, purpuric rash, and renal disease. Although HSP can follow an upper respiratory tract infection, it most commonly affects boys between the ages of 2 and 11 years.

Answer D is incorrect. Idiopathic thrombocytopenic purpura may cause petechiae, nonpalpable purpura, or ecchymoses, but not nodules. Mucosal bleeding resulting in epistaxis and menorrhagia are also common. The lesions in this case do not appear to be bruises, and there are no petechiae or purpuric lesions present.

Answer E is incorrect. The rash of secondary syphilis is characteristically papular and involves palms and soles.

8. **The correct answer is D.** From the history, it is possible that this is the patient's first exposure to herpes simplex virus (HSV). In patients with HIV, a 7-day course of oral acyclovir has been shown to reduce the duration and morbidity associated with HSV infection, and there may also be a role for acyclovir in prophylaxis if administered soon after exposure.

Answer A is incorrect. This is not an available therapy for herpes simplex virus-1 infection.

Answer B is incorrect. If the patient develops severe disease, this is appropriate therapy. However, he is asymptomatic at this time, and this treatment plan may be more harmful (line infection, nosocomial infection) than beneficial.

Answer C is incorrect. Acyclovir therapy is effective if initiated within 72 hours of infection. This patient is still within the window for initiation of therapy.

Answer E is incorrect. This would be an inappropriate course of action. This patient is immunosuppressed and is therefore at risk for developing severe disease.

9. **The correct answer is D.** This is a case of actinic keratosis (AK), which can be differenti-

ated from seborrheic keratosis by the presence of an erythematous base. In addition, seborrheic keratoses are typically darker, ranging from brownish-pink to black. The primary risk factor for development of AK is sun exposure. The risk of an AK progressing to squamous cell carcinoma (SCC) is small; however, approximately half of cutaneous SCCs arise from AK.

Answer A is incorrect. Actinic keratoses may enlarge and progress to squamous cell carcinoma, but actinic keratoses themselves do not invade locally. Actinic keratoses often present as erythematous scaly macules (as in this case), or they may be hyperkeratotic plaques or papules closely resembling squamous cell carcinoma.

Answer B is incorrect. An actinic keratosis is not a risk factor for development of basal cell carcinoma. Risk factors for basal cell carcinoma include sun exposure, arsenic exposure, immunosuppression, a history of nonmelanoma skin cancer, and inherited disorders such as xeroderma pigmentosum, nevoid basal cell carcinoma syndrome, and Bazex syndrome.

Answer C is incorrect. Though sun exposure (particularly a history of severe sunburns in childhood) is also a risk factor for development of malignant melanoma, the lesion shown is an example of actinic keratosis, which is not a precursor of malignant melanoma. Dysplastic nevi are precursor lesions for melanoma.

Answer E is incorrect. Though actinic keratosis is not a malignant lesion, a small proportion of cases may undergo malignant transformation and should therefore be evaluated by biopsy.

10. **The correct answer is C.** Lichen sclerosus (LS, also called lichen sclerosus et atrophicus) is most common in postmenopausal women, and causes itching of the anogenital region. However, it can occur in all ages and both sexes and can be found anywhere on the skin. Though the etiology is unknown, chronic inflammation is thought to play a role in causing the labia to become white, wrinkled, and fragile. The tissue may be so fragile that minor trauma may cause petechial bleeding or fis-

sures, as seen in this case. The patient described here has early disease. More advanced disease may cause loss of labial distinction and fusing of the prepuce, obscuring the urethra and clitoris. Definitive diagnosis is made by biopsy, and treatment is with an ultrapotent topical corticosteroid applied daily for several weeks and then less frequently in the long term.

Answer A is incorrect. Candidiasis can cause white plaques, intense itching, and some pain with fissure formation. However, the surrounding mucosa is typically intensely erythematous and may be edematous.

Answer B is incorrect. Estrogen deficiency may cause atrophy of the vaginal mucosa and many of the same symptoms as seen in lichen sclerosus, such as atrophic changes and loss of architecture, dyspareunia, and labial adhesion. However, estrogen deficiency should respond to application of estrogen cream within 2 weeks.

Answer D is incorrect. Sexual abuse may manifest as whitish scarring and disruption of architecture, and fissure formation is suggestive of trauma. However, in a postmenopausal woman the symptoms of intense itching and white, wrinkled mucosa are suggestive of other diagnoses.

Answer E is incorrect. Vitiligo has a predilection for orifices (mouth, eyes, and anus) and acral areas and can cause whitening of the vaginal mucosa. However, vitiligo is not typically associated with symptoms of itching, pain, or architectural changes.

CHAPTER 3

Endocrinology

1. A 41-year-old woman presents to the emergency department (ED) with palpitations. On questioning, she notes heat intolerance, nervousness, and insomnia. On physical examination, the physician notes a fine tremor, diffuse nonpitting edema of the anterior lower leg, and bulging of both of her eyes. What finding on blood test would confirm the diagnosis?

(A) Anti-thyroid-stimulating hormone receptor antibodies
(B) Decreased thyroid-stimulating hormone levels
(C) Increased creatine kinase–myocardial bound fraction
(D) Increased thyroid-stimulating hormone levels
(E) Positive antinuclear antibody

2. A 17-year-old girl presents to the obstetrics and gynecology clinic with her mother. The mother says that she became concerned about a year ago because her daughter had not yet menstruated and she did not have significant breast development. There is no significant family history, except for some cousins who are color blind. With the mother out of the examination room, the patient denies ethanol, tobacco, and illicit drug use and sexual activity. Physical examination reveals a normal-appearing girl in no acute distress with minimal breast development and a lack of pubic hair. She is 168 cm (5 ft 6 in) tall, and weighs 61.2 kg (135 lb). Cardiac examination reveals no murmurs, rubs, or gallops, with point of maximal impulse at the right midclavicular line between the third and fourth intercostal space. Gynecologic examination reveals a vagina without rugae and a cervix that is easily visualized. There is no discharge. Laboratory results reveal a negative pregnancy test. What is the most likely diagnosis in this patient?

(A) Androgen insensitivity syndrome
(B) Gonadal dysgenesis
(C) Kallmann's syndrome
(D) Kartagener's syndrome
(E) Pregnancy

3. A 26-year-old man presents with increased thirst, urinary frequency, and nocturia over the past several months. Physical examination is unremarkable. Twenty-four-hour urine osmolarity is < 300 mOsm/L. A fluid deprivation test does not result in an increased urine osmolarity. Administration of 0.03 µg/kg of desmopressin results in a urine osmolarity of 450 mOsm/L after 2 hours. What is this patient's diagnosis?

(A) Central diabetes insipidus
(B) Diabetes mellitus
(C) Nephrogenic diabetes insipidus
(D) Psychogenic polydipsia
(E) Syndrome of inappropriate secretion of antidiuretic hormone

4. A 6-year-old boy presents to his pediatrician for a routine checkup. He has not been seen by a physician for the past 3 years. Recently, he has developed some patchy areas of hair loss on his scalp. The mother also notes that he has had many colds over the past year. The mother states that he has had a normal development, although he started walking later than her other two children. On physical examination, his wrists appear enlarged, and he has bowing of the forearms and legs. X-ray of the boy's legs is shown in the image. Laboratory testing reveals a Ca^{2+} level of 7.1 mg/dL, phosphorus of 1.8 mg/dL, and parathyroid hormone of 130 pg/mL. Vitamin D is normal. Treatment with vitamin D does not correct the patient's hypocalcemia. Which of the following disorders explains this patient's findings?

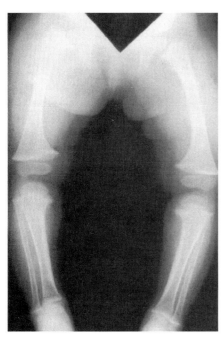

Reproduced, with permission, from Skinner HB. *Current Diagnosis & Treatment in Orthopedics*, 4th ed. New York: McGraw-Hill, 2006: Figure 11-3.

(A) Dietary vitamin D deficiency
(B) Hypoalbuminemia
(C) Primary hyperparathyroidism
(D) Pseudohypoparathyroidism
(E) Vitamin D–resistant rickets

5. A 53-year-old woman presents with complaints of headache and blurred vision for the past several months. She also says that her family has commented that her face "looks different," and her nose is bigger than it used to be. In addition, she notes that her shoes feel tighter. On physical examination, she has coarse facial features with a prominent mandible and widely spaced incisors. An MRI of the brain reveals a mass in the pituitary. This patient may be at increased risk of developing which of the following malignancies?

(A) Colon cancer
(B) Hepatocellular carcinoma
(C) Lung cancer
(D) Malignant brain tumor
(E) Pancreatic adenocarcinoma

6. A 13-year-old boy is brought to the pediatrician by his mother because of increasing body hair. Several months earlier, he had been diagnosed with 17α-hydroxylase deficiency and treated with hydrocortisone. Physical examination reveals an overweight boy with a moderate amount of both chest and genital hair, and some facial hair growth. His physical examination is otherwise unremarkable. What is the best treatment for this patient?

(A) Add cosyntropin
(B) Add dexamethasone
(C) Add spironolactone
(D) Increase hydrocortisone
(E) Keep the current dose of hydrocortisone

7. A 72-year-old man with a history of atrial fibrillation presents with complaints of fatigue and feeling cold. He also notes constipation and dry skin. His daughter states that he has seemed more forgetful over the past several months. His temperature is 37.3°C (99.1°F), heart rate is 48/min, and blood pressure is 130/82 mm Hg. Cardiac examination shows bradycardia but normal rhythm, and normal S1 and S2 with no murmurs; the lungs are clear to auscultation bilaterally, and the abdomen is soft and nontender. The patient's extremities are noted to be cool and puffy with dry, coarse skin. Laboratory studies show thyroid-stimulating hormone is 32 μU/L, free thyroxine is 0.3 ng/dL, and total triiodothyronine is 30 ng/dL. What medication is the patient likely taking for treatment of atrial fibrillation?

(A) Amiodarone
(B) Flecainide
(C) Lithium
(D) Methimazole
(E) Sotalol

8. A 45-year-old woman with chronic alcohol abuse admitted 3 days ago for nausea and severe diarrhea now complains of perioral and finger tingling. She was admitted for hydration after 1 week of severe watery diarrhea. She has been receiving intravenous hydration and dex-

trose but has not been able to take oral nutrition secondary to continued nausea. Her blood pressure is 130/74 mm Hg, pulse is 68/min, and respiratory rate is 16/min. She is afebrile. Physical examination is significant for facial twitching on percussion of her facial nerve just anterior to the ear, as well as the induction of carpal spasm after the inflation of a blood pressure cuff on her arm. Which of the following abnormalities is likely to have caused these findings?

(A) Azotemia
(B) Hypernatremia
(C) Hypomagnesemia
(D) Hypophosphatemia
(E) Hypouricemia

9. A 17-year-old girl has never had a menstrual period. On physical examination, she has minimal breast development and no axillary or pubic hair. She is color blind and has had a diminished sense of smell since birth. Laboratory evaluation would reveal which of the following?

Choice	Gonadotropin-Releasing Hormone	Follicle-Stimulating Hormone	Luteinizing Hormone
A	↓	↓	↓
B	↑	↓	↑
C	↓	↑	↑
D	↑	↓	↓
E	↑	↑	↑

(A) A
(B) B
(C) C
(D) D
(E) E

10. A 28-year-old woman presents to her gynecologist for her annual examination. She mentions that she and her husband have been trying to conceive for 9 months without success and that her menstrual cycles have become irregular. Her gynecologist suggests that she and her husband continue to try and that the woman return in 3 months for some laboratory studies if she still has not become pregnant. In the interim, a routine visit to the ophthalmologist reveals bitemporal hemianopsia. What is the most likely cause of this woman's infertility?

(A) Ectopic endometrial tissue
(B) Failure of implantation
(C) Hostile cervical mucus
(D) Ovarian unresponsiveness to gonadotropins
(E) Suppression of ovulation

11. A 4-year-old boy is brought to the pediatrician by his worried mother. She notes that he "urinates 10 times a day and is always drinking water." She also reports that despite eating more than either of his brothers did at the same age, he is not gaining any weight. Which of the following human leukocyte antigen (HLA) types is associated with the most likely diagnosis for this child?

(A) HLA-B27
(B) HLA-B51
(C) HLA-D11
(D) HLA-DR2
(E) HLA-DR3

12. A 48-year-old woman presents with a chief complaint of 2 weeks of neck pain that is a constant, sharp pain in the anterior portion of her neck, rated at 10/10 in severity. She also notes several weeks of loose stools and fatigue. Past medical history is significant for a viral upper respiratory infection about a month ago. She has a temperature of 37.9°C (100.2°F), a heart rate of 96/min, and a blood pressure of 136/82 mm Hg. On neck examination, there is diffuse enlargement of the thyroid and it is exquisitely tender to even mild palpation. Relevant laboratory findings include a total triiodothyronine level of 280 ng/dL, total thyroxine of 25 μg/dL, and thyroid-stimulating hormone of 2 μU/mL. Which of the following is the most likely diagnosis?

(A) Acute infectious thyroiditis
(B) Drug-induced thyroiditis
(C) Hashimoto's thyroiditis
(D) Riedel's thyroiditis
(E) Subacute granulomatous thyroiditis

13. A 26-year-old G1P1 woman presents to a family practice clinic with a chief complaint of cloudy, milky nipple discharge for 4–5 weeks. She has a past medical history significant for both obesity and schizophrenia. Her schizophrenia was diagnosed when she was 19 years old and has been well managed by a local psychiatrist. She does not remember what medications she takes; her mother, who is her primary caregiver, is "in charge of all that stuff." However, she does recall her psychiatrist mentioning that he recently put her on a new antipsychotic medication because her old one caused her to develop a blood disorder. Her last normal menstrual period was 6 weeks ago. Review of systems is positive for occasional mild headaches and feelings of restlessness, but she denies changes in vision or sensation. What is the most likely cause of her symptoms?

(A) Central nervous system sarcoidosis
(B) Idiopathic prolactinemia
(C) Medication effect
(D) Pregnancy
(E) Prolactinoma

14. An 18-year-old woman presents to the ED with acute mental status changes, rapid and deep breathing, abdominal pain, and vomiting. On examination, she is tachypneic and tachycardic, her abdomen is soft and nontender, and her mucous membranes are dry. Laboratory values are notable for potassium of 5.5 mEq/L, bicarbonate of 12 mEq/L, and serum glucose of 400 mg/dL. Which of the following are appropriate therapies in the first 24 hours?

(A) Diuresis and ventilatory support
(B) Diuresis, strict potassium restriction, and insulin
(C) Intravenous fluids, insulin, and potassium
(D) Intravenous fluids, insulin, and strict potassium restriction
(E) Intravenous fluids, loop diuretic, and potassium

15. A 56-year-old woman presents to the outpatient clinic for a routine visit. On physical examination, a 1-cm nodule is palpated in her thyroid. Her physical examination is otherwise unremarkable. Her heart rate is 70/min and regular, blood pressure is 126/82 mm Hg, and her temperature is 36.7°C (98.0°F). She is very anxious to know the seriousness of her abnormal physical examination finding. Which of the following symptoms or factors is a poor prognostic indicator for the thyroid nodule?

(A) Female gender
(B) Her age of 56 years
(C) Hoarseness
(D) Palpitations
(E) Slow growth of nodule
(F) Tender nodule

16. A 26-year-old man with a history of kidney stones presents with 1 week of severe burning epigastric pain. He also notes several days of diarrhea and nausea but denies emesis or fever. His family history is remarkable for a paternal uncle with pancreatic cancer. His temperature is 37°C (98.6°F), heart rate is 88/min, respiratory rate is 16/min, and blood pressure is 125/85 mm Hg. Abdominal examination is significant for tenderness in the mid-epigastrium. Upper endoscopy reveals a 1-cm ulceration in the first part of the duodenum. This is the third episode of confirmed peptic ulcers in this patient. Laboratory evaluation results are shown below. Which of the following may also be found in this patient?

Na^+	140 mEq/L
K^+	4.9 mEq/L
Cl^-	105 mEq/L
HCO_3^-	25 mEq/L
Ca^{2+}	12.0 mg/dL
Phosphorus	1.4 mg/dL
Mg^{2+}	2.0 mg/dL
Blood urea nitrogen	10 mg/dL
Creatinine	1.0 mg/dL
Glucose	87 mg/dL

(A) Medullary thyroid carcinoma
(B) Pheochromocytoma
(C) Prolactinoma
(D) Papillary thyroid carcinoma
(E) Squamous cell lung cancer

17. An obese 18-year-old woman is brought to the ED by her mother, who noted that she had been lethargic all day, and suffered a brief, seizure-like episode. One month earlier, the patient had been started on medication for type 2 diabetes. Lactic acid levels are normal. Which of the following medications most likely played a role in the patient's current presentation?

    (A) An α-glucosidase inhibitor
    (B) A statin
    (C) A sulfonylurea
    (D) A thiazolidinedione
    (E) Metformin

18. A 75-year-old woman is brought to the ED after being found unresponsive at her home. She was last spoken to by her daughter on the phone 24 hours earlier, at which time she complained of chills, lethargy, and weakness. The woman has had a heart attack in the past, she has high blood pressure, and she had a total thyroidectomy performed a decade ago for cancer. The daughter had returned from several months out of town and is unsure if the patient was taking her medications. Vital signs in the ED are temperature 34.9°C (94.9°F), pulse 48/min, blood pressure 110/65 mm Hg, oxygen saturation 99% on fraction of inspired oxygen of 100%, and glucose 85 mg/dL. On examination the patient is unresponsive, obese, and edematous with periorbital edema. Her cardiac and pulmonary examinations are normal. Head CT scan demonstrates no signs of trauma or increased intracranial pressure, and ECG demonstrates no acute ischemic changes. Blood is drawn for laboratory testing. Which of the following interventions is most appropriate in treating the patient's mental status change?

    (A) Aspirin
    (B) Glucagon
    (C) Hemodialysis
    (D) Levothyroxine
    (E) Metoprolol
    (F) Norepinephrine

19. A 52-year-old African-American woman with diabetes mellitus type 2 presents to her physician's office and states that she has been "feeling lousy in the morning." She notes that she

reliably checks her blood glucose levels, and is frustrated at the fact that she often has a blood sugar level in the 120s at night, followed by a level in the 170s to 180s the following morning. The patient's primary care physician increased her nightly dose of neutral protamine Hagedorn insulin 1 month ago, but her morning glucose levels have only become more elevated. She has recently begun to limit her carbohydrate intake at night, with no effect. This patient's morning hyperglycemia might be alleviated by which of the following means?

    (A) Decreasing neutral protamine Hagedorn insulin at night
    (B) Increasing neutral protamine Hagedorn insulin at night
    (C) Increasing neutral protamine Hagedorn insulin in the morning
    (D) Increasing regular insulin at night
    (E) Increasing regular insulin in the morning

20. A 26-year-old G1P0 woman who is 12 weeks pregnant presents to her obstetrician for her first visit. Her pregnancy thus far has been notable only for some mild nausea and vomiting that lasted throughout her first trimester. She reports feeling overly tired lately and very weak. Her past medical history is significant for pernicious anemia. On physical examination, she is an anxious-appearing, thin woman. Her blood pressure is 130/85 mm Hg, heart rate 115/min, and respiratory rate 18/min. Fetal heart tones are present at 135/min. The uterine fundus is at 12 cm. The woman has a diffuse, nontender goiter, a resting tremor, and poor global muscle strength. Which is the most likely mechanism underlying this woman's condition?

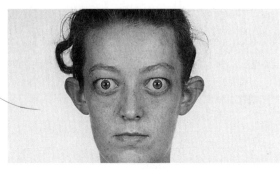

Reproduced, with permission, from Kasper DL, Braunwald E, Fauci AS, Hauser SL, Longo DL, Jameson LJ, Isselbacher KJ, eds. *Harrison's Online.* New York: McGraw-Hill, 2005: Figure 320-6.

(A) Autoantibodies against thyroid-stimulating hormone receptor
(B) Iodine overdose
(C) The mechanism of this disease is unknown
(D) Uncontrolled cell growth
(E) Viral infection

21. A 60-year-old woman recently diagnosed with type 2 diabetes complains of daily headaches and double vision that have gradually worsened over the previous month. An MRI shows a large pituitary adenoma. Which of the following hormones is most likely being secreted by this tumor?

(A) Adrenocorticotropic hormone (ACTH)
(B) Growth hormone
(C) Luteinizing hormone
(D) Prolactin
(E) Thyroid-stimulating hormone

22. A 14-year-old boy presents at the pediatric clinic for a routine checkup. The patient had developed end-stage renal disease over the previous 2 years, and was successfully treated with a renal transplant 6 months prior. Since his operation, he has developed purple striae on his back and arms, central obesity, and an increasingly round face. During the subsequent blood analysis, which of the following results would be most likely?

CHOICE	ACTH	URINARY FREE CORTISOL
A	↓	↓
B	↓	normal
C	↓	↑
D	↑	↓
E	↑	↑

(A) A
(B) B
(C) C
(D) D
(E) E

23. A 64-year-old man presents to the ED after a motor vehicle crash and receives a CT of the abdomen that shows a finding of a unilateral mass in the left adrenal gland. He is unharmed from the accident, feels well, and has never smoked. His blood pressure is 155/90 mm Hg, deep tendon reflexes are 3/4, and muscle strength is 4/5. Laboratory studies indicate:

Na^+	150 mEq/L
K^+	3.0 mEq/L
Cl^-	105 mEq/L
HCO_3^-	33 mEq/L

Plasma renin activity is decreased. Which of the following is most likely to be increased?

(A) Aldosterone
(B) Anion gap
(C) Carcinoembryonic antigen
(D) Prostate-specific antigen
(E) Troponin

24. A 28-year-old patient with known Addison's disease presents with abdominal pain and is hypotensive to a systolic pressure of 88 mm Hg. He presents with a 2-week history of progressively worse nonproductive dry cough, sore throat, malaise, and headache. He has not checked his temperature at home but complains of constant chills. What is the first mode of management?

(A) Azithromycin
(B) Check serum glucose
(C) Hydrocortisone
(D) Intravenous fluids
(E) X-ray of the chest

25. A generally healthy 74-year-old woman who recently moved into the area visits the physician's office for her first well visit. She states that her previous doctor had been treating her with propylthiouracil (PTU) for subclinical hyperthyroidism, but that her prescription ran out several months ago. Laboratory studies reveal that her free thyroxine and triiodothyronine levels are normal, but her thyroid-stimulating hormone is depressed. PTU therapy is most important in this patient to prevent the development of which disorder?

(A) Cardiac dysrhythmias
(B) Hypothyroidism
(C) Pretibial myxedema
(D) Thyroid cancer
(E) Thyroid storm

26. A 67-year-old man seeks evaluation from his physician for chronic cough. He denies any sputum production or hemoptysis. He also complains of feeling more weak and fatigued than usual. He says he has lost about 4.5 kg (10 lb) in the past month and that he has been constipated recently. Physical examination revealed coarse breath sounds. X-ray of the chest showed hilar lymphadenopathy and infiltrative disease. Routine serum chemistries are notable for an isolated elevation in calcium to 12.2 mg/dL. Which of the following laboratory abnormalities is also likely to be present in a patient with these findings?

(A) Decreased thyroid hormone
(B) Decreased vitamin D
(C) Elevated amylase and lipase
(D) Elevated angiotensin-converting enzyme (ACE)
(E) Elevated citrate

27. A 49-year-old woman presents to her physician's office with a long-standing history of polydipsia, polyuria, central obesity, and hyperlipidemia. She is currently taking metformin, a sulfonylurea, and an ACE inhibitor. ACE inhibitors are most beneficial in preventing or slowing the progression of which of the following diabetic complications?

(A) Diabetic ketoacidosis
(B) Diabetic nephropathy
(C) Diabetic neuropathy
(D) Diabetic retinopathy
(E) Peripheral vascular disease

28. A 42-year-old woman presents to her physician with complaints of fever (38.2°C [100.8°F]) and mild-to-moderate anterior neck pain. On examination, the physician finds her to be tachycardic and sweating, and to have an exquisitely tender thyroid gland. Her blood work shows a depressed thyroid-stimulating hormone level and increased free thyroxine. What is the appropriate treatment at this time?

(A) Acetaminophen
(B) Ibuprofen
(C) Levothyroxine
(D) Prednisone
(E) Radioactive iodine

29. A 24-year-old woman presents to her gynecologist's office because of irregular menstrual cycles. She is otherwise healthy and takes no medication. She began menstruating at the age of 12 and has never had regular intervals between cycles, which range from 5 weeks to 3 months. She is not sexually active. On physical examination, she is overweight, with moderate acne on her forehead and chin. Her blood pressure is 115/85 mm Hg, heart rate is 95/min, and respiratory rate is 18/min. A pelvic examination reveals a smooth, nontender, appropriately sized uterus and slightly enlarged ovaries bilaterally. Laboratory studies are ordered. Which of the following are the most likely laboratory results?

CHOICE	FOLLICLE-STIMULATING HORMONE	LUTEINIZING HORMONE	ESTROGEN
A	↓	↓	↑
B	↓	↑	↑
C	↑	↑	↓
D	↑	↑	↑

(A) A
(B) B
(C) C
(D) D

30. A 35-year-old G4P4 woman presents for follow-up to the obstetrics and gynecology clinic with the chief complaint of amenorrhea. She says that she is concerned because she was not able to breast-feed and has not had a menstrual period since the birth of her last child 1 year ago. She has no medical problems and takes no medications. The only medications she has ever taken are oral contraceptives, which she has used between pregnancies. Her obstetric history reveals three spontaneous vaginal deliveries without complications. Her last delivery was by cesarean section because of fetal intolerance of labor complicated by maternal hypotension. She denies any sexual activity in the past year because her husband has been working abroad. Physical examination reveals a

well-developed female in no acute distress. Head and neck examination reveals no ophthalmoplegia. Vision is intact in all four quadrants by confrontation bilaterally. Neck examination reveals no thyroid enlargement. Examination of the extremities reveals normal capillary refill and no edema. Gynecologic examination allows easy visualization of the cervix, and a normal-sized uterus and ovaries are palpated on internal examination. Laboratory tests show a prolactin level of 2 ng/mL. What is the most likely diagnosis in this patient?

(A) Craniopharyngioma
(B) Empty sella syndrome
(C) Pregnancy
(D) Previous oral contraceptive use
(E) Sheehan's syndrome

31. A 42-year-old man with a long-standing history of diabetes mellitus type 1 presents to his physician for his yearly checkup. On examination, the physician notes decreased sensation in both of his feet. Although he insists otherwise, the physician suspects that he has not been adequately monitoring and controlling his blood glucose level. Which of the following tests would be best for letting the physician know how well the patient's blood glucose has been controlled over the past 3 months?

(A) Dilated eye examination
(B) Fasting blood glucose level
(C) Hemoglobin A_{1c}
(D) Microalbumin screening
(E) Random blood glucose level

32. A moderately overweight 34-year-old woman presents to the ED with excessive sweating, flushing, tachycardia, and nervousness. Presuming that she might be suffering from thyrotoxicosis, the physician checks her blood levels of thyroid hormones, and finds that her free thyroxine and triiodothyronine are elevated, while her thyroid-stimulating hormone is de-

creased. Her radioactive iodine uptake test shows a complete absence of iodine uptake. What is the most likely diagnosis?

(A) Factitious thyrotoxicosis
(B) Graves' disease
(C) Thyroid-stimulating hormone–secreting pituitary tumor
(D) Toxic adenoma
(E) Toxic multinodular goiter

33. A 42-year-old woman with no significant past medical history presents for a routine health maintenance visit. On physical examination, a solitary nodule is palpated in the thyroid. She denies pain, dysphagia, or hoarseness. She denies fatigue, weight change, heat or cold intolerance, diarrhea, or constipation. There is no family history of thyroid cancer. Her serum thyroid-stimulating hormone is normal. Which of the following is the most appropriate next step in evaluation?

(A) Fine-needle aspiration
(B) MRI
(C) Radionuclide scan
(D) Thyroid lobectomy
(E) Ultrasonography

34. A 60-year-old man presents to his primary care physician for routine medical care. He has no complaints, takes no medications, and has a family history of diabetes. Examination is unremarkable. A screening laboratory test reveals fasting blood glucose 152 mg/dL. One week later, the test is repeated and a value of 144 mg/dL is obtained. Which is the most likely cause of these findings?

(A) Autoimmune destruction of pancreatic islet cells
(B) Pancreatitis
(C) Peripheral insulin resistance
(D) Surreptitious insulin injection
(E) The patient's findings represent normal laboratory values

35. A 65-year-old man presents with a 1-day history of hematuria and sharp 10 of 10 flank pain radiating toward the groin on the right side. He has had three prior episodes of nephrolithiasis over the past 5 years, which all presented with a similar clinical picture. He is not taking any medication. There is no family history of renal calculi, renal disease, or endocrine disorders. His temperature is 36.9°C (98.5°F), heart rate is 125/min, and blood pressure is 132/86 mm Hg. He is in obvious distress and cannot sit still on the bed. Physical examination reveals a soft, nontender abdomen but extreme costovertebral angle tenderness on the right. Laboratory values are shown. Tests show:

Na^+	142 mEq/L
K^+	4.8 mEq/L
Cl^-	104 mEq/L
HCO_3^-	24 mEq/L
Ca^{2+}	11.0 mg/dL
Phosphorus$^+$	1.4 mg/dL
Mg^{2+}	2.0 mg/dL
Blood urea nitrogen	12 mg/dL
Creatinine	1.0 mg/dL
Glucose	118 mg/dL
Parathyroid hormone	300 pg/mL

Which of the following is the most likely diagnosis?

(A) Malignancy
(B) Milk-alkali syndrome
(C) Primary hyperparathyroidism
(D) Sarcoidosis
(E) Secondary hyperparathyroidism

36. A 72-year-old woman presents complaining of fatigue, malaise, weight loss, and salt cravings. The patient has chronic obstructive pulmonary disease (COPD) and is intermittently treated with corticosteroids but is not on home oxygen. In the office, her oxygen saturation is 97% on room air with a blood pressure of 115/65 mm Hg, which is significantly lower than her baseline of 125/78 mm Hg. On auscultation she has good breath sounds bilaterally without wheeze, although the expiratory phase is slightly prolonged. Her last corticosteroid treatment occurred 5 weeks ago for an acute COPD exacerbation for which she was hospi-talized and placed on 3 L of oxygen via nasal cannula. However, she admits that after discharge she was having continued difficulty breathing and did not follow the taper of the corticosteroids. The patient has smoked a pack of cigarettes per day for the past 51 years. What is the appropriate first step in the management of this patient?

(A) CT scan of the chest
(B) Intravenous fluids
(C) 3 L of oxygen via nasal cannula
(D) Restart corticosteroids and follow a strict taper
(E) X-ray of the chest

37. An obese patient with a long-standing history of type 2 diabetes presents to his primary care physician. On examination, he is found to have decreased sensation in both lower extremities. Upon questioning of his compliance with his prescribed medications, he reports that he has stopped taking one medication because it gave him flatulence and abdominal pain. Which of the following drugs or drug classes did this man most likely stop taking?

(A) α-Glucosidase inhibitor
(B) Meglitinide
(C) Metformin
(D) Sulfonylurea
(E) Thiazolidinedione

38. A 38-year-old woman presents with several months of decreased libido and a 4.5-kg (10-lb) weight gain. She has not had her menstrual period in the past 3 months. Physical examination is unremarkable, except that a small amount of white discharge is manually expressed from the nipples bilaterally. The serum prolactin level is 300 ng/mL. What is the appropriate first-line treatment for this patient?

(A) Bromocriptine
(B) Cortisol
(C) Methyldopa
(D) Metoclopramide
(E) Octreotide

39. A 6-year-old boy presents to his pediatrician for a routine physical examination. His mother reports no problems over the past year other than that he seems to be shorter than the other boys

in his class. His mother is 163 cm (5 ft 4 in) tall and experienced menarche at age 12, and his father is 178 cm (5 ft 10 in) tall and went through puberty at approximately age 14. On his growth curve, the boy's height was at the 10th percentile at birth, at the sixth percentile by age 3, and at the third percentile right now. His weight is currently at the 25th percentile. Which of the following should be performed in the evaluation of this patient?

(A) Chromosomal analysis
(B) Colonoscopy
(C) Growth hormone level
(D) Insulin-like growth factor-1 level
(E) No further evaluation is necessary

40. A 32-year-old man presents to his primary care physician complaining of diffuse muscle weakness, dry and puffy skin, and patchy areas of hair loss on his scalp. He also notes numbness around his mouth and a tingling sensation in his hands and feet. He has a history of seizure disorder, and has been taking carbamazepine for the past 5 years. On physical examination, he has dry skin and coarse, brittle hair with patchy alopecia. Upon tapping his right cheek, muscles at the corner of his mouth, nose, and eye on the right side contract. Which of the following measures may have prevented the development of the patient's current problem?

(A) Magnesium supplementation
(B) Parathyroidectomy
(C) Thyroid hormone
(D) Vitamin C supplementation
(E) Vitamin D supplementation

41. A 16-year-old obese Hispanic girl presents to her physician's office complaining of "ugly skin around my neck" and having to wear turtlenecks. On examination the physician notes darkening and thickening of the skin, which has a velvety appearance. What is the most appropriate course of action?

(A) Obtain a CT scan of the abdomen
(B) Obtain a punch biopsy of the affected skin
(C) Obtain a serum glucose test
(D) Obtain a shave biopsy of the affected skin
(E) Obtain liver function tests

42. A 24-year-old woman comes into the ED with recurrent episodes of palpitations, headache, and tremor. Her blood pressure is 155/95 mm Hg, heart rate is 135/min, temperature is 37.9°C (100.2°F), and respiratory rate is 12/min. A CT of the abdomen shows a suprarenal mass. After confirming the diagnosis with a laboratory test, the physician informs the patient that she will require immediate therapy and surgical resection of the mass within the next few weeks. In order to achieve short-term control of her blood pressure, which of the following agents is most appropriate?

(A) Furosemide
(B) Hydralazine
(C) Phenylzine
(D) Prazosin
(E) Propranolol

43. A 49-year-old man presents in clinic for a health maintenance visit. He has a family history of type 2 diabetes mellitus. His medical history is significant for gastroesophageal reflux disease, for which he takes omeprazole and over-the-counter antacids. He smokes 1 pack of cigarettes per day and drinks an average of two beers per night. The patient's body mass index is 32 kg/m². Which of the following single interventions most greatly reduces the patient's risk of future coronary artery disease, renal failure, and retinopathy?

(A) Alcohol avoidance
(B) Daily multivitamin
(C) Diet rich in fruit and vegetables
(D) Smoking cessation
(E) Weight loss and exercise

44. A 72-year-old man with end-stage renal disease secondary to hypertension presents with several months of back pain. He denies fever, weight loss, difficulty walking, altered sensation in his legs, or incontinence. He was diagnosed with renal disease 20 years ago and was managed medically for many years. However, 2 years ago he began hemodialysis because of a progressive decline in renal function. There is no family history of renal disease or malignancy. Physical examination is unremarkable. X-ray of the chest shows a "rugger-jersey" spine with ill-defined bands of increased bone density adjacent to the vertebral endplates. What laboratory abnormalities would be expected in this patient?

(A) Bence Jones protein in urine
(B) Decreased parathyroid hormone
(C) Decreased phosphorus
(D) Elevated bone-specific alkaline phosphatase
(E) Elevated parathyroid hormone

45. A 32-year-old G2P1 woman at 16 weeks' gestation presents to her obstetrician complaining of fatigue, anxiety, and palpitations. She notes that she has been feeling warm, even in her air-conditioned home, and has been having three or four loose stools per day, as compared to one or two prior to her pregnancy. She has a temperature of 37.1°C (98.8°F), a heart rate of 105/min, and a blood pressure of 128/76 mm Hg. Neck examination reveals mild diffuse enlargement of the thyroid gland with no lymphadenopathy. Relevant laboratory findings include a total triiodothyronine level of 400 ng/dL, a free thyroxine of 6.8 ng/dL, and a thyroid-stimulating hormone of 0.01 μU/mL. Results of a thyroid-stimulating hormone-receptor antibody test are positive. Which of the following is appropriate therapy for this patient?

(A) High-dose iodine therapy
(B) Methimazole
(C) Propylthiouracil
(D) Radioiodine ablation
(E) Surgical resection

46. A 32-year-old woman undergoes a cesarean section for failure of labor to progress, and delivers a healthy baby boy. The procedure is complicated by significant intraoperative blood loss and hypotension, but the patient is successfully resuscitated. Postoperatively, she experiences dull, aching, nonlocalized abdominal pain and nausea, but denies headache, visual changes, or abnormal edema. On postoperative day three she is passing flatus and remains afebrile, but becomes hypotensive to the 90s systolic over the 40s diastolic. She has not begun lactating despite her attempts to breast-feed her infant. Laboratory values indicate that she is hyponatremic and mildly hyperkalemic. Urinalysis and liver enzymes are normal. What is a likely cause of her symptoms?

(A) Appendicitis
(B) HELLP syndrome
(C) Postoperative infection
(D) Sheehan's syndrome
(E) Toxic shock syndrome

47. A 52-year-old man presents to the primary care clinic for the first time. He states that he has been in good health throughout his life and takes no medications. He was once athletic but has noted a dramatic decrease in his muscle strength and exercise tolerance over the past year. On examination, the physician finds that the patient is moderately hypertensive, with a tanned, round, plethoric face; large supraclavicular fat pads; and significant truncal obesity. He has no focal cardiovascular, pulmonary, or neurologic findings. His fasting blood sugar is 200 mg/dL. Which of the following is the most common etiology of this condition?

(A) ACTH-secreting pituitary adenoma
(B) Adrenal tumor
(C) Ectopic ACTH-secreting tumor
(D) Primary adrenal hyperplasia
(E) Small cell lung cancer

48. A 48-year-old high school teacher with no prior medical history presents to his primary care physician after feeling extremely fatigued for more than 1 month. Previously an avid runner, he has recently experienced dyspnea on moderate exertion. Although he denies vomiting, he admits to intermittent episodes of diarrhea. His blood pressure is 73/37 mm Hg, and he is afebrile. On physical examination, his skin is warm and erythematous, and his jugular

venous pressure is elevated. Cardiac examination reveals a systolic murmur near the right border of the sternum that is accentuated with inspiration. Which of the following is most consistent with these findings?

(A) Elevated urinary excretion of 5-hydroxyindoleacetic acid
(B) Elevated urinary excretion of vanillylmandelic acid
(C) Peaked T waves on ECG
(D) *Pseudomonas* species grown from blood cultures
(E) Severe pulmonary congestion on x-ray of the chest

49. During a well-visit checkup, a 1-month-old baby girl who was born at home with midwife assistance is evaluated. Her mother states that she has been feeding poorly and is constipated, with poor weight gain. The child's heart rate is 145/min, blood pressure is 82/52 mm Hg, and respiratory rate is 40/min. On physical examination, the child appears jaundiced and demonstrates large anterior and posterior fontanelles and poor muscle tone. An umbilical hernia, in addition to mild genital swelling, is also noted. What is the most likely diagnosis for this 1-month-old baby girl?

(A) α_1-Antitrypsin deficiency
(B) Congenital herpes
(C) Congenital hypothyroidism
(D) DiGeorge's syndrome
(E) Pheochromocytoma

50. A 3010-g (6.6-lb) boy was born to a 37-year-old primagravida by spontaneous vaginal delivery after an uncomplicated pregnancy. On examination, he has cyanotic extremities and a significant right precordial heave, a single S2, and a harsh systolic ejection murmur along the sternal border. He also has a prominent squared nose and cleft palate. An echocardiogram is subsequently performed and demonstrates tetralogy of Fallot. Corrective surgery is performed without complications. At 2 months of age, the infant is diagnosed with *Pneumocystis jiroveci* (formerly *carinii*) pneumonia and at 3 months, he is diagnosed with fungal septicemia. Additional workup of this child should include which of the following tests?

(A) Hemoglobin electrophoresis
(B) Nitroblue tetrazolium
(C) Renal ultrasound
(D) Quantitative immunoglobulin levels
(E) Serum calcium

1. **The correct answer is A.** Anti–thyroid-stimulating hormone receptor antibodies are pathognomonic for Graves' disease, as is suggested by this patient's symptoms of thyrotoxicosis with exophthalmos and pretibial myxedema. These antibodies mediate the disease by provoking a continuous and inappropriate release of thyroid hormone, which results in the clinical picture described. Common modalities of treatment include surgical removal of the gland, radioactive iodine gland ablation, and antithyroid medication such as propylthiouracil.

Answer B is incorrect. While thyroid-stimulating hormone (TSH) levels are decreased in Graves' disease, they are also decreased in all other forms of hyperthyroidism, so a decreased TSH level would be suggestive of, but not diagnostic for, Graves' disease.

Answer C is incorrect. An increased creatine kinase–myocardial bound fraction is sometimes seen in conjunction with hypothyroidism. In this case, this patient most likely has Graves' disease, a form of hyperthryoidism.

Answer D is incorrect. This patient most likely has Graves' disease, and as a form of hyperthyroidism, her TSH level will be decreased, not increased.

Answer E is incorrect. Antinuclear antibody (ANA) is a nonspecific test that generally indicates autoimmune disease. It is commonly used in conjunction with other diagnostic and clinical tests in the diagnosis of systemic lupus erythematosus, Sjögren's syndrome, and rheumatoid arthritis. While Graves' disease is an autoimmune disease, it is not commonly associated with ANA.

2. **The correct answer is C.** Kallmann's syndrome is a disorder of gonadotropin-releasing hormone (GnRH) synthesis and is associated with primary amenorrhea without secondary sexual characteristics due to the lack of pulsatile GnRH release, which is the initiating event of puberty. It is associated with anosmia or hyposmia due to olfactory bulb agenesis or hypoplasia. It is also associated with color blindness, optic atrophy, nerve deafness, cleft palate, renal abnormalities, cryptorchidism, and neurologic abnormalities such as mirror movements. Multiple mechanisms of inheritance have been observed, including autosomal recessive, autosomal dominant, and X-linked. Treatment is with oral contraceptives. To become pregnant, patients with Kallmann's syndrome require further treatment with a GnRH pump. This syndrome would account for this patient's symptoms of amenorrhea and lack of secondary sexual characteristics.

Answer A is incorrect. Androgen insensitivity syndrome is characterized by the presence of breasts and lack of axillary hair growth. This occurs when a patient is genetically XY, but has female external genitalia. Usually there is the presence of undescended testes, which generally must be removed due to the increased risk of testicular cancer in these patients. This diagnosis would account neither for the lack of breast development or the presence of a cervix. This would not be the correct diagnosis in this patient.

Answer B is incorrect. Gonadal dysgenesis or Turner's syndrome is a possibility in this patient with amenorrhea. It would account for both the amenorrhea and the lack of secondary sexual characteristics because, although growth hormone is present if there is no response from the ovaries, estrogen and testosterone are not released in sufficient amounts to affect puberty. However, the patient lacks the dysmorphic features classically seen in patients with Turner's syndrome, including short stature, square-shaped chest, webbed neck, high palate, and short fourth metacarpal. Turner's syndrome patients also can have autoimmune diseases, including chronic autoimmune thyroiditis; morphologic defects of cardiovascular, urologic, and bone structure; and hearing loss.

Answer D is incorrect. Kartagener's syndrome is an autosomal recessive defect of cilial movement. It has been known to cause bronchiectasis, situs inversus, chronic sinusitis, and infertility in men due to defective sperm movement.

Answer E is incorrect. Pregnancy causes amenorrhea, but this patient denies sexual activity and has a negative pregnancy test.

3. **The correct answer is A.** Central diabetes insipidus (DI) is a deficiency of production of antidiuretic hormone (ADH) in the posterior pituitary. ADH acts in the distal nephron and collecting tubule of the kidney to concentrate the urine and reabsorb water. Central DI can be a primary condition due to a genetic disorder or may be idiopathic; it can also be a secondarily acquired disorder due to trauma, neoplasm, infection, inflammatory conditions, and toxins. A deficiency in ADH leads to decreased water reabsorption in the kidney that results in hypernatremia and increased volumes of dilute urine.

Answer B is incorrect. Diabetes mellitus also causes increased thirst, increased urinary frequency, and nocturia. However, the mechanism is through a solute (glucose) diuresis, not an inability to concentrate the urine. The urine osmolarity in diabetes mellitus will be elevated. The fact that the urine osmolarity is decreased excludes the diagnosis of diabetes mellitus.

Answer C is incorrect. Nephrogenic diabetes insipidus (DI) has the same clinical presentation as central DI. However, patients with nephrogenic DI secrete a normal amount of ADH from the pituitary, but they have a mutation in the receptor for ADH in the kidney. Desmopressin (or DDAVP) is a synthetic form of ADH. If administration of desmopressin increases urine osmolarity by ≥ 50% in 1–2 hours, the diagnosis of central DI is confirmed, as occurred in this patient. If administration of desmopressin fails to increase urine osmolarity, this indicates a nephrogenic source of DI, because even though ADH levels are increased, the kidney cannot respond.

Answer D is incorrect. Psychogenic polydipsia is a condition in which the patient consumes excessive amounts of water. This also leads to increased urinary frequency and nocturia. However, in patients with psychogenic polydipsia, the urine osmolarity should normalize after a water deprivation test.

Answer E is incorrect. Syndrome of inappropriate secretion is a condition in which the pituitary secretes excessive amounts of ADH. This leads to hyponatremia and concentrated urine.

4. **The correct answer is E.** This patient's presentation is consistent with rickets. Rickets is a disorder of bone mineralization that can be due to hypocalcemia or hypophosphatemia. Hypocalcemic rickets is typically due to a deficiency of vitamin D from dietary insufficiency, lack of exposure to sunlight, lack of enzymes to convert vitamin D to active metabolites, or end-organ resistance to vitamin D. In this patient with normal vitamin D levels, it is one of the later etiologies, and treatment with exogenous vitamin D will not correct the hypocalcemia. Clinical presentation may include tetany, convulsions, alopecia, and skeletal abnormalities. Skeletal findings include widened growth plates, frontal bossing, enlargement of the wrists, bowing of the distal forearm, lateral bowing of the femur and tibia, and delay in closure of the fontanelles. Children may present with dental enamel hypoplasia, delay in motor milestones, and frequent infectious diseases. Laboratory findings will include hypocalcemia, hypophosphatemia, and secondary hyperparathyroidism.

Answer A is incorrect. Dietary deficiency of vitamin D can also cause the clinical presentation seen in this patient. However, the vitamin D level would be decreased, and the disorder would correct with exogenous administration of vitamin D.

Answer B is incorrect. Hypoalbuminemia is a common cause of hypocalcemia in malnourished adults. Normally 40% of calcium is bound to albumin. When a patient has hypoalbuminemia, he or she has decreased total serum calcium, even though there is a normal amount of free calcium. The correction is that a 1-g/dL reduction in albumin will decrease total serum calcium by 0.8 mg/dL. In an otherwise healthy pediatric patient, this is an extremely unlikely etiology.

Answer C is incorrect. Primary hyperparathyroidism will cause hypophosphatemia and elevated parathyroid hormone, but patients will have hypercalcemia, not hypocalcemia. Furthermore, the bony abnormalities seen with hyperparathyroidism include osteitis fibrosa cystica and brown tumors, not rickets. These patients develop subperiosteal bone resorption due to excessive osteoclast activity, which classically affects the clavicle, phalanges, and vertebral bodies.

Answer D is incorrect. Pseudohypoparathyroidism is a disorder caused by end-organ resistance to parathyroid hormone (PTH). Patients present with signs of hypoparathyroidism, including hypocalcemia, but the PTH level will be elevated, not decreased, as would be expected with true hypoparathyroidism. Unlike in this patient, patients with pseudohypoparathyroidism have hyperphosphatemia.

5. **The correct answer is A.** This patient has acromegaly, a condition caused by excessive levels of growth hormone, most commonly due to a pituitary adenoma. Blurred vision is due to compression of the optic chiasm by the pituitary mass, and patients may also exhibit frontal bossing, mandibular growth, coarsened facial features, and increased hand and foot size due to bony overgrowth and soft tissue swelling. Patients with acromegaly may be at increased risk for developing colonic polyps and colonic malignancy. Patients with acromegaly are also at increased risk for coronary artery disease, cardiomyopathy, hypertension, diabetes mellitus, and sleep apnea.

Answer B is incorrect. There is no association between growth hormone hypersecretion and hepatocellular carcinoma.

Answer C is incorrect. Although there are rare cases of lung tumors producing ectopic growth homone (GH), this patient has hypersecretion of GH due to a pituitary adenoma. These patients are not at increased risk of developing lung malignancies.

Answer D is incorrect. Pituitary adenomas are usually benign tumors that do not result in increased risk of other malignant brain tumors.

Answer E is incorrect. There are rare cases of excessive ectopic GH secretion by tumors of the pancreas. However, this patient has evidence of a pituitary adenoma, which is the source of the GH hypersecretion. These patients are not at increased risk of developing pancreatic cancer.

6. **The correct answer is B.** In individuals with 17α-hydroxylase deficiency, adrenocorticotropic hormone (ACTH) secretion is elevated secondary to decreased cortisol levels. The goal of treatment with hydrocortisone is not only to replenish cortisol, but also to suppress ACTH secretion. The reason for this is that if ACTH remains high, it will stimulate androgen production and lead to premature virilization and growth plate ossification. Nightly dexamethasone treatments may be necessary to more completely suppress ACTH secretion in adolescents.

Answer A is incorrect. Cosyntropin stimulates ACTH production, and cosyntropin levels are used to diagnose 21-hydroxylase deficiency.

Answer C is incorrect. Spironolactone is a potassium-sparing diuretic and would not affect ACTH levels.

Answer D is incorrect. Increased hydrocortisone alone may not be sufficient to suppress ACTH secretion in this patient.

Answer E is incorrect. This individual is exhibiting signs of increased virilization and likely needs further suppression of ACTH secretion to prevent premature skeletal maturation.

7. **The correct answer is A.** The patient is presenting with signs and symptoms consistent with hypothyroidism which include fatigue, weakness, cold intolerance, dry skin, constipation, bradycardia, coarse hair and skin, and puffy, cool extremities. Hypothyroidism can be a primary disorder of the thyroid gland, a secondary disorder due to deficient production of TSH by the pituitary, or a tertiary disorder due to deficient production of thyrotropin-releasing hormone (TRH) by the hypothalamus. This patient's laboratory results confirm a diagnosis of primary hypothyroidism because the thyroid

hormone levels are low in the presence of an elevated TSH. Amiodarone, an antiarrhythmic agent commonly used in atrial fibrillation, can cause hypothyroidism by inhibiting production of triiodothyronine, by direct toxicity to thyroid follicular cells, and by effects due to amiodarone's iodine content.

Answer B is incorrect. Flecainide is a class IC antiarrhythmic agent sometimes used in the treatment of atrial fibrillation; however, it is not known to cause hypothyroidism.

Answer C is incorrect. Lithium is used primarily in the therapy of bipolar disorder. Hypothyroidism is a common side effect of lithium; however, it is not used to treat atrial fibrillation.

Answer D is incorrect. Methimazole is an agent used to treat hyperthyroidism. If given in excessive amounts, it can cause iatrogenic hypothyroidism. However, methimazole is not used to treat atrial fibrillation.

Answer E is incorrect. Sotalol is a β blocker that is used to maintain sinus rhythm in patients with atrial fibrillation, but it is not known to cause thyroid toxicity.

8. **The correct answer is C.** This patient is displaying classic signs of hypocalcemia, including hyperexcitability of her facial nerve (Chvostek's sign), induced carpal spasm (Trousseau's sign), and tingling of the extremities and lips. Calcium homeostasis is a complicated process involving parathyroid hormone, vitamin D, albumin, and numerous electrolytes. Acquired hypoparathyroidism is the most common form of true hypocalcemia, most often occurring transiently after thyroid surgery or after the removal of a parathyroid adenoma. Occasionally, hypomagnesemia can produce hypocalcemia by decreasing both the body's production of parathyroid hormone and its sensitivity to the hormone. In this case, it is likely that the patient became magnesium depleted from her course of watery diarrhea, likely baseline poor nutritional status, and alcohol abuse.

Answer A is incorrect. Azotemia is not a cause of hypocalcemia. Chronic kidney disease, however, can lead to hypocalcemia in the setting of secondary hyperparathyroidism, but there is no evidence of renal failure in this patient.

Answer B is incorrect. Fluid balance (hyper- or hyponatremia) does not play a role in calcium homeostasis.

Answer D is incorrect. Hypophosphatemia is not a cause of hypocalcemia. Actually, hypocalcemia often leads to hyperphosphatemia secondary to increased parathyroid hormone-mediated bone resorption. Elevations in phosphorus may also contribute to hypocalcemia by complexing with circulating calcium and suppressing conversion of 25-OH to 1,25-OH vitamin D.

Answer E is incorrect. Urate levels do not affect calcium homeostasis.

9. **The correct answer is A.** The patient's findings are consistent with Kallmann's syndrome, a congenital deficiency of GnRH synthesis in the hypothalamus. Women present with primary amenorrhea and failure to develop secondary sexual characteristics. Laboratory evaluation will show low or absent levels of GnRH. Because GnRH is required for release of gonadotropins from the anterior pituitary, there will also be diminished levels of luteinizing hormone and follicle-stimulating hormone. This syndrome is associated with anosmia or hyposmia due to hypoplasia or agenesis of the olfactory bulb, color blindness, cleft palate, renal disorders, and nerve deafness.

Answer B is incorrect. In Kallmann's syndrome, both luteinizing hormone (LH) and follicle-stimulating hormone (FSH) are decreased. A situation in which both gonadotropin-releasing hormone and LH are increased, but FSH may be decreased, is polycystic ovarian syndrome.

Answer C is incorrect. In Kallmann's syndrome, both LH and FSH are decreased. A situation in which GnRH is decreased, but LH/FSH are increased, is one in which there is a mutation constitutionally activating the GnRH receptor in the anterior pituitary.

Answer D is incorrect. In Kallmann's syndrome, there is a deficiency, not an excess of GnRH. One situation in which there would be elevated GnRH but decreased gonadotropins would be a mutation in the receptor for GnRH in the anterior pituitary.

Answer E is incorrect. Kallmann's syndrome is a deficiency of GnRH. A situation in which one might see amenorrhea with elevated gonadotropins would be primary ovarian failure.

10. **The correct answer is E.** This woman has a pituitary prolactinoma, which is associated with amenorrhea, infertility, and galactorrhea. Prolactin inhibits the secretion of gonadotropins and suppresses ovulation. Dopamine is used to suppress prolactin and thus restore fertility.

Answer A is incorrect. Ectopic endometrial tissue, as seen with endometriosis, is a common cause of infertility. Patients experience severe dysmenorrhea and irregular menstrual cycles. Infertility typically results from adhesions caused by scarring of the ectopic endometrial tissue. However, endometriosis is not likely to cause the visual field defects seen in this patient.

Answer B is incorrect. This woman has a prolactinoma and is therefore most likely not ovulating. As a result, failure of implantation cannot be the cause of her infertility because a zygote cannot be formed in the first place.

Answer C is incorrect. At the beginning of the menstrual cycle, the cervical mucus is viscous and very cellular. Around ovulation, the salt and water concentration of the mucus increases, making it thinner and allowing sperm to penetrate it. If this fails to occur, infertility can result due to the hostile cervical mucus. However, this would not be associated with this patient's visual symptoms.

Answer D is incorrect. Prolactin inhibits the secretion of gonadotropins and suppresses ovulation. The ovaries are still responsive to gonadotropins, as demonstrated by treatment with dopamine, which suppresses prolactin and restores ovulation. Because the patient is still menstruating, although irregularly, her ovaries are still functioning.

11. **The correct answer is E.** Given that diabetes mellitus type 1 (DM-1) is most likely an autoimmune disease, it is not surprising that it is associated with certain human leukocyte antigen (HLA) types. HLA-DR3 is associated with DM-1 and is found in about 4% of patients. It is also associated with systemic lupus erythematosus and Graves' disease.

Answer A is incorrect. HLA-B27 is strongly associated with ankylosing spondylitis, as well as Reiter's syndrome (arthritis, urethritis, and conjunctivitis).

Answer B is incorrect. HLA-B51 is associated with Behçet's syndrome.

Answer C is incorrect. HLA-D11 is associated with Hashimoto's disease.

Answer D is incorrect. HLA-DR2 is associated with Goodpasture's syndrome and multiple sclerosis.

12. **The correct answer is E.** Painful thyroiditis limits the differential to subacute granulomatous thyroiditis, acute infectious thyroiditis, and palpation- or trauma-induced thyroiditis. In this case the diagnosis is subacute granulomatous thyroiditis, otherwise known as de Quervain's thyroiditis, which typically follows an acute viral illness, typically an upper respiratory infection. Inflammation leads to destruction of thyroid follicles, causing release of thyroid hormone stores, leading to a transient period of hyperthyroidism until the stores are exhausted. There may be a transient period of hypothyroidism that follows, but as inflammation subsides, the follicles will regenerate and the patient will return to a euthyroid state. Because of the increased thyroid hormone in the serum, the thyroid-stimulating hormone will be low due to negative feedback on the pituitary.

Answer A is incorrect. Acute infectious thyroiditis is a cause of painful thyroiditis. However, it can be differentiated from subacute granulomatous thyroiditis by the clinical presentation. Acute infectious disease is typically unilateral as opposed to diffuse as seen in this patient. Patients will have acute onset of pain with fever and chills. Many will have a unilateral neck mass, which may be fluctuant. In addition, thyroid function is typically normal in patients with acute infectious thyroiditis.

Answer B is incorrect. Drugs can cause painless, not painful, thyroiditis. Examples include lithium, interferon alfa, interleukin-2, and amiodarone.

Answer C is incorrect. Hashimoto's thyroiditis is a chronic autoimmune disorder causing hypothyroidism. Hashimoto's very rarely causes a painful thyroid gland. In addition, serum thyroid hormone would be low and thyroid-stimulating hormone elevated. Patients will have symptoms of hypothyroidism including weight gain, cold intolerance, and constipation.

Answer D is incorrect. Riedel's thyroiditis is a nonpainful type of thyroiditis. Patients with this disorder have extensive fibrosis of the thyroid, causing the gland to become enlarged, hard, and fixed. Patients may complain of neck discomfort, dysphagia, and hoarseness due to compression of adjacent structures, but they do not have tenderness to palpation. Typically they are euthyroid, although some patients may be hypothyroid.

13. **The correct answer is C.** Under normal conditions, dopamine is delivered from the hypothalamus to the pituitary in a tonic fashion, constitutively inhibiting the release of prolactin into the bloodstream. Typical antipsychotics, such as haloperidol, block dopamine receptors on the surface of prolactin-secreting cells in the anterior pituitary. This leads to inappropriate release of prolactin. She is also predisposed to the galactorrheic effect of prolactin by virtue of her parity. Another clue to this answer is her history of a "blood disorder." It is possible that she was on an atypical antipsychotic such as clozapine, which can cause agranulocytosis. This may have prompted her psychiatrist to switch to a typical antipsychotic such as haloperidol, which generally does not produce that adverse effect.

Answer A is incorrect. Central nervous system sarcoidosis may cause galactorrhea, but this is an uncommon manifestation of the disease.

Answer B is incorrect. Idiopathic prolactinemia is a diagnosis of exclusion, and there are other explanations available.

Answer D is incorrect. Pregnancy may present with irregularities in the menstrual cycle, and it is possible that the patient is pregnant, but that is probably not the cause of her presenting symptom. Pregnancy does not generally present as galactorrhea.

Answer E is incorrect. A prolactinoma does not always cause vision and sensation changes, but the lack of those symptoms makes the diagnosis less likely.

14. **The correct answer is C.** This patient is in a state of diabetic ketoacidosis. Lack of insulin is the primary disorder, and insulin administration will allow glucose to enter cells and reverse the metabolic starvation that is driving the production of ketoacids. It is also important to immediately administer intravenous fluids because the patient is severely dehydrated. Finally, even though she is hyperkalemic, her potassium levels will decrease rapidly once the insulin is given because it will cause the potassium to enter the cells. Therefore, it is important to give additional potassium to ensure that the patient does not become hypokalemic.

Answer A is incorrect. The patient is dehydrated, and therefore needs additional fluid; diuresis would only make her diabetic ketoacidosis (DKA) worse. Ventilatory support is usually not needed because the tachypneic Kussmaul breathing seen in DKA is driven by metabolic acidosis, not hypoxia. Correction of the metabolic acidosis through insulin administration will reduce the need for this respiratory compensation.

Answer B is incorrect. As insulin is administered, potassium shifts from extracellular to intracellular, exposing what had been a concealed whole body hypokalemia. Potassium restriction would make the ensuing drop in the measured extracellular potassium even more pronounced and dangerous, given the possibility of fatal arrhythmias in hypokalemia. Diuresis would also be inappropriate in a diabetic ketoacidosis patient, who is likely dehydrated.

Answer D is incorrect. Potassium restriction would make the patient likely to become hypokalemic once the insulin is administered because he will probably have very low intracellular potassium. If potassium levels are extremely high, calcium gluconate can be administered to prevent hyperkalemia-induced arrhythmias.

Answer E is incorrect. The patient is dehydrated, so not only will diuresis make the situation worse, but the loop diuretic would also cause additional depletion of whole body potassium levels, which are low in diabetic ketoacidosis.

15. **The correct answer is C.** Hoarseness generally implies vocal cord impairment due to tumor involvement of the recurrent laryngeal nerve. This suggests a malignant tumor that has extended beyond the thyroid and invaded local structures. This is a poor prognostic indicator. Local invasion is particularly common with papillary carcinoma.

Answer A is incorrect. Female gender is a good prognostic indicator because thyroid nodules in men have a higher risk of malignancy.

Answer B is incorrect. Age is an important prognostic indicator. Nodules are more likely to be malignant in patients older than 60 and younger than 30. So, a patient at age 50 has a better chance of having a benign nodule.

Answer D is incorrect. Palpitations may be a symptom of hyperthyroidism. Typically, functioning nodules that produce thyroid hormone are more likely to be benign. These lesions are seen as "hot" on radionuclide scans, whereas malignant lesions tend to be nonfunctioning and therefore are seen as "cold."

Answer E is incorrect. Slow growth is also a good prognostic factor because malignant nodules tend to grow rapidly.

Answer F is incorrect. Malignant thyroid nodules are classically painless. A tender nodule usually suggests a benign disorder such as subacute viral thyroiditis or hemorrhage into a benign cyst.

16. **The correct answer is C.** This patient's current symptoms and past medical and family histories are highly suspicious for type I multiple endocrine neoplasia (MEN-I), an autosomal dominant condition consisting of pancreatic tumors, hyperparathyroidism, and pituitary adenomas. Zollinger-Ellison syndrome causes recurrent peptic ulcers due to excessive gastrin secretion by a gastrinoma, either in the pancreas or elsewhere in the gastrointestinal tract. Hyperparathyroidism causes hypercalcemia, hypophosphatemia, and elevated levels of serum parathyroid hormone. The most common pituitary tumor found in MEN-I is prolactinoma, but other tumors include ACTH-secreting and GH-secreting adenomas.

Answer A is incorrect. Medullary thyroid cancer is found in association with type IIA multiple endocrine neoplasia, type IIB multiple endocrine neoplasia, and familial medullary thyroid cancer. It is not found in patients with type I multiple endocrine neoplasia.

Answer B is incorrect. Pheochromocytomas are found in patients with type IIA multiple endocrine neoplasia (medullary thyroid cancer, pheochromocytoma, and hyperparathyroidism) and type IIB multiple endocrine neoplasia (medullary thyroid cancer, pheochromocytoma, and mucosal neuromas).

Answer D is incorrect. Papillary thyroid cancer is the most common type of thyroid cancer. However, it is not found in association with the inherited multiple endocrine neoplasia syndromes.

Answer E is incorrect. Squamous cell lung cancer can cause hypercalcemia and hypophosphatemia by secretion of parathyroid hormone–related protein. However, lung cancer is rare in such a young patient and there is no association with recurrent peptic ulcer disease.

17. **The correct answer is C.** Sulfonylureas (glipizide, glyburide) treat diabetes mellitus type 2 by increasing the amount of insulin secretion. The obvious potential adverse effect of this is hypoglycemia. Weight gain is another adverse effect.

Answer A is incorrect. α-Glucosidase inhibitors (acarbose) work by decreasing intestinal absorption of carbohydrates. Hypoglycemia is not a common adverse effect, but flatulence and abdominal pain are often complaints.

Answer B is incorrect. Statins (HMG CoA-reductase inhibitors) will reduce cholesterol levels, and therefore may be helpful as an adjunct treatment to oral hyperglycemic medications for patients with diabetes mellitus type 2. Hypoglycemia is not an adverse effect of statins.

Answer D is incorrect. The thiazolidinediones (glitazones) increase peripheral insulin sensitivity. Adverse effects include weight gain, edema, and potential hepatotoxicity.

Answer E is incorrect. Metformin inhibits hepatic gluconeogenesis and increases peripheral sensitivity to insulin, and although hypoglycemia is a possible adverse effect, it is rare and mild. More common adverse effects include weight loss, gastrointestinal upset, and metabolic lactic acidosis.

18. **The correct answer is D.** It is highly likely that this patient has myxedema coma. She has a history of thyroidectomy, making her dependent on thyroid hormone supplementation, and she may have ran out of medications. Myxedema coma most often presents as depressed mental status and hypothermia, and can also involve bradycardia, hypotension, hypoglycemia, and hyponatremia. It is often brought on by a precipitating illness, ischemic insult, or administration of sedatives. Management includes blood thyroid function tests prior to administration of levothyroxine (T_4) and triiodothyronine (T_3).

Answer A is incorrect. Aspirin would be given if an acute thrombotic event were suspected, such as a stroke or myocardial infarction.

Answer B is incorrect. Glucagon can be used in cases of refractory hypoglycemia, but this patient has an acceptable blood glucose level.

Answer C is incorrect. The indications for urgent hemodialysis include demonstrated renal failure plus metabolic **A**cidosis, life-threatening **E**lectrolyte abnormalities, toxic **I**ngestion, fluid **O**verload, or symptoms of **U**remia ("**A E I O U**"). Periorbital edema may be seen in renal failure, but hypothyroidism is a more likely cause in this patient.

Answer E is incorrect. Metoprolol would be first-line therapy if an acute myocardial infarc-

tion were suspected, but this is less likely given the ECG results.

Answer F is incorrect. Norepinephrine is a peripheral venoconstrictor used in the treatment of hypotension. While norepinephrine may be used to treat this patient's hypotension, especially if it worsens, it will not treat the underlying cause of the myxedema coma.

19. **The correct answer is A.** This patient's morning hyperglycemia may be her body's reaction to nocturnal hypoglycemia. Reactive hyperglycemia following hypoglycemia is known as the Somogyi effect. To approach this question, the actions of regular and neutral protamine Hagedorn (NPH) insulin should be understood. Compared to NPH, regular insulin has a shorter duration of onset, a peak action at 3–4 hours (versus 6–8 hours for NPH), and a shorter overall duration (6–8 hours for regular insulin versus 18–20 hours for NPH). If the dose of NPH insulin given at night causes the morning glucose to be too low, then the body may release stress hormones in response. The release of these stress hormones then causes the morning glucose to be high. The correct response is to decrease insulin at night.

Answer B is incorrect. Although morning hyperglycemia may be secondary to insufficient insulin at night, the patient's history suggests that this is not the case. Her morning hyperglycemia did not resolve after attempts at diet modification or after increasing her nighttime insulin dose. Further increasing her nighttime insulin would only exacerbate the problem.

Answer C is incorrect. Increasing morning insulin would not help decrease this patient's morning glucose.

Answer D is incorrect. Increasing nighttime insulin would worsen the Somogyi effect.

Answer E is incorrect. Increasing morning insulin would not help decrease this patient's morning glucose.

20. **The correct answer is A.** This woman likely has Graves' disease, an autoimmune disease in which antibodies against the thyroid-stimulating hormone receptor activate the thyroid into overproduction of thyroxine. It is associated

with other autoimmune disorders such as pernicious anemia. The photograph displays the ophthalmopathy and diffuse goiter seen with Graves' disease. Her fetus is at risk of developing thyrotoxicosis because thyroid-stimulating autoantibodies can cross the placenta and activate the fetal thyroid. Hence, fetal heart rate and maternal thyroid-stimulating immunoglobulin levels should be monitored during the pregnancy.

Answer B is incorrect. Ingestion of iodine can result in hyperthyroidism, but given this woman's history of pernicious anemia, Graves' disease is more likely.

Answer C is incorrect. This woman likely has Graves' disease, an autoimmune disease in which antibodies against the TSH receptor activate the thyroid into overproduction of thyroxine.

Answer D is incorrect. Thyroid adenomas can cause hyperthyroidism but usually do not result in a uniform goiter.

Answer E is incorrect. Viral hyperthyroidism is seen in acute and subacute thyroiditis. However, the thyroid is usually tender and is accompanied by or follows an upper respiratory tract infection.

21. **The correct answer is B.** GH has both direct effects, and effects mediated by release of insulin-like growth factor-1 (IGF-1) from the liver. Most of the long-term growth-promoting effects of GH are mediated by IGF-1. GH itself acts as an insulin antagonist, which may account for the existence of a feedback mechanism that inhibits GH release in response to a high-glucose meal in healthy persons. It also explains the high incidence of diabetes in patients with GH-secreting pituitary tumors, such as this patient.

Answer A is incorrect. ACTH tumors cause Cushing's disease, which is marked by truncal obesity, moon facies, abdominal striae, hypertension, and hyperpigmenation.

Answer C is incorrect. LH–producing tumors may cause symptoms similar to polycystic ovarian syndrome, such as amenorrhea, hirsutism, and obesity.

Answer D is incorrect. Prolactinomas cause galactorrhea, amenorrhea, and decreased libido.

Answer E is incorrect. TSH-secreting tumors produce symptoms of hyperthyroidism including tachycardia, tremor, diaphoresis, nervousness, weight loss, and increase blood pressure.

22. **The correct answer is A.** Given his history of recent renal transplantation and the symptoms of Cushing's syndrome, it is most likely that this child is currently taking corticosteroids as a means of immunosuppression. Exogenous corticosteroids such as prednisolone and dexamethasone have similar effects to those of cortisol, and the high levels used in posttransplant immunosuppression cause feedback suppression of ACTH release from the pituitary, as well as cushingoid symptoms. ACTH suppression causes suppression of endogenous cortisol production from the adrenal. This explains the seemingly paradoxical laboratory findings of hypothalamic-pituitary-adrenal axis suppression in the setting of hyperglucocorticoid symptoms (although note that specific exogenous glucocorticoids occasionally may cross-react with some cortisol assays).

Answer B is incorrect. Cortisol levels are unlikely to be normal in a cushingoid patient, since cortisol would be elevated if the cause were endogenous, and suppressed if the cause were exogenous steroid administration, as in this case.

Answer C is incorrect. These findings would occur in a state of primary adrenal hyperfunction, such as in adrenal carcinoma. Primary adrenal hyperfunction is uncommon, and there is a far more likely explanation for this patient's symptoms. This laboratory profile could fit with the patient described, but exogenous steroids do not reliably cross-react in a urinary cortisol assay, and the urinary cortisol level is more likely to be calculated as depressed than elevated.

Answer D is incorrect. An increased level of ACTH and decreased level of urinary free cortisol could be seen in a situation of adrenal insufficiency (the increased ACTH is a feedback response to decreased glucocorticoid levels).

This patient's symptoms suggest high, not low levels of glucocorticoids.

Answer E is incorrect. Increased ACTH and increased urinary free cortisol would be seen in conditions where the body releases an increased amount of ACTH, such as in an ACTH-secreting pituitary adenoma (Cushing's disease) or an ectopic ACTH-secreting tumor, such as small cell carcinoma of the lung or a carcinoid tumor. Exogenous steroid administration is a more likely explanation for this patient's symptoms.

23. **The correct answer is A.** The patient is presenting signs and symptoms of primary hyperaldosteronism: hypertension, hyperreflexia, weakness, hypernatremia, hypokalemia, alkalosis, and decreased plasma renin suggest the unilateral mass seen on CT is an adrenal adenoma hypersecreting mineralocorticoids.

Answer B is incorrect. Anion gap is calculated as $Na - (Cl^- + HCO_3^-)$ and when this formula is used the normal anion gap is 8–12 mEq/L. For this patient, using this equation yields a normal anion gap of 12 mEq/L: $150 - (105 + 33)$. This patient is alkalemic as a consequence of primary aldosteronism.

Answer C is incorrect. Carcinoembryonic antigen (CEA) could be elevated in smokers, as well as patients with liver disorders or adenocarcinomas of the colon, pancreas, breast, lung, or ovary. CEA levels are not used for diagnostic purposes; instead they are usually used to monitor the recurrence of cancer.

Answer D is incorrect. Increased prostate-specific antigen (PSA) may be seen in a variety of conditions that affect the prostate, including prostatitis and prostate cancer. An increased PSA would not cause hypernatremia, hypokalemia, or increased blood pressure. Look for elevated PSAs in elderly male patients with urinary symptoms.

Answer E is incorrect. Troponin would be elevated during an acute cardiac event. Troponins T and I are most specific for cardiac tissue. Look for elevated troponin in patients presenting with acute substernal chest pain and cardiac risk factors.

24. **The correct answer is D.** Intravenous fluids should first be administered prior to any other treatment. Although hydrocortisone is indicated to prevent an adrenal crisis in patients with primary adrenal insufficiency, Airway, Breathing, and Circulation (the ABCs) must first be addressed. As the patient is able to speak comfortably, his airway and breathing are intact and stable. However, the systolic blood pressure of 88 mm Hg requires fluid resuscitation.

Answer A is incorrect. Azithromycin or a macrolide antibiotic is indicated in atypical mycoplasma pneumonia or walking pneumonia commonly seen in adolescents and young adults. X-ray of the chest would help to confirm this diagnosis. Although the adrenal crisis in this scenario was likely triggered by infection and the patient could not mount a normal glucocorticoid stress response, his more urgent need is fluid resuscitation for hypotension.

Answer B is incorrect. Although diabetes may initiate an adrenal crisis, in this instance the patient has a clear source of infection which is likely the cause of the crisis. Therefore, checking serum glucose ultimately has no diagnostic or therapeutic benefit in this scenario.

Answer C is incorrect. Since the patient is in adrenal crisis due to primary adrenal insufficiency, hydrocortisone should be administered expediently. However, although the steroids address the issue of primary adrenal insufficiency, and the patient's hypotension will eventually be reversed, their effect is not evident immediately. The hypotension requires immediate treatment with intravenous fluids.

Answer E is incorrect. X-ray of the chest would be helpful to determine if the patient had a pneumonia or respiratory infection, but given this patient's past medical history it is important to address the hypotension and begin management before imaging.

25. **The correct answer is A.** Patients with subclinical hyperthyroidism who are > 60 years old have a three- to fivefold increased risk of developing atrial fibrillation. There is some controversy regarding the best way to treat subclinical hyperthyroidism, but antithyroid med-

ications such as propylthiouracil (PTU) are commonly used. In addition to cardiac dysrhythmias, there is an increased risk of bone density abnormalities in patients who are noted to have subclinical hyperthyroidism.

Answer B is incorrect. Although hypothyroidism can subsequently follow hyperthyroidism (subclinical or otherwise), antithyroid medications such as PTU are more likely to lead to hypothyroidism than they are to prevent it.

Answer C is incorrect. Pretibial myxedema is a common symptom of Graves' disease, and although subclinical hyperthyroidism can progress to Graves' disease, the most common concerns are in regard to cardiac dysrhythmias and bone density abnormalities.

Answer D is incorrect. Thyroid cancer is not commonly associated with hyperthyroidism.

Answer E is incorrect. Thyroid storm is an exacerbation of hyperthyroidism, and would be seen much more commonly in patients with hyperthyroidism with increased levels of free thyroxine and triiodothyronine than it would in patients with subclinical hyperthyroidism.

26. **The correct answer is D.** This patient has isolated hypercalcemia. An important cause of hypercalcemia is sarcoidosis and other granulomatous diseases, malignancies, and bony metastases. Of the choices listed, only elevation in angiotensin-converting enzyme (ACE) levels is commonly found in patients with hypercalcemia due to sarcoidosis. Sarcoidosis leads to hypercalcemia secondary to increased production of $1,25\ (OH)_2$ vitamin D by macrophages within the granulomas. Isolated hypercalcemia, however, is most often caused by a parathyroid adenoma.

Answer A is incorrect. Low thyroid hormone levels have little effect on calcium homeostasis. Hyperthyroidism, in contrast, and myxedema can be associated with hypercalcemia, believed to be due to increased bone turnover.

Answer B is incorrect. Whereas hypervitaminosis D is associated with hypercalcemia, vitamin D deficiency (rickets) is one of the most prevalent causes of acquired hypocalcemia.

Answer C is incorrect. Elevations in amylase and lipase levels are sensitive indications of pancreatitis. In severe cases of pancreatitis, hypocalcemia may be caused by free calcium complexing with free fatty acids that have been liberated by pancreatic enzymes from retroperitoneal fat. Interestingly, pancreatitis itself is a complication of hypercalcemia, especially if long-standing, secondary to biliary obstruction by calcium precipitate.

Answer E is incorrect. Citrate is a calcium chelator commonly used in blood products to inhibit the calcium-dependent coagulation cascade. In patients who receive multiple blood transfusions, elevated citrate levels may lead to hypocalcemia via chelation of calcium within the blood circulation.

27. **The correct answer is B.** ACE inhibitors such as captopril have been shown to decrease blood pressure and prevent and slow the progression of diabetic nephropathy in patients with diabetes. It is believed that ACE inhibitors play a renoprotective role by reducing glomerular filtration rate and reducing macroproteinuria.

Answer A is incorrect. DKA is a serious, potentially fatal complication of diabetes mellitus type 1, but it is rarely seen in diabetes mellitus type 2. Adequate control of blood glucose levels, as well as avoiding physiologic stressors such as infections, trauma, and alcohol, are important in preventing the onset of DKA.

Answer C is incorrect. Diabetic neuropathy is a common complication of diabetes and is best prevented by adequate control of blood glucose levels.

Answer D is incorrect. Diabetic retinopathy is a complication of long-standing diabetes mellitus, and although blood pressure control with drugs such as ACE inhibitors can slow the onset of retinopathy, ACE inhibitors are specifically renoprotective, even in normotensive patients.

Answer E is incorrect. Peripheral vascular disease is a common complication of diabetes mellitus, and is the underlying cause of diabetic neuropathy and other cardiovascular complications. Although adequate blood pressure control is important, ACE inhibitors are most effective in preventing diabetic nephropathy.

28. **The correct answer is B.** This patient presents with the classic symptoms of subacute (de Quervain's) thyroiditis, which is typically tender to palpation. Also, increased TSH and thyroxine indicate that the patient also has primary hyperthyroidism. It is most commonly due to viral infection of the thyroid gland and is self-limited in 90% of cases. Other causes of hyperthyroidism, such as Graves' disease, do not lead to anterior neck pain. Nonsteroidal anti-inflammatory drugs are the most appropriate treatment at this time.

Answer A is incorrect. Although acetaminophen would likely reduce the patient's temperature, subacute thyroiditis is an inflammatory process, and acetaminophen has analgesic and antipyretic properties, but not anti-inflammatory ones.

Answer C is incorrect. Although the patient is currently hyperthyroid (based on both her symptoms and her decreased TSH level), patients with subacute thyroiditis can fluctuate between hyper- and hypothyroidism. If her symptoms and TSH levels indicated that she was currently hypothyroid, then administration of levothyroxine would be appropriate.

Answer D is incorrect. The patient's fever and pain are relatively mild. If either were more severe, prednisone would be an appropriate addition, but her current presentation does not warrant the prednisone, and it would never be appropriate as a sole treatment.

Answer E is incorrect. Radioactive iodine is the appropriate first-line treatment for conditions such as a solitary toxic adenoma, but not in subacute thyroiditis, which is self-limited in 90% of cases.

29. **The correct answer is B.** This woman displays several characteristics of polycystic ovarian syndrome, which is a high-estrogen, high-androgen state, resulting in virilization (hair growth and acne) and menstrual irregularities. Increased levels of androgens lead to high estrogen levels, which suppress FSH and lead to increased LH levels.

Answer A is incorrect. This hormone profile would be seen in the case of an estrogen-secreting tumor, with synthesis of gonadotropin suppressed due to the high estrogen levels. Estrogen-secreting tumors can be found in the ovaries, testicles, and pituitary.

Answer C is incorrect. This hormone profile represents the findings in ovarian failure. Although FSH and LH are both elevated, the estrogen level remains low due to the resistance of the ovaries to secreted gonadotropins.

Answer D is incorrect. This hormone profile would be the result of increased gonadotropin secretion, leading to a high-estrogen state. This may be seen in some liver cancers and in hyperprolactinemic hypothyroidism.

30. **The correct answer is E.** Sheehan's syndrome is a disorder of anterior pituitary function. It occurs as the result of an insult to the anterior pituitary. The insult is low blood flow secondary to childbirth or trauma. It frequently presents as failure to lactate postpartum. Damage to the pituitary results in a lack of prolactin. Patients may also fail to ovulate, accounting for the amenorrhea. Given this patient's failure to lactate, history of low blood pressure during childbirth, and failure to menstruate, Sheehan's diagnosis is likely. The low prolactin level also supports this diagnosis. There are many disorders of the pituitary gland, such as empty sella syndrome and craniopharyngioma, but Sheehan's syndrome is the only one with lower-than-normal prolactin levels following hypotension.

Answer A is incorrect. Craniopharyngioma is the most common nonpituitary tumor implicated in hyperprolactinemia. This patient has elevated prolactin levels and complains of difficulty with lactation, so this diagnosis is ruled out. In addition, this is more commonly a pediatric-oncologic diagnosis.

Answer B is incorrect. Empty sella syndrome is caused by herniation of the subarachnoid membrane into the sella turcica through an incompetent sella diaphragm. This herniation causes compression of the pituitary gland. Secondary empty sella syndrome usually occurs in a patient that is postradiation or postsurgery.

The condition is usually asymptomatic. If symptoms do occur, they may mimic pituitary insufficiency, but this patient's symptomatic state and suggestive history makes Sheehan's syndrome the correct diagnosis.

Answer C is incorrect. Pregnancy causes amenorrhea, but this patient is not sexually active. This diagnosis is ruled out by the presence of a negative pregnancy test.

Answer D is incorrect. Previous oral contraceptive pill (OCP) use is an unlikely cause of amenorrhea and lack of lactation in this patient. OCP use may cause amenorrhea while the patient takes the drug and for up to 5 months afterward, but it would not cause amenorrhea later on in life. In addition, it would not account for the fact that she was unable to lactate.

31. **The correct answer is C.** When hemoglobin is exposed to increased levels of glucose circulating in the blood, a higher percentage of glucose binds to the hemoglobin. This glycosylated hemoglobin can be measured with the HbA_{1c} blood test. Target HbA_{1c} levels for diabetics are < 7.0% to 6.5% in diabetic patients. Because the average lifetime of an RBC is 120 days, this test is best for determining average blood glucose levels over the previous 3–4 months.

Answer A is incorrect. Although a dilated eye examination is recommended yearly for diabetic patients to monitor the presence and progression of diabetic retinopathy, it does not reliably indicate how well the patient's blood glucose levels have been controlled in the past 3–4 months.

Answer B is incorrect. Although a fasting blood glucose level will indicate what the blood glucose level is at that moment, it does not reflect what the levels have been over the past 3–4 months because the blood glucose level changes very rapidly. It is useful for diagnosing diabetes if the fasting blood glucose level is ≥ 126 mg/dL on separate occasions.

Answer D is incorrect. Microalbumin screening is recommended on a yearly basis to monitor for diabetic nephropathy, but it does not reliably indicate how well the patient's blood

glucose levels have been controlled in the past 3–4 months.

Answer E is incorrect. A random blood glucose level is similar to a fasting blood glucose level in that, although it will accurately reflect the current blood glucose status, it does not reflect what the status has been over the past 3–4 months. It is useful for diagnosing diabetes, and is diagnostic if any sample is ≥ 200 mg/dL and the patient is symptomatic.

32. **The correct answer is A.** Factitious thyrotoxicosis involves the administration of exogenous thyroid hormone, commonly in an attempt to lose weight. The distinguishing factor between factitious thyrotoxicosis and the other choices is the result of the radioactive iodine uptake test. By exhibiting no uptake, it shows that the administration of exogenous T_3 and thyroxine T_4 has downregulated uptake by the thyroid gland. The other conditions involve primary or secondary overactivity of the thyroid gland, thereby resulting in increased levels of T_3 and T_4.

Answer B is incorrect. The antithyroid-stimulating hormone receptor antibodies in Graves' disease continually activate the thyroid gland, resulting in hyperthyroidism with increased activity on the radioactive iodine uptake test.

Answer C is incorrect. A TSH-secreting pituitary tumor will produce unregulated amounts of TSH, thereby stimulating the thyroid gland and resulting in hyperthyroidism with increased activity in the radioactive iodine uptake test.

Answer D is incorrect. A toxic adenoma will most commonly show a "hot nodule" on the radioactive uptake test with increased uptake in the area of the nodule, and commonly an absence of uptake in the unaffected lobe.

Answer E is incorrect. A toxic multinodular goiter will show increased uptake on a radioactive iodine uptake test and is thereby differentiated from factitious thyrotoxicosis.

33. **The correct answer is A.** Palpable thyroid nodules are more common in women, older patients, and people in iodine-deficient parts of the world. The initial step in evaluation should

be measuring a TSH level, which is usually normal. However, in a "functional nodule" that is producing excess hormone, it can be decreased. If the TSH is decreased, the next step is a radionuclide scan to determine if the nodule is "hot" (i.e., absorbs the radioactive iodide readily). If it is "hot," the risk of malignancy is very low. If the TSH is normal, as in this case, the next step is fine-needle aspiration of the nodule. Those nodules found to be malignant should be surgically removed. Radionuclide scans can be helpful to identify "cold" nodules, which should be removed surgically due to increased risk of malignancy or simply to help localize the nodule prior to surgery.

Answer B is incorrect. MRI is not typically used in the workup of thyroid nodules.

Answer C is incorrect. Radionuclide scan is the next step in a patient with a decreased TSH level, as there is an increased likelihood that the patient has a functioning nodule that is unlikely to be malignant. However, in a patient with a normal TSH, fine-needle aspiration should be performed first and a radionuclide scan performed only if the biopsy is indeterminate.

Answer D is incorrect. Surgical excision should be reserved for patients with documented malignancy on biopsy or evidence of a "cold" nodule on radionuclide scanning.

Answer E is incorrect. Ultrasound can provide anatomic detail about the nodule but does not give information on the functional status of the nodule. Ultrasound is frequently used to assist with fine-needle aspiration, but alone is not considered the next step in the workup of a thyroid nodule.

34. **The correct answer is C.** The finding on two separate occasions of a fasting blood glucose level of ≥ 126 mg/dL indicates that the patient has diabetes mellitus type 2 (DM-2). Etiology of DM-2 includes relative paucity of insulin secretion, often in the presence of increased body weight, peripheral insulin resistance, and impaired regulation of gluconeogenesis in the liver.

Answer A is incorrect. Autoimmune destruction of pancreatic islet cells is the pathophysiologic mechanism of diabetes mellitus type 1, which is not a likely diagnosis in a previously healthy man of this age.

Answer B is incorrect. Pancreatitis is incorrect. Although hyperglycemia of ≥ 200 mg/dL in the setting of pancreatitis can be a poor prognostic sign on admission, this patient is not presenting with abdominal pain, as would be expected in either acute or chronic pancreatitis.

Answer D is incorrect. Insulin injections would be expected to lower the patient's blood glucose levels, not to raise them.

Answer E is incorrect. This answer is incorrect because the finding on two separate occasions of a fasting blood glucose level of ≥ 126 mg/dL is diagnostic of diabetes mellitus.

35. **The correct answer is C.** This patient's condition is consistent with primary hyperparathyroidism, most commonly due to a parathyroid adenoma. Patients may present with recurrent renal calculi, mental status changes, or abdominal pain, but many asymptomatic patients are diagnosed incidentally by findings of elevated serum calcium. Laboratory findings include elevated PTH, hypercalcemia, and hypophosphatemia. The elevated level of PTH causes hypercalcemia via increased bone resorption, increased distal tubular reabsorption of calcium in the kidney, and stimulation of renal hydroxylation of 25-hydroxyvitamin D, which increases dietary calcium absorption in the gastrointestinal tract. Elevated PTH causes hypophosphatemia by inhibiting proximal tubular reabsorption of phosphorus in the kidney.

Answer A is incorrect. Malignancy can cause hypercalcemia and hypercalciuria by many mechanisms, including local resorption of bone induced by metastases, production of humoral osteoclast activators such as parathyroid hormone–related protein (PTHrP), or increases in calcitriol production in patients with some lymphomas. In patients with humorally mediated hypercalcemia, PTHrP mimics the action of PTH, and patients will have hypercalcemia and hypophosphatemia, but PTH levels will not be elevated.

Answer B is incorrect. Milk-alkali syndrome is a type of hypercalcemia due to excess intake of calcium and absorbable antacids. However, PTH will not be elevated.

Answer D is incorrect. Sarcoidosis can cause hypercalcemia as a result of excess 1,25-dihydroxyvitamin D synthesis by macrophages in granulomas. However, parathyroid hormone will not be elevated.

Answer E is incorrect. Secondary hyperparathyroidism is caused by chronic renal disease. Diminished ability to excrete phosphorus leads to hyperphosphatemia. Excess phosphorus binds calcium, causing hypocalcemia. The parathyroid reacts by undergoing hyperplasia to increase release of PTH. Therefore, laboratory values will show elevated PTH, low calcium, and high phosphorus. In addition, there would be an elevated creatinine in a patient with end-stage renal disease.

36. **The correct answer is D.** Patients who take corticosteroids may develop secondary hypoadrenalism and may become unable to mount an appropriate response to ACTH. This can result in renal failure, hypotension, and hyponatremia. Thus restarting steroids is the first priority in this patient. Gradually tapering off of steroids allows the suppressed adrenals time to return to full function.

Answer A is incorrect. Radiologic imaging is appropriate to rule out lung pathology as a contributor to this patient's symptoms, but she should have an x-ray of the chest before proceeding to a CT of the chest.

Answer B is incorrect. Although the first steps in management are always the **ABC**s (Airway, Breathing, and Circulation), and fluids are an important component of maintaining circulation, the patient is not currently hypotensive enough to require resuscitation. Intravenous fluids are important if the patient develops hypotension as a component of the adrenal insufficiency, but is not the current first step in management.

Answer C is incorrect. The patient is currently well saturated on room air and there is no indication for oxygen supplementation. Before starting a patient with chronic obstructive

pulmonary disease on oxygen, one should obtain an arterial blood gas so not to suppress their ventilatory drive.

Answer E is incorrect. X-ray of the chest to rule out lung pathology as the cause of possible constitutional symptoms may be appropriate in this patient, but is not necessary immediately.

37. **The correct answer is A.** α-Glucosidase inhibitors are medications that reduce the amount of carbohydrates absorbed from the intestine. They are not commonly used because of the bothersome adverse effect of gastrointestinal upset and flatulence.

Answer B is incorrect. Meglitinides are short-acting insulin secretagogues. They can cause hypoglycemia, and are generally better tolerated, from a gastrointestinal standpoint, than α-glucosidase inhibitors.

Answer C is incorrect. Metformin is an oral hyperglycemic that works by inhibiting hepatic gluconeogenesis and increasing peripheral sensitivity to insulin. Though it can cause some gastrointestinal upset, this is usually transient at the beginning of treatment and is not associated with flatulence. A serious adverse effect of metformin is lactic acidosis. Metformin does not cause hypoglycemia.

Answer D is incorrect. Sulfonylureas are insulin secretagogues—they increase the amount of insulin that is secreted. This class of drugs can commonly cause hypoglycemia.

Answer E is incorrect. Thiazolidinediones ("glitazones") increase peripheral insulin sensitivity. They cause edema and weight gain and typically do not cause gastrointestinal distress.

38. **The correct answer is A.** This patient is presenting with signs and symptoms consistent with hyperprolactinemia. The most likely cause is a prolactin-secreting pituitary adenoma because the serum prolactin level is > 200 ng/mL. When the prolactin level is between 20 and 200 ng/mL, other causes of hyperprolactinemia such as drugs, hypothyroidism, and renal failure should be considered. Bromocriptine is a dopamine agonist that can decrease both prolactin secretion and the size of the adenoma.

Answer B is incorrect. Cortisol is used to treat patients with a deficiency of ACTH. Although a prolactinoma can suppress the secretion of other hormones in the anterior pituitary, including ACTH, the patient is not currently presenting with evidence of hypocortisolemia. Therefore, cortisol would not be considered as first-line therapy for this patient.

Answer C is incorrect. Methyldopa is an α-adrenergic antagonist used in the treatment of hypertension. Because it is known to elevate serum prolactin levels, methyldopa would therefore worsen this patient's signs and symptoms.

Answer D is incorrect. Metoclopramide is an antiemetic and gastrointestinal prokinetic drug that is known to increase prolactin levels and would therefore worsen this patient's signs and symptoms.

Answer E is incorrect. Octreotide is a somatostatin analog used to decrease growth hormone levels in patients with gonadotropin hormone–secreting pituitary adenomas.

39. **The correct answer is D.** The most concerning type of short stature is attenuated growth, in which the patient starts off at a normal height but falls off of his growth curve as he gets older, as this pattern is always pathologic and requires further evaluation. Causes of attenuated growth include renal disease, hypothyroidism, Crohn's disease, cancer, glucocorticoid therapy, and growth hormone deficiency (GHD). GHD is typically idiopathic, but can also be caused by tumors, particularly craniopharyngiomas, or rarely a genetic mutation in the GH-releasing hormone receptor in the pituitary. To diagnose growth hormone deficiency, serum insulin-like growth factor-1 (IGF-1) levels should be measured as opposed to GH levels, because GH is secreted in a pulsatile fashion and a random measurement is not a reliable indicator of growth hormone status, whereas IGF-1 is produced by the liver under GH stimulation and is a more reliable measurement of GH levels.

Answer A is incorrect. Chromosomal analysis is an important tool in evaluating females with short stature, because Turner's syndrome is a common cause of short stature in girls. These patients will typically be short from birth but will continue to grow along their growth curve, as opposed to having attenuated growth, as seen in this patient.

Answer B is incorrect. Colonoscopy can be used to evaluate for inflammatory bowel disease, a frequent cause of attenuated growth. However, this patient has no complaints of diarrhea, bloody stool, or abdominal pain. In addition his weight is normal. Patients with short stature due to malabsorption will typically be underweight for their height. Patients with endocrine disease, such as growth hormone deficiency, will typically be overweight for their height.

Answer C is incorrect. Because GH is secreted in a pulsatile manner, a random GH level is not a reliable indicator as to whether a patient has GH deficiency.

Answer E is incorrect. Because this patient has continued to fall off his growth curve, further evaluation should be performed. It is not safe to assume that his height is due to familial short stature, in which both parents are typically short and the patient starts off low on the growth chart, but maintains a normal curve and growth rate. Nor is it safe to assume that his height is due to constitutional delay, in which the child will eventually attain a normal adult height but develops later than other children. Parents will typically be of average height but report a delayed age of puberty.

40. **The correct answer is E.** This man has signs and symptoms that indicate hypocalcemia. His complaints of weakness, dry skin, alopecia, circumoral numbness, and paresthesias are all consistent with hypocalcemia. These patients can also develop cataracts, myocardial dysfunction, osteomalacia, and seizures. This patient has a positive Chvostek's sign, which is ipsilateral contraction of the facial muscles following tapping the facial nerve. The most likely cause of this patient's hypocalcemia is vitamin D deficiency due to therapy with carbamazepine. Carbamazepine and other medications including phenytoin, rifampin, and theophylline increase the activity of cytochrome P450 enzymes in the liver that inactivate vitamin D.

Deficient vitamin D leads to decreased absorption of calcium from the gut.

Answer A is incorrect. Hypomagnesemia can be a cause of hypocalcemia, but this patient's hypocalcemia is more likely due to vitamin D deficiency, as he is on a medication, carbamazepine, that is known to suppress vitamin D levels.

Answer B is incorrect. Parathyroidectomy may be used to treat patients with hyperparathyroidism due to a parathyroid adenoma. Resection of the parathyroids would cause hypocalcemia, which would worsen this patient's clinical presentation.

Answer C is incorrect. Hypothyroidism can cause dry skin and alopecia. However, patients with hypothyroidism do not typically have signs of tetany as seen in this patient. Therefore thyroid hormone administration would not have prevented this condition.

Answer D is incorrect. This patient has symptoms of vitamin D deficiency, not vitamin C deficiency. Vitamin C deficiency leads to impaired collagen synthesis. This causes scurvy, which is characterized by mucosal bleeding, bruising, petechiae, arthralgias, and vasomotor instability.

41. **The correct answer is C.** Acanthosis nigricans is a velvety dark thickening of the skin around the neck, axillae, and groin areas. It is related to diabetes, malignancy, obesity, drugs, and various endocrine disorders, and is not uncommonly found in young Hispanic women. Diabetes should be suspected in this case, as well as in other conditions associated with insulin resistance such as polycystic ovarian syndrome.

Answer A is incorrect. Acanthosis nigricans is associated with visceral malignancies, particularly gastric cancer, in adults. However, this is very unlikely in a 16-year-old patient, so a CT is probably not warranted.

Answer B is incorrect. A punch biopsy would be appropriate for diagnosis of a primary skin disorder. Acanthosis nigricans is usually a dermatologic manifestation of a systemic disease. It is the underlying disease, not the skin lesion, that merits further investigation.

Answer D is incorrect. A shave biopsy would be appropriate for diagnosis of a primary skin disorder. Acanthosis nigricans is usually a dermatologic manifestation of a systemic disease. It is the underlying disease, not the skin lesion, that merits further investigation.

Answer E is incorrect. Liver function tests may be elevated but are not diagnostic of a particular condition.

42. **The correct answer is D.** The symptoms of headache, palpitations, and tremor are all consistent with a pheochromocytoma, as is the CT finding of a suprarenal mass. The confirming laboratory test was likely an elevated urinary catecholamine level; also, serum calcium and glucose may well have been high. A pheochromocytoma secretes excessive amounts of epinephrine and norepinephrine, resulting in both peripheral vasoconstriction (α-mediated effect) and increased cardiac contractility (β-mediated effect). An α-adrenergic blocker such as prazosin is the principal means of relieving hypertension in these patients.

Answer A is incorrect. Furosemide, a loop diuretic, will decrease blood pressure by decreasing electrolyte and fluid resorption in the thick ascending tubule and resulting in diuresis. While diuretics are commonly used to treat primary hypertension, they are a poor choice in pheochromocytoma since these patients are generally already volume-contracted. In fact, patients should be encouraged to take in ample salt and water to restore volume once α-blockade is established.

Answer B is incorrect. Hydralazine, a direct vasodilator, does not address the underlying cause of hypertension in pheochromocytoma and is not commonly used in these patients.

Answer C is incorrect. Although monoamine oxidase (MAO) inhibitors such as phenylzine can reduce blood pressure in normal persons, they are not typically used as antihypertensives. In particular, they are contraindicated in pheochromocytoma, since inhibition of MAO can lead to increased levels of adrenergic monoamines and lead to a hypertensive crisis.

Answer E is incorrect. β-Adrenergic blockade is useful for controlling tachycardia and palpitations in pheochromocytoma patients, but only after α-adrenergic blockade has been established, since β-blockade will exacerbate peripheral vasoconstriction, thereby worsening hypertension in the setting of unopposed α-adrenergic stimulation.

43. **The correct answer is E.** Reduction in weight by just 7% and incorporating 30 minutes of daily activity reduced diabetes by 58% in a landmark study.

    Answer A is incorrect. Alcohol avoidance will not lower the patient's diabetes risk; although alcohol excess can lead to either acute or chronic pancreatitis, it is not necessary to remove alcohol from the diet completely.

    Answer B is incorrect. Use of a daily multivitamin is not necessary if one's diet is adequate, but it can serve as an "insurance policy" for vitamin and mineral intake. Its use, however, is not linked to diabetes reduction.

    Answer C is incorrect. Dietary changes, including incorporation of fruits and vegetables, are important, as they may contribute to weight loss, but it is the weight loss that reduces diabetes risk by reducing the body's total insulin requirements.

    Answer D is incorrect. Smoking cessation, while important for overall health, has not been shown to reduce diabetes incidence.

44. **The correct answer is E.** This patient has radiographic findings consistent with bone disease caused by secondary hyperparathyroidism. Patients with end-stage renal disease have impaired excretion of phosphorus. Excess phosphorus complexes with calcium, leading to a secondary increase in PTH secretion. PTH acts on the bone to increase osteoclastic resorption in an attempt to normalize serum calcium. Over time this can lead to the pathologic condition osteitis fibrosa cystica. Patients develop subperiosteal bone resorption, which classically affects the clavicle, phalanges, and vertebral bodies. X-ray of the chest may show a classic "rugger-jersey" (striped like a rugby jersey) spine due to ill-defined bands of increased bone density adjacent to the vertebral endplates.

Answer A is incorrect. Bence Jones protein is found in the urine of patients with multiple myeloma. Multiple myeloma is a malignancy of plasma cells in which patients develop lytic lesions of the skeleton. Radiographs show the classic finding of multiple punched-out, round lesions within the skull, spine, and pelvis.

Answer B is incorrect. Patients with end-stage renal disease develop secondary hyperparathyroidism, not decreased levels of parathyroid hormone PTH. Hypoparathyroidism is usually acquired after surgical resection of the parathyroid glands for adenoma or inadvertently during thyroidectomy. Patients can also have genetic deficiencies of PTH.

Answer C is incorrect. Patients with end-stage renal disease tend to have elevated serum phosphorus levels due to decreased excretion by the kidney. The elevated phosphorus contributes to the development of secondary hyperparathyroidism.

Answer D is incorrect. Elevated bone-specific alkaline phosphatase is found in patients with Paget's disease, a disorder of increased bone turnover. Patients have excessive bone resorption and new bone formation. Radiographic findings include a "cotton-wool" appearance of the skull due to multifocal areas of sclerosis. In the spine, vertebrae can develop a thickened cortical margin, causing a "picture-frame" appearance.

45. **The correct answer is C.** This patient has clinical symptoms and laboratory evidence consistent with hyperthyroidism and the presence of TSH-receptor antibodies is consistent with Graves' disease, which is the most common cause of hyperthyroidism in both normal patients and pregnant women. If left untreated, maternal hyperthyroidism can lead to spontaneous abortion, premature labor, preeclampsia, and maternal heart failure. The thionamides are considered first-line therapy in pregnant women, including methimazole and PTU. Although both cross the placenta and can cause fetal goiter and hypothyroidism, PTU is the preferred drug because it has a lower risk of severe congenital anomalies.

HIGH-YIELD SYSTEMS

Endocrinology

Answer A is incorrect. Although low-dose iodine may be safe for pregnant women with mild hyperthyroidism, high-dose therapy is associated with an increased risk of fetal goiter, so it should not be used in pregnant patients.

Answer B is incorrect. Methimazole, along with the other thiocarbamide drugs, blocks thyroid hormone synthesis by inhibiting thyroid peroxidase. It has been associated with a higher risk of aplasia cutis, a rare fetal scalp disorder. There has also been a suggested association with tracheoesophageal fistulas and choanal atresia. Therefore, PTU is typically chosen over methimazole in pregnant patients.

Answer D is incorrect. Radioiodine ablation is absolutely contraindicated in pregnancy. Because fetal thyroid tissue is present by 10–12 weeks' gestation, radioiodine therapy can destroy fetal thyroid tissue.

Answer E is incorrect. Surgical resection may be necessary in a pregnant patient with hyperthyroidism, but surgery is associated with an increased risk of spontaneous abortion and premature delivery. As with nonpregnant patients, medical therapy should be attempted first. If the patient cannot tolerate thionamide therapy, then surgery may be the next treatment option.

46. **The correct answer is D.** Sheehan's syndrome is postpartum pituitary necrosis, usually in the setting of obstetric hemorrhage and circulatory collapse. Sheehan's syndrome is a secondary cause of hypoadrenalism, which would explain the patient's hyponatremia. Also common are abdominal pain, weakness, fatigue, and hypotension. The patient with Sheehan's will often have an inability to breast-feed secondary to deficient prolactin production and have other endocrine abnormalities associated with loss of anterior pituitary hormone production (the posterior pituitary is usually preserved), such as hypothyroidism.

Answer A is incorrect. The patient is experiencing a dull, aching abdominal pain that is not localized and accompanied by nausea, but she remains afebrile and has a nonsurgical abdomen on examination. While appendicitis is still a possibility, the patient's electrolyte abnormalities and inability to lactate suggest another cause.

Answer B is incorrect. HELLP syndrome is defined by **H**emolysis, **E**levated **L**iver enzymes, and **L**ow **P**latelets. Other important diagnostic criteria include hypertension, visual disturbance, headache, 2+ proteinuria, and severe edema. HELLP syndrome is seen in patients experiencing eclampsia. Definitive treatment is delivery. This patient has none of the classic signs and is hypotensive.

Answer C is incorrect. Postoperative infection should always remain on the differential, but this patient is afebrile and the surgical site is unremarkable. Additionally her inability to lactate and electrolyte abnormalities cannot be explained by infection.

Answer E is incorrect. Toxic shock syndrome (TSS) would be unlikely in this case, as the patient is afebrile and has no rash. *Staphylococcus aureus* is the most common pathogen associated with TSS, and this is a common postoperative pathogen, but the patient would likely present with fever and erythema, edema, and warmth around the surgical incision site.

47. **The correct answer is A.** This patient has the classic symptoms of Cushing's syndrome, which most directly results from an excess of cortisol. ACTH is secreted by the anterior pituitary and stimulates the adrenal cortex to secrete cortisol. The most common cause of Cushing's syndrome is exogenously administered corticosteroids; however, the patient was not on any medication, and the most common noniatrogenic etiology is Cushing's disease, an ACTH-secreting pituitary adenoma. In addition, hyperpigmentation with hypercortisolism is only seen in Cushing's disease, due to increased production of melanocyte-stimulating hormone induced by the tumor.

Answer B is incorrect. Although adrenal tumors can potentially lead to oversecretion of cortisol, they are not as common as ACTH-secreting pituitary adenomas.

Answer C is incorrect. An ectopic ACTH-secreting tumor will present in a manner similar to an ACTH-secreting pituitary adenoma because it is secreting ACTH out of the control of the hypothalamus-pituitary-adrenal axis. It is not, however, as common as the ACTH-secreting pituitary adenoma.

Answer D is incorrect. Adrenal hyperplasia, which is most commonly bilateral, can lead to oversecretion of cortisol and Cushing's syndrome. Primary disease (in the absence of elevated ACTH) is extremely rare and is most appropriately treated by bilateral adrenalectomy.

Answer E is incorrect. Small cell lung cancers can be ACTH secreting and are a possible cause of Cushing's syndrome, although not the most common.

48. **The correct answer is A.** Increased levels of urine 5-hydroxyindoleacetic acid (5-HIAA) are a by-product of serotonin metabolism and are consistent with carcinoid syndrome. Carcinoid tumors often affect the right heart due to fibrous deposits on the right-sided valves that can induce right-sided heart failure. The carcinoid syndrome includes flushing, diarrhea, and hypotension. The murmur is likely due to tricuspid regurgitation, although pulmonary valve involvement is also common. Patients with cardiac involvement have higher levels of plasma serotonin and urine 5-HIAA.

Answer B is incorrect. Urinary catecholamines and metanephrine are found in association with pheochromocytomas, which would present with hypertension, not hypotension.

Answer C is incorrect. Peaked T waves are a common finding in hyperkalemia but are not associated with carcinoid heart disease. The ECG in carcinoid may show low QRS voltage.

Answer D is incorrect. Sepsis can cause hypotension and would be associated with fatigue (and a murmur if due to endocarditis). However, the time course is unusual given an otherwise healthy individual, and *Pseudomonas* bacteremia would be unlikely outside the hospital setting.

Answer E is incorrect. Carcinoid syndrome typically affects the right heart (except in the case of a primary carcinoid tumor in the bronchus), and congestion, if present, is usually mild. X-ray of the chest may reveal a prominence of the right heart border.

49. **The correct answer is C.** Congenital hypothyroidism commonly consists of the constellation of signs and symptoms described, with constipation, prolonged jaundice secondary to delayed maturation of glucuronide conjugation, failure to thrive, and open fontanelles. Many children have umbilical hernias with genital swelling, and some may present with hypothermia. The condition affects girls twice as often as boys. Newborn screening catches most cases before clinical manifestations occur, but this child, being born at home, was not likely screened. Testing will likely show elevated TSH with a low T_4 level. Untreated cases of congenital hypothyroidism can lead to severe mental retardation, neurologic complications, and growth failure. Treatment aims to maintain the T_4 and TSH within normal ranges, and L-thyroxine is usually administered.

Answer A is incorrect. α_1-Antitrypsin deficiency is a relatively rare condition and infrequently presents early in life. α_1-Antitrypsin is produced by the hepatocytes, and therefore this disease may present as neonatal hepatitis during the first 3 months of life. Hepatosplenomegaly may be found on physical examination. It often results in respiratory abnormalities with early-onset obstructive respiratory disease. Diagnosis is made by quantifying levels of α_1-antitrypsin. Treatment consists of infusions of α_1-antitrypsin or liver transplant in serious cases of cirrhosis that may result.

Answer B is incorrect. Congenital herpes is a devastating and potentially life-threatening illness that is caused by herpes simplex virus (HSV) type 2. Congenital HSV infection usually presents with central nervous system (CNS) disease, usually encephalitis. Vesicles can be seen within the first 2 weeks of life and commonly arise at sites of trauma (i.e., the fetal scalp or after a circumcision). Disseminated disease within the first few days of life is characterized by hypotonia, thrombocytopenia, and disseminated intravascular coagulation. Two weeks postnatally, generalized disease with CNS involvement consists of fever, lethargy, and difficult-to-manage seizures. Intranuclear inclusion bodies and multinucleated giant cells can be seen on blood smear (Tzanck smear). Treatment should be with antivirals such as acyclovir.

Answer D is incorrect. DiGeorge's syndrome is a genetic syndrome caused by a microdeletion on chromosome 22q11. This syndrome is characterized by cardiac anomalies, thymic hypoplasia, hypocalcemia, and abnormal facies. Patients will often present with an increased susceptibility to upper respiratory viral infections and viral gastroenteritis. Infants may experience feeding difficulties due to palatal abnormalities and heart defects. Abnormal facies include hypertelorism, low-set ears, micrognathia, and a short philtrum. Complete blood count will show a low absolute lymphocyte count, and further workup will indicate a diminished total T lymphocyte count.

Answer E is incorrect. Pheochromocytoma is a catecholamine-secreting tumor that arises from chromaffin cells and often originates in the adrenal medulla. Patients typically present with paroxysmal hypertension. Older patients will experience headaches and palpitations. Urine vanillylmandelic acid and plasma catecholamines will be elevated. Treatment consists of and α-antagonist.

50. **The correct answer is E.** This child has DiGeorge's syndrome, with deletion of chromosome 22q11. This chromosomal anomaly causes the third and fourth pharyngeal pouches to develop abnormally, resulting in midline defects. Abnormal facies, cleft palate, congenital heart defects, thymic aplasia, and parathyroid hypoplasia with hypocalcemia characterize DiGeorge's syndrome. Patients are identified by physical examination, tetany in the neonatal period, and frequent infections, especially with fungus and/or *Pneumocystis jiroveci* pneumonia. Evaluation should include measurement of serum calcium, echocardiogram, and absolute lymphocyte count. The diagnosis is made by detection of the deletion on fluorescent in situ hybridization.

Answer A is incorrect. Hemoglobin electrophoresis is diagnostic for sickle cell disease and thalassemia. These disorders are not associated with congenital cardiac anomalies, facial dysmorphisms, or cleft palate. Children with sickle cell disease are at increased risk of infection from encapsulated organisms because of functional asplenism from either dysfunction and/or autoinfarction of the spleen, which can present with life-threatening infection(s) as early as 4 months of age.

Answer B is incorrect. This test is used to detect chronic granulomatous disease (CGD). Recurrent mucous membrane infections with catalase-positive organisms, abscesses, and poor wound healing characterize CGD. CGD is not associated with cardiac anomalies, facial anomalies, or cleft palate.

Answer C is incorrect. Congenital cardiac anomalies can be associated with renal anomalies as part of the **VACTERL** syndrome, which includes anomalies of the **V**ertebrae, **A**nus, **C**ardiovascular tree, **T**rachea, **E**sophagus, **R**enal system, and **L**imb buds. However, this patient does not have signs or symptoms of the other anomalies, and the VACTERL syndrome does not explain his frequent infections, facial anomalies, or cleft palate.

Answer D is incorrect. This test is useful in diagnosing B-lymphocyte deficiencies. B-lymphocyte deficiencies rarely present in patients younger than 6 months because maternally derived antibodies are protective against infection until they clear from the infant's circulation at approximately 6 months of age. They are not associated with congenital cardiac malformations or cleft palate.

CHAPTER 4

Epidemiology and Preventive Medicine

1. A 53-year-old woman presents to the clinic for her yearly physical. She is concerned about heart disease because her mother recently had a myocardial infarction at age 74 and her father passed away from heart disease at the age of 63. She is a high school teacher who smokes a half-pack per day. Her blood pressure during the last two office visits was 122/69 and 128/73 mm Hg. Her last HDL was 63 mg/dL. On physical examination, she is close to her ideal body weight, and there are no abnormalities. Which of the following is an appropriate goal for this patient's LDL?

(A) Direct therapy at raising HDL, not reducing LDL
(B) ≤ 100 mg/dL
(C) ≤ 130 mg/dL
(D) ≤ 160 mg/dL
(E) ≤ 200 mg/dL

2. A healthy 26-year-old man presents for his annual physical examination. He has no significant medical history, and his surgical history is only significant for an arthroscopic procedure on his left knee 3 years prior. He takes no daily medications and has no known drug allergies. He is married and currently attends business school in Philadelphia. He admits to occasional tobacco and social alcohol use but denies other drug use. He had a lipid panel drawn last year that was normal. Which of the following is an important annual screening measure in all patients 25 years and older?

(A) Cholesterol
(B) Complete blood count and erythrocyte sedimentation rate
(C) Depression and alcohol abuse
(D) ECG
(E) Fecal occult blood

3. A 3-year-old boy is brought to the clinic by his mother. She is concerned because the patient has complained of a sore throat over the past 4 days. He is not in day care and has had no known sick contacts. His 7-year-old sister is currently healthy. The physician does a throat swab for a rapid streptococcal test and sends a second specimen for culture. Why does the physician perform both tests?

(A) The culture may grow strains of bacteria which are not detected by the rapid test
(B) The rapid streptococcal test and culture both have high sensitivity
(C) The rapid streptococcal test and culture both have high specificity
(D) The rapid streptococcal test has a high sensitivity, while the culture has high specificity
(E) The rapid streptococcal test has a high specificity, while the culture has high sensitivity

4. A 34-year-old woman presents to a surgeon to discuss the possibility of an elective splenectomy. Several weeks ago, she was diagnosed with idiopathic thrombocytopenic purpura. A complete blood cell count was performed at that time and revealed a platelet count of 24,000/mm^3. Her primary care doctor started her on 50 mg oral prednisone daily. At presentation today, she continues to have lower extremity petechiae along with mucosal bleeding. Her repeat platelet count is 29,000/mm^3. An elective splenectomy is scheduled. Infection with which of the following organisms is most likely to result in postsplenectomy sepsis?

(A) Haemophilus influenzae
(B) Moraxella catarrhalis
(C) Pseudomonas aeruginosa
(D) Staphylococcus aureus
(E) Streptococcus viridans

5. A 64-year-old woman presents to the clinic wanting to know if she should take a daily 81-mg aspirin tablet. She has a family history of cardiac disease and her mother died of an aneurysm. In reviewing her chart, the physician notes that she has not had a pneumococcal vaccine or flu shot in the past year, although she has diabetes. Which is the most frequent cause of death among all women in this age group?

(A) Cardiac disease
(B) Chronic obstructive pulmonary disease

(C) Diabetes
(D) Influenza
(E) Pneumonia
(F) Stroke

6. A 65-year-old woman presents with 3 months of unintentional weight loss, jaundice, and upper abdominal pain that radiates to her back. Her gallbladder is palpable on physical examination, and an ultrasound demonstrates dilated bile ducts with no visible stones. Which of the following is a known risk factor for this patient's condition?

(A) Chronic gastritis
(B) Diabetes insipidus
(C) Diabetes mellitus
(D) History of cholecystitis
(E) Smoking

7. A 29-year-old woman presents with fatigue and lymphadenopathy, and is diagnosed with nodular-sclerosing Hodgkin's lymphoma. She is treated with a chemotherapy regimen including doxorubicin (Adriamycin), bleomycin, vinblastine, and dacarbazine (ABVD), as well as radiation to her mediastinum and neck. She achieves a full remission following her therapy. Her risk of developing which of the following is equal to that of the general population?

(A) Acute myelogenous leukemia
(B) Addison's disease
(C) Breast cancer
(D) Coronary artery disease
(E) Hypothyroidism
(F) Infertility
(G) Lhermitte's syndrome

8. A 78-year-old woman in otherwise good health schedules a visit with her primary care physician because she has been experiencing blood in her stool that she describes as "maroon" in color. Her past medical history is only significant for psoriasis and mild degenerative joint disease. In thinking about the possible causes of her lower gastrointestinal bleed, which of the following lists is in order of most common to least common?

(A) Angiodysplasia > cancer/polyp > diverticulosis
(B) Angiodysplasia > diverticulosis > cancer/polyp

(C) Cancer/polyp > diverticulosis > angiodysplasia
(D) Diverticulosis > angiodysplasia > cancer/polyp
(E) Diverticulosis > cancer/polyp > angiodysplasia

9. A hypothetical study is created to examine the effect of cigarette smoking on the development of lung cancer. Patients who smoke at least one pack per day are matched with an appropriate group of nonsmokers. Ten years later, information on the development of lung cancer is collected, and the following data are observed. What is the relative risk (risk ratio) of developing lung cancer for cigarette smokers?

Exposure to cigarettes	(+) Lung cancer (no. of pts.)	(-) Lung cancer (no. of pts.)
History of exposure	a = 20	b = 80
No history of exposure	c = 1	d = 100
Total patients	21	180

Reproduced, with permission, from USMLERx.com.

(A) 1
(B) 1/20
(C) 19/100
(D) 20
(E) 20/(80/99)

10. A study is performed to assess the relationship of dietary cholesterol and myocardial infarction. Participants are assigned to either an experimental group, which eats a low-cholesterol diet, or a control group, which eats a standard American diet. Dietary analysis later reveals that the group assigned a low-cholesterol diet ended up also consuming less fat than the control group. In analyzing the relationship between dietary cholesterol and myocardial infarction, the amount of dietary fat consumed represents what type of study characteristic?

(A) Confounding variable
(B) Enrollment bias
(C) Measurement bias
(D) Recall bias
(E) Self-selection bias

11. A 5-year-old boy presents to his pediatrician because his mother notices that he has been complaining of fatigue and headache for several weeks. On examination, he is found to have enlarged lymph nodes and is sent for a bone marrow biopsy. The biopsy shows large lymphoblasts with prominent nucleoli and light blue cytoplasm, and the patient is diagnosed with acute lymphoid leukemia. He is treated with high-dose glucocorticoids, intravenous and intrathecal methotrexate, cyclophosphamide, doxorubicin, and vincristine. He achieves a full remission. Which of the following accurately matches the causative drug with the possible side effect that he may experience now or in the future?

(A) Cyclophosphamide: hearing loss
(B) Glucocorticoids: cataracts
(C) Glucocorticoids: peripheral neuropathy
(D) Methotrexate: cognitive deficit
(E) Methotrexate: pulmonary fibrosis

12. A 72-year-old man presents to his primary physician with complaints of fatigue, weight loss, dyspnea on exertion, abdominal pain, and dark blood in the stool. Although the patient had a negative sigmoidoscopy on routine examination 6 months ago, colon cancer is strongly suspected. Which is the best diagnostic modality to use in this patient?

(A) Colonoscopy
(B) CT scan of abdomen
(C) Double-contrast barium enema
(D) Sigmoidoscopy
(E) Upper gastrointestinal series

13. A 23-year-old woman presents to her gynecologist for a refill of her oral contraceptive prescription. She denies recent sexual activity, although she has been sexually active in the past and is currently on oral contraceptives to regulate her menstrual cycle and control acne. Her last Papanicolaou (or Pap) smear was 13 months prior. She says that her 31-year-old sister just went for her annual examination and was told that she did not need an annual Pap smear. In which of the following populations may an annual Pap smear be deferred?

(A) HIV-positive women with no documented history of cervical pathology
(B) Women > 30 years old who have had three consecutive conventional cytology negative Pap smears
(C) Women > 60 years old with positive human papillomavirus DNA
(D) Women who have had a hysterectomy and documented cervical intraepithelial neoplasia II/III
(E) Women with two or more negative conventional cytology smears

14. A 53-year-old man presents to his physician's office in tears. A close friend of his was recently diagnosed with lung cancer, so the patient is concerned because he has smoked a pack of cigarettes daily for 39 years and his father died of lung cancer. He recalls that he had a productive cough 2 months prior that resolved after several weeks. He is concerned that he might have lung cancer or might develop it in the future. He asks whether there is a test he can undergo on a regular basis to "catch the cancer early." What is the appropriate screening test for this patient?

(A) Annual x-ray of the chest
(B) Annual x-ray of the chest and biannual sputum cytology
(C) Biannual low-dose helical CT scan
(D) Biannual sputum cytology
(E) Bronchoscopy
(F) None; advise the patient to quit smoking, and monitor for clinical signs of lung cancer

15. A 34-year-old man was diagnosed with type 1 diabetes mellitus (DM) as a child and has been presenting for annual examinations since he was in his early 20s. Which of the following screening tests is indicated more than once a year?

(A) Hemoglobin A_{1c}
(B) Lipid profile
(C) Microalbuminuria
(D) Ophthalmologic examination
(E) Podiatric examination
(F) Serum fructosamine

16. A bariatrics researcher wants to study the relative impact of diet alone and exercise alone on weight loss. Two study groups are established, one of which will follow a supervised reduction diet, and the other will run 2 miles daily. After 1 month, the researcher determines the amount of weight lost via each method. Which of the following would be a confounding variable?

    (A) Both groups knew the study was being done
    (B) Dieters were given culturally sensitive nutritional advice
    (C) Runners had instruction from a track-and-field coach on running efficiently
    (D) Runners who became injured and could no longer run were excluded from the study
    (E) The running group was instructed to drink more water than usual

17. The cutoff value of normal prostate-specific antigen (PSA) levels is 4.0 ng/dL. If this value were to be decreased to 3.7 ng/dL, the sensitivity and specificity of the test for detecting prostate cancer will change. How would lowering the normal value of PSA in cancer screening alter the number of false positives and false negatives?

    (A) Decrease both false positives and false negatives
    (B) Decrease the number of false negatives and increase the number of false positives
    (C) Increase both false positives and false negatives
    (D) Increase the number of false negatives and decrease the number of false positives
    (E) It would not change either parameter

18. A 24-year-old man presents with notably slurred speech, stating that "I don't want to live anymore, I just want to take pills and make the pain go away." A psychiatric history reveals that the patient has suffered from major depression for 9 years, has had numerous psychiatric admissions for violent behavior, and has attempted suicide twice by overdose. The patient currently has a blood alcohol level of 0.012 mg/mL. Which of the following is this patient's most significant risk factor for a completed suicide attempt?

    (A) Antisocial behavior
    (B) Depression
    (C) Male gender
    (D) Past suicide attempts
    (E) Substance abuse

19. A study to evaluate the relationship of caffeine consumption and gastric cancer is conducted. Patients with gastric cancer are enrolled in the study, and researchers seek to match each patient with an individual similar to him or her in as many ways as possible, except that the control subject does not have a diagnosis of gastric cancer. Both case and control subjects are then surveyed to examine possible exposures, including caffeine exposure. Of 500 patients, 250 are cases and an equal number are controls. Of cases, 150 met the minimum caffeine consumption limit set by the study, whereas only 50 controls did. What is the odds ratio defining the relationship of exposure and disease in this study?

    (A) 0.17
    (B) 0.375
    (C) 1.7
    (D) 2.7
    (E) 3
    (F) 6

20. A 4-year-old girl with a rash is brought by her mother to the pediatrician. She had a fever and headache yesterday, and this morning broke out in a rash on her torso. She is in day care and has been otherwise healthy. On examination her temperature is 38.9°C (102°F) and she appears tired but otherwise well. The lesions are erythematous macules and vesicles in different stages, distributed diffusely over her trunk but most prominent on her left upper chest and right flank. A diagnosis of chickenpox is made. Of note, there is a 16-year-old sibling in the household who has not been vaccinated and has never had chickenpox. Which of the following interventions will most successfully prevent infection of susceptible household contacts?

(A) Administration of intravenous acyclovir to the patient
(B) Administration of oral acyclovir to the patient and household contacts
(C) Administration of vaccine and intramuscular varicella zoster immunoglobulin to household contacts
(D) Administration of varicella vaccine to household contacts
(E) No prophylaxis is necessary for household contacts under age 25 years

21. A researcher wants to examine the relationship of childhood cigarette exposure and subsequent asthma diagnosis. She designs a study in which telephone interviewers contact randomly chosen study participants with questions regarding their childhoods and whether they have asthma. Which type of study is this researcher conducting?

(A) Case-control study
(B) Cohort study
(C) Cross-sectional study
(D) Meta-analysis
(E) Randomized controlled clinical trial

22. A researcher studying the impact of drug A on hypertension assigns patients randomly to either a treatment group or a control group. The treatment group receives drug A, and the control group receives the current standard medication for its situation. Neither study staff nor the patients know what drug a given patient is receiving. What type of study is the researcher conducting?

(A) Case-control study
(B) Cohort study
(C) Cross-sectional survey
(D) Meta-analysis
(E) Randomized controlled clinical trial

23. A 34-year-old G4P3 woman presents to the clinic with her husband desiring contraception. She has a past medical history significant for endometriosis, for which she was prescribed oral contraceptive pills as a teenager. Her past surgical history includes an exploratory laparotomy with laser ablation and resection of an endometrioma at the age of 26 years as part of an infertility workup. She subsequently delivered three healthy children with no obstetric complications. She denies any history of sexually transmitted disease and is sexually active with her husband only. She states that she and her husband do not desire any further children. Which of the following is the most effective contraceptive option and will therefore have the lowest failure rate for this couple?

(A) Bilateral tubal ligation
(B) Bilateral vasectomy
(C) Combination oral contraceptive pill
(D) Diaphragm
(E) Intrauterine device
(F) Male condom
(G) Progestin-only oral contraceptive pill

24. A researcher wants to study outcomes after exposure to a particular drug. Participants will be randomized into an exposed group and an unexposed group, and observations will be made and data collected regarding the outcome of each study participant. What does it mean for the researcher to "single-blind" the study?

(A) Neither participants nor researchers know whether a participant is assigned to the study group or the control group
(B) Participants do not know if they are assigned to the study group or the control group
(C) Researchers do not know if a participant is assigned to the study group or the control group

(D) Researchers do not know if the drug will be efficacious

(E) Researchers do not know if the drug will be safe

25. A 27-year-old primigravida at 35 weeks' gestation presents to her obstetrician with the chief complaint of a long bump on her leg. She denies ever having had a problem like this before. Her pregnancy has been without complication. Prior to her pregnancy, she used only barrier protection. Age of menarche was 12 years. She denies any travel history, and has been "mainly in bed" since 1 week ago. On physical examination, she in no acute distress, with a pulse of 78/min, respiratory rate of 10/min, and temperature of 37.2°C (99°F). Her lungs are clear to auscultation bilaterally, and her extremities are warm and well perfused. Examination of the extremities reveals a long, firm, cordlike mass on the lateral aspect of her left leg. It is subcutaneous, erythematous, and tender. Compression ultrasonography of the lower extremity shows normal compressibility and normal Doppler flow. How should the physician advise this patient?

(A) The patient should be advised to take heparin if the mass does not resolve

(B) The patient should be advised to take ibuprofen only with caffeine

(C) The patient should be advised to take warfarin if the mass does not resolve

(D) The patient should be advised to use warm compresses and elevation of the affected area

(E) The patient should be reassured that ibuprofen is safe in pregnancy

26. A group of researchers at the state university conduct a study investigating the relationship of cigarette smoking and vascular dementia. Retrospective data are obtained from a cross-sectional survey on smoking habits and later neurologic symptoms as observed by close relatives. Researchers find that smokers are four times as likely as nonsmokers to suffer from vascular dementia and that they also consume twice as much alcohol as nonsmokers in their study. Which of the following statements could be accurately made on the basis of the available information?

(A) Both alcohol and cigarettes independently increase the risk for vascular dementia

(B) Drinking alcohol increases the risk for vascular dementia

(C) Smoking cigarettes increases the risk for vascular dementia

(D) Smoking increases the risk for vascular dementia, but alcohol has no effect on the risk

(E) Smokers are more likely to drink than nonsmokers

27. A cardiologist wishes to compare outcomes of medical management and cardiac catheterization for myocardial infarct presentation to the emergency department. She conducts a literature search and statistically combines the data from seven published studies. Which of the following is an advantage of this type of study?

(A) Ability to overcome poor study design in individual studies

(B) Less bias than other types of studies

(C) May allow detection of small differences between outcomes

(D) Pooled data already represent sufficiently similar populations and interventions

(E) Statistical analysis of pooled data is straightforward

28. A 26-year-old G2P1 woman at 19 weeks' gestation comes into the clinic for her scheduled prenatal visit. She complains only of mild fatigue. Past obstetric history is notable for a prior pregnancy 2 years ago. Although that pregnancy was without complications, the child has significant developmental delay. The patient takes no medications other than prenatal vitamins. Her family history is significant for two maternal aunts with mental retardation. The patient is an only child. Physical examination reveals a well-developed gravid female in no acute distress. The uterus is appreciated well above the pubic symphysis. A triple screen test is ordered. What other test would be ordered at this visit?

(A) Amniocentesis

(B) Biophysical profile

(C) Chorionic villus sampling

(D) α-Fetoprotein

(E) Nonstress test

(F) Percutaneous umbilical blood sampling

(G) Ultrasound

29. A 55-year-old woman presents to her gynecology clinic for a routine checkup. She says she has been too busy for the past 3–4 years to come to the clinic. She is G2P2, and both children were delivered by spontaneous vaginal delivery without complications. She is currently sexually active with her husband, and has no other partners. She says she has an occasional glass of wine with dinner, and has smoked about half a pack per day for the past 25 years. To her knowledge, there is no family history of cancer, heart disease, or diabetes. Her blood pressure is 115/75 mm Hg and heart rate is 80/min. She is 170 cm (5 ft 7 in) tall and weighs 65.8 kg (145 lb). Skin examination reveals no suspicious moles. Breast examination reveals no masses. Pelvic and bimanual examinations are likewise within normal limits. A sample is taken for a Pap smear without significant cervical bleeding. Mammography from 3 years ago shows no suspicious masses. A Pap smear from 3 years prior showed no atypical cells. Relevant laboratory findings are:

WBC count	7500/mm^3
Hemoglobin	12.4 g/dL
Platelet count	220,000/mm^3
Total cholesterol	195 mg/dL
LDL	125 mg/dL
HDL	45 mg/dL

What is the next appropriate step in the management of this patient?

(A) Cancer antigen-125
(B) Endometrial biopsy
(C) Mammogram
(D) Transvaginal ultrasound
(E) X-ray of the chest

30. A 48-year-old man is admitted to the hospital with fulminant hepatitis leading to liver failure following consumption of raw oysters. He is treated with immediate liver transplantation, which is performed successfully. Following a prolonged hospital stay, he is discharged in excellent condition. In addition to his antirejection medications, which of the following is recommended for prophylaxis in this patient?

(A) Acyclovir
(B) Ketoconazole

(C) Niacin
(D) Nystatin swish and swallow
(E) Trimethoprim-sulfamethoxazole

31. A 17-year-old girl with a history of refractory B-lymphocyte lymphoma undergoes a bone marrow transplant from a matched unrelated donor. On day 19 posttransplant, an erythematous, maculopapular rash is noted on her trunk and extremities. Within 3 days, she has developed diffuse bullae and severe diarrhea. She requires vigorous hydration and narcotic pain medication. Jaundice is noted, and her serum total bilirubin is found to be 10 mg/dL. Which of the following interventions gives the patient the best chance of survival?

(A) Hepatic transplantation
(B) The patient has little chance of survival; donor T lymphocytes should have been removed from the stem cells prior to infusion
(C) Total body irradiation to remove the graft
(D) Treatment with monoclonal antibodies directed at T lymphocytes
(E) Treatment with thalidomide

32. In a hypothetical case-control study meant to associate presence of acute coronary syndrome (ACS) with use of rofecoxib, the data shown in the table were collected. What is the odds ratio that ACS is linked to exposure to rofecoxib?

Exposure to rofecoxib	(+) Acute coronary syndromes (no. of pts.)	(-) Acute coronary syndromes (no. of pts.)
History of exposure	a = 10	b = 5
No history of exposure	c = 10	d = 15
Total patients	20	20

Reproduced, with permission, from USMLERx.com.

(A) 1/15
(B) 1
(C) 5/3
(D) 3
(E) 60

33. A 75-year-old man presents to his physician with a 4-week history of exertional shortness of breath. He worked as a pipe fitter for 45 years, quitting 5 years ago. He denies chest pain, palpitations, swelling in his legs, cough, hemopty-

sis, and weight loss. He smokes 1 pack per day and has done so for the past 45 years. His temperature is 36.7°C (98°F), pulse is 85/min, blood pressure is 120/80 mm Hg, respiratory rate is 14/min, and oxygen saturation is 99% on room air. Physical examination is unremarkable. Pulmonary function testing shows a mild restrictive pattern with a normal diffusing capacity. X-ray of the chest shows linear opacities at the lung bases and pleural plaques. Which of the following is the most appropriate intervention?

(A) High-resolution CT scan
(B) Pulmonary function testing
(C) Repeat sputum cytologies every 6 months
(D) Repeat x-ray films of the chest every 6 months
(E) Smoking cessation

34. A male infant presents to his pediatrician's office for a well-child visit. On physical examination, he has a temperature of 37.2°C (99°F) and clear nasal drainage. The examination is otherwise unremarkable. The infant is able to lift his head when prone, track past the midline, and coo. His immunization record indicates that he received his first hepatitis B vaccination at birth. Which immunizations should this infant receive today?

Vaccine	Birth	1 month	2 months	4 months	6 months	12 months	15 months
Hepatitis B	HepB #1		HepB #2			HepB #3	
Diphtheria, Tetanus, Pertussis			DTaP	DTaP	DTaP		DTaP
Haemophilus influenzae type b			Hib	Hib	Hib	Hib	
Inactivated Poliovirus			IPV	IPV		IPV	
Measles, Mumps, Rubella						MMR #1	
Varicella						Varicella	
Pneumococcal			PCV	PCV	PCV	PCV	
Influenza						Influenza (Yearly)	

Reproduced, with permission, from USMLERx.com.

(A) Administer hepatitis B vaccine
(B) Administer hepatitis B vaccine and diphtheria-tetanus-pertussis vaccine
(C) Administer hepatitis B vaccine, diphtheria-tetanus-pertussis vaccine, and inactivated poliomyelitis vaccine
(D) Administer hepatitis B vaccine, diphtheria-tetanus-pertussis vaccine, *Haemophilus influenzae* type b vaccine, inactivated po-

liomyelitis vaccine, and pneumococcal conjugate vaccine
(E) Schedule a return visit when the child's nasal congestion subsides, and administer the immunizations the

35. A 36-year-old G2P1 woman at 19 weeks' gestation presents to the obstetrics clinic for her scheduled prenatal visit. She has no complaints except for some fatigue. Past obstetric history is notable for a pregnancy 2 years ago. Although that pregnancy was without complications, the child has significant developmental delay. The patient takes no medications other than prenatal vitamins. Family history is significant for two maternal aunts with mental retardation. She is an only child. Physical examination reveals a well-developed female in no acute distress. The uterus may be appreciated well above the pubic symphysis. Laboratory results are notable for an ultrasound performed 1 week ago, which revealed no abnormalities. The physician orders a triple screen test. What other test would be the next most appropriate test for this patient?

(A) Amniocentesis
(B) Biophysical profile
(C) Chorionic villus sampling
(D) Maternal serum α-fetoprotein
(E) Nonstress test
(F) Percutaneous umbilical blood sampling
(G) Ultrasound

36. A man approaches his physician about his target cholesterol level. He is 29 years old with no personal or family history of cardiac disease. He does not smoke, denies high blood pressure and diabetes, and has a body mass index of 26 kg/m². The man says he has heard that there are multiple types of cholesterol, but wants to know just one marker that will be the best for him to follow. The physician tells the man that following the LDL cholesterol would be a reasonable option. At what LDL level should pharmacologic therapy be considered?

(A) LDL >100 mg/dL
(B) LDL >130 mg/dL
(C) LDL >160 mg/dL
(D) LDL >190 mg/dL
(E) LDL >200 mg/dL

37. A 22-year-old woman from sub-Saharan Africa comes to her primary care physician to be tested for HIV. She denies illicit drug use and has not been sexually active since she moved to the United States 3 years ago. Her initial enzyme-linked immunosorbent assay is positive. Which of the following would confirm the diagnosis of HIV?

(A) A positive Western blot test
(B) A repeat enzyme-linked immunosorbent assay
(C) Clinical evidence of an opportunistic infection such as thrush or Kaposi's sarcoma
(D) History of unprotected sex with an HIV-positive partner
(E) Lymphopenia

38. A 57-year-old man comes to his primary care physician complaining of increasing fatigue in the past few months. He is unable to walk up to his third floor apartment without becoming short of breath. The physician orders a basic blood test. Laboratory tests show:

WBC count	5000/mm³
Hemoglobin	10.2 g/dL
Hematocrit	37%
Platelet count	221,000/mm³
Mean corpuscular volume	70 fL

Additionally, the patient's stool is guaiac-positive. The physician sends the patient for a colonoscopy which is shown in the image. With the new diagnosis the patient is concerned about his 35-year-old son. What recommendations should the physician make?

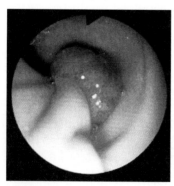

Reproduced, with permission, from Kasper DL, Braunwald E, Fauci AS, Hauser SL, Longo DL, Jameson LJ, Isselbacher KJ, eds. *Harrison's Online.* New York: McGraw-Hill, 2005: Figure 272-14.

(A) His son should be screened with a colonoscopy every 1–2 years starting now
(B) His son should be screened with a colonoscopy every 5 years starting at the age of 40
(C) His son should be screened with a colonoscopy every 5 years starting at the age of 50
(D) His son should be screened with a colonoscopy every 5 years starting now
(E) His son should be screened with a fecal occult blood test every year starting at the age of 50

EXTENDED MATCHING

Questions 39 and 40

Select the mechanism of action of the antihypertensive drug that would be the best choice to treat each of the following patients.

(A) Antagonizes aldosterone receptors
(B) Antagonizes β_1-adrenergic receptors
(C) Antagonizes β_1- and β_2-adrenergic receptors
(D) Blocks α_1-adrenergic receptors
(E) Blocks angiotensin II formation
(F) Blocks calcium influx into vascular smooth muscle and myocardium
(G) Blocks distal convoluted tubule sodium and chloride reabsorption
(H) Blocks loop of Henle sodium and chloride reabsorption
(I) Directly relaxes smooth muscle
(J) Stimulates α_2-adrenergic receptors
(K) Stimulates aldosterone formation
(L) Stimulates angiotensin II formation

39. A 52-year-old man with a history of diabetes and hypertension presents to a new primary care provider. He currently uses insulin to control his diabetes and hydrochlorothiazide (HCTZ) to control his hypertension. On physical examination, he is an overweight man with no concerning findings, except for a blood pressure of 171/93 mm Hg. His creatine is 1.7 mg/dL with a urinalysis that shows proteinuria. His physician wants to add another antihypertensive in addition to his HCTZ.

40. A 63-year-old woman with a history of osteoporosis presents for a second opinion regarding hypertension management because she is worried about starting any medication that might worsen her osteoporosis. Her only medication is calcium supplements. She smokes 1 pack per day for 15 years. Her physical examination is normal, except for a blood pressure of 165/90 mm Hg. Laboratory work shows total serum calcium of 7.0 mg/dL and mild hypercalciuria. She wonders if an antihypertensive exists that would not cause her calcium to decrease further and that might even increase it.

1. **The correct answer is D.** According to the most recent report from the National Cholesterol Education Program, the goal LDL should take into account the individual's risk factors. This patient's smoking history is her only risk factor. In addition, her relatively high HDL level is protective. Therefore, she should be considered in the group with a zero to one risk factor, and her optimal LDL is ≤ 160 mg/dL.

Answer A is incorrect. Although HDL is an important risk factor for coronary artery disease, both HDL and LDL should be considered when formulating a treatment plan. This is because HDL is a negative risk factor for heart disease.

Answer B is incorrect. The lowest goal for LDL is reserved for those with known coronary heart disease or equivalent risk factors. This includes all patients with diabetes mellitus.

Answer C is incorrect. Patients with two or more risk factors should be treated with at least lifestyle modification at an LDL of ≥ 130 mg/dL. Risk factors include age (men > 45 years, women > 55 years), smoking, low HDL (< 40 mg/dL), hypertension, and family history of premature coronary heart disease (first-degree female relatives < 65 years old or first-degree male relatives < 55 years old).

Answer E is incorrect. Individuals with no risk factors are still recommended to undergo lifestyle modifications at any LDL > 160 mg/dL.

2. **The correct answer is C.** Depression and alcohol abuse screening are important in all patients 25 years and older. The physician can ask both the **CAGE** (**C**ut down [on drinking], **A**nnoyance, **G**uilt [about drinking], [need for] **E**ye-opener) questions and questions to evaluate for depression.

Answer A is incorrect. Cholesterol levels should be checked every 5 years in patients 25 years or older.

Answer B is incorrect. A complete blood count (CBC) and erythrocyte sedimentation rate are not necessary for screening. In female patients, a CBC is often checked to evaluate for anemia at a physical or gynecologic examination.

Answer D is incorrect. A baseline electrocardiogram (ECG) may be helpful in establishing the patient's normal cardiac patterns but is not a necessary part of the annual physical examination until the patient reaches 40 years of age.

Answer E is incorrect. Fetal occult blood is not needed annually until a patient reaches 50 years of age or, in high-risk patients, 40 years of age.

3. **The correct answer is D.** Screening tests, such as the rapid streptococcal test, have high sensitivity and low specificity. If the rapid streptococcal test is positive, this indicates but does not prove that the patient's pharyngitis may be due to group A streptococcal infection. If the rapid streptococcal test is negative, then no further testing is needed, because sensitive tests effectively rule out disease. The throat culture is highly specific and thus is able to confirm (rule in) the disease. It may also indicate exactly which organism is involved and narrow treatment options.

Answer A is incorrect. Because detection of β-hemolytic streptococci is the goal of this testing series, other bacteria which may be incidentally identified through culture are generally not significant.

Answer B is incorrect. The critical property of culture is its high positive predictive value resulting from the high specificity of the test, combined with the fact that most cultured patients have tested positive on the rapid test and thus are already likely to have the disease. Sensitivity is less important since most uninfected individuals will have already been identified by the rapid test.

Answer C is incorrect. The critical property of the rapid streptococcal test is its high sensitivity; a negative result is considered definitive, while a positive result requires culture to confirm. A confirmatory test will have high specificity, such as the culture.

Answer E is incorrect. As a general rule, a rapid screening test will be highly sensitive, while a confirmatory test will have a high specificity and positive predictive value.

4. **The correct answer is A.** Asplenic patients are at an increased risk of developing infections compared to those patients with functional spleens. These patients may develop overwhelming postsplenectomy sepsis in which encapsulated organisms (including *Streptococcus pneumoniae*, *Neisseria meningitidis*, and *Haemophilus influenzae*) may cause fever, lethargy, or upper respiratory infection that leads to coma and death in up to 50% of patients. The capsule that surrounds these organisms is an antiphagocytic factor that permits these organisms to survive and cause bacteremia. It is vital for these patients to receive vaccination against these encapsulated organisms to prevent the development of postsplenectomy sepsis.

Answer B is incorrect. *Moraxella catarrhalis* is one of the organisms that frequently causes otitis media in pediatric patients. It has not been associated with postsplenectomy sepsis in asplenic patients.

Answer C is incorrect. *Pseudomonas aeruginosa* causes pneumonia, external otitis media, urinary tract infection, folliculitis, and wound and burn infections. This organism has not been associated with the development of overwhelming postsplenectomy sepsis in asplenic patients.

Answer D is incorrect. *Staphylococcus aureus* has been associated with food poisoning, skin infections, organ abscesses, pneumonia, toxic shock syndrome, and scalded skin syndrome. However, this organism is not encapsulated and has not been associated with overwhelming postsplenectomy sepsis.

Answer E is incorrect. *Streptococcus viridans* are part of the normal flora of the mouth. *Streptococcus viridans* is involved in subacute bacterial endocarditis and can cause dental caries but not overwhelming postsplenectomy sepsis in asplenic patients.

5. **The correct answer is F.** Although cardiac disease is a leading cause of death among adults 45–64 years old, stroke is responsible for more deaths among women in this age group. Recent studies indicate that a daily 81-mg aspirin tablet doesn't reduce the risk of cardiac events in women, but can lower the risk of stroke.

Answer A is incorrect. Cardiac disease is the second leading cause of death in all patients aged 45–64 years old, but stroke is responsible for a higher mortality among female patients in this age group.

Answer B is incorrect. Chronic obstructive pulmonary disease (COPD) is the sixth leading cause of death in this age group. COPD is responsible for more deaths in those > 64 years of age.

Answer C is incorrect. Diabetes is the fifth leading cause of death in all patients in this age group, behind stroke, neoplasm, heart disease, and injury.

Answer D is incorrect. Influenza is a leading cause of death in patients > 65 years old.

Answer E is incorrect. Pneumonia is a major cause of death in patients > 65 years old.

6. **The correct answer is E.** Patients with pancreatic cancer can present with weight loss, jaundice, abdominal pain, dark urine, acholic stools, and pruritus. On physical examination the gallbladder or other abdominal mass is palpable. Diagnosis is usually made with ultrasound with findings of dilated bile ducts or visible mass, or CT scan which demonstrates the pancreatic mass. The associated risk factors for pancreatic cancer include smoking, chronic pancreatitis, a first-degree relative with pancreatic cancer, and high-fat diet.

Answer A is incorrect. Chronic pancreatitis, not chronic gastritis, is a risk factor for pancreatic cancer.

Answer B is incorrect. Diabetes insipidus is not a pathology of the pancreas and is not a risk factor for pancreatic cancer.

Answer C is incorrect. Diabetes mellitus can result from neoplasm in the body of the pancreas, but it is not a risk factor for pancreatic cancer.

Answer D is incorrect. History of cholecystitis is not a risk factor for pancreatic cancer. Post-operative biliary stricture should be on the differential diagnosis in a patient with a history of cholecystectomy who presents with symptoms suggestive of pancreatic neoplasm.

7. **The correct answer is B.** No evidence exists to suggest that patients are at increased risk for development of Addison's disease after having been treated for Hodgkin's disease with radiation to the chest alone. Adrenocortical insufficiency may result from subdiaphragmatic irradiation, but this patient did not receive this treatment.

Answer A is incorrect. Patients treated with alkylating agents in combination with radiotherapy are at risk for development of acute leukemias in the 10 years following their therapy.

Answer C is incorrect. Because of the very high long-term cure rates associated with Hodgkin's disease, observation of long-term sequelae of treatment has been possible. Patients treated with irradiation to the chest are at increased risk of development of carcinomas following treatment. Breast carcinomas may develop > 10 years after therapy. For this reason, women treated with thoracic radiotherapy should undergo mammography 5–10 years after treatment and every year thereafter.

Answer D is incorrect. Patients with a history of thoracic irradiation are at increased risk for coronary artery disease, and are three times as likely to have a fatal myocardial infarction as their age-matched counterparts. They should be encouraged to minimize risk factors by avoiding smoking and monitoring cholesterol levels.

Answer E is incorrect. Patients who receive thoracic radiotherapy are at high risk for development of hypothyroidism, and should be observed closely for this.

Answer F is incorrect. All patients, male and female, treated for Hodgkin's disease are at risk for infertility that may be permanent due to effects of cytotoxic chemotherapy. This risk is decreased with modern chemotherapeutic regimens, but is still significant.

Answer G is incorrect. Lhermitte's syndrome, manifested by shock-like sensations traveling to the lower extremities on flexion of the neck, occurs in 15% of patients who receive thoracic radiotherapy.

8. **The correct answer is E.** Diverticulosis accounts for 42–55% of lower gastrointestinal bleeding, followed by cancer/polyps accounting for 8–26%, and bleeding and angiodysplasia which accounts for 3–12%. Other causes include inflammatory bowel disease (2–8%), anorectal disease (3–9%), small bowel disease (3–5%), infectious colitis (1–5%), radiation colitis (1–5%), and vasculitis (1–3%).

Answer A is incorrect. The correct order is diverticulosis, cancer/polyp, and then angiodysplasia.

Answer B is incorrect. The correct order is diverticulosis, cancer/polyp, and then angiodysplasia.

Answer C is incorrect. The correct order is diverticulosis, cancer/polyp, and then angiodysplasia.

Answer D is incorrect. The correct order is diverticulosis, cancer/polyp, and then angiodysplasia.

9. **The correct answer is D.** This is an example of a prospective cohort study. Using the letters from the table, the relative risk is calculated as $(a / (a + b)) / (c / (c + d)) = 20$, so smokers have 20 times the risk of nonsmokers of developing lung cancer.

Answer A is incorrect. The relative risk would be 1 if there were no difference between smokers and nonsmokers, which is not the case.

Answer B is incorrect. The reciprocal of the relative risk is 1/20, and it represents the relative risk of nonsmokers developing lung cancer as compared to that of smokers developing lung cancer.

Answer C is incorrect. The attributable risk (or risk difference), calculated as the risk in the exposed population minus the risk in the unexposed population for a particular risk factor, is 19 / 100. This would be $a / (a + b) - c / (c + d) = 1/10$.

Answer E is incorrect. The odds ratio, which is typically calculated for case-control studies as (a/c) / (b/d), is 20/(80/99). It is close to the relative risk when the prevalence of a disease is very small.

10. **The correct answer is A.** A confounding variable is a characteristic associated with both the exposure of interest and the disease or condition being studied that may have an independent effect on the relationship between the exposure and disease of interest. In the study, dietary cholesterol may influence the risk of myocardial infarction (MI), but dietary fat may also influence MI risk and thus it is difficult to tell what proportion of decreased MI risk is due to which dietary factor.

Answer B is incorrect. Enrollment bias occurs when group assignment of participants is not random, for example, when a sicker set of participants on average is assigned to the experimental group than to the control group.

Answer C is incorrect. Measurement bias refers to systematic (whether intentional or unintentional) error in data collection such that the true relationship between the variables under study is distorted.

Answer D is incorrect. Recall bias refers to bias introduced by relying on participants' memory in retrospective studies. For example, participants who believe a given exposure had negative consequences may be more likely to remember the exposure than those who experienced no problems afterward.

Answer E is incorrect. Self-selection bias refers to the decision of the participant whether to enroll in the study. Those who choose to participate may have different characteristics as a group than those who choose not to enroll.

11. **The correct answer is B.** Chronic use of high-dose steroids, as those used to treat acute lymphoid leukemia, may result in formation of bilateral cataracts. Patients should be monitored closely, particularly those that are school-aged, because they may suffer from visual defects.

Answer A is incorrect. Cyclophosphamide is not implicated in hearing loss; however, cis-platin and carboplatin have been associated with this effect. Common side effects of cyclophosphamide use include alopecia, infertility, nausea, vomiting, leukopenia, and potentially fatal acute hemorrhagic cystitis.

Answer C is incorrect. No evidence suggests that glucocorticoids cause peripheral neuropathy. Common side effects of glucocorticoids include cataracts, cushingoid body habitus, increased incidence of cardiovascular disease, gastric ulcer, and osteoporosis, among many others.

Answer D is incorrect. Systemic methotrexate is not implicated in the development of cognitive deficits. Common toxicities of methotrexate use include nausea, loose stools, stomatitis, alopecia, and rash. Methotrexate can also cause pulmonary, renal, and hepatic toxicity.

Answer E is incorrect. Methotrexate is not associated with an increased risk of pulmonary fibrosis. Common toxicities of methotrexate use include nausea, loose stools, stomatitis, alopecia, and rash. Methotrexate can also cause pulmonary, renal, and hepatic toxicity.

12. **The correct answer is A.** Colonoscopy is the method of choice in this individual because the lesion is most likely right sided, as suggested by a negative sigmoidoscopy 6 months ago. With colonoscopy, the entire large bowel can be visualized, and it also allows the biopsy of lesions or removal of polyps found on examination.

Answer B is incorrect. A CT scan of the abdomen is not the diagnostic method of choice in diagnosing right-sided colon cancers, although CT colonoscopy (high-resolution CT also known as virtual colonoscopy) is currently being explored. This is because current resolution may miss some polyps and other lesions. Also, colonoscopy allows for biopsy of potential lesions.

Answer C is incorrect. Double-contrast barium enema can be used to make a radiographic diagnosis of colonic cancer if it is not possible to perform a colonoscopy (e.g., tortuosity of the colon). Colonoscopy is the preferred method.

Answer D is incorrect. Sigmoidoscopy would not be helpful here because the patient had a negative sigmoidoscopy 6 months ago, suggesting that the lesion is not on the left side of the colon. To visualize the right side of the colon, a colonoscopy should be performed.

Answer E is incorrect. The lesion is most likely a right-sided colonic adenocarcinoma, and this area would not be well visualized by an upper gastrointestinal series.

13. **The correct answer is B.** Current recommendations are that a Pap smear be done once every 1–3 years based on risk factors and cytology method. In 2003, the American College of Obstetricians and Gynecologists recommended that women younger than 30 years be screened annually, regardless of liquid or conventional culture method. However, the U.S. Preventive Services Task Force recommends that women of any age extend time between screening to every 2–3 years if they meet certain criteria. Women may extend the time between Pap smears to every 2–3 years if they have no risk factors and have had three consecutive negative cytologies by conventional method. Risk factors include diethylstilbestrol exposure in utero, prior cervical intraepithelial neoplasia II/III or abnormal Pap smear, smoking, or immunocompromised state. Gonorrhea and chlamydia screening may be recommended if the patient is sexually active.

Answer A is incorrect. All women should have a Pap smear once they are determined to be HIV-positive because immunocompromised states are a risk factor for human papillomavirus (HPV). Of note, condoms do not protect against HPV transmission because any skin-to-skin contact with an infected individual may lead to infection.

Answer C is incorrect. Women > 70 (not 60) years old with no abnormal Pap smear cytologies in the past 10 years and no new risk factors may elect to cease having a Pap smear done. However, any patient with positive human papillomavirus DNA would benefit from continued screening. Of note, screening does not need to continue in patients who have a limited life expectancy or who would be unable to tolerate cervical cancer therapy.

Answer D is incorrect. Women who have had a hysterectomy without removal of the cervix should continue to be screened. In women with documented cervical intraepithelial neoplasia II/III, a screening should be done regardless of whether the patient had a total hysterectomy. The cytologic screening of women after total hysterectomy should include the vaginal, vulvar, and perianal epithelium at 4- to 6-month intervals until she has three consecutive negative results, after which point she can be screened annually.

Answer E is incorrect. Current recommendations are annual screening if conventional cytology is used and biannual screening if liquid cytology is used in healthy patients without risk factors or prior disease. The American Cancer Society and American College of Obstetricians and Gynecologists support the use of liquid-based cytology because it is more sensitive and increases the number of adequate Papanicolaou (or Pap) smear readings, while reducing the false-negative rate among patients with HIV and chronic cervicitis, obscuring blood and repetitive atypical squamous cells of undetermined significance (or ASCUS) Pap reports.

14. **The correct answer is F.** Lung cancer is not hereditary but is based on environmental exposures to radon, asbestos, or cigarette smoke. There is evidence to suggest that a patient's risk of developing lung cancer from tobacco exposure decreases somewhat after the patient quits smoking, depending on the patient's smoking history and medical status. The patient should be counseled about smoking cessation, and appropriate adjustments to medications should be made if the patient is started on nicotine gum or patch. In 2004, the U.S. Preventive Services Task Force determined that "the evidence is insufficient to recommend for or against screening asymptomatic persons for lung cancer with either low-dose computed tomography, plain chest radiographs, sputum cytology, or a combination of these tests."

Answer A is incorrect. X-rays of the chest are not recommended as a screening measure. X-rays of the chest or CT scans of the lungs are necessary in the diagnosis of lung cancer and should be pursued once the index of suspicion for lung cancer increases.

Answer B is incorrect. In the Memorial-Sloan Kettering Lung Project, there was no significant difference in 5-year survival rate among patients who had sputum cytology and plain films versus patients who just had plain films to screen for lung cancer.

Answer C is incorrect. Initial results of the Early Lung Cancer Action Project showed that low-dose spiral CT of the chest screening of 1000 asymptomatic patients with ≥ 10 pack-year smoking history found more malignant nodules than plain films (2.7% vs. 0.7%). However, many of the detected nodules were ultimately found to be benign (20.6%), and no survival benefit of this screening has been proven.

Answer D is incorrect. Studies reviewed by the U.S. Preventive Services Task Force demonstrated that lung cancer screening with sputum cytology can detect cancer at an earlier stage than in the unscreened population but had no effect on mortality.

Answer E is incorrect. Bronchoscopy and/or fine-needle aspiration may be necessary for further diagnosis of suspected lung nodules but have no role in screening.

15. **The correct answer is A.** A hemoglobin A_{1c} should be checked every 3 months to assess the average serum glucose levels over that period. This is important in adjusting medications and to follow the disease progression.

Answer B is incorrect. Patients with either type 1 or type 2 DM are at increased risk for hyperlipidemia and should be screened on an annual basis. Patients with type 1 DM should be screened during puberty if they have a positive family history of coronary artery disease in order to prevent silent ischemic damage.

Answer C is incorrect. Approximately 30–40% of patients with type 1 DM will develop renal failure. In patients > 10 years old who have had diabetes for > 3 years, a microalbuminuria will help assess kidney function. This should be checked annually. Current studies have shown that an angiotensin-

converting enzyme inhibitor is beneficial in reversing or delaying renal impairment in diabetics who have no renal artery stenosis.

Answer D is incorrect. Approximately 30–40% of patients with type 1 DM will eventually develop loss of vision, so it is important to screen these patients annually to assess for vision loss and possible retinal tear.

Answer E is incorrect. A podiatry examination is important for screening associated diabetic neuropathies. Patients with type 1 DM are also at increased risk for peripheral vascular disease, so peripheral pulses should be checked often. These screens should be checked at the patient's annual visit unless he is developing signs or symptoms.

Answer F is incorrect. This indicates the patient's glycemic control over the previous 2 weeks. This test would be helpful in the case of abnormal hemoglobins or to determine glycemic control at time of conception in women with diabetes. This test is not necessary on a regular basis.

16. **The correct answer is E.** Confounding variables are variables that could affect the outcome, are not evenly distributed between the study groups, and are not part of the primary intervention. The researcher is looking to compare the contributions of diet and exercise to weight loss, thus the running group should eat the diet to which they are accustomed, and the diet group should not change their usual activity level. Instructing the runners to drink more water may decrease their consumption of other drinks, like sports drinks, juice, milk, or soda—beverages that contain calories. Changing fluid calorie intake changes the diet of the exercise group and may confound the results, as it wouldn't be possible to tell what portion of the runners' weight loss occurred due to physical activity and what portion due to calorie reduction. Confounders can be controlled for either by study design or by data analysis.

Answer A is incorrect. Subjects' awareness of a study means it is unblinded, but is not automatically a confounder in the absence of a feasible relationship between awareness of the study and increased performance.

Answer B is incorrect. Variations in the recommended diet for the dieting group are unlikely to affect the outcome if basic nutritional composition and calorie and fat intake for dieters are comparable. Confounding variables are variables which could affect the outcome, are not evenly distributed between the study groups, and are not part of the primary intervention. Since all the recommended diets are part of the primary intervention for the diet group, they are not confounding variables.

Answer C is incorrect. While it is possible that running instruction might affect weight loss, it can be considered a component of the primary intervention (exercise) for this group, and is therefore not a confounding variable.

Answer D is incorrect. Excluding injured members from the study might be considered a form of selection bias, but is not confounding.

17. **The correct answer is B.** By lowering the cutoff value, the number of people who will be diagnosed as having prostate cancer will increase. This will decrease the number of false negatives (those who are told they do not have the disease when they in fact do), and increase the number of false positives (those told they have the disease when they in fact do not).

    Answer A is incorrect. False positives and false negatives could both decrease if the test were made more valid, perhaps through averaging the results from several samples taken on different days, but this question asks what would happen if the cutoff value were lowered.

    Answer C is incorrect. False positives and false negatives could both rise if the test were made less precise, perhaps through laboratory errors, but this question asks what will happen if a cutoff value is lowered.

    Answer D is incorrect. The number of false positives would decrease and false negatives increase if the cutoff value were raised, but the cutoff value was lowered.

    Answer E is incorrect. This is not correct, because lowering the cutoff value will decrease the number of false negatives and increase the number of false positives.

18. **The correct answer is D.** Many studies have found that the greatest risk factor for a completed suicide attempt in any patient is whether they have attempted suicide in the past. In fact, some research shows that past attempts may increase the risk of suicide by 22 times. It is also important to assess whether the patient has a plan for suicide and whether the suicide attempt was by lethal means.

    Answer A is incorrect. Antisocial behavior increases the risk of suicide, but significantly less so than previous suicide attempts.

    Answer B is incorrect. Depression increases suicide risk more than antisocial behavior, but significantly less so than previous suicide attempts.

    Answer C is incorrect. Male gender is a risk factor for completed suicide, but is not as significant a risk factor as previous attempts.

    Answer E is incorrect. Substance abuse is a risk factor for violence and suicide, but it is not as significant as previous suicide attempts. Substance abuse may increase the risk of suicide by a factor of eight.

19. **The correct answer is F.** The odds ratio can be calculated as (number exposed who have disease/number not exposed who have disease) / (number exposed without disease/number not exposed without disease), which in this scenario yields $(150/100) / (50/200) = 6$. Odds ratios are used in studies employing a case-control design (typically retrospective) and can be used as an approximation of the relative risk only when the disease being studied is very rare in the overall population from which the controls are drawn.

    Answer A is incorrect. Reversing the relationship of the variables by mistake yields 1/6, or 0.17.

    Answer B is incorrect. Calculation error.

    Answer C is incorrect. Erroneously calculating the relative risk for this retrospective case-control study yields 1.7. Relative risk is a statistical measure of the influence of an exposure on the risk of a disease. It is used in studies employing a cohort design (typically prospective).

    Answer D is incorrect. Calculation error.

    Answer E is incorrect. Calculation error.

20. The correct answer is D. Varicella develops in approximately 90% of susceptible household contacts with significant exposure. The vaccine, if given in the first 3 days postexposure, has been shown to prevent or modify the course of illness in susceptible individuals. Seventy-eight percent of adults seroconvert after the first dose; a cumulative 99% have converted after the second dose.

Answer A is incorrect. In an otherwise healthy child, treatment with oral acyclovir may be indicated under special circumstances (such as in the case of a child with susceptible household contacts at increased risk of serious disease), but treatment with intravenous acyclovir is appropriate only in cases of severe infection or immunocompromised hosts.

Answer B is incorrect. Postexposure oral acyclovir may be appropriate as prophylaxis instead of varicella zoster immunoglobulin or vaccine, but there are insufficient data to support routine use. Oral acyclovir, if administered within the first 3 days of infection, has been shown to lessen the duration and severity of disease in healthy children, but is recommended only in cases involving household contacts who are at increased risk for severe disease (e.g., immunosuppression, extremes of age, and pregnant women).

Answer C is incorrect. Administration of varicella zoster immunoglobulin to adults after exposure is indicated for pregnant women, health care professionals with significant exposure, and immunocompromised individuals.

Answer E is incorrect. Because individuals > 13 years old are at risk for more serious disease, prophylaxis with varicella vaccine is indicated and safe for the older sibling.

21. The correct answer is C. Cross-sectional study involves assessing variables at one given point in time. Exposure and outcome are measured simultaneously. It is useful for estimating disease prevalence and distribution within a population, but cannot establish causal relationships, although these can be estimated with chi-square analysis.

Answer A is incorrect. Case-control studies involve identifying two populations: one of cases, which are persons with the disease or condition of interest, and another population of controls, which are individuals similar to the case subjects in relevant parameters other than the disease or condition under study. Potential exposures or etiologic factors are then examined to determine if there is a common denominator in the background of the cases that the controls tend not to share.

Answer B is incorrect. Cohort studies involve identifying a group of subjects, or "cohort," as well as a matched control group, that are followed for a period of time to assess whether the disease or condition of interest develops.

Answer D is incorrect. Using existing individual studies, but combining their data statistically to maximize power and minimize study limitations, is known as a meta-analysis.

Answer E is incorrect. Randomized controlled clinical trial is a study in which subjects are assigned to either control or treatment groups and then treatment groups are exposed to some factor that control groups do not experience. Outcomes are measured in both groups to determine the effects of the exposure or treatment.

22. The correct answer is E. The researcher is conducting a randomized controlled clinical trial. Patients have been assigned randomly to minimize bias. In this instance, the control group is not receiving placebo; this does not mean that this study is not a randomized controlled clinical trial. For diseases and conditions where the patient would be unduly harmed by remaining untreated for the study duration, it is customary to compare the study drug or procedure to the current standard of care for that disease or condition and not to placebo. In this scenario, the study is also double blinded because neither the study staff nor patients know who receives what treatment.

Answer A is incorrect. A case-control study involves matching each person in a study with another patient who is similar in all disease-relevant aspects aside from the factor under study. These studies are not randomized and thus are subject to a variety of biases; however, they are useful for initial hypothesis testing.

Answer B is incorrect. A cohort study involves following a group of patients and a group of controls over time to see whether a given disease or condition afflicts one group disproportionately.

Answer C is incorrect. A cross-sectional survey is an assessment of a given population where information on the disease or condition of interest and possible past risk factors or events is collected simultaneously.

Answer D is incorrect. A meta-analysis, or literature review, is the mathematical combination of prior studies and does not involve the collection of new data.

23. **The correct answer is B.** Bilateral male sterilization has theoretical and actual failure rates of 0.15% and 0.1%, respectively, the lowest failure rates of any contraceptive option other than complete abstinence. Unlike nonsurgical contraceptive options, however, sterilization is a permanent intervention and thus must be preceded by sufficient patient counseling. This couple states that they do not desire any further children, and thus while other contraceptive options could be prescribed, male sterilization remains the most effective option for them.

Answer A is incorrect. Female sterilization has failure rates only slightly higher than male sterilization, with both theoretical and actual failure rates of 0.5%. Like male sterilization, this option is also permanent and must be performed only after sufficient patient counseling. Additionally, female sterilization in this couple is less desirable, as surgical interventions should be minimized in a patient with a previous history of abdominal surgery, as she is already at increased risk for adhesions.

Answer C is incorrect. Both the combination and the progestin-only oral contraceptive pill have actual failure rates of 5% and thus are less effective than the more invasive options. However, if this patient were symptomatic from her endometriosis, she could be started on the combination pill for symptom relief.

Answer D is incorrect. The diaphragm has an actual failure rate of 12–18% and thus would not be a good option for this patient. The diaphragm should be used in patients who are unable to tolerate more effective surgical or medical contraception.

Answer E is incorrect. An intrauterine device (IUD) would be a good contraceptive option for this patient, given that she is monogamous with her husband and does not have a history of sexually transmitted diseases. A copper IUD could be placed at an office visit, and would last for ~10 years (progesterone IUDs last for ~5 years). However, failure rates for these devices are higher (0.8% actual failure rate for the copper IUD and 2.0% for the progesterone IUD) than those for sterilization, making this option less effective.

Answer F is incorrect. The male condom has a 14% actual failure rate. The benefit to the male condom over other forms of contraception is its protection from sexually transmitted diseases; the male condom is thus particularly useful in high-risk populations and would not be necessary in this couple.

Answer G is incorrect. Both the combination and the progestin-only oral contraceptive pill have actual failure rates of 5% and thus are less effective than the more invasive options.

24. **The correct answer is B.** A "blinded" or "single-blinded" study is one in which the participant does not know whether he or she is an experimental subject or a control subject. "Double blinded" means that neither the participants nor the researchers know who is assigned to which group.

Answer A is incorrect. If neither the study participants nor the researchers know the group assignments, the study is "double blinded."

Answer C is incorrect. Single blinding refers to blinding study participants. Blinding researchers would limit observational bias but would not limit reporting bias on the part of the participants if they know whether they are the experimental group or the control group. Sometimes it is not possible to double blind a study; for example, a study comparing outcomes of two surgical procedures could not blind the surgeons, who would have to know which procedure they were to perform on which participant.

Answer D is incorrect. Phase II and III drug trials assess drug efficacy, but this is a separate issue from blinding.

Answer E is incorrect. Phase I, II, and III drug trials assess safety of drugs under study, but this is a separate study characteristic from blinding. Phase II and III studies focus on efficacy of drugs shown to be safe in Phase I studies.

25. **The correct answer is D.** This patient is suffering from a superficial thrombosis, which does not require anticoagulation. This is a non-life-threatening condition and it does not increase the risk of pulmonary embolus. First-line treatment is warm compresses applied so the clot does not extend to the deep veins. Treatment should last for 5–7 days.

Answer A is incorrect. Anticoagulation is not necessary for superficial vein thrombosis. A deep vein thrombosis would have shown decreased Doppler flow and lack of compressibility on ultrasonography.

Answer B is incorrect. There have been no large, controlled trials regarding the use of caffeine during pregnancy. Although it has not been linked to congenital birth defects, the standard recommendation is to avoid caffeine, or limit intake to no more than 1–2 caffeine-containing beverages per day. Any medications with caffeine should also be avoided if at all possible.

Answer C is incorrect. Warfarin may cause birth defects such as stippling of bone epiphyses, intrauterine growth restriction, nasal hypoplasia, and mental retardation. The sensitive period for birth defects due to warfarin is in the first trimester, but nevertheless it should be avoided in this case since anticoagulation is contraindicated.

Answer E is incorrect. Ibuprofen is a non-steroidal anti-inflammatory drug (NSAID) with analgesic properties. NSAIDs may be used as therapy for a superficial vein thrombosis in conjunction with warm compresses and elevation. When used in the first two trimesters of pregnancy, ibuprofen has not been linked to any congenital defects. During the third trimester of pregnancy, however, it has been linked to persistent pulmonary hypertension of the newborn. In addition, it has tocolytic properties.

26. **The correct answer is E.** Without controlling for the difference in alcohol consumption between smokers and nonsmokers, it is difficult to know which is responsible for the observed difference in vascular dementia incidence. What can be definitively stated is that, among the study population, smokers are more likely to be drinkers than nonsmokers.

Answer A is incorrect. Smoking and alcohol have not been evaluated independently in this study.

Answer B is incorrect. Alcohol may be the cause for the increase in vascular dementia, but unless the smoking disparity is controlled for by study design or multivariate analysis, this statement cannot be conclusively made.

Answer C is incorrect. Smoking may be the cause for the increase in vascular dementia, but unless the disparity in alcohol consumption is controlled for by study design or multivariate analysis, this statement cannot be conclusively made.

Answer D is incorrect. Although the observed result may be due to smoking, with no effect from alcohol consumption, this statement cannot be conclusively made. The presence of the confounding variable, in this case, alcohol consumption, precludes a definitive answer as to which variable accounts for the increased incidence of vascular dementia.

27. **The correct answer is C.** The type of study described is known as a meta-analysis. Combining results from several studies enhances statistical precision and may allow a statistically significant result from the combined analysis that did not reach a significant level when each smaller study was analyzed alone.

Answer A is incorrect. Meta-analyses are limited by the quality of individual studies and do not resolve flaws in those studies, although the impact of any single flawed study may be lessened.

Answer B is incorrect. Performing a meta-analysis does not remove or decrease the bias inherent in each study, and may have a compounding effect of each study's individual bias.

Answer D is incorrect. Since there is usually significant variation in the populations, methods, and interventions used in separately conducted studies, researchers must strike a difficult balance between including the greatest number of studies and excluding those whose differences would cloud the overall validity of the analysis.

Answer E is incorrect. Statistical analysis of multiple studies is inherently more complex than analysis of a single study.

28. **The correct answer is G.** Ultrasound would be an appropriate test for this patient at this visit. Ultrasound may be done at 18–20 weeks in order to determine gestational age if it cannot be determined by last menstrual period. It may also be done to survey fetal anatomy, amniotic fluid volume, and placental location. As she gave a history significant for possible birth defects, ultrasound is likely to be helpful in this patient. She would also benefit from a visit to a genetic counselor in addition to the ultrasound.

Answer A is incorrect. In general, amniocentesis is indicated in conjunction with a positive triple screen in patients that are > 35 years of age at the time of delivery. The risk of chromosomal abnormality in children born of women > 35 years old is 1 in 200. Amniocentesis carries a similar risk of about 1 in 200 for fetal loss and so is usually considered too risky for a 26-year-old patient. This patient is < 35 years old, but has a history of possible chromosomal abnormalities, which may make her a candidate for amniocentesis. Amniocentesis would still follow ultrasound evaluation and the results of her triple screen, making ultrasound evaluation the correct answer.

Answer B is incorrect. A biophysical profile is performed in the third trimester of a high-risk pregnancy. This would include patients who are post-dates, have diabetes, experience decreased fetal movement, or with known intrauterine growth restriction. A biophysical profile is a combination of a real-time ultrasound used to assess four parameters of fetal

well-being in addition to a nonstress test. The four ultrasound parameters are fetal tone, breathing, movement, and amniotic fluid volume, each with a 2-point maximum. A reassuring biophysical profile has a score of 8–10. A score of 0–2, however, is grounds for immediate delivery.

Answer C is incorrect. Chorionic villus sampling is performed at 10–12 weeks of gestation for an earlier assessment of chromosomal abnormalities, with diagnostic accuracy comparable to that of amniocentesis.

Answer D is incorrect. Maternal serum α-fetoprotein (MSAFP) is already part of the triple screen test. It is used to screen for neural tube defects (including anencephaly and spina bifida), abdominal wall defects (including gastroschisis and omphalocele), and is elevated in multiple gestation, fetal death, and chromosomal defects (trisomies 18, 21, and 13). The triple screen test of β-human chorionic gonadotropin, estriol, and MSAFP provides increased sensitivity for chromosomal abnormalities compared to MSAFP alone.

Answer E is incorrect. A nonstress test (NST) is a measurement of the fetal heart rate by external Doppler in correlation with spontaneous fetal movement as reported by the mother. A normal response is heart rate accelerations of > 15/min over baseline for ≥ 15 seconds. A normal NST shows two such accelerations in a 20-minute period. An NST is performed in two clinical scenarios. It may be performed at 32–34 weeks of gestation in high-risk patients as described above, or in pregnant patients presenting in acute distress as part of the triage evaluation of fetal well-being. An NST can be done as early as 28 weeks' gestation since 85% of fetuses will be reactive at this time.

Answer F is incorrect. Percutaneous umbilical blood sampling (PUBS) is performed by puncturing the umbilical cord vessels, which are not large enough for the procedure until the late second/early third trimesters. PUBS is useful in the evaluation of fetal anemia that occurs in erythroblastosis fetalis late in pregnancy.

29. The correct answer is C. The recommendations for mammography are screening every year when the patient is ≥ 50 years old.

Answer A is incorrect. Cancer antigen-125 (CA-125) is a serum tumor marker associated with ovarian, lung, breast, uterine tube, and gastrointestinal cancer. It had been proposed in the past as a possible screening tool for ovarian cancer, but it has been determined to be ineffective in detecting ovarian carcinoma in asymptomatic women. According to the U.S. Preventive Services Task Force, sensitivity has been shown to range from 55% to 85%. CA-125 levels may be elevated in noncancerous states such as infection (e.g., peritonitis and pleuritis), menstruation, pregnancy, endometriosis, and liver disease. CA-125 testing would not therefore be appropriate for this patient.

Answer B is incorrect. Endometrial biopsy is not recommended as a screening test. An endometrial biopsy would be performed on a patient presenting with postmenopausal bleeding.

Answer D is incorrect. Like cancer antigen-125, transvaginal ultrasound is only used to screen patients who are at high risk for ovarian cancer.

Answer E is incorrect. In spite of this patient's smoking history, x-ray of the chest is not recommended as a screening test.

30. The correct answer is E. Trimethoprim-sulfamethoxazole is indicated as prophylactic treatment against *Pneumocystis jiroveci* (formerly *carinii*) pneumonia in immunosuppressed patients for the duration of immunosuppression.

Answer A is incorrect. Raw oysters have been associated with various viral and bacterial infections. Hepatitis A virus is the likely cause of this patient's fulminant hepatitis. This cause of liver failure does not necessarily increase the patient's risk for posttransplant viral infections. Therefore, without history of another underlying disease, prior cytomegalovirus infection, prior HIV infection or risks, or underlying malnourished state, this middle-age man is a low-risk posttransplant patient. Antiviral therapy is not indicated for prophylaxis in low-risk patients but would be indicated for certain high-risk posttransplant patients and treatment of viral infections in posttransplant patients.

Answer B is incorrect. Antifungal therapy is not indicated for prophylaxis in this case. An indication for antifungal therapy in transplant patients would be candidiasis.

Answer C is incorrect. Niacin is generally not used as a prophylactic drug and has been associated with hepatotoxicity. Therefore, niacin would not be indicated.

Answer D is incorrect. Nystatin is used to treat oral infection by *Candida albicans*. Although this condition may arise in patients who are immunosuppressed, prophylaxis is generally not indicated.

31. The correct answer is D. The patient is experiencing severe acute graft-versus-host disease (GVHD), caused by allogeneic T lymphocytes that were transferred with the donor's stem cells reacting with antigenic targets on her own cells. Acute GVHD is usually experienced within 4 weeks of the initial transplant. It is characterized by rash, diarrhea, and decreased liver function, and is graded from I through IV. Significant GVHD develops in up to 60% of patients receiving stem cells from unrelated donors, and 30% of those receiving transplants from siblings. It is usually treated with glucocorticoids, antithymocyte globulin, or monoclonal antibodies targeted against T lymphocytes.

Answer A is incorrect. Hepatic transplantation might be considered if the patient's overall condition improved and lasting effects of GVHD left her with impaired hepatic function. However, a recent bone marrow transplant patient would not be considered a candidate for hepatic transplantation.

Answer B is incorrect. Although removal of T lymphocytes from the stem cell inoculum has been proposed as a method of preventing GVHD, it is associated with increased incidence of graft failure, as well as increased risk of tumor recurrence. No evidence exists suggesting that this method should be instituted.

Answer C is incorrect. Total body irradiation may be performed prior to the transplant. It is not indicated as therapy for GVHD, as it would most likely be fatal, and at the very least would leave the patient requiring a second transplant.

Answer E is incorrect. Thalidomide is an experimental therapy for chronic GVHD. It is not indicated as therapy for acute GVHD.

32. **The correct answer is D.** The odds ratio, which is used primarily in case-control studies, is the ratio of the odds of exposure in those with a disease to the odds of exposure in those without a disease. In terms of the letters shown, the odds ratio is calculated as (a/c) / (b/d) = 3.

    Answer A is incorrect. This is the attributable risk (AR), also called the risk difference, that is used in cohort studies: AR = (a / (a + b)) − (c / (c + d)) = 1/15.

    Answer B is incorrect. An odds ratio of 1 represents no difference, which is not the case from the data presented.

    Answer C is incorrect. This is the relative risk (RR), which is not calculated for case-control studies but rather for cohort studies: RR = (a / (a + b)) / (c / (c + d)) = 5/3.

    Answer E is incorrect. This is the attributable risk percent in the exposed, calculated as ((RR − 1) / RR) × 100 = 60%. RR represents relative risk.

33. **The correct answer is E.** Squamous cell carcinoma and adenocarcinoma are the most common cancers associated with asbestos exposure, which is associated with a sixfold increase in lung cancer. This risk increases to 59-fold with a concurrent smoking history. Therefore the most appropriate intervention is smoking cessation. The average time between the exposure to asbestos and the development of lung cancer is 15 years. The patient has signs and symptoms of asbestosis (shortness of breath, restrictive pattern on pulmonary function testing, and x-ray of the chest that shows linear opacities and pleural plaques). Specific therapy, such as steroids or immunosuppressive or antifibrotic agents, may also be warranted.

Answer A is incorrect. To date, no randomized trial has confirmed the benefit of lung cancer screening using high-resolution CT to reduce lung cancer mortality.

Answer B is incorrect. Pulmonary function testing (PFT) in patients with asbestosis shows a restrictive pattern with a decrease in lung volumes (decreased FEV_1; normal or increased FEV_1:FVC; and decreased FVC, vital capacity, and total lung capacity). PFTs play no role in lung cancer screening. They are warranted in lung cancer patients when surgical resection is considered.

Answer C is incorrect. Unfortunately, surveillance studies such as sputum cytology repeated at intervals of 4–6 months have not been shown to improve early detection or prolong lung cancer survival in high-risk individuals. The most appropriate intervention is smoking cessation.

Answer D is incorrect. Unfortunately, surveillance studies such as chest x-ray repeated at intervals of 4–6 months have not been shown to improve early detection or prolong lung cancer survival in high-risk individuals. The most appropriate intervention is smoking cessation.

34. **The correct answer is D.** The developmental milestones this infant has reached suggest that the child is 2 months old. A mild illness and low-grade fever are not contraindications to receiving immunizations. The standard immunizations given at the 2-month visit are hepatitis B (Hep B) vaccine, diphtheria-tetanus-pertussis (DTaP) vaccine, *Haemophilus influenzae* type b (HiB) vaccine, inactivated poliomyelitis vaccine (IPV), and pneumococcal conjugate vaccine (PCV). The Hep B vaccine is a hepatitis B surface antigen. The DTaP vaccine is a combined vaccine against diphtheria, tetanus, and pertussis. The diphtheria and tetanus portions are toxoids, whereas the pertussis is an acellular pertussis component (DTaP vs. DTP). The HiB vaccine contains killed portions of the *Haemophilus influenzae* type B bacterium. IPV contains three forms of inactivated polio virus. PCV is the pneumococcal conjugate vaccine containing seven strains of *Streptococcus pneumoniae*.

Answer A is incorrect. A child would only receive the Hep B vaccine at birth and at 1 month.

Answer B is incorrect. There is no time when the child would just receive the Hep B and DTaP vaccines.

Answer C is incorrect. There is no time when the child would just receive the Hep B, DTaP, and IPV vaccines.

Answer E is incorrect. A mild illness and low-grade fever are not contraindications to receiving immunizations.

35. **The correct answer is A.** The risk of chromosomal abnormalities in children of women over the age of 35 is 1 in 200. For that reason, amniocentesis, which carries a risk of about 1 in 200 for fetal loss, is recommended for women who will be > 35 years of age at the time of delivery. In conjunction with a triple screen test, amniocentesis has a sensitivity of 65% for trisomy 21, which makes it the next appropriate test for this patient after triple screen.

Answer B is incorrect. A biophysical profile (BPP) is performed in the third trimester if the nonstress test is not reassuring. A BPP can also be done in patients who are postdates, and those who have diabetes, decreased fetal movement, or intrauterine growth restriction. A biophysical profile is a combination of a real-time ultrasound used to assess four parameters of fetal well-being in addition to a nonstress test. The four ultrasound parameters are fetal tone, breathing, movement, and amniotic fluid volume. A reassuring biophysical profile has a score of 8–10. A score of 0–2, however, is grounds for immediate delivery.

Answer C is incorrect. Chorionic villus sampling is performed at 10–12 weeks' gestation, for an earlier assessment of chromosomal abnormalities, with diagnostic accuracy comparable to that of amniocentesis.

Answer D is incorrect. Maternal serum α-fetoprotein (MSAFP) would not add any additional information here; it is already part of the triple screen. It is used to screen for neural tube defects (including anencephaly and spina

bifida), abdominal wall defects (including gastroschisis and omphalocele), multiple gestation, fetal death, and placental abnormalities such as abruption and chromosomal defects (trisomy 18, 21, and 13). The triple screen test (β-human chorionic gonadotropin and estriol in addition to MSAFP) provides increased sensitivity for chromosomal abnormalities.

Answer E is incorrect. A nonstress test (NST) is performed in two clinical scenarios. It may be performed at 32–34 weeks of gestation in high-risk patients. An NST can be done as early as 28 weeks' gestation since 85% of fetuses will be reactive. This test should be considered later on in the pregnancy. Also, all patients who present for evaluation in triage during pregnancy will get an NST, not only high-risk patients.

Answer F is incorrect. Percutaneous umbilical blood sampling (PUBS) is performed by puncturing the umbilical cord vessels, which are not large enough for the procedure until the late second/early third trimesters. PUBS is useful for evaluation of fetal karyotype, or conditions such as infection or erythroblastosis fetalis late in pregnancy.

Answer G is incorrect. Ultrasound was performed in the week prior; it would not be necessary to repeat it at this time.

36. **The correct answer is D.** The National Cholesterol Education Program guidelines recommend that those with low risk for cardiac disease (0–1 risk factor) maintain an LDL cholesterol under 160 mg/dL, but pharmacologic treatment is only recommended if LDL levels go above 190 mg/dL. An LDL cholesterol in between 160 and 190 mg/dL can be treated with therapeutic lifestyle changes. Risk factors include older age, heart disease, diabetes, hypertension, and smoking.

Answer A is incorrect. This level of LDL does not require pharmacologic therapy.

Answer B is incorrect. This level of LDL does not require pharmacologic therapy.

Answer C is incorrect. This is the recommended level above which therapeutic lifestyle changes are recommended.

Answer E is incorrect. This level is too high to be ideal.

37. **The correct answer is A.** Because the enzyme-linked immunosorbent assay (ELISA) test has a false-positive rate of approximately 2%, the results need to be confirmed with a Western blot analysis.

    Answer B is incorrect. If the ELISA test is positive, it will likely be positive again, regardless of whether the positive is false or true. The diagnosis should be confirmed by an independent method.

    Answer C is incorrect. Clinical evidence of an opportunistic infection would support the diagnosis, but is not used as part of the definition of HIV status. Opportunistic infections are part of the definition of AIDS, but may also be indicative of immunosuppression from another source.

    Answer D is incorrect. While unprotected sex is a significant risk factor for HIV infection, this history alone is not diagnostic of active HIV infection in the patient.

    Answer E is incorrect. While a patient with an untreated HIV infection will develop a low CD4+ count, a number of other conditions may lead to generalized lymphopenia, including congenital immunodeficiencies, bone marrow disorders, and hematologic malignancies.

38. **The correct answer is B.** The patient in the question has colon cancer. His presentation and blood tests are consistent with microcytic anemia. The colonoscopy reveals an exophytic mass in the colon consistent with adenocarcinoma. The current American Gastroenterological Association guidelines state that people with first-degree relatives diagnosed with colon cancer or adenomatous polyps diagnosed at an age of < 60 years should be screened with a colonoscopy every 5 years beginning at the age of 40, or 10 years younger than the earliest diagnosis in the family, whichever comes first. Since the patient was diagnosed with colon cancer at the age of 57 the son should be screened at the age of 40 since that is earlier than 10 years younger than his father's diagnosis.

Answer A is incorrect. Since the patient was diagnosed with colon cancer at the age of 57 the son should be screened at the age of 40, since that is earlier than 10 years younger than his father's diagnosis. Furthermore, every 1–2 years is too frequent for screening.

Answer C is incorrect. Screening colonoscopy beginning at the age of 50 is recommended for average-risk individuals and should be repeated every 10 years.

Answer D is incorrect. Since the patient was diagnosed with colon cancer at the age of 57 the son should be screened at the age of 40, since that is earlier than 10 years younger than his father's diagnosis.

Answer E is incorrect. Fecal occult blood testing beginning at the age of 50 is recommended for average-risk individuals and should be repeated every year.

Questions 39 and 40

39. **The correct answer is E.** First-line treatment for hypertension in diabetics with proteinuria is an angiotensin-converting enzyme (ACE) inhibitor such as captopril and enalapril. ACE inhibitors have been shown to decrease mortality and the risk for stroke in diabetic, hypertensive patients. ACE inhibitors have also been shown to slow the progression of renal disease in diabetic, hypertensive patients with proteinuria. ACE inhibitors act by blocking ACE, the enzyme necessary for conversion of angiotensin I to angiotensin II. Angiotensin II causes increased aldosterone production, increased retention of sodium and water, increased output of the sympathetic nervous system, and vasoconstriction of vascular smooth muscle, all leading to increased blood pressure. Therefore, if angiotensin II synthesis is blocked, this leads to a decrease in blood pressure.

40. **The correct answer is G.** First-line treatment for hypertension in patients with osteoporosis is a thiazide diuretic, such as hydrochlorothiazide. Thiazide diuretics act by inhibiting a sodium/chloride cotransporter in the distal tubule, thereby decreasing sodium reabsorp-

tion, which leads to decreased blood pressure. Thiazide diuretics increase the secretion of sodium and potassium, and the reabsorption of calcium. Therefore, patients with hypocalcemia, hypercalciuria, and osteoporosis may benefit from thiazide diuretics in terms of calcium balance.

Answer A is incorrect. Spironolactone antagonizes aldosterone receptors.

Answer B is incorrect. Selective β-blockers antagonize β_1-adrenergic receptors.

Answer C is incorrect. Nonselective β-blockers antagonize β_1- and β_2-adrenergic receptors.

Answer D is incorrect. α_1-Adrenergic blockers antagonize α_1-adrenergic receptors.

Answer F is incorrect. Calcium channel blockers inhibit calcium inflow into vascular smooth muscle and myocardium.

Answer H is incorrect. A loop diuretic blocks loop of Henle sodium and chloride reabsorption.

Answer I is incorrect. Hydralazine directly relaxes smooth muscle.

Answer J is incorrect. Centrally acting adrenergic agonists stimulate α_2-adrenergic receptors.

Answer K is incorrect. ACE inhibitors block, not stimulate, aldosterone formation.

Answer L is incorrect. ACE inhibitors block, not stimulate, angiotensin II formation.

CHAPTER 5

Ethics
and Legal Issues

1. A 65-year-old man presents to the physician's office with his daughter, who is a resident in internal medicine. She encouraged her father to come in because he has experienced a 4.5-kg (10-lb) weight loss in 2 months, as well as decreased appetite and occasional night sweats. She thinks his eyes appear somewhat icteric. After the physician conducts the interview, the physician and the patient's daughter leave so the patient can undress for the examination. Once in the hallway, the daughter says to the physician in a low voice, "I am really afraid that he might have pancreatic cancer, and he would be devastated to find out. Can you please discuss his test results with me first so that we can decide what to tell him together?" How should the physician respond?

(A) "As long as your father agrees to have me discuss his health situation with you privately, I would be happy to do that, and we can decide together what information to give your father. Remember your HIPAA (Health Insurance Portability and Accountability Act) training."

(B) "Don't worry, I doubt that he has pancreatic cancer."

(C) "I am ashamed of you. An internal medicine resident should know better than to ask me that."

(D) "I appreciate your concern, but your father has a right to full disclosure, and it would be inappropriate for me to withhold information from him. Perhaps we can explore with him what information he might like to hear and if he would like for you to be present when we discuss his examination findings and results."

(E) "If this is really important to you, I can tell you the results before I tell your father."

(F) "I would be happy to do that, but first we have to have a full family meeting and discuss together what would be best for your father."

2. A 74-year-old woman with dementia has been in the intensive care unit (ICU) for 14 days following acute respiratory decompensation and renal failure. She is receiving continuous hemodialysis, and her electrolytes have been stable. Her oxygen saturation has been maintained on mandatory mechanical ventilation. She remains in critical condition, but the ICU team believes that she has a reasonable chance of recovering. A living will shows that she has agreed to intubation and resuscitation if necessary. However, her daughter, who is her designated health care proxy and who until now has been in contact with the medical team only by phone, arrives stating that she has power of attorney and asking that her mother be taken off the ventilator. What is the best course of action?

(A) Discuss with the daughter her reasons for withdrawing care

(B) Maintain current management based on the patient's prognosis

(C) Obtain a court order mandating continuation of ventilatory support

(D) Obtain an ethics consultation

(E) Withdraw ventilatory support based on the daughter's power of attorney

3. A 45-year-old woman is scheduled to undergo elective bilateral tubal ligation. The gynecology resident, covering for a colleague, greets the patient in the preoperative area with the consent paper, which outlines the nature and indications of intervention, risks and benefits, and potential alternatives. The physician, however, finds the patient to be a Laotian-speaking woman with limited English skills, and does not seem to understand the resident's explanations. The patient's husband, who speaks some English, offers to translate the physician's explanation and appears to be eager for his wife to undergo the procedure. How should the resident proceed to obtain consent?

(A) Allow the patient's husband to translate

(B) Ask the husband to be a surrogate decision maker and sign the consent

(C) Ask the husband to step out and again explain, slowly and clearly, the informed consent with the patient

(D) Draw an "X" next to the signature line and ask the patient to sign the form

(E) Obtain a translator or translation services for the patient and conduct proper discussion for informed consent

4. An 87-year-old man with prostate cancer, Gleason grade 9, is now receiving palliative care following failure of hormonal therapy and chemotherapy. He has severe bone pain from multiple metastases, despite receiving both bisphosphonate and radiation therapy. His oxygenation is borderline on room air, and he has required supplemental oxygen by face mask. The patient and his family are distraught that he is in so much pain, and they ask the physician to "make the pain stop." The physician explains that raising the dose of opiates will suppress the patient's breathing, but the family repeats their request. What is the best course of action?

(A) Give strong nonsteroidal anti-inflammatory drugs to avoid respiratory depression, even if the pain is not well controlled

(B) Increase the dose of bisphosphonate

(C) Intubate the patient

(D) Medicate the patient with sufficient opioids to control his pain, regardless of respiratory response

(E) Obtain an ethics consultation

5. A patient in clinic has a positive HIV test, first by enzyme-linked immunosorbent assay antibody test and then confirmed by Western blot. She is married, has three children, and is sexually active with her husband. After explaining what the results mean, she is advised that it is important for the husband to be informed of these test results. She appears stunned and frightened by this suggestion. What would be the most appropriate course of action?

(A) Call up the husband and suggest he stop in for an appointment so that he can be informed of the results of the test

(B) Contact the public health department and ask that they inform the husband

(C) Continue persuading the patient of the importance and necessity of informing her husband and offer support and resources to enable her to have this discussion

(D) Send an anonymous letter informing the husband of the exposure

(E) Tell her that it is illegal for her not to inform her husband and other sexual contacts who have been potentially exposed

6. An 85-year-old mentally competent patient is brought to the emergency department (ED) in respiratory distress. No living will is brought with the patient, and before contact is made with the family, the patient requires intubation and pressors and is transferred to the ICU. Broad-spectrum antibiotics are started for a presumed pneumonia. The family, including the patient's wife and children, arrive the next day. A discussion is initiated with the family regarding the patient's wishes as they relate to Do Not Resuscitate (DNR) and Do Not Intubate orders. During this time the patient's wife is declared the surrogate, and she states that she would like the antibiotics continued, but her husband should be DNR. The patient begins to recover and is able to be extubated on day 3 of his hospital care. On CT scan of the chest to evaluate the extent of his pneumonia, he is found to have a pulmonary embolism. A recommendation is made by the hospital staff that he receive an inferior vena cava (IVC) filter. In this situation, under whose authority can the IVC filter be placed?

(A) A court of law

(B) The patient

(C) The patient's children

(D) The patient's doctor

(E) The patient's spouse

7. An 89-year-old woman is diagnosed with metastatic breast cancer to the lungs, bone, and brain. Four months after diagnosis, the patient is admitted to the hospital with excruciating bone pain and changes in her mental status. What term refers to the administration of morphine to relieve this pain with the incidental consequence of causing respiratory depression and death?

(A) Indirect euthanasia

(B) Involuntary active euthanasia

(C) Nonvoluntary active euthanasia

(D) Passive euthanasia

(E) Voluntary active euthanasia

8. A physician is a pediatrician with many adolescents in his practice. One of the patients arrives for an athletic checkup. On examination, he observes needle tracks on the patient's arms. On questioning, the patient admits to recent heroin use. When asked if he would consider treatment, he says yes, but only if he can tell his parents that he is going to an academic camp. What is the most appropriate course of action?

   (A) Detain the boy and admit him to treatment under minor law
   (B) Inform the boy's parents and leave the decision about treatment up to them
   (C) Inform the boy's parents and refer him to a treatment center
   (D) Refer him to a treatment center only
   (E) Refer the patient to another pediatrician

9. A 93-year-old man is transferred to the ED after staff at the long-term care facility note confusion and agitation. He takes many medications, including insulin and a glipizide for diabetes and a β-blocker for hypertension. On examination, the patient mumbles incoherently when not spoken to and yells at the speaker when directly addressed. His temperature is 38.2°C (100.8°F), respiratory rate is 28/min, blood pressure is 135/88 mm Hg, and pulse is 58/min. His oxygen saturation is 72%. A hospital staff member reminds the physician that the patient's chart contains a signed Do Not Resuscitate order. Which of the following is the most appropriate next step in patient management?

   (A) Culture of blood, urine, and sputum
   (B) Haloperidol administration
   (C) No intervention out of respect for the Do Not Resuscitate order
   (D) Oxygen by nasal cannula
   (E) Serum glucose measurement

10. A child is brought into the ED after a trauma. The patient is 10 years old and is bleeding profusely. His parents arrive soon afterward and state that they are Jehovah's Witnesses and do not consent to giving blood to their child, even though to not do so threatens the life of their child. The child, awake and receiving pain medications, agrees with his parents, requesting that he receive no blood. What is the next step in treatment?

    (A) Attempt to save the child, but honor the child's wishes and give no blood
    (B) Attempt to save the child, but honor the parent's wishes and give no blood
    (C) Get a court order, then give the child blood
    (D) Give the child blood immediately, as needed
    (E) Refuse to treat the child with those restrictions placed

11. A 32-year-old woman presents to her primary care physician's office complaining of dysuria, urgency, and frequency. The physician quickly scribbles a prescription for antibiotics, and the patient takes it to the pharmacist, saying "Darn UTI again." A few hours later, the pharmacist contacts the physician's office because she notices that the amount of antibiotics the physician prescribed is 10 times the usual dose given for urinary tract infection. The physician admits that she was distracted by having so many patients waiting to be seen and must have accidentally added an extra zero. What is the most appropriate next step for the physician?

    (A) Ask the pharmacist to explain the error to the patient
    (B) Call the patient, explain what happened, and apologize for the error
    (C) Make a note to be more careful about double-checking prescriptions in the future
    (D) Thank the pharmacist and return to seeing patients; she can tell the patient about the error next time she sees her because no harm was done
    (E) Thank the pharmacist and return to seeing patients; the pharmacist will tell the patient about the error

12. A 75-year-old man is in a persistent vegetative state following a large intracranial bleed secondary to an arteriovenous malformation. Two advance directives are in the chart. One is a living will stating that the patient requests withdrawal of life-sustaining treatment if he were to ever be in a vegetative state. The other is a durable power of attorney form stating that

his brother is the legally designated surrogate health care decision maker. After reading these forms, the brother approaches the physician and requests that the medical team continue to treat, feed, and hydrate the patient. How should the medical team proceed?

(A) The medical team should consult the hospital ethics committee
(B) The medical team should continue to feed and hydrate the patient but not provide additional care (e.g., antibiotics if the patient develops an infection)
(C) The medical team should continue to treat, feed, and hydrate the patient
(D) The medical team should let a court decide how to proceed
(E) The medical team should seek out the opinion of the next closest family member to resolve the issue
(F) The medical team should withdraw all treatment

13. A primary care physician is caring for a patient with stage IV ovarian cancer. The woman, who has chosen to participate in hospice care, asks the physician to give her "something to end it all." What is the most appropriate next step for the physician?

(A) Call the patient's daughter and explain her mother's request
(B) Discuss with the patient her feelings and identify why she is asking for life-ending medication
(C) Provide the patient with a prescription for narcotics
(D) Refer the patient to a psychiatrist
(E) Tell the patient that her request is shocking and such medication will not be provided

14. A 48-year-old woman presents to her gynecologist for evaluation of irregular menses, dyspareunia, and bloating. Her symptoms have been present approximately 4 months. Review of systems uncovers shortness of breath and persistent cough that the patient attributed to her 10 pack-year smoking habit. Pelvic examination is significant for a fixed, nontender left adnexal mass. CT of the pelvis demonstrates a 5.5-cm (2.2-in) ovarian mass, and x-ray of the chest reveals pleural effusion. A surgical staging laparotomy is performed, and frozen sections are consistent with a malignancy of epithelial origin. Of 12 inguinal nodes, 10 are positive for carcinoma. Thoracentesis yields effusion fluid for cytologic diagnosis, which is also positive for carcinomatous cells. The patient is diagnosed with stage IV ovarian cancer. Which of the following characteristics of the patient's disease defines her condition as "terminal"?

(A) Duration of symptoms
(B) Expected survival of < 6 months
(C) Five-year survival is < 5%
(D) Size of primary tumor
(E) Young age at presentation

15. A 46-year-old man with advanced pancreatic cancer is hospitalized following a pancreatic duct stent placement. He has recently been told that he is not a candidate for a Whipple procedure. His previously marked jaundice has improved, but he is experiencing ongoing 8 of 10 abdominal pain. The patient was divorced 6 years ago, and his parents are his only family. Since his procedure, the patient has asked several members of the medical team to help him end his life. What is the appropriate next step?

(A) Admit this patient to hospice care
(B) Call the patient's family and inform them of the patient's request
(C) Consult the psychiatry service about patient's ability to make medical decisions
(D) Evaluate pain management
(E) Increase opioid dosage with the intent of causing respiratory depression

1. **The correct answer is D.** Patients have a right to full disclosure of their medical status, and family members cannot request that the physician withhold information from a patient. Furthermore, without the patient's explicit permission, the physician cannot discuss the patient's health status with anyone else.

Answer A is incorrect. The Health Insurance Portability and Accountability Act of 1996 mandates complete confidentiality in patient care, although patients may allow their physicians to discuss their health situation with specified individuals. Regardless of this, however, the physician still cannot withhold information from the patient at the request of a family member.

Answer B is incorrect. Without the patient's explicit permission, the physician cannot discuss the patient's health status with family members.

Answer C is incorrect. Rather than being dismissive, the physician should address the daughter's concerns, but remind her gently that his obligation is to the patient whose right to full disclosure must be respected.

Answer E is incorrect. Without the patient's explicit permission, the physician cannot discuss the patient's health status with family members.

Answer F is incorrect. A family meeting may be appropriate some time in the future, but first and foremost the patient should be asked what information he wants to hear himself and if he would like to involve his family in decision making.

2. **The correct answer is A.** Before any decision regarding this patient's care is undertaken, the daughter's reasoning must be elucidated. Although she has durable power of attorney, the daughter's decision clearly disagrees with the patient's living will. Patients reserve the right to change their decision within a given set of circumstances. However, when a proxy does so, it must be determined whether the patient might have made the same decision. This determina-

tion is difficult but must be done to rule out any conflict of interest or ulterior motives by the daughter.

Answer B is incorrect. Maintaining current management without first addressing the daughter's concerns is inappropriate.

Answer C is incorrect. If, after questioning, any conflicts of interest are found and the daughter continues to insist on withdrawal of care, it may be necessary to obtain a court order to maintain support.

Answer D is incorrect. Although an ethics consultation may eventually be necessary, the daughter's motives must be delineated first.

Answer E is incorrect. Durable power of attorney allows a surrogate to make decisions on the patient's behalf in cases of incapacity. However, because this patient has a living will that contradicts the choice made by the daughter, the daughter's choice should not be automatically accepted.

3. **The correct answer is E.** The patient must be informed of all components of an informed consent in a language that she understands. The only appropriate way to discuss the informed consent is through a translator.

Answer A is incorrect. Although it would be convenient to ask the husband to translate, the husband is untrained in translation. Due to his intimate relationship with the patient and potentially biased views, an independent, professional translator should be used.

Answer B is incorrect. The patient is not incapacitated but needs proper translation to understand the situation and the risks and benefits of the procedure.

Answer C is incorrect. The patient does not understand English and therefore a repeated discussion will be of no additional benefit. Translator service is needed for proper informed consent.

Answer D is incorrect. The patient needs to be informed properly before signing the consent paperwork.

4. **The correct answer is D.** Treating a patient's pain with the risk of hastening death has been addressed and supported by both the U.S. Supreme Court and the Catholic Church. In *Vacco v. Quill* (1997), Justice O'Connor stated that a patient has no legal barrier to receiving relief from pain "even to the point of causing unconsciousness and hastening death." The Catholic Church has adopted the principle of double effect, whereby the hastening of death as an adverse effect of pain relief is morally acceptable if there was no intention of doing so by the treating physician.

Answer A is incorrect. Providing inadequate pain relief to prevent respiratory depression is inappropriate unless it is the desire of the patient.

Answer B is incorrect. The first step in relieving chronic pain is to attempt to remove or lessen the inciting factor. However, because that treatment has failed, the physician should directly relieve the sensation of pain. In this case, the patient is already on palliative care.

Answer C is incorrect. Although intubating the patient would secure the airway and allow full use of opioids, it would entail taking the patient off palliative care, a decision that must be made first by either the patient or the family.

Answer E is incorrect. In this case, both the law and moral consensus support the principle of double effect, which holds that a physician may relieve pain even if it hastens death. The case is clear enough that an ethics consultation would probably not be necessary.

5. **The correct answer is C.** The patient should be convinced to disclose this information personally to her husband and the practitioner should not directly contact the husband; this is the best way to maintain a trusting and open doctor-patient relationship. Support should be made available to the patient so that she can inform the husband. Disease intervention specialists or HIV partner counseling and referral services, operating out of the department of health, may serve as valuable resources to help patients contact their partners. These services vary from state to state, but they can be offered to patients to facilitate this process.

Answer A is incorrect. Going behind the patient's back is inappropriate; however, in some states there are laws that protect the physician from legal liability for breach of confidentiality if they do inform third parties of HIV exposure. The physician is protected, however, only after efforts by the physician have failed to convince the primary patient to disclose this information to his or her sexual contacts.

Answer B is incorrect. The ideal situation is one in which the patient informs her husband, and so the most appropriate response is to continue persuading the patient to reveal this information. However, if the patient does not feel comfortable revealing this information, especially in settings of domestic violence, a public health agency may be asked, with consent of the patient, to intervene and attempt to contact the spouse.

Answer D is incorrect. If the patient refuses to inform her husband, then depending on the state there might be other avenues by which sexual partners may be contacted. Sending an anonymous letter informing the husband of the exposure, however, would likely damage the doctor-patient and husband-wife relationships.

Answer E is incorrect. As a rule, partner notification is confidential and voluntary. Disease intervention specialists cannot inform third parties without the consent of the infected persons. Contacts are also typically not informed of the identity of the source.

6. **The correct answer is B.** Whenever possible, consent for any treatment or procedure should be obtained from the patient. In this situation, although the patient's wife was the surrogate, her decision-making capacity ended when the patient was extubated and was able to speak for himself.

Answer A is incorrect. A court of law is only utilized when a disagreement occurs among members of a patient's family and/or the physician is in charge of the patient's care.

Answer C is incorrect. The patient's children are not in a position to make decisions on behalf of the patient because the patient has the capacity to make his own decisions and his wife is his surrogate.

Answer D is incorrect. The patient's doctor can suggest the best treatment, but when family members are present they make decisions for the patient if the patient does not have the ability to make decisions himself.

Answer E is incorrect. The patient's spouse, although she is the surrogate decision maker, can no longer make decisions when the patient is extubated and able to communicate for himself.

7. **The correct answer is A.** The administration of morphine or other medications to relieve pain with the incidental consequence of causing respiratory depression leading to death is known as indirect euthanasia and is legal everywhere in the United States.

Answer B is incorrect. Involuntary active euthanasia involves intentionally giving medications or interventions to cause a patient's death when the patient is competent to consent but does not.

Answer C is incorrect. Nonvoluntary active euthanasia involves providing these medications or interventions to a patient who is incapable of consent.

Answer D is incorrect. Passive euthanasia is the withholding or withdrawing of life-sustaining treatments to let a patient die.

Answer E is incorrect. Voluntary active euthanasia is defined as the intentional administration of medication or of an intervention to cause a patient's death with their informed consent.

8. **The correct answer is D.** Just as minors are exempt from parental consent or involvement when they are treated for sexually transmitted diseases and pregnancy counseling, they may also undergo drug rehabilitation without parental knowledge.

Answer A is incorrect. Patients may not be forcibly detained except when they are an immediate risk to themselves or others.

Answer B is incorrect. The boy has the right to confidentiality when seeking drug rehabilitation.

Answer C is incorrect. Inform the boy's parents and refer him to a treatment center.

Answer E is incorrect. Referring the patient to another pediatrician would be unethical and nonbeneficial for this patient. It is important to communicate with the patient and allow him to make decisions for himself.

9. **The correct answer is D.** Attention in the emergency department must first be directed to the **ABCs** (**A**irway, **B**reathing, and **C**irculation). Because he is conversant, the patient's airway is intact. His respiration rate indicates some distress, and his oxygen saturation is low. Oxygen supplementation via mask or nasal cannula is in order, and it is possible that this may be sufficient to begin to improve the patient's mental status while other problems are sought and addressed. Do Not Resuscitate (DNR) does not mean "do not treat." Taken literally, a DNR order only applies after cardiac arrest has occurred, although in practice some actions that may be undertaken prior to cardiac arrest (e.g., endotracheal intubation) may be considered resuscitative. DNR orders may sometimes be written as DNR/DNI (Do Not Intubate), if that is the patient's wish, to help ease confusion.

Answer A is incorrect. Multiple cultures may reveal an underlying infection, but attention must first be paid to the ABCs.

Answer B is incorrect. Haloperidol administration may be necessary later in the patient's treatment, but in this patient attention to and stabilization of the ABCs should be addressed first.

Answer C is incorrect. The patient requires evaluation and treatment, not resuscitation. Therefore, the Do Not Resuscitate order is not yet in force.

Answer E is incorrect. Serum glucose measurement would be warranted and could be instructive, but attention must first be paid to the ABCs.

10. **The correct answer is D.** Treatment can be initiated on the basis of legal precedent. This patient is 10 years old, and is not emancipated. Legally, he does not have the ability to refuse

treatment. His parents cannot refuse treatment for him if that refusal will pose a serious health risk.

Answer A is incorrect. Not giving blood is withholding life-saving treatment. Legally, a physician can give blood to a minor against his and his parents' wishes when to not do so would be hastening the child's death.

Answer B is incorrect. Not giving blood is withholding life-saving treatment. Legally, a physician can give blood to a minor against his and his parents' wishes when to not do so would be hastening the child's death.

Answer C is incorrect. In a less life-threatening situation, a court order should be obtained to treat the minor against his parent's wishes. Under these emergent circumstances, it is necessary to treat the patient first, and is legal to do so.

Answer E is incorrect. Refusing to treat would be to give in to the parents' demands, thus hastening the child's death.

11. **The correct answer is B.** The physician has an obligation to fully disclose any errors made in patient care. The most effective and responsible way to do this is to call the patient immediately, explain what happened, and apologize. This is particularly easy in this case because no harm was done. Furthermore, acknowledgment of an error and an apology can help the physician avoid litigation.

Answer A is incorrect. It is the physician's responsibility to disclose the error directly to the patient.

Answer C is incorrect. Although this is a good practice, the physician should also inform the patient of the error.

Answer D is incorrect. Even though no harm was done with this error, it is appropriate and responsible to inform the patient about the error. By doing this, the physician can also enlist the help of the patient in preventing further errors because the patient can be more vigilant about her care and detect future errors. Medical errors due to human faults are inevitable, and it is appropriate to do anything possible to help prevent errors in the future.

Answer E is incorrect. It is the physician's responsibility to disclose the error directly to the patient; she should not rely on someone else to do so.

12. **The correct answer is F.** A living will is a legal document written by the patient dictating the patient's wishes about withholding or withdrawing life-sustaining treatment in the event of a terminal disease or a persistent vegetative state. In this case, the patient meets criteria for persistent vegetative state and therefore the medical team should follow the patient's written request and withdraw life-sustaining treatment. If the living will were not present, the surrogate health care decision maker would have had authority to dictate how to proceed with treatment. Although surrogates should typically make decisions consistent with the stated wishes of the patient, this case highlights the importance of patients making their wishes known in a format such as the living will.

Answer A is incorrect. The hospital ethics committee does not need to be consulted because the living will clearly states the appropriate course of action for the given clinical situation.

Answer B is incorrect. According to the living will, all life-sustaining treatment should be withdrawn.

Answer C is incorrect. In this case, the patient meets criteria for persistent vegetative state and therefore the medical team should follow the patient's written request and withdraw life sustaining treatment.

Answer D is incorrect. The court does not need to be involved because the living will clearly states the appropriate course of action for the given clinical situation.

Answer E is incorrect. Although a close family member should be consulted for decision making if a living will or designated health care proxy is not present, both are available and the living will in this case dictates care.

13. **The correct answer is B.** Taking time to understand a patient's emotions and reasons for asking for life-ending measures is the correct answer. Understanding why the patient has

made such a request will help address the underlying problem.

Answer A is incorrect. Calling the woman's daughter without her permission violates patient privacy rights and should not be the physician's next step. The physician should discuss the problem with the patient and call family members only with the patient's permission.

Answer C is incorrect. Physician-assisted suicide is unethical and illegal throughout the United States, except in the state of Oregon. The physician should not provide the patient with medication that is intended to be life-ending.

Answer D is incorrect. Before immediately referring the patient to another physician, it is most appropriate to understand her emotional state and identify her underlying problem.

Answer E is incorrect. Passing judgment on the patient is not the most appropriate step and should be avoided. The physician should gain an understanding of the woman's position in a nonthreatening, nonjudgmental manner.

14. **The correct answer is B.** "Terminal" illness is that which is expected to cause the demise of the patient within the next 6 months. The distinction may be critical for such administrative matters as admittance to hospice or early pension benefits from employers.

Answer A is incorrect. Duration of symptoms may suggest the progression of the disease over time but does not indicate patient life expectancy.

Answer C is incorrect. Although the 5-year survival rate for stage IV ovarian cancer is in fact < 5%, population survival rates do not, by themselves, define terminal illness. Each patient has individual factors that contribute to his or her survival and must be individually evaluated.

Answer D is incorrect. Although the size of the primary tumor is important in disease staging, it is not the definitive factor in patient survival.

Answer E is incorrect. Some ovarian and breast cancers do tend to be more aggressive when presenting in younger individuals; however, age is not a component of the 'terminal illness' definition.

15. **The correct answer is D.** Inadequate pain control and comorbid depression are the two most common causes of such a request by a patient, and both should be evaluated in this situation.

Answer A is incorrect. Although admission to hospice care may be necessary for this patient to control pain and provide adequate support for the patient, such major decisions should not be made in the setting of poor pain management.

Answer B is incorrect. The patient's family should not be informed of this unless the patient has made an active attempt on his life and a medical decision that the patient is not able to make is necessary. It is illegal to comply with a patient's requests for euthanasia.

Answer C is incorrect. The patient may be temporarily unable to make medical decisions but psychiatry's involvement should be focused on the patient's ability to cope with his diagnosis.

Answer E is incorrect. Pain control should be appropriate to the disease process. It is ethical to provide palliative care even if it may hasten the patient's death, but it should not be the cause of death. Physician-assisted suicide involves a physician's writing a prescription for a drug that will allow the patient to end his or her own life. Currently, this is legal only in Oregon and only after specific legal procedures have been followed.

CHAPTER 6

Gastrointestinal

1. A 54-year-old man presents to his primary care provider with the complaint of upper abdominal fullness and pain. He states that he has lost 2.3–4.6 kg (5–10 lb), but denies other symptoms. Physical examination reveals a firm mass in the epigastric area. Ultrasonography reveals an echoic mass in the gastric antrum. A salivary gland biopsy reveals the pathology shown in the image. Which of the following therapies is expected to be part of his treatment plan?

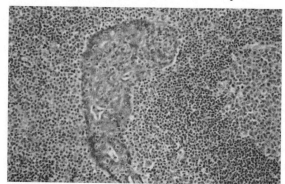

Reproduced, with permission, from Lichtman MA, Beutler E, Kipps TJ, Seligsohn U, Kaushansky K, Prchal JT. *Williams Hematology*, 7th ed. New York: McGraw-Hill, 2006: Plate XXII-21.

(A) Antibiotic therapy
(B) Bone marrow transplantation
(C) Gene therapy
(D) Liver transplantation
(E) Multiagent chemotherapy
(F) Resection of mass and gastric antrum

2. A 55-year-old white man with a 20-year history of gastroesophageal reflux visits the clinic for worsening reflux symptoms over the past 18 months. His last visit was 7 years ago and he claims to be otherwise in good health. He has been compliant with his antireflux medications, including an H₂-blocker and a proton pump inhibitor. At this visit, it is most appropriate to perform which of the following?

(A) Double the dose of his H₂-blocker and schedule him for follow-up in 4 weeks
(B) Double the dose of his proton pump inhibitor and schedule him for follow-up in 4 weeks
(C) Perform an esophagoscopy
(D) Schedule him for elective esophagectomy
(E) Schedule him for emergent Nissen fundoplication

3. The physician on call is paged to the well-baby nursery because a full-term, 3-hour-old boy has had green emesis twice. He has vomited after each of his feedings. He is being breast-fed. He was born by spontaneous vaginal delivery following a pregnancy complicated by polyhydramnios. His Apgar scores were 8 and 9 at 1 and 5 minutes, respectively. His temperature is 37°C (98.6°F), blood pressure is 70/50 mm Hg, pulse is 150/min, and respiratory rate is 24/min. His upper abdomen is distended, soft, and without palpable masses. Air is visualized in the duodenum and the stomach on x-ray. Which of the following is the most likely diagnosis?

(A) Duodenal atresia
(B) Hirschsprung's disease
(C) Intussusception
(D) Malrotation with volvulus
(E) Pyloric stenosis

4. A 68-year-old African-American man presents to his primary care physician for a checkup. He has not been to the physician's office in over 15 years. He reports that he is fine but that his wife keeps telling him that he has to "go see the doctor." He tells us that he has never been sick, and this despite smoking 3 packs a day for over 40 years. He also says that he drinks 2–3 beers a night but never had a problem with that either. He's as healthy "as a bull," he says. His wife is in the room and says that he recently has had some problems swallowing food and that he is losing weight. He laughs and says, "I just need to chew more and eat more." His vitals are normal, as are his lab-

oratory values. The physician is concerned and orders an endoscopy, which reveals a biopsy positive for squamous cell carcinoma of the esophagus. Which of the following is most likely to have prevented this condition?

(A) Alcohol and smoking cessation
(B) Eating more meats, especially smoked meats
(C) Getting a colonoscopy every 5 years
(D) Eating fewer fruits and vegetables
(E) Taking proton pump inhibitors regularly

5. A 58-year-old man comes to the emergency department (ED) complaining of colicky abdominal pain over the past 3 days that suddenly became more severe and constant over the past 6 hours. A contrast study is performed (see image). What is the first-line treatment after fluid resuscitation and nasogastric tube placement?

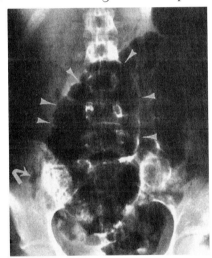

Reproduced, with permission, from Chen MYM, Pope TL, Ott DJ. *Basic Radiology.* New York: McGraw-Hill, 2004: Figure 8-29.

(A) Colonoscopy
(B) Hemicolectomy
(C) Proximal colostomy with delayed resection
(D) Sigmoid colectomy
(E) Sigmoidoscopy

6. A full-term 6-day-old boy presents to a physician's office for routine care. He is tolerating breast milk well. He is urinating, defecating, and sleeping normally. Physical examination reveals an alert newborn with mild eczema, good skin turgor, normal reflexes, and a musty odor. His newborn laboratory screen is notable for phenylketones in the urine. What advice should the parents be given about his diet?

(A) Increase iron
(B) Increase niacin
(C) Increase phenylalanine
(D) Increase tyrosine
(E) Increase vitamin D

7. A 59-year-old woman with a known history of renal cell carcinoma presents to the ED with severe right upper quadrant (RUQ) pain. On physical examination, she is afebrile, acutely tender in the RUQ, and has shifting dullness and a palpable liver edge. Murphy's sign is negative. Laboratory studies reveal a normal complete blood count and:

Na$^+$	138 mEq/L
K$^+$	3.6 mEq/L
Glucose	80 mg/dL
Aspartate aminotransferase	50 U/L
Alanine aminotransferase	43 U/L
Alkaline phosphatase	138 U/L
Total protein	64 g/dL
Albumin	3.8 g/dL
Total bilirubin	1.1 mg/dL

Imaging demonstrates a spider web of collateral veins in the liver. Although extensive measures are taken, the patient expires 6 hours after arriving. What was the most likely initial treatment?

(A) β-Blocker followed by lactulose
(B) Cholecystectomy
(C) Endoscopic retrograde cholangiopancreatography with dilation of the common bile duct
(D) Exploratory laparotomy
(E) Tissue plasminogen activator followed by anticoagulation

8. A 74-year-old man presents to the ED with abdominal pain. The pain is deep and aching in quality and is localized to the left lower quadrant. The man reports multiple episodes of diarrhea over the preceding week. He reports having multiple similar episodes of abdominal pain in the past. On physical examination he is febrile and has tenderness to palpation of the left lower quadrant. His WBC count is 23,000/mm^3. X-ray of the abdomen is shown in the image. What is the most likely diagnosis?

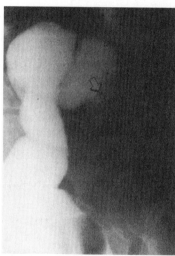

Reproduced, with permission, from Chen MYM, Pope TL, Ott DJ. *Basic Radiology.* New York: McGraw-Hill, 2004: Figure 10-58.

(A) Angiodysplasia
(B) Carcinoid syndrome
(C) Carcinoma of the colon
(D) Diverticulitis
(E) Infectious colitis

9. A 60-year-old man with no past medical history undergoes upper endoscopy and biopsy for an upset stomach that is worsened by eating and is found to have inflammation predominantly in the antrum of the stomach. Which of the following is the most likely etiology of this condition?

(A) Alcohol abuse
(B) Cigarette smoking
(C) Iatrogenic
(D) Infection
(E) Spicy foods

10. A 21-year-old man presents to the Medicaid clinic feeling tired and generally unwell. He has fallen several times over the past month and has developed a slight tremor in both hands. Physical examination is significant for scleral icterus, ankle edema, and a distended and tense abdomen. Laboratory studies show:

Hemoglobin	7 g/dL
Reticulocyte count	7%
Total bilirubin	3.1 mg/dL
Aspartate aminotransferase	84 U/L
Alanine aminotransferase	92 U/L
Ceruloplasmin (normal: 20–45 mg/dL)	5 mg/dL
Coombs test	Negative

What is an appropriate preventive management step after chelation therapy?

(A) Blood protein electrophoresis
(B) Colonoscopy
(C) Electrocardiogram (ECG)
(D) Schilling test
(E) Upper endoscopy

11. A 45-year-old HIV-positive woman comes to her primary care physician complaining of a 2-day history of bloody diarrhea. She states that she has been feeling well until 2 days ago when she developed abdominal pain. She denies fevers, chills, night sweats, nausea, or vomiting. She admits to feeling tired over the last couple of weeks and has had a 2.3-kg (5-lb) weight loss over the last 2 weeks. Her stool sample shows leukocytes and RBCs. Her Gram stain reveals gram-negative rods. Her CD4+ count is 201/mm^3. What is the most likely cause of this woman's symptoms?

(A) *Escherichia coli*
(B) Kaposi's sarcoma
(C) *Legionella*
(D) *Mycobacterium avium* complex
(E) *Mycobacterium tuberculosis*

12. A 76-year-old man who has had multiple episodes of pancreatitis presents to his physician's office with mild epigastric pain and 9.1-kg (20.0-lb) weight loss over the last 6 months. The patient also describes daily foul-smelling stools that "float" in the toilet bowl. The physician pulls up his electronic medical record and finds that the patient presented to the ED last week for the same symptoms. During that visit, he had a CT scan of the abdomen (see image). What is the appropriate treatment for this patient?

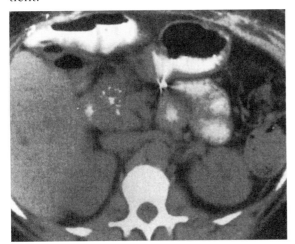

Reproduced, with permission, from Chen MYM, Pope TL, Ott DJ. *Basic Radiology*. New York: McGraw-Hill, 2004: Figure 11-62.

(A) Endoscopic retrograde cholangiopancreatography
(B) Pancreatic enzyme replacement
(C) Pancreaticogastrostomy
(D) Surgical resection of pancreas
(E) Whipple procedure

13. A 62-year-old woman is transferred to the medical service with an appendiceal mass serendipitously picked up at the edge of an x-ray taken of a broken femur in the emergency department. Otherwise, the patient has no significant past medical history and no current symptoms. Which of the following studies is most likely to be useful?

(A) Arterial blood gas
(B) CT of the chest and abdomen
(C) Immediate ECG
(D) MRI of the chest and abdomen
(E) Room air oxygen saturation

14. A 55-year-old white woman with a history of iron deficiency anemia has had intermittent trouble swallowing solids for the past few years. She denies alcohol or tobacco use. Her vital signs are stable. Her iron panel shows that her iron level is 40 µg/dL (normal: 50–175 µg/dL) and total iron binding capacity is 500 µg/dL (normal: 350–460 µg/dL). Other laboratory tests are within normal limits. Which of the following is the most likely diagnosis?

(A) Achalasia
(B) Barrett's esophagus
(C) Esophageal carcinoma
(D) Mallory-Weiss syndrome
(E) Plummer-Vinson syndrome
(F) Reflux esophagitis
(G) Symptomatic diffuse esophageal spasm

15. A premature newborn is being treated in the neonatal intensive care unit. He is noted on the sixth day of life to be lethargic and is experiencing mild respiratory distress. His heart rate is 162/min, blood pressure is 55/38 mm Hg, and respiratory rate is 56/min. In addition to a distended abdomen, he has guaiac-positive stools on physical examination. An x-ray of the abdomen shows gas bubbles within the bowel wall. From what potentially life-threatening condition is this patient most likely suffering?

(A) Bowel obstruction
(B) Intussusception
(C) Meconium ileus
(D) Meningitis
(E) Necrotizing enterocolitis

16. A 45-year-old white man with unknown history is brought to the emergency department by ambulance. He is waving wildly, trying to hit the "flying bats" that are all around him. He is very agitated and strongly smells of alcohol. The ambulance crew informs the physician that the patient was found bleeding from the mouth outside a bar. They could not find any laceration on his mouth or lips and believe that the bleeding is internal. The patient screams that he will not stand for this maltreatment any longer and tries to stand up, at which point he begins to vomit. Blood pours out of his mouth, and the patient says, "Here we go again." The ambulance crew tells the physician that there was also a lot of vomit at the bar where he was found. The physician is able to subdue the patient to obtain his vital signs. His blood pressure is 118/78 mm Hg, pulse is 98/min, respiratory rate is 22/min, and temperature is 37.2°C (98.9°F). The physician is unable to obtain a history on the patient or contact any relatives or friends. No signs of obvious trauma are observed. What is the next best step in diagnosis?

(A) Barium swallow
(B) Electrocardiogram
(C) Endoscopy
(D) Esophageal manometry
(E) X-ray of the chest

17. A 65-year-old man comes to the ED complaining of left lower abdominal pain that began the prior morning. He became concerned when he developed bloody diarrhea overnight. He has experienced similar pain, although to a lesser degree, over the past 2 months, especially after eating. The pain usually resolved within 1–2 hours, and he never had bloody diarrhea. His past medical history is significant for coronary artery disease and hypertension. He has smoked 1 pack of cigarettes per day for the past 30 years. On physical examination, he is afebrile. He has a heart rate of 90/min, and his blood pressure is 135/85 mm Hg. He is visibly uncomfortable but in no apparent distress. His abdominal examination is significant for left lower quadrant tenderness but no guarding or rebound. What is the most likely diagnosis?

(A) Acute mesenteric ischemia
(B) Colon cancer
(C) Diverticulitis
(D) Infectious colitis
(E) Inflammatory bowel disease

18. A 70-year-old man with a history of constipation has been experiencing intermittent left-sided abdominal pain and fevers for 2 days. He came to the ED immediately after he noticed blood in his toilet this morning. His heart rate is 110/min, blood pressure is 90/50 mm Hg, respiratory rate is 18/min, and his oxygen saturation is 95% on room air. On physical examination the physician notes copious amounts of bright red blood per rectum. The physician immediately places two large-bore intravenous lines, administers fluid, and sends blood for type and screen. What is the next step in the management of this patient?

(A) Arteriography
(B) Colonoscopy
(C) Endoscopy
(D) Nasogastric tube aspiration
(E) Surgical consultation

19. A 3-year-old boy is brought to the pediatrician because his mother has noticed a reddish-purple rash on his buttocks, thigh, and legs (shown in the image). She notes that he has not seemed well since he had a mild cold 2

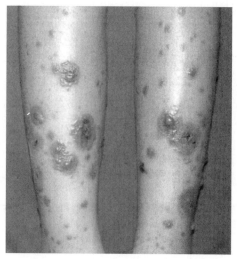

Reproduced, with permission, from Lichtman MA, Beutler E, Kipps TJ, Seligsohn U, Kaushansky K, Prchal JT. *Williams Hematology*, 7th ed. New York: McGraw-Hill, 2006: Figure XXV-15.

weeks earlier; he has been complaining of aches and pains in his legs and a stomach ache. Urinalysis shows 10–20 RBCs/hpf and 2+ proteinuria. Which of the following is associated with this patient's disease process?

(A) Hemoptysis
(B) High antistreptolysin O titer
(C) Impaired glucose tolerance
(D) Intussusception
(E) Malar rash

20. A 63-year-old man with a history of diabetes is called by his primary care physician because of abnormal liver function test results. Relevant laboratory findings are:

Aspartate aminotransferase	85 U/L
Alanine aminotransferase	102 U/L
Alkaline phosphatase	180 U/L
Total bilirubin	1.9 mg/dL

On physical examination his liver is enlarged. His skin has a slightly yellow hue, especially on his face. The review of symptoms is significant for some weight loss, weakness, arthritis in his hands, and decreased libido. What test would generate the most likely diagnosis and should be done first?

(A) Blood smear
(B) CT scan of the abdomen
(C) Endoscopic retrograde cholangiopancreatography
(D) Fasting transferrin saturation levels
(E) Liver biopsy

21. A 50-year-old woman undergoes screening colonoscopy at her primary care physician's recommendation. She has no family history of colorectal cancer. A single lesion is removed during the procedure and sent for pathologic examination. Which of the following findings carries the greatest risk of malignancy?

(A) Lymphoid polyp
(B) Peutz-Jeghers polyp
(C) Tubular adenoma
(D) Tubulovillous adenoma
(E) Villous adenoma

22. A 61-year-old man in previously excellent health presents to his physician with complaints of hematochezia, tenesmus, and rectal pain. On workup, the physician discovers that he has a rectal tumor that is 5 cm from the anal verge. Given the location of the tumor, what is the most appropriate treatment?

(A) Abdominoperineal resection
(B) Imatinib
(C) Low anterior resection
(D) Radiation alone
(E) Radiation plus chemotherapy

23. A full-term 5-day-old African-American girl is taken to the pediatrician because her "eyes look yellow." She is being exclusively formula fed with an iron-rich formula. She has six wet diapers a day and stools twice a day. The pregnancy was uncomplicated and she was delivered by spontaneous vaginal delivery. Her Apgar scores were 9 and 10 at 1 and 5 minutes, respectively. On examination, her temperature is 37°C (98.6°F), her head circumference is in the 50th percentile, and her weight is 3420 g (3 g below her birth weight). Her sclerae are icteric. There is no hepatomegaly or splenomegaly. Her total bilirubin is 9 mg/dL and her conjugated bilirubin is 0.2 mg/dL. Hemoglobin is 15 g/dL. Which of the following is the most likely diagnosis?

(A) α_1-Antitrypsin deficiency
(B) Biliary atresia
(C) Dubin-Johnson syndrome
(D) Physiologic jaundice
(E) Rotor syndrome

24. A 64-year-old white woman with a history of breast cancer treated with lumpectomy and radiation, hypertension, high cholesterol, and ovarian polyps presents to her primary care physician complaining of difficulty and pain with swallowing, as well as occasional chest pain. She indicates that her problem started with liquids, but has progressed to solids, and that the food "just gets stuck in my throat." The chest pain was once so bad that she took one of her husband's nitroglycerin pills and the pain subsided, but it has since occurred many times. The physician orders an x-ray of the chest, but it is not diagnostic. Manometry is conducted, and it shows uncoordinated contractions. Which of the following is the most likely diagnosis?

(A) Breast cancer relapse
(B) Diffuse esophageal spasm
(C) Esophageal cancer
(D) Myocardial infarction
(E) Nutcracker esophagus

25. A 32-year-old man with a history of Crohn's disease presents to the ED with acute-onset diffuse abdominal pain and emesis. The patient states that these symptoms are different than his usual Crohn's disease flare-ups. The pain is severe (10/10) and is cramping in nature. The patient states that his abdomen feels larger than usual. His Crohn's disease has been well managed on 6-mercaptopurine for the past 6 months. The patient denies any recent sick contacts or eating underprepared foods. He states that he has had a bowel movement and flatus since the abdominal pain began. In addition to Crohn's disease, the patient has a past medical history significant for appendicitis for which he underwent an appendectomy 12 years ago. His temperature is 37.1°C (98.7°F), blood pressure is 135/86 mm Hg, pulse is 84/min, and respiratory rate is 14/min. On physical examination, the abdomen is distended and diffusely tender with high-pitched bowel sounds. There is rebound tenderness throughout the abdomen along with guarding. The remainder of the physical examination is noncontributory. An x-ray of the abdomen was obtained in which dilated small loops of bowel were noted along with absence of gas in the colon. What is the next step in the management of this patient?

(A) Bowel rest only
(B) Intravenous fluids and antibiotics only
(C) Laparotomy
(D) MRI of the abdomen
(E) Ultrasound

26. A 39-year-old Japanese-American woman with a history of insulin-dependent diabetes and asthma presents to her primary care physician complaining of trouble swallowing for the past few months. She explains that it started with solids, which she noticed when she could not swallow sandwiches for lunch, and then progressed to liquids. She states it now is hard even to swallow water and that she is often very thirsty. She says she has lost about 3.2 kg (7 lb), but says she is working out frequently. Her blood pressure is 118/76 mm Hg, pulse is 86/min, respiratory rate is 16/min, and temperature is 37.2°C (98.9°F). Laboratory tests show:

Na^+	144 mEq/L
K^+	4.0 mEq/L
Cl^-	100 mEq/L
Carbon dioxide (normal: 22–28 mmol/L)	22 mmol/L
Blood urea nitrogen	18 mg/dL
Creatinine	1.0 mg/dL
Glucose	88 mg/dL

Her hemoglobin A_{1c} level, measured 3 months earlier, was 6.1 g/dL. A barium swallow is performed, which reveals a dilated esophagus, especially distally, that flares out near the lower esophageal junction. Still not completely sure of the diagnosis, esophageal manometry is performed, which reveals abnormal peristalsis and increased lower sphincter pressure. Which of the following is the best management option for this patient?

(A) Cholinergic agents
(B) Glucose pharmacotherapy
(C) Instruct patient to elevate the bed, avoid fatty foods, and consider a histamine blocker
(D) Pneumatic dilation
(E) Surgery to remove diverticula

27. A 75-year-old woman with a history of diabetes and coronary heart failure presents to the ED because of increasing abdominal girth. In recent months, she has been feeling increasingly fatigued, and although she has had decreased appetite, she has gained weight. On physical examination, she has a heart rate of 100/min and blood pressure of 112/70 mm Hg. She has scleral icterus; the skin over her face, neck, and lower legs is slightly bronze in color; she has palmar erythema; and she has numerous ecchymoses over her body. Her abdominal examination is significant for the presence of ascites. Her laboratory values are significant for:

Aspartate transaminase	102 U/L
Alanine transaminase	97 U/L
Alkaline phosphatase	300 U/L
Total bilirubin	1.9 mg/dL
Albumin	2.9 g/dL
Prothrombin time	22 seconds
Partial thromboplastin time	42 seconds

An ultrasound of her abdomen shows a shrunken and nodular liver. Based on the patient's most likely diagnosis, what is a likely complication of her disease?

(A) Acute pancreatitis
(B) Amyloidosis
(C) Bone marrow failure
(D) Hepatocellular carcinoma
(E) Splenomegaly

28. A term baby boy with Apgar scores of 9 and 9 at 1 and 5 minutes, respectively, has failed to pass meconium at 72 hours of life. He has had no episodes of emesis, and his abdomen is only mildly distended to palpation. The patient's mother reports that her older son had the same problem at birth. A plain radiograph of the abdomen shows a small bowel obstruction with numerous air-filled loops of bowel. The patient is treated with a Gastrografin enema with good results. What is the mechanism for this infant's acute intestinal problem?

(A) Congenital aganglionosis of the colon
(B) Deficiency of pancreatic enzymes
(C) Intussusception of the large bowel
(D) Total absence of the small bowel
(E) Volvulus of the transverse colon

29. A 75-year-old woman comes to the ED with complaints of nausea and nonbilious, nonbloody vomiting over the past 4 days. The patient reports that both the nausea and vomiting come in "waves"; that is, several hours will pass during which she feels well before the vomiting suddenly recurs. A detailed history reveals that the woman was told several months ago that she "has stones in her gallbladder," but she has been too frightened to undergo surgery. She has not had a bowel movement for 7 days. Her physical examination reveals a temperature of 38.4°C (101.1°F) and a distended abdomen with high-pitched bowel sounds. What is the most appropriate initial test for a patient with suspected gallstone ileus?

(A) Abdominal ultrasound
(B) Diagnostic laparoscopy
(C) Endoscopic retrograde cholangiopancreatography
(D) Hepatic iminodiacetic acid scan
(E) Plain x-ray of the abdomen

30. A 62-year-old woman with a history of diabetes mellitus presents to the ED complaining of severe abdominal pain for the past 12 hours, first beginning as dull pain near the umbilicus but now localized to the right lower quadrant. She initially thought she was suffering from heartburn, but decided to come to the hospital because of the unrelenting pain. The patient reports that just prior to examination by the physician, she experienced a sudden decrease in intensity of pain, but she remains feeling very uncomfortable and must remain on the stretcher. On examination, the patient appears in distress secondary to pain, tachycardic, slightly hypotensive, and febrile at 39°C (102°F). She has a diffusely tender abdomen with point tenderness over her right lower quadrant, accompanied by guarding and rebound. Laboratory values showed a leukocytosis of 20,000/mm^3 with 95% polymorphonuclear lymphocytes. After confirming the diagnosis with imaging, what is the most appropriate management of this patient?

(A) Emergent appendectomy and postoperative antibiotics
(B) Give nothing by mouth with intravenous hydration
(C) Percutaneous drainage and interval appendectomy
(D) Serial abdominal examinations
(E) Urgent ECG and cardiac enzymes

31. A 40-year-old man with a recent history of exploratory laparotomy for a stabbing injury presents to the ED with diffuse cramping abdominal pain for 1 day, accompanied by nausea, multiple episodes of brown-colored vomitus, and lack of stool, but he reports some flatulence. He denies any fever. On physical examination, the patient has stable vital signs, and there is diffuse distention in the abdomen with guarding and tenderness but no rebound, as well as high-pitched bowel sounds. Rectal examination reveals no fecal impaction in the rectal vault, and the stool was guaiac negative. Complete blood cell count reveals no significant abnormalities and serum chemistry shows a mild metabolic alkalosis. CT demonstrates a noticeable difference in the diameter of proxi-

mal and distal small bowel. What is the most appropriate management for this patient?

(A) Broad-spectrum antibiotics
(B) Colonoscopy
(C) Exploratory laparotomy with lysis of adhesions
(D) Give the patient nothing by mouth, insert a nasogastric tube, and perform intravenous correction of electrolyte abnormalities
(E) Serial abdominal examinations

32. A 65-year-old woman presents with 3 months of unintentional weight loss, jaundice, and upper abdominal pain that radiates to her back. Her gallbladder is palpable on physical examination, and an ultrasound demonstrates dilated bile ducts with no visible stones. Which of the following is a known risk factor for this patient's condition?

(A) Chronic gastritis
(B) Diabetes insipidus
(C) Diabetes mellitus
(D) History of cholecystitis
(E) Smoking

33. A 2-year-old boy is brought to the ED. His mother reports that the patient had been well until 3 days ago, when he developed a fever and nasal congestion. He was diagnosed with otitis media in his right ear, and was started on amoxicillin with clavulanic acid by his pediatrician. He appeared to be improving until this morning, when he began to complain of abdominal pain. The pain has been intermittent, with episodes occurring every 20 minutes for several minutes each time. However, the episodes appear to be worsening and lasting longer with increasing pain. Thirty minutes ago he had an episode of nonbloody nonbilious emesis that was followed by passage of blood- and mucus-stained stools. He is currently in no acute distress, and his vital signs are normal. A firm sausage-shaped mass is palpable in the right upper quadrant of his abdomen. A rectal examination yields bloody mucus. He does not have any skin lesions or rashes. X-ray of the abdomen is shown in the image below. What is the most likely diagnosis?

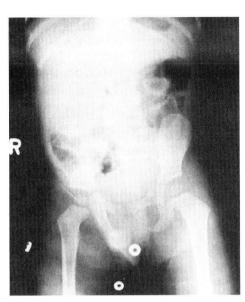

Reproduced, with permission, from Tintinalli JE, Kelen GD, Stapczynski S, Ma OJ, Cline DM. *Tintinalli's Emergency Medicine: A Comprehensive Study Guide*, 6th ed. New York: McGraw-Hill, 2004: Figure 127-2.

(A) Cystic fibrosis
(B) Enterocolitis
(C) Henoch-Schönlein purpura
(D) Idiopathic intussusception
(E) Meckel's diverticulum
(F) Pyloric stenosis

34. A 59-year-old man presents for his routine colonoscopy and during his visit he has numerous large adenomas removed from his colon. In terms of follow-up, what should be recommended to the patient?

(A) Elective colectomy
(B) Repeat colonoscopy in 3 years
(C) Repeat colonoscopy in 10 years
(D) Sigmoidoscopy in 10 years
(E) Urgent colectomy

35. A 22-year-old man is starting medical school. He received a hepatitis B vaccination series several years ago and needs serology to verify his immune status. What serology results would indicate continuing immunity to hepatitis B?

(A) Negative hepatitis B surface antigen and hepatitis B surface antibody
(B) Positive hepatitis B core antibody
(C) Positive hepatitis B e antibody
(D) Positive hepatitis B surface antibody
(E) Positive hepatitis B surface antigen

36. A baby girl is delivered at 37 weeks' gestation via cesarean section for breech presentation. The pregnancy was complicated by polyhydramnios. The 34-year-old mother is rubella immune and has blood type B. She is negative for Rh antibody, group B streptococci, rapid plasma reagin, hepatitis B surface antigen, gonorrhea, and chlamydia. At delivery, there is no meconium. He has a birth weight of 2.7 kg (6 lb). The baby has a weak cry and is pale and frothing at the nose and mouth. He has nasal flaring and retractions, with a respiratory rate of 56/min. He has a heart rate of 140/min with a regular rhythm and a harsh 2/6 holosystolic murmur that is best heard at the left sternal border. On auscultation, he has fine diffuse crackles in his lungs bilaterally. The infant is missing both thumbs and has fusion of the remaining digits of his upper extremities bilaterally. The pediatric resident is able to suction secretions from the patient's nasopharynx and oropharynx; however, she is unable to pass a nasogastric or orogastric tube more than 10 cm down. X-ray of the chest is shown in the image. Which of the following is the most likely diagnosis?

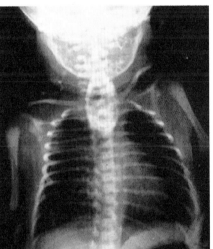

Reprinted, with permission, from Brunicardi FC, Andersen DK, Billiar TR, Dunn DL, Hunter JG, Matthews JB, Pollock RE, Schwartz SI. *Schwartz's Principles of Surgery*, 8th ed. New York: McGraw-Hill, 2005: Figure 38-10.

(A) Congenital diaphragmatic hernia
(B) Pyloric stenosis
(C) Respiratory distress syndrome
(D) Tracheoesophageal fistula
(E) Transient tachypnea of the newborn

37. The physician on call is called to the well-baby nursery because a full-term, African-American boy who is 49 hours old has not passed meconium. The pregnancy was uncomplicated. The neonate's blood pressure is 70/50 mm Hg, heart rate is 140/min, and respiratory rate is 36/min. The neonate is crying but is easily consolable. His abdomen is markedly distended. A barium enema is ordered, which shows dilated proximal bowel and a narrowed distal segment. Which of the following would provide a definitive diagnosis in this child?

(A) Absent ganglion cells on rectal biopsy
(B) Absent ligament of Treitz on upper gastrointestinal series
(C) Air bubbles in the stomach and duodenum on x-ray film of the abdomen
(D) Positive sweat test
(E) Telescoping of bowel on air contrast barium enema

38. A 73-year-old comes to his primary care physician for his yearly checkup. His medical history is significant for obesity, new-onset diabetes mellitus, and a remote history of tobacco use. The patient has noticed that his stool has been darker for the past 3 months, although he has only seen gross blood in his stool once, a week ago. He also complains of recent fatigue and occasional lightheadedness when standing up from sitting. The patient had a colonoscopy 1 year ago that did not reveal any pathology. On examination, the patient is found to have fecal occult blood and a hematocrit of 32%. Suspecting a very low output bleed, what is the best diagnostic test to locate this bleed?

(A) Angiography
(B) Barium enema
(C) Colonoscopy
(D) CT scan with contrast
(E) Tagged RBC scan

39. A pregnant 16-year-old girl with no prior prenatal care presents to the ED in labor. A baby boy is delivered precipitously. Prenatal laboratory test results are unknown. There is no meconium. He has a birth weight of 3 kg (6 lb, 10 oz). He is pink and is crying, his heart rate is 130/min, and his respiratory rate is 36/min, with good respiratory effort. The emergency medicine resident notices the infant has ascites and a membrane-covered anterior abdominal mass at the base of his umbilical cord. Which of the following is the most likely diagnosis?

(A) Duodenal atresia
(B) Gastroschisis
(C) Hirschsprung's disease
(D) Meckel's diverticulum
(E) Omphalocele

40. A 35-year-old white woman comes to her physician's office complaining of loose, bloody stools. Her vital signs are temperature 36.4°C (97.5°F), heart rate 70/min, and blood pressure 114/74 mm Hg. Her physical examination is unremarkable. Further workup, including stool examination, colonoscopy, and rectal biopsy, leads to the diagnosis of ulcerative colitis. Which of the following can exacerbate ulcerative colitis?

(A) An emotional and stressful life event
(B) Consumption of alcohol
(C) Oral contraceptives
(D) Smoking cigarettes
(E) Upper respiratory infection

41. A 47-year-old woman presents to the ED with an 8-day history of left lower quadrant pain and semiformed stools. Starting this afternoon, she has noticed blood in her stool as well as dizziness when she gets up from sitting. Otherwise, she denies fever, nausea, vomiting, weight loss, and night sweats. She had a temperature of 38.9°C (102°F); a heart rate of 104/min; a

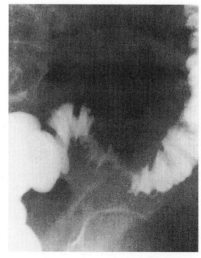

Reproduced, with permission, from Chen MYM, Pope TL, Ott DJ. *Basic Radiology*. New York: McGraw-Hill, 2004: Figure 10-54.

blood pressure of 120/82 mm Hg supine, which falls to 103/63 mm Hg when she sits up; and a respiratory rate of 18/min. Physical examination reveals no peritoneal signs and is remarkable only for fecal occult blood on rectal examination. Laboratory results reveal a WBC count of 13,000/mm^3 and hematocrit of 29%. Results of an x-ray of the abdomen are shown in the image. What is the next best step in managing this patient?

(A) Angiography with embolization
(B) Immediate surgery for partial colectomy
(C) Intravenous hydration and blood transfusion
(D) Nothing by mouth, nasogastric tube, and broad-spectrum antibiotics
(E) Place the patient on a high-fiber diet

42. A middle-aged woman presents to the gastrointestinal clinic with crampy abdominal pain and blood-tinged diarrhea. She reports that she has recently been to see an ophthalmologist who told her she has uveitis. She smokes cigarettes and has seasonal allergies; her medical and social history is otherwise unremarkable. Her gastroenterologist has a strong clinical suspicion of inflammatory bowel disease. Which of the following would be more suggestive of ulcerative colitis than Crohn's disease?

(A) Absence of gross bleeding
(B) Perianal disease
(C) Presence of fistulae
(D) Sparing of the rectum
(E) Sparing of the small bowel

43. A 61-year-old woman is brought to the ED drowsy and disoriented, only able to follow simple commands. On examination, her abdomen is distended and nontender, her skin has a yellow hue, and there are multiple spider nevi on her chest. In her purse, the physician finds prescriptions for peginterferon and ribavirin. When asked to raise her hands, the physician notices a coarse tremor. Significant laboratory values include:

Blood urea nitrogen	17 mg/dL
Creatinine	1.1 mg/dL
Aspartate aminotransferase	89 U/L
Alanine aminotransferase	93 U/L
Total bilirubin	3.1 mg/dL
Ammonia	124 μg/dL

What is the most likely diagnosis?

(A) Bleeding esophageal varices
(B) Hepatic encephalopathy
(C) Hepatocellular carcinoma
(D) Hepatorenal syndrome
(E) Spontaneous bacterial peritonitis

44. A 38-year-old man is diagnosed by his primary care physician with diverticulitis. The patient is afebrile, is experiencing minimal abdominal pain, and has a WBC count of 6500/mm^3. He has no other medical problems and no allergies. What is the most appropriate choice of antibiotics in this patient?

(A) Cefotetan
(B) Intravenous ampicillin/sulbactam (Unasyn)
(C) Intravenous ampicillin/sulbactam (Unasyn) followed by metronidazole
(D) Metronidazole alone
(E) Metronidazole and ciprofloxacin

45. Three months ago a 56-year-old former alcoholic with chronic pancreatitis presented to the ED complaining of pruritus of several weeks' duration. Since then he has been maintained on total parenteral nutrition. He has recently developed mild watery diarrhea. Today his temperature is 37.2°C (98.9°F), blood pressure is 118/64 mm Hg, and pulse is 88/min. Physical examination reveals a normally developed man in no acute distress, with slight temporal wasting. Numerous areas of irritation with several vesiculobullous lesions and mild alopecia are noted on his skin and head. Cardiac and pulmonary examinations are normal, and there are no focal neurologic findings. Relevant laboratory findings are:

Na$^+$	143 mEq/L
K$^+$	4.4 mEq/L
Cl$^-$	97 mEq/L
HCO$_3$$^-$	23 mEq/L
Blood urea nitrogen	18 mg/dL
Creatinine	0.8 mg/dL

Deficiency of what mineral is a likely cause of this patient's symptoms?

(A) Chromium
(B) Cobalt
(C) Copper
(D) Selenium
(E) Zinc

46. An 82-year-old woman is in the surgical intensive care unit after a carotid endarterectomy. She has been taking clindamycin and ciprofloxacin for the past 13 days. On postoperative day two, the patient is noticed to be febrile and tachycardic with a high WBC count and a low RBC count. She is also noted to be dehydrated and hypotensive. On physical examination, she is distended and has abdominal tenderness with rebound and guarding. A barium enema reveals colonic dilatation of 8 cm. Stool is sent for Gram stain, fecal leukocytes, fecal occult blood, and *Clostridium difficile* toxin. Which of the following is most likely present in the stool sample of this patient?

    (A) *Clostridium difficile* toxin
    (B) Gram-negative rods
    (C) Gram-positive cocci
    (D) No fecal occult blood
    (E) Spores and hyphae

47. A 40-year-old Asian woman presents to the ED complaining of intermittent epigastric pain. The pain is severe, lasts for a few hours, and is sometimes accompanied by nausea and vomiting. Her bowel movements have been normal. Her temperature is 38.3°C (100.9°F), pulse is 100/min, blood pressure is 150/80 mm Hg, and respiratory rate is 22/min. On examination, she is in moderately obese; sclerae are mildly icteric; bowel sounds are normal, with an abrupt halt of inspiration with palpation of the right upper quadrant (RUQ); and RUQ guarding. Laboratory tests show a WBC count of 13,000/mm^3, total bilirubin of 3.3 mg/dL, and normal liver enzymes and alkaline phosphatase. Which of the following is the first diagnostic imaging study that should be performed?

    (A) CT scan
    (B) Flat and upright plane x-rays of the abdomen
    (C) Hepatobiliary iminodiacetic acid scan
    (D) MRI
    (E) Right upper quadrant ultrasound

Questions 48–50

For each patient with diarrhea, select the most likely etiology.

    (A) *Bacillus cereus*
    (B) *Campylobacter jejuni*
    (C) Carcinoid
    (D) Celiac disease
    (E) *Clostridium difficile*
    (F) Crohn's disease
    (G) *Entamoeba histolytica*
    (H) *Escherichia coli*
    (I) *Giardia*
    (J) Irritable bowel syndrome
    (K) Lactose intolerance
    (L) Ulcerative colitis
    (M) *Vibrio parahaemolyticus*
    (N) Whipple's disease

48. A 25-year-old Asian man, recently immigrated, presents with watery diarrhea, cramping, and flatulence after attending a picnic, where he ate corn on the cob and ice cream cake. Stool guaiac is negative. One day after the picnic, his symptoms resolve.

49. A 2-year-old boy presents with history of smelly, bulky diarrhea and poor weight gain. A small bowel biopsy shows villous atrophy.

50. A 79-year-old woman presents with 2 days of fever, dehydration, and bloody diarrhea. She was recently hospitalized and finished a course of antibiotics for pneumonia. Stool sample is positive for WBCs.

ANSWERS

1. The correct answer is A. The patient's biopsy shows a proliferation of lymphocytes consistent with a mucosa-associated lymphoid tissue (MALT) lymphoma. This type of small cell lymphoma makes up approximately 8% of non-Hodgkin's lymphoma, and may occur in the stomach, orbit, intestine, lung, thyroid, or salivary gland; however, it most often arises in the stomach. Patients generally present with complaints of abdominal pain or fullness. Ninety-five percent of gastric MALToma cases are associated with *Helicobacter pylori* infection and the majority of cases achieve remission with simple antibiotic eradication of *H. pylori*. Patients with very extensive disease are occasionally treated with single-agent chemotherapy with chlorambucil.

Answer B is incorrect. Bone marrow transplantation is generally not required for mucosa-associated lymphoid tissue lymphomas. Even widespread disease is generally responsive to much more mild chemotherapy.

Answer C is incorrect. Although certain genetic alterations have been identified in mucosa-associated lymphoid tissue lymphomas, such as t(11;18) and trisomies of chromosomes 3, 7, 12, and 18, gene therapy is not a standard of care for any cancer currently. In addition, because cure rates are so high with known therapies, any physician should be reluctant to propose that a patient with this disease be exposed to the inherent risks of gene therapy.

Answer D is incorrect. Liver transplantation would not be required in a patient with mucosa-associated lymphoid tissue lymphoma that would most likely be responsive to mild therapy. Even in patients with metastatic cancer to the liver, transplantation is generally not indicated because of the comorbidities associated with major surgery and immunosuppression in cancer patients.

Answer E is incorrect. Multiagent chemotherapy is not required to treat mucosa-associated lymphoid tissue lymphoma.

Answer F is incorrect. Patients with gastric carcinoma may be treated with resection of the mass and gastric antrum. However, the pathology of this patient's tumor is clearly not a carcinoma. Surgical procedures used to treat mucosa-associated lymphoid tissue lymphomas generally include only resection of the tumor itself, not the gastric antrum.

2. The correct answer is C. A one-time esophagoscopy is recommended in patients 50 years or older to evaluate for the development of esophageal metaplasia (Barrett's esophagus). There is a direct correlation between the development of Barrett's esophagus and history of gastroesophageal reflux disease. If metaplasia is present, these patients are 30 to 125 times more likely to develop adenocarcinoma. An esophagoscopy and biopsy could help discern whether this patient has a Barrett's esophagus or has already progressed to an early stage cancer that has yet to cause dysphagia and weight loss.

Answer A is incorrect. Although doubling the medication dose may provide symptomatic relief of the gastroesophageal reflux disease, it does not tell us anything about the damage that has been done to the esophagus as a result of the condition. To properly manage the disease, it is necessary to evaluate for metaplasia.

Answer B is incorrect. Changing the medication dose may provide further symptomatic relief of the gastroesophageal reflux disease, but this patient is in need of an esophagoscopy to evaluate for metaplasia in order to properly manage the disease.

Answer D is incorrect. Esophagectomy is typically indicated for the removal of long segments of metaplasia in patients with Barrett's esophagus. In this patient, it is unknown if there is any metaplasia, so an esophagoscopy should be performed first.

Answer E is incorrect. There is no indication for any emergent surgical procedure. Nissen fundoplication is typically used for active reflux that is refractory to medical management.

3. The correct answer is A. Duodenal atresia is the most likely diagnosis because it presents with bilious vomiting following any feeding in the first few hours of life. Constipation often develops after meconium is passed. Physical examination is notable for abdominal distention of predominantly the upper abdomen. Polyhydramnios is often the earliest sign. Infants with Down's syndrome are at increased risk of having duodenal atresia. A double-bubble sign, air bubbles in the stomach and duodenum on x-ray of the abdomen, is diagnostic of duodenal atresia.

Answer B is incorrect. Hirschsprung's disease usually presents with delayed passage of meconium and abdominal distention. Other symptoms include poor feeding and bilious vomiting. Patients with this disease usually pass meconium after rectal stimulation. A barium enema that shows dilated proximal bowel and a narrowed distal segment is highly suggestive of Hirschsprung's disease, while the lack of ganglion cells on rectal biopsy is diagnostic.

Answer C is incorrect. Intussusception is a common cause of bowel obstruction in infants younger than 2 years. It presents with bouts of irritability, colicky abdominal pain, and vomiting. If it is not diagnosed at this point, infants become lethargic and pass red currant jelly–like stools. Physical examination is notable for a palpable right lower quadrant mass. Air contrast barium enema showing telescoping of the bowel is diagnostic for intussusception and often therapeutic as well.

Answer D is incorrect. A malrotation with volvulus is the most critical cause of bowel obstruction. It presents in the first week of life with bilious emesis and constipation. Rectal hemorrhage and peritonitis can occur. An upper gastrointestinal series with an absent or abnormal position of the ligament of Treitz confirms the diagnosis of malrotation.

Answer E is incorrect. Pyloric stenosis presents with nonbilious projectile vomiting during the first weeks to months of life. Physical examination is classically notable for a palpable olive-shaped, mobile, nontender epigastric mass. Laboratory values reveal a hypochloremic-hypokalemic metabolic alkalosis. Barium study shows a narrow pyloric channel, which is sometimes called a "string sign" or a "pyloric beak."

4. The correct answer is A. Smoking and alcohol consumption are the two most prominent risk factors for esophageal squamous cell carcinoma, which can present with dysphagia and weight loss.

Answer B is incorrect. Smoked meats are a risk factor for carcinoma and one of the leading reasons why this disease is so prevalent in other countries. Patients should stay away from smoked foods.

Answer C is incorrect. While it is true that colonoscopies are suggested as regular preventive measures, this test would not have helped detect the esophageal changes he was undergoing.

Answer D is incorrect. To the contrary, anecdotal evidence suggests that these foods actually have a protective effect against squamous cell carcinoma.

Answer E is incorrect. Squamous cell carcinoma is not due to reflux. Barrett's esophagus is more likely due to this problem and results in adenocarcinoma.

5. The correct answer is B. The image shows a cecal volvulus. The image shows a distended cecum and right colon (arrowheads) at the midabdomen, with the terminal ileun (curved arrow) lateral to the cecal volvulus. Cecal volvulus typically displays a classic "kidney bean" appearance. After fluid resuscitation and large bowel decompression have been achieved, the first-line therapy is hemicolectomy with second-line treatment being colonoscopy.

Answer A is incorrect. Colonoscopy is the second-line treatment for cecal volvulus, after hemicolectomy.

Answer C is incorrect. This is the second-line treatment for splenic flexure volvulus. It is only indicated if extended hemicolectomy cannot be performed.

Answer D is incorrect. The obstruction here involves the cecum, not the sigmoid. Sigmoid volvulus may present as abdominal distention with minimal tenderness or severe pain, vomiting, and absolute constipation. Sigmoid colectomy is the removal of the sigmoid section of the colon. It may be performed open or laparoscopically. Sigmoid colectomy is the second-line treatment for sigmoid volvulus, after sigmoidoscopy.

Answer E is incorrect. The obstruction involves the cecum, not the sigmoid. Sigmoid volvulus may present as abdominal distension with minimal tenderness or severe pain, vomiting, and absolute constipation. Sigmoidoscopy refers to the insertion of a scope into the colon to examine the rectum, the sigmoid, and descending portions of the colon. The procedure is indicated for temporary decompression of sigmoid volvulus (recurrence of the volvulus is common without prompt surgery).

6. **The correct answer is D.** This child has phenylketonuria (PKU). In PKU, phenylalanine cannot be converted to tyrosine. It is screened for at birth, and is detected by phenylketones (phenylacetate, phenyllactate, and phenylpyruvate) in the urine. Classic features of PKU are fair skin, eczema, musty body odor, and mental retardation. Mental retardation can be prevented by reducing phenylalanine (not one of the answer choices) and increasing tyrosine in the diet.

Answer A is incorrect. Symptoms of iron deficiency include pallor and lethargy. Iron deficiency is an acquired deficiency; it does not result from an inborn error of metabolism.

Answer B is incorrect. Niacin deficiency also known as pellagra, is characterized by dermatitis, diarrhea, and dementia. In children, this occurs most commonly in developing countries where the diet is high in corn. Niacin deficiency is acquired; it does not result from an inborn error of metabolism.

Answer C is incorrect. In phenylketonuria, phenylalanine needs to be reduced rather than increased.

Answer E is incorrect. Vitamin D deficiency leads to rickets. Rickets is characterized by bowlegs, a pigeon-breast deformity (in which the sternum projects forward), kyphosis, scoliosis, and enlargement of wrist joints. Vitamin D is an acquired deficiency; it does not result from an inborn error of metabolism.

7. **The correct answer is E.** This patient suffers from Budd-Chiari syndrome, a condition caused by hepatic vein thrombosis that is typically secondary to a hypercoagulable state such as cancer, pregnancy, oral contraceptive use, or hematologic disease. Chronic hepatic vein thrombosis is a cause of postsinusoidal portal hypertension, and acute thrombosis will cause right upper quadrant pain, hepatomegaly, and ascites. Liver function tests may be slightly elevated, but laboratory values are otherwise typically normal. Ultrasound will often show collateral vessels in a spider web pattern and decreased hepatic venous blood flow. Mortality is high at 40–90%. Initial medical treatment is thrombolysis followed by anticoagulation, especially in patients presenting with acute symptoms. However, the TIPS procedure (transjugular intrahepatic portosystemic shunt) or hepatic transplantation is a more definitive treatment.

Answer A is incorrect. β-Blocker therapy is used to medically treat portal hypertension due to its effect on the systemic and splanchnic circulations, whereas lactulose is used to treat hepatic encephalopathy associated with liver dysfunction. Neither are appropriate treatments for Budd-Chiari syndrome.

Answer B is incorrect. Emergent cholecystectomy should be performed if the patient is suffering from acute cholecystitis. However, signs of portal hypertension, negative Murphy's signs, and evidence of collateral venous flow on imaging suggest hepatic vein thrombosis, not cholecystitis.

Answer C is incorrect. Nonsurgical treatment for common bile duct stones includes endoscopic retrograde cholangiopancreatography with dilation of the common bile duct, removal of existing stones, and stent placement. This is not an appropriate treatment for this patient.

Answer D is incorrect. An exploratory laparotomy would be performed for various reasons, including whether a bowel obstruction was suspected or whether debulking of tumor was necessary. However, the information provided suggests hepatic vein thrombosis, which would not require an exploratory laparotomy.

8. **The correct answer is D.** The radiograph demonstrates multiple diverticuli of the sigmoid colon. The arrow points to a near complete colonic obstruction. The sigmoid colon is the most common site for diverticuli due to the narrower diameter of the colon in that region. Left lower quadrant abdominal pain is present in > 90% of patients with diverticulitis, while fever and leukocytosis occur in more than 50% and 83% of patients, respectively. Treatment includes intravenous antibiotics and fluid resuscitation.

Answer A is incorrect. Although angiodysplasia is the most common cause of lower GI tract bleeding in the elderly, there is no evidence of an arteriovenous malformation (AVM) on the CT image. AVM bleeding tends to be self-limited and painless, without significant leukocytosis.

Answer B is incorrect. Carcinoid syndrome may present with chronic diarrhea, but fever and leukocytosis would not likely be present.

Answer C is incorrect. Carcinoma of the colon is unlikely to present acutely with diarrhea, fever, and high leukocytosis.

Answer E is incorrect. Infectious colitis is a possibility, but given the CT scan showing inflamed diverticuli, it is a less likely diagnosis.

9. **The correct answer is D.** Infection with *Helicobacter pylori* is a cause of type B or antral-dominant, chronic gastritis. The most common cause of chronic type B gastritis is use of nonsteroidal anti-inflammatory drugs, but our patient lacks this history. The incidence of chronic gastritis increases with age and the histologic appearance improves with the treatment of *H. pylori*. Symptoms of chronic gastritis may include pain, nausea, vomiting, anorexia, and upper gastrointestinal bleeding; however, this condition is frequently asymptomatic. Diagnosis is confirmed by *H. pylori* antibody test and breath urease test, as well as a direct gastric biopsy and culture. Treatment of *H. pylori* gastritis is with triple therapy, which includes two antibiotics (metronidazole and clarithromycin), bismuth compound, and a proton pump inhibitor. Type A gastritis is autoimmune-mediated, affecting the fundus, and is associated with vitamin B_{12} deficiency.

Answer A is incorrect. Severe alcohol abuse may have negative effects on the gastric mucosa, including the development of acute (stress) gastritis; however, in a patient with no history of alcoholism and with inflammation confined to the antrum, alcohol abuse would not be the most likely cause of gastritis.

Answer B is incorrect. Cigarette smoking may promote atrophic gastritis in *Helicobacter pylori*–positive patients, but it has not been shown to cause inflammation of the gastric mucosa by itself.

Answer C is incorrect. Although there is some erythema associated with endoscopy, gastritis is defined as the histologic appearance of inflammation of the gastric mucosa.

Answer E is incorrect. Spicy foods may lead to increased gastric acid production, but would not be the most likely cause of the inflammation in this case.

10. **The correct answer is E.** This patient's presentation and laboratory tests all point to Wilson's disease, a disease characterized by copper accumulation in multiple organs, especially the liver and brain, due to defective excretion of this metal. Along with basal ganglia dysfunction and hemolytic anemia, this patient is showing signs of portal hypertension due to cirrhosis caused by copper accumulation in the liver. This increase in pressure in the portal circulation leads to variceal formation at the junctions of the portal and systemic circulations. An upper endoscopy should be performed to monitor for esophageal varices that could be treated prophylactically or closely monitored to prevent life-threatening bleeding.

Answer A is incorrect. A protein electrophoresis should be performed if multiple myeloma, a neoplastic proliferation of plasma cells, is suspected. Although this patient has evidence of anemia, the other clinical and laboratory findings clearly support the diagnosis of Wilson's disease, making a protein electrophoresis unnecessary.

Answer B is incorrect. While a colonoscopy is an important screening measure for all individuals starting at the age of 50, this test would not be particularly revealing in a patient suffering from Wilson's disease. However, hemorrhoids, a condition associated with portal hypertension, should be considered in such individuals.

Answer C is incorrect. Although cardiac dysfunction should be monitored in diseases involving abnormal accumulation of substances, such as hemochromatosis, this is not the case in Wilson's disease.

Answer D is incorrect. In the Schilling test radioactive vitamin B_{12} is given orally with a parenteral dose of unlabeled vitamin B_{12} in order to measure the ability of the enteric tract to absorb vitamin B_{12} in the setting of megaloblastic anemia. Hemolytic anemia, not megaloblastic anemia, is found in Wilson's disease. Therefore the Schilling test would be unnecessary.

11. **The correct answer is A.** The Gram stain shows gram-negative rods, which make *Escherichia coli* the only possible correct answer. The patient's symptoms are characteristic for enterohemorrhagic *E. coli* infection. The illness develops 3–5 days after infection and is characterized by bloody diarrhea without fever.

Answer B is incorrect. Kaposi's sarcoma lesions can be found in the gastrointestinal tract, where they can be asymptomatic or cause symptoms such as abdominal pain, weight loss, hemorrhage, and diarrhea. Since Gram stain revealed gram-negative organisms, Kaposi's sarcoma is a less likely cause of the patient's symptoms.

Answer C is incorrect. *Legionella* generally appears as small coccobacilli that stain weakly gram-negative, and the infection presents clinically as a pneumonia with high fevers and accompanying gastrointestinal symptoms.

Answer D is incorrect. *Mycobacterium avium* complex (MAC) infection can involve the large bowel and cause symptoms similar to this patient's. MAC infection, however, is unlikely with a CD4+ count > 200/mm^3; it is more common with a CD4+ count < 50/mm^3.

Answer E is incorrect. Similarly to *Mycobacterium avium* complex, *Mycobacterium tuberculosis* infection can also involve the gastrointestinal tract in AIDS patients. This is unlikely, though, with CD4+ counts > 200/mm^3.

12. **The correct answer is B.** This patient has chronic pancreatitis; the image shows an atrophic, calcified pancreas. He now has exocrine insufficiency, which leads to malabsorption, fatty stools with diarrhea, and weight loss. This patient will need to take pancreatic enzymes with each meal for the remainder of his life.

Answer A is incorrect. Endoscopic retrograde cholangiopancreatography or endoscopic retrograde pancreaticoduodenostomy is used to diagnose stones and strictures in the biliary tract. It can also be therapeutic for choledocholithiasis.

Answer C is incorrect. A pancreaticogastrostomy can be used to internally drain pancreatic pseudocysts. Another option is percutaneous surgical drainage.

Answer D is incorrect. Surgical resection of the pancreas is neither necessary nor helpful for this patient's pancreatic insufficiency.

Answer E is incorrect. A Whipple procedure is a pancreaticoduodenectomy and reanastomosis of the digestive tract to itself and with the pancreas. It is performed for pancreatic tumors and tumors of the ampulla of Vater. The Whipple is theoretically curative if further spread of the tumor has not yet occurred; however, the 5-year postsurgical survival rate is a mere 5%.

13. **The correct answer is B.** The most common tumors of the appendix are carcinoid tumors. Remembering the "rule of one-thirds," you know that one-third metastasize, one-third are accompanied by a second malignancy, and one-third present with multiple carcinoid tumors. Since treatment will be based on tumor location, tumor size, and metastases, a CT scan of both the chest and abdomen will give you most of the information you need. This imaging modality will also possibly reveal a second malignancy.

Answer A is incorrect. With an asymptomatic tumor, there should be no pulmonary compromise secondary to late carcinoid heart syndrome, so an arterial blood gas study would not be helpful. Patients with carcinoid heart syndrome may develop shortness of breath from right heart failure, secondary to tricuspid valve stenosis.

Answer C is incorrect. Carcinoid tumors may cause carcinoid syndrome, which presents with flushing, diarrhea, bronchospasm, and hypotension. This syndrome progresses to carcinoid heart syndrome in up to 50% of patients, characterized by endocardial plaques in the right heart that can lead to right heart failure. Late carcinoid heart syndrome can produce diffuse low-voltage ECG changes. Since this patient's tumor was asymptomatic, there is no need to suspect that it has damaged the right side of her heart enough to produce ECG changes. While there is no need for an immediate ECG, she should get a standard admission ECG when the nursing staff is able to get her one.

Answer D is incorrect. An MRI is not the imaging modality appropriate for this type of screening image for solid tumors.

Answer E is incorrect. Again, since the tumor is asymptomatic, there should be no pulmonary complications, so room air oxygen saturation would not be helpful.

14. **The correct answer is E.** Plummer-Vinson syndrome is the name given for the association of dysphagia, upper esophageal webs, and iron deficiency anemia. Its etiology is uncertain, and it is actually a rare phenomenon in the United States. Diagnosis is made by laboratory assessment, esophageal imaging, and the exclusion of other competing explanations. Its components, anemia and esophageal anatomic irregularities, are treated in the same manner they would if they presented independently.

Answer A is incorrect. Achalasia is commonly associated with dysphagia of both solid and liquids and is not associated with iron deficiency. It is a rare disease of unclear etiology that is truly a functional pathology: unlike the anatomic impairment of Plummer-Vinson syndrome, achalasia is due to a failure of the lower esophageal sphincter to work properly.

Answer B is incorrect. Barrett's esophagus is defined by columnar epithelium replacing squamous epithelium due to continuous inflammation associated with reflux. It is an indication for surgical intervention, which generally means a Nissen fundoplication, as it carries an elevated risk of esophageal carcinoma.

Answer C is incorrect. Carcinoma is usually due to smoking, alcohol consumption, or Barrett's esophagus. It is characterized by dysphagia of solids but would not present with the iron studies given and with no identifiable risk factors.

Answer D is incorrect. Mallory-Weiss syndrome is secondary to heavy vomiting causing a tear in the lining of the esophagus. It is a source of upper gastrointestinal bleeding that should be considered when the clinical history involves a recent history of retching. Diagnosis is made by endoscopy.

Answer F is incorrect. Reflux esophagitis is caused by reflux of gastric contents into the esophagus. Patients present with a classic presentation of "heartburn" that is worse when recumbent. It is typically managed first with proton pump inhibitor or histamine blocker therapy.

Answer G is incorrect. Symptomatic diffuse esophageal spasm usually will present with both solid and liquid dysphagia. The diagnosis is made by manometry, and initial treatment generally involves anticholinergics, nitroglycerin, and long-acting nitrates. Surgical intervention is often ultimately required.

15. **The correct answer is E.** Necrotizing enterocolitis (NEC) is the most common life-threatening condition of the newborn gastrointestinal tract. Risk of NEC is significantly increased for premature infants. Symptoms usually beg in within the first 2 weeks of life, and initial signs often include abdominal distention with delayed gastric emptying. Bloody stools can be seen, and patients may develop respiratory distress as the illness progresses. On x-ray of the abdomen, hepatic portal venous gas and a bubbly appearance of pneumatosis intestinalis (gas within the bowel wall) are pathognomonic for NEC. Treatment of NEC includes nasogastric suction, but surgical resection of the affected section of bowel may be

required in infants that develop pneumoperitoneum, obstruction, or other serious complications. The overall survival of infants afflicted with NEC is approximately 70–80%.

Answer A is incorrect. Bowel obstruction could produce the abdominal distention and delayed gastric emptying. However, the x-ray findings are most consistent with the diagnosis of necrotizing enterocolitis.

Answer B is incorrect. Although intussusception would cause guaiac-positive stools, the infant lacks apparent risk factors or clinical manifestations (i.e., vomiting). Also, because intussusception results in a loss of gas, the x-ray findings are most consistent with the clinical picture of necrotizing enterocolitis.

Answer C is incorrect. Meconium ileus often presents in a manner similar to bowel obstruction, and vomiting is often present. X-ray findings for meconium ileus include varying width loops of bowel with an uneven gas filling pattern.

Answer D is incorrect. Meningitis is not likely given the abdominal findings in addition to the x-ray demonstrations.

16. **The correct answer is C.** This patient is suffering from a Mallory-Weiss tear, which is caused by excessive vomiting. Hematemesis is very common at presentation and may also be associated with endoscopy and hiatal hernias, which predispose to this condition. The bleeding is often self-limited but may persist, recur, and be life threatening. It is important to diagnose it quickly, preferably with endoscopy. Although endoscopy may cause hematemesis, it will not exacerbate it.

Answer A is incorrect. A barium swallow should not be completed because it will interfere with the endoscopy procedure and has a low diagnostic yield.

Answer B is incorrect. ECG might help if the patient was more hypotensive/tachycardic and showing signs of failing because fatal arrhythmias may occur, but it is a better test for treatment than for diagnosis.

Answer D is incorrect. Manometry would be of no value in this case.

Answer E is incorrect. X-ray of the chest does not help in the diagnosis.

17. **The correct answer is A.** Acute mesenteric ischemia is often seen in individuals who are > 60 years old and who have a history of atherosclerotic disease. The patients may describe symptoms consistent with abdominal angina (e.g., postprandial abdominal pain that resolves in a few hours). Its presentation can be either acute or chronic, with abdominal pain and bloody diarrhea usually developing 24 hours after the abdominal pain. Early on, the pain is severe with frequent passage of bloody stools. The blood loss is not significant enough to necessitate a transfusion. As the ischemia continues, the pain diminishes, and the abdomen becomes more tender and distended. Finally, the bowel may become gangrenous with fluid and protein leaking through the damaged mucosa, causing shock and metabolic acidosis. At this point, rapid surgical intervention is necessary

Answer B is incorrect. In the absence of constitutional symptoms and due to the acute nature of his abdominal pain and bloody diarrhea, the diagnosis of colon cancer is unlikely. Although the possibility of colon cancer cannot be excluded in this patient, it is not the most likely diagnosis.

Answer C is incorrect. Bleeding is usually more consistent with diverticulosis than diverticulitis. Although the presence of diverticular disease cannot be ruled out in this patient, it is unlikely to be the cause of his current symptoms.

Answer D is incorrect. The chronicity of this patient's symptoms does not support a diagnosis of infectious colitis. Infectious colitis presents with mild to moderate diarrhea but is not bloody. Other symptoms include acute onset of fever, malaise, and abdominal pain.

Answer E is incorrect. Postprandial pain that resolves in 1–2 hours is not commonly described in patients with inflammatory bowel disease (IBD). Additionally, the acute onset of this presentation is not consistent with IBD, which typically presents in much younger patients and has chronic symptoms.

18. **The correct answer is D.** The patient in the question has symptoms consistent with a lower gastrointestinal (GI) bleed in the context of diverticulitis. Although the symptoms described are suggestive of a lower GI bleed, a massive upper GI bleed can also present as rectal bleeding. Therefore it is important to perform nasogastric tube aspiration and rule out an upper GI bleed.

Answer A is incorrect. Arteriography should be done if the colonoscopy is not possible because of the severity of the bleeding or if it was not able to identify the site of the bleed. This technique, however, is limited, as the patient must be bleeding briskly during the scan in order to localize the site of the bleeding.

Answer B is incorrect. Colonoscopy should be performed once an upper GI bleed has been ruled out. Colonoscopy not only allows you to localize the site of the bleeding, but can also be a therapeutic intervention.

Answer C is incorrect. Endoscopy should be performed if the nasogastric tube yields frank blood. This finding suggests that the source of the bleeding could be in the upper GI tract. That suspicion can be confirmed and possibly treated with endoscopy.

Answer E is incorrect. Surgical consultation should be obtained if the patient remains unstable despite aggressive resuscitation.

19. **The correct answer is D.** This patient has the characteristic tetrad of Henoch-Schönlein purpura (HSP), including the purpuric rash, arthralgias ("aches and pains"), abdominal pain, and glomerular renal involvement. HSP is a systemic vasculitis most commonly seen in children. It is associated with numerous gastrointestinal complications, most classically intussusception (typically ileo-ileal in HSP versus the more common terminal ileum, ileocecal valve, and ascending colon involvement seen otherwise), but also pancreatitis and cholecystitis.

Answer A is incorrect. Hemoptysis would be expected in Wegener's granulomatosis or Goodpasture's syndrome, both inflammatory diseases presenting with symptoms of nephritic syndrome such as edema and hypertension.

Answer B is incorrect. Patients with postinfectious glomerulonephritis often have a high antistreptolysin O titer due to association with recent group A β-hemolytic streptococcal infection. These patients present with oliguria, edema, hypertension, and brown urine.

Answer C is incorrect. Impaired glucose tolerance would be expected in a patient with diabetes mellitus (DM). Patients with longstanding, poorly controlled DM often have glomerular disease with proteinuria; however, they do not present with the symptoms of HSP such as purpuric rash and abdominal pain.

Answer E is incorrect. A malar rash would be seen in systemic lupus erythematosus and may be associated with lupus nephritis.

20. **The correct answer is D.** The diagnosis of hemochromatosis should be suspected when a patient presents with diabetes, hepatomegaly, skin pigmentation changes, arthritis, and hypogonadism. Three tests used in diagnosis of iron overload states include serum iron, serum ferritin, and transferrin concentration. An increase in iron stores in normal subjects leads to an increase in plasma iron levels, a rise in plasma transferrin saturation (ratio of iron to transferrin), and a rise in the concentration of ferritin. A fasting transferrin saturation ≥ 60% in men or ≥ 50% in women will detect about 90% of patients with homozygous hypogonadotropic hypogonadism. Often, a lower cutoff will be used to minimize the number of patients with the condition who are missed.

Answer A is incorrect. Many diseases of the blood can cause iron overload syndromes. In such disease a blood smear can lead to a diagnosis, but without any other symptoms the possibility of a blood disorder is unlikely in our patient.

Answer B is incorrect. CT scan of the abdomen can show increased density of the liver due to iron deposition, but this test is not used to diagnose hemochromatosis.

Answer C is incorrect. Endoscopic retrograde cholangiopancreatography is used in the diagnosis of choledocholithiasis, tissue sampling in patients with pancreatic or biliary cancer, diagnosing ampullary cancer, and many others. It is not used in the diagnosis of hemochromatosis.

Answer E is incorrect. A liver biopsy is the only reliable method for establishing or excluding the presence of liver cirrhosis in the setting of hemochromatosis. This is an invasive test and should not be used as the first test in the diagnosis of hemochromatosis.

21. **The correct answer is E.** These large, broad-based polyps carry the highest potential for malignant change.

    Answer A is incorrect. Lymphoid polyps are inflammatory polyps and are non-neoplastic.

    Answer B is incorrect. Hamartomatous polyps, such as Peutz-Jeghers polyps, are non-neoplastic, although the Peutz-Jeghers syndrome in which they appear does confer additional risk for malignancy in other organs including the stomach, breasts, and ovaries.

    Answer C is incorrect. Tubular adenoma is incorrect, as these polyps less frequently undergo malignant change than villous adenomas do.

    Answer D is incorrect. Villous adenomata have less malignant potential than their solely villous counterparts.

22. **The correct answer is A.** Given that the lesion is < 10.0 cm from the anal verge, it is not possible to preserve the anal sphincter, and surgical treatment requires an abdominoperineal resection, which involves resection of the rectum and anus with placement of a permanent colostomy.

    Answer B is incorrect. Imatinib, an inhibitor of certain oncogenic tyrosine kinases, is useful for gastrointestinal stromal tumors. A rectal lesion of this type requires surgical resection.

    Answer C is incorrect. If the lesion had been > 10.0 cm from the anal verge, it would have likely been possible to perform a low anterior resection, which would preserve the anus and distal rectum, allowing for resection and primary anastomosis, thereby avoiding the need for a colostomy.

    Answer D is incorrect. Radiation is a useful adjunct to surgical resection in rectal cancer but is not adequate as the only treatment modality.

    Answer E is incorrect. Radiation is used as an adjuvant to surgical resection, but without surgery (even when followed by chemotherapy) it is insufficient treatment.

23. **The correct answer is D.** This is a typical presentation of physiologic jaundice. Physiologic jaundice affects most newborns; it results in a mild unconjugated hyperbilirubinemia after day of life three and resolves by 1 week in full-term neonates and 2 weeks in preterm neonates. Notably, the conjugated bilirubin is always normal and total bilirubin is always < 14 g/dL in physiologic jaundice.

    Answer A is incorrect. α_1-Antitrypsin deficiency can present as conjugated hyperbilirubinemia. This child has an unconjugated hyperbilirubinemia and no known family history, making this an incorrect diagnosis.

    Answer B is incorrect. Biliary atresia is the most common structural abnormality of the biliary tree in infants, and one of the two most common causes of conjugated hyperbilirubinemia. Lack of a gallbladder and presence of a triangular cord sign on ultrasound are suggestive of biliary atresia. However, this child has an unconjugated hyperbilirubinemia, making this diagnosis incorrect.

    Answer C is incorrect. Dubin-Johnson syndrome is an inborn disorder of bilirubin metabolism that leads to a conjugated hyperbilirubinemia. Since this child has an unconjugated hyperbilirubinemia, this diagnosis is incorrect. The inborn disorders of bilirubin metabolism that cause an unconjugated hyperbilirubinemia are Gilbert's syndrome and Crigler-Najjar syndrome.

    Answer E is incorrect. Rotor syndrome is an inborn disorder of bilirubin metabolism that leads to a conjugated hyperbilirubinemia. Since this child has an unconjugated hyperbilirubinemia, this diagnosis is incorrect.

24. **The correct answer is B.** Spasms of the esophagus are characterized by problems with both solids and liquids, causing odynophagia and dysphagia, as well as noncardiac angina.

Globus pharyngeus, or the feeling of food stuck in one's throat, is also very common. Nitroglycerin may actually confuse the diagnosis because it acts to relax the smooth muscle, thereby relieving the pain. X-rays may be helpful in diagnosis by showing what is known as a corkscrew formation of the esophagus. The anatomy of the esophagus may be divided into three parts, and when these three do not contract in a uniform manner as with spasms, then a food bolus may become trapped and cause pain. Manometry establishes the diagnosis by showing these uncoordinated contractions.

Answer A is incorrect. Although this patient has had cancer in the past, she does not seem to be suffering from it again. Her symptoms do not indicate any such etiology.

Answer C is incorrect. Usually, cancer will cause dysphagia only for solids and may not cause the pain this patient is experiencing unless it has spread beyond the walls of the esophagus.

Answer D is incorrect. A myocardial infarction will not present with the given history of progressive dysphagia. Remember that chest pain does not always translate into a cardiac etiology.

Answer E is incorrect. Very similar to spasms, nutcracker esophagus differs in the fact that it is characterized by continuous, coordinated contractions on manometry. This difference is important with treatment because spasms may ultimately be treated with a myotomy, while nutcracker cannot.

25. **The correct answer is C.** This patient presents with symptoms of a small bowel obstruction with peritoneal signs and thus needs surgical management. His presenting symptoms along with the radiographic findings support this diagnosis. Small bowel obstruction is the most common indication for surgery in a patient with Crohn's disease. Although patients with incomplete small bowel obstructions can be initially treated conservatively with bowel rest, a nasogastric tube, and intravenous fluids, patients who develop peritoneal signs with a small bowel obstruction should be taken to the operating room for surgical management.

Answer A is incorrect. Like all patients with small bowel obstruction, this patient should be put on bowel rest, resuscitated with intravenous fluids, and have a nasogastric tube placed. However, since he has developed peritoneal signs, he should be taken to the operating room for surgical management.

Answer B is incorrect. Although some patients with small bowel obstructions can be initially treated with conservative measures (intravenous fluids and a nasogastric tube for bowel decompression), this patient has peritoneal signs and should therefore be taken to the operating room for surgical management.

Answer D is incorrect. The clinical history, physical examination, and radiographic findings are diagnostic of a small bowel obstruction. Further workup with an MRI is not indicated at this time. Since this patient has developed peritoneal signs, he should be taken to the operating room for surgical management.

Answer E is incorrect. The clinical history, physical examination, and radiographic findings are diagnostic of a small bowel obstruction. Further workup with an ultrasound is not indicated at this time. Since this patient has developed peritoneal signs, he should be taken to the operating room for surgical management.

26. **The correct answer is D.** Dysphagia is the number one symptom of achalasia, which is characterized by a neuronal deficit that results in incomplete lower esophageal sphincter relaxation. It affects both solids and liquids. Her weight loss is almost assuredly due to this problem. The "bird's-beak" appearance seen on barium swallow is due to the dilated distal esophagus. Manometry is the definitive study and the results are as described in the question. Pneumatic dilation works in 80–90% of patients, though it may cause perforation. Botulinum toxin also may be given, as can anticholinergic agents, calcium channel blockers, and prostaglandins.

Answer A is incorrect. Cholinergic agents such as pilocarpine and bethanechol are not indicated for treatment of achalasia. In fact, there is minimal evidence that anticholinergic agents may be of some benefit, though this is largely anecdotal. Few patients are managed successfully with exclusively medical management.

Answer B is incorrect. Although this patient has a history of diabetes, dysphagia is rarely a symptom. Her hemoglobin A_{1c} level is also below the cutoff.

Answer C is incorrect. These are all remedies for reflux esophagitis, not achalasia. Patients with reflux typically present with complaints of indigestion, regurgitation, an acidic taste in the mouth, or chronic cough. Progressive dysphagia should raise suspicions of an anatomic or functional defect in peristalsis and lower esophageal sphincter (LES) function. Manometry in reflux generally shows decreased LES tone.

Answer E is incorrect. This patient does not have diverticula, which would be seen on barium swallow. An uncommon esophageal diverticulum that is nonetheless worth knowing for Step 2 questions is Zenker's diverticulum, which is an outpouching of the esophageal mucosa between the cricopharyngeus and the lower inferior constrictor. It forms after years of high intrapharyngeal pressure during swallowing (possibly secondary to upper esophageal sphincter dysfunction) and usually doesn't present until the patient's seventh decade. It predisposes patients to aspiration pneumonia, and should be treated surgically.

27. **The correct answer is D.** Hemochromatosis is the pathologic accumulation of iron in parenchymal organs. The patient in question has ascites, a coagulopathy (evident from the extensive bruising and elevated prothrombin time and partial thromboplastin time), and a nodular, shrunken liver on ultrasound giving her a diagnosis of liver cirrhosis. Additionally, with her history of diabetes, coronary heart failure, and skin pigmentation changes, the diagnosis of hemochromatosis is likely. Other potential symptoms include hypogonadism, fatigue, and arthralgias. Diagnosis could be confirmed based on Perls Prussian blue stain of a liver biopsy specimen. Hepatocellular carcinoma is a late sequela in these patients, especially if they are cirrhotic on presentation. Treatment is through phlebotomy and restriction of iron intake.

Answer A is incorrect. Acute pancreatitis is not a likely complication of hemochromatosis, although some reports show that hemochromatosis can cause chronic pancreatitis. Acute pancreatitis typically presents as acute epigastric pain radiating to the back, often associated with nausea, emesis, and fever. Diagnosis is usually through abnormal amylase and lipase serum levels, although CT imaging can also be useful, particularly if abscesses or pseudocysts are suspected. Treatment is typically supportive, involving food restriction, fluid resuscitation, and further investigation into underlying causes such as alcoholism or cholic sources.

Answer B is incorrect. Amyloidosis is not a complication of hemochromatosis. Amyloidosis can present in a wide variety of ways, depending on which organ system is involved. However, the most common complications are renal, so symptoms of renal failure such as peripheral edema typically present first. Other symptoms include coronary heart failure, peripheral neuropathy, arthritis, and carpal tunnel syndrome. Definitive diagnosis is typically through biopsy of the involved organ system, although CT imaging may also show some hints of disease.

Answer C is incorrect. Bone marrow failure is not a known complication of hemochromatosis. Patients with bone marrow failure present with low blood counts. The types of cell counts that are low depend on which cell lines have failed. Symptoms of fatigue and malaise typically follow from red cell aplasia, fever and other signs of infection from neutropenia, and bruising and bleeding from thrombocytopenia. Diagnosis can be done through laboratory tests such as a complete blood count with differential, but the gold standard test is bone marrow biopsy. Treatment is with bone marrow transplantation, although treatment with antithymocyte globulin or antilymphocyte globulin can be used for severe aplastic anemia.

Answer E is incorrect. Although several blood diseases that result in iron overload disease can cause splenomegaly, hemochromatosis does not cause splenomegaly.

28. **The correct answer is B.** Meconium ileus is nearly pathognomonic for cystic fibrosis (CF) but can less commonly be caused by volvulus, intestinal pseudo-obstruction, or other rarer causes of pancreatic insufficiency. CF is especially likely in this case with a positive family history for a sibling with meconium ileus. Meconium ileus occurs in CF because of a deficiency in pancreatic secretions, which causes the meconium to become mucilaginous and viscid, sticking to the walls of the intestine.

Answer A is incorrect. Congenital aganglionosis of the colon (Hirschsprung's disease) typically presents with constipation in the first month of life following the normal passage of meconium.

Answer C is incorrect. Intussusception occurs in infants between 5 and 10 months of age and presents with intermittent, colicky abdominal pain. Radiographs typically show small bowel obstruction with absence of gas in the right colon.

Answer D is incorrect. Total absence of the small bowel is a rare condition typically associated with volvulus and gastroschisis.

Answer E is incorrect. Volvulus may occur shortly after birth but presents with bilious vomiting and poor feeding.

29. **The correct answer is E.** Gallstone ileus is an unusual complication of cholelithiasis and occurs when a gallstone enters the bowel through a biliary-enteric fistula and creates an obstruction, usually at the ileocecal valve. In all patients with suspected small bowel obstruction, rapidly obtainable supine and erect plain films are the first diagnostic test of choice. They may demonstrate air under the diaphragm due to perforation, air in the biliary tree, or signs of partial or complete obstruction. Direct visualization of the gallstone tends to occur only 15% of the time because most gallstones are radiolucent. CT of the abdomen is a useful confirmatory test in these patients and would provide better anatomic detail prior to surgery.

Answer A is incorrect. Abdominal ultrasound may demonstrate enterobiliary fistulas but is limited due to reflection from bowel gas.

Answer B is incorrect. The diagnosis of gallstone ileus is made preoperatively in about 50% of patients and is often made at laparotomy or laparoscopy. However, noninvasive diagnostic tests, such as plain x-ray and CT, should be attempted first.

Answer C is incorrect. Endoscopic retrograde cholangiopancreatography is only useful in demonstrating a fistula if the gallbladder is able to be filled at the time of diagnosis.

Answer D is incorrect. Hepatic iminodiacetic acid scan is a nuclear medicine study that is used to assess the gallbladder and biliary tree for obstruction. It is most useful in acute cholecystitis and would not provide information about the patient's suspected bowel obstruction, although it might demonstrate a biliary-enteric fistula.

30. **The correct answer is A.** For perforated appendicitis with no clear loculations, the recommended management is emergent appendectomy with postoperative intravenous antibiotics and delayed primary closure.

Answer B is incorrect. Bowel rest with nothing-by-mouth status and intravenous hydration are appropriate in the setting of acute pancreatitis, not acute appendicitis.

Answer C is incorrect. Percutaneous drainage and interval appendectomy are appropriate for perforated appendicitis with a well-loculated abscess in patients who may need temporizing measures or have contraindications such as cardiovascular instability. Our patient is stable and does not have a loculated abscess, and therefore percutaneous drainage is unlikely to be the primary management for this patient.

Answer D is incorrect. Serial abdominal examinations along with antimicrobial treatment are appropriate management steps for diverticulitis, not appendicitis.

Answer E is incorrect. The patient's pain is more typical of acute appendicitis and not an acute myocardial infarction, thus ECG and cardiac enzymes would not be appropriate.

31. The correct answer is D. Patients with partial small bowel obstructions (SBOs) may complain of crampy abdominal pain, with or without passage of feces or flatus. Those with malignancies, hernias, or previous intra-abdominal surgeries may be prone to bowel obstructions. Presentation may include fever, tachycardia, hypotension, dry mucous membranes, high pitched or hypoactive bowel sounds, and abdominal tenderness or distention. For a partial SBO, supportive care may be enough under close supervision. Nasogastric suction should be used for decompression, and the patient should be maintained on nothing by mouth with intravenous hydration and correction of electrolyte abnormalities.

Answer A is incorrect. The patient does not have signs of infection or necrotic bowel. With infection or peritonitis, the patient will present with abdominal wall tenderness and rigidity, rebound tenderness, and decreased bowel sounds. These patients will most likely minimize their movement to decrease pain. Mesenteric ischemia, which can lead to necrotic bowel, will present with acute abdominal pain and pain out of proportion to examination results. Look for risk factors such as atrial fibrillation, congestive heart failure, peripheral vascular disease, or hypercoagulability. Diagnosis is made with an angiogram, which identifies vascular compromise.

Answer B is incorrect. Colonoscopy may be helpful in a stable patient with large bowel obstruction, but it is inappropriate for small bowel obstructions. Clinical symptoms are similar to those of small bowel obstruction, but x-ray of the abdomen may demonstrate dilated loops of small bowel.

Answer C is incorrect. Complete SBOs will present with vomiting and crampy abdominal pain with or without passage of feces or flatus, since 12–24 hours are usually required before the colon has become vacant. Surgery is appropriate for complete SBO, SBO with vascular compromise such as necrotic bowel, or symptoms lasting > 3 days without resolution.

Answer E is incorrect. While serial abdominal examinations are useful to mark the progress of patients recovering from partial small bowel obstruction, such examinations alone are inappropriate for management because the bowels still need to be decompressed and relieved of volume load by nasogastric suction and nothing-by-mouth status.

32. The correct answer is E. Patients with pancreatic cancer can present with weight loss, jaundice, abdominal pain, dark urine, acholic stools, and pruritus. On physical examination the gallbladder or other abdominal mass is palpable. Diagnosis is usually made with ultrasound with findings of dilated bile ducts or visible mass, or CT scan which demonstrates the pancreatic mass. The associated risk factors for pancreatic cancer include smoking, chronic pancreatitis, a first-degree relative with pancreatic cancer, and high-fat diet.

Answer A is incorrect. Chronic pancreatitis, not chronic gastritis, is a risk factor for pancreatic cancer.

Answer B is incorrect. Diabetes insipidus is not a pathology of the pancreas and is not a risk factor for pancreatic cancer.

Answer C is incorrect. Diabetes mellitus can result from neoplasm in the body of pancreas, but it is not a risk factor for pancreatic cancer.

Answer D is incorrect. History of cholecystitis is not a risk factor for pancreatic cancer. Postoperative biliary stricture should be on the differential diagnosis in a patient with a history of cholecystectomy who presents with symptoms suggestive of pancreatic neoplasm.

33. The correct answer is D. Intussusception is the most common abdominal emergency in children younger than 2 years, and the second most common cause of intestinal obstruction (pyloric stenosis is first). The image shows loss of bowel pattern in the right upper quadrant. Intussusception occurs most commonly near the ileocolic junction, and 75% of these cases are idiopathic. Mucosal bleeding leads to bloody, sometimes mucus-containing, stool known as "currant jelly stools." The onset is typically abrupt with severe, recurrent, colicky abdominal pain. Episodes typically last 15–20 minutes and the child may act normally between episodes. Nonbloody nonbilious emesis may also be observed. As the intussusception worsens, it may become bilious.

Answer A is incorrect. Cystic fibrosis (CF) is a fatal autosomal recessive disease that is more common in whites. CF may have respiratory, gastrointestinal, sinus, and/or musculoskeletal manifestations and can cause infertility. Pancreatic insufficiency affects 85% of CF patients, and leads to steatorrhea with the passage of bulky, foul-smelling, floating stools. This thick stool can act as a lead point for intussusception in patients with CF.

Answer B is incorrect. Enterocolitis is inflammation of the mucosa of the small and large intestine, which may result from infection, diet, or other etiologies. Intussusception may complicate enterocolitis; however, there is usually diarrhea and less severe, less regular pain associated with enterocolitis. The child also remains noticeably ill between episodes of abdominal pain.

Answer C is incorrect. HSP is a systemic vasculitic syndrome characterized by the deposition of IgA-containing immune complexes in tissues. There is a classic tetrad of rash (palpable purpura), arthralgias, abdominal pain (often colicky, associated with emesis), and renal disease that can manifest over days to several weeks in any order. Intussusception is a rare complication of HSP that may result from intestinal hemorrhage and hematoma formation serving as a lead point.

Answer E is incorrect. A Meckel's diverticulum is a vestigial remnant of the embryonic yolk sac, typically seen as an outpouching of the ileum. Intussusception may also complicate Meckel's diverticulum; however, these diverticuli typically manifest with painless rectal bleeding within the first 2 years of life, secondary to mucosal ulceration of ectopic gastric tissue within the diverticulum. Intussusception associated with Meckel's is often seen in older male children.

Answer F is incorrect. Pyloric stenosis often presents at age 3–6 weeks with nonbilious projectile vomiting immediately after meals. Patients exhibit a characteristic desire to be re-fed soon after ("hungry vomiter"). On physical examination, an olive-like mass may be palpated in the mid-epigastrium. Laboratory tests may show a hypochloremic metabolic alkalosis due to a loss of gastric hydrochloric acid and fluid from vomiting.

34. **The correct answer is B.** It is recommended that if a patient has numerous large adenomas removed from the colon, they should return for colonoscopy in 3 years.

    Answer A is incorrect. Those who have had ulcerative colitis for > 10 years or those with familial adenomatous polyposis are candidates for prophylactic colectomy. This patient's situation does not warrant such treatment.

    Answer C is incorrect. Ten years is the regular interval for routine screening colonoscopies. In this situation, with the presence of numerous large adenomas, waiting 10 years is too long, since that would be enough time for cancer to develop and then spread.

    Answer D is incorrect. Ten years is too long to wait in this situation. Moreover, the less sensitive nature of sigmoidoscopies leads to their use in screening more often than every 10 years.

    Answer E is incorrect. This is not the correct answer, as this intervention is not appropriate for this patient's presentation. Urgent colectomy is generally performed in cases of acute colitis secondary to ulcerative colitis, Crohn's colitis, colonic inertia, and familial adenomatous polyposis. Colonic ischemia and perforation are also potential indications.

35. **The correct answer is D.** Positive hepatitis B surface antibody (HBsAb) indicates that the patient has acquired immunity, either via a now-resolved infection or vaccination. The end of the window period usually is marked by the rise in HBsAb.

    Answer A is incorrect. Negative hepatitis B surface antigen and hepatitis B surface antibody occur together during the window phase of recovery from infection, but may also be seen in a patient who is neither infected nor immune.

    Answer B is incorrect. Hepatitis B core antibody (HBcAb) is positive during the window period and IgM HBcAb indicates a recent disease state. The window period usually occurs 5–6 months after exposure and HBcAb is commonly the most positive serologic marker during this period.

Answer C is incorrect. Positive hepatitis B e antibody may be seen during ongoing infection, but indicates a low likelihood of spreading the disease. It is the other serologic marker, besides hepatitis B core antibody that may be present during the window period.

Answer E is incorrect. Positive hepatitis B surface antigen indicates an acute or chronic unresolved infection. Its continued presence indicates a carrier state.

36. **The correct answer is D.** Tracheoesophageal fistula (TEF) is a relatively common congenital anomaly involving the respiratory tract. It occurs in approximately 1 in 4000 live births. TEF occurs with esophageal atresia (EA) in > 90% of cases. In the most common form of TEF and EA, the esophagus ends in a blind pouch, and the TEF is connected to the distal esophagus. TEF and EA result from a defect in lateral septation of the foregut into the esophagus and trachea. TEF and EA often occur with the **VACTERL** (**V**ertebral, **A**norectal, **C**ardiovascular, **T**racheal, **E**sophageal, **R**enal, and **L**imb abnormalities) syndrome, as seen in this patient with the holosystolic murmur of a ventricular septal defect and limb abnormalities. In cases with EA, there is polyhydramnios in utero. These babies present with excessive secretions that cause frothing at the mouth and nose, drooling, choking, cyanosis, and respiratory distress immediately after birth. If the trachea is connected to the distal esophagus, gastric distention can occur. The symptoms of respiratory distress are exacerbated by feeding, which may result in regurgitation and reflux of gastric contents through the TEF, sometimes resulting in aspiration pneumonia. Patients with TEF and no EA (H-type TEF) account for 5% of cases of TEF. If the defect is large, they may also present early, with coughing and choking with feeding. Smaller defects may present with chronic respiratory problems such as bronchospasm and recurrent pneumonia later in life, and may not be diagnosed until as late as age 4 years. In the presence of EA, a naso- or orogastric tube can only be passed 10–15 cm down the airway and cannot be passed into the stomach. The tube is seen coiled in the up-

per esophageal pouch on an anteroposterior x-ray of the chest. With a distal TEF, a distended gas-filled stomach is seen on x-ray of the chest, and the TEF may be seen on a lateral view. Fluoroscopy can confirm the diagnosis of EA.

Answer A is incorrect. Congenital diaphragmatic hernia (CDH) results from a defect in the diaphragm that allows herniation of abdominal contents into the thorax. Approximately 85% of the defects occur on the left. Intestinal malrotation and pulmonary hypoplasia are associated with almost all cases of CDH. Most affected infants present within the first few hours of life with severe respiratory distress. They also have a scaphoid abdomen, absence of breath sounds, and shifted heart sounds. In left-sided CDH, bowel sounds are heard over the left hemithorax. CDH is usually diagnosed in utero by prenatal ultrasound. X-ray of the chest postnatally shows the intestine passing through the diaphragm and confirms the diagnosis.

Answer B is incorrect. Pyloric stenosis often presents at age 3–6 weeks with nonbilious projectile vomiting immediately after meals and a desire to be fed again soon after ("hungry vomiter"). On physical examination, an olive-like mass may be palpated in the mid-epigastrium. Laboratory values can show a hypochloremic metabolic alkalosis due to a loss of gastric hydrochloric acid and fluid from vomiting. The diagnosis of pyloric stenosis can be confirmed by ultrasound or upper gastrointestinal study.

Answer C is incorrect. Respiratory distress syndrome (RDS) most often occurs in premature infants with an incidence that is inversely proportional to gestational age and birth weight. Infants of diabetic mothers, delivery before 37 weeks' gestation, delivery via cesarean section, precipitous delivery, asphyxia, and multigestational pregnancies have an increased incidence of RDS. RDS results from surfactant deficiency that leads to high surface tension, collapse of alveoli, and less compliant lungs. RDS presents within minutes of birth with tachypnea (respiratory rate > 60/min), grunting, nasal flaring, retractions, shallow rapid breathing, and cyanosis. The cyanosis is progressive and is minimally responsive to oxygen therapy. Tubular breath sounds may be present, and rales may be heard at the lung bases on inspiration. Laboratory tests initially show a respiratory and metabolic acidosis. Hypoxemia and hypercapnia may develop. X-ray of the chest shows lung parenchyma with a reticulogranular ground-glass appearance and air bronchograms, especially in the left lower lobe because of the cardiac shadow.

Answer E is incorrect. Transient tachypnea of the newborn (TTN) is a benign self-limited condition that usually occurs after a normal vaginal or cesarean delivery of a preterm or term infant. It is believed to result from slow absorption of lung fluid in the fetus. It is more common in infants of mothers who are diabetic or asthmatic. TTN presents with an early onset of tachypnea, usually within 2 hours of delivery, which may be associated with grunting and retractions. Occasionally, cyanosis also occurs but is relieved with administration of < 40% oxygen. Mild hypoxemia, hypercapnia, or acidosis may be present on laboratory evaluation. X-ray of the chest shows perihilar streaking in the interlobular fissures due to excess lung fluid filling up the alveoli and spilling over into the extra-alveolar interstitium, especially the perivascular tissue and interlobar fissures.

37. **The correct answer is A.** It is considered pathologic for a full-term infant not to pass meconium within the first 48 hours of life. Hirschsprung's disease, or congenital megacolon, usually presents with delayed passage of meconium and abdominal distention. This is a condition that arises when neural crest cells fail to migrate to the colon during embryonic development, leaving the patient without peristalsis. A barium enema that shows dilated proximal bowel and a narrowed distal segment is highly suggestive of Hirschsprung's disease. The lack of ganglion cells on rectal biopsy is also diagnostic of Hirschsprung's disease.

Answer B is incorrect. A volvulus with malrotation is the most critical cause of bowel obstruction. It presents in the first week of life with bilious emesis and constipation. An upper GI series with an absent or abnormal position of the ligament of Treitz confirms the diagnosis of malrotation.

Answer C is incorrect. A double-bubble sign (air bubbles in the stomach and duodenum) is diagnostic of duodenal atresia, a condition classically associated with Down's syndrome. Duodenal atresia can cause constipation, but that is usually after meconium has been passed. Duodenal atresia presents clinically with bilious emesis within the first few hours of life. Physical examination is notable for abdominal distension of predominantly the upper abdomen.

Answer D is incorrect. A positive sweat test is the definitive way to diagnose cystic fibrosis (CF). Delayed passage of meconium for > 48 hours can be an initial sign of CF, but there are no dilated or narrowed loops of bowel in patients with CF. CF is most prevalent in white subjects.

Answer E is incorrect. Intussusception is a common cause of bowel obstruction in infants < 2 years old. It presents with bouts of irritability, colicky abdominal pain, and vomiting. If it is not diagnosed at this point, infants become lethargic and pass red currant jelly–like stools. Physical examination is sometimes notable for a palpable right lower quadrant mass. Air contrast barium enema showing telescoping of the bowel is both diagnostic and therapeutic for intussusception.

38. **The correct answer is E.** Technetium-labeled RBCs can detect bleeding rates as low as 0.1 mL/min, although higher rates provide for optimal localization. No other method can detect bleeding rates lower than this. After administration of the tagged RBCs, the body is scanned to detect the location of the bleeding.

Answer A is incorrect. Angiography can detect bleeding rates as low as 0.5 mL/min. This is a higher rate than a tagged RBC scan can detect, so this would not be the ideal diagnostic test.

Answer B is incorrect. Barium enema can show the architecture of the colon, but would not be expected to show colonic bleeding.

Answer C is incorrect. Colonoscopy can detect gross bleeding but would not pick up the low level of bleeding that this patient has.

Answer D is incorrect. CT scanning is not the modality used to detect colonic bleeding.

39. **The correct answer is E.** Omphalocele is a congenital defect in which there is herniation of abdominal viscera through the abdominal wall into the base of the umbilical cord. Unlike an umbilical hernia, the viscera herniate into a sac that is covered by amniotic membrane and peritoneum but no skin. Omphalocele typically presents with polyhydramnios in utero, and the infant is often born prematurely and has other gastrointestinal and cardiac defects. Ninety-five percent of these defects are accurately diagnosed on prenatal ultrasound. Ten percent of infants with omphalocele have Beckwith-Wiedemann syndrome (exophthalmos, macroglossia, gigantism, hyperinsulinemia, and hypoglycemia). The exposed intestine should be wrapped sterilely to minimize insensible fluid losses and loss of heat. An oro- or nasogastric tube should be inserted to decompress the stomach, the airway should be stabilized, and peripheral intravenous (IV) access should be established for initiation of IV fluids and antibiotics. The omphalocele is emergently repaired with surgery.

Answer A is incorrect. Duodenal atresia is complete obstruction of the lumen of the duodenum. It is a cause of bowel obstruction during the neonatal period. Up to 30% of patients with duodenal atresia have Down's syndrome. Other congenital abnormalities have also been associated with duodenal atresia. It typically presents with bilious emesis on the first day of life. Polyhydramnios in utero is associated with 50% of cases, and one-third of the cases are associated with jaundice. A double-bubble sign is seen on x-ray of the abdomen due to gaseous distention of the stomach and proximal duodenum. Initial management includes withholding feedings, decompressing the stomach by the placement of a naso- or orogastric tube to suction, starting intravenous fluid replacement, and antibiotics. The duodenal atresia is then repaired surgically.

Answer B is incorrect. Gastroschisis is also a congenital defect that involves herniation of abdominal viscera through the abdominal wall next to the umbilicus. There is no sac covering the herniated viscera. It is typically located to the right of a normally positioned umbilical cord. It usually presents with polyhydramnios in utero and is usually detectable on prenatal ultrasound. The affected infant is typically delivered spontaneously, preterm, and has malrotation, stenosis, or atresia of the gastrointestinal tract. An oro- or nasogastric tube should be inserted to decompress the stomach, the airway should be stabilized, and peripheral intravenous (IV) access should be established for initiation of IV fluids and antibiotics. Emergency surgery is necessary to correct the defect.

Answer C is incorrect. Hirschsprung's disease, also known as congenital aganglionic megacolon, results from abnormal innervation of the bowel. It is the most common cause of obstruction of the lower intestine in neonates. It is often associated with other congenital defects. It typically presents in full-term infants with delayed passage of meconium (meconium is normally passed within the first 48 hours of birth in full-term babies), bilious emesis, and abdominal distention. Some affected infants may pass meconium normally during the neonatal period, and then present later with a history of chronic constipation and failure to thrive. Patients with Hirschsprung's have normal anal tone on rectal examination, and the examination is often followed by explosive release of gas and feces (blast sign). Hirschsprung's may be diagnosed by rectal manometry if rectal distention results in a failure of rectal pressure to drop or a paradoxical rise in pressure. Barium enema may reveal a cone-shaped transition zone between the normal dilated proximal intestine and the smaller-caliber obstructed distal colon, which results from nonrelaxation of the aganglionic segment. Absence of ganglion cells on rectal biopsy is the gold standard for diagnosis. Hirschsprung's disease is treated with surgery.

Answer D is incorrect. Meckel's diverticulum is a vestigial remnant of the embryonic yolk sac, also known as the vitelline or omphalomesenteric duct, which is typically seen as an outpouching of the ileum. These diverticula typically manifest as painless rectal bleeding within the first 2 years of life, secondary to mucosal ulceration of ectopic gastric tissue within the diverticulum. They can also present with diverticulitis or with intestinal obstruction from intussusception or volvulus. It is the most common congenital anomaly of the gastrointestinal tract and has been associated with the rule of twos: two times as many men are affected, it often occurs 2 feet from the ileocecal valve, two types of mucosa (gastric and pancreatic) may be located within the diverticula, and it occurs in 2% of infants.

40. **The correct answer is A.** A stressful event, such as divorce or death of a loved one, can lead to an exacerbation of underlying inflammatory bowel disease (IBD). Ulcerative colitis is an IBD characterized by recurrent episodic inflammation of the mucosal layer of the colon. It frequently involves the rectum, and may extend in a proximal and continuous fashion to involve other areas of the colon. The mainstay of treatment is topical or oral 5-aminosalicylic acid or topical/systemic corticosteroids. Surgical intervention is reserved for patients who are intractable to medical therapy or who develop an acute complication (e.g., hemorrhage, perforation).

Answer B is incorrect. Alcohol has not been shown to exacerbate IBD.

Answer C is incorrect. According to studies, oral contraceptive use leads to a relative risk of 1.9 in the development of Crohn's disease. However, again no evidence exists that the use of oral contraceptive pills in a patient with IBD will exacerbate symptoms.

Answer D is incorrect. Unlike Crohn's disease, where smoking appears to increase risk, cigarette smoking lessens the risk of a patient developing ulcerative colitis.

Answer E is incorrect. An upper respiratory infection has no relation to the development of IBD symptoms. In Crohn's disease, a gastrointestinal infection can cause symptoms of diarrhea and abdominal pain, which are often treated with antibiotics.

41. **The correct answer is C.** This patient presents with typical signs and symptoms of diverticular bleeding. She has signs of hypovolemia and blood loss. The best treatment is to rehy-

drate the patient and transfuse her to bring her hematocrit up. Most diverticular bleeding will stop on its own.

Answer A is incorrect. If the patient has persistent bleeding that does not stop on its own, this is a reasonable option. But before moving to this invasive procedure, it is preferable to treat by hydration and transfusion and see if the bleeding will spontaneously stop.

Answer B is incorrect. If there is significant bleeding that does not self-resolve and is not able to be embolized, surgery is the next option. The patient in this question has not yet gone through a trial of conservative treatment of rehydration and blood transfusion, so it is incorrect to go straight to surgery.

Answer D is incorrect. This is appropriate treatment for diverticulitis, but this patient does not appear to have diverticulitis, as she is afebrile with no nausea or vomiting, no marked abdominal cramping pain, and only a relatively mild leukocytosis. When treating for diverticulitis, the choice of antibiotics would include metronidazole and a second- or third-generation cephalosporin or fluoroquinolone.

Answer E is incorrect. This is a treatment used for people with uncomplicated diverticular disease. This patient is showing signs of dehydration and anemia and should be treated for those conditions. After the patient is stable, she can be discharged with instructions to eat a high-fiber diet.

42. **The correct answer is E.** Involvement of the small bowel occurs only in Crohn's disease, and involvement of the small intestine excludes ulcerative colitis as a diagnosis. While both diseases are chronic inflammatory processes of the bowel wall, ulcerative colitis progresses in a stereotyped pattern from the rectum proximally along the colon. Crohn's disease notoriously appears at any possible site along the entire length of the gastrointestinal tract. Its proclivity is to attack the terminal ileum. While rates of ulcerative colitis have been steady in recent decades, the incidence of Crohn's is rising, suggesting a distinct etiology. Both diseases are best diagnosed by biopsy, generally via colonoscopy.

Answer A is incorrect. Gross bleeding is common in ulcerative colitis, although it can also be seen in Crohn's. Bleeding from inflammatory bowel disease is typically self-limited and not life threatening, and may be managed conservatively or via colonoscopy. Because of the increased risk of colon cancer in patients with ulcerative colitis, a high suspicion for malignancy is prudent.

Answer B is incorrect. The presence of perianal disease and fistulae are rare in ulcerative colitis and are suggestive of Crohn's. One-third of Crohn's patients develop perianal disease. Examples of perianal pathologies include skin tags, fissures, perirectal abscesses, and fistulae.

Answer C is incorrect. Fistulae are common in Crohn's, but are very rare in ulcerative colitis. This distinction may be made intuitive by reflecting on the fistula as a direct consequence of the transmural inflammation typical of Crohn's. The inflammation in ulcerative colitis is superficial and thus less predisposing to such structural sequelae.

Answer D is incorrect. Sparing of the rectum almost never occurs in ulcerative colitis, and is therefore suggestive of Crohn's disease. One caveat is that application of a topical medication, such as mesalamine, in ulcerative colitis patients may give the impression of rectal sparing.

43. **The correct answer is B.** This patient suffers from hepatic encephalopathy secondary to hepatitis C cirrhosis. Hepatic encephalopathy is a neuropsychiatric condition caused by the inability of the liver to filter nitrogenous compounds and other toxins out of the systemic circulation. Ammonia is believed to play a role in pathogenesis, but several other toxins have also been implicated. Symptoms include disturbed intellectual function, consciousness, and neuromuscular function (asterixis, hyperreflexia, and myoclonus). Management strategies include reducing protein consumption, as well as treating with lactulose and metronidazole.

Answer A is incorrect. Because this patient shows signs of portal hypertension secondary to hepatitis C virus cirrhosis, esophageal varices must be considered. However, although all patients with signs of portal hypertension should be monitored for variceal formation, this patient's acute clinical presentation is consistent with hepatic encephalopathy.

Answer C is incorrect. Although this patient's likely hepatitis C diagnosis puts her at risk for hepatocellular carcinoma, the acute clinical presentation is most consistent with hepatic encephalopathy.

Answer D is incorrect. Hepatorenal syndrome, a diagnosis of exclusion, is defined as a liver disease, such as cirrhosis, complicated by functional renal failure. Glomerular filtration rate is decreased and blood urea nitrogen-to-creatinine ratio is typically elevated. Although this diagnosis must be ruled out in the setting of decompensated cirrhosis, this patient's presentation is more consistent with hepatic encephalopathy.

Answer E is incorrect. Spontaneous bacterial peritonitis (SBP) is an infection of the ascitic fluid, typically with *Enterobacteriaceae*, pneumococcus, or gram-negative bacteria. SBP typically occurs in the setting of cirrhosis. Physical examination findings can include fever and abdominal pain and tenderness, or the infection may be silent clinically. The clinical presentation, along with an ascitic fluid polymorphonuclear leukocyte count > 250 cells/mL, is diagnostic of SBP.

44. **The correct answer is E.** In this patient with minimal symptoms, broad-spectrum antibiotic coverage, including anaerobic coverage, is appropriate.

Answer A is incorrect. Cefotetan alone would provide inadequate coverage against many of the gram-negative organisms found in the gut.

Answer B is incorrect. Broad-spectrum intravenous antibiotics would be appropriate in a more severe episode of diverticulitis but should always be followed by oral antibiotics to ensure adequate length of treatment.

Answer C is incorrect. The patient presents with uncomplicated diverticulitis. Intravenous ampicillin/sulbactam followed by metronidazole is inappropriate because it is used to treat more severe diverticulitis.

Answer D is incorrect. Metronidazole alone would provide inadequate coverage against many of the gram-negative organisms found in the gut.

45. **The correct answer is E.** This patient presents with dermatitis, diarrhea, and alopecia while on long-term total parenteral nutrition (TPN) therapy. In this setting, it is important to consider both common and uncommon vitamin deficiencies, especially with unenriched TPN or in patients with malabsorptive pathology. Specifically, patients on chronic TPN therapy are at risk for deficiencies in several minerals, including selenium, gold, zinc, and copper, among others. In this case, the triad of diarrhea, dermatitis, and alopecia suggests zinc deficiency. Niacin deficiency can also present with diarrhea and dermatitis but rarely alopecia. Moreover, such patients commonly demonstrate altered level of consciousness or dementia. Niacin deficiency is not seen in patients on TPN therapy.

Answer A is incorrect. Chromium is believed to play a role in glucose tolerance and increase insulin sensitivity when administered to diabetics. Deficiencies can contribute to glucose intolerance and lipid disturbances.

Answer B is incorrect. Cobalt deficiency is not a pathologic state and poses no risk to patients. In excess, however, cobalt can lead to damage to cardiac myocytes and result in dilated cardiomyopathy.

Answer C is incorrect. Copper plays an important role in multiple metabolic pathways, including the hepatic cytochrome system; erythropoiesis; and catecholamine processing in the brain. Patients receiving total parenteral nutrition often receive free amino acids, which increases urinary copper loss. When deficient, patients are at risk of developing anemia and neutropenia.

Answer D is incorrect. Selenium affects enzyme and membrane activity, especially in myocytes, and deficiency can lead to cardiomyopathy and skeletal muscle dysfunction. This patient displays no evidence of muscle pathology.

46. **The correct answer is A.** This patient has been on an extended course of antibiotics and is most likely suffering from toxic megacolon. This is diagnosed by three of the following: anemia, an elevated WBC count, tachycardia, and a fever. There needs to also be one of the following present: change in mental status, dehydration, hypotension, and electrolyte abnormalities. A stool sample will most likely reveal *Clostridium difficile* toxin, which is the most common culprit in situations of toxic megacolon such as this in which a patient has been exposed to a long course of an antibiotic active against the gram-negative bacteria in commensal intestinal flora.

Answer B is incorrect. While several gram-negative organisms including *Klebsiella* and *Proteus* can cause changes in bowel habits, usually diarrhea, this clinical picture is most likely associated with toxic megacolon brought on by *Clostridium difficile*.

Answer C is incorrect. The most likely culprit is *Clostridium difficile*, and its toxin is most readily picked up on stool sample. Gram-positive cocci including enterococci may prove problematic in the colon in the context of diverticulitis. This condition may present with abdominal pain, tenderness in the left lower quadrant, fever, nausea, vomiting, chills, cramping, and constipation.

Answer D is incorrect. Patients with toxic megacolon often have bloody diarrhea, so we would expect to see blood in the stool. Intestinal bleeding results in anemia, one of the diagnostic criteria for toxic megacolon.

Answer E is incorrect. Spores and hyphae are consistent with a fungal infection, but this is most likely toxic megacolon caused by *Clostridium difficile*, not a fungus. *Candida* has been found in stool samples of patients on chronic antibiotics experiencing diarrhea, though such patients would not experience the other toxic effects noted above.

47. **The correct answer is E.** This patient is presenting with signs and symptoms that should direct the physician's attention to the biliary tree and, more specifically, to the gallbladder. She has three of the "4 F's" (Fat, Forty, Female, and Fertile) for typical cholelithiasis patients, and her pain as described is suspicious for biliary colic. On physical examination,

mild icterus, low fever, positive Murphy's sign, and tenderness/guarding in the RUQ should prompt evaluation for acute cholecystitis. The imaging study of choice in initial evaluation of acute cholecystitis is an ultrasound of the RUQ. This has been demonstrated to be 95% sensitive for stones of any type in the gallbladder. It can detect stones as small as 3 mm in diameter, and is excellent at detecting inflammation in the gallbladder and dilation of intra- and extrahepatic ducts.

Answer A is incorrect. CT scanning is not the first-line choice for imaging in suspected cholecystitis due to its lower sensitivity (vs. ultrasound), its higher cost, and the involvement of radiation exposure. CT is useful in the evaluation of neoplasms in the pancreas and hepatobiliary tree.

Answer B is incorrect. Plane x-rays of the abdomen are rarely diagnostic for stones because only 10–15% are radiopaque. This imaging modality is useful in the evaluation of acute emphysematous cholecystitis, pneumobilia secondary to a gastrointestinal-biliary fistula, and small bowel obstruction. However, in this case, these diagnoses are not likely.

Answer C is incorrect. Hepatobiliary iminodiacetic acid scanning (radionuclide biliary scanning) is sensitive and specific for detection of acute cholecystitis and for detection of a bile leak after surgery. It is a good technique for imaging of the gallbladder; however, it is more expensive and time consuming than an ultrasound and is therefore used if ultrasound is inconclusive.

Answer D is incorrect. MRI is not commonly used in the evaluation of acute cholecystitis, due to its high cost and the presence of other highly effective imaging for this purpose.

Questions 48–50

48. **The correct answer is K.** Lactose intolerance is most prominent in Asians and African-Americans, and the incidence is lowest in whites of northern European descent. The symptoms described occur after ingestion of milk or milk-containing foods and reliably stop with a lactose-free diet. They are caused by an osmotic

diarrhea secondary to the inability to break down lactose (a protein found in milk). Laboratory findings may include low fecal pH or presence of reducing substances in the stool. However, diagnosis should be confirmed by a positive lactose breath hydrogen test.

49. **The correct answer is D.** Celiac disease is classically a disease of infancy, which presents with failure to thrive and malabsorption, associated with ingestion of wheat gluten. However, due to evolving recommendations of when to introduce wheat-containing foods during infancy and early childhood, celiac disease can also present later in childhood. Histopathology shows villous atrophy.

50. **The correct answer is E.** Although the presentation of pseudomembranous colitis following usage of clindamycin is classic, many different classes of antibiotics can alter the intestinal flora and lead to overgrowth of *Clostridium difficile*. Furthermore, most antibiotic-associated diarrhea is osmotic in nature and does not result from *C. difficile* infection. The mechanism involves decreased breakdown of carbohydrates in the gut due to reduced bacterial counts. This causes a greater concentration of complex carbohydrates within the intestinal lumen, leading to higher osmotic pressure and watery diarrhea.

Answer A is incorrect. *Bacillus cereus* is gram-positive rod that produces exotoxins that are very heat stable. It can lead to both diarrheal and emetic illness, which are caused by distinct exotoxins. The diarrheal illness produces a watery diarrhea with abdominal cramps 6–15 hours after consumption and is limited to about 24 hours' duration. Emetic illness causes vomiting within 0.5–6 hours of consumption that lasts < 24 hours. Diagnosis rests on identification of disease-causing serotypes of *B. cereus* in the suspect food (classically reheated rice).

Answer B is incorrect. *Campylobacter jejuni* is a curved gram-negative rod that is the leading cause of bacterial diarrheal illness in the United States. It is often contracted from raw chicken or milk and from nonchlorinated water. Symptoms of the illness include watery or mucoid diarrhea, which may contain occult blood, along with fever, nausea, abdominal pains, and headache. The illness is usually self-limiting and passes within 7–10 days. *C. jejuni* is identified in stool samples through Gram stain and culture on special media.

Answer C is incorrect. Carcinoid syndrome is a constellation of symptoms resulting from hormone-producing tumors most commonly found in the gut. The carcinoid cells produce serotonin derivatives, which are normally metabolized to an inactive form by the liver. Carcinoid syndrome occurs when the tumor metastasizes to the liver so the hormonal products can bypass hepatic metabolism. The serotonin-like compounds enter the systemic circulation and cause a number of symptoms, most commonly secretory diarrhea, flushing, and wheezing. Diagnosis is based on urinary 5-hydroxyindoleacetic acid, a breakdown product of serotonin.

Answer F is incorrect. Crohn's disease is a chronic inflammatory disease that affects any portion of the gastrointestinal tract. It causes mucoid nonbloody diarrhea that is recurrent, as well as constitutional symptoms and abdominal pain. It commonly affects individuals in their 20s with another peak in the sixth and seventh decades of life. Intestinal biopsy shows transmural inflammation with noncaseating granulomas.

Answer G is incorrect. *Entamoeba histolytica* is a protozoan that exists in two life stages: the trophozoite and cyst. The trophozoites infect humans and cause disease, while the cysts survive outside the host in water and soil and on foods. When cysts are swallowed, the protozoa excyst and progress to the trophozoite phase. Infection is often subclinical but can present with bloody mucoid stools. Diagnosis depends on finding cysts in three separate stool samples.

Answer H is incorrect. *Escherichia coli* is a gram-negative bacillus that is part of the normal bacterial flora of the gut. There are four different classes of *E. coli* that are recognized to cause disease in humans, each with a different mechanism: enteroinvasive, enterohemorrhagic, enterotoxigenic, and enteropathogenic. Disease presents as either watery or bloody diarrhea with crampy abdominal pain. Diagnosis rests on identifying disease-causing serotypes in the stool.

Answer I is incorrect. *Giardia*, similar to *Entamoeba*, has both cystic and trophoblastic phases of its life cycle, with the trophozoites causing disease in humans. The protozoan is contracted through drinking contaminated water and sometimes through ingestion of raw vegetables. *Giardia* causes a watery nonbloody diarrhea that is often limited to 1–2 weeks but may establish itself as a chronic infection in some individuals. Diagnosis depends on visualization of the organism in stool samples.

Answer J is incorrect. Irritable bowel syndrome is a functional GI disorder that can cause abdominal pain and changes in bowel habits. It commonly occurs in individuals younger than 35 years, and postulated etiologic factors include enteric infection and hyperactivity of N-methyl-D-aspartate glutamate receptors. Diagnosis is by exclusion of other causes of chronic diarrhea.

Answer L is incorrect. Ulcerative colitis is a type of inflammatory bowel disease that is limited to the colon and produces a chronic bloody diarrhea with crampy abdominal pain. Colonic involvement is continuous, involves the rectum, and progresses proximally. Biopsy shows a friable mucosa with superficial microulcerations and crypt abscesses.

Answer M is incorrect. *Vibrio parahaemolyticus* is a free-living bacterium that is found in saltwater and is contracted by eating raw seafood. Gastroenteritis is the most common presentation, with crampy abdominal pain and often guaiac-positive stool. The disease is generally self-limiting and treatment is supportive, with antibiotics considered only for severe infection.

Answer N is incorrect. Whipple's disease is a systemic illness linked to a gram-positive bacillus, *Tropheryma whippelii*. GI manifestations include a malabsorptive syndrome, with cachexia, distended abdomen, and signs of vitamin deficiency such as glossitis and night blindness. Other organ systems may be affected such as the central nervous system, heart, joints, and skin. Biopsy of the small bowel shows expanded villi containing macrophages that stain positively with periodic acid-Schiff.

CHAPTER 7

Hematology/Oncology

1. A 56-year-old man presents to his physician complaining of severe fatigue. He began to feel increasingly tired about 6 months ago, but believes that his fatigue has been worsening over the past 3 weeks. He also notes that he has had a nonproductive cough for about 2 weeks, and has experienced several episodes of drenching night sweats. On examination, he has several large bruises on his extremities but recalls no injuries. Abdominal examination reveals massive enlargement of both the liver and the spleen, without any lymphadenopathy. Laboratory tests show:

WBC count	12,000/mm^3
Neutrophils	58%
Eosinophils	7%
Lymphocytes	30%
Monocytes	0%
Basophils	5%
RBC count	3.0/mm^3
Hemoglobin	7.5 mg/dL
Platelet count	18,000/mm^3

Peripheral blood smear reveals irregular nuclei and cell membranes, as well as cytoplasmic projections. What is the patient's most likely diagnosis?

(A) Acute lymphocytic leukemia
(B) Hairy cell leukemia
(C) Idiopathic thrombocytopenic purpura
(D) Infectious mononucleosis
(E) Nodular sclerosing Hodgkin's lymphoma

2. A 42-year-old woman who smokes tobacco is found to have acute-onset respiratory distress and tachycardia 4 hours after a nonemergent cholecystectomy. She is subsequently treated for a symptomatic pulmonary embolism. She is begun on low-molecular-weight heparin and warfarin while in the hospital and is supplied with subcutaneous doses of low-molecular-weight heparin to take at home for a total course of 5 days, in addition to the warfarin that she will take for at least 6 months. The initial 5 days of overlap of both heparin and warfarin is necessary because at the beginning of treatment, warfarin actually leads to hypercoagulability. What is the underlying reason for this?

(A) There is an initial increase in vitamin K–dependent coagulation factors
(B) Venous valvular insufficiency is exacerbated during the first 3 days of warfarin therapy
(C) Warfarin causes a more rapid drop in the levels of proteins C and S than factors II, VII, IX, and X
(D) Warfarin induces resistance of factor V to degradation by activated protein C
(E) Warfarin leads to an initial increase in platelet aggregation

3. A 23-year-old woman is diagnosed with stage IIIA Hodgkin's lymphoma after an extensive workup. As her physician is explaining the recommended treatment regimen for her disease, the patient confesses that she has been hoping to become pregnant in the next few years. However, she states that she is willing to wait until she has completed her treatment. She wants to know the consequences of both her primary disease of Hodgkin's lymphoma and her treatment regimen, as well as what effects they may have on a potential pregnancy. Which of the following complications is the least likely?

(A) An increased risk of second malignancy
(B) Ovarian failure that will preclude pregnancy
(C) Pericarditis that may cause congestive heart failure during the pregnancy
(D) Recurrence of the patient's disease due to increased estrogen
(E) Restrictive lung disease that may be exacerbated by pregnancy

4. A 97-year-old man was admitted to the hospital for weakness and rectal bleeding for the previous 24 hours. Questioning reveals a decrease in stool caliber over the past several months. Examination reveals a nontender mass in the left lower quadrant. Stool heme is positive. Serum hemoglobin is 8.8 g/dL. Further workup reveals colon cancer, Dukes stage D. The patient's spouse and only child are no longer living, but the patient's 50-year-old granddaughter pleads with the physician not to

inform her grandfather of the diagnosis, stating that he is an anxious man and that she wants him to enjoy his remaining time. Which of the following is the most appropriate next step?

(A) Agree not to reveal the diagnosis to the patient
(B) Ask the granddaughter to contact her brother to obtain other family members' opinions and try to reach consensus
(C) Ask the patient how much information he wants to know
(D) Request a consult from the hospital's ethics team
(E) Request psychiatric evaluation of the patient

5. A 10-year-old girl is brought to the pediatrician due to a limp. She has been complaining of fatigue and pain in her right leg for months. Physical examination reveals multiple bruises on different sites of her body, enlarged anterior cervical and axillary lymph nodes, and hepatosplenomegaly. A blood smear is shown in the image. What is the next best step?

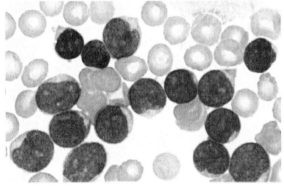

Reproduced, with permission, from Lichtman MA, Beutler E, Kipps TJ, Seligsohn U, Kaushansky K, Prchal JT. *Williams Hematology*, 7th ed. New York: McGraw-Hill, 2006: Plate XX-11.

(A) Call child protective services for suspected child abuse
(B) Obtain a bone marrow biopsy
(C) Obtain a liver biopsy
(D) Perform a test for serum heterophile antibodies
(E) Recommend a diet higher in vitamin C

6. A 69-year-old woman has been in the intensive care unit for 7 days following complicated hip replacement surgery. The patient is currently receiving heparin subcutaneously and wears intermittent pneumatic compression devices on her lower extremities bilaterally. The patient has developed new-onset right calf pain, edema, tenderness, and a positive Homans' sign. A doppler ultrasound was performed in which a deep vein thrombosis was noted. Her complete blood cell count was notable for a platelet count of 78,000/mm^3, and there has been no evidence of spontaneous bleeding. Which of these will best help prevent further complications?

(A) Beginning warfarin therapy
(B) Discontinuation of bilateral pneumatic compression devices
(C) Discontinuation of heparin
(D) Performing venography
(E) Placing an inferior vena cava filter
(F) Transfusing platelets

7. A 62-year-old woman is found to have an abnormal Papanicolaou (or Pap) smear finding of low-grade squamous intraepithelial lesion (LSIL) on routine screening. She does not have a significant past medical history, and she is immunocompetent. Her last Pap smear 3 years ago was normal. She has never had an abnormal Pap smear and has always complied with obtaining routine screening tests. She is entirely asymptomatic and postmenopausal. She is referred for colposcopy, and biopsy of a satisfactory specimen confirms LSIL. What is the most appropriate next step in the management of this patient?

(A) Endocervical curettage
(B) Loop electrosurgical excision procedure
(C) Observation consisting of colposcopy and repeat Pap smears every 4 months for up to a year
(D) Observation consisting of a repeat Pap smear in 1 year
(E) Repeat colposcopy in 1 year, even if repeat Pap smear is normal

8. A 32-year-old woman develops a progressive idiopathic cardiomyopathy and eventually undergoes a cardiac transplant. She is placed on a rigorous protocol for immunosuppression. Two years later she develops right-sided sinus fullness, and imaging reveals a mass filling the right paranasal sinus. She is treated with a reduction in immunosuppression and acyclovir. She achieves a full recovery. Why is acyclovir part of her therapeutic regimen?

(A) Acyclovir has also been shown to have antineoplastic properties
(B) Acyclovir is necessary for prophylaxis against cytomegalovirus in any immunosuppressed patient
(C) Acyclovir will reduce the risk of infection due to radiation of the mucous membranes and subsequent breakdown
(D) Eradication of Epstein-Barr virus may contribute to resolution of the paranasal sinus mass
(E) Since the patient's immunosuppressive regimen must be decreased, protection against viruses that might infect the patient's new heart is particularly important

9. A 22-year-old man presents to the emergency department (ED) with right-sided lower abdominal pain that began yesterday afternoon. The pain had started in the periumbilical region and has since migrated to the right lower quadrant of the abdomen. Soon after the onset of abdominal pain, the patient began to feel nauseous and has vomited twice. He states that he has no appetite despite not being able to eat anything since yesterday. His temperature is 38.4°C (101.1°F), his heart rate is 84/min, his blood pressure is 125/78 mm Hg, and his respiratory rate is 14/min. Physical examination is significant for right lower quadrant pain upon palpation of the left lower quadrant as well as pain upon extension of the right leg. A complete blood cell count is obtained in which the WBC count is 21,000/mm³, hemoglobin is 15 g/dL, and platelet count is 252,000/mm³. A CT scan is obtained and shows a distended appendix with an enhancing wall and stranding in the periappendiceal fat. What is the next step in management?

(A) Intravenous fluid and antibiotics
(B) Obtain an MRI
(C) Obtain an x-ray film of the abdomen
(D) Operative management
(E) Perform a colonoscopy

10. A 58-year-old man with a history of psoriasis presents for his annual examination. He was first diagnosed with psoriasis 3 years ago and has shown little improvement despite numerous therapeutic regimens. His plaques are primarily distributed around his waist and buttocks and have recently begun to itch. Skin biopsy reveals atypical lymphocytes aligned along the basal layer and epidermal microabscesses (see image). Which of the following is the most likely diagnosis?

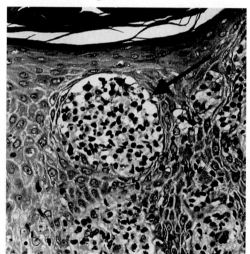

Reproduced, with permission, from Armed Forces Institute of Pathology.

(A) Contact dermatitis
(B) Eczema
(C) Inverse psoriasis
(D) Mycosis fungoides
(E) Plaque psoriasis

11. A 47-year-old man presents to his primary care physician complaining of fatigue for the past several months. A review of systems reveals that the man has had poor sleep due to sweating at night and has lost 4.5 kg (10 lb) recently, although he has not been trying to lose weight. In addition, he has been suffering from severe headaches and blurry vision recently. On examination, he is pale and thin, with multiple ecchymoses. Cardiac examination is significant for a II/VI systolic flow murmur. He has

an enlarged spleen on abdominal examination. Laboratory tests show:

WBC count	95,000/mm^3
15% Blasts	
15% Bands	
47% Polymorphonuclear cells	
7% Basophils	
10% Lymphocytes	
Hemoglobin	7.2 g/dL
Platelet count	90,000/mm^3

Which of the following is the next best step in establishing a diagnosis?

(A) Coagulation studies
(B) Cytogenetic studies
(C) Detection of serum leukocyte alkaline phosphatase levels
(D) Iron studies
(E) No further studies are necessary for establishing the diagnosis

12. A 28-year-old man presents complaining of heaviness in his testicle for 2 weeks. He states that he feels as though his testicle is enlarged. The man has a temperature of 37.2°C (98.9°F), a heart rate of 60/min, and a blood pressure of 115/70 mm Hg. He has a normal abdominal examination with no palpable masses. The right testicle is noticeably larger than the left testicle. There are no discrete nodules. Testicular ultrasound is performed, followed by an orchiectomy. He is found to have a seminoma and a retroperitoneal lymph node that is enlarged at 1.8 cm. He is given a diagnosis of stage IIA testicular seminoma (T2N1M0). What additional treatment is needed?

(A) Contralateral orchiectomy
(B) Platinum-based chemotherapy and bilateral orchiectomy
(C) Prophylactic mediastinal radiation
(D) Retroperitoneal lymph node dissection
(E) Retroperitoneal radiation

13. A 28-year-old woman with a history of refractory promyelocytic leukemia is admitted to the hospital to undergo a bone marrow transplant from a matched unrelated donor. In the week prior to the transplant, she receives myeloabla-

tive chemotherapy. She remains stable on antibacterial prophylaxis for 9 days following her transplant. On day 10, she develops large bullae on her palms and soles and is diagnosed with graft-versus-host disease, which requires long-term therapy. She is discharged home with nursing care on trimethoprim-sulfamethoxazole, glucocorticoids, and tacrolimus. On day 45, she develops spiking fevers and rigors. She states that she has been compliant with her prescribed medications. Given her history, which of the following immunocompromised infectious associations describes the most prominent infectious risk at this time?

(A) Acute bacterial infection with *Staphylococcus aureus* 6 weeks following transplant
(B) Fungal infection due to prolonged immunosuppression
(C) Gram-negative bacteremia in the first 6 weeks following transplant
(D) *Pneumocystis jiroveci* (formerly *carinii*) after being treated for hematogenous malignancy
(E) Reactivation of herpes simplex virus in the posttransplant period
(F) *Salmonella* infection, given patient history of promyelocytic leukemia

14. A 45-year-old man presents to his primary care physician with a complaint of patchy dry areas on his skin. After several trials of skin emollients and corticosteroid therapies without improvement, the lesions are biopsied by a dermatologist. Pathologic examination reveals a monoclonal population of B lymphocytes infiltrating the dermis and epidermis. A complete blood count is normal, and no atypical cells are observed on peripheral blood smear. The patient states that he feels quite well. Which of the following management options would be appropriate as recommended by the patient's dermatologist?

(A) Anticipation of bone marrow transplant
(B) Observation alone
(C) Systemic chemotherapy
(D) Systemic corticosteroids
(E) Treatment of the affected areas of skin with topical nitrogen mustard
(F) Treatment of the entire skin surface via total skin electron beam therapy

15. A 70-year-old man who was admitted to an in-patient unit 7 days ago for lower gastrointestinal bleeding develops chest pain, a cough, and a fever to 38.3°C (100.9°F). The chest pain is not positional or exertional but hurts every time he takes a breath. Physical examination reveals mild tachycardia and tachypnea, no jugular venous distention or edema, consolidation over the right lower lobe with dull breath sounds in this area, and a nontender abdomen. A review of systems reveals that the patient had a negative purified protein derivative 3 months ago. An anteroposterior x-ray of the chest reveals patchy infiltrate in the right lower lobe. The right lateral decubitus film is shown in the image. What is the next best step in managing this patient?

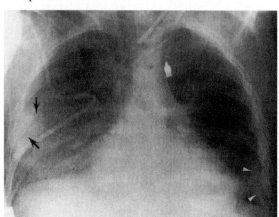

Reproduced, with permission, from Chen MYM, Pope TL, Ott DJ. *Basic Radiology*. New York: McGraw-Hill, 2004: Figure 4-55B.

(A) Oral piperacillin-clavulanate
(B) Pleurodesis
(C) Surgery to remove the left lower lung lobe
(D) Therapeutic thoracentesis
(E) Tube thoracostomy and intrapleural thrombolytics

16. A 32-year-old woman presents to the ED with edema and pain of the right lower extremity that began after a 6-hour car ride. A Doppler ultrasound was completed in which a deep vein thrombosis was noted. The patient has no prior history of deep vein thrombosis or pulmonary emboli. The patient has been taking oral contraceptive pills for the past 2 years and is currently compliant with her medication. Her family history is significant for a maternal grandmother, mother, and sister with recurrent deep vein thrombosis. Her temperature is 36.2°C (97.2°F), her blood pressure is 112/78 mm Hg, her heart rate is 86/min, and her respiratory rate is 14/min. There is no clinical evidence indicating a pulmonary embolism. What is the most likely cause of her deep vein thrombosis?

(A) Antithrombin deficiency
(B) Coagulation factor V gene mutation
(C) Protein C excess
(D) Protein S deficiency
(E) Prothrombin gene mutation

17. A 55-year-old woman with a history of alcoholism and chronic pancreatitis (last exacerbation 2 years ago) presents to her primary care physician with weight loss, pruritus, anorexia, dark urine, jaundice, yellow sclerae, and vague abdominal pain. Which of the following physical findings is most likely to be seen in this patient to support her likely diagnosis?

(A) Chandelier sign
(B) Courvoisier's sign
(C) Cullen's sign
(D) Grey Turner sign
(E) Positive Murphy's sign

18. A 51-year-old woman undergoes a successful bone marrow transplant from a matched unrelated donor for refractory Hodgkin's disease. She is discharged from the hospital on no medications and is feeling well. At an appointment 6 months posttransplant, she is well with no evidence of malignancy. Three weeks later, she travels to Florida with her family. She is cautious of the sun but develops sunburn on her face, despite wearing sunscreen and a protective hat. When she returns from her trip 5 days later, she presents with persistent erythema of her face. She also states that her wrists and hands have been sore for the past 2–3 weeks. On examination, her face is mildly tender to touch, and a rash is present. Her hands are diffusely swollen. She is afebrile, and the remainder of her physical examination is benign. What is the most likely diagnosis?

(A) Graft-versus-host disease
(B) Hypersensitivity to sunlight due to the patient's antirejection regimen

(C) New-onset systemic lupus erythematosus

(D) Rosacea

(E) Staphylococcal skin infection acquired during travel

(F) Sun poisoning

19. A 33-year-old man presents with complaints of headaches and blurred vision for the past 3 months. He also notes decreased libido. Past medical history is significant for peptic ulcer disease for which he takes omeprazole. Family history is significant for a mother with recurrent peptic ulcers and an uncle who died of a pancreatic tumor. Physical examination is unremarkable. MRI of the brain reveals a mass in the pituitary. In addition to managing the pituitary mass, which of the following studies should be done in this patient?

(A) Calcitonin

(B) Parathyroid hormone

(C) Renal ultrasound

(D) Thyroid ultrasound

(E) Urinary metanephrines

20. A 14-month-old boy with no known medical history presents to his pediatrician with a black eye. He has had the injury for at least a week, but his mother is uncertain as to when or how it happened, although she does report that he has had a low-grade fever and has been sleeping "all the time" for the last 6 days. On examination, he is pale and ill appearing with temperature 38°C (100.4°F), blood pressure 120/72 mm Hg, heart rate 86/min, and respiratory rate 22/min. He is in the 10th percentile for weight, the 10th percentile for height, and the 50th percentile for head circumference. There is periorbital bruising and proptosis of the right eye, petechiae on his legs, and cervical lymphadenopathy. There is no hepatomegaly, splenomegaly, or palpable masses. Laboratory tests show:

Blood urea nitrogen	7 mg/dL
Creatinine	0.4 mg/dL
WBC count	12,000/mm^3
Hemoglobin	8 g/dL
Platelet count	190,000/mm^3
Activated partial thromboplastin time	25 seconds
Prothrombin time	23 seconds
Alanine aminotransferase	16 U/L
Aspartate aminotransferase	14 U/L
Urine vanillylmandelic acid	Elevated
D-dimer	Normal

Which of the following is the most likely diagnosis?

(A) Acute lymphoid leukemia

(B) Aplastic anemia

(C) Child abuse

(D) Neuroblastoma

(E) Pheochromocytoma

21. A 62-year-old woman presents to her gynecologist for vaginal bleeding. She had her last menstrual cycle at age 45 and has not had any episodes of vaginal bleeding since then. She states that she first noticed some spotting on her underwear approximately 3 months ago; this spotting continues "off and on" but has not increased in amount. She is sexually active with her husband of 40 years but has not noticed a relationship between sexual activity and bleeding. She has hypertension for which she takes "a water pill" but is otherwise healthy. A speculum examination reveals an atrophic vaginal vault, with no evidence of blood. The cervix is small and nonfriable. A pelvic examination reveals a small, nontender uterus, and her ovaries are not palpable. Which of the following is the appropriate next course of action?

(A) Abdominal ultrasound

(B) Endometrial biopsy

(C) Follow-up examination in 6 months

(D) Luteinizing hormone and follicle-stimulating hormone serum levels

(E) Prescription of testosterone cream

22. A 59-year-old man presents with a 6.8-kg (15-lb) unintentional weight loss over 2 months, with occasional night sweats. He notices some abdominal fullness but no pain, and his last colonoscopy was negative for polyps. He has never smoked tobacco, but he has had prior radiation exposure as an x-ray technician. Physical examination is significant for splenomegaly, with no signs of jaundice. Fecal occult blood is negative. X-ray of the chest is clear. A complete blood count shows a WBC count of 126,000/mm^3, and a peripheral smear shows a leukocytosis with all stages of maturation seen and 3% blasts. Which of the following tests would confirm the diagnosis?

(A) Bone marrow biopsy with hypercellularity and elevated proportion of blasts
(B) Cytogenetic identification of t(9;22)
(C) Elevated α-fetoprotein
(D) Lymph node biopsy showing Reed-Sternberg cells
(E) Repeat colonoscopy showing colonic polyps

23. A 65-year-old previously healthy Ashkenazi Jewish woman presents with complaints of tenderness throughout her ribs and spine. She has noted increasing fatigue and weight loss over the past 6 months, and has missed several days of work due to minor infections. Physical examination is within normal limits aside from point tenderness near her posterior ribs and thoracic spine. Laboratory studies reveal WBC count of 8400/mm^3, hemoglobin 7.9 mg/dL, platelet count 200,000/mm^3, and 3+ protein in the urine. X-ray of the chest reveals lytic lesions in several areas of the ribs and spine. Bone scan is within normal limits. What is the most likely pathology behind her fractures?

(A) Anorexia nervosa
(B) Bony infarcts resulting from Gaucher's disease
(C) Congenital osteoporosis
(D) Domestic abuse
(E) Increased osteoclastic activity secondary to multiple myeloma
(F) Metastatic disease to bone from an unidentified breast cancer

24. A 67-year-old woman is seen in the doctor's office for a cough productive of bloody sputum and an 11.3-kg (25-lb) unintentional weight loss, both occurring within the past 6 months. In addition, the patient notes that over the past 3 months she has become increasingly lethargic and experienced bouts of nausea. She has smoked two packs per day for the past 50 years. She denies a history of heart failure or liver cirrhosis. She currently takes no medications. Her temperature is 36.7°C (98.1°F), blood pressure is 125/85 mm Hg, pulse is 78/min and regular, respiratory rate is 15/min, and oxygen saturation is 99% on room air. Examination reveals crackles at the left lower lung field; no lower extremity edema is present. Laboratory tests show:

WBC count	6000/mm^3
Hemoglobin	14.7 g/dL
Platelet count	210,000/mm^3
Na$^+$	125 mEq/L
K$^+$	4 mEq/L
Cl$^-$	102 mEq/L
CO$_2$	24 mmol/L
Blood urea nitrogen	8 mg/dL
Creatinine	1 mg/dL
Glucose	120 mg/dL
Urine osmolality	125 mOsm/kg
Urinary Na$^+$	35 mEq/L

X-ray of the chest shows a focal 5-cm mass lesion in the right lower lung that is corroborated by CT scan. Which of the following is the most likely histologic type of lung cancer present in this patient?

(A) Adenocarcinoma
(B) Bronchoalveolar cell carcinoma
(C) Large cell carcinoma
(D) Small cell carcinoma
(E) Squamous cell carcinoma

25. A 68-year-old man has been treated for non-Hodgkin's lymphoma for the past 3 weeks, and now complains of weakness and fatigue for the past day. His temperature is 38.5°C (101.3°F), blood pressure is 140/88 mm Hg, and heart rate is 78/min. The remainder of the examination is normal. Laboratory tests show:

Na$^+$	136 mEq/L
K$^+$	5.8 mEq/L

Cl$^-$	99 mEq/L
Ca^{2+}	7.9 mg/dL
HCO$_3^-$	25 mg/dL
Blood urea nitrogen	9 mg/dL
Creatinine	0.9 mg/dL
Urate	9.1 mg/dL

What is the most likely cause of this patient's hyperkalemia?

(A) Increased gastrointestinal absorption
(B) Lysis of neoplastic cells
(C) Metabolic acidosis
(D) Pseudohyperkalemia
(E) Renal failure

26. A 68-year-old woman presents to her primary care office for a routine visit. She is generally in good health, and her only medications are hydrochlorothiazide and metoprolol for high blood pressure. She has had no recent changes in her health, and review of systems is negative. Examination shows occasional enlarged cervical and inguinal lymph nodes. The liver and spleen are not enlarged. An electrolyte panel is within normal limits, a peripheral smear shows smudge cells, and a complete blood count shows a WBC count of 47,000/mm^3 (with 89% lymphocytes), a hemoglobin of 12.9 g/dL, and a platelet count of 213,000/mm^3. What is the best treatment for this patient?

(A) Chemotherapy
(B) Imatinib therapy
(C) No treatment is indicated at this time
(D) Radiation therapy
(E) Splenectomy

27. A 69-year-old man with congestive heart failure and chronic obstructive pulmonary disease has palpable adenopathy in the neck and inguinal region. He feels perfectly well and has normal blood counts. Lymph node biopsy shows follicular small cleaved lymphocytic lymphoma. Bone marrow biopsy shows peritrabecular infiltrates of small cleaved lymphocytes. Which of the following describes the most reasonable management?

(A) Arrange for bone marrow transplant
(B) Arrange for immediate hospice care
(C) Begin palliative radiation therapy to involved lymph node beds

(D) Initiate an aggressive multiagent chemotherapy regimen
(E) Manage symptoms conservatively with close follow-up

28. A 63-year-old postmenopausal woman is referred to the gynecologic clinic by her primary care physician for evaluation of genital pruritus. A month-long history of vulvar pruritus is obtained. She has a remote history of human papillomavirus. She denies changes in vaginal discharge or vaginal bleeding. She also denies constitutional symptoms or weight loss. On examination, she is in no apparent distress. Her heart rate is 70/min, blood pressure is 100/58 mm Hg, and respiratory rate is 10/min. Genital examination reveals an ulcerative white lesion approximately 1 cm in diameter on her labia majora. What is the next most appropriate step in the management of this patient?

(A) Obtain a biopsy of the lesion
(B) Prescribe estrogen cream to be applied to the area
(C) Treat with acyclovir
(D) Treat with cryotherapy
(E) Treat with fluconazole
(F) Treat with metronidazole

29. A 9-year old African-American boy is brought in by his mother after she noticed a droop on the left side of his face and difficulty moving his left arm. There was no preceding head trauma or aura, and he was conscious throughout. The deficit lasted for about 3 hours and he returned to baseline activity except for some residual weakness of the left hand. He has a maternal grandfather who had a heart attack at age 63, and the child's father has hypertension. Review of systems is significant for easy fatiguing with exercise, but negative for fevers, loss of appetite, weight loss, vomiting, or diarrhea. Significant findings on examination include mild pallor and modestly decreased left hand strength. On laboratory studies, his total cholesterol is 140 mg/dL. Which of the following diagnoses could unify these findings?

(A) Familial hypercholesterolemia
(B) Hypertension
(C) Multiple myeloma
(D) Sickle cell disease
(E) Simple partial seizure

30. A 30-year-old woman presents to a primary care physician for a new patient visit. She reports recurrent episodes of pneumonia, bronchitis, and otitis over the past 4 years. Although her vaccinations were up to date, she developed tetanus following a foot laceration last year. Her lymph nodes and tonsils are enlarged. Laboratory testing reveals low IgG, IgA, and IgM levels. After referral to a hematologist, who rules out other acquired and genetic causes of her hypogammaglobulinemia, she is diagnosed with common variable immunodeficiency. This woman is at the highest risk of developing which of the following condition?

(A) Cardiovascular disease
(B) Lymphoma
(C) Miscarriage
(D) Renal disease
(E) Splenic autoinfarction

31. A 72-year-old man with a 40 pack-year smoking history presents with a 9-kg (20-lb) weight loss and fatigue. He has no other complaints. He is not taking any medication. His physical examination and vital signs are unremarkable. Laboratory tests show:

Na^+	138 mEq/L
K^+	4.6 mEq/L
Cl^-	101 mEq/L
HCO_3^-	24 mEq/L
Ca^{2+}	11.2 mg/dL
PO_4	1.6 mg/dL
Mg^{2+}	2.0 mg/dL
Blood urea nitrogen	11 mg/dL
Creatinine	1.1 mg/dL
Glucose	94 mg/dL
Parathyroid hormone	12 pg/mL

What is the next best step in the evaluation of this patient?

(A) CT scan of the chest
(B) MRI of the brain
(C) Parathyroid ultrasound
(D) Renal biopsy
(E) Serum vitamin D levels

32. A 29-year-old woman presents to an obstetrics clinic asking for a pregnancy test. Her last menstrual period was 7 weeks ago. She took a home pregnancy test and it was positive. She says that this is a highly desired pregnancy, and that she and her partner have been attempting to become pregnant for almost a year. She says that she has no other complaints, and says that she "has never felt better." Her pulse is 78/min, blood pressure is 110/70 mm Hg, and she is afebrile. Pelvic examination is within normal limits. The physician notices, however, an abnormality on breast examination, which reveals a 3-cm mass palpated just above the nipple. The mass is mobile and well circumscribed. The patient says that she noticed it before, and that it has gotten larger recently. However, she didn't think it was important because it didn't hurt. What is the most likely diagnosis?

(A) Carcinoma of the breast
(B) Fibroadenoma
(C) Fibrocystic change
(D) Galactocele
(E) Mammary duct ectasia

33. A 6-year-old boy presents with 5 days of nosebleeds and a rash. The nosebleeds have increased in frequency to three times a day. The mother reports no fevers at home, though he did have 4–5 days of cough and runny nose 2 weeks ago. His past medical history is unremarkable and he takes no medications. On physical examination, he is afebrile with a petechial rash and some crusted blood on the nares. There is no splenomegaly. A complete blood cell count shows a platelet count of 127,000/mm^3 and normal hemoglobin. A peripheral smear shows megathrombocytes. Initial treatment should consist of which of the following?

(A) Corticosteroids
(B) Dialysis
(C) Intravenous gamma-globulin
(D) Observation
(E) Platelet transfusion

34. A 22-year-old man who has recently moved to the United States from east Africa presents to the ED with severe abdominal pain. He states that the pain began 30–40 minutes earlier and that it is currently 10 of 10 on the pain scale. He denies vomiting or diarrhea. While in the ED, he passes a bloody stool. Examination demonstrates an acute abdomen, and the patient is taken to the operating room. On laparotomy, an intussusception caused by tremendous swelling of the intestinal wall is discovered. A large section of intestine is resected. Pathologic examination of frozen sections reveals lymphoid tissue. What is the most likely diagnosis?

(A) Burkitt's lymphoma
(B) Chronic lymphocytic leukemia
(C) Chronic myelogenous leukemia
(D) Ewing's sarcoma
(E) Sézary syndrome

35. A 47-year-old African-American woman presents to her primary care doctor complaining of lightheadedness when rising from bed and swelling of her feet and ankles over the last 6 weeks. She also reports some bone pain. Her temperature is 37.2°C (99°F), pulse is 93/min, and blood pressure is 100/80 mm Hg seated and 80/70 mm Hg standing. Further evaluation reveals jugular venous pressure of 11 cm H_2O, 3+ proteinuria, and hepatomegaly. The physician suspects amyloid cardiomyopathy. The presence of which finding would support this diagnosis most?

(A) A prominent systolic heart murmur
(B) A thickened interventricular septum
(C) Atrial fibrillation
(D) A wide pulse pressure
(E) Lytic bone lesions on x-ray of the chest

36. A 53-year-old woman with history of polycystic kidney disease undergoes a renal transplant from a cadaveric donor. She experiences several bouts of acute rejection that are controlled by appropriate increases in immunosuppression during the first year posttransplant. During her fourth posttransplant year, her creatinine is rising gradually. Transcutaneous biopsy reveals architectural distortion and sclerosis of the renal tubules. What is the most likely outcome of the patient's condition?

(A) Development of lymphoproliferative tumors requiring decreased immunosuppression
(B) Gradual onset of renal failure and return to dialysis

(C) Requirement of chronic antibiotic prophylaxis against urinary tract infection
(D) Response to a short course of high-dose steroids
(E) Response to increased chronic immunosuppression

37. A 3-year-old sickle cell patient is brought to the ED complaining of pain in his lower arms for 3 days. On physical examination, both arms are swollen, tender, and erythematous. He is febrile, and complains of chills. Leukocytosis is seen on blood count, with prominent neutrophils. Which of the following will be the most appropriate pharmacology?

(A) Calcitonin
(B) Ceftriaxone
(C) Ciprofloxacin
(D) Etidronate
(E) Vitamin D

38. A 4-year-old boy presents with increased fatigue over the past 4 months. He also has intermittent fevers that resolve on their own and progressively more frequent nosebleeds, up to three times a week. His mother notes that he has generally stopped walking, but when he tries to walk he seems to favor his left leg. Examination shows pallor, cervical lymphadenopathy, hepato- and splenomegaly, and crusted blood on the nares. A complete blood count shows a WBC count of 28,000/mm³, with hemoglobin of 8.3 g/dL and a decreased platelet count. A bone marrow biopsy shows increased cellularity and lymphoblast predominance. Which of the following is true of this patient's likely diagnosis?

(A) Children with trisomy 21 are at increased risk of developing this disease
(B) Presence of the Philadelphia chromosome means that there is no current treatment
(C) Survival with chemotherapy is approximately 20–30% in children
(D) The central nervous system is usually spared from metastatic spread
(E) Tumor lysis syndrome is uncommon

39. A 66-year-old postmenopausal white woman presents to her physician with a 1-month history of painless gross hematuria. She works as a hairdresser, is an avid coffee drinker, and has been a 50 pack-year smoker. Her physical examination is entirely normal. Based on the physician's suspicions, which of the following below would best confirm the diagnosis?

(A) CT scan of the pelvis
(B) Cystoscopy
(C) Serum creatine kinase levels
(D) Ultrasound
(E) Urine culture

40. A 53-year-old woman presents with diffuse back and rib pain that is worsened with movement. She states that her periods have recently stopped, but denies experiencing hot flashes or other menopausal symptoms. She also notes a 6.8-kg (15-lb) weight gain over the past 3–4 months. On further questioning she states that she has noted tingling in her fingers and toes for the past 7 months, and has recently found that she has been tripping frequently and having trouble opening doors and buttoning her shirts. On physical examination, diffuse lymphadenopathy is noted. Abdominal examination reveals hepatomegaly. Her skin is warm and dry; hyperpigmentation is noted in the regions of the neck and shoulders, and her digits are noted to be clubbed. Laboratory testing and peripheral blood smear results reveal large numbers of plasma cells; other findings are:

WBC count	13,000/mm^3
Hemoglobin	9.8 g/dL
Platelet count	340,000/mm^3
Erythrocyte sedimentation rate	64 mm/hr
Blood urea nitrogen	35 mg/dL
Creatinine	2.1 mg/dL
Thyroid-stimulating hormone	25 U/mL
Blood glucose level	384 mg/dL
Serum calcium	15.4 mg/dL

Which of the following tests is most likely to confirm the patient's underlying diagnosis?

(A) Complete thyroid evaluation
(B) Dexamethasone suppression test
(C) Hemoglobin A$_{1c}$
(D) Pulse oximetry

(E) Urine and serum protein electrophoresis
(F) WBC differential

41. A 63-year-old African-American man with no past medical history presents with a recent increase in prostate-specific antigen from 2.2 to 4.3 ng/mL. Digital rectal examination reveals a 0.5-cm nodule on the left lobe of prostate. What is the next step in the evaluation of this patient?

(A) CT scan and bone scan
(B) Prostate biopsy
(C) Radical prostatectomy
(D) Treat patient with a 7-day course of antibiotics and recheck prostate-specific antigen level in 3 months
(E) Urinalysis

42. A 37-year-old woman gives birth to her third healthy child. He is discharged from the hospital with her, at 2 days of life. For the first 3 months of his life, however, his parents note poor weight gain, chronic diarrhea, and persistent diaper rash. Complete blood count reveals a paucity of lymphocytes, and antibody staining demonstrates a deficiency of the X-linked interleukin-2 receptor chain. The baby is diagnosed with X-linked severe combined immunodeficiency. His parents are told that the standard of care for him is a bone marrow transplant from a major histocompatibility complex–matched related donor. His two sisters are tested and are not matches. His parents are interested in exploring the option of gene therapy. Which of the following concerns is unique to the use of gene therapy for treatment of severe combined immunodeficiency?

(A) Graft-versus-host disease
(B) Increased risk of failure
(C) Increased susceptibility to viral illness in the future
(D) Inefficient response to vaccines in the future
(E) Leukemia

43. A 6-year-old African-American girl presents with intense pain in both feet after jumping in a cold swimming pool. There was no trauma reported, and the pain seems to decrease with warming of the feet. Physical examination shows scleral icterus and splenomegaly. There is no point tenderness of the ankles or feet, but the toes are cool and appear dusky. A complete blood count shows hemoglobin of 10.2 g/dL, and a liver panel shows increased indirect bilirubin. A peripheral smear is shown in the image. What is the long-term medical treatment needed to minimize the recurrence of her condition?

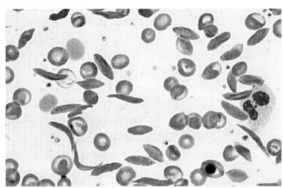

Reproduced, with permission, from Lichtman MA, Beutler E, Kipps TJ, Seligsohn U, Kaushansky K, Prchal JT. *Williams Hematology*, 7th ed. New York: McGraw-Hill, 2006: Plate III-5.

(A) Avoidance of sulfa drugs and fava beans
(B) Corticosteroids
(C) Hematopoietic stem cell transplant
(D) Hydroxyurea
(E) Serial transfusions

44. A 52-year-old woman presents to the surgery clinic 6 days after lumpectomy with axillary node dissection for invasive ductal-type breast carcinoma. She is presenting for evaluation for postprocedure radiation therapy. She is postmenopausal, and her cancer, by histology, is hormone sensitive. Although her pain is well controlled, she is having some problems lifting objects above her head, and her husband says that her shoulder looks "pointy," especially when her arms are raised. On physical examination, the physician notes that when the patient is leaning forward with her hands pressed against the wall, her scapula seems to move laterally and posteriorly, away from the posterior thoracic cage. The physician also confirms that she cannot abduct her arm above the horizontal. What is the most likely cause of her symptoms?

(A) Axillary nerve damage
(B) Conversion disorder
(C) Long thoracic nerve damage
(D) Poland syndrome
(E) Thoracodorsal nerve damage

45. A 30-year-old man presents to his physician for a routine physical. On questioning, he comments that his father was diagnosed with colon cancer at 45 years of age. The patient has never had polyps and does not suffer diarrhea, constipation, or bloody stools. The patient is nervous about screening and wants to delay as long as possible. According to current recommendations, when should he have his first colonoscopy?

(A) 30 years old
(B) 35 years old
(C) 40 years old
(D) 45 years old
(E) 50 years old

46. A 2-year-old girl presents to the pediatrician because her mother noticed a mass while dressing her. Aside from the mass, the child's mother has no concerns. She reports that the child is otherwise well and denies any fever, weight loss, or fatigue. On examination, her temperature is 37°C (98.6°F), blood pressure is 100/60 mm Hg, heart rate is 80/min, and respiratory rate is 25/min. A smooth, firm, left-sided nontender flank mass is palpated. There is no hepatomegaly, no splenomegaly, and no lymphadenopathy. A CT scan reveals only an encapsulated left-sided mass and no other abnormalities. Laboratory studies show:

Blood urea nitrogen	8 mg/dL
Creatinine	0.4 mg/dL
Alanine aminotransferase	20 U/L
Aspartate aminotransferase	20 U/L
Total bilirubin	0.4 mg/dL
Alkaline phosphatase	70 U/L
Urine vanillylmandelic acid	Negative
WBC count	6200/mm³
Hemoglobin	14 g/dL
Platelet count	190,000/mm³
Urine RBCs	1+
Urine protein	0
Urine WBC esterase	Negative

What is the most appropriate therapy?

(A) Chemotherapy only
(B) Local excision of tumor without nephrectomy
(C) Nephrectomy and chemotherapy
(D) Nephrectomy only
(E) Radiation

47. A 55-year-old woman presents to her primary care physician with complaints of pain in her hands in the cold. On further questioning, she states that she notices that her hands have a bluish hue when she is outside, and that they become pale and then quite red when warm. Her physician, concerned that Raynaud's phenomenon may indicate the presence of an autoimmune illness, initiates an autoimmune workup that is entirely negative. Three weeks later, the patient returns to the office with reports of visual "floaters." She states that she feels fine otherwise. Her physical examination is negative aside from several large bruises on her legs. What is the most appropriate course of action to be taken by the physician?

(A) Begin a course of prednisone to alleviate the patient's autoimmune symptoms in the absence of concrete diagnosis
(B) Discuss the possibility of domestic violence with the patient
(C) Order plasma electrophoresis
(D) Reassure the patient and reevaluate in 3 months
(E) Resend the patient's serum for antinuclear antibody tests

48. A 60-year-old man presented with dysphagia, facial flushing, and diarrhea. On examination he was noted to have a goiter and mild cervical lymphadenopathy. His physician orders thyroid function tests and refers him to a surgeon. It is now 8 months later and the patient is status post total thyroidectomy, where the pathology indicated medullary carcinoma. He is currently being treated with thyroid hormone suppression therapy. Which of the following is the most significant risk factor for this form of thyroid cancer?

(A) Alcohol
(B) Genetic risk factor
(C) Iodine exposure
(D) Radiation to the neck for enlarged tonsils as a child
(E) Smoking
(F) Viral infection

49. A 55-year-old woman who was successfully treated with chemotherapy for breast cancer several years ago presents to her primary care physician complaining of 2 months of easy bruising, bleeding gums, fatigue, and shortness of breath. On physical examination, she has a low-grade fever and several bruises in different locations on her body. She does not have jugular venous distention. No masses are palpable on breast examination. Heart and lung examination are within normal limits. Abdominal examination is significant for hepatosplenomegaly. A complete blood count is sent out, and her WBC count is 35,000/mm³. Her WBCs are myeloperoxidase positive. Which of the following is true for patients carrying this diagnosis?

(A) Incidence decreases with increasing age

(B) Patients with this disease are at increased risk for stroke

(C) Previous chemotherapy does not affect risk for developing the disease

(D) Prognosis is not affected by the cytogenetics of the disease

(E) Retinoic acid was once used to treat this disease but is no longer part of the current treatment

50. Which of the following laboratory findings listed in the table below are characteristic of von Willebrand's disease? PT refers to prothrombin time, and aPTT refers to activated partial thromboplastin time.

(A) A

(B) B

(C) C

(D) D

(E) E

51. A 7-year-old boy presents to his pediatrician with increased gingival bleeding after brushing his teeth. The patient's mother denies a history of easy bruising or prolonged bleeding. The boy also reports an episode of prolonged and painful knee swelling after a fall in which he hit his knee. The patient's family history is significant for a maternal grandfather who died of

a massive hemorrhage after a minor surgical procedure. On examination there are no ecchymoses or petechiae. His conjunctivae are pink, and a full physical examination is noncontributory. His activated partial thromboplastin time is 63 seconds, prothrombin time is 12 seconds, bleeding time is 4 seconds, and coagulation time is prolonged. Which of the following additional laboratory results is most likely to be seen in this patient?

(A) Decreased factor VIII concentrations

(B) Decreased platelet concentrations

(C) Decreased WBC count

(D) Increased factor V concentrations

(E) Increased hemoglobin

52. A 64-year-old woman with a history of cardiac disease, multiple strokes, and progressive osteoarthritis is admitted to the hospital for bilateral total knee replacement surgery. Routine blood chemistries the morning after surgery reveal a platelet count of 9000/mm³. Which of the following medications is most likely to be responsible for this finding?

(A) Aspirin

(B) Clopidogrel

(C) Heparin

(D) Streptokinase

(E) Warfarin

Choice	Bleeding Time (min)	PT (sec)	aPTT (sec)	Platelet Count (mm³)	Factor IX	Factor VIII
A	3	17	45	202,000	abnormal	normal
B	9	20	29	67,000	normal	normal
C	4	12	45	230,000	normal	abnormal
D	8	13	27	58,000	normal	normal
E	9	12	45	143,000	normal	abnormal

53. A 67-year-old man presents with flulike symptoms and cough. He also reports a 2.3-kg (5-lb) weight loss over the past 2 months. The patient has a 40 pack-year history of smoking but quit 10 years ago. His past medical history and physical examination are unremarkable. Complete blood cell count and liver function tests are normal. His stool is negative for occult blood. X-ray of the chest revealed a 3.5-cm right lobe mass and widening of the mediastinum. CT scan shows a right middle lobe mass, and in addition two mediastinal lymph nodes are seen that measure 1.5 and 2 cm in diameter, respectively. Biopsies of the lung nodule obtained by bronchoscopy indicate malignancy. What is the appropriate next best step in management of this patient?

(A) Mediastinoscopy
(B) Pulmonary function tests
(C) Thoracentesis
(D) Ventilation-perfusion lung scan
(E) Video-assisted thoracoscopic surgery

54. A 12-year-old boy presents with pain and swelling of his left thigh, and is diagnosed with osteosarcoma. He has no other medical problems; however, his family history reveals that his mother has been treated for bilateral breast cancer and that his sister and two uncles died of "brain tumors." He is treated with multiagent chemotherapy and recovers from his disease. Several years later, a complete blood count sent on routine follow-up reveals abnormalities consistent with myelodysplastic syndrome. Within weeks, he has developed a refractory form of acute myelogenous leukemia that is rapidly fatal. Which of the following syndromes should this family's physician be most concerned about?

(A) Ataxia telangiectasia
(B) Familial Li-Fraumeni syndrome
(C) Von Hippel–Lindau syndrome
(D) Wiskott-Aldrich syndrome
(E) Xeroderma pigmentosa

55. A 37-year-old woman presents with 3 days of fever, fatigue, and rash. Her medications include oral contraceptives. On physical examination, she has a temperature of 38.7°C (101.7°F), a nonpalpable petechial rash, and splenomegaly. Coagulation studies and fibrino-

gen are normal, but complete blood count shows hemoglobin of 9.7 g/dL and platelet count of 135,000/mm³. A peripheral blood smear shows schistocytes. What is the most likely diagnosis?

(A) Disseminated intravascular coagulation
(B) HELLP syndrome
(C) Henoch-Schönlein purpura
(D) Idiopathic thrombocytopenic purpura
(E) Thrombotic thrombocytopenic purpura

56. A 56-year-old woman with a history of diabetes and proteinuria presents to the ED complaining of right groin pain and decreased urine output for the past day. She denies any trauma, fever, or history of kidney stones or urinary tract infections. Her temperature is 37.2°C (99.0°F), blood pressure is 146/90 mm Hg, pulse is 104/min, and respiratory rate is 16/min. Heart and lung examinations are normal; she has no visible rashes and no costovertebral angle tenderness. There is trace ankle edema bilaterally. Laboratory tests show:

Na⁺	134 mEq/L
K⁺	4.9 mEq/L
Cl⁻	100 mEq/L
HCO₃⁻	24 mEq/L
Blood urea nitrogen	38 mg/dL
Creatinine	1.6 mg/dL
Albumin	2.2 g/dL
Urinalysis	3+ blood, 4+ protein, no WBCs, no stones

What is the most appropriate next step in management of this patient's condition?

(A) Analgesics and angiotensin-converting enzyme inhibitors
(B) Kidney biopsy and high-dose corticosteroids
(C) Renal vein ultrasound and heparin
(D) Thiazides and spiral CT of the pelvis
(E) Urine culture and oral quinolones

57. A 49-year-old man with a history of several dysplastic nevi presents for an annual examination. He mentions that one of the moles on his left shoulder seems larger than usual. It has also started to itch. He denies anorexia, weight changes, or malaise, though he admits to feeling somewhat tired in the past couple of months. On examination he is well appearing

and has no lymphadenopathy. The mole is dark brown, 7 mm in diameter, nodular, and round with an irregular shape. There is no ulceration or bleeding. Which of the following is the most appropriate next step in managing this patient?

(A) Excision of the lesion
(B) Excision of the lesion with sentinel lymph node biopsy
(C) Local radiation therapy
(D) Oral antihistamines for symptomatic relief
(E) Reassurance, with follow-up in 6 months

58. Which of the following laboratory findings shown in the table below are characteristic of hemophilia B?

(A) A
(B) B
(C) C
(D) D
(E) E

59. A 28-year-old woman is diagnosed with acute promyelocytic leukemia after experiencing severe fatigue and malaise for several weeks. She and her parents have done extensive reading on the Internet and expect that she will be treated with intensive multiagent chemotherapy. To their surprise, her physician suggests an oral agent that is not used to treat other forms of acute leukemia. Why might the physician be concerned about using standard intensive multiagent chemotherapy in this patient?

(A) A desire to allow the patient to preserve her fertility
(B) A higher incidence of chemotherapy-related death in patients with acute

promyelocytic leukemia as compared to other leukemias
(C) An observation that acute promyelocytic leukemia does not respond to conventional chemotherapeutics
(D) A personal preference to treat acute promyelocytic leukemia with homeopathic agents
(E) An understanding that acute promyelocytic leukemia is so sensitive to oral agents that intravenous chemotherapy is simply not required in its treatment

60. A 31-year-old man with history of idiopathic pulmonary fibrosis undergoes a successful lung transplant. An immunosuppressive regimen is instituted. Six months following the transplant, the patient presents with cough and low-grade fever. On examination, he is febrile to 38.9°C (102.1°F). His vital signs are heart rate 135/min, respiratory rate 50/min, and blood pressure 145/98 mm Hg. Oxygen saturation is 82% on room air. Lung examination reveals diffuse inspiratory crackles. The remainder of the examination is within normal limits. An x-ray of the chest shows diffuse bilateral opacities. Following stabilization, what is the next step in terms of appropriate management of the patient?

(A) Expectant therapy with broad-spectrum antibiotics, antivirals, and antifungals
(B) Immediate treatment with high-dose steroids
(C) Pulmonary function tests
(D) Reduction of the immunosuppressive regimen
(E) Transbronchial biopsy

CHOICE	BLEEDING TIME (MIN)	PT (SEC)	APTT (SEC)	PLATELET COUNT (/MM³)	FACTOR VIII	FACTOR IX
A	3	17	27	202,000	Normal	Normal
B	4	12	42	190,000	Normal	Abnormal
C	4	12	45	230,000	Abnormal	Normal
D	8	13	27	58,000	Normal	Normal
E	9	12	45	212,000	Abnormal	Normal

1. **The correct answer is B.** Hairy cell leukemia is a rare malignancy of B lymphocytes. It is most common between the ages of 50 and 60 years, and shows a 5:1 male predominance. Patients generally present with the symptoms of pancytopenia, namely fatigue, easy bruising, and recurrent infection, as well as splenomegaly (and hepatomegaly in 50% of patients). Mycobacterial infections are common due to a striking monocytopenia that is nearly universal in these patients. Lymphadenopathy is rare. Examination of the spleen shows infiltration of the red pulp by these cells, which demonstrate the characteristic "hairy cell" cytoplasmic projections and are typically tartrate-resistant acid phosphatase positive. Although patients may demonstrate markedly abnormal blood counts at presentation, > 90% of patients will live longer than 10 years with treatment.

Answer A is incorrect. Acute lymphoid leukemia (ALL) affects children much more often than adults. It may result in pancytopenia, as is seen in this patient, but would not cause such a striking monocytopenia. Immature blasts are evident on the peripheral smear of ALL patients.

Answer C is incorrect. Idiopathic thrombocytopenic purpura is an antibody-mediated thrombocytopenia caused by antibody response to platelets. It does not affect other cell lines, so is an unlikely cause of this patient's illness.

Answer D is incorrect. Infectious mononucleosis (Epstein-Barr virus) may affect patients of any age, although it is most common in adolescents. It may cause splenomegaly and a peripheral smear not unlike that shown. It does not, however, cause pancytopenia, a hallmark of hairy cell leukemia.

Answer E is incorrect. Although the possibility of other lymphoid malignancies must be considered in any patient with leukemia or lymphoma, this patient's presentation is not consistent with Hodgkin's lymphoma, nor is his laboratory evaluation. Fatigue and night

sweats may affect patients with newly diagnosed Hodgkin's disease, but splenomegaly is not a common finding, and lymphadenopathy is almost universally found. In addition, the peripheral blood smear is generally normal in Hodgkin's disease.

2. **The correct answer is C.** Along with the coagulation factors (II, VII, IX, and X), the anticoagulant proteins C and S are also vitamin K–dependent, and therefore affected by warfarin, which is a vitamin K analog. Proteins C and S have shorter half-lives than the coagulation factors, and therefore a faster turnover in the body. Thus, for a brief window of approximately 3 days after the initiation of warfarin therapy, the body has normal function of its coagulation factors, but loss of anticoagulant proteins C and S, rendering the patient hypercoagulable. Negative consequences of this are avoided by administering heparin with warfarin for the first 5 days.

Answer A is incorrect. Warfarin inhibits the synthesis of the vitamin K–dependent factors, including factors II, VII, IX, and X, and proteins C and S; it never increases the amount of the factors, but the shorter half-life of the anticoagulants protein C and S lead to the initial hypercoagulable state.

Answer B is incorrect. Venous valvular insufficiency is a common factor that contributes to venous stasis, one of the three elements of Virchow's triad (along with endothelial injury and a hypercoagulable state). Warfarin, however, has no effect on venous valvular insufficiency.

Answer D is incorrect. Factor V Leiden is the most common inherited hypercoagulable state and results from a point mutation that causes resistance of factor V to protein C degradation. Warfarin does not induce a condition similar to factor V Leiden.

Answer E is incorrect. Warfarin is a vitamin K analog, and therefore inhibits the production of the vitamin K–dependent factors (both coagulants and anticoagulants). Therefore, it has no effect on platelets.

3. The correct answer is D. The patient is presenting with stage IIIA disease, which implies that her disease has spread to nodal sites on both sides of her diaphragm. This disease stage will require therapy with both systemic chemotherapy and radiation to the mediastinum, and potentially the abdomen and pelvis. This patient should be concerned about many effects of her disease and its treatment that may prevent or complicate her pregnancy; however, there is no evidence that the hormonal milieu of pregnancy promotes recurrence of Hodgkin's disease. Importantly, this type of evidence does exist in breast cancer, where increased estrogen may promote the growth of tumor cells.

Answer A is incorrect. The risk of a second cancer is substantially increased in patients with Hodgkin's lymphoma, particularly if systemic chemotherapy is required as treatment. The risk of leukemia may be elevated almost 100-fold in this case.

Answer B is incorrect. Ovarian failure is a risk for this patient who will receive systemic chemotherapy. In some cases, ovarian tissue can be removed surgically and frozen to preserve a patient's fertility. Should the patient need to undergo pelvic irradiation, her risk of ovarian failure would be almost 100%.

Answer C is incorrect. Mediastinal irradiation that is required to treat Hodgkin's lymphoma may cause pericarditis that can result in fibrosis and congestive heart failure. Because pregnancy requires increased cardiac output, heart failure or worsening of underlying heart failure may result.

Answer E is incorrect. Patients treated with radiation to the mediastinum are at risk for restrictive lung disease that may follow radiation pneumonitis. During pregnancy, when the diaphragm is displaced superiorly and breathing is somewhat restricted, asymptomatic lung disease may become clinically important.

4. The correct answer is C. With rare exceptions, patients are entitled to know their diagnosis and prognosis, even if they are old, their condition is probably terminal, and they have anxious personalities and/or psychiatric diag-

noses. Exceptions to the physician's obligation to discuss the diagnosis with the patient include the previous request of the patient to not be informed or the belief of the physician that disclosure would severely harm the patient.

Answer A is incorrect. It would be unethical to acquiesce to the family's request. If nondisclosure is the patient's request as well, then the physician will be able to honor it.

Answer B is incorrect. Even if the entire family wants to keep the diagnosis from the patient, if the patient him- or herself wants to be informed, the physician is obligated to tell the patient the diagnosis.

Answer D is incorrect. Rarely will consultation be a correct answer on a USMLE examination. The physician has the information needed to act and should do so.

Answer E is incorrect. Psychiatric evaluation is not warranted at this time. All physicians can judge decision-making capacity, and if the patient has the capacity to decide whether he or she wants to be informed of the diagnosis, the obligation then exists to abide by that wish.

5. The correct answer is B. This child's symptoms of bone pain, easy bruising, and fatigue, as well as examination findings of hepatosplenomegaly and lymphadenopathy, suggest a malignancy, which is confirmed by the presence of blasts on the blood smear. The most common leukemia in children is acute lymphoid leukemia (ALL), and this diagnosis is supported by the lymphocytes on the smear. A bone marrow biopsy is recommended for all patients with ALL.

Answer A is incorrect. Child abuse should always be suspected in cases of children with multiple bruises and/or bone pain. However, this child's other systemic symptoms and blood smear results suggest another etiology for her bruises.

Answer C is incorrect. Although the patient does have signs of liver dysfunction, including hepatomegaly and easy bruising, her smear suggests a hematologic malignancy.

Answer D is incorrect. A test for serum heterophile antibodies is helpful in diagnosing infectious mononucleosis, which would explain this patient's lymphadenopathy, fatigue, and hepatosplenomegaly. However, given the patient's easy bruising and blood smear, mononucleosis is not high on the list of differential diagnoses.

Answer E is incorrect. Although vitamin C deficiency does cause easy bruising, it would not explain the patient's bone pain, hepatosplenomegaly, lymphadenopathy, or blood smear.

6. **The correct answer is C.** The patient in this clinical scenario most likely has heparin-induced thrombocytopenia (HIT), which commonly occurs within 4–10 days after the initiation of unfractionated heparin treatment. Unlike other drug-induced thrombocytopenia, HIT is associated with thrombosis due to platelet activation rather than bleeding. Because platelet counts typically remain above 20,000/mm³, spontaneous bleeding is rarely seen. Pathophysiology of this disorder includes the presence of platelet antibodies that cause limb- and life-threatening thrombosis, often at unusual sites including arteries. The first intervention in cases of HIT is immediate cessation of any heparin and immediate initiation of a direct thrombin inhibitor such as argatroban or lepirudin.

Answer A is incorrect. Warfarin therapy should be avoided in patients with heparin-induced thrombocytopenia until the platelet count rises to > 100,000/mm³. Initiation of warfarin therapy may cause a transient hypercoagulable state due to a decline in protein C levels, thereby increasing the risk of limb ischemia.

Answer B is incorrect. Patients with heparin-induced thrombocytopenia are at an increased risk for thrombosis. The noninvolved contralateral leg is at increased risk for developing a deep venous thrombosis. Discontinuation of the pneumatic compression devices bilaterally might lead to an increase in mortality and would not prevent further complications.

Answer D is incorrect. Ultrasound has an accuracy rate of 80–90% in the detection of deep vein thrombosis (DVT). Therefore, Doppler ultrasound in conjunction with the physical symptoms and presentation of pain, edema, tenderness, and a positive Homans' sign (calf pain on dorsiflexion of the foot) are sufficient to make a diagnosis of DVT. A further DVT workup consisting of venography is not indicated in this case and would not prevent further complications.

Answer E is incorrect. Although patients with a history of deep venous thrombosis may be at increased risk for pulmonary embolism, the first step in management is cessation of heparin exposure rather than placement of an inferior vena cava filter.

7. **The correct answer is C.** Recent evidence suggests that most low-grade squamous intraepithelial lesions (LSILs) will regress spontaneously. Current guidelines indicate observation of a biopsy-confirmed LSIL is appropriate management for a reliable patient that is also immunocompetent.

Answer A is incorrect. Endocervical curettage is reserved for abnormal Pap smear findings of high-grade squamous intraepithelial lesion.

Answer B is incorrect. Loop electrosurgical excision procedure is reserved for abnormal Pap smear findings of high-grade squamous intraepithelial lesion.

Answer D is incorrect. Repeat Pap smear in 1 year following a biopsy-confirmed LSIL is not an acceptable form of management.

Answer E is incorrect. Repeat colposcopy in 1 year is not an acceptable form of management.

8. **The correct answer is D.** This patient has developed a posttransplant lymphoproliferative disorder (PTLD). Any patient who is chronically immunosuppressed is at risk for development of lymphoproliferative malignancy, and a cardiac transplant patient is at intermediate risk (4.6% incidence) compared to kidney (1.0%) or liver (3.0%) transplant patients. PTLDs generally occur in extranodal locations, and may respond completely to reduction in immunosuppression; however, since immunosuppression is necessary for protection of grafted organs, radiotherapy is also often employed. In addition, most PTLDs are related to

primary or reactivation infection with Epstein-Barr virus. Some evidence demonstrates that the use of acyclovir during treatment for PTLD contributes to eradication of the virus and resolution of the malignancy caused by it. The majority of centers thus employ acyclovir as an adjuvant therapy to radiotherapy/surgery coupled with a reduction in immunosuppression.

Answer A is incorrect. The purpose of acyclovir in treatment of posttransplant lymphoproliferative disorder is to eliminate the Epstein-Barr virus that is causative in the development of the malignancy, not to eradicate the neoplastic cells themselves; this is left to the host immune system and radiation therapy, if employed.

Answer B is incorrect. Although severe infection with cytomegalovirus is a risk for any immunosuppressed patient, antiviral therapy is generally not employed in patients undergoing cancer therapy. Acyclovir prophylaxis is employed in some bone marrow transplant centers.

Answer C is incorrect. Radiation to mucous membranes will indeed cause inflammation and decreased barrier protection. This is generally not held to be an indication for antiviral prophylaxis, however.

Answer E is incorrect. If anything, decreasing the patient's immunosuppressive regimen will assist her immune system in preventing viral infection.

9. **The correct answer is D.** This patient is presenting with acute appendicitis that began approximately 24 hours ago. Although the clinical findings of a positive Rovsing's sign (right lower quadrant pain when palpating the left lower quadrant) as well as a psoas sign (pain upon extension of the right leg) are not specific for appendicitis, they support the diagnosis when considering the overall clinical history. Pain that begins in the periumbilical region (visceral peritoneal irritation) and localizes to the right lower quadrant (parietal peritoneal irritation) along with nausea, vomiting, and anorexia that follow the onset of pain are characteristic of appendicitis. The patient pre-

sents with an elevated WBC count (indicative of an infectious process) and fever. Finally, the CT scan shows a distended appendix with an enhancing wall and stranding in the periappendiceal fat. These radiographic findings are consistent with acute appendicitis. The treatment of appendicitis is surgical removal of the inflamed appendix in order to avoid appendiceal rupture. The risk of appendiceal perforation increases from 25% to 75% after the first 24–48 hours of presentation, respectively. Patients presenting within 24–72 hours of the onset of abdominal pain (as in this case) can be treated with appendectomy. If, on the other hand, appendiceal perforation is suspected or the patient has had symptoms for 5 days, medical management with antibiotics, intravenous fluids, and bowel rest are indicated.

Answer A is incorrect. The treatment of appendicitis is surgical removal of the inflamed appendix prior to its rupture. Patients presenting within 24–72 hours of the onset of abdominal pain (as in this case) can be treated with appendectomy. If, on the other hand, appendiceal perforation is suspected or the patient has had symptoms for 5 days, medical management with antibiotics, intravenous fluids, bowel rest, and close follow-up are indicated. There is no reason to suspect rupture in this patient.

Answer B is incorrect. The CT scan that was obtained has sensitivities above 90% for the diagnosis of appendicitis. The CT scan shows a distended appendix with stranding in the periappendiceal fat, which is pathognomonic for acute appendicitis. These radiographic findings in conjunction with the clinical presentation support a diagnosis of appendicitis without the need for further studies.

Answer C is incorrect. The CT scan that was obtained has sensitivities above 90% for the diagnosis of appendicitis. The CT scan above shows a distended appendix with stranding in the periappendiceal fat (pathognomonic for acute appendicitis). These radiographic findings in conjunction with the clinical presentation support a diagnosis of appendicitis without the need for further studies.

Answer E is incorrect. The CT scan that was obtained has sensitivities above 90% for the diagnosis of appendicitis. The CT scan above shows a distended appendix with stranding in the periappendiceal fat (pathognomonic for acute appendicitis). These radiographic findings in conjunction with the clinical presentation support a diagnosis of appendicitis without the need for further studies.

10. **The correct answer is D.** The arrow in the image indicates an epidermal cluster of atypical lymphocytes (Pautrier's abscess). This is pathognomonic for mycosis fungoides (MF), a subtype of cutaneous T-lymphocyte lymphoma, which is unrelated to fungal infection in spite of the name. This disease is most frequently found in men in their mid-50s and is often misdiagnosed for years. Skin lesions may progress from patch phase to plaque phase to cutaneous tumor, and subcutaneous deposits in the face may lead to the classic (though rarely seen) "leonine facies." Sézary syndrome is MF with erythroderma, lymphadenopathy, and the presence of atypical T lymphocytes in the blood.

Answer A is incorrect. While contact dermatitis may develop in this distribution in reaction to clothing or local irritants, the biopsy points to another diagnosis.

Answer B is incorrect. This is a very late and atypical presentation for eczema and should not be the primary consideration in this case.

Answer C is incorrect. Inverse psoriasis typically presents as erythematous plaques in intertriginous areas. It has minimal scaling in comparison to the more common plaque psoriasis and tends to spare extensor surfaces. Like plaque psoriasis, it is a chronic, relapsing disorder with an inflammatory basis.

Answer E is incorrect. The histology of psoriasis is characterized by infiltration of skin by activated lymphocytes and epidermal hyperproliferation.

11. **The correct answer is B.** Given this patient's clinical picture and laboratory results, he likely has chronic myelogenous leukemia (CML). The differential diagnosis includes acute myelogenous leukemia and myelodysplastic syndrome. A definitive diagnosis can be made by cytogenetic studies that reveal the Philadelphia chromosome (9,22 translocation), which is pathognomonic for CML. Ninety percent of CML patients will demonstrate this translocation, and in the 10% that do not, a bone marrow biopsy will be definitive.

Answer A is incorrect. Coagulation studies are helpful in assessing for liver disease or in bruising of unknown etiology; however, this patient's easy bruising is likely due to thrombocytopenia, which in turn is likely due to his leukemia.

Answer C is incorrect. While low levels of leukocyte alkaline phosphatase are seen in chronic myelogenous leukemia, this information alone cannot make a definitive diagnosis.

Answer D is incorrect. Iron studies are helpful in evaluating microcytic anemia of unknown etiology; however, this patient's anemia is likely due to his leukemia.

Answer E is incorrect. While chronic myelogenous leukemia is the suspected diagnosis based on the clinical picture, further studies are needed to confirm this diagnosis.

12. **The correct answer is E.** Seminoma is a tumor type that is extremely sensitive to radiation. Stage I and IIA can be successfully treated with orchiectomy and irradiation of the retroperitoneum. The low dose of radiation that is required is usually well tolerated with minimal gastrointestinal side effects. Chemotherapy can be used as salvage therapy for patients who relapse following irradiation. The staging of seminomas is as follows: stage I: disease confined to the testis; stage II: retroperitoneal nodal involvement (IIA if < 2 cm and IIB if > 2 cm); stage III: supradiaphragmatic nodal involvement or involvement of the viscera.

Answer A is incorrect. At this point there is no need to remove the man's other testicle.

Answer B is incorrect. Platinum-based chemotherapy is used to treat patients that have metastatic nonseminomatous germ cell tumors after treatment by orchiectomy or with bulky retroperitoneal disease. In the case of unilateral testicular cancer, a bilateral orchiectomy is not warranted.

Answer C is incorrect. Prophylactic mediastinal radiation had been practiced in the past but it is no longer used. The myelosuppression that may result can compromise the patient's ability to receive chemotherapy at a later date.

Answer D is incorrect. Retroperitoneal lymph node dissection (RPLND) is used in treating low-stage nonseminomatous germ cell tumors and has significant morbidity. RPLND often damages the sympathetic innervation of the seminal vesicle, which can lead to retrograde ejaculation and infertility. The case presented here is a seminoma and does not warrant this surgical procedure.

13. **The correct answer is B.** Fungal infections become increasingly important in bone marrow transplant after the first 7 days posttransplant. Patients with graft-versus-host disease who require long-term immunosuppression are at high risk of infection by organisms such as *Candida* and *Aspergillus*. These infections can occur even after engraftment and resolution of neutropenia (which would be expected at posttransplant day 45). Other infections that are important during this time frame are cytomegaloviral pneumonia, parasitic infection, and human herpes virus 6 infection of the skin and mucous membranes.

Answer A is incorrect. The risk of bacterial infection is high for bone marrow transplant patients in the first 20–30 days following transplant. This is due to the 1 to 4 weeks of neutropenia that follows the transplantation and renders patients susceptible to aerobic bacteria found in the gut and on the skin. Infection with *Nocardia* is a concern during the 30–90 days after transplantation. Infections with *Staphylococcus aureus* are generally limited to the pre-engraftment period 1–3 weeks posttransplant. This type of infection would not be expected in a patient 45 days posttransplant.

Answer C is incorrect. Patients are most at risk for gram-negative bacteremia in the 1–3 weeks following transplant. These infections are usually caused by intestinal flora such as *Escherichia coli*, *Pseudomonas*, and *Klebsiella*.

Answer D is incorrect. Patients being treated for hematogenous malignancy are indeed at increased risk of *Pneumocystis carinii* pneumonia. However, they are treated with trimethoprim-sulfamethoxazole prophylaxis, which prevents 100% of cases when taken correctly. Provided this patient has been compliant with her medications as stated, her risk of acquiring this disease is quite low.

Answer E is incorrect. The risk of herpes simplex virus (HSV) reactivation is highest in the 2 weeks following transplant. It causes severe mucositis that has been shown to occur with lower incidence if HSV-seropositive patients are treated with prophylactic acyclovir.

Answer F is incorrect. Patients with Hodgkin's disease are at an unexplained increased risk for *Salmonella* infection. No such known risk exists for patients with promyelocytic leukemia.

14. **The correct answer is E.** The patient is presenting with cutaneous T-cell lymphoma (CTCL), or mycosis fungoides. This disease is a B-lymphocyte lymphoma that is generally indolent. The malignant process involves B-lymphocyte that normally inhabit the dermis and epidermis, and may not affect the lymph nodes themselves at all. CTCL may affect patients in several different stages, although one stage does not necessarily lead to another. Patients may live for 20+ years without progression of disease. The phases of disease are as follows: The phase of least severity is a patch stage, involving only the epidermis in discrete areas of the skin. This phase may or may not progress to a plaque stage, affecting discrete skin areas but invading the dermis as well as the epidermis. The tumor phase may follow the plaque stage, and involves deep involvement of the dermis with growth in height, forming discrete tumors. The final and most severe stage of disease is a systemic illness generally called Sézary's syndrome. During this phase the entire skin is involved with lymphoma cells, and telltale Sézary cells are found in the circulation. This is the only phase of CTCL that affects the systemic circulation. This patient's disease is consistent with the plaque stage of disease, since the dermis is invaded by lym-

phomatous cells. Several treatments exist for CTCL and vary according to stage. Early (patch or plaque) stage disease may be treated with topical nitrogen mustards on an outpatient basis. More advanced disease may be treated with conventional radiation therapy or total skin electron beam therapy.

Answer A is incorrect. Bone marrow transplant may be considered in cases of Sézary's syndrome. It would not be anticipated in a patient with plaque stage disease because of the relatively small chance that the disease might progress to systemic illness.

Answer B is incorrect. Although observation is appropriate for certain patients, it is rarely relied upon because of the real chance that disease might progress to disfigurement or death. Because topical treatments have relatively benign adverse effect profiles, they are generally used for even mild early-stage disease.

Answer C is incorrect. Occasionally, systemic chemotherapy is required to treat CTCL; however, it is generally used only after the onset of systemic disease (Sézary's syndrome).

Answer D is incorrect. Systemic corticosteroids are not generally used to treat CTCL.

Answer F is incorrect. More advanced or refractory CTCL may be treated with total skin electron beam therapy. This method of treatment is generally reserved for patients with involvement of large areas of skin, or with disease refractory to less expensive and more convenient therapies.

15. **The correct answer is E.** This patient has a loculated parapneumonic effusion likely resulting from a nosocomial pneumonia. The loculation is shown by the arrowheads. Because the effusion is loculated, a tube thoracostomy with intrapleural thrombolytics is indicated. It is important to note that loculated pleural effusions cannot be diagnosed only by x-ray, but rather a CT is needed. Although simple, nonloculated effusion may be treated with thoracentesis, a complicated, loculated effusion may need thoracoscopy, chest tube, and thrombolytics.

Answer A is incorrect. Oral antibiotics can be used to treat pneumonia alone or to treat an uncomplicated parapneumonic effusion. However, complicated effusions, loculated effusions, and empyema require both drainage and antibiotics.

Answer B is incorrect. Pleurodesis, or injection of an irritant between the visceral and parietal pleura causing them to scar together, is the treatment of choice for malignant pleural effusions that are refractory to other treatments.

Answer C is incorrect. Surgery is generally not indicated in instances of acute pleural effusions but may be indicated for lung parenchymal malignancies.

Answer D is incorrect. Therapeutic thoracentesis is used to treat symptomatic pleural effusions; however, the underlying disease process must also be addressed. Thoracentesis is indicated for free-flowing effusions or effusions that layer.

16. **The correct answer is B.** This patient is a young female presenting with a DVT. Although DVTs in this population are often attributed to the use of oral contraceptives, there is a strong family history of recurrent DVTs and therefore we must consider hereditary disorders of the coagulation system. Factor V Leiden is an autosomal dominant disorder in which coagulation factor Va (the activated form of coagulation factor V) is resistant to degradation by activated protein C. Factor Va remains active and allows for the conversion of prothrombin to thrombin, thereby promoting a hypercoagulable state in patients. Factor V Leiden accounts for 40–50% of venous thromboemboli in cases in whom a genetic predisposition is found. The relative risk of venous thrombosis in a patient with a heterozygous mutation of the gene encoding factor V is 7, and that in a patient with the mutation in conjunction with concomitant oral contraceptive use is 35.

Answer A is incorrect. Factor V Leiden is the most common cause of inherited thrombophilia. Antithrombin is an inhibitor of thrombin and of coagulation factors IXa and Xa. Although antithrombin deficiency would lead to a hypercoagulable state, a mutation in the gene encoding coagulation factor V is more common and thus is more likely to be the underlying cause of a venous thrombotic event than is antithrombin deficiency.

Answer C is incorrect. Protein C excess would lead to inactivation of coagulation factors Va and VIII, and decreased propensity for the formation of thrombi.

Answer D is incorrect. Factor V Leiden is the most common cause of inherited thrombophilia. Protein S is a cofactor of the protein C system in which factor Va and factor VIIIa are inactivated and clot formation is thereby inhibited. Although protein S deficiency leads to a severely hypercoagulable state, a mutation in the gene encoding coagulation factor V is more common and thus is more likely to be the underlying cause of a venous thrombotic event than is protein S deficiency.

Answer E is incorrect. Factor V Leiden is the most common cause of inherited thrombophilia. The increased relative risk of developing venous thrombosis with factor V Leiden is 7, whereas that of a prothrombin gene mutation is 2.8.

17. **The correct answer is B.** Courvoisier's sign is a palpable nontender gallbladder as a result of common bile duct obstruction/compression by pancreatic adenocarcinoma at the head of the pancreas. Biliary obstruction below the level of the cystic duct is unlikely to be caused by stone disease.

Answer A is incorrect. Chandelier sign refers to the pain on manipulation of the cervix and uterus during a pelvic examination in a patient with pelvic inflammatory disease.

Answer C is incorrect. Cullen's sign refers to ecchymosis in the periumbilical region suggestive of retroperitoneal hemorrhage in severe acute pancreatitis.

Answer D is incorrect. Grey Turner sign refers to ecchymosis in the flank that suggests retroperitoneal hemorrhage accompanying severe acute pancreatitis.

Answer E is incorrect. Murphy's sign refers to the inspiratory arrest during deep palpation of the right upper quadrant in patients with acute cholecystitis.

18. **The correct answer is A.** Twenty to fifty percent of patients with a history of allogeneic bone marrow transplant develop chronic graft-versus-host disease (GVHD). GVHD is caused by a proliferation of grafted donor T lymphocytes that ultimately reject the host's foreign proteins, leading to end-organ damage. This disease is a separate entity from acute GVHD and resembles an autoimmune disorder. It may result in maculopapular rash, as seen in this patient; sicca syndrome; arthritis; and bile duct degeneration, leading to jaundice. The chronic form of GVHD may occur months or even years after transplant and is likely due to vascular damage by the proliferated T lymphocytes. Patients who are older than 40 years at the time of transplant are at the greatest risk of developing chronic GVHD. This complication is irreversible, but prednisone is the standard of care.

Answer B is incorrect. Following bone marrow transplant, patients are not placed on an immunosuppressive regimen in the absence of GVHD. It is stated that the patient was discharged on no medications 6 months prior to her trip.

Answer C is incorrect. Although the patient certainly could be suffering from new-onset systemic lupus erythematous, in a patient with a history of bone marrow transplant, chronic GVHD is much more likely.

Answer D is incorrect. Rosacea is a possible diagnosis for this patient, particularly because rosacea is often exacerbated by sun exposure. However, chronic GVHD is much more likely.

Answer E is incorrect. Staphylococcal skin infections include impetigo and abscesses. The patient's rash does not resemble either of these. In addition, she feels well and is afebrile.

Answer F is incorrect. The patient may simply have sunburn. From her account, however, she avoided much direct sunlight and applied sunscreen. Regardless, a patient at risk for chronic GVHD deserves a full workup when presenting with these symptoms. In addition, it seems that her hands and wrists were sore and inflamed, leading away from the diagnosis of sun poisoning.

19. **The correct answer is B.** This patient has a pituitary mass causing headaches and blurred vision due to compression of the optic chiasm. It is most likely a prolactin-secreting adenoma because the patient is complaining of decreased libido, a common finding in men with hyperprolactinemia, along with possible impotence, infertility, gynecomastia, and galactorrhea. Given his history of peptic ulcer disease as well as a family history of peptic ulcer disease and pancreatic tumors, type I multiple endocrine neoplasia (MEN) should be considered in this patient since the autosomal dominant disorder consists of **P**ituitary tumors, **P**ancreatic tumors, and **P**rimary hyperparathyroidism (the "3 P's"). Parathyroid hormone as well as serum calcium and phosphate should be checked to evaluate for hyperparathyroidism and resultant hypercalcemia and hypophosphatemia.

Answer A is incorrect. Calcitonin is a hormone secreted by thyroid C cells. Serum levels may be elevated in patients with medullary thyroid cancer. This malignancy is associated with type II MEN syndromes, not type I MEN.

Answer C is incorrect. Renal ultrasound would not be indicated in this patient, as there is no association of renal pathology with any of the multiple endocrine neoplasias.

Answer D is incorrect. Thyroid ultrasound could be used to evaluate for a mass if there was concern for thyroid malignancy. Although medullary thyroid cancer is found in patients with type II MEN syndromes, it is not associated with pituitary adenomas and pancreatic tumors.

Answer E is incorrect. Plasma and/or urinary metanephrines are used to evaluate for pheochromocytoma, an adrenal tumor that produces catecholamines. Pheochromocytomas are found in association with type IIA MEN, which also includes medullary thyroid cancer and hyperparathyroidism, and type IIB MEN, which also may include medullary thyroid cancer, mucosal neuromas, intestinal ganglioneuromas, and marfanoid habitus. Pheochromocytoma is not typically associated with pancreatic and pituitary tumors.

20. **The correct answer is D.** This child has metastatic neuroblastoma, which is common in children < 2 years old. Primary neuroblastoma most commonly presents as a painless abdominal mass, hypertension, respiratory distress, Horner's syndrome, or cord compression. Often, however, neuroblastoma is not diagnosed until after it has metastasized. Tumor infiltration of the bone marrow causes pancytopenia. Tumor infiltration of the periorbital bones causes periorbital ecchymoses and proptosis, an appearance often referred to as "raccoon eyes." Low-grade fever, fatigue, and failure to thrive (which is evidenced by his small size) occur with metastatic disease. Urinary catecholamines are elevated in neuroblastoma, but definitive diagnosis requires biopsy. Treatment involves chemotherapy and surgical excision of local disease. Prognosis varies with age at presentation: infants with metastatic disease respond favorably to treatment, while most children older than 1 year with advanced neuroblastoma will die from progressive disease despite intensive multimodality therapy.

Answer A is incorrect. Acute lymphoid leukemia (ALL) is the most common form of cancer in children. ALL can cause pancytopenia, lymphadenopathy, fever, failure to thrive, petechiae, and pallor. ALL does not cause periorbital ecchymoses, proptosis, hypertension, or elevated urinary catecholamines.

Answer B is incorrect. Aplastic anemia, characterized by pancytopenia and hypocellular marrow, is usually due to injury to the pluripotent stem cell. The initial insult may be congenital or acquired. Congenital causes are uncommon, including Fanconi's anemia and Shwachman-Diamond syndrome. Acquired causes are more common, including a wide variety of drugs and chemicals, ionizing radiation, and viruses. Petechiae, pallor, fatigue, and fever are consistent with this diagnosis. However, aplastic anemia would not cause hypertension, lymphadenopathy, periorbital bruising, proptosis, or elevated urinary catecholamines.

Answer C is incorrect. Child abuse should be considered if a child sustains injuries incompatible with normal activities. His periorbital bruise might resemble a bruise from an eye being punched by a fist. However, proptosis would not occur in this situation. Child abuse could explain failure to thrive if physical abuse was accompanied by neglect. However, it would not explain any of his other symptoms, his hypertension, or his laboratory values.

Answer E is incorrect. Pheochromocytomas is a catecholamine-secreting neoplasm of chromaffin cells that causes intermittent hypertension and can result in elevated urinary catecholamines. Other symptoms of a pheochromocytoma include headache, perspiration, palpitations, pallor, and diaphoresis. A pheochromocytoma does not cause lethargy, abnormal complete blood count, fever, lymphadenopathy, or periorbital bruising, and is thus unlikely in this child.

21. **The correct answer is B.** In a postmenopausal woman whose menses ceased more than 1 year ago, vaginal bleeding must be met with a high level of suspicion for a pathologic process, especially cancer. The standard of care is that all vaginal bleeding in these instances must be evaluated by an endometrial biopsy.

Answer A is incorrect. An abdominal ultrasound could be used to visualize the uterine cavity and measure the thickness of the endometrial tissue, but it could not be used to rule out endometrial cancer, which should be considered in this woman.

Answer C is incorrect. In postmenopausal women in whom menses ceased more than 1 year ago, vaginal bleeding must be worked up immediately.

Answer D is incorrect. In a postmenopausal woman, luteinizing hormone and follicle-stimulating hormone levels would be expected to be high. These tests are not useful because they would not provide information about what is causing this woman's vaginal bleeding.

Answer E is incorrect. Vaginal atrophy is a common cause of vaginal bleeding in postmenopausal women, and the atrophy can be remedied by use of topical (or systemic) estro-

gens or topical testosterone cream. However, the standard of care is that all vaginal bleeding in these instances must be evaluated by an endometrial biopsy.

22. **The correct answer is B.** Chronic myelogenous leukemia (CML), in its chronic phase, presents with constitutional symptoms along with abdominal fullness due to splenomegaly. Diagnosis is most common in the fourth to sixth decades of life, and irradiation increases the risk of developing CML. Because it is a proliferation of mature myeloid cells, peripheral smear should show predominant leukocytosis with cells in all stages of maturation. Definitive diagnosis relies on identification of the Philadelphia chromosome or the bcr-abl fusion product. However, approximately 5% of patients have atypical CML without presence of bcr-abl and show a poor response to therapy.

Answer A is incorrect. A bone marrow biopsy may be part of the workup of leukemia. CML may show hypercellularity of the bone marrow, as well as differentiated cells rather than blasts. A bone marrow biopsy will not, however, differentiate the type of leukemia. The diagnosis of CML depends on cytogenetics.

Answer C is incorrect. α-Fetoprotein is a marker for liver cancer, which normally presents with jaundice, elevated liver enzymes, and abdominal fullness. It is most common in individuals with cirrhosis, either from hepatitis infection or alcohol use.

Answer D is incorrect. Reed-Sternberg cells can be seen in Hodgkin's lymphoma, which typically presents as lymphadenopathy rather than an elevated WBC count.

Answer E is incorrect. Colon cancer may be consistent with the constitutional symptoms of this patient but would not explain the hematologic findings.

23. **The correct answer is E.** The patient's most likely diagnosis is multiple myeloma. This malignancy of plasma cells leads to proliferation of a single plasma cell clone. This plasmacytosis leads to secretion of osteoclast-activating factor by myeloma cells, increasing osteoclastic activity and causing lytic lesions. The plas-

macytosis also contributes to immunosuppression (because one antibody clone dominates rather than the hundreds of thousands that are found in a normal patient) and anemia. The proliferation of plasma cells also causes a proliferation of antibody clones that spill into the urine, known as Bence Jones proteins, and may eventually cause renal failure.

Answer A is incorrect. Anorexia nervosa may cause increased susceptibility to fracture through osteopenia. However, this would not cause lytic lesions on radiograph.

Answer B is incorrect. Type 1 Gaucher's disease is due to a genetic deficiency of glucocerebrosidase, and can cause osteopenia, osteolytic lesions, and pathologic fractures. It is usually diagnosed in childhood or, rarely, early adulthood. Gaucher's disease is most often found in the Ashkenazi Jewish population, but it is a rare disease that is much less common than multiple myeloma. A patient with Gaucher's disease would not be at increased susceptibility to infection, and would normally have splenomegaly and growth delay in addition to the bone symptoms.

Answer C is incorrect. Congenital osteoporosis would cause multiple fractures, but would be expected to cause diffuse low bone density, not lytic lesions.

Answer D is incorrect. Domestic abuse should always be considered in cases of multiple fractures; however, it does not account for the patient's other symptoms or her lytic lesions.

Answer F is incorrect. One method of differentiating multiple myeloma from other malignancies is through bone scan. Osteoclastic metastases from breast cancer can appear as hot spots on bone scan, although osteoblastic lesions would be invisible. Malignancy is less likely in the setting of increased protein in the urine, especially if there is a high M spike on protein electrophoresis. A biopsy can be done on the lytic lesion to confirm the diagnosis if there are few Bence Jones proteins.

24. **The correct answer is D.** An 11.3-kg (25-lb) unintentional weight loss, hemoptysis, lesion

visible on CT scan, and a significant smoking history should raise concern for lung cancer. The patient is suffering from euvolemic hyponatremia due to syndrome of inappropriate secretion of antidiuretic hormone, a paraneoplastic syndrome seen in small cell carcinoma of the lung. Small cell carcinoma, along with sarcoidosis, pneumonia, head injury, and antipsychotics or antidepressants can cause nonosmotically stimulated release of antidiuretic hormone (ADH), resulting in euvolemic hyponatremia. Diagnosis is based on urine osmolality > 50–100 mOsm/kg with concurrent serum hyposmolality in the absence of a physiologic reason for increased ADH (chronic heart failure or cirrhosis). Urine sodium > 20 mEq/L is used to show that the patient is not hypovolemic. Of the bronchogenic carcinomas of the lung, small cell carcinoma carries the worst prognosis and is assumed to be metastatic at time of diagnosis.

Answer A is incorrect. Adenocarcinomas typically cause the paraneoplastic syndromes of digital clubbing, hypertrophic pulmonary osteoarthropathy, thrombophlebitis, and nonbacterial verrucous endocarditis. Adenocarcinoma and the other non–small cell lung cancers carry a better prognosis than small cell.

Answer B is incorrect. Bronchoalveolar cell carcinoma is most often associated with multiple nodules on imaging studies, interstitial infiltration, and prolific sputum production. It may be confused with interstitial pneumonia on x-ray of the chest. Bronchoalveolar cell carcinoma and the other non–small cell lung cancers carry a better prognosis than small cell.

Answer C is incorrect. Large cell carcinoma is a very uncommon type of lung cancer that is associated with gynecomastia. Large cell carcinoma carries a slightly worse prognosis than the other non–small cell lung cancers.

Answer E is incorrect. Squamous cell carcinomas typically cause the paraneoplastic syndrome of hypercalcemia via production of parathyroid hormone–related peptide. Squamous cell carcinoma and the other non–small cell lung cancers carry a better prognosis than small cell.

25. The correct answer is B. This patient displays classic signs of hyperkalemia, including lethargy and weakness. In the context of normal kidney function as well as hyperuricemia and hypocalcemia, this hyperkalemia is likely the result of the chemotherapeutic effect on his tumor. This phenomenon, known as tumor lysis syndrome, presents shortly after commencement of chemotherapy with elevations in serum urate, and can progress to urate-induced kidney failure. Along with urate elevations, potassium may climb to dangerously high levels.

Answer A is incorrect. Potassium is readily absorbed from ingested food in the gastrointestinal tract. However, increased potassium intake is rarely a cause of significant hyperkalemia in the setting of normal renal function.

Answer C is incorrect. Acidosis can lead to extracellular potassium shifts, causing a transient increase in plasma potassium levels. The patient's electrolyte panel reveals a normal anion gap, and acidosis would not explain his uric acid and calcium abnormalities.

Answer D is incorrect. Pseudohyperkalemia is due to in vitro hemolysis of red cells, causing them to release their potassium-rich contents. It occurs most frequently when there is a long delay between specimen collection and analysis. This patient displays symptoms of true hyperkalemia, making pseudohyperkalemia less likely.

Answer E is incorrect. Renal failure is a cause of hyperkalemia, especially when filtration levels fall or the distal tubule fails to function normally due to nephrotoxins or decreased distal delivery of filtrate. This patient, however, displays a normal creatinine and is unlikely to be experiencing significant renal failure.

26. The correct answer is C. This patient most likely has chronic lymphocytic leukemia, which mainly affects individuals > 60 years old and accounts for 30% of all leukemias in the United States. The patients are often asymptomatic at presentation, and the disease is only detected on laboratory tests. In this case, the patient has an increased WBC count consisting predominantly of lymphocytes. This pa-

tient has a predicted median life expectancy of 7 years. Early treatment does not improve the outcome, and management is symptomatic rather than aimed at a cure. Because this patient is asymptomatic, no treatment is indicated at this time.

Answer A is incorrect. This patient most likely has chronic lymphocytic leukemia, which mainly affects individuals older than 60 years and accounts for 30% of all leukemias in the United States. The patients are often asymptomatic at presentation, and the disease is only detected on laboratory tests. In this case, the patient has an increased WBC count consisting predominantly of lymphocytes. This patient has a predicted median life expectancy of 7 years. Early treatment does not improve the outcome, and management is symptomatic rather than aimed at a cure. Because this patient is asymptomatic, no treatment is indicated at this time.

Answer B is incorrect. Imatinib is an inhibitor of the bcr-abl gene product that is the hallmark of chronic myelogenous leukemia and would not be indicated in this patient.

Answer D is incorrect. Radiation therapy is reserved for patients with symptoms secondary to mass effects of large lymphoid masses.

Answer E is incorrect. Splenectomy is useful when there is marked splenomegaly and anemia or thrombocytopenia refractory to medical treatment.

27. The correct answer is E. The patient has been diagnosed with follicular lymphoma, a low-grade disease of B-lymphocyte origin that is a result of a t(14;18) translocation. Such disease is almost always stage III (involved nodes above and below the diaphragm) or intravenous (disseminated disease) at diagnosis, as was the case for this patient. Rarely, low-grade lymphomas are curable with intensive chemotherapy; however, they are generally indolent, with most patients surviving 7–10 years with no therapy. The "watch and wait" approach has become the standard of care for patients with low-grade lymphomas, with palliative chemotherapy started only on progression of the disease. Histologic transformation may occur in 30–50% of follicular lymphomas to a large B-lymphocyte lymphoma. Median survival is less than 1 year after transformation occurs.

Answer A is incorrect. In an patient who is elderly with other medical problems, bone marrow transplant would not be indicated for a low-grade lymphoma.

Answer B is incorrect. This patient will most likely survive for several years before his disease progresses. Hospice care is generally reserved for terminally ill patients with a life expectancy of less than 6 months. It is not indicated for this patient's current health status.

Answer C is incorrect. Because the natural history of follicular lymphoma is such that the patient may live for 7–10 years without disease progression, palliative radiation is not indicated in the patient who is asymptomatic. It would only be considered in the presence of severe pain or obstructive symptoms.

Answer D is incorrect. The **CHOP** protocol (**C**yclophosphamide, doxorubicin [**H**ydroxydaunomycin], **O**ncovin [vincristine], and **P**rednisone) is an intensive multiagent chemotherapeutic regimen that is often used to treat intermediate- and high-grade lymphomas. It would not be indicated in treatment of low-grade disease because it has a severe adverse effect profile with low success in indolent disease.

28. **The correct answer is A.** This is a common presentation of vulvar carcinoma. Typically, it presents in women 65–70 years old, and the most common presenting complaint is vulvar pruritus. Previous human papillomavirus infection is a major risk factor for the development of vulvar carcinoma. Definitive diagnosis requires a biopsy. Spread is by local invasion and then to regional lymph nodes, so treatment includes wide surgical excision and regional lymph node excision.

Answer B is incorrect. Topical estrogen treats atrophic vaginitis, which results from a reduction of endogenous estrogens in postmenopausal women. Symptoms include vaginal soreness, dyspareunia, and burning. On examination, the vaginal mucosa is thin, with a decrease in the number of vaginal folds.

Answer C is incorrect. Acyclovir is used to treat herpes simplex virus. Primary infection is characterized by malaise and systemic symptoms, whereas genital involvement results in painful vesicular eruptions that progress to painful ulcers.

Answer D is incorrect. Cryotherapy is used to treat condyloma acuminata, or anogenital warts. Diagnosis of condyloma acuminata can usually be made by clinical inspection. Lesions are typically exophytic and not ulcerative. Although they are caused by human papillomavirus (HPV) infections (HPV types 6 and 11), they do not cause vulvar pruritus.

Answer E is incorrect. Fluconazole is used to treat infections with *Candida albicans*. Candida vulvovaginitis can present with genital pruritus, as well as burning, dysuria, and dyspareunia. A thick, cottage cheese–like, odorless discharge is characteristic. When there is vulvar involvement, it results in diffuse erythema, not discrete ulcerative lesions.

Answer F is incorrect. Metronidazole is used to treat bacterial vaginosis, which is an infection of the vaginal canal, not the external genitalia. Women typically complain of a fishy odor and increased vaginal discharge. Diagnosis is made via microscopic examination of vaginal secretions obtained by speculum examination, which will show the characteristic "clue cells," epithelial cells with cocci attached to their surface.

29. **The correct answer is D.** A stroke or transient ischemic attack in a child should prompt a search for causes other than those commonly seen in adults. Sickle cell disease is often thought of in African-Americans, but should also be considered in individuals from Central or South America. Approximately 11% of children with sickle cell disease have a stroke before the age of 20, and transient ischemic attacks can often be the first sign of an impending stroke. The pallor and fatiguing can also be clues pointing toward anemia. Chronic red blood cell transfusion in sickle cell patients has been shown to reduce the risk

of cerebral thrombotic events as well as pain crises and acute chest syndrome.

Answer A is incorrect. Familial hypercholesterolemia would certainly raise the possibility of developing strokes, but this would be unusual given the negative family history and lack of other physical findings such as xanthomas (lipid deposits in soft tissues).

Answer B is incorrect. Hemorrhagic strokes secondary to hypertension occur only after an individual has had the disease for many years. It is unlikely that a 9-year-old boy would already have a complication of hypertension.

Answer C is incorrect. Multiple myeloma can cause both anemia due to myelophthisis and stroke secondary to hyperviscosity syndrome. However, this patient is much too young to consider this diagnosis, which usually presents after age 40 with a median age of 66 years.

Answer E is incorrect. Simple partial seizures may cause transient focal deficits without change in consciousness, but would not explain the clinical picture of anemia. Additionally, seizures do not leave residual neurologic deficits.

30. **The correct answer is B.** Common variable immunodeficiency (CVID) is a syndrome characterized by hypogammaglobulinemia in combination with phenotypically normal B lymphocytes. The disease presents suddenly in the third or fourth decade after recurrent infections and lack of response to vaccines. It is a diagnosis of exclusion, and its pathogenesis is not well understood. Women in their fifth and sixth decades of life with CVID are at a 438-fold increased risk of developing lymphoma. In addition to malignancy, patients with CVID are at increased risk of chronic lung disease, autoimmune phenomenon, and chronic diarrhea.

Answer A is incorrect. Patients with CVID are not at increased risk of cardiovascular disease, although they are at greater risk for chronic lung disease (most commonly, bronchiectasis).

Answer C is incorrect. There is not an associated increased risk of miscarriage in patients with CVID.

Answer D is incorrect. There is no association between CVID and renal disease.

Answer E is incorrect. Twenty-five percent of patients with CVID have splenomegaly. However, there is no evidence that patients with CVID are more likely to autoinfarct their spleens.

31. **The correct answer is A.** This patient has hypercalcemia and hypophosphatemia. This is consistent with hyperparathyroidism; however, the parathyroid hormone (PTH) level is low to normal. In addition to parathyroid adenomas, malignancy can cause hypercalcemia by the release of parathyroid hormone–related protein (PTHrP). PTHrP mimics the action of PTH, and causes hypercalcemia by increased bone resorption and increased distal tubular reabsorption of calcium in the kidney. It causes hypophosphatemia by inhibiting proximal tubular reabsorption of phosphate. Malignancy (particularly lung cancer, breast cancer, and multiple myeloma) should be suspected in patients with unexplained hypercalcemia and low or normal PTH. This is especially true in this patient who has a significant smoking history and weight loss.

Answer B is incorrect. MRI of the brain may be used to evaluate patients with suspected central nervous system malignancy. However, brain tumors are less likely to secrete parathyroid hormone–related protein. Lung cancer is a much more common cause of tumor-induced hypercalcemia, especially in a patient who has a significant smoking history.

Answer C is incorrect. A parathyroid ultrasound may be used to localize a parathyroid adenoma in a patient with suspected primary hyperparathyroidism. These patients will also present with hypercalcemia and hypophosphatemia, but they will have **elevated** levels of parathyroid hormone.

Answer D is incorrect. Chronic renal disease can lead to phosphate retention, which binds calcium and leads to a secondary hyper-parathyroidism. Patients would have an elevated creatinine, hyperphosphatemia, and elevated parathyroid hormone. End-stage renal disease would not be expected to show hypercalcemia and hypophosphatemia. Renal tumors rarely produce PTH-related protein. Thus, a renal biopsy would not be helpful in identifying the source of this patient's problem.

Answer E is incorrect. Hypercalcemia with low to normal PTH can be due to vitamin D intoxication as a result of excessive ingestion of vitamin D. The vitamin D metabolites calcidiol and calcitriol should be measured if there is no obvious source of malignancy and neither PTH nor PTH-related protein is elevated. In a patient who is not taking any medication, vitamin D intoxication is less likely. In addition, vitamin D intoxication would cause elevated phosphorus levels.

32. **The correct answer is B.** A fibroadenoma is a benign and slow-growing breast tumor with epithelial and stromal components. It is the most common lesion in women < 30 years old. This patient's presentation of a sharply demarcated, mobile, nontender mass is classic for fibroadenoma. In addition, these lesions often get larger with pregnancy. These tumors are usually removed when they reach 2–4 cm in diameter.

Answer A is incorrect. Carcinoma of the breast is unlikely in this patient. Although the mass is nontender, which is typical of carcinoma, her age and the mass's mobility and location make this diagnosis less likely.

Answer C is incorrect. Although fibrocystic changes are common in premenopausal women, patients normally experience bilateral breast swelling and pain. Also, there is usually fluctuation in symptoms with the menstrual cycle.

Answer D is incorrect. Galactocele is also a dilatation of the duct in which a cyst becomes filled with a viscous milky fluid. However, it usually presents during or shortly after lactation.

Answer E is incorrect. Mammary duct ectasia usually occurs in patients in their 40s, and presents as a new breast mass, with nipple discharge and breast tenderness. These symptoms are caused by blockage and subsequent dilatation of the mammary duct.

33. **The correct answer is D.** Idiopathic (or immune) thrombocytopenic purpura (ITP) is a disorder of primary immune platelet destruction. The clinical presentation is of insidious onset of mucocutaneous bleeding. The diagnosis is one of exclusion; a complete blood cell count usually shows isolated thrombocytopenia, and large platelets may be apparent on peripheral smear. Other tests may include a bone marrow biopsy to exclude aplastic anemia or drug-induced suppression of megakaryocytes. In children, this disease is usually self-limiting and requires no treatment, but adults generally require medical (through immunosuppression or dialysis) or surgical (through splenectomy) management. Children with chronic ITP have platelet counts from 20,000 to 75,000/mm^3 and typically do not require treatment. Pulse or short-course corticosteroids may be used in refractory cases, but long-term daily steroid use should be avoided.

Answer A is incorrect. Corticosteroids are the initial treatment of choice if the disease proves not to be self-limiting. Fifty to seventy-five percent of adults will respond, but less than 20% of those patients will achieve long-term remission.

Answer B is incorrect. Dialysis has been used to treat idiopathic (or immune) thrombocytopenic purpura, but it is not a first-line treatment.

Answer C is incorrect. Intravenous gammaglobulin is the next step for relapse of disease after a course of steroids. It is not used as an initial treatment.

Answer E is incorrect. Platelet transfusion is indicated for active bleeding, particularly if platelet levels fall below 20,000/mm^3.

34. **The correct answer is A.** The presence of intussusception in an adult or older child should raise suspicion for Burkitt's lymphoma. This disease is more common in patients living in Africa, an association believed to be due to the high rate of infection with Epstein-Barr virus.

The African form tends to involve the maxilla and mandible rather than the abdomen. However, the African form of Burkitt's lymphoma can affect the Peyer's patches of the intestine, causing tremendous swelling that leads to foci for intussusception. The 8;14 translocation, which is associated with the *c-myc* oncogene, is commonly found in Burkitt's lymphoma. This disease is a high-grade lymphoma that is very responsive to chemotherapy.

Answer B is incorrect. The median age for presentation of chronic lymphocytic leukemia (CLL) is 60 years. When symptomatic, this condition classically presents with lymphadenopathy, hepatosplenomegaly, and lymphocytosis. Additionally, CLL rarely involves the gastrointestinal mucosa. Therefore, CLL is not the most likely diagnosis.

Answer C is incorrect. Chronic myelogenous leukemia (CML) typically affects patients older than 50 years. CML is a myeloproliferative disorder that is often discovered on routine blood tests where leukocytosis and thrombocytosis are discovered. When symptomatic, fatigue, weight loss, malaise, abdominal discomfort, and bleeding due to platelet dysfunction are common. The t(9;22) translocation creates the Philadelphia chromosome, which is often seen in CML. Because CML is less likely to cause intussusception or to affect a patient in his or her 20s, this answer is not the best answer.

Answer D is incorrect. Ewing's sarcoma may develop in any bone or soft tissue, but is most common in the flat and long bones. This condition is characterized by localized pain and swelling rather than intestinal involvement, so this is not the most likely diagnosis.

Answer E is incorrect. Sézary's syndrome is a term used to describe a systemic form of cutaneous T-cell lymphoma (CTCL), during which Sézary cells are visible in the peripheral blood and the entire skin surface is affected by erythematous lesions. This patient's presentation is not consistent with Sézary's syndrome, the most advanced stage of CTCL. Sézary syndrome usually occurs after the more localized stages (patch, plaque, and tumor) have persisted for several years. Sézary cells are recog-

nizable for their convoluted or cerebriform nuclei and scant cytoplasm.

35. **The correct answer is E.** Amyloid cardiomyopathy is most often caused by deposition of monoclonal light chain fragments in the myocardium forming stiff, β-pleated sheets. Thus, primary amyloidosis is seen in plasma cell dyscrasias such as multiple myeloma, which characteristically causes "punched-out" lytic bone lesions on x-ray. Amyloid cardiomyopathy in the setting of multiple myeloma might also present with hypercalcemia and bone pain.

Answer A is incorrect. Mitral and tricuspid regurgitation are common in amyloid cardiomyopathy and would cause systolic murmurs. However, the presence of the murmur alone, even with the stated findings, does not necessarily suggest amyloid cardiomyopathy.

Answer B is incorrect. Uncommonly, amyloid can cause isolated thickening of the interventricular septum. However, this finding is usually suggestive of hypertrophic cardiomyopathy.

Answer C is incorrect. Although atrial fibrillation is common in advanced cases of amyloid cardiomyopathy, it does not necessarily indicate the diagnosis, especially since this patient's symptoms have been present for only 6 weeks.

Answer D is incorrect. Infiltration of the myocardium by amyloid causes impaired relaxation, which leads to diastolic dysfunction. In turn, diastolic dysfunction leads to a narrowed pulse pressure, mostly as a result of decreased stroke volume.

36. **The correct answer is B.** The patient is experiencing chronic rejection of her graft, a process of gradual decline in renal function. The underlying immune mechanism of chronic rejection is poorly understood but is assumed to be humoral in origin. Unfortunately, chronic rejection is unresponsive to steroids and other immunosuppressives, and it is the single most important cause of late graft failure. Factors implicated in chronic rejection are cadaveric source, past episodes of acute rejection, ischemic injury to the donor kidney,

prolonged warm ischemic time prior to the transplant of the kidney, and poor compliance with drug therapy.

Answer A is incorrect. Any transplant patient is at risk for posttransplant lymphoproliferative disorder (PTLD), which presents with a mass comprised of B lymphocytes that rarely causes a rise in creatinine levels. However, this patient shows no sign of PTLD.

Answer C is incorrect. The patient has no sign of infection (characterized by fever and inflammation but rarely fibrosis or architectural distortion), so further infectious prophylaxis is not indicated.

Answer D is incorrect. Acute rejection would be characterized by a rapid rise in creatinine levels and histologically is characterized by inflammation without fibrosis. Chronic rejection does not respond to high-dose steroids in the way that acute rejection does.

Answer E is incorrect. Chronic rejection is not resolved by increased immunosuppression.

37. **The correct answer is B.** In patients with sickle cell anemia the primary agents of osteomyelitis are *Salmonella paratyphi* and *Staphylococcus aureus*. Osteomyelitis is a common complication of sickle cell disease, as sickle cell crises may stop blood flow to portions of bones, allowing those segments of bone to become foci for infection. Any antibiotic regimen will need to cover both organisms. A third-generation cephalosporin, such as ceftriaxone, is an acceptable choice.

Answer A is incorrect. Calcitonin is a hormone involved in bone metabolism. It can be used for osteoporosis, Paget's disease, and some cancers. The patient's bone lesions are not associated with hormonal abnormalities, but rather with sickle cell osteomyelitis.

Answer C is incorrect. The patient is 3 years old; therefore, while fluoroquinolones are very effective against *Salmonella* osteomyelitis, their use in a child may cause problems with bone development, and should be substituted for less morbid, but still effective, medications.

Answer D is incorrect. Etidronate is a bisphosphonate useful in the treatment of Paget's dis-

ease, osteoporosis, myeloma, and metastatic disease to bone (from breast and prostate), among others. The patient in this question most likely has an infectious process, given the history of sickle cell disease, fever, and leukocytosis with left shift, and will require an antibiotic to cure it.

Answer E is incorrect. Vitamin D is a vitamin with a pivotal role in the prevention of rickets and osteomalacia; however, the diagnosis in this case is more likely to be osteomyelitic lesions.

38. **The correct answer is A.** Acute lymphocytic leukemia is a disease of hyperproliferative immature lymphocytes and occurs mainly in children, with a second peak in persons who are elderly. It is associated with a number of other diseases, including Down's syndrome, Fanconi's anemia, and ataxia-telangiectasia.

Answer B is incorrect. Immunohistochemistry usually shows positive terminal deoxynucleotidyl transferase in 95% of patients with acute lymphocytic leukemia (ALL), but a subset of adults have the Philadelphia chromosome on cytogenetics. These patients are able to be treated with imatinib mesylate (Gleevec), which is effective in decreasing the burden of ALL.

Answer C is incorrect. In children, acute lymphocytic leukemia (ALL) is treated with combination chemotherapy, including daunorubicin, vincristine, prednisone, and L-asparaginase, and survival rates exceed 75%. However, adults who have ALL have a lower survival rate of between 35% and 40%.

Answer D is incorrect. The central nervous system (CNS) is actually a sanctuary site for acute lymphocytic leukemia, and any patient with this disease should have a lumbar puncture to rule out metastasis to the CNS.

Answer E is incorrect. Tumor lysis syndrome is an oncologic emergency commonly seen in patients with acute lymphocytic leukemia, due to the fast turnover of leukemic cells.

39. **The correct answer is B.** The presence of otherwise unexplained hematuria in an individual over 40 denotes bladder cancer until proven

otherwise. The patient also has numerous risk factors that raise suspicion for bladder cancer, such as her smoking history, possible exposure to dyes, and coffee drinking. Cystoscopy is the mainstay of diagnosis and staging of bladder cancer. A cystoscope is inserted into the bladder, and any tumor is then biopsied and resected.

Answer A is incorrect. A CT scan of the pelvis is neither sensitive nor specific in the diagnosis of bladder cancer. However, this is important in staging the cancer after diagnosis has been made.

Answer C is incorrect. Serum creatine kinase level is the most important test in evaluating for rhabdomyolysis, which may lead to myoglobinuria that mimics hematuria. This patient, however, has no indication that she is breaking down muscle tissue (such as muscle pain, aches, or a history of recent trauma).

Answer D is incorrect. Ultrasound may be useful in evaluating the upper tracts for renal parenchymal disease, hydronephrosis, or a soft tissue mass. However, it cannot determine the depth of invasion and is not useful in the diagnosis of bladder cancer.

Answer E is incorrect. Urine culture may help to establish infection as the cause of hematuria; however, the lack of pyuria, fever, and pain makes a urinary tract infection an unlikely cause of gross hematuria.

40. **The correct answer is E.** This patient is presenting with **POEMS** syndrome, a constellation of symptoms associated with osteosclerotic multiple myeloma. Symptoms include **P**olyneuropathy, **O**rganomegaly, **E**ndocrinopathy, **M**ultiple myeloma, and **S**kin changes. Polyneuropathies are generally progressive sensorimotor deficits. Hepatosplenomegaly is generally seen, in contrast to other myeloma patients. Endocrine manifestations include amenorrhea, diabetes mellitus, hypothyroidism, and adrenal insufficiency. Skin changes are diverse, but may include hyperpigmentation, hypertrichosis, thickening, and digital clubbing. Although this patient's symptoms seem unrelated, her peripheral blood smear demonstrates a large number of plasma cells,

as are seen in multiple myeloma. In addition, her laboratory work reveals anemia, hyperuricemia, and hypercalcemia, all consistent with a diagnosis of multiple myeloma. This diagnosis can be confirmed by the presence of an M spike on protein electrophoresis of urine and serum.

Answer A is incorrect. The patient has symptoms of hypothyroidism, and her elevated thyroid-stimulating hormone level supports this diagnosis. However, her other symptoms prompt a multisystem evaluation.

Answer B is incorrect. The dexamethasone suppression test is used to assess the presence of Cushing's syndrome. Although this patient has some of the manifestations of Cushing's, including weight gain and hyperglycemia, her other symptoms and abnormal peripheral blood smear are indicative of another process.

Answer C is incorrect. A hemoglobin A_{1c} level would allow the clinician to assess how long the patient has been hyperglycemic. It would not, however, aid in the diagnosis of multiple myeloma.

Answer D is incorrect. Although the patient's clubbed digits might promote a pulmonary evaluation, pulse oximetry would do nothing to confirm a diagnosis of multiple myeloma.

Answer F is incorrect. A differential of the patient's WBCs might aid in the diagnosis of a malignancy. It would not confirm the diagnosis, however.

41. **The correct answer is B.** Patients with a recent elevation of prostate-specific antigen (PSA) levels and a positive digital rectal examination are at high risk for prostate cancer. The next appropriate step is a biopsy to assess whether cancer is present. Prostate cancer is the most common cancer in men in the United States and the second largest cause of cancer-related death in men. However, most men diagnosed with prostate cancer do not die from the disease and in the early stages most men have no symptoms. Later signs and symptoms can include nocturia, dysuria, hesitancy, sexual dysfunction, or bone pain (if disease is advanced). Once diagnosed, more tests and analyses are performed to determine the stag-

ing and grading of the disease (using the Gleason system which assigns a score of 1–5 for the two most common patterns of tumor found in the biopsy). Treatment can include watchful waiting, surgery, radiation therapy, high-intensity focused ultrasound, chemotherapy, cryosurgery, hormonal therapy, or some combination of these. Ultimately the plan is based on stage of the disease, the Gleason score, the PSA level, the man's age, his general health, and his comfort about potential treatments.

Answer A is incorrect. Although CT scan and bone scan are important components in evaluation of the disease, these tests are ordered after a prostate biopsy confirms that cancer is present.

Answer C is incorrect. Radical prostatectomy is one treatment for prostate cancer. This would be one of the options to consider if a biopsy is positive.

Answer D is incorrect. The patient displays no signs and symptoms of prostatitis, which presents with signs of infection and a painful digital rectal examination. Getting a recheck of the PSA level in 3 months would be inappropriate with this patient, who is highly at risk of prostate cancer.

Answer E is incorrect. An urinalysis may help in distinguishing between urinary tract infection or prostatitis, which may increase PSA levels, and prostate cancer. This patient, however, has both a positive digital rectal examination and increased PSA, and no signs of infection. A urinalysis, therefore, is not needed to rule out infection.

42. **The correct answer is E.** Patients with X-linked severe combined immunodeficiency (X-SCID) and no matched related donor are very good candidates for stem cell gene therapy. The defect in the X-linked interleukin-2 receptor chain gene is known, making this disease a prototype for gene treatment. The first gene therapy in SCID patients was performed in 1991, and involved transduction with a retroviral vector with clinical improvements documented in all patients. Trials have continued and several patients have been successfully treated in this fashion. A significant number, however, have developed a rapidly fatal

leukemia, a transformation thought to result from the gene insertion into patient cells with oncogenic action.

Answer A is incorrect. Graft-versus-host disease is not a risk in gene therapy patients, as they are not undergoing bone marrow transplant.

Answer B is incorrect. Both gene therapy and bone marrow transplant carry a 30–40% risk of failure. Gene therapy is much less studied, but has had similar success rates to bone marrow transplant in the small population in question.

Answer C is incorrect. No difference in susceptibility to illness has been demonstrated.

Answer D is incorrect. Patients treated with gene therapy have been shown to respond well to clinical vaccinations, as have those treated with bone marrow transplant.

43. **The correct answer is D.** Sickle cell anemia is a recessive genetic disease that often presents with painful microocclusive crises due to sickling of RBCs in capillaries. Chronic hemolysis is evident with jaundice and elevated unconjugated bilirubin. Blood smear shows sickle-shaped RBCs and nuclear fragments called Howell-Jolly bodies. Acute treatment is symptomatic pain control, increasing oxygen tension to reduce future sickling (oxygen), and reducing the occlusive crisis through hydration. Long-term treatment includes hydroxyurea. Hydroxyurea stimulates the production of fetal hemoglobin, which will not sickle with low oxygen tension.

Answer A is incorrect. Glucose-6-phosphate dehydrogenase (G6PD) deficiency is a genetic disorder common in individuals of African and Mediterranean descent. Hemolysis is induced by exposure to certain drugs or foods, including sulfa compounds and fava beans, and by infections. These substances have no effect on individuals with sickle cell anemia. In G6PD deficiency, a peripheral smear will show bite cells and Heinz bodies (oxidized hemoglobin).

Answer B is incorrect. Patients with autoimmune hemolytic anemia would have spherocytes on a peripheral blood smear and a positive Coombs test. These patients would benefit from a course of corticosteroids, but this treatment has no role in management of sickle cell disease.

Answer C is incorrect. Allogeneic hematopoietic stem cell transplant is an emerging therapy for patients with severe refractory sickle cell disease.

Answer E is incorrect. Serial transfusion is a treatment for the thalassemia, a family of genetic disorders of the blood found in people of Mediterranean descent. Thalassemia usually presents with anemia and small, pale RBCs on a peripheral smear.

44. **The correct answer is C.** The patient is suffering from a "winged scapula." This is a common source of surgical morbidity and results from damage to the long thoracic nerve (C5–7), which innervates the serratus anterior muscle. The serratus anterior is responsible for lifting the glenoid cavity so the arm can be raised above the shoulder and for keeping the scapula flat against the back of the thoracic cage so other muscles may move the arm. Damage to this nerve causes a "winged scapula."

Answer A is incorrect. The anterior deltoid, innervated by the axillary nerve, is responsible for flexing and medially rotating the arm. Damage to the muscle or its innervation would lead to disability in those functions.

Answer B is incorrect. Conversion disorder is a somatoform disorder characterized by motor or sensory deficits that suggest a neurologic or medical condition but that cannot be reasonably attributed to one. Because there is a more plausible explanation in this case, conversion disorder is unlikely.

Answer D is incorrect. Poland syndrome is the absence of part the pectoralis major and generally does not result in a disability.

Answer E is incorrect. The thoracodorsal nerve innervates the latissimus dorsi muscle. Damage would lead to difficulty adducting, extending, and medially rotating the humerus.

45. **The correct answer is B.** The current recommendations are for patients to receive their first colonoscopy at age 50 years if there is no family history of colorectal cancer. If there is a family history of cancer in a first-degree relative or multiple second-degree relatives, colonoscopy is recommended at 40 years of age, or 10 years before the age when the youngest first-degree relative was diagnosed with colon cancer (whichever is earlier). Repeat colonoscopy should be performed every 10 years. Patient nervousness should be dealt with by educational counseling by the doctor and does not change the recommended screening age.

Answer A is incorrect. Although the patient has a family history of colorectal cancer, it would not be recommended that he have his first colonoscopy until 10 years before his father was diagnosed, or 35 years of age.

Answer C is incorrect. If his father had been 50 years of age or older at the time of his colorectal cancer diagnosis, it would be recommended that the patient in question have his first colonoscopy at 40 years.

Answer D is incorrect. The age of the patient's relative at the time of his diagnosis was 45 years. It is recommended that patients with a family history of colorectal cancer have their first colonoscopy 10 years before the age when the family member was diagnosed.

Answer E is incorrect. If the patient had no family history of colon cancer, 50 years would be the recommended age for his first colonoscopy.

46. **The correct answer is C.** This child has Wilms' tumor. Wilms' tumor usually presents between 2 and 4 years of age with a painless flank mass that does not cross the midline. Some children, such as this one, also present with hypertension and microscopic hematuria. Others can present with fever, weight loss, polyuria, dysuria, bone pain, nausea, and vomiting. The diagnosis is made by abdominal CT. Stage 1 is treated with nephrectomy and chemotherapy. If metastasis is present, radiation therapy is added. This child has no evidence of metastasis.

Answer A is incorrect. Chemotherapy without excision is palliative therapy for advanced, bilateral, unresectable Wilms' tumor.

Answer B is incorrect. Excising the tumor is appropriate therapy for localized neuroblastoma. Neuroblastoma is commonly confused with Wilms' tumor on physical examination because it can present with a painless abdominal mass and hypertension. However, neuroblastoma causes elevated urine catecholamines and does not cause hematuria. Most important, on imaging neuroblastoma does not originate from the kidney.

Answer D is incorrect. Chemotherapy must also be used in treating Wilms' tumor.

Answer E is incorrect. Radiation is used as adjuvant therapy for treatment of more advanced Wilms' tumor but has no role in this patient without evidence of metastasis.

47. **The correct answer is C.** The most likely diagnosis for this patient is Waldenström's macroglobulinemia, a low-grade malignant lymphoma of plasmacytoid lymphocytes that secrete excessive amounts of IgM. Most patients with this disease present with symptoms of hyperviscosity (Raynaud's phenomenon and visual disturbances), and protein-protein interaction (platelet dysfunction). Diagnosis requires the demonstration of an IgM spike on plasma electrophoresis, as well as infiltration of bone marrow with plasmacytoid lymphocytes. Plasmapheresis is used to control hyperviscosity initially because response to chemotherapy can take several weeks. Treatment regimens involve the same chemotherapeutics as those used for multiple myeloma, including alkylating agents and prednisone. Overall mean survival is 5 years.

Answer A is incorrect. Beginning a course of prednisone without a final diagnosis could be deadly to this patient. Beginning low-dose steroids may initially cause her disease to respond, but treatment outside a chemotherapeutic regimen puts her at risk for relapse with refractory, rapidly fatal disease.

Answer B is incorrect. Domestic violence is an important issue of which to be mindful when treating any patient, specifically one with repeated, vague complaints and suspicious lesions. However, this patient's symptoms indicate a disease that requires diagnosis. Her

safety should be assessed by her physician, but domestic violence is unlikely to account for this constellation of symptoms.

Answer D is incorrect. The patient has symptoms that require an active workup and diagnosis. They are unlikely to resolve without treatment, and waiting to diagnose and treat her disease will increase the likelihood of a fatal outcome.

Answer E is incorrect. Although the possibility of autoimmune disease exists, it would be rare following a complete and extensive workup with no abnormalities. Generally, resending tests in anticipation of laboratory error is futile without an indication of abnormality.

48. **The correct answer is B.** Medullary carcinoma accounts for about 5% of all thyroid cancers and is familial in up to 25% of cases. Multiple endocrine neoplasia (MEN) consists of three syndromes featuring tumors of endocrine glands, each with its own characteristic pattern. Specifically, medullary thyroid cancer is associated with MEN type IIA, as well as pheochromocytoma and parathyroid hyperplasia/tumor causing hyperparathyroidism. In MEN type IIA and familial medullary thyroid carcinoma, most patients present in the third decade of life, but screening of family members is important at an early age so patients can inform their children of the condition. Mutations in the *RET* proto-oncogene are responsible for approximately > 90% of cases of MEN type IIA. Papillary and anaplastic carcinomas have not been found to have a genetic risk factor to date.

Answer A is incorrect. Although it is difficult to separate the effects of alcohol from those of tobacco as risk factors in head and neck cancer, neither has been directly linked to thyroid cancer. Alcohol is a risk factor for upper aerodigestive tract cancers, with greatest risk at ingestion rates > 50 g/day.

Answer C is incorrect. Iodine exposure prior to radiation exposure can be preventative for thyroid cancer.

Answer D is incorrect. Radiation to the neck for enlarged tonsils is a risk factor for all types of thyroid cancer. Between 1920 and 1960 radiation was used to treat several benign diseases including enlarged tonsils, enlarged lymph nodes in the neck, enlarged thymus, acne, and scalp ringworm. However, this is not specific to medullary carcinoma of the thyroid.

Answer E is incorrect. Thus far there has been a negative correlation between smoking and thyroid cancer. There has been speculation as to whether or not this may be secondary to the higher incidence of thyroid carcinoma among female patients.

Answer F is incorrect. Chronic viral infections such as herpes, HIV, Epstein-Barr, and human papillomavirus are risk factors for head and neck squamous cell carcinoma. This is likely secondary to suppression of the tumor suppressor gene.

49. **The correct answer is B.** This patient presents with a thrombocytopenic picture and with leukocytosis. Her positive myeloperoxidase test is diagnostic for acute myelogenous leukemia (AML). Complications of this disease include leukostasis leading to hyperviscosity retinopathy, transient ischemic attacks/cerebrovascular accidents, tumor lysis syndrome (while undergoing treatment), gingival hyperplasia, central nervous system involvement, recurrent infection, and disseminated intravascular coagulation (especially with M3 subtype).

Answer A is incorrect. The incidence of AML increases with age. Persons with AML who are > 60 years old have a poor prognosis.

Answer C is incorrect. Environmental risk factors for developing leukemia include radiation, chemotherapy (especially with alkylating agents and topoisomerase inhibitors), benzene exposure, and smoking.

Answer D is incorrect. Cytogenetics and subtype are extremely important in determining prognosis and effectiveness of treatment in AML. Poor prognostic factors include monosomies of chromosomes 5 or 7, deletion of 5q, and complex karyotype.

Answer E is incorrect. Retinoic acid will often help induce remission in the promyelocytic form of acute myelogenous leukemia (M3 subtype).

50. **The correct answer is E.** Von Willebrand's disease is a bleeding disorder in which there is a deficiency in von Willebrand's factor (vWF). vWF stabilizes coagulation factor VIII and allows for normal platelet function to occur. A deficiency in vWF leads to increased degradation of coagulation factor VIII and increased bleeding time. Thrombocytopenia is not usually seen with von Willebrand's disease because the platelet dysfunction is usually qualitative. Deficiency of coagulation factor VIII affects the intrinsic coagulation pathway and therefore leads to a prolonged aPTT. Von Willebrand's disease has no effect on the extrinsic coagulation pathway and therefore a normal PT is expected to be seen.

Answer A is incorrect. This set of values is most consistent with hemophilia B. Deficiency of von Willebrand's factor leads to increased factor VIII degradation and has no effect on factor IX. Von Willebrand's disease is associated with prolonged bleeding time in addition to factor VIII deficiency and prolonged aPTT. The PT would not be prolonged in von Willebrand's disease because the extrinsic coagulation pathway remains intact.

Answer B is incorrect. This set of values is most consistent with disseminated intravascular coagulation. Deficiency of von Willebrand's factor leads to increased factor VIII degradation and has no effect on factor IX. In addition, von Willebrand's disease is associated with a prolonged bleeding time and prolonged aPTT.

Answer C is incorrect. This set of values is most consistent with hemophilia A. Von Willebrand's disease is associated with a prolonged bleeding time in the context of a normal platelet count along with factor VIII deficiency and prolonged aPTT.

Answer D is incorrect. This set of values is most consistent with thrombocytopenia. A deficiency in von Willebrand's factor leads to increased degradation of coagulation factor VIII with an increased aPTT. Although bleeding time is increased in von Willebrand's disease due to decreased platelet function, thrombocytopenia is not necessarily a finding of von Willebrand's disease.

51. **The correct answer is A.** This patient has hemophilia. This diagnosis is based on a history of mucosal bleeding and hemarthrosis along with a family history of a bleeding disorder that is consistent with an X-linked recessive inheritance pattern (the patient's mother is a carrier of the disease). Patients with hemophilia do not present with ecchymoses or petechiae as may be seen in other bleeding disorders such as von Willebrand's disease. Hemophilia presents with an increased activated partial thromboplastin time because of deficiencies in components of the intrinsic pathway. The prothrombin time is normal in these patients because their extrinsic coagulation pathway remains intact. Finally, bleeding time is normal in these patients because neither their platelet concentration nor function is altered.

Answer B is incorrect. Patients with hemophilia do not typically present with low platelet concentrations. One would expect that a patient with a decreased platelet concentration may have prolonged bleeding time and may have spontaneous bleeding. Low platelet concentration would not explain a prolonged activated partial thromboplastin time, as seen in this patient.

Answer C is incorrect. Leukopenia, or a decreased WBC count, is not a finding associated with hemophilia. This may be seen with immunodeficiencies.

Answer D is incorrect. Factor V Leiden is a disorder in which coagulation factor V is resistant to degradation by activated protein C. Increased factor V concentrations are not associated with hemophilia, but rather with an increased tendency to clot, leading to strokes, pulmonary embolism, and frequent miscarriages.

Answer E is incorrect. Hemophilia is not associated with increased hemoglobin. The deficiency that leads to hemophilia involves coagulation factors (either VIII or IX).

52. **The correct answer is C.** Heparin-induced thrombocytopenia (HIT) is a well-established adverse effect of treatment and may occur in as many as 20% of patients receiving heparin therapy. Thrombocytopenia most commonly occurs after 4–10 days of treatment. The more severe form of HIT, or type II HIT, is caused by antibodies against the heparin–platelet factor 4 complex. Patients on chronic warfarin therapy (e.g., those with a history of cardiac disease and multiple strokes) are transitioned to the shorter-acting heparin prior to major surgery, thus explaining the time course of this patient's reaction.

Answer A is incorrect. Aspirin is a nonsteroidal anti-inflammatory drug that also inhibits platelet activation, although it does not cause thrombocytopenia. Aspirin may cause bleeding, gastrointestinal ulcer, or dyspepsia. Aspirin is commonly used as an antiplatelet agent in patients at risk for stroke or myocardial infarction and for pain and inflammatory relief in arthritis.

Answer B is incorrect. Although clopidogrel does interfere with platelet activation, it does not cause thrombocytopenia. The main adverse effects of clopidogrel are mild bleeding, rash, and dyspepsia. Clopidogrel is commonly used as an antiplatelet agent in patients at risk for stroke or myocardial infarction.

Answer D is incorrect. Streptokinase is a thrombolytic agent that is not associated with thrombocytopenia. The main adverse effects of streptokinase are hypotension, shivering, and occasional fever. There is no apparent indication for streptokinase in this patient, although thrombolytic agents may be used in the acute setting for the treatment of acute stroke, myocardial infarction, pulmonary embolism, or deep vein thrombosis in selected patients.

Answer E is incorrect. Warfarin is a common anticoagulant used, for example, in patients with deep venous thromboses, history of atrial fibrillation, or artificial heart valves. It does not cause thrombocytopenia. Its major adverse hematologic effect is hemorrhage; other major adverse effects include hypersensitivity reaction and skin necrosis.

53. **The correct answer is A.** This patient is symptomatic, a smoker, and has a right lobe mass and mediastinal lymph node involvement that require immediate evaluation. Nodes that are smaller than 2 cm in diameter are typically be-

nign nodes, whereas nodes > 2 cm are more likely to be malignant. The status of his nodes would provide critical information necessary for this patient's management. Therefore, the next appropriate step would be to evaluate the nodes by mediastinoscopy. If the nodes are benign, the patient would be a good candidate for surgical resection. However, if the nodes are malignant, other modalities of treatment would be indicated.

Answer B is incorrect. Pulmonary function tests are used to evaluate the risk of perioperative complications following lung resection. Patients considered for lung surgery undergo spirometry in order to provide important information regarding the management of the patient. Preoperative testing would not be a priority until a staging procedure has established the patient's candidacy for surgery.

Answer C is incorrect. Thoracentesis is used to evaluate pleural effusions. This procedure would not be used in this case.

Answer D is incorrect. Ventilation-perfusion (V/Q) lung scans are used to detect pulmonary emboli, evaluate lung function for advanced cases of chronic obstructive pulmonary disease, and detect the presence of shunts in pulmonary blood vessels. V/Q scans would not be used to evaluate mediastinal lymph nodes.

Answer E is incorrect. For solitary pulmonary nodules with intermediate probability of malignancy, video-assisted thoracoscopic surgery offers a more aggressive approach to diagnosis. In this case, a bronchoscopy has already been performed and indicated malignancy.

54. **The correct answer is B.** Li-Fraumeni syndrome is a syndrome characterized by a mutation in one copy of the *p53* tumor suppressor gene. It is inherited in an autosomal dominant fashion, and predisposes patients to sarcomas, central nervous system tumors, and carcinomas. Patients are at a 100-fold risk of acquiring treatment-related acute myelogenous leukemias (t-AML) following treatment with cytotoxic drugs. t-AML is universally refractory to known therapies.

Answer A is incorrect. Ataxia-telangiectasia is an autosomal recessive disorder that is charac-

terized by progressive ataxia, telangiectasias of the conjunctiva and ears, and predisposition to malignancy.

Answer C is incorrect. Von Hippel-Lindau syndrome is an autosomal dominant disease characterized by hemangioblastomas of the retina and central nervous system. Bilateral renal cysts are also common. It is caused by a mutation in the tumor suppressor gene *VHL*, located on chromosome 3p25, the same gene that is mutated in sporadic renal cell carcinoma. Forty to seventy percent of patients develop renal cell carcinoma at some point.

Answer D is incorrect. Wiskott-Aldrich syndrome is an X-linked disorder of T lymphocytes that presents as immune deficiency. Patients have an increased risk of leukemia and/or lymphoma.

Answer E is incorrect. Xeroderma pigmentosum is an autosomal recessive disorder that results from a defect in DNA repair mechanisms. Patients are at very high risk for basal and squamous cell carcinomas, as well as melanoma.

55. **The correct answer is E.** Thrombotic thrombocytopenic purpura is a disorder of increased platelet aggregation leading to mucocutaneous bleeding (petechiae or purpura) and hemolysis. Most cases are idiopathic, but the condition is associated with certain medications such as cyclosporine and clopidogrel, oral contraceptive use, HIV infection, and autoimmune disease. The classic pentad is thrombocytopenia, microangiopathic hemolytic anemia, mental status changes, fever, and renal failure, although the last three may not be present. Diagnosis is confirmed with unexplained thrombocytopenia and microangiopathic hemolysis; peripheral smear shows schistocytes.

Answer A is incorrect. Disseminated intravascular coagulation can also present with thrombocytopenia and hemolysis due to massive thrombosis, and peripheral smears may also show schistocytes. Coagulation studies, however, should show an elevated prothrombin time, and the fibrinogen level should be low.

Answer B is incorrect. HELLP syndrome is a constellation of findings, including Hemolysis, Elevated Liver enzymes, and Low Platelets. It is a variant of preeclampsia that occurs during pregnancy.

Answer C is incorrect. Henoch-Schönlein purpura is the most common systemic vasculitis in children and is caused by immune complex deposition in vessel walls. The clinical presentation includes palpable purpura beginning on the extensor surfaces and buttocks, polyarthralgia of the lower extremity joints, colicky abdominal pain, and nephritis. Platelet count is normal, whereas serum IgA levels are usually increased.

Answer D is incorrect. Idiopathic thrombocytopenic purpura also presents with a petechial rash and thrombocytopenia. It is more common in children than thrombotic thrombocytopenic purpura, but it does not present with fever or splenomegaly.

56. **The correct answer is C.** This patient has diabetes with proteinuria and likely has nephrotic syndrome. Among the many sequelae of nephrotic syndrome is hypercoagulability secondary to the loss of antithrombotic proteins in the urine (protein C, S, and antithrombin). These patients are at increased risk for arterial and venous thrombotic complications, including myocardial infarction, pulmonary embolism, deep vein thrombosis, and, as is the case with this patient, unilateral renal vein thrombosis (RVT). Classically, patients with RVT present with flank pain (secondary to distention of the renal capsule), hematuria, and evidence of renal impairment. Timely diagnosis via renal ultrasound, CT, or direct venography, as well as treatment with heparin, is crucial. The disruption of renal blood flow can lead to permanent damage.

Answer A is incorrect. Analgesics and angiotensin-converting enzyme (ACE) inhibitors would do little to address the underlying pathology in this patient. Moreover, ACE inhibition may worsen this patient's renal failure by decreasing the contralateral kidney's hyperfiltration.

Answer B is incorrect. These modalities are important tools for the diagnosis and treatment of nephrotic syndrome. High-dose corticosteroids are used to treat minimal change disease, among other causes of nephrotic syndrome, but they will do little to address this patient's acute complication.

Answer D is incorrect. Spiral CT is useful in diagnosing renal calculi, and administration of a thiazide diuretic is helpful in treating chronic stone formation by decreasing hypercalciuria. This patient does not have findings that are consistent with nephrolithiasis; thus, these treatments would not be helpful.

Answer E is incorrect. Urine culture and antibiotics are appropriate diagnostic and treatment modalities to address acute pyelonephritis. This patient is afebrile, lacks costovertebral angle tenderness, and does not have dysuria or pyuria.

57. **The correct answer is A.** Any description of a changing mole is concerning for occurrence of melanoma. The **ABCDE** mnemonic is often used to remember the key changes that indicate development of malignancy (**A**symmetry, irregular **B**orders, **C**olor changes or irregularity, **D**iameter increasing, and **E**volution or changing of the mole). Several features of this mole are particularly concerning, including the size (> 6 mm) and presence of itching. The treatment of choice is excisional biopsy, with margins determined by apparent depth of the lesion.

Answer B is incorrect. Identification of the sentinel lymph node with excisional biopsy is indicated in patients with clinical evidence of lymph node involvement or with deep lesions.

Answer C is incorrect. Radiation therapy is not an accepted treatment modality for malignant melanoma. Furthermore, biopsy and pathologic diagnosis of the lesion should be obtained prior to the initiation of therapy.

Answer D is incorrect. Because this lesion is concerning for malignant transformation, symptomatic treatment alone is not appropriate.

Answer E is incorrect. While dysplastic nevi may be irregular in shape and color, the enlarging size and patient's complaint of itching are concerning for malignancy and should be further evaluated immediately.

58. The correct answer is B. This profile is consistent with hemophilia B. Hemophilia B (Christmas disease) is an X-linked recessive coagulopathy involving a deficiency of coagulation factor IX that may lead to mild to severe bleeding, depending on the factor activity. A prolonged activated partial thromboplastin time is seen with hemophilia. Prothrombin time, bleeding time, and platelet count are expected to be normal in a patient with hemophilia.

Answer A is incorrect. This is a normal profile and is not consistent with the diagnosis of hemophilia.

Answer C is incorrect. This profile is consistent with hemophilia A. Hemophilia A is an X-linked recessive coagulopathy involving a deficiency in coagulation factor VIII that may lead to mild to severe bleeding, depending on the factor activity. A prolonged activated partial thromboplastin time is seen with hemophilia. Prothrombin time, bleeding time, and platelet count are expected to be normal in a patient with hemophilia.

Answer D is incorrect. This profile is consistent with thrombocytopenia, as seen with disorders such as idiopathic thrombocytopenic purpura or heparin-induced thrombocytopenia.

Answer E is incorrect. This profile is consistent with von Willebrand's disease (vWD). vWD is a genetic defect in von Willebrand factor, which both mediates platelet binding to damaged endothelium and binds/stabilizes factor VIII. Patients with vWD typically present with a prolonged bleeding time, a prolonged activated partial thromboplastin time, and a factor VIII deficiency.

59. The correct answer is B. Although acute promyelocytic leukemia (APL) is generally responsive to the chemotherapeutics used to treat acute myelogenous leukemia, cytarabine and daunorubicin, approximately 10% of APL patients treated on this regimen die from disseminated intravascular coagulation. This phenomenon occurs when dying leukemic promyelocytes release their granule components. Modern protocols use tretinoin, an oral drug that promotes maturation of leukemic cells bearing the t(15;17) abnormality, the best known genetic marker for APL. Tretinoin is often used in combination with anthracycline chemotherapy, with a period during which tretinoin is used alone.

Answer A is incorrect. Few data are available on the effects of tretinoin on long-term fertility; however, as it is a derivative of retinoic acid, it is a major teratogen and could be devastating to a fetus during maternal treatment. Women of childbearing age being treated with tretinoin are strongly urged to avoid pregnancy for this reason.

Answer C is incorrect. Acute promyelocytic leukemia is a subtype of acute myelogenous leukemia (AML), and is generally responsive to the chemotherapeutics used to treat AML (cytarabine and daunorubicin). Older protocols did involve the use of these medications; however, the emergence of tretinoin as a treatment option has allowed a decrease in the risk of chemotherapy-associated disseminated intravascular coagulation.

Answer D is incorrect. No physician should recommend homeopathic agents as first-line therapy for a potentially treatable cancer. Tretinoin is an FDA-approved agent that has been tested in multiple clinical trials for safety and efficacy.

Answer E is incorrect. In fact, clinical trials have shown that tretinoin is not sufficient as a single agent to treat acute promyelocytic leukemia (APL). For this reason current protocols involve the use of tretinoin in combination with intravenous anthracycline chemotherapy (daunorubicin or doxorubicin). Although the understanding of the sensitivity of cells with t(15;17) to tretinoin has allowed major treatment advances and increased the therapeutic:toxicity ratio in APL, tretinoin has not proven to produce durable remission when used alone.

60. The correct answer is E. This patient is likely experiencing an episode of acute rejection. This is an immunologic response to foreign antigens in the graft that leads to bronchiolar lymphocytic inflammation. Acute rejection is experienced by at least 50% of lung transplant patients within the first year posttransplant, and is characterized by cough, low-grade fever, dyspnea, hypoxia, and interstitial infiltrates and edema. It can be treated effectively with high-dose steroids and increased immunosuppression. However, the symptoms may mimic those of infections such as cytomegalovirus, so the diagnosis should be confirmed by biopsy.

Answer A is incorrect. Antimicrobial therapy in immunosuppressed patients should be specific whenever possible. A "shotgun" approach may promote resistance in this at-risk population. Because acute rejection is more statistically likely than infection in this patient, confirmation by biopsy is warranted before antimicrobial therapy is initiated. Therefore, immediate expectant therapy with empiric antimicrobial therapy is not warranted until an infectious cause is found.

Answer B is incorrect. Treatment with high-dose steroids is indicated once rejection is confirmed. However, because the symptoms of acute rejection may overlap with those of infection, initiating steroid therapy without biopsy confirmation of rejection and the absence of infection is dangerous.

Answer C is incorrect. Although pulmonary function tests are important maintenance tests that should be performed periodically on transplant patients, they are more useful in assessing chronic rejection than acute rejection.

Answer D is incorrect. If the patient has an infection, reduction of the immunosuppressive regimen might be warranted; however, reducing immunosuppression in the case of acute rejection would be extremely dangerous and might lead to irreversible graft rejection.

CHAPTER 8

Infectious Disease

QUESTIONS

1. An 18-month-old baby girl presents to the emergency department (ED) with a fever. She was the product of a normal pregnancy. Her parents state that the patient has had a cough and rhinorrhea for the past 24 hours. She also has a decreased appetite and has been fussy. She had been afebrile until this morning, when she appeared flushed and uncomfortable and had a temperature of 40°C (104°F). In the ED, the patient begins to have generalized tonic-clonic movements of her face, neck, and extremities for 1 minute. She is conscious but drowsy immediately after the seizure. Her temperature is 40.5°C (104.9°F), respiratory rate is 24/min, pulse is 120/min, and blood pressure is 100/54 mm Hg. Her pupils are round and equally reactive to light. Her mucous membranes are moist, and her pharynx is mildly erythematous. She is able to move her extremities spontaneously and has normal tone throughout. Kernig's and Brudzinski's signs are absent. The patient has no prior history of seizures. Which of the following is the most appropriate next step in management?

(A) Acetaminophen
(B) Electroencephalogram
(C) Lumbar puncture
(D) Phenobarbital
(E) Valproic acid

2. A 36-year-old man comes to his primary care physician with a rapidly expanding rash under his right arm. The rash is round with central clearing. Upon questioning, the man admits that he has been feeling somewhat lethargic and "achy" lately, but had attributed this to fatigue after a recent hike in the Shenandoah Valley in Virginia. What is the most likely diagnosis?

(A) Lyme disease
(B) Meningitis
(C) Myocarditis
(D) Rocky Mountain spotted fever
(E) *Staphylococcus aureus* infection

3. A 33-year-old man who has AIDS is brought to the ED after he collapses outside his apart-ment. The patient is found to have *Pneumocystis jiroveci* pneumonia and his current CD4+ count is < 170/mm^3. The patient is intubated and intravenous fluids are started. The patient's brother arrives and states that the patient has expressed wishes to withhold treatment at this stage of his disease. According to the brother, the patient had created an advance directive during his last hospitalization. The patient has not taken his medication regimen for the past month. Assuming the patient remains unconscious, which of the following would compel the physician to withhold medical treatment?

(A) An acquaintance to whom the patient granted power of attorney for the duration of his previous hospital stay requests that interventions be withheld
(B) A signed advance directive stating that the patient wishes to refuse all treatment
(C) A statement by the patient's brother indicating that the patient wishes to refuse treatment
(D) A statement by the patient's primary care physician indicating that the patient wishes to refuse treatment
(E) Initial paperwork for an advance directive in conjunction with the brother's statement
(F) The brother's statements alone are sufficient to withhold new interventions, but ventilation and fluid treatment should continue

4. A 28-year-old white woman with HIV comes to the ED with a headache, mild fevers, and night sweats. The headache developed slowly but became more noticeable 2 weeks ago. Occasionally, she feels mild pain in her neck as well. Results of lumbar puncture and India ink stain are shown in the image. She is taking trimethoprim-sulfamethoxazole. Her CD4+ count is 51/mm^3. Her vital signs are: temperature 38°C (100°F), pulse 74/min, respiratory rate 24/min, and blood pressure 130/80 mm Hg. Which of the following is the most likely diagnosis?

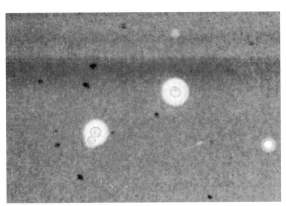

Reproduced, with permission, from Brooks GF, Carroll KC, Butel JS, Morse SA. *Jawetz, Melnick, & Adelberg's Medical Microbiology*, 24th ed. New York: McGraw-Hill, 2007: Figure 45-21.

(A) Cryptococcal meningitis
(B) HIV encephalopathy
(C) Migraine
(D) *Neisseria meningitidis* infection
(E) Toxoplasmosis

5. An 18-year-old girl presents to her obstetrician/gynecologist with dysuria and frequency. Urine culture demonstrates *Escherichia coli*, and the patient is placed on a 3-day course of ciprofloxacin. Which of the following adverse reactions occurs most commonly with this class of medication?

(A) Allergic reactions and rashes
(B) Gastrointestinal upset with anorexia, nausea, and vomiting
(C) Mild headache and dizziness
(D) QT prolongation of ECG
(E) Tendonitis and tendon rupture

6. A 45-year-old white woman with type 2 diabetes mellitus originally admitted for a pulmonary embolism develops a cough and fever while in the hospital. She was admitted 4 days ago and had started warfarin the day prior to the onset of her cough and fever. On day two of admission she was advanced to a normal diet and maintenance intravenous fluids were discontinued. The nurses say she has been eating and drinking normally. On examination she is febrile, her neck veins are flat, her skin is warm to the touch, and her blood pressure is 80/40 mm Hg. Urine output was 20 mL/hr for the last 3 hours. A CT is ordered and shows a right lower lobe pneumonia. Laboratory work also shows a blood urea nitrogen (BUN) of 35 mg/dL and creatinine of 4.3 mg/dL. Her BUN and creatinine the day before had been 23 mg/dL and 1.5 mg/dL, respectively. WBC count is 25,000/mm³ and blood cultures grow *Pseudomonas aeruginosa*. There is tenderness upon palpation of the costovertebral angle region. Which of the following mechanisms would most likely account for the worsening kidney function?

(A) Contrast administration during the course of her treatment in the hospital
(B) Diabetic kidney failure secondary to angiotensin II–induced vasoconstriction
(C) Hematogenous spread of the pulmonary infection to the kidney leading to pyelonephritis
(D) Insufficient intravascular volume secondary to discontinuation of maintenance intravenous fluids
(E) Respiratory acidosis secondary to pulmonary infection

7. A 2-week-old infant is brought to the ED with fever, increased irritability, anorexia, and decreased responsiveness. The infant did not improve after administration of the appropriate dose of infant acetaminophen. When the infant is examined, he is centrally pink, lethargic, and has shallow respirations. The fontanelle is soft and flat, and heart sounds, breath sounds, and abdominal examination are all normal. Capillary refill is adequate. Neurologic examination shows decreased tone and a weak, intermittent cry. While the physician examines the child, the mother tells him that she delivered the baby at home with a midwife and did not receive prenatal care. A lumbar puncture performed in the ED reveals a pleocytosis with a neutrophil predominance, and a low glucose and high protein content. Which of the following is the most common cause of the infant's symptoms?

(A) Group B *Streptococcus*
(B) Influenza
(C) Overdose of acetaminophen
(D) Varicella-zoster virus
(E) Viridans streptococcus

8. A 3-month-old girl presents to her general pediatrician's office with a rash. She is the product of a normal uncomplicated pregnancy, and was born at 40 weeks' gestation. Her mother reports that she was well until this morning, when she suddenly developed a fever to 41°C (105.8°F) with no other symptoms. In the pediatrician's office, the patient begins to seize and is rushed to a nearby hospital. She is hospitalized and continues to have seizures whenever her temperature spikes above 40°C (104°F). After 3 days, her fever breaks and she develops a maculopapular rash on her trunk that then spreads to her face and extremities. Which of the following is the most likely pathogen?

(A) Human herpesvirus-6
(B) Measles virus
(C) Parvovirus B19
(D) Rubella virus
(E) Varicella-zoster virus

9. A 4-month-old infant born at 32 weeks' gestation is taken to her pediatrician's office for evaluation of a respiratory illness. The patient's mother says her daughter developed a low-grade fever (38.5°C [101°F]) with sneezing and clear rhinorrhea 3 days prior to this visit, after her 5-year-old brother had a similar illness. Now her symptoms include wheezing, cough, and irritability. The infant is hemodynamically stable but tachypneic with a respiratory rate of 68/min. Head, ears, eyes, nose, and throat examination is notable for clear rhinorrhea with nasal flaring, but her tympanic membranes are nonerythematous and nonbulging bilaterally. Lung auscultation demonstrates wheezing bilaterally, with prolongation of the expiratory phase. What is the next step that should be taken in managing this patient?

(A) Antibiotic administration and release to home
(B) Hospitalization with supportive care
(C) Palivizumab administration and release to home
(D) Respiratory syncytial virus intravenous immunoglobin administration and release to home
(E) X-ray of the chest and WBC count with differential

10. A 34-year-old African-American diabetic man is brought to the ED after collapsing on the bus on his way home from work. His blood sugar was 20 mg/dL on admission. After resuscitative measures, his blood sugar is 90 mg/dL; he is awake, alert, oriented, and appears stable. His insulin dosage had recently been adjusted, and physical examination reveals white patches in his mouth. A contrast-enhanced CT study done in the ED is normal. Which of the following is the most appropriate step to manage his condition and prevent morbidity?

(A) Administer amphotericin B
(B) Administer glucose
(C) Administer mannitol
(D) Do nothing; this represents normal oral flora
(E) Manage blood sugars and insulin medication

11. A concerned father takes his 6-year-old son to the pediatrician's office after he notices a target-shaped rash on his son's back several days after returning home from a camping trip. In addition to the rash, the boy has had a low-grade fever (temperature 38.3°C [100.9°F]) for the past 3 days, recurrent headaches, and generalized malaise. While talking with the pediatrician, the father recalls he noticed a black bump where his son's rash began, which he scraped off at the time. Suspicious of Lyme disease, the pediatrician prescribes a course of amoxicillin. The boy's father questions why the pediatrician did not prescribe doxycycline, which he was treated with when he had Lyme disease 2 years earlier. What potential adverse effect of doxycycline is the pediatrician avoiding by prescribing amoxicillin for this patient?

(A) Cartilage damage
(B) Ototoxicity
(C) Red man syndrome
(D) Renal toxicity
(E) Tooth discoloration

12. An 8-year-old boy is brought to the ED with a fever, myalgias, and a rash (see image) involving his trunk, limb, and extremities. His mother states that the patient had a temperature of 39.4°C (103°F) on the morning of his presentation. His temperature in the ED is

38.9°C (102°F). His mother states that the trunk was the last place to be involved by the rash. The patient states that about a week ago he found a stray dog and returned it to its owner after he saved the dog from many "vampire ticks." Which of the following is the most likely diagnosis?

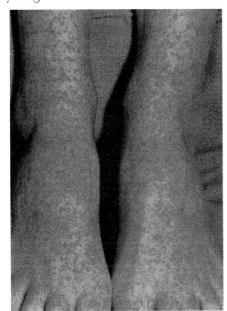

Reproduced, with permission, from Wolff K, Johnson RA, Surmond D. *Fitzpatrick's Color Atlas & Synopsis of Clinical Dermatology*, 5th ed. New York: McGraw-Hill, 2005: 759.

(A) Ehrlichiosis
(B) Lyme disease
(C) Rocky Mountain spotted fever
(D) Tick-borne encephalitis
(E) Tularemia

13. A 3-year-old girl complaining of fever is brought to the ED by her parents. The girl has had a tactile fever for the last 24 hours and is now complaining of a painful mouth. She has no significant past medical history, and her social, family, and travel histories are noncontributory. Her parents deny that she has been coughing or has had any upper respiratory infection symptoms. Her heart rate is 89/min, blood pressure is 96/58 mm Hg, respiratory rate is 22/min, and temperature is 38.2°C

(100.8°F). On physical examination, her oropharynx is inflamed, with multiple vesicles scattered throughout her tongue, buccal mucosa, posterior pharynx, palate, and lips. Additionally, she has maculopapular and vesicular lesions on both of her hands, her buttocks, and her groin. What viral agent is most likely responsible for this clinical presentation?

(A) Coxsackie A
(B) Human herpesvirus-6
(C) Paramyxovirus
(D) Parvovirus B19
(E) Varicella-zoster virus

14. A 49-year-old man seeks evaluation of a recent skin infection. He is otherwise healthy and has never had a similar episode. He has a noncontributory social and family history. During the interview, he mentions he really enjoys working out at the community gym each day. On physical examination he has no symptoms other than a localized infection that is pruritic and mildly malodorous (see image). A potassium hydroxide preparation of scrapings from the lesion confirms the diagnosis. Which of the following is the most likely diagnosis?

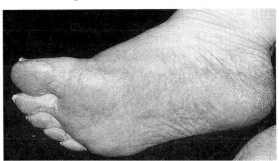

Reproduced, with permission, from Wolff K, Johnson RA, Surmond D. *Fitzpatrick's Color Atlas & Synopsis of Clinical Dermatology*, 5th ed. New York: McGraw-Hill, 2005: 695.

(A) Contact dermatitis
(B) Hand-foot-and-mouth disease
(C) Scabies
(D) Stevens-Johnson syndrome
(E) Tinea pedis

15. A 10-month-old baby girl is brought to her pediatrician's office because she has been febrile and irritable. She is the product of a normal pregnancy. She has been healthy since birth. Yesterday, her parents noticed that she was fussy, less active, and did not eat as much as usual. Overnight she developed a temperature of 38.5°C (101.3°F) and was awake crying for most of the night. Her parents report that she has also been tugging on her left ear. Her temperature is 39°C (102.2°F), respiratory rate 24/min, and pulse 140/min. She is not toxic appearing but continues to be irritable. Her pupils are equally reactive to light bilaterally. She has moist mucous membranes, and her pharynx is nonerythematous. The left tympanic membrane is bulging, erythematous, and immobile on pneumatic otoscopy. The right tympanic membrane is mobile and non-erythematous. She does not have a rash or a history of ear infections. Her immunizations are up to date. What is the most appropriate next step in management of this infant?

(A) Observe the patient
(B) Refer the patient to a surgeon for myringotomy and placement of tympanostomy tubes
(C) Refer the patient to the ED of a tertiary care facility
(D) Start amoxicillin at 80 to 90 mg/kg/d for 10 days
(E) Start amoxicillin-clavulanate at 90 mg/kg/d of amoxicillin and 6.4 mg/kg/d of clavulanate for 10 days
(F) Start erythromycin and sulfisoxazole at 50 to 150 mg/kg/d for 10 days

16. A 2-day-old baby girl, the product of a 34-week gestation, develops a fever of 39°C (102.2°F), poor feeding, and a maculopapular rash on her extremities. Her mother did not receive prenatal care but had no complications or abnormal findings on delivery. Cerebrospinal fluid analysis reveals 28 WBCs/mm^3, a glucose of 17 mg/dL, and a protein of 170 mg/dL. Gram stain is positive. Which of the following is the most likely organism?

(A) Group B *Streptococcus*
(B) *Haemophilus influenzae*
(C) Herpes simplex virus

(D) *Mycobacterium tuberculosis*
(E) *Neisseria meningitidis*
(F) *Streptococcus pneumoniae*

17. A 23-year-old patient with a past medical history of type 1 diabetes and recent outpatient treatment for pelvic inflammatory disease with oral antibiotics returns to the emergency department with a chief complaint of fevers and lower abdominal pain for 1 day. Her temperature is 39.6°C (103.3°F), pulse is 125/min, blood pressure is 88/48 mm Hg, and respiratory rate is 18/min. She confirms that she took her entire course of oral antibiotic therapy and has regularly been taking her insulin. On examination her skin is warm to the touch and her abdomen is rigid and diffusely tender to light palpation. Laboratory tests show:

Hemoglobin	13.4 g/dL
WBC count	24,000/mm^3
Platelet count	247,000/mm^3
Plasma glucose	224 mg/dL

Urinalysis results are negative for β-human chorionic gonadotropin. What is the most likely underlying cause of her symptoms?

(A) Acute cholecystitis
(B) Diabetic ketoacidosis
(C) Gonorrheal cervicitis after reinfection by an untreated sexual partner
(D) Ruptured ectopic pregnancy
(E) Ruptured tubo-ovarian abscess

18. A 27-year-old woman presents to her primary care physician with a complaint of several days of dysuria, vaginal pruritus, and increased vaginal discharge. She has never experienced similar symptoms. A pregnancy test is negative. She is currently sexually active with only one male partner and uses barrier contraception. Gynecologic examination reveals a thick white discharge. The patient has a vaginal pH of 4, and a 10% potassium hydroxide preparation reveals branching hyphae with budding yeast. Which of the following oral medication is the most appropriate treatment?

(A) Azithromycin
(B) Ciprofloxacin
(C) Clindamycin
(D) Fluconazole
(E) Metronidazole

19. A former full-term, 4-year-old boy presents to his pediatrician's office. He has had a cough and clear nasal discharge for the past 2–3 days, with fevers ranging from 38°C to 40°C (100.4–104°F) over the past 48 hours. On examination, he is febrile and appears tired but responsive. He has small red spots with grey centers on his buccal mucosa, as well as an erythematous, blanching, maculopapular rash on his face that appeared within the past hour. His examination is otherwise unremarkable. The patient and his 6-month-old sister have not received any immunizations since birth because, after his mother had an adverse reaction to the influenza vaccine, the parents consider immunizations to be more harmful than helpful. Which of the following immunizations should be administered to the 6-month-old sister as soon as possible?

(A) Diphtheria-tetanus-pertussis vaccine
(B) *Haemophilus influenzae* type b vaccine
(C) Influenza vaccine
(D) Measles-mumps-rubella vaccine
(E) Varicella vaccine

20. A 30-year-old man begins an antibiotic regimen that includes isoniazid for treatment of pulmonary tuberculosis. One month after initiation of therapy, the man visits his primary care physician with complaints of fatigue, anorexia, and nausea. The following laboratory values are obtained:

WBC count	8000/mm^3
Hemoglobin	15.2 g/dL
Hematocrit	49.7%
Aspartate aminotransferase	240 U/L
Alanine aminotransferase	285 U/L
Alkaline phosphatase	405 U/L

Which of the following places this patient at increased risk for developing this complication of isoniazid therapy?

(A) Active injection drug use
(B) Age < 35 years
(C) First-time treatment with isoniazid
(D) Male gender
(E) White race

21. A 55-year-old man with Hodgkin's lymphoma on CHOP (cyclophosphamide, hydroxydaunomycin [doxorubicin], vincristine [Oncovin], and prednisone) chemotherapy is brought to the ED with a history of worsening headaches for 5 weeks; blurred vision, double vision and persistent hearing loss for 3 days; and mild confusion on the morning of admission. His brother, who brought him in, said the patient also had difficulty walking earlier that morning. On admission he has a fever of 38.3°C (101°F). The physician is worried about an intracranial infection. Which of the following is the most appropriate initial step in diagnosis?

(A) Administer tissue plasminogen activator
(B) Central nervous system imaging
(C) Urgent lumbar puncture and culture
(D) Urgent lumbar puncture and India ink stain
(E) Urgent lumbar puncture and serology

22. A 36-year-old woman brings her 2-month-old child for a pediatric checkup. The baby has been developing normally. The woman has a 29-year-old brother with autism. She is very concerned that her baby will develop this condition as well. She has read many alarming reports that vaccinations have been linked to higher incidence of autism in the United States and refuses to put her child at risk. What is the next most appropriate action?

(A) Ask the mother to step out of the room to speak further about the issue and have the nurse administer the vaccine to the child while no one else is in the room
(B) Contact the baby's father to ask him to convince his wife that immunizations are necessary
(C) Educate the mother about the benefits of vaccines and the lack of evidence linking autism and vaccinations, but leave the decision to her
(D) Obtain a court order to administer the vaccine
(E) Report the mother for child endangerment

23. Which of the following measures would help to prevent Lyme disease?

    (A) Avoidance of travel to the western region of the United States
    (B) Lyme vaccine, consisting of recombinant OspA in adjuvant, rebooted at 1 and 2 months
    (C) Minimizing exposure to people with active Lyme disease
    (D) Prevention of animal bites
    (E) Prophylactic antibiotics when traveling to endemic areas

24. A 4-year-old Asian boy presents to the ED with a fever of 40.6°C (105.1°F). He presented 5 days ago to his pediatrician's office with bilateral injected conjunctivae and a fever of 39°C (102.2°F). He has been a healthy child and his immunizations are up to date. His respiratory rate is 22/min, his heart rate is 130/min, and his blood pressure is 105/63 mm Hg. He has a nonexudative injection of his bulbar conjunctivae bilaterally. His lips are erythematous, dry, and cracked, and his tongue is bright red. He has a nonvesicular polymorphous rash on his trunk. He does not have cervical, occipital, or inguinal lymphadenopathy. He has a normal S1 and S2 with no murmurs. He has normal bowel sounds and a nontender, nondistended abdomen without organomegaly. His hands and feet are edematous and his palms and soles are erythematous. Physical examination findings are shown below. Which of the following is the most likely diagnosis?

    (A) Adenovirus infection
    (B) Kawasaki's disease
    (C) Measles
    (D) *Staphylococcus aureus* infection
    (E) Stevens-Johnson syndrome

25. Initially, screening tests for hepatitis C infection include enzyme immunoassay (EIA). If the EIA is positive, recombinant immunoblot assay or polymerase chain reaction may be used for confirmation of results. To minimize the chance that persons who are not infected with hepatitis C test positive, which of the following is the most important?

    (A) The EIA must have a high positive predictive value
    (B) The EIA must have high sensitivity
    (C) The EIA must have high specificity
    (D) The recombinant immunoblot assay or polymerase chain reaction must have high sensitivity
    (E) The recombinant immunoblot assay or polymerase chain reaction must have high specificity

26. A 33-year-old man with HIV with a CD4+ count of 54/mm^3 presents to the ED with a nonproductive cough, fever, and exertional dyspnea. An x-ray of the chest is shown in the image. Which of the following is the most appropriate pharmacotherapy?

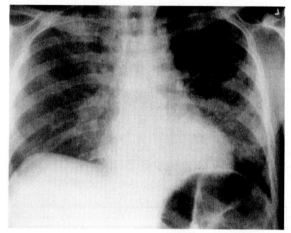

Reproduced, with permission, from Kasper DL, Braunwald E, Fauci AS, Hauser SL, Longo DL, Jameson LJ, Isselbacher KJ, eds. *Harrison's Online.* New York: McGraw-Hill, 2005: 1195.

    (A) Amphotericin B
    (B) Ceftriaxone
    (C) Fluconazole
    (D) Metronidazole
    (E) Nystatin swish and swallow
    (F) Pyrazinamide
    (G) Trimethoprim-sulfamethoxazole

27. An otherwise healthy 20-year-old woman presents to the ED with complaints of 1 day of headache and fever with associated nausea, vomiting, and a diffuse red rash. She reports that she has been on spring break for the past week, has been drinking heavily, and has been

spending most of each day in the sun, but she has used SPF 30 sunblock and does not remember getting sunburned. Her last menstrual period began 3 days ago. She reports that she forgot her tampons at home and borrowed one from her friend, which she has left in for the past 2 days. She denies any recent sexual activity. Examination is notable for a diffuse macular erythematous rash resembling sunburn that covers the majority of her body, including her palms and soles. Her neck is supple, and she does not exhibit any photophobia or signs of intoxication. Twenty minutes after initial presentation, she becomes lethargic, and her vital signs are temperature 39.6°C (103.3°F), heart rate 115/min, blood pressure 84/48 mm Hg, and respiratory rate 18/min. What is the most likely diagnosis?

(A) Alcohol poisoning
(B) Heatstroke
(C) *Neisseria* meningococcemia
(D) Rocky Mountain spotted fever
(E) Toxic shock syndrome

28. A 22-year-old man with cystic fibrosis presents to the ED with the acute onset of fever, chills and dyspnea. Blood cultures are positive for *Pseudomonas aeruginosa*, and the patient is started on a multiple-antibiotic regimen of a β-lactam antibiotic and gentamicin. Ten days later, the patient's bacteremia has resolved but his creatinine is 2.0 mg/dL. Urinalysis demonstrates muddy brown granular casts, and the fractional excretion of sodium in his urine is 2.5%. What is the most likely mechanism of this patient's renal disease?

(A) Decreased perfusion of the kidney secondary to volume depletion
(B) Deposition of antibody and/or antibody-antigen complexes on the glomerular basement membrane
(C) Direct toxic effect on renal tubule cells
(D) Decreased perfusion of the kidney secondary to volume depletion
(E) Renal arterial and arteriolar vasoconstriction

29. A new blood test for *Plasmodium falciparum* is developed. Initial screening indicates that the test is much more sensitive for the parasite, and is just as specific. What effect would a switch to the new test have in screening a certain population for *Plasmodium* infection?

(A) A lower false-negative ratio and a higher negative predictive value
(B) A lower false-negative ratio and a lower positive predictive value
(C) A lower false-positive ratio and a higher positive predictive value
(D) A lower false-positive ratio and a lower negative predictive value
(E) The effect on positive predictive value and negative predictive value cannot be known without knowledge of the disease prevalence

30. A 7-year-old boy is brought to the ED for evaluation of neck pain. His mother reports he first started complaining of the pain approximately 3 days ago, and she noted a mass along his left neck earlier today. The child has been healthy previously and has never had a similar episode. His immunizations are up to date. There is no family history of lymphoma or other cancers. He has had no recent travel and has not been exposed to any sick contacts. There are no pets in the house, but the mother does report noticing several small scratches on the boy's face after he played with the neighbor's cats a few weeks ago. His heart rate is 102/min, blood pressure is 96/62 mm Hg, and respiratory rate is 22/min. Physical examination is normal except for three red papules (~3 mm each) on the left neck with two 3-cm lymph nodes in the anterior cervical chain. He has no lymphadenopathy elsewhere. What organism is most likely responsible for this infection?

(A) *Bartonella henselae*
(B) *Brucella*
(C) *Clostridium botulinum*
(D) *Francisella tularensis*
(E) *Staphylococcus aureus*

31. A patient with HIV and CD4+ counts of less than 100/mm³ who is a cat lover developed lesions on his hands and arms about 2 weeks ago (see image). Biopsy of the lesions reveals tiny clumps of bacilli on Warthin-Starry silver stain. What can this disease can be treated with?

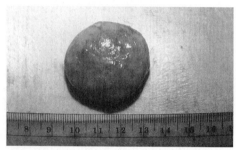

Reproduced, with permission, from Kasper DL, Braunwald E, Fauci AS, Hauser SL, Longo DL, Jameson LJ, Isselbacher KJ, eds. *Harrison's Online.* New York: McGraw-Hill, 2005: 931.

(A) Acyclovir
(B) Dexamethasone cream
(C) Erythromycin
(D) Ganciclovir
(E) Highly active antiretroviral therapy

32. A 21-year old HIV-positive man with a CD4+ count of 42/mm³ presents to his ophthalmologist with blurry vision and floaters in his right eye, but denies pain. What is the most important disease to rule out?

(A) Blepharitis
(B) Conjunctivitis
(C) Cytomegalovirus retinitis
(D) Open-angle glaucoma

33. A 21-year-old G0P0 woman with no significant past medical history presents to the ED with a 2-day history of bilateral lower abdominal pain and vaginal discharge. She began having unprotected sexual intercourse with her new boyfriend 4 weeks ago. Her temperature is 39.1°C (102.4°F), her blood pressure is 131/73 mm Hg, her heart rate is 98/min, and her respiratory rate is 13/min. On examination she has adnexal tenderness, purulent cervical discharge, and extreme pain during the bimanual examination. Which diagnostic test is most useful in guiding the treatment of her condition?

(A) Diagnostic laparoscopy
(B) DNA probes for *Chlamydia trachomatis* and *Neisseria gonorrhoeae*
(C) Gram stain of discharge
(D) β-Human chorionic gonadotropin test
(E) WBC count

34. A 3-year-old boy is brought to his family pediatrician for evaluation of chronic low-grade fevers, decreased appetite, and nonproductive cough. He has previously been healthy, with no past similar episodes. The pediatrician learns that the patient has been visiting his grandparents in a retirement living facility on weekends. The physician wants to rule out all possibilities and orders an x-ray of the chest, which appears to be normal. A purified protein derivative test is performed and 48 hours later demonstrates 12-mm induration. The diagnosis of pulmonary tuberculosis is made, and the child is started on isoniazid, rifampin, and pyrazinamide. Which of the following is a known adverse reaction of rifampin that should be monitored during this child's treatment?

(A) Angioedema
(B) Hepatotoxicity
(C) Hyperuricemia
(D) Peripheral neuritis
(E) Stevens-Johnson syndrome

35. A 33-year-old smoker is being treated for chronic cavitary histoplasmosis. He lives in rural Missouri and works at a farm where he cleans chicken coops. He also owns a small farm where he plants and harvests corn. He makes occasional long trips to Baltimore to sell his corn and buy more seeds. He states that his only hobby is swimming and he swims in local public swimming pools. Which of the following is most likely to have prevented the condition?

(A) Avoiding cigarette smoke
(B) Avoiding corn fields
(C) Avoiding swimming in public pools
(D) Avoiding the chicken droppings
(E) Avoiding travel to Baltimore

36. A 45-year-old veteran is seen in the clinic for poor impulse control. Over the last month, he has spent all of his savings on business ventures and is currently estranged from his wife. He admits a decreased need for sleep, a new sense of grandiosity, and increased energy spent on researching projects to make money. He has no prior psychiatric history, and his only medical history includes treatment for gonorrhea during his military service and an appendectomy at age 36 years. Physical examination reveals a thin, middle-age man with pressured speech. His pupillary examination is normal, except that the pupils are reactive to convergence but not to light. Infection with which of the following organisms could be the most likely etiology of his symptoms?

    (A) *Chlamydia trachomatis*
    (B) Herpes simplex virus
    (C) *Neisseria gonorrhoeae*
    (D) *Toxoplasma*
    (E) *Treponema pallidum*

37. A 25-year-old primigravida at 38 weeks' gestation presents to the ED in labor. Her labor started about 6 hours ago, and her cervix is effaced and 2 cm dilated. She has not received prenatal care. She has no known drug allergies. What medication should be begun empirically?

    (A) Ampicillin
    (B) Doxycycline
    (C) Magnesium sulfate
    (D) Oxytocin
    (E) Terbutaline

38. A 13-year-old boy with sickle cell disease is brought to the emergency department for evaluation of leg pain. He says he developed significant leg pain approximately 2 days ago that prohibited his participation in gym class and even created marked pain on walking. He took acetaminophen for the pain and had mild improvement. However, he has noticed within the past 24 hours that the area of pain is now showing redness of the skin with some mild swelling. His heart rate is 92/min, blood pressure is 108/68 mm Hg, respiratory rate is 19/min, and temperature is 38.5°C (101.3°F). Physical examination is normal, except for a painful right tibia with mild edema and erythema of the overlying skin. He is sent for a radiologic evaluation and is found to have no lytic lesions but does demonstrate edema of the deep muscle. What organism is most likely responsible for this child's condition?

    (A) *Escherichia coli*
    (B) *Haemophilus influenzae*
    (C) *Mycoplasma*
    (D) *Salmonella*
    (E) *Staphylococcus aureus*

39. A 27-year-old sexually active African-American woman presents to the ED complaining of low-grade fevers, chills, night sweats, and burning chest pain that is worse with swallowing. The physician immediately notices white patches consistent with oral candidiasis on the patient's tongue. She has never had this before. Further examination reveals extension of thrush into the esophagus. Which of the following conditions does the patient most likely have?

    (A) Cardiac chest pain
    (B) HIV
    (C) Mallory-Weiss tear
    (D) Nothing; healthy patients can get candidal esophagitis
    (E) Severe combined immunodeficiency syndrome
    (F) Vaginal candidiasis

40. A 2.5-year-old girl was diagnosed with a viral upper respiratory infection last week and now presents to her physician with a brassy cough and purulent airway secretions. Her parents believed that she may have croup and attempted mist therapy without success. The patient has been febrile to 39.0°C (102.2°F) for the past 24 hours and has had difficulty breathing during the past hour. Her review of systems is otherwise negative, and the mother denies that the patient has had any drooling or difficulty/pain when swallowing. Vital signs are stable with a heart rate of 92/min, blood pressure of 92/60 mm Hg, respiratory rate of 21/min, and temperature of 38.9°C (102°F). A Gram stain of secretions obtained in the office is shown in the image. What organism is most likely responsible for this patient's condition?

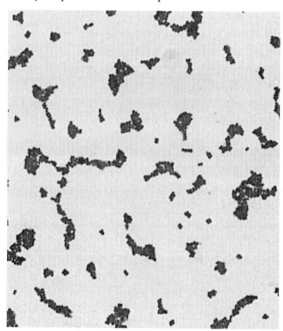

Reproduced, with permission, from Brooks GF, Carroll KC, Butel JS, Morse SA. *Jawetz, Melnick, & Adelberg's Medical Microbiology*, 24th ed. New York: McGraw-Hill, 2007: Figure 14-1.

(A) Anaerobic organisms
(B) *Moraxella catarrhalis*
(C) Nontypeable *Haemophilus influenzae*
(D) *Pseudomonas aeruginosa*
(E) *Staphylococcus aureus*

41. A 2-year-old boy is brought to the clinic for evaluation of "acne." His mother describes a recent onset of pain in his left foot and in his right hand. She says he has been hospitalized once for lymphadenitis, but he has been otherwise healthy. His review of systems is otherwise negative. He as two maternal uncles who died in childhood from pneumonia. The child is afebrile, with a heart rate of 64/min, blood pressure of 108/70 mm Hg, and respiratory rate of 15/min. Physical examination reveals multiple scarred lesions on his skin, two of which are 1 cm in diameter and filled with purulent material. Pain is elicited by palpation of the purulent lesions, and they are somewhat warm to the touch. From which immunodeficiency disorder is this patient most likely suffering?

(A) Ataxia-telangiectasia
(B) Chédiak-Higashi syndrome
(C) Chronic granulomatous disease
(D) Hyper IgE syndrome
(E) Wiskott-Aldrich syndrome

42. A 30-year-old woman comes to her primary care physician complaining of episodes of an "irregular heartbeat," muscle weakness, joint swelling, and headaches. The symptoms began in early October and have lasted for approximately 5 weeks; she was unable to get an earlier appointment. The headaches and irregular rhythm fluctuated throughout the day. Now the arrhythmia has resolved, but she is still bothered by the weakness and headaches. She had no precipitating illness, condition, or unusual exposures. Her only recent travel was a camping trip with her daughter in West Virginia this past summer. What is the most likely diagnosis?

(A) Gonococcal disease
(B) Gout
(C) Lyme disease
(D) Migraines
(E) Sjögren's syndrome
(F) Systemic lupus erythematosus

43. A 49-year-old quarry worker undergoes her yearly employee physical. Screening x-ray of the chest reveals a 1.5-cm (0.6-in) subpleural parenchymal lesion in the lateral aspect of the right lung, as well as enlarged hilar nodes, eggshell hilar calcifications, and multiple small nodules scattered throughout the upper lung fields. The patient denies cough, weight loss, and night sweats. In fact, she states that she feels perfectly well. Sputum culture is positive for acid-fast bacilli. Exposure to which of the following substances increased this patient's chance of contracting tuberculosis?

(A) Asbestos
(B) Beryllium
(C) Carbon
(D) Coal
(E) Silica

44. A 27-year-old man with a history of sickle cell disease comes to the ED with a 3-day history of fever and chills but no pain. On physical examination, his temperature is 38.5°C (101.3°F). A peripheral blood smear shows Howell-Jolly bodies. Which of the following organisms is the patient at increased risk for because of his underlying sickle cell disease?

(A) *Chlamydia trachomatis*
(B) *Escherichia coli*
(C) *Staphylococcus aureus*
(D) *Streptococcus pneumoniae*
(E) Viridans streptococcus

45. A 50-year-old man presents to the ED with a fever, productive cough, dyspnea, and pleuritic chest pain. He states that the symptoms started suddenly last night. X-ray of the chest demonstrates a confluent left lower lobe. The border of the minor fissure is visible. Quellung reaction identifies the infection as pneumococcal pneumonia. Susceptibility and culture show resistance to penicillin. Which of the following is the most appropriate antibiotic treatment?

(A) Aztreonam
(B) Ceftriaxone
(C) Doxycycline
(D) Gentamicin
(E) Metronidazole

46. A 4-year-old child presents to the clinic for evaluation of a recent-onset illness. He developed a fever (39.0°C [102.1°F]) 2 days before presenting. Simultaneous to his fever, he developed a headache with generalized malaise and had a decreased appetite. He has now developed a generalized rash all over his body as shown in the image. Which of the following is the most likely diagnosis?

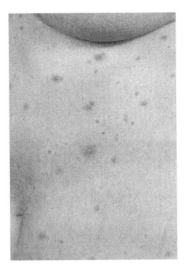

Reproduced, with permission, from Wolff K, Johnson RA, Surmond D. *Fitzpatrick's Color Atlas & Synopsis of Clinical Dermatology*, 5th ed. New York: McGraw-Hill, 2005: 819.

(A) Chickenpox
(B) Contact dermatitis
(C) Hand-foot-and-mouth disease
(D) Herpes zoster
(E) Smallpox
(F) Stevens-Johnson syndrome

47. A 67-year-old man is brought to the ED by his daughter, who reports that her father has been acting "strangely." She indicates that he is usually quiet and considerate. However, for the past day he has been argumentative, irresponsible, and increasingly confused. She decided to bring him to the ED when an elderly neighbor called to complain that he had made overt sexual advances toward her. The patient is alert but disoriented and uncooperative. Notably, his temperature is 38.2°C (100.8°F), and he is sensitive to light. There are no focal neurologic deficits, but cerebrospinal fluid contains 50 WBCs, normal protein, and normal glucose. Which of the following would most likely confirm the diagnosis?

(A) Draw blood to check blood alcohol level
(B) Obtain CT of the head with contrast
(C) Perform herpes simplex virus DNA polymerase chain reaction of the cerebrospinal fluid
(D) Perform urinalysis and begin empiric antibiotics
(E) Repeat lumbar puncture to measure opening pressure

48. A 43-year-old man with HIV who has declined antiretroviral therapy is undergoing a corticosteroid taper for *Pneumocystis jiroveci* pneumonia. He presents to his primary care physician with the lesions shown in the image and complains of nausea, abdominal pain, and foul-smelling stools. The patient's skin lesions are not pruritic or painful. What treatment could have prevented this development?

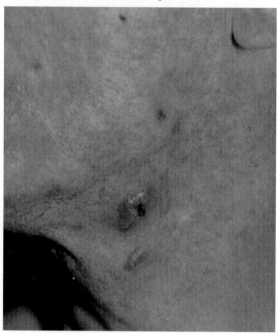

Reproduced, with permission, from Wolff K, Johnson RA, Surmond D. *Fitzpatrick's Color Atlas & Synopsis of Clinical Dermatology*, 5th ed. New York: McGraw-Hill, 2005: Figure 1e-HIV6.

(A) Dapsone
(B) Highly active antiretroviral therapy
(C) Trimethoprim-sulfamethoxazole
(D) Zidovudine/lamivudine combination therapy
(E) Zidovudine monotherapy

49. A 26-year-old sexually active woman who recently spent a year in East Africa presents to her gynecologist with bilateral nontender inguinal lymphadenopathy. Serology confirms the diagnosis of lymphogranuloma venereum. Which of the following is the most appropriate pharmacotherapy?

(A) Acyclovir
(B) Ceftriaxone
(C) Doxycycline
(D) Gentamicin
(E) Penicillin

50. A patient sustained an open tibial fracture of his left leg in a motor vehicle accident and is taken to the operating room for surgical repair. The patient undergoes an intramedullary nail fixation of the tibial fracture. Five days after the reconstructive procedure, the patient is still complaining about swelling, redness, and tenderness in his left leg. The leg feels warm, and is visibly swollen and erythematous. The patient is febrile and a complete blood cell count reveals 87% polymorphonuclear cells and 5% bands. A bone aspirate is performed and reveals purulent material. An x-ray of the tibia and fibula is shown in the image. Which of the following is the most appropriate initial pharmacotherapy?

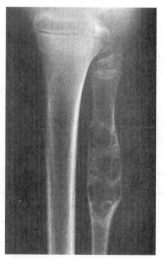

Reproduced, with permission, from Chen MYM, Pope TL, Ott DJ. *Basic Radiology.* New York: McGraw-Hill, 2004: Figure 6-19.

(A) Ampicillin or amoxicillin
(B) Aztreonam
(C) Ciprofloxacin
(D) Methicillin
(E) Nafcillin
(F) Nafcillin and gentamicin

51. A 25-year-old primigravida woman presents to the obstetrician's office for her first prenatal visit. Which of the following titers is routinely obtained at the first prenatal visit?

(A) Cytomegalovirus and hepatitis B
(B) Cytomegalovirus and rubella

(C) Rubella and syphilis

(D) Rubella, syphilis, HIV, hepatitis B, cytomegalovirus, and toxoplasmosis

(E) Toxoplasmosis and HIV

(F) Toxoplasmosis, syphilis, and rubella

52. A 41-year-old white man from rural Maryland presents to his primary care physician complaining of muscle aches and severe headaches of 12 months' duration. The patient's wife, who accompanies him, reports that the patient has been irritable and lethargic for "quite a while now." The patient works outdoors most days, and says he occasionally has tick bites. He does not recall any recent rashes, but his wife confirms that he did have a rash last summer after working outside. Physical examination reveals the lesions shown in the image. Which of the following could have prevented this?

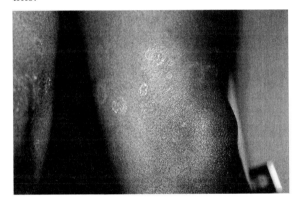

Reproduced, with permission, from Wolff K, Johnson RA, Surmond D. *Fitzpatrick's Color Atlas & Synopsis of Clinical Dermatology*, 5th ed. New York: McGraw-Hill, 2005: 682.

(A) A 3-week course of amoxicillin followed by 3 weeks of doxycycline

(B) Ibuprofen 600 mg three times a day until the muscle aches subsided

(C) Immunization against meningococci

(D) Latex condom prophylaxis during sexual intercourse

(E) No treatment is necessary; the symptoms will be self-limited

53. An 18-year-old swimmer arrives at the ED and is complaining of ear pain and discharge for the last 2 days. He denies any fever or headache, but states that he does feel some pressure in his head, and pulling on his pinna elicits pain. Which of the following is the most appropriate next step for the patient's condition?

(A) CT scan of the head

(B) Intravenous antibiotics for *Naegleria fowleri*

(C) MRI of the head

(D) Surgery

(E) Topical medication and cleaning

54. A 14-year-old girl presents to her family practitioner with a 2-day history of profuse vaginal discharge and pruritus. She admits that she has recently become sexually active with her new boyfriend. The physician performs a potassium hydroxide prep of the vaginal discharge and sees many leukocytes, but no hyphae. The pH of the discharge is higher than normal. What is the physician obligated to do next?

(A) Inform the patient's mother that she is engaging in unsafe sex

(B) Recommend abstaining from sexual intercourse for 2 weeks

(C) Report the case to the county department of health

(D) Recommend treatment of her boyfriend

(E) Screen the patient for diabetes

55. A number of common bacterial, viral, and parasitic infections can cause neutropenia. Which of the following is usually the most appropriate therapy for patients with postinfectious neutropenia?

(A) Empiric antibiotics

(B) Granulocyte transfusions

(C) Recombinant granulocyte colony-stimulating factor

(D) Supportive care with subglottic narrowing

EXTENDED MATCHING

Questions 56–58

For each of the following patients, select the most appropriate treatment.

(A) Acyclovir
(B) Amantadine
(C) Amphotericin B
(D) Dapsone
(E) Doxycycline
(F) Foscarnet
(G) Fluconazole
(H) Gentamicin
(I) No treatment is necessary
(J) Penicillin

56. A 12-year-old boy presents to the ED with a fever of 39°C (102°F), myalgias, headaches, and petechial rash after returning from Boy Scout camp in western North Carolina. His mother states that the rash started at his feet and hands and then spread to his trunk.

57. A 2-year-old boy who attends day care has a fever for 3 days. The fever finally subsides, but a maculopapular pink rash develops over his trunk and spreads to his arms and face. His mother has not noticed the child scratching at the rash, but says that the boy does seem more irritable.

58. A 9-year-old boy is brought to his doctor's office with a headache, fever, vomiting, and extremely sore throat. He also has a red rash that feels like "sandpaper." Physical examination reveals a bright pink tongue and erythematous oropharynx with white patches on his tonsils.

Questions 59–61

For each of the following patients, select the most likely sexually transmitted disease.

(A) *Candida albicans*
(B) *Chlamydia trachomatis*
(C) *Escherichia coli*
(D) *Haemophilus ducreyi*
(E) Herpes simplex virus
(F) HIV
(G) Human papillomavirus
(H) *Neisseria gonorrhea*
(I) *Proteus*
(J) *Treponema pallidum*

59. A 28-year-old African-American man presents with penile discharge, frequent urination, and pain on urination. His left knee is swollen, red, and tender. He was recently sexually active without protection.

60. A 28-year-old African-American man presents with penile discharge, frequent urination, and pain on urination. He was recently sexually active without protection. Gram stains of a urethral specimen show no gram-negative diplococci.

61. A 28-year-old African-American man presents with penile discharge, frequent urination, and pain on urination. There are multiple vesicles on the patient's penis.

Questions 62–64

For each of the following patients, choose the most appropriate diagnostic test.

(A) Acid-fast stain of induced sputum
(B) Basic metabolic panel
(C) Bone scan
(D) Cardiac stress test
(E) Complete metabolic panel (electrolytes, proteins, glucose, and kidney and liver tests)
(F) CT scan
(G) HIV enzyme-linked immunosorbent assay
(H) Lumbar puncture
(I) Muscle biopsy
(J) Psychiatric evaluation
(K) Transthoracic echocardiogram
(L) X-ray of the chest

62. An 87-year-old woman has a 3-week history of fever and anorexia. Cultures of blood, urine, and sputum are negative.

63. A 37-year-old man with a history significant for heavy alcohol consumption presents to the ED with a 3-week history of fever and anorexia. Cultures of blood, urine, and sputum are negative.

64. An 87-year-old man with a history of a low-pitched diastolic murmur presents to the ED

with a 3-week history of fever and anorexia. Cultures of blood, urine, and sputum are negative.

Questions 65 and 66

For each of the following patients, select the most likely cause of congenital infection.

- (A) *Chlamydia trachomatis*
- (B) Cytomegalovirus
- (C) Epstein-Barr virus
- (D) Hepatitis B
- (E) Hepatitis E
- (F) Herpes simplex virus
- (G) Herpes zoster
- (H) *Neisseria gonorrhoeae*
- (I) Parvovirus
- (J) Rubella
- (K) Syphilis
- (L) Toxoplasmosis

65. At an infant's 1-month checkup with the pediatrician, the baby is noted to have a vesicular rash on the skin, eyes, and mouth. The mother reportedly had a history of vesicles in her genital region.

66. A jaundiced infant is noted to have cutaneous lesions on his palms and soles. He occasionally snuffles. Abdominal examination reveals hepatosplenomegaly. The blood count is remarkable for anemia.

Questions 67 and 68

For each of the following patients, select the most appropriate prophylactic and/or treatment regimen to institute.

- (A) Hepatitis B vaccine
- (B) Isoniazid and pyridoxine
- (C) No new treatment or prophylaxis is needed at this time
- (D) Papanicolaou smears every 6 months
- (E) *Pneumocystis jiroveci* pneumonia prophylaxis
- (F) Suppressive acyclovir
- (G) Toxoplasmosis prophylaxis
- (H) X-ray of the chest

67. A 34-year-old HIV-positive man whose most recent CD4+ count was 196/mm^3.

68. A 26-year-old HIV-positive woman who has had two outbreaks of painful genital lesions in the last 6 months.

Questions 69 and 70

For each patient with urinary symptoms, select the most likely diagnosis.

- (A) Acute cystitis
- (B) Acute pyelonephritis
- (C) Acute urinary retention
- (D) Carcinoma of the bladder
- (E) Carcinoma of the prostate
- (F) Diabetes insipidus
- (G) Diabetes mellitus
- (H) Hypercalcemia
- (I) Interstitial cystitis
- (J) Neurogenic bladder
- (K) Psychogenic polydipsia
- (L) Renal cell carcinoma
- (M) Urethral stricture

69. A 19-year-old woman presents to her primary care provider with symptoms of urinary urgency, hesitancy, frequency, painful urination, and incomplete voids. Abdominal and pelvic examinations are unremarkable. The patient recently became sexually active. Gram stain of a centrifuged mid-void urine specimen shows a coagulase-negative, gram-positive coccus resistant to novobiocin.

70. A 41-year-old woman presents with a 1-day history of dysuria, moderate back pain, nausea, and vomiting. Her temperature is 38.4°C (101.1°F). Abdominal examination reveals costovertebral angle tenderness, and pelvic examination is unremarkable. A urine β-human chorionic gonadotropin test is negative.

HIGH-YIELD SYSTEMS

Infectious Disease

1. **The correct answer is A.** The patient has had a simple febrile seizure, which is a brief, generalized, tonic-clonic seizure associated with a febrile illness (temperature > 38°C [100.4°F]), without an underlying serious infection or neurologic cause. Febrile seizures occur within 24 hours of the onset of fever and can be simple or complex. In contrast to complex febrile seizures, simple febrile seizures last less than 15 minutes, have no focal features during the seizure or postictal period, and, if they occur in series, do not last longer than 30 minutes total. Febrile seizures are most common in the 12- to 18-month age group. Febrile seizures may occur with viral infections, such as human herpesvirus 6 infection (roseola), upper respiratory tract infections, and acute otitis media, and after immunization with diphtheria-tetanus-pertussis or measles-mumps-rubella vaccine. Antipyretics such as acetaminophen and sponging with tepid water can be used to control the fever. A short-acting benzodiazepine such as lorazepam can be given intravenously if the seizure lasts longer than 5 minutes.

Answer B is incorrect. An electroencephalogram is unnecessary in the setting of a simple febrile seizure and cannot predict the likelihood of recurrent febrile seizures or development of other types of seizures.

Answer C is incorrect. A lumbar puncture should be performed in children who are younger than 12 months after their first febrile seizure. It should also be considered if the seizure occurs after the second day of illness and if the clinician cannot confidently rule out meningitis. Because this patient has no focal neurologic symptoms, meningismus, or Brudzinski's or Kernig's signs, and has an upper respiratory infection that explains her fever, meningitis is very unlikely.

Answer D is incorrect. Phenobarbital is another antiepileptic medication that is effective in decreasing recurrent febrile seizures. The risks and potential adverse effects, however, outweigh the benefits, and it is not recommended by the American Academy of Pediatrics.

Answer E is incorrect. Valproic acid is an antiepileptic medication that is effective in decreasing recurrent febrile seizures. However, the risks and potential adverse effects outweigh the benefits. Valproic acid can lead to valproate-induced hepatotoxicity, especially in children who are younger than 2 years. There are also no data to suggest that preventing recurrent febrile seizures decreases the risk of developing afebrile seizures.

2. **The correct answer is A.** This patient's rash, erythema chronicum migrans, is suggestive of Lyme disease, caused by the pathogen *Borrelia burgdorferi*, which is transmitted by the bite of the *Ixodes* tick. It is endemic in the northeastern United States. Treatment is with oral doxycycline, amoxicillin, or cefuroxime axetil. Patients with certain neurologic or cardiac forms of the illness may require intravenous treatment with drugs such as ceftriaxone or penicillin.

Answer B is incorrect. Meningitis typically presents with a headache and can sometimes include a rash, typically with meningococcus, but this is more prevalent in children. Also, the history of recent hiking in an area endemic for Lyme disease is highly suggestive of a tick-borne illness. Ceftriaxone is generally the antibiotic of choice for staphylococcal infections.

Answer C is incorrect. Myocarditis is inflammation of the myocardium with myocyte necrosis. It often follows viral infection and can present like an upper respiratory tract infection, featuring fever, dyspnea, and chest pain. Only rarely would it present with such a localized rash. Treatment is focused on reducing the demands placed on the myocardium. Immunosuppression and anti-inflammatory drug use is controversial.

Answer D is incorrect. Rocky Mountain spotted fever, like Lyme disease, presents with a headache and rash, but the rash described in the stem is more typical of Lyme disease. The rash suggestive of Rocky Mountain spotted fever is more diffuse, appearing on the wrists, ankles, soles, and palms, rather than in one isolated location. This disease is endemic to the southeastern United States. Treatment is with doxycycline and chloramphenicol.

Answer E is incorrect. Though *Staphylococcus aureus* may superinfect a skin lesion such as a tick bite, it generally produces an ulcerating lesion with a more evenly erythematous surrounding area. Erythema chronicum migrans is thus inconsistent with this infection. Treatment is generally with penicillin or vancomycin, though resistance patterns for this agent are evolving rapidly.

3. **The correct answer is B.** A patient and family have the right to withhold treatment for ventilation, antibiotics, or fluids. There is no distinction between withholding and withdrawing life-supporting treatment. However, when the patient is not conscious it is important to confirm the patient's wishes through prior legal documentation and to ensure that the relative is aware of the most recent decisions of the patient.

Answer A is incorrect. Power of attorney can be granted by the patient to any person for a specific period of time, or permanently (durable power of attorney). A person previously granted power of attorney holds no special decision-making rights once that specific period of time (previous hospitalization) has ended.

Answer C is incorrect. In the absence of a signed legal document, the patient's family is the first line of contact for decision making regarding the patient's management.

Answer D is incorrect. Although the patient's primary care physician may be called upon to help make choices in management after family members have been contacted, the physician's prior interactions with the patient alone are not enough to withdraw care.

Answer E is incorrect. The advance directive does not become a legal document until it is signed. Any prior paperwork may be used to help a power of attorney.

Answer F is incorrect. The patient has the right to refuse life-supporting treatment. Withholding and withdrawing life-supporting care

from a patient are currently considered ethically identical.

4. **The correct answer is A.** Cryptococcal meningitis is commonly seen in AIDS patients. Typical presenting symptoms are headache, fever, nausea, vomiting, stiff neck, sensitivity to light, and mental status changes. The India ink stain shows *Cryptococcus* blastocysts in the cerebrospinal fluid, which are often coupled with an elevated opening pressure in cryptococcal meningitis.

Answer B is incorrect. HIV encephalopathy is a type of subcortical dementia that evolves over weeks to months. Some of the common symptoms include slowing of reasoning, forgetfulness, difficulty concentrating, lack of energy, mild depressive symptoms, and emotional blunting. Impairment of alertness, neck stiffness, and focal or lateralizing neurologic signs (e.g., hemiparesis and aphasia) are not typical for HIV encephalopathy.

Answer C is incorrect. A migraine can present with symptoms that mimic meningitis; however, the blastocysts seen in the cerebrospinal fluid and immunocompromised status make the diagnosis of cryptococcal meningitis.

Answer D is incorrect. Pneumococcal meningitis is caused by a bacterium, which would render more neutrophils in the cerebrospinal fluid (CSF); however, the infection described is a unquestionably a fungal infection because of the cryptococcal blastocysts in the CSF.

Answer E is incorrect. Toxoplasmosis is an infection from cats that is known to infect HIV patients. It is caused by the parasite *Toxoplasma gondii*. The patient is taking trimethoprim-sulfamethoxazole, which prevents *Pneumocystis jiroveci* pneumonia and toxoplasmosis. The picture shown is that of *Cryptococcus*.

5. **The correct answer is B.** Up to 17% of patients taking fluoroquinolones experience some degree of gastrointestinal upset.

Answer A is incorrect. Allergic reactions, including rash occur in < 2% of patients taking fluoroquinolones.

Answer C is incorrect. Neurologic manifestations such as mild headache and dizziness are the second most common adverse reaction of patients taking fluoroquinolones, affecting up to 11% of patients.

Answer D is incorrect. QT prolongation is also a rare complication of treatment and very uncommonly leads to ventricular arrhythmias.

Answer E is incorrect. Tendonitis and Achilles tendon rupture are exceedingly rare in patients taking fluoroquinolones but have increased incidence in children and pregnant women.

6. **The correct answer is C.** Patients with urinary tract infections and hospital-acquired pneumonias can quickly become bacteremic. With hematogenous spread, the infecting agents can potentially infect other organs. In this case, the sudden onset of fever, bacteremia, x-ray findings, and acute kidney failure are suggestive of sepsis. The costovertebral angle tenderness also suggests pyelonephritis.

Answer A is incorrect. Contrast nephropathy may be contributing, as it can occur a few days after the administration of contrast and is more likely in patients with diabetic nephropathy, but it would not explain the clinical picture of fever and low blood pressure. Had hypotension and decreased urine output immediately followed the administration of intravenous contrast, it would be characterized as an anaphylactoid reaction due the activation of mast cells.

Answer B is incorrect. Diabetic nephropathy causes a more chronic renal failure. Given the patient's baseline creatinine of 1.5 mg/dL, it is likely that diabetic nephropathy is the etiology of her underlying chronic renal insufficiency. This patient presents with acute renal failure.

Answer D is incorrect. Insufficient intravascular volume may cause acute renal failure(prerenal azotemia). Although maintenance fluids had been discontinued, the patient was not restricted to nothing by mouth and presumably was eating and drinking normally. While still a possible explanation, this is less likely, as there is an infectious source as well as clinical findings compatible with pyelonephritis. Furthermore, classically, the blood urea nitrogen:creatinine ratio in prerenal azotemia is > 20; here the ratio is < 10. Further tests to determine the etiology of the renal failure would be urine osmolality, urine sodium, and fractional excretion of sodium.

Answer E is incorrect. Acidosis will not explain the costovertebral angle tenderness or the entire clinical picture. Furthermore, the most common acid-base disturbance in sepsis is combined metabolic acidosis and respiratory alkalosis.

7. **The correct answer is A.** Group B *Streptococcus* (GBS) is the most common cause of neonatal meningitis, transmitted vertically from the mother to the patient. Late-onset GBS infection usually occurs between postpartum weeks 2 and 3. This mother did not receive prenatal care and was most likely GBS-positive but this was not recognized. Normally at 36 weeks' gestation, many institutions perform screening for GBS, and patients who have a positive culture receive intravenous penicillin when they present in labor.

Answer B is incorrect. Meningitis due to influenza is rare in neonates compared to rates of group B streptococcal infection. Though the examination would likely be similar for infection by either agent, the cerebrospinal fluid glucose level would likely be normal to increased in influenza infection.

Answer C is incorrect. The child received an appropriate dose of acetaminophen based on the history.

Answer D is incorrect. Varicella-zoster virus is not the most likely cause, as neither the classic stigmata of skin rash/skin scar or eye abnormalities (chorioretinitis and cataracts) is present.

Answer E is incorrect. Viridans streptococcus is the etiologic agent of subacute bacterial endocarditis, not meningitis in neonates. Systemic infection with this organism presents most commonly with fever and chills. Physical examination is notable for petechiae, splinter hemorrhages, Osler nodes, Janeway lesions, and Roth spots.

8. **The correct answer is A.** Roseola (or exanthema subitum or sixth disease) is most commonly caused by human herpesvirus-6 (HHV-6), and less commonly HHV-7. It is a mild febrile illness that occurs predominantly in infants. There may be mild symptoms such as mild rhinorrhea and mild erythema of the pharynx and conjunctivae. The acute onset of high fever, often > 40°C (104°F), heralds clinical illness and may be accompanied by seizures. The fever resolves abruptly after 3–5 days, and a rose-colored maculopapular rash with discrete 2- to 5-mm lesions begins as the fever breaks. The rash starts on the trunk and then spreads to the face and extremities. It typically remains nonconfluent and disappears in 24 hours or less.

Answer B is incorrect. Measles is characterized by a 3-day prodrome of low-grade to moderate fever, Cough, Coryza, and Conjunctivitis (the "3 C's"). Koplik's spots, small red spots with grey centers on the buccal mucosa, occur 2–3 days later. A high fever ≥ 40°C (104°F) typically accompanies a blanching, maculopapular rash that begins on the head and then descends over the rest of the body. It can become confluent and fades in a cranial-to-caudal fashion, leaving behind desquamation and brownish discoloration that lasts 7–10 days.

Answer C is incorrect. Parvovirus B19 infection causes erythema infectiosum (fifth disease). The prodrome may include low-grade fever, headache, and symptoms of upper respiratory tract infection. There is a "slapped-cheek" erythematous rash on the face, which rapidly spreads as a diffuse, erythematous, maculopapular rash to the trunk and proximal extremities. There is then central clearing of the lesions, resulting in a lacy reticular rash. The rash worsens with fever, exposure to the sun, exercise, and/or stress.

Answer D is incorrect. Rubella causes an erythematous, tender, maculopapular rash that begins on the face and descends over the rest of the body. Tender cranial lymphadenopathy precedes the rash by at least 24 hours. The rash usually lasts 3 days but evolves rapidly. As it becomes visible on the trunk, it may have faded from the face. Discrete maculopapules and large areas of flushing are often present. The rash may coalesce, especially on the face, and may become pinpoint, especially on the trunk. There may be low-grade fever.

Answer E is incorrect. The prodromal stage of varicella (chickenpox) manifests with fever of 37.8–38.9°C (100–102°F), anorexia, malaise, and headache that occurs 24–48 hours before the rash. The rash begins on the scalp, face, or trunk, and spreads peripherally. It is a generalized, pruritic, macular rash that evolves into clear, fluid-filled, teardrop-shaped vesicles. The vesicles become cloudy and umbilicated and then crust over, and appear at different stages.

9. **The correct answer is B.** This child's presentation is characteristic for bronchiolitis. Acute bronchiolitis is commonly a viral disease with > 50% of cases being caused by respiratory syncytial virus. This patient has presented in respiratory distress with tachypnea (normal respiration rate for an infant of this age is 30–40/min) and nasal flaring. Bronchiolitis is generally self-limited, although in severe cases or in high-risk patients complications include apnea and severe respiratory distress, requiring hospitalization for further monitoring. Guidelines for hospitalization for infants with bronchiolitis are not fixed but usually include toxic appearance; oxygen saturation < 95%; atelectasis or consolidation on x-ray of the chest; tachypnea > 70/min or other signs of respiratory distress, such as nasal flaring, intercostal retraction, or cyanosis; and gestational age < 34 weeks or age < 3 months. Treatment is largely supportive because common interventions (e.g., epinephrine, bronchodilators, and corticosteroids) have not been proven effective in randomized controlled trials.

Answer A is incorrect. Because most cases of bronchiolitis are viral in nature, antibiotics have no role in the treatment of this condition. Given the ineffectiveness of antibiotics in this patient's condition in addition to her respiratory distress, the patient's release to home after antibiotic administration would be unwise.

Answer C is incorrect. Palivizumab (Synagis) is a monoclonal antibody to the respiratory syncytial virus (RSV) F protein that is given intramuscularly and is effective in preventing severe RSV disease. It is most effective when given to high-risk infants before and during the RSV season. Palivizumab should be given to children younger than 2 years of age with chronic lung disease (e.g., bronchopulmonary dysplasia) or prematurity. Although prophylactic administration of palivizumab would have been a reasonable action for this child prior to illness, administration during an acute illness is not recommended and release to home is not reasonable.

Answer D is incorrect. Respiratory syncytial virus intravenous immunoglobin (RSV-IVIG) is a pooled hyperimmune IVIG that is also effective in preventing severe RSV disease. Some studies have demonstrated an increase in mortality when given to symptomatic cyanotic congenital heart disease patients. Given her respiratory distress, release to home is not advisable.

Answer E is incorrect. X-ray of the chest would reveal hyperinflated lungs with patchy atelectasis. The WBC count and differential are usually normal in cases of bronchiolitis, and neither test would be definitive for a diagnosis or necessary for determining a course of treatment.

10. **The correct answer is E.** The patient has acute pseudomembranous candidiasis, which can be precipitated by changes in immune status, antibiotics, and abnormal glucose levels in diabetics. In the setting of abnormal blood sugars, thrush is likely to resolve with improved management of his blood sugars.

Answer A is incorrect. Amphotericin B is an effective antifungal, but it has several serious side effects such as nephrotoxicity, fever, and rigors, that reserve its use for more serious fungal infections.

Answer B is incorrect. This patient's blood sugar has been normalized and insulin levels adjusted. Adding sugar would actually feed the yeast, and create further instability of the blood sugar levels, further complicating this patient's thrush.

Answer C is incorrect. Mannitol is used as a diuretic, especially in the setting of increased intracranial pressure from cerebral edema, classically after traumatic head injury and associated epidural bleed.

Answer D is incorrect. While *Candida albicans* can be a normal inhabitant of the oral mucosa, the patient has an overgrowth of *C. albicans*, as evidenced by the abnormal white patches in his mouth.

11. **The correct answer is E.** The rash described is classic for a case of Lyme disease. Patients typically present in the early stage with erythema migrans with or without systemic symptoms, including fever, myalgia, malaise, and/or headache. Early-stage Lyme disease is treated with one of a number of antibiotics, including tetracycline, doxycycline, amoxicillin, and cefuroxime. Doxycycline (as well as other tetracyclines) should be avoided in children < 8 years old because of the risk that permanent tooth discoloration may occur.

Answer A is incorrect. Cartilage damage is an adverse effect associated with quinolones.

Answer B is incorrect. Ototoxicity is an adverse effect of aminoglycosides.

Answer C is incorrect. Red man syndrome is an adverse effect attributed to vancomycin.

Answer D is incorrect. Renal toxicity can be observed as an adverse effect of aminoglycosides and cyclosporine, among other drugs.

12. **The correct answer is C.** The American dog tick is one of the vectors for Rocky Mountain spotted fever (RMSF). RMSF classically has the rash described in the stem, starting on the hands and feet and spreading to the trunk.

Answer A is incorrect. Also transmitted by the dog tick, the presentation of ehrlichiosis is very similar to that of Rocky Mountain spotted fever, as it is transmitted by a dog tick bite and symptoms include high fever and headache. It rarely has a rash, however.

Answer B is incorrect. Lyme disease is transmitted by the deer tick or white-footed mouse tick and presents with fever, fatigue, and a erythema chronicum migrans, a target-like rash. Consider it in persons who have been camping or otherwise outdoors in Connecticut, even if they don't report a tick bite, as only a minority of patients give a history of tick bite.

Answer D is incorrect. There is no encephalitis in Rocky Mountain spotted fever. Tick-borne encephalitis is a viral (Flavivirus) disease carried by ticks that manifests as meningitis. There is no specific treatment for tick-borne encephalitis.

Answer E is incorrect. Tularemia is usually acquired by the handling of infected rabbits, and from the bites of ticks and deerflies. Initial presentation is an acute febrile illness that progresses to pneumonia, but it may also lead to pharyngitis, pleural effusion, hilar lymphadenopathy, and pneumonitis.

13. **The correct answer is A.** This vignette is a classic presentation of hand-foot-and-mouth disease caused by coxsackie A virus. Patients typically present with a mild illness that may or may not have the presence of fever. The oropharynx is inflamed, with vesicles scattered on the tongue, buccal mucosa, posterior pharynx, gums, palate, and lips. Hands and fingers, feet, buttocks, and groin may also demonstrate maculopapular, vesicular, or pustular lesions. Hands and fingers are affected more often than feet, and most commonly it is the dorsal surfaces that demonstrate the lesions of the disorder.

Answer B is incorrect. Human herpesvirus-6 is the virus associated with roseola infantum, which manifests with a prodrome of an acute-onset high fever (> 40°C [104°F]) preceding a maculopapular rash that appears as the fever breaks. The rash is classically described as manifesting on the trunk with a rapid spread to the face and extremities. There are no associated oropharynx lesions.

Answer C is incorrect. Paramyxovirus is responsible for measles, which presents with a low-grade fever prodrome with Cough, Coryza, and Conjunctivitis (the "**3 C's**") and later development of an erythematous, maculopapular rash that spreads from the head to the feet.

Answer D is incorrect. Parvovirus B19 is associated with erythema infectiosum (fifth disease), which manifests with a characteristic "slapped cheek" rash in addition to a pruritic, erythematous, maculopapular rash that manifests on the arms and spreads to the trunk and legs.

Answer E is incorrect. Varicella-zoster virus is responsible for causing varicella (chickenpox), characterized by the classical "teardrop" vesicular rash with vesicles in multiple stages of healing; the virus also causes zoster, which manifests with a pruritic "teardrop" vesicular rash distributed in a dermatomal fashion.

14. **The correct answer is E.** Tinea pedis (athlete's foot) is a common cutaneous fungal infection that is often acquired secondary to occlusive footwear. It is often transmitted in swimming pool and shower facility areas. Although rare in younger children, it is common in preadolescents and adolescents. The infection often affects the lateral toe webs and the subdigital crevices. A potassium hydroxide preparation will reveal branching hyphae. Treatment involves the application of topical antifungals.

Answer A is incorrect. Although contact dermatitis often presents as a localized pruritic rash, a potassium hydroxide preparation of scrapings from the lesion would not yield any findings.

Answer B is incorrect. This presentation is not consistent with hand-foot-and-mouth disease, which typically presents with constitutional symptoms and white-grey maculopapular vesicles with a characteristic peripheral distribution on the hands, feet, buttocks, and buccal mucosa/palate/tongue/tonsils (herpangina). Coxsackie A virus is the most common causative agent and would not be visible on a potassium hydroxide preparation.

Answer C is incorrect. Scabies (*Sarcoptes scabiei*) is a mite that burrows in the skin and causes characteristic pruritic lesions (small erythematous papules with excoriations and blood crusts). When the feet are affected, the scabies typically burrow on the lateral/posterior aspects of the feet. The diagnosis can be made by identifying mites or eggs in scrapings from the lesions. Treatment involves topical permethrin cream.

Answer D is incorrect. This presentation is not classic for Stevens-Johnson syndrome, which typically presents as a diffuse, desquamating rash (erythema multiforme) involving the mucous membranes and/or conjunctivae. In most cases, Stevens-Johnson syndrome is drug induced, although infection (especially in children) may also cause disease. A potassium hydroxide preparation of scrapings from the lesion would not yield any findings.

15. **The correct answer is D.** Otitis media (OM) is an infection of the middle ear. Children have a shorter, more horizontal eustachian tube than adults, which predisposes them to OM. The peak age range for OM is 6 to 18 months. The most common pathogens are *Streptococcus pneumoniae, Haemophilus influenzae,* and *Moraxella catarrhalis.* OM can also occur with viral infections. It may present with ear pain, hearing loss, and vertigo. On otoscopic examination, the tympanic membrane is erythematous due to inflammation and bulges due to fluid in the middle ear. Pneumatic otoscopy reveals an immobile tympanic membrane because the middle ear is filled with fluid instead of air. Swelling around the ear suggests that the mastoid is involved. Amoxicillin, a β-lactam, is the initial antimicrobial treatment of choice in acute OM. The usual course of treatment is 10 days. Even when treated with the appropriate antimicrobial therapy, fluid can still persist in the patient's ears for months. Other possible complications include perforation of the tympanic membrane from pressure of the fluid on the membrane, acute mastoiditis, petrositis, and labyrinthitis from contiguous spread of infection.

Answer A is incorrect. Observation is reserved for patients who are older than 2 years who have nonsevere illness and close follow-up. Antimicrobial therapy may then be initiated if the patients worsen or do not improve over 48 to 72 hours.

Answer B is incorrect. Myringotomy, with placement of tympanostomy tubes to drain middle ear fluid and prevent abscess formation, is reserved for treatment of chronic or recurrent acute otitis media.

Answer C is incorrect. The patient is not toxic appearing and does not have meningismus. Her fever can be explained by the acute OM. It is unlikely that she has meningitis, sepsis, or a more serious infection that would require referral to a tertiary care facility.

Answer E is incorrect. Signs of illness usually resolve in 24–48 hours with appropriate antimicrobial therapy. Amoxicillin-clavulanate is reserved for patients who fail to show improvement after 48–72 hours on amoxicillin therapy and still have symptoms.

Answer F is incorrect. Erythromycin plus sulfisoxazole is a macrolide combination used in patients who have had anaphylaxis or urticaria with previous β-lactam therapy.

16. **The correct answer is A.** Group B *Streptococcus* (GBS), or *Streptococcus agalactiae,* is part of the normal flora of the gut and vagina and can cause serious illness and sometimes death in infants that acquire the infection from their mother during childbirth. Therefore good prenatal care involves culturing mothers late in their pregnancies so they can be treated during labor if positive for the organism. Given the symptoms of the infant and the fact that the patient's mother received no prenatal care, the most likely diagnosis is group B streptococcal meningitis. Treatment is with intravenous penicillin.

Answer B is incorrect. *Haemophilus influenzae* is a gram-negative bacteria with most strains being opportunistic pathogens. *H. influenzae* type B (HIB) causes bacteremia and acute bacterial meningitis in infants and young children. Since 1990, the routine use of the HIB conjugate vaccine in the United States has decreased the incidence of invasive HIB disease significantly. Treatment involves antibiotics (ceftriaxone and chloramphenicol are effective) and often systemic steroids to minimize the complication of hearing loss.

Answer C is incorrect. Herpes simplex virus (HSV) is more likely to cause meningitis or encephalitis in older adult patients following primary genital HSV-2 infection. Infants can be at risk during labor and delivery if the mother has active lesions. There was no description of this on delivery in this case, making HSV meningitis less likely. Treatment is with acyclovir.

Answer D is incorrect. Tuberculosis can be a rare cause of meningitis, but is not likely to show up as being gram-positive as in this case.

Answer E is incorrect. *Neisseria meningitidis* is a gram-negative bacteria that can cause sepsis and meningitis. It is more likely in young adult patients who live in close quarters, such as college dorm residents and military recruits. Treatment is with intravenous penicillin.

Answer F is incorrect. *Streptococcus pneumoniae* is a more typical cause of meningitis in early childhood, the elderly, and immunocompromised patients. The patient in this case would be very young for this type of infection. Treatment of pneumococcal meningitis is with high-dose intravenous penicillin.

17. **The correct answer is E.** This patient was recently treated with outpatient antibiotics for pelvic inflammatory disease (PID). Given her immunocompromised state secondary to her diabetes mellitus, more aggressive treatment as an inpatient with intravenous antibiotics would have been more appropriate. It is most probable that this patient developed a tubo-ovarian abscess (TOA) as a result of her inadequately treated PID, which subsequently ruptured. Patients who have a TOA will often be febrile, nauseated, tachycardic, and complain of abdominal and pelvic pain.

Answer A is incorrect. Acute cholecystitis presents with fever and pain in the upper right quadrant of the abdomen, especially after fatty meals. However, this patient is presenting with lower abdominal pain and symptoms of septic shock, which would be uncommon in cholecystitis. Rupture of the gallbladder is possible with cholecystitis, and is more common in diabetic patients, but has not usually occurred at the time of initial development of cholecystitis symptoms.

Answer B is incorrect. Diabetic ketoacidosis (DKA) occurs in diabetics who have inadequate insulin levels or after a precipitating event such as an infection has led to a high-catecholamine state. Patients present with hyperglycemia, polydipsia, polyuria, abdominal pain, and lethargy. Fever would be unlikely to result purely from DKA; a fever could be caused by an underlying infectious precipitant such as pelvic inflammatory disease or TOA. Additionally, it would be expected for a patient in DKA to have urine positive for ketone bodies. Thus, while a TOA would make this diabetic patient at risk for DKA, it is unlikely that DKA is the primary cause of this patient's illness.

Answer C is incorrect. Reinfection from an untreated sexual partner is a significant risk after treatment for any sexually transmitted disease. However, this patient has symptoms of vasodilatory shock, which would be inconsistent with gonorrheal cervicitis.

Answer D is incorrect. Ruptured ectopic pregnancy often presents with vaginal bleeding, abdominal pain, and hypotension. However, this patient has a negative (-human chorionic gonadotropin test, indicating that she is not pregnant at this time. In addition, a ruptured ectopic pregnancy would present with hypovolemic shock and cool, clammy skin rather than vasodilatory shock with warm skin.

18. **The correct answer is D.** The constellation of this patient's symptoms, normal vaginal pH, and hyphae on potassium hydroxide preparation likely indicates that the patient has vaginal candidiasis, a fungus. Most antibiotics are not effective against fungus, which needs to be treated with antifungal medications. Because this is presumably her first infection by history, she may be treated with a single 150-mg dose of fluconazole, the drug of choice for uncomplicated vaginal candidiasis infections.

Answer A is incorrect. Azithromycin is a macrolide antibiotic that inhibits RNA synthesis by binding to the 50S ribosomal RNA subunit. It is used to treat *Chlamydia* infections but is not therapeutic for vaginal candidiasis.

Answer B is incorrect. Ciprofloxacin is a fluoroquinolone with a wide spectrum of antibiotic activity. It is a first-line agent for the treatment of gonorrhea but is not effective against *Candida*.

Answer C is incorrect. Clindamycin is a 50S ribosome inhibitor that is effective against gram-positive bacteria and many anaerobes. It is largely ineffective against gram-negative bacteria. It is used to treat bacterial vaginosis and has no activity against *Candida* species.

Answer E is incorrect. Metronidazole is an antibiotic effective in treating anaerobic bacteria and some protozoa. It is used to treat bacterial vaginosis and *Trichomonas* infections but is ineffective against *Candida*.

19. **The correct answer is D.** The child has measles, which present with a 3-day prodrome of low-grade fever; Cough, Coryza, Conjunctivitis (the "**3 C's**"); and Koplik's spots (small red spots with grey centers on the buccal mucosa), which last for 12–24 hours followed by an erythematous, blanching, maculopapular rash that begins on the face and then descends over the rest of the body. Complications include otitis media, pneumonia, laryngotracheitis, and rarely subacute sclerosing panencephalitis. Treatment of measles is supportive and mainly consists of antipyretics and hydration; however, unimmunized contacts should receive the measles-mumps-rubella vaccine to prevent the spread of the disease.

Answer A is incorrect. The diphtheria-tetanus-pertussis vaccine is an important standard childhood immunization. However, it does not need to be administered as soon as possible to the patient's sister.

Answer B is incorrect. The *Haemophilus influenzae* type b vaccine is another standard childhood immunization that children should receive. However, it does not need to be administered as soon as possible to the patient's sister.

Answer C is incorrect. The patient has measles; therefore, the influenza vaccine is not the vaccine that is needed as soon as possible.

Answer E is incorrect. Varicella is not usually associated with the "3 C's"; Koplik's spots; or high fever; thus, the varicella vaccine is not indicated at this time.

20. **The correct answer is A.** This patient suffers from isoniazid-induced hepatitis, a complication that has varying rates in different population groups but can be fatal. Treatment with isoniazid more commonly causes mild, asymptomatic hepatotoxicity characterized by minor elevations in transaminases (< 100 U/L). Active intravenous drug use (largely via viral hepatitis infection), as well as chronic alcohol use, increases the risk of developing symptomatic isoniazid-induced hepatitis. Each of the other answer choices decreases the risk for this complication. Also of note, isoniazid inhibits the cytochrome P450 hepatic enzyme system, thus increasing the effective serum concentrations of medications such as warfarin, phenytoin, theophylline, and carbamazepine.

Answer B is incorrect. Older age is associated with an increased rate of isoniazid-induced hepatitis.

Answer C is incorrect. Previous intolerance of isoniazid is associated with an increased rate of isoniazid-induced hepatitis.

Answer D is incorrect. Female gender is associated with an increased rate of isoniazid-induced hepatitis.

Answer E is incorrect. African-Americans experience increased rates of isoniazid-induced hepatitis.

21. **The correct answer is B.** The most serious complication of lumbar puncture is cerebral herniation. In patients with increased risk factors for herniation, cranial imaging in the form of a CT scan should be performed prior to lumbar puncture. These include patients suspected to have increased intracranial pressure (focal neurologic deficits or papilledema), patients with impaired cellular immunity, patients with altered mental status, and patients with recent seizures. MRI is another imaging option, but CT is most often performed due to the acuity of these situations.

Answer A is incorrect. Thrombolytic therapy (such as tissue plasminogen activator [t-PA]), if given within 3 hours of an ischemic stroke, greatly improves functional outcome. The patient's symptoms developed well over 3 hours ago. While all the patient's symptoms could indicate a cerebrovascular accident, the time course is not consistent with this diagnosis. Embolic and hemorrhagic stroke symptoms occur acutely, while ischemic stroke symptoms may occur over the course of a few hours or even a few days. However, stroke symptoms rarely develop over the course of weeks. Furthermore, t-PA should not be administered without cranial imaging to exclude hemorrhagic stroke. t-PA is strictly contraindicated for hemorrhagic strokes.

Answer C is incorrect. Urgent lumbar puncture and culture would be the test of choice for diagnosing bacterial, fungal, mycobacterial, or viral meningitis and is warranted in this immunocompromised patient, but lumbar puncture should await cranial imaging in patients with risk factors for herniation. Though this delays the lumbar puncture, medical treatment should not be withheld in cases with a high index of suspicion for infectious etiology.

Answer D is incorrect. Urgent lumbar puncture and India ink stain would be the quickest method for evaluating a patient for cryptococcal meningoencephalitis. It is most common in patients with AIDS with CD4+ counts < 100/mm^3. Symptoms (fever, malaise, and headache) are indolent and begin over the course of 1–2 weeks, consistent with this patient's presentation. However, given his immunocompromised state, a CT scan should be done prior to lumbar puncture to reduce the chances of herniation. While staining with India ink is highly suggestive of cryptococcal disease, definitive diagnosis is based on culture of organisms from cerebrospinal fluid.

Answer E is incorrect. A CT scan would be the first test in this patient, but further analysis of cerebrospinal fluid (CSF) from a lumbar puncture would be helpful in discerning the etiology of the patient's symptoms. Analysis of cells, protein, and glucose in CSF can narrow down the differential. The presence of WBCs is not specific for infection, but the absence of WBCs makes infection an unlikely diagnosis. The presence of RBCs could indicate subarachnoid hemorrhage (or a traumatic tap). A low CSF glucose supports the diagnosis of bacterial meningitis over viral meningitis. A high CSF protein suggests bacterial meningitis over viral meningitis. Finally, cytology can be sent if malignancy is suspected.

22. **The correct answer is C.** The documented decrease in life-threatening childhood infections is ample justification for routine immunizations. Several large studies have failed to find evidence that autism is increased in immunized children. The physician must ensure that a parent is well informed about the benefits of immunization.

Answer A is incorrect. Although it may seem that the physician is acting in the best interest of the child, it is the parents' right to withhold treatment that is not necessary in the immediate term to keep the child alive. Acting without the parent's consent is extremely unethical.

Answer B is incorrect. This is not an appropriate or effective response.

Answer D is incorrect. The court will not authorize forced immunization. Parents have the right to withhold treatment that is not necessary in the immediate term to keep the child alive.

Answer E is incorrect. Refusal to vaccinate a child does not fall under the category of child endangerment.

23. **The correct answer is B.** The commercially available Lyme vaccine prevents the development of Lyme disease in 49% of patients after one booster shot and in 76% after two boosters. The first booster should be administered at a 1-month follow-up appointment. The second may be administered between 2 and 12 months after the initial injection; it should be administered in April if at all possible. Other protective measures include protective clothing, insect repellant, and tick checks when in endemic areas.

Answer A is incorrect. Lyme disease is most common in the northeast United States, with 95% of cases reported in Massachusetts, Connecticut, Maine, New Hampshire, Rhode Island, New York, New Jersey, Pennsylvania, Delaware, Maryland, Michigan, and Wisconsin. Although Lyme disease has been reported in the western United States, avoidance of that area will obviously not minimize exposure to infected ticks in the northeast United States. Infections with high prevalence to the western

United States include coccidioidomycosis, hantavirus, and tularemia.

Answer C is incorrect. Lyme disease is caused by infection with the spirochete *Borrelia burgdorferi*, carried by the *Ixodes* tick. *Ixodes* ticks feed on mammals, predominantly the white-tailed deer, then wait on low-lying brush for another animal on which to feed. Spending time in forests or brush where white-tailed deer live increases one's chances of exposure to ticks, and therefore becoming infected with Lyme disease. There are no other proven modes of transmission, including human-to-human transmission.

Answer D is incorrect. Animal bites will not increase one's likelihood of contracting Lyme disease, as *Borrelia burgdorferi* is carried by infected ticks. A common infectious agent associated with animal bites is *Pasteurella multocida*. *Pasteurella* infections begin as erythema, swelling, and pain around the site of the bite, which progress proximally as the infection develops.

Answer E is incorrect. Antibiotics should only be used if there is evidence of a tick bite in an endemic area. The use of prophylactic antibiotics has not been shown to decrease the infection rate, and may contribute to antibiotic resistance.

24. **The correct answer is B.** Kawasaki's disease is an acute, febrile, multisystemic vasculitis that occurs predominantly in young children (80% of the cases are in children < 5 years old). It has a much higher incidence in Asians. The diagnostic criteria for Kawasaki's disease are fever for a minimum of 5 days and at least four of the following five signs: (1) bilateral nonexudative conjunctivitis, (2) a polymorphous nonvesicular rash that is primarily truncal, (3) cervical lymphadenopathy that is usually unilateral, (4) changes of the extremities (edema or erythema of the hands and feet and desquamation of the fingertips), and (5) mucous membrane changes (injected/fissured lips, injected oropharynx, and strawberry tongue [as shown in the image]).

Answer A is incorrect. Adenoviruses are responsible for a vast array of clinical syndromes including acute respiratory disease, conjunctivitis, myocarditis, gastrointestinal infections, hemorrhagic cystitis, and Reye's syndrome. Pharyngoconjunctival fever is a respiratory adenoviral infection which manifests with high fever for 4–5 days, pharyngitis, nonpurulent conjunctivitis, rhinitis, and lymphadenopathy. A rash may also be present.

Answer C is incorrect. Measles presents with a 3-day prodrome of low-grade fever, Cough, Coryza, Conjunctivitis (the "3C's") and Koplik's spots (small red spots with grey centers on the buccal mucosa) that last for 12–24 hours. The prodrome is followed by an erythematous, blanching, maculopapular rash that begins on the face, descends over the rest of the body, and rarely also involves the palms and soles.

Answer D is incorrect. Toxic shock syndrome is an acute desquamating disorder with multisystem involvement which typically presents with an abrupt onset of high fever, diarrhea, vomiting, pharyngitis, headache, and myalgias. A diffuse, erythematous, macular scarlatiniform rash that resembles sunburn appears within 24 hours, and can be subtle or fleeting but typically involves the hands and feet. There may be erythema of the pharynx, conjunctiva, and vaginal mucosa, and commonly a strawberry tongue.

Answer E is incorrect. Stevens-Johnson syndrome (SJS) is a blistering mucocutaneous syndrome that can be induced by drugs or infections. Drug-induced SJS usually manifests 1–3 weeks after the initiation of the drug, with fever and constitutional symptoms 1–3 days before the mucocutaneous lesions develop. These lesions include painful, confluent purpuric macules that progress to blisters and epidermal detachment. They are symmetrically distributed on the face and trunk with sparing of the scalp. There is mucosal erosion of at least two surfaces.

25. **The correct answer is E.** The recombinant immunoblot assay or polymerase chain reaction is used as a confirmatory test for persons whose blood tests are positive on the EIA. These tests have high specificities, or probability of a negative test in subjects without the disease, reducing most of the false-positive from

the initial EIA screen and thereby minimizing the chance that a hepatitis-free person will be erroneously informed that he or she is infected with hepatitis C.

Answer A is incorrect. Positive predictive value is the proportion of persons with a positive screening test result who are diseased.

Answer B is incorrect. Sensitivity is the proportion of diseased persons who have a positive test. If all patients with a given disease have a positive test, the test sensitivity is 100%. The EIA should approach high sensitivity to initially detect hepatitis C infection.

Answer C is incorrect. Although a high specificity on the screening test is not undesirable, it is far more important to optimize this test for maximum sensitivity to reduce the number of false-negatives.

Answer D is incorrect. Having a high sensitivity on the confirmatory test will not reduce the number of false positives because the ratio of false positives to genuinely uninfected patients is only affected by specificity.

26. **The correct answer is G.** The most likely diagnosis is *Pneumocystis carinii* pneumonia (PCP). *Pneumocystis carinii*, now renamed *Pneumocystis jiroveci*, is presently classified as a fungus. PCP occurs almost exclusively in the immune-compromised (primarily AIDS) population. The classic triad of nonproductive cough, fever, and exertional dyspnea is seen in about 50% of cases. Diagnosis is usually through imaging, either x-ray of the chest or CT of the chest when x-ray is inconclusive. The first-line chemotherapeutic and chemo-prophylactic agent is trimethoprim-sulfamethoxazole.

Answer A is incorrect. Amphotericin B is a potent antifungal with serious adverse effects that is used in the treatment of severe fungal disease. Amphotericin B functions by binding to membrane sterols in fungal cells, disrupting the membrane, and causing lysis.

Answer B is incorrect. *Pneumocystis carinii* pneumonia is caused by what is presently classified as a fungus. Ceftriaxone is a β-lactam class drug for use against bacterial infections.

Answer C is incorrect. Fluconazole is an antifungal used for mild fungal disease or meningitis. It can also be used for maintenance therapy. It acts through inhibition of the ergosterol synthesis pathway, as do all of the azoles.

Answer D is incorrect. Metronidazole is an antiprotozoal drug commonly used against flagellated protozoans. It works well against anaerobic bacteria, among others; however, trimethoprim-sulfamethoxazole is the first-line treatment for *Pneumocystis carinii* pneumonia. Metronidazole acts by disrupting the helical structure of DNA, causing it to fragment. It is metabolized into an active form by the enzyme ferredoxin in bacteria.

Answer E is incorrect. Nystatin swish and swallow is an antifungal predominantly used for oral candidal infections that appear as white plaques and occur primarily in the immune-compromised population. Nystatin acts by altering cell membrane permeability.

Answer F is incorrect. Pyrazinamide is used for treatment of tuberculosis (TB) in combination with isoniazid and rifampin. It acts through inhibition of fatty acid synthase I. TB classically presents as a prolonged cough associated with hemoptysis, fever, rigors, night sweats, and weight loss. TB usually occurs in a population with a history of exposure (i.e., those who live in endemic areas).

27. **The correct answer is E.** This patient is suffering from the effects of toxic shock syndrome (TSS), which is most often caused by *Streptococcus aureus* or group A streptococci. Factors that increase the risk of TSS include high-absorbency tampons and using a single tampon for multiple days. Nonmenstrual causes of TSS include a variety of infections, as well as both vaginal and cesarean childbirth. Symptoms of TSS include high fevers, headaches, gastrointestinal distress, neurologic symptoms, hypotension, and erythematous macular rash. Treatment is supportive, with admission to an intensive care unit, removal of any foreign material such as tampons, and pressure support with fluids and vasopressors as needed. There is no firm evidence supporting the use of antibiotics, intravenous immunoglobulin, or cor-

ticosteroids in TSS, although these treatment measures are often employed.

Answer A is incorrect. Although this patient is clearly at risk for alcohol poisoning as a result of binge drinking, her symptoms are worsening after several hours of abstinence from alcohol use. Although alcohol could account for her change in mental status, it would not be expected to cause a febrile illness or a diffuse erythematous rash.

Answer B is incorrect. Heatstroke is a condition in which the body's core temperature rises above 40.6°C (105°F), with associated neurologic dysfunction. Other findings in heatstroke include cutaneous vasodilation, disseminated intravascular coagulation, rhabdomyolysis, and seizures. Macular rash is not expected. Although this patient is febrile, her core body temperature does not meet the requirements for heatstroke.

Answer C is incorrect. *Neisseria* meningococcemia is another febrile illness that can rapidly progress to shock. However, it is usually accompanied by meningitis and meningeal signs such as photophobia and a stiff neck. In addition, the rash of meningococcemia is petechial, not diffuse and macular.

Answer D is incorrect. Rocky Mountain spotted fever (RMSF) is another febrile illness with a rapid course. However, in RMSF, the rash typically appears several days after the onset of the fever. In addition, the rash is petechial and begins at the distal extremities before moving centripetally.

28. **The correct answer is C.** This patient suffers from aminoglycoside nephrotoxicity secondary to treatment with gentamicin. Nephrotoxicity from aminoglycosides most commonly manifests as acute tubular necrosis, with toxic damage and death of the proximal tubule cells, resulting in exposed gaps and exposure of the basement membrane.

Answer A is incorrect. This choice describes a prerenal etiology of renal failure, which would result in a fractional excretion of sodium < 1%.

Answer B is incorrect. This choice describes the pathology of several renal diseases, including rapidly progressive glomerulonephritis and post-streptococcal glomerulonephritis, but it is not the mechanism behind aminoglycoside nephrotoxicity.

Answer D is incorrect. This choice describes the pathophysiology of membranoproliferative glomerulonephritis, which is typically idiopathic, autoimmune, or infectious in etiology.

Answer E is incorrect. This choice describes another prerenal etiology that would result in a fractional excretion of sodium < 1%. Renal arterial and arteriolar vasoconstriction occurs in hepatorenal syndrome and with medications such as nonsteroidal anti-inflammatories, but not with the use of aminoglycosides.

29. **The correct answer is A.** A more sensitive test will have a low false-negative ratio, calculated as the number of patients who test negative but have the disease, divided by the total number of patients with the disease. The false-negative ratio is equal to 1 − sensitivity. Negative predictive value (NPV) is calculated as the number of patients with the disease who test positive (which increases with sensitivity) over the total number of patients who test positive. A high NPV indicates that the patient with a negative test result has a very low likelihood of having the disease.

Answer B is incorrect. A more sensitive test will lower the false-negative ratio, since the false-negative ratio equals 1 − sensitivity. A higher positive predictive value (PPV) would be expected since a higher number of the diseased individuals would be detected with the test. A lower PPV would only be seen in that setting if the prevalence of the disease dropped very significantly.

Answer C is incorrect. Specificity is defined as the number of healthy individuals with a negative test result divided by the total number of healthy individuals. A specific test is good for ruling in. A highly specific test is a good confirmatory test. Consider that the equation for the false-positive ratio is 1 − specificity. A more specific (not sensitive) test will have fewer false-positive results. Thus, a positive result will be more meaningful (higher positive predictive value).

Answer D is incorrect. A more specific test will lower the false-positive ratio, since the false-positive ratio equals 1 − specificity. A higher negative predictive value (NPV) would be expected since more of the healthy individuals test negative. A lower NPV would only be seen in that setting if the prevalence of the disease increased very significantly.

Answer E is incorrect. Disease prevalence is not necessary to calculate either negative predictive value (NPV) or positive predictive value (PPV). However, for diseases with low prevalence, the NPV for a test will be higher, and for diseases with high prevalence, the PPV will be higher.

30. **The correct answer is A.** The patient described has cat scratch disease, caused by *Bartonella henselae*. Patients typically present after an incubation period of 7–12 days with one or more red papules at the site of inoculation. Lymphadenopathy often manifests after a period of 1–4 weeks. The patient's exposure to neighborhood cats should provide a hint to the diagnosis.

Answer B is incorrect. *Brucella* species are responsible for a variety of zoonotic diseases that cause a classic triad of fever, arthritis/arthralgia, and hepatosplenomegaly. They can be acquired from cattle, goats, sheep, swine, and dogs.

Answer C is incorrect. *Clostridium botulinum* is responsible for botulism, which results in a symmetric, descending, flaccid paralysis that can be life threatening if not diagnosed and treated promptly.

Answer D is incorrect. *Francisella tularensis* is the microorganism responsible for tularemia. This disease often manifests with lymphadenopathy and fever, with significant numbers of patients developing ulcers/eschars/papules, pharyngitis, myalgias, nausea/vomiting, and hepatosplenomegaly. *F. tularensis* may be transmitted by cat scratch or bite, although it is classically transmitted by handling rabbits. However, overall, tularemia is less common than cat scratch disease, so *F. tularensis* is less likely to be responsible for this infection. Serologic testing would be useful to rule out tularemia.

Answer E is incorrect. *Staphylococcus aureus* is responsible for large numbers of osteomyelitis and cellulitis cases, in addition to other infectious illnesses. However, it is not implicated commonly in cases of lymphadenopathy.

31. **The correct answer is C.** The disease is bacillary angiomatosis, caused by *Bartonella henselae* infection. It is caused by vascular proliferation and neutrophilic inflammatory response to the bacteria and can look similar to Kaposi's sarcoma. Biopsy of the lesions often shows tiny clumps of bacilli on Warthin-Starry silver stain, which are diagnostic. It can be treated with antibiotics; erythromycin and doxycycline are effective. For cutaneous bacillary angiomatosis, 2–4 months of therapy is recommended; if there are other manifestations, including osteomyelitis, splenitis, or endocarditis, therapy should be extended for 4–6 months.

Answer A is incorrect. Acyclovir is used to treat herpes zoster reactivation, commonly known as shingles, in HIV-positive patients. These lesions are not typical of shingles in that they cross the midline and occupy more than one dermatome.

Answer B is incorrect. Corticosteroids are not useful in *Bartonella* infection, which is causing this patient's bacillary angiomatosis. Also steroids should not be given to patients with compromised immune systems.

Answer D is incorrect. Ganciclovir is an antiviral medication effective against both herpes viruses and cytomegalovirus (CMV). CMV commonly causes ocular disease in immunocompromised patients, and rarely presents with only cutaneous manifestations.

Answer E is incorrect. Highly active antiretroviral therapy should be considered in eligible patients with CD4+ counts < 350/mm^3, and treatment with antiretroviral drugs can prevent bacillary angiomatosis. To treat bacillary angiomatosis, however, antibiotic therapy is needed.

32. **The correct answer is C.** In this untreated HIV-positive patient, it is important to rule out

cytomegalovirus (CMV) retinitis, as it can lead to blindness if left untreated. A polymerase chain reaction assay is the test of choice, as serologic tests could be unreliable in this patient. An ophthalmologic examination would reveal a "pizza-pie" pattern retinopathy with exudates and perivascular hemorrhage. Therapy for CMV retinitis consists of oral valganciclovir, intravenous ganciclovir, or intravenous foscarnet, with cidofovir as an alternative.

Answer A is incorrect. Blepharitis is infection of the eyelids, characterized by swelling, redness, and dry crusting, but it is not typically painful. Instead, it often presents with a foreign body sensation. Also, if left untreated, it will not lead to vision loss.

Answer B is incorrect. Conjunctivitis is characterized by discharge, irritation (but not frank pain), and itching.

Answer D is incorrect. Open-angle glaucoma is not an ophthalmologic emergency; acute closed-angle glaucoma is an emergency. Open-angle glaucoma has no symptoms in the early stages with a gradual loss of peripheral vision over a period of years resulting in tunnel vision.

33. **The correct answer is D.** This patient likely has pelvic inflammatory disease (PID). When pregnant, patients with PID are managed as inpatients. Empiric outpatient therapy for PID is recommended only when physical examination and risk factors are consistent with PID and a pregnancy test is negative. Therefore, a negative pregnancy test will cause the patient to meet this threshold. PID is rare in pregnancy, and thus a positive pregnancy test would cause the likelihood of PID to be much lower on the differential.

Answer A is incorrect. Diagnostic laparoscopy is useful in establishing a definitive diagnosis of PID. However, laparoscopy is specific but not sensitive for the diagnosis of PID. Laparoscopy is usually indicated in patients who remain symptomatic after treatment for PID or in whom another diagnosis, such as appendicitis, is likely.

Answer B is incorrect. DNA probes for *Chlamydia trachomatis* and *Neisseria gonor-*

rhoeae are useful as a confirmatory test for pelvic inflammatory disease. However, empiric therapy is often started before the results of these tests are available, and therefore they are rarely useful in guiding therapy.

Answer C is incorrect. Gram stain of cervical discharge is useful only when positive for *Neisseria gonorrhoeae*, which makes a diagnosis of PID significantly more likely. A negative test is not useful in ruling out PID.

Answer E is incorrect. WBC counts are of limited utility in the diagnosis of pelvic inflammatory disease, and would not be expected to change the management. The number of patients with the disease who manifest an increased WBC count is less than 50%.

34. **The correct answer is B.** Rifampin is a commonly employed anti-tuberculosis (TB) agent that is used in combination with isoniazid (for 6 months) and pyrazinamide (for the first 2 months) for treating TB. The multidrug approach is used to minimize the likelihood of development of secondary drug resistance during therapy. Adverse effects of rifampin include orange discoloration of the urine and tears, gastrointestinal disturbances, and hepatotoxicity, which often manifests as an asymptomatic elevation in transaminase levels.

Answer A is incorrect. Angioedema is not a recognized adverse reaction to rifampin.

Answer C is incorrect. Hyperuricemia is an adverse effect that is well recognized in adults taking pyrazinamide. In such patients, the increased uric acid levels often manifest as gout. Children on pyrazinamide who develop hyperuricemia are often asymptomatic. Other adverse effects of pyrazinamide include arthralgias and arthritis.

Answer D is incorrect. Peripheral neuritis is a principal toxic effect of isoniazid. Most commonly, it manifests as tingling or numbness in the hands or feet. Vitamin B6 (pyridoxine) is often administered concurrently to prevent the symptoms of peripheral neuropathy. It is important to mention that hepatotoxicity is also a common toxic effect of isoniazid.

Answer E is incorrect. Stevens-Johnson syndrome often occurs in the setting of beginning a new medication and results in a severe, desquamating rash (erythema multiforme) that involves the mucous membranes and/or conjunctiva. Although clinical responses to various drugs will differ and some patients may develop a mild rash or experience pruritus while taking rifampin, these are uncommon adverse effects and rarely progress to the severity of Stevens-Johnson syndrome. However, as with the initiation of any new medications, any change in the patient's condition, including the development of a rash, should be monitored and reported to the physician.

35. **The correct answer is D.** Exposure to bird and bat droppings or soil contaminated with bird or bat droppings is a well known cause of histoplasmosis. Histoplasmosis is also more common in the vast areas that drain into the Mississippi River. Histoplasmosis is an indolent fungal infection, and the acute lung form of the disease usually presents with chest pain, dyspnea, and dry cough. The chronic form of the disease usually occurs in those who already have lung disease and may present similarly to tuberculosis. Symptoms occur within 10 days of exposure. Immunocompromised patients may develop a potentially fatal disseminated form of the disease. Treatment is with ketoconazole or voriconazole. In disseminated disease, particularly meningitis, patients may be treated with intravenous amphotericin followed by long-term suppression with itraconazole.

Answer A is incorrect. Avoiding cigarette smoke will not reduce the risk of histoplasmosis infection.

Answer B is incorrect. Avoiding corn fields will not reduce the risk of histoplasmosis infection.

Answer C is incorrect. Avoiding swimming in public pools would not reduce the risk of histoplasmosis infection. There is no person-to-person transmission of the infecting agent, *Histoplasma capsulatum.*

Answer E is incorrect. Histoplasmosis is not common in Baltimore, so avoiding travel to Baltimore will not reduce the risk of infection.

36. **The correct answer is E.** The Argyll Robertson pupil in the presence of acute mania is the clinical finding suggestive of neurosyphilis in this patient. Other central nervous system manifestations, such as gait abnormalities (i.e., tabes dorsalis) are now rare. A remote history of sexually transmitted disease and a solitary presentation of a manic episode without a prior psychiatric history are also important in this case. Often patients may have been infected years earlier and only present to the physician during this stage of infection. Confirmation can be done with a Venereal Disease Research Laboratory test on the patient's cerebrospinal fluid.

Answer A is incorrect. Patients with *Chlamydia trachomatis* infections usually present with urethritis, epididymitis, and urethral discharge.

Answer B is incorrect. Herpes simplex virus can cause altered mental status, seizures, and meningitis in young children but is unlikely in an immune-competent adult host.

Answer C is incorrect. *Neisseria gonorrhoeae* may cause monarticular arthritis and genital symptoms, but is unlikely to result in acute psychiatric symptoms such as in this patient.

Answer D is incorrect. Toxoplasmosis is usually transmitted by contact with cat feces and is also unusual in an immune competent host.

37. **The correct answer is A.** Intravenous intrapartum ampicillin appears to prevent the colonization of infants whose mothers carry group B streptococci (GBS). GBS infection in the first month of life can present as fulminant sepsis, meningitis, or neonatal respiratory distress syndrome. This woman, who has not received prenatal care, may be one of the 5–25% of women who carry GBS as part of their normal vaginal flora and prophylaxis is indicated.

Answer B is incorrect. Doxycycline is contraindicated in pregnancy and during lactation, as it has a safety class rating D. It can cause permanent tooth staining.

Answer C is incorrect. Magnesium sulfate is useful to prevent seizures associated with preeclampsia. This patient has made it to 38 weeks of gestation without complications, and is currently in labor. Magnesium sulfate can also be used in tocolysis, but this patient is full-term at 38 weeks, and labor should be allowed to progress.

Answer D is incorrect. The patient is already in labor, so pitocin (oxytocin), normally used to induce or augment labor, has no role in this patient's empiric management. She may need it if labor fails to progress or if she has excessive postpartum bleeding.

Answer E is incorrect. Terbutaline is useful in tocolysis, but the infant is mature and its lungs have a sufficient amount of surfactant to sustain life; therefore, the pregnancy should be allowed to proceed.

38. **The correct answer is D.** *Salmonella* is the most common cause of osteomyelitis in patients with sickle cell disease. This patient's presentation is classic for a case of osteomyelitis with marked pain, erythema, edema, and the systemic manifestation of fever. The radiograph can show displacement of the deep muscle secondary to deep tissue edema. Lytic bone lesions do not commonly manifest on plain films until 30–50% of the bone matrix is destroyed.

    Answer A is incorrect. *Escherichia coli* is not a commonly acknowledged cause of osteomyelitis in any patient population.

    Answer B is incorrect. *Haemophilus influenzae* type B was responsible for > 50% of all cases of bacterial arthritis in infants before universal vaccination was implemented. It is no longer a common cause of bacterial arthritis or osteomyelitis.

    Answer C is incorrect. *Mycoplasma* is also not recognized as a cause of osteomyelitis.

    Answer E is incorrect. Although *Staphylococcus aureus* is the organism most commonly implicated in cases of osteomyelitis in healthy patients in all age groups, the fact that this patient has sickle cell makes him acutely sensitive to *Salmonella* infection.

39. **The correct answer is B.** Oral candidiasis most often presents as white patches in the oral mucosa. Candidiasis is present only in the immunocompromised, which would make HIV the most likely comorbidity in this case. Treatment is usually simple nystatin swish and swallow. Prognosis is excellent and candidal thrush usually resolves without complications as long as the condition is appropriately diagnosed and treated.

    Answer A is incorrect. Candidal esophagitis is not associated with cardiac chest pain. Both may present with chest pain, but the history states that the patient's chest pain is retrosternal and worse with swallowing, suggesting esophagitis. No other symptoms are suggestive of cardiac chest pain.

    Answer C is incorrect. Mallory-Weiss tear is a condition producing hematemesis following esophageal mucosal tear. It is predisposed by vomiting, coughing, and retching. It is certainly in the differential for esophagitis, but it is not the correct answer here.

    Answer D is incorrect. Candidiasis does not infect the esophagus in immunocompetent hosts.

    Answer E is incorrect. Severe combined immunodeficiency syndrome (SCID) is a condition in which children have a total deficiency of T and B lymphocytes, resulting in immunocompromise from birth. This patient could have SCID; however, this condition is less likely than HIV and would have affected the patient from birth.

    Answer F is incorrect. Candidal esophagitis and vaginal candidiasis are separate entities. The former is seen only in immunocompromised hosts, while the latter can be seen in healthy females.

40. **The correct answer is E.** Bacterial tracheitis is an acute bacterial infection of the upper airway that can cause a potentially fatal airway obstruction. The condition affects patients who are generally < 3 years old and is often seen in the setting of a recent viral respiratory infection. Bacterial tracheitis is characterized by a brassy cough with high fever and possible respiratory distress. Treatments aimed at croup (mist and racemic epinephrine) are ineffective against bacterial tracheitis. The most common pathogen responsible for bacterial tracheitis is *Staphylococcus aureus*.

Answer A is incorrect. Anaerobic organisms are grouped with *Moraxella catarrhalis* and nontypeable *Haemophilus influenzae* as significant contributors to cases of bacterial tracheitis, but all three pathogens are less common than *Staphylococcus aureus*.

Answer B is incorrect. *Moraxella catarrhalis* is a pathogen commonly associated with bacterial tracheitis but is not as common a cause of the condition as *Staphylococcus aureus*.

Answer C is incorrect. Nontypeable *Haemophilus influenzae* has also been associated with bacterial tracheitis cases but trails behind *Staphylococcus aureus* as the most common cause of the condition.

Answer D is incorrect. *Pseudomonas aeruginosa* is largely implicated in ventilator-associated pneumonias, central nervous system infections, osteomyelitis/septic arthritis, urinary tract infections, and primary and secondary skin infections. However, it is not a common pathogen in cases of bacterial tracheitis.

41. **The correct answer is C.** The patient described in the vignette has chronic granulomatous disease (CGD). Although the presentation of CGD is variable, the diagnosis should be suspected in patients with recurrent lymphadenitis, multiple-site osteomyelitis, cutaneous abscesses (confused with "acne"), hepatic abscesses, a family history of recurrent infections, or unusual infections with catalase-positive organisms such as *Staphylococcus aureus* or *Aspergillus*. In many of these cases, the patient is asymptomatic or with much fewer signs and symptoms (e.g., lack of fever) than would otherwise be expected given the infectious burden. The disease is caused by mutations in genes encoding proteins involved in generating a respiratory burst. One of these, *phox91*, is on the X chromosome, providing an X-linked pattern of inheritance as demonstrated by the family history.

Answer A is incorrect. Ataxia-telangiectasia is a T-lymphocyte disorder that manifests as oculocutaneous telangiectasias and progressive cerebellar ataxia. It is caused by a DNA repair defect resulting from a mutation in the ATM gene encoding a protein critical for repair of DNA breaks. Ataxia generally begins when the child learns to walk, and the telangiectasias generally become apparent between 3 and 6 years of age.

Answer B is incorrect. Chédiak-Higashi syndrome includes neutropenia, neuropathy, and oculocutaneous albinism. It is inherited in an autosomal-recessive manner. The disorder is caused by a defect in neutrophil chemotaxis resulting from mutations in the *LYST* gene required for sorting of lysosomal granule contents. Patients have albinism due to abnormal melanosomes and inappropriate delivery of melanin in the skin.

Answer D is incorrect. Hyper IgE syndrome (HIES) is characterized by recurrent bacterial infection and cavitating pneumonia. It is typically associated with impaired inflammation giving rise to so-called "cold abscesses." Although abscesses are found in HIES, granulomas are generally not. Furthermore, HIES occurs in an autosomal dominant or autosomal recessive pattern of inheritance and not in the X-linked pattern suggested by the case history.

Answer E is incorrect. Wiskott-Aldrich syndrome is an X-linked disorder with B- and T-lymphocyte dysfunction. Affected patients typically present with eczema and thrombocytopenia. Although patients have abnormalities of their skin, these are heralded by petechiae (from the thrombocytopenia) and eczema. The disease results from mutations of the Wiskott-Aldrich syndrome protein (WASp) gene on the X chromosome. WASp is important for rearranging the actin cytoskeleton in immune cells and thus enables responsiveness.

42. **The correct answer is C.** The history is typical of disseminated Lyme disease. After the acute phase of the illness, cardiac, neurologic, and musculoskeletal symptoms become prominent. Typical cardiac symptoms include fluctuating second- or third-degree atrioventricular block, which resolves completely after a few weeks, and myocarditis. Neurologic complaints can include meningitis, cranial neuritis, and rarely, encephalitis. Musculoskeletal symptoms include intermittent joint swelling and sometimes chronic arthritis.

Answer A is incorrect. Gonococcal disease can cause joint swelling, but the cardiac and neurologic symptoms are not commonly caused by *Neisseria gonorrhoeae.*

Answer B is incorrect. Gout can cause joint pain and swelling, but the neurologic and cardiac symptoms cannot be attributed to gout. Also, the patient is not in a demographic group in which gout is usually seen; she is too young.

Answer D is incorrect. The headaches are not typical of migraines. They have an acute onset and last longer than typical migraines, fluctuating throughout the day, rather than being steadily progressive and then resolving. Also, the muscle aches and arrhythmia are not associated with migraines.

Answer E is incorrect. Sjögren's syndrome is possible, but again, the recent travel to an endemic area and the time course of the symptoms makes Lyme disease the more likely diagnosis.

Answer F is incorrect. While the patient's symptoms could be caused by systemic lupus erythematosus, the recent travel to an area endemic for Lyme disease and the time course of the symptoms makes it the more likely diagnosis.

43. **The correct answer is E.** Patients with silicosis are particularly susceptible to tuberculosis infection, and the risk increases with increasing lung dust burden. In one study, miners with silicosis were 30 times more likely to be infected with tuberculosis than miners without diagnosable silicosis. Regular tuberculin screening is especially important for patients with silicosis.

Answer A is incorrect. Asbestos exposure can lead to bronchogenic carcinoma and malignant mesothelioma, and the risk of cancer is further increased in smokers.

Answer B is incorrect. Beryllium inhalation causes berylliosis, which does not increase the risk of tuberculosis infection.

Answer C is incorrect. Exposure to carbon dust causes anthracosis, a usually harmless pigmentation of the lungs noted at autopsy among city dwellers and, to a much greater extent, in smokers.

Answer D is incorrect. Coal workers' pneumoconiosis results from coal dust inhalation and is not linked to an increased risk of tuberculosis. Coal dust contains both carbon and silica and causes more cellular reaction (and thus more pathology) than carbon dust alone.

44. **The correct answer is D.** Patients who are functionally asplenic, like patients with sickle cell anemia, are at increased risk for infection with encapsulated organisms, including *Streptococcus pneumoniae, Neisseria meningitidis,* and *Haemophilus influenzae.* This is because the spleen is responsible for processing foreign material to stimulate production of opsonizing antibodies important for the clearance of encapsulated organisms. In addition, the splenic macrophages are responsible for phagocytosing bacteria and for the removal of aged blood cells (therefore an asplenic patient would be expected to have Howell-Jolly bodies, which are nuclear remnants in old RBCs, on a peripheral blood smear).

Answer A is incorrect. *Chlamydia trachomatis* is a small gram-negative rod that is also an obligate intracellular organism. It not an encapsulated organism.

Answer B is incorrect. *Escherichia coli* is gram-negative rod. It not an encapsulated organism.

Answer C is incorrect. *Staphylococcus aureus* is gram-positive coccus. It not encapsulated.

Answer E is incorrect. Viridans streptococcus is a gram-positive coccus. It not an encapsulated organism, and therefore does not pose an increased risk of infection in people with sickle cell disease.

45. **The correct answer is B.** Streptococcal pneumonia is the most common cause of community-acquired pneumonia in this age group. In those over 40 years of age, the most common causes are *Streptococcus pneumoniae, Haemophilus influenzae,* anaerobes, viruses, and *Mycoplasma* spp. Streptococcal pneumonia causes a lobar pneumonia, but diagnosis cannot be made on radiographic findings alone. Diagnosis depends on sputum Gram stain and culture. Macrolides (erythromycin and clarithromycin) are first-line empiric treatment for

unidentified community-acquired pneumonia, but in this patient with rapid-onset symptoms and lobar consolidation characteristic of pneumococcal infection, oral ampicillin would be used in penicillin-sensitive strains. If the strain is resistant to penicillin, a β-lactam (such as ceftriaxone) can be used.

Answer A is incorrect. Aztreonam is ineffective against the gram-positives and would be ineffective against streptococcal pneumonia. Aztreonam is a monobactam used against gram-negative bacteria, and is indicated in hospital-acquired pneumonia.

Answer C is incorrect. Doxycycline is mostly used for *Chlamydia pneumoniae*, *Mycoplasma pneumoniae*, *Rickettsia*, and *Brucella*. Patients affected by these microbes are relatively asymptomatic and disease usually manifests as gradual onset of headache, malaise, and low-grade fever. *M. pneumoniae* is most common in school-aged children, military recruits, and college students in fall and winter. *C. pneumoniae* is most common in elderly patients. Azithromycin and erythromycin are commonly used for atypical pneumonia and would cover *Streptococcus pneumoniae* as well. Doxycycline can be used for atypical pneumonia but would not cover *S. pneumoniae*.

Answer D is incorrect. Gentamicin is effective against gram-negatives and even covers pseudomonads; it is usually combined with a penicillin-based drug for broader-spectrum coverage. Gentamicin is used for treatment of pneumonia when *Staphylococcus aureus* is isolated. *S. aureus* is easy to grow in culture, but oftentimes represents contamination.

Answer E is incorrect. Metronidazole is used as an alternative regimen for pneumonia caused by anaerobes such as *Bacteroides fragilis*, *Peptostreptococcus*, and *Fusobacterium* (first-line therapy is clindamycin or amoxicillin-clavulanate). These agents are more commonly indicated in aspiration pneumonia caused by anaerobes that are part of the normal flora of the mouth and nasopharynx. Aspiration pneumonia is most common in patients with decreased consciousness and those with dysphagia due to neurologic deficits or upper gastrointestinal disorders. Patients present with

typical symptoms of cough, fever, purulent sputum, and dyspnea that occurs over days to weeks (instead of hours). Sputum is characteristically putrid.

46. **The correct answer is A.** Chickenpox (varicella) is an acute febrile illness associated with a rash that is common in children who have not been immunized. The illness has a wide spectrum of clinical severity but is generally self-limited. The prodromal phase often consists of fever, malaise, headache, and anorexia, which usually manifest 1–2 days before the outbreak of the rash. The rash of varicella often first appears on the scalp, face, and trunk. Pruritic erythematous macules comprise the primary exanthem, with progression through the papular stage to form clear, fluid-filled vesicles. New areas of lesions develop while initial lesions are crusting. The characteristic rash of varicella has lesions in multiple stages of evolution as opposed to smallpox, in which all lesions advance through development at the same rate.

Answer B is incorrect. This presentation is not consistent with contact dermatitis, which is typically pruritic, has a pattern that suggests external causes (i.e., a linear distribution), and does not have an associated viral prodrome. An inciting exposure can usually be identified.

Answer C is incorrect. This presentation is not consistent with hand-foot-and-mouth disease, which typically presents with fever and constitutional symptoms, and then as white-grey maculopapular vesicles with a characteristic peripheral distribution on the hands, feet, buttocks, and buccal mucosa/palate/tongue/tonsils (herpangina). Coxsackie A virus is the most common causative agent.

Answer D is incorrect. This presentation is not normal for herpes zoster, which typically presents as vesicular lesions distributed along a dermatome, usually in patients who are immunocompromised or elderly. Herpes zoster occurs after reactivation of latent virus in the dorsal root ganglia.

Answer E is incorrect. This presentation is not consistent with smallpox infection (variola major), which typically presents as a confluent rash with discrete, firm vesicles and nodules that are characteristically all at the same stage of development.

Answer F is incorrect. This presentation is not classic for Stevens-Johnson syndrome, which typically presents as a diffuse, desquamating rash (erythema multiforme) involving the mucous membranes and/or conjunctiva. In most cases, Stevens-Johnson syndrome is drug induced, although infection (especially in children) may also cause disease.

47. **The correct answer is C.** The patient has herpes simplex virus encephalitis, characterized by bizarre behavior, hypersexuality, fever, and aseptic cerebrospinal fluid. He should be started on intravenous acyclovir after diagnosis is confirmed with a cerebrospinal herpes simplex virus DNA polymerase chain reaction.

Answer A is incorrect. The presence of WBCs in the patient's cerebrospinal fluid is not consistent with alcohol intoxication.

Answer B is incorrect. This case is inconsistent with a large stroke that could be visualized on CT scan of the head. Instead, the patient may have had a frontal lobe stroke or be experiencing multi-infarct dementia, but this does not explain the WBCs in the patient's cerebrospinal fluid.

Answer D is incorrect. The patient is not quite old enough or sick enough to be at a high risk of developing urosepsis. Urosepsis also does not cause appearance of WBCs in the cerebrospinal fluid.

Answer E is incorrect. This could be hydrocephalus; however, the onset is too acute, and WBCs should not be in the cerebrospinal fluid (CSF) with hydrocephalus. The patient is also not in a high-risk demographic. Hydrocephalus is an increase in the volume of CSF within the central nervous system. Symptoms of hydrocephalus in the adult population include cognitive disturbances, headaches, nausea, difficulty walking, blurred vision, and incontinence. Definitive treatment is usually surgical, with shunt placement required in all but 25% of cases.

48. **The correct answer is B.** Kaposi's sarcoma (KS) is a low-grade vascular tumor associated with infection by human herpesvirus 8. There are four forms of KS, but the one most common in HIV-positive patients is AIDS-related Kaposi's sarcoma, an opportunistic infection that afflicts patients with AIDS 20,000 times more commonly than the U.S. population in general. Cutaneous involvement is common, but the disease can cause extracutaneous manifestations, including disease in the oral cavity, gastrointestinal tract, and the respiratory tract. The lesion depicted here is classic for KS. The development and progression of KS can be halted with highly active antiretroviral therapy.

Answer A is incorrect. Dapsone is an alternative drug for prophylaxis of *Pneumocystis jiroveci* pneumonia, given as second-line therapy to patients allergic to sulfa drugs.

Answer C is incorrect. Trimethoprim-sulfamethoxazole is useful in prophylaxis of *Pneumocystis jiroveci* pneumonia, but will not prevent Kaposi's sarcoma.

Answer D is incorrect. Zidovudine/lamivudine combination therapy can be a useful part of a highly active antiretroviral therapy regimen, but they would not be recommended without a third antiretroviral drug.

Answer E is incorrect. Zidovudine, or AZT, was the first available antiretroviral drug, but current recommendations do not advise monotherapy with AZT for Kaposi's sarcoma.

49. **The correct answer is C.** Lymphogranuloma venereum is caused by *Chlamydia trachomatis* serotypes L1, L2, and L3. It is uncommon in the United States, but is endemic in parts of East and West Africa, India, Southwest Asia, and the Caribbean. HIV seropositivity is the strongest risk factor. Primary infection with lymphogranuloma venereum is characterized by a genital ulcer that heals within a few days. Inguinal lymphadenopathy occurs 2–6 weeks later, and represents direct extension of the infection to inguinal lymph nodes. Diagnosis is usually made through serologic testing in the setting of a compatible clinical scenario. Doxycycline is the recommended therapy for both

lymphogranuloma venereum and other sero-types of *Chlamydia trachomatis*.

Answer A is incorrect. Acyclovir is an antiviral therapy, and is the treatment of choice for genital herpes. Herpes is characterized by painful genital ulcers and is diagnosed using polymerase chain reaction testing of the ulcerated tissue.

Answer B is incorrect. Ceftriaxone is the recommended treatment for gonorrhea. In women, gonorrhea is often asymptomatic, but it may present as vaginal pruritus with a mucopurulent discharge. If left untreated, gonorrhea may develop into pelvic inflammatory disease and concomitant infertility.

Answer D is incorrect. Gentamicin is an aminoglycoside associated with nephrotoxicity and ototoxicity. Doxycycline is a safer therapy for lymphogranuloma venereum.

Answer E is incorrect. Penicillin remains the standard of care for syphilis. The clinical presentation of syphilis begins as a painless chancre in the primary infection, later progressing to a systemic infection that includes a maculopapular rash involving the palms and soles, raised white-grey lesions of the mucous membranes termed condyloma lata, and diffuse lymphadenopathy. Later stages of syphilis include cardiac and neurologic manifestations if left untreated.

50. **The correct answer is F.** This patient most likely suffers from osteomyelitis. Plain radiographs of osteomyelitis may show destructive changes, osteosclerosis, periosteal new bone formation, and occasional fracture. For patients with osteomyelitis due to trauma, *Staphylococcus aureus*, coliform bacilli, and *Pseudomonas aeruginosa* are the primary infecting agents. Nafcillin and gentamicin will be effective against *S. aureus* as well as *P. aeruginosa*. Vancomycin and antipseudomonal third-generation cephalosporins (e.g., carbenicillin, piperacillin, and ticarcillin) will also be effective.

Answer A is incorrect. Ampicillins are anti-enterococcal and are effective against organisms such as *Escherichia coli* and *Salmonella*, but they are ineffective against *Pseudomonas aeruginosa*, which is one of the likely infecting organisms in osteomyelitis due to trauma.

Answer B is incorrect. Aztreonam is effective against *Pseudomonas aeruginosa*, but has no activity against *Staphylococcus aureus*, one likely infecting organism in this case of osteomyelitis due to trauma.

Answer C is incorrect. Ciprofloxacin use is no longer encouraged in cases of *Staphylococcus aureus* infection, due to a rapidly increasing incidence of resistance. *S. aureus* is a likely infecting organism in this case of osteomyelitis due to trauma.

Answer D is incorrect. Methicillin is effective against *Staphylococcus aureus*, but it has a narrow spectrum and will not cover *Pseudomonas aeruginosa*, a likely infecting organism in this case of osteomyelitis due to trauma.

Answer E is incorrect. Nafcillin can cover *Staphylococcus aureus*, but it has a narrow spectrum and will not cover *Pseudomonas aeruginosa*, which are the likely infecting organisms in osteomyelitis due to trauma.

51. **The correct answer is C.** The **ToRCHes** infections include **To**xoplasmosis, **R**ubella, **C**ytomegalovirus, **H**erpes simplex virus/HIV, and **S**yphilis. Infections in utero or during birth are associated with significant fetal and neonatal morbidity and mortality. These infections have been grouped together because they feature similar presentations, including a rash and ocular findings. The American College of Obstetricians and Gynecologists currently recommends that rubella and syphilis serologies be checked during the first prenatal visit.

Answer A is incorrect. Cytomegalovirus is not routinely checked during prenatal visits.

Answer B is incorrect. Cytomegalovirus is not routinely checked during prenatal visits.

Answer D is incorrect. The utility of checking the ToRCHeS titers during routine prenatal care has not been cost effective in controlled studies. Diagnosis is more accurately made with rubella and syphilis titers, cytomegalovirus urine cultures, and fetal ultrasound.

Answer E is incorrect. Toxoplasmosis is not routinely checked during prenatal visits.

Answer F is incorrect. Toxoplasmosis is not routinely checked during prenatal visits.

52. **The correct answer is A.** The patient's symptoms are characteristic of secondary Lyme disease, which results when Lyme disease is not treated promptly with antibiotics. Lyme disease is caused the spirochete *Borrelia burgdorferi* and is treated with amoxicillin and doxycycline as first-line agents.

Answer B is incorrect. The patient's neurologic symptoms argue against an isolated musculoskeletal process.

Answer C is incorrect. The patient's duration of symptoms is not consistent with meningitis, which would be more likely in a patient with photophobia, changes in mental status, and nuchal rigidity.

Answer D is incorrect. The patient's illness is not caused by a sexually transmitted infection, which would probably present with a penile discharge or genital pain/pruritus, depending on its etiology.

Answer E is incorrect. The patient's symptoms haven't resolved over a year. This is Lyme disease, which can progress further without treatment.

53. **The correct answer is E.** Pain elicited by gently pushing/pulling the pinna is classic for otitis externa. In diabetic patients, otitis externa is usually due to *Pseudomonas*, and can be chronic in patients with seborrhea. The treatment of choice is antibiotic ear drops.

Answer A is incorrect. CT is a relatively costly test that may do nothing to alter the treatment plan. The patient is afebrile, and it is unlikely that the infection has spread into the bone to become osteomyelitis.

Answer B is incorrect. Naegleria fowleri is an unrelated infection in which people swimming in colonized ponds get a cerebral infection via the nose. It can be fatal after about a week.

Answer C is incorrect. MRI is a fairly costly test that may do nothing to alter the treatment

plan. The patient is afebrile, and it is unlikely that the infection has spread past the external ear. If osteomyelitis (malignant otitis externa) was suspected an imaging study would be appropriate.

Answer D is incorrect. Surgical debridement would only be necessary if the patient had malignant otitis externa. Malignant otitis externa is almost exclusively seen in immunocompromised patients. If this patient had a fever or signs of systemic toxicity, then more concern would be raised, and further investigation would be warranted.

54. **The correct answer is D.** This patient likely has *Trichomonas* infection. This is distinguished from candidiasis by the lack of hyphae on the KOH prep and increased pH of the vaginal fluid. The disease classically "bounces" between partners as they reinfect each other, making treatment of the partner simultaneously an important aspect of management.

Answer A is incorrect. As a minor seeing her physician for a sexually transmitted disease (STD), the patient has the right to confidentiality. However, fully educating the patient about effective strategies for STD and pregnancy prevention, including abstinence, would be appropriate.

Answer B is incorrect. This is not necessary for effective treatment.

Answer C is incorrect. Reportable sexually transmitted diseases are chlamydia, gonorrhea, and syphilis. The patient may have one of these conditions and should be tested for them, but *Trichomonas* is not necessary to report per se.

Answer E is incorrect. Candida infection can be a presenting symptom of diabetes. However, the lack of hyphae in the vaginal discharge makes this diagnosis unlikely.

55. **The correct answer is D.** The majority of postinfectious neutropenic patients will experience only a transient neutropenia and will recover without infection or specific therapy.

Answer A is incorrect. Empiric antibiotics are seldom indicated in neutropenic patients unless they have neutropenia and a fever of greater than 38°C (100.4°F).

Answer B is incorrect. Granulocyte transfusions are indicated for patients with gram-negative sepsis who have not shown a clinical response to antibiotics within 48 hours of t reatment. Granulocyte colony-stimulating factor is often used in place of granulocyte transfusions in patients capable of making granulocytes.

Answer C is incorrect. In cases of severe neutropenia, granulocyte colony-stimulating factor has been shown to increase absolute neutrophil counts, but this should be reserved for patients at high risk for infection, such as patients with bone marrow disorders or those undergoing chemotherapy. Patients with postinfectious neutropenia are seldom at such a risk.

Questions 56–58

56. **The correct answer is E.** Rocky Mountain spotted fever (RMSF) is caused by infection with *Rickettsia rickettsii*, an organism carried by the American dog tick. Patients such as the one in this case, who have exposure to the wilderness and tick bites in the mid-atlantic region, are at highest risk of infection. RMSF is characterized by a rash that begins on the wrists and ankles and spreads centrally. Headache, fever, and malaise can also be present along with disseminated intravascular coagulation or altered mental status in severe cases. Treatment should be initiated as soon as possible with doxycycline, even in younger populations, since the condition is rapidly fatal if untreated. Short courses of doxycycline to treat RMSF do not cause significant dental staining.

57. **The correct answer is I.** Roseola, also called sixth disease, is caused by human herpesvirus 6. It usually affects children from 6 months to 3 years of age and manifests as a rosy rash after 3 days of high fevers. It is a self-limited disease requiring no treatment.

58. **The correct answer is J.** Scarlet fever is caused by group A β-hemolytic streptococci and can occur if streptococcal pharyngitis is left untreated. It is characterized by findings such as strawberry tongue and a sandpaper-like rash on the trunk which desquamates after a few days. Treatment is with penicillin to prevent rheumatic fever and its complications which can include irreversible damage to the heart and its valves.

Answer A is incorrect. Acyclovir is an antiviral agent which preferentially inhibits viral DNA polymerase. It is most effective against herpes simplex virus (mucocutaneous and genital herpes lesions), but is also effective against varicella-zoster virus and Epstein-Barr virus.

Answer B is incorrect. Amantadine was initially developed to treat Parkinson's disease, but was found to have antiviral activity and is used for prophylaxis of influenza A. It works by blocking viral penetration and uncoating but has a lot of unwanted side effects including ataxia, slurred speech, and depression, since it can cross the blood-brain barrier.

Answer C is incorrect. Amphotericin B is an antifungal agent used in treatment of a wide spectrum of systemic mycoses. It binds ergosterol, a compound unique to fungi, and forms pores that allow leakage of electrolytes.

Answer D is incorrect. Dapsone inhibits bacterial synthesis of dihydrofolic acid and is used in the treatment of leprosy and other skin conditions. It is also sometimes used as prophylaxis against *Pneumocystis jiroveci* pneumonia in patients with HIV (if trimethoprim-sulfamethoxazole is not tolerated) and to treat idiopathic thrombocytopenic purpura.

Answer F is incorrect. Foscarnet inhibits the pyrophosphate binding site on viral DNA polymerases and is used in the treatment of herpes simplex virus (HSV)-1 and HSV-2 and cytomegalovirus retinitis.

Answer G is incorrect. Fluconazole is an antifungal which inhibits the synthesis of ergosterol. It is used in treatment of systemic mycoses including cryptococcal meningitis in AIDS patients and candidal infections (oral thrush and yeast infections).

Answer H is incorrect. Gentamicin is an aminoglycoside, a bactericidal class of antibiotics that inhibits the initiation complex, thereby causing misreading of mRNA transcripts. It is used for treatment of severe gram-negative rod infections along with β-lactam antibiotics, which help break down the cell walls, allowing the aminoglycoside to be effective.

Questions 59–61

59. **The correct answer is H.** Sexually transmitted disease with septic monarthritis is gonorrhea until proven otherwise. Gonorrhea typically presents with urethral discomfort, dysuria, and discharge. Risk factors include unprotected sex with multiple partners. It is treated by antibiotics such as third-generation cephalosporins or ciprofloxacin and usually fully resolves with treatment.

60. **The correct answer is B.** Nongonococcal urethritis comprises the most common sexually transmitted diseases. Because the Gram stain does not show the presence of gonorrhea, chlamydia remains the most likely cause. Although chlamydia can present asymptomatically, it can also present as dysuria, urethral discomfort, discharge, scrotal swelling in men, and pelvic inflammatory disease in women. Risk factors include unprotected sex with multiple partners. Treatment is with antibiotics such as doxycycline or azithromycin.

61. **The correct answer is E.** Herpes infection is a viral infection that can be caused by herpes simplex virus type 1 or type 2, and its spectrum of diseases includes gingivostomatitis, keratoconjunctivitis, encephalitis, genital disease, and newborn infection. Genital herpes typically presents with multiple vesicles that can erupt, dysuria, urethral discharge, and cervicitis in women. Risk factors include unprotected sex with multiple partners. Suppressive treatment is through antiviral medications such as acyclovir. Symptomatic relapses are common throughout the patient's life.

Answer A is incorrect. *Candida albicans* is a fungus that can cause yeast infections. It is relatively common in women and is not a sexually transmitted disease. It can cause itching and white discharge. Treatment is through antifungal medications.

Answer C is incorrect. *Escherichia coli* is a member of the family Enterobacteriaceae, the enteric family of bacteria. It can cause a urinary tract infection, and the clinical picture is one of dysuria, including frequent urination, burning on urination, fever, and high WBC counts. Treatment is through antibiotics.

Answer D is incorrect. *Haemophilus ducreyi*, a gram-negative rod and relative of *Haemophilus influenzae*, causes chancroid characterized by painful genital ulcers. It must be distinguished from syphilis, herpes, and lymphogranuloma venereum (LV). Syphilis and LV are painless, but misdiagnosis with herpes is possible because both conditions cause painful blisters. Because herpes simplex virus (HSV) is far more common than chancroid in the United States, it is the usual diagnosis of painful genital blisters. If syphilis serology and HSV cultures are negative, chancroid is the diagnosis of exclusion. Chancroid is treated through antibiotics, particularly macrolides.

Answer F is incorrect. HIV is a lentivirus, a subgroup of the retroviruses. It is particularly known for its latency (it may manifest several years after infection) and its persistent viral titer. It has a high affinity for the CD4+ cells and weakens the host's immune system. It is typically diagnosed after the occurrence of an infection that predominantly occurs only in the immune-compromised population. Treatment is through antiretroviral medications.

Answer G is incorrect. Human papillomavirus is a virus that can cause epithelial tumors of the skin and mucosa. It can also cause cervical cancer, so routine Papanicolaou smears are recommended in sexually active women. Treatment is through immune-modifying medications such as imiquimod or surgical resection.

Answer I is incorrect. *Proteus* is a member of the family Enterobacteriaceae, the enteric family of bacteria. It can cause a urinary tract infection, and the clinical picture is one of dysuria, including frequent urination, burning on urination, fever, and high WBC counts. It is also associated with kidney stones. Treatment is through antibiotics such as β-lactams.

Answer J is incorrect. *Treponema pallidum* is associated with the sexually transmitted disease syphilis. It is a member of the Spirochaetaceae family of bacteria. Symptoms depend on the stage of the disease, but syphilis initially presents as a painless genital ulceration. Treatment is through antibiotics, particularly penicillin.

Questions 62–64

62. **The correct answer is F.** In a patient in this demographic, the predominant cause of a fever of unknown origin is an occult malignancy.

63. **The correct answer is E.** In this patient with a history of heavy alcohol use and fever of unknown origin, alcoholic hepatitis is the most likely diagnosis. Alcoholic hepatitis is a syndrome of progressive inflammatory liver injury associated with long-term heavy intake of ethanol. The pathogenesis is not completely understood. Patients who are severely affected present with subacute onset of fever, hepatomegaly, leukocytosis, marked impairment of liver function (e.g., jaundice and coagulopathy), and manifestations of portal hypertension (e.g., ascites, hepatic encephalopathy, and variceal hemorrhage). Disease that is sufficiently severe to cause the acute development of encephalopathy is associated with substantial early mortality, which may be ameliorated by treatment with glucocorticoids. Alcoholic hepatitis usually persists and progresses to cirrhosis if heavy alcohol use continues. If alcohol use ceases, alcoholic hepatitis resolves slowly over weeks to months, sometimes without permanent sequelae, but often with residual cirrhosis. Liver function tests in a patient with this condition will show disproportionate elevation of aspartate aminotransferase with respect to alanine aminotransferase in a ratio of 2:1.

64. **The correct answer is K.** This patient with a classic mitral stenosis murmur likely has rheumatic heart disease. In this population, infective endocarditis is the most likely cause of a fever of unknown origin, and it should be evaluated via blood cultures and an echocardio-

gram to seek mitral vegetations. Infective endocarditis is defined as an infection of the endocardial surface of the heart, which may include one or more heart valves, the mural endocardium, or a septal defect. Infective endocarditis generally occurs as a consequence of nonbacterial thrombotic endocarditis, which results from turbulence or trauma to the endothelial surface of the heart. Transient bacteremia then leads to seeding of lesions with adherent bacteria, and infective endocarditis develops. Pathologic effects due to infection can include local tissue destruction and embolic phenomena. Fever and chills are the most common presenting symptoms. Physical examination is notable for petechiae, splinter hemorrhages, Osler nodes, Janeway lesions, and Roth spots. Definitive diagnosis of infective endocarditis is generally made using the Duke criteria. Major criteria include (1) multiple positive blood cultures for the infecting organism and (2) echocardiographic evidence of endocardial involvement or a new regurgitant murmur on physical examination. Treatment may include penicillin G, gentamicin, nafcillin, vancomycin, and/or rifampin, depending on the presentation of disease and risk factors of the patient.

Answer A is incorrect. Acid-fast stain is often used to identify tuberculosis (TB) infection. TB can be a cause of fever of unknown origin, but in these patients without the risk factors of travel to endemic regions or living in close quarters such as in prisons or barracks, other etiologies are more likely.

Answer B is incorrect. In these seriously ill patients, you need complete baseline liver, renal, and metabolic data to follow. A basic panel (chem-7) is not enough.

Answer C is incorrect. A bone scan may be useful to look for osteomyelitis or neoplastic bone lesions, but it is not the most immediate test to order.

Answer D is incorrect. Cardiac stress tests are employed to assess the ability of the heart to function under physiologic stress. Though a patient with endocarditis may exhibit increased ischemia and reduced exercise tolerance, more direct clinical examinations and laboratory tests exist to gain information similarly valuable in defining and characterizing the disease state. Additionally, stress test results are not a component of the Duke criteria, the gold standard endocarditis diagnostic guidelines. There are no other indications for this test in the work-up for a fever of unknown origin.

Answer G is incorrect. None of the three patients seems to have risk factors for HIV infection.

Answer H is incorrect. There is no suspicion of central nervous system involvement in any of the patients. If there are changes in neurologic status or another locus of infection cannot be found, then a lumbar puncture may be indicated.

Answer I is incorrect. Muscle biopsies are used to distinguish between neurogenic and myopathic disorders, to identify specific muscular disorders such as muscular dystrophy or congenital myopathy, to identify metabolic defects of the muscle, to diagnose diseases of the connective tissue and blood vessels (such as polyarteritis nodosa), and to diagnose infections that affect the muscles (such as trichinosis or toxoplasmosis). There are no direct indications for this painful procedure to evaluate a fever of unknown origin.

Answer J is incorrect. These symptoms are real and are probably indicative of organic disease. Do not presume that a fever of unknown origin is factitious until other diagnoses have been excluded.

Answer L is incorrect. X-ray of the chest, though providing an image of the heart and a common region of cancer development, as well as potential complications of hepatitis and cirrhosis, is of lower yield than the other diagnostic modalities for all three patients. Any relevant findings produced would be nonspecific, and the tests identified by the correct answer choices will need to be performed regardless.

Questions 65 and 66

65. **The correct answer is F.** Herpes simplex virus (HSV) is transmitted to an infant during birth primarily through an infected maternal genital tract or by an ascending infection. When primary genital herpes occurs in the third trimester of pregnancy, the risk of fetal and neonatal involvement is high. Most newborns with perinatally acquired HSV appear normal at birth, although many are born prematurely. HSV infection in newborns usually develops in one of three patterns within 4 weeks of birth: (1) localized to the skin, eyes, and mouth (40%), (2) localized central nervous system disease (35%), and (3) fulminant, disseminated disease involving multiple organs (25%).

66. **The correct answer is K.** Congenital syphilis occurs when the spirochete *Treponema pallidum* is transmitted from a pregnant woman to her fetus. Two-thirds of live-born neonates with congenital syphilis are asymptomatic at birth. Overt infection can manifest in the fetus, the newborn, or later in childhood. Clinical manifestations after birth are divided into early (< 2 years) and late (> 2 years). Syphilis has many possible fetal manifestations, including stillbirth, neonatal death, and overt infection at birth, such as hydrops fetalis. Early manifestations can be quite variable and often appear within the first 5 weeks of life. Cutaneous lesions occur on the palms and soles. Other early manifestations include hepatosplenomegaly, jaundice, anemia, and snuffles. Metaphyseal dystrophy and periostitis often are noted on radiographs at birth. Late manifestations develop from scarring related to early infection, but can be prevented by treatment of the infant within the first 3 months of birth. Late findings can include frontal bossing, short maxilla, high palatal arch, Hutchinson's triad (Hutchinson's teeth [blunted upper incisors], interstitial keratitis, and eighth nerve deafness), saddle nose, and perioral fissures.

Answer A is incorrect. *Chlamydia trachomatis* is a gram-negative, aerobic, intracellular organism that causes a cervicitis. It is the most common bacterial sexually transmitted infection. Approximately half of those infected have no symptoms. Those that do have symptoms may not see them until 1–3 weeks after infection, at which point genital discharge and dysuria may be noted. Up to 40% of women with untreated chlamydia may develop pelvic inflammatory disease. Treatment is with a single dose of azithromycin or a 7-day course of doxycycline, most commonly.

Answer B is incorrect. Cytomegalovirus, a member of the herpesvirus family, rarely presents with symptoms; however, it may rarely present with symptoms of fatigue, fever, and sore throat. In most cases, there is no effective treatment, although ganciclovir prophylaxis may be used in immunocompromised patients. An effective vaccine has not yet been developed.

Answer C is incorrect. Epstein-Barr virus (EBV) is a member of the herpesvirus family. Infection with EBV presents with fatigue, lymphadenopathy, fever, and sore throat. A swollen spleen and lymph nodes may develop, requiring a patient to rest for several weeks to prevent the complication of splenic rupture. There is no specific treatment for EBV other than control of the symptoms.

Answer D is incorrect. Hepatitis B is caused by the hepatitis B virus and presents in much the same way as hepatitis E. Chronic infection, in contrast to hepatitis E, is a possibility (90% of infants, 30% of 1–5 year olds, and 6% of those infected after the age of 5). Death from liver failure occurs in 15–25% of those affected with chronic infection. Transmission of hepatitis B is via body fluids. An effective hepatitis B vaccine exists; however, treatment for infants who are infected is hepatitis B immune globulin and the first vaccine of the series, followed by the other two injections in the series. Those able to tolerate the drugs should be placed on a regimen of adefovir dipivoxil, interferon alfa, lamivudine, and entecavir.

Answer E is incorrect. Hepatitis E is caused by the hepatitis E virus, and is most severe among pregnant women. It is spread by fecal-oral contact. Presenting symptoms include jaundice, fatigue, abdominal pain, nausea/vomiting, and dark urine. Treatment is supportive.

Answer G is incorrect. Herpes zoster is an acute, localized infection with varicella-zoster virus that causes a dermatomal painful, blistering rash. Treatment is with acyclovir to reduce pain and complications and shorten the course of the infection.

Answer H is incorrect. *Neisseria gonorrhoeae* is a sexually transmitted infection caused by a gram-negative aerobic bacteria. This bacterium usually causes an urethritis that may result in purulent discharge and dysuria. Complications include prostatitis and orchitis in males and salpingitis or ovaritis in females. As many as 15% of females with cervical involvement may progress to pelvic inflammatory disease. Uncomplicated infections are treated with a third-generation cephalosporin or fluoroquinolone, along with an antibiotic effective against possible co-infection with *Chlamydia trachomatis*, such as erythromycin or doxycycline.

Answer I is incorrect. Parvovirus is a childhood infection typically diagnosed in patients with a "slapped cheek" rash that appears several days after the onset of coldlike symptoms. It is caused by human parvovirus B19, and the condition may cause anemia. The only treatment required is occasional hospitalization and blood transfusions in those with severe anemia. Most patients may simply observe self-care treatment at home.

Answer J is incorrect. Clinical manifestations of congenital rubella syndrome include sensorineural deafness (60–75%), cataracts and glaucoma (10–25%), cardiac malformations such as patent ductus arteriosus or peripheral pulmonary artery stenosis (10–20%), and neurologic sequelae, ranging from meningoencephalitis to behavior disorders and mental retardation (10–25%). At birth, many infants with this congenital infection are growth retarded and have radiolucent bone disease (not pathognomonic for congenital rubella), hepatosplenomegaly, thrombocytopenia, and purpuric skin lesions (classically described as "blueberry muffin" lesions) that represent extramedullary hematopoiesis, and hyperbilirubinemia.

Answer L is incorrect. Toxoplasmosis is caused by the single-celled parasite *Toxoplasma gondii* and is usually asymptomatic; however, pregnant women and the immunocompromised must be aware that the disease may cause brain lesions (typically appearing as ring-enhancing lesions on cerebral imaging) in newborns. Infection is usually from exposure to cat feces from an infected feline.

Questions 67 and 68

67. **The correct answer is E.** This is a general recommendation for all HIV-positive females due to the increased risk of cervical cancer caused by their immunocompromised state. The patient in question two should already be having this screening, and her herpes outbreaks mean that she should be started on acyclovir, making that the most correct answer. Primary prophylaxis against *Pneumocystis jiroveci* pneumonia is indicated for patients with CD4+ counts below 200/mm^3. The prophylaxis of choice is one double-strength tablet of trimethoprim-sulfamethoxazole per day.

68. **The correct answer is F.** This is a general recommendation for all HIV-positive females due to the increased risk of cervical cancer caused by their immunocompromised state. The patient in this question should already be having this screening, and her herpes outbreaks mean that she should be started on acyclovir, making that the most correct answer. Any patient with HIV and recurrent genital herpes outbreaks should be placed on 400 mg acyclovir twice a day to prevent further sequelae.

Answer A is incorrect. Any patient who has a CD4+ count < 100/mm^3 and is seronegative for hepatitis B should be given the vaccine series.

Answer B is incorrect. Any patient with a purified protein derivative test which is larger than 5 mm, but who is found not to have active infection (by x-ray of the chest and three negative cultures) should receive this tuberculosis prophylactic regimen for 6 months to prevent reactivation.

Answer C is incorrect. Each of these patients requires a change in management.

Answer D is incorrect. This is a general recommendation for all HIV-positive females due to the increased risk of cervical cancer caused by their immunocompromised state. The 26-year-old HIV-positive patient should already be having this screening, and her herpes out-

breaks mean that she should be started on acyclovir, making that the most correct answer.

Answer G is incorrect. Patients with anti-*Toxoplasma* antibodies are at risk for reactivated toxoplasmosis when their CD4+ counts are < 100/mm^3. The prophylaxis of choice is one double-strength tablet of trimethoprim-sulfamethoxazole per day. Patients with CD4+ counts in this range should already be on trimethoprim-sulfamethoxazole for *Pneumocystis jiroveci* pneumonia prophylaxis.

Answer H is incorrect. Any patient with a purified protein derivative test larger than 5 mm, or who is considered to be at high risk for tuberculosis exposure should receive x-ray of the chest.

Questions 69 and 70

69. **The correct answer is A.** Dysuria, hesitancy, urgency, and frequency are the hallmarks of urinary tract infection. So-called "honeymoon cystitis" caused by *Staphylococcus saprophyticus* is common when acquiring a first or new sexual partner, or when intercourse is frequent. Microscopic examination reveals bacteriuria in addition to pyuria.

70. **The correct answer is B.** Symptoms of systemic illness, including fever, nausea, and vomiting, differentiate pyelonephritis from uncomplicated urinary tract infection. The classic triad of costovertebral angle tenderness, fever, and nausea/vomiting suggests pyelonephritis.

Answer C is incorrect. Acute urinary retention typically presents with suprapubic pain on palpation and without symptoms of infection.

Answer D is incorrect. The classic presentation of bladder cancer is painless gross hematuria.

Answer E is incorrect. Prostate cancer may be asymptomatic and discovered via digital rectal examination and prostate-specific antigen screening; alternatively, patients may present with urinary dribbling, nocturia, and difficulty initiating a urine stream. Prostate cancer affects only men.

Answer F is incorrect. Diabetes insipidus is marked by polyuria, nocturia, and polydipsia, and is caused by decreased ADH secretion or ADH resistance.

Answer G is incorrect. Diabetes mellitus is marked by polyuria, polydipsia, and polyphagia, and is caused by autoimmune destruction of β cells in pancreas or insulin resistance.

Answer H is incorrect. Classic presentation of hypercalcemia includes "stones, bones, abdominal groans, and psychic overtones" (nephrolithiasis, joint and muscle aches, abdominal pain, nausea and vomiting, constipation, and depression). Polyuria may also be present.

Answer I is incorrect. Interstitial cystitis presents with similar symptoms to uncomplicated urinary tract infection, but no bacteria are found on urinalysis, and the symptoms do not respond to antibiotic therapy.

Answer J is incorrect. Neurogenic bladder may present with either urinary overflow leakage or urinary retention.

Answer K is incorrect. Psychogenic polydipsia involves drinking excess water, and may present with polyuria and nocturia. Diagnosis is via a water deprivation test.

Answer L is incorrect. Renal cell carcinoma often presents with flank pain, palpable abdominal mass, and hematuria.

Answer M is incorrect. Urethral stricture presents with obstructive symptoms, including dribbling, intermittency, incomplete emptying of the bladder, and weak urine stream.

CHAPTER 9

Musculoskeletal

1. A 48-year-old woman presents to her primary care physician with swelling of her hands for the past 3 months. She says that her fingers and hands appear swollen, and her skin feels firm and tight. For the past 5 years, she notes that her hands turn very pale when she goes outside in cold weather, then turn blue, and then return to a red color. She has a history of gastroesophageal reflux disease and is on omeprazole. Recently, she has begun having pain while swallowing solid foods. On physical examination, she has bilaterally swollen fingers and hands. The overlying skin appears very smooth, but on palpation the hands are firm and indurated. On the finger pads there are several subcutaneous hard nodules. Which of the following autoantibodies will be elevated in this patient?

(A) Anti-centromere autoantibody
(B) Antineutrophil cytoplasmic autoantibody
(C) Anti-Scl-70 autoantibody
(D) Anti-Smith autoantibody
(E) Anti-SSA autoantibody

2. A 32-year-old man with a history of Wolff-Parkinson-White syndrome presents complaining of a rash on his face and joint aches that started about a month ago, but got much worse after spending a long day at the beach a few days ago. He also has had pain, warmth, and swelling of his knees for the past few weeks, as well as low-grade fevers to 37.9–38.3°C (100.2–100.9°F) daily for the past 2 weeks. He is taking a medication to prevent atrial fibrillation. Family history is negative for any rheumatologic disorders or malignancy. He has a temperature of 38.3°C (100.9°F), a heart rate of 84/min, and a blood pressure of 118/76 mm Hg. He has an area of erythema on his cheeks bilaterally that extends across his nasal bridge. His knees are edematous, red, and warm bilaterally with decreased flexion. Neurologic examination is nonfocal. Laboratory evaluation reveals a positive antinuclear antibody titer. Which of the following medications taken for the treatment of Wolff-Parkinson-White syndrome is likely causing this patient's symptoms?

(A) Amiodarone
(B) Hydralazine
(C) Isoniazid
(D) Procainamide
(E) Sotalol

3. A 4-year-old boy is brought to the pediatrician for evaluation of frequent falls. His mother says that for the past 6 months he seems to be moving more slowly than usual, and he can't run as quickly and can't climb stairs. The boy was born at 39 weeks' gestation via normal spontaneous vaginal delivery with no complications. He has been otherwise healthy and achieved all of his appropriate motor and speech milestones. Family history is significant for a maternal uncle who died at age 20 from respiratory failure. On physical examination, the patient has hyperlordosis of the spine. His calves are very prominent bilaterally. When asked to lie on his back and stand up, he first rolls over onto his stomach and then uses his hands to climb up his legs until he is standing. He has 3/5 strength in his shoulders and thighs bilaterally, but 5/5 strength in his hands, calves, and feet. The rest of the neurologic examination is unremarkable. Serum creatine kinase is 1500 U/L. How was this boy's disorder most likely inherited?

(A) Autosomal dominant
(B) Autosomal recessive
(C) Autosomal trisomy
(D) Mitochondrial
(E) X-linked recessive

4. An 83-year-old woman is admitted after being found on the floor in her apartment. She was found by her daughter, who estimates that the patient may have been there for several days. Initial workup shows that the patient had suffered a left middle cerebral artery stroke and was unable to move from her position to call for help. On examination, she is slightly obtunded and unable to talk but responsive to simple commands. Her vital signs are blood pressure 158/68 mm Hg and pulse 90/min. Although she lacks feeling in the right side of her body, she complains of diffuse muscle pain, es-

pecially in her back, buttocks, and thigh on the left side. Initial laboratory studies are ordered and straight catheterization produces 40 mL of dark brown urine. Dipstick urinalysis is positive for blood, but RBCs are absent on microscopic evaluation. Which of the sets of laboratory findings in the table below is this patient most likely to demonstrate?

(A) A
(B) B
(C) C
(D) D
(E) E

5. A 69-year-old woman presents to her primary care physician complaining of fatigue and achiness in her shoulders and hips. She says that over the past 2 months, she has lost 4.5 kg (10 lb) and feels tired all the time. Her whole body feels stiff in the morning for at least half an hour. She has trouble getting dressed because it is difficult to put on a shirt or pull up her pantyhose. On physical examination, she has decreased active range of motion of her shoulders and hips. She has no muscle tenderness. Strength is 5/5 in all four extremities. Neurologic examination is nonfocal. Relevant laboratory findings are as follows:

WBC count	8600/mm^3
Hemoglobin	10.4 g/dL
Platelet count	160,000/mm^3
Erythrocyte sedimentation rate	120 mm/h
Creatine kinase	52 U/L

A short course of prednisone leads to almost complete resolution of symptoms. What is the most likely diagnosis in this patient?

(A) Fibromyalgia
(B) Osteoarthritis
(C) Polymyalgia rheumatica
(D) Polymyositis
(E) Rheumatoid arthritis

6. A 15-year-old soccer player runs into a goal post, protecting his body with an outstretched left hand. After the game he complains to his father that his wrist hurts and they stop by the local emergency department (ED) on their way home. The boy screams in pain when the emergency physician palpates the floor of the anatomic snuffbox. An x-ray of the left wrist and hand is obtained that shows no fracture. What is the next best step in management?

(A) Operative exploration for the source of pain
(B) Removable plaster splint and physical therapy
(C) Rest, ice, and nonsteroidal anti-inflammatory medications
(D) Short arm cast and physical therapy in 4–6 weeks
(E) Thumb spica cast and repeat x-rays of the left wrist and hand in 2–3 weeks

CHOICE	K$^+$	PHOSPHATE	URIC ACID	CREATININE	CA^{2+}
A	↓	↓	↓	↓	↑
B	↓	↓	↑	↓	↑
C	Normal	↑	Normal	↑	↑
D	↑	↑	↓	↑	↓
E	↑	↑	↑	↑	↓

7. A 24-year-old man presents to the ophthalmologist complaining of blurred vision. He notes that his left eye has been red and painful for the past 3 days, and he has not been able to look at bright lights. On further questioning, he also notes that he has had pain and swelling of the right knee for about 1 week, and for the past month his hips have felt very stiff, especially in the morning. On physical examination, his vital signs are normal, the conjunctiva of his left eye is severely injected and his right knee is edematous, erythematous, and warm to touch, with limited flexion and extension of the leg. Additionally, his hips are tender to palpation, and he has limited forward and lateral flexion of the spine. On genitourinary examination, the patient is an uncircumcised male. Upon retraction of the foreskin, there is a 1 × 1 cm shallow nontender ulcer with well-defined margins adjacent to the urethral meatus. Which of the following laboratory tests will confirm the most likely diagnosis?

(A) Serum rheumatoid factor
(B) Serum Venereal Disease Research Laboratory test
(C) Stool bacterial culture
(D) Urethral swab for gonococcus
(E) Urine polymerase chain reaction for *Chlamydia trachomatis*

8. A 57-year-old man presents to his primary care physician complaining of shortness of breath that has been worsening over the past 6 months. Initially, he had dyspnea on exertion but this evolved into dyspnea at rest, as well as a nonproductive cough for the last month. He denies weight loss, fevers, or night sweats. On further review of systems, he complains of pain and swelling in his hands. He also notes that his body feels stiff in the morning. He has no other significant past medical history and is taking no medication except for occasional ibuprofen for his hand pain. He has never smoked. On physical examination, he has crackles at the lung bases bilaterally. He has enlarged metacarpophalangeal joints bilaterally. They are red, warm, and tender to palpation. He also has slight ulnar deviation of the fingers. What will pulmonary function tests on this patient most likely show?

(A) Decreased ratio of FEV_1:FVC
(B) Increased residual volume
(C) Increased total lung capacity
(D) Normal or increased ratio of FEV_1:FVC and decreased carbon monoxide diffusion capacity
(E) Normal or increased ratio of FEV_1:FVC and normal carbon monoxide diffusing capacity

9. A 72-year-old man presents to the ED with pain in his right big toe. The pain started this morning and is getting progressively worse, and he is unable to bear weight on that foot. This is his fifth presentation to the ED in the past 7 years for similar complaints. He says his doctor gave him a medication to prevent the attacks, but he does not remember the name and hasn't taken it in many months. He is febrile, has a pulse of 90/min, and has a blood pressure of 136/86 mm Hg. The first metatarsophalangeal joint of the right foot is swollen, warm, and erythematous. It is exquisitely tender to palpation and there is decreased movement. He also has several nontender nodules on the medial aspect of the big toes bilaterally, alongside the first metacarpophalangeal joints bilaterally, and on his ears. Which of the following is the best agent for acute management of this patient's condition?

(A) Acetaminophen
(B) Allopurinol
(C) Indomethacin
(D) Intravenous colchicines
(E) Probenecid

10. A 57-year-old woman presents to her primary care physician complaining of shortness of breath. These symptoms first began after strenuous exercise approximately 6 months ago, but over the past month she has felt short of breath after climbing 10 steps and sometimes at rest. She has no known medical problems, but has not seen a physician in 5 years. She is not taking any medication and is a nonsmoker. Cardiac examination is notable for a loud P_2 component of S_2 but no murmurs. Her fingers are shiny, swollen, and indurated. She also has several telangiectasias on her hands and hard, subcutaneous nodules on her finger pads. Laboratory evaluation is significant for elevated an-

ticentromere antibody but normal antitopoiso-merase I antibody. What is the most likely diagnosis in this patient?

(A) Diffuse cutaneous systemic sclerosis
(B) Limited cutaneous systemic sclerosis
(C) Rheumatoid arthritis
(D) Systemic lupus erythematosus
(E) Wegener's granulomatosis

11. A physician suspects that his patient might have gouty arthritis. To confirm his clinical suspicion, the physician orders a microscopic evaluation of the joint fluid for the presence of negatively birefringent, needle-shaped crystals. This is known to be a highly specific test. Relative to the physician's clinical diagnosis alone, a highly specific test will greatly reduce which of the following?

(A) False negatives
(B) False positives
(C) Prevalence
(D) True negatives
(E) True positives

12. A 26-year-old jogger presents to her primary care physician complaining of left lower leg pain when she exercises. She states that when she is not jogging, she is pain free, but when she jogs over 3 miles, she begins to note pain and tightness in her left lower leg. She states that she often has concurrent numbness and tingling in the top of her foot during these episodes of pain. When she ceases strenuous activity, all symptoms slowly subside over the course of half an hour. Physical examination is unremarkable and demonstrates a neurovascularly intact left lower extremity with supple compartments, and no focal areas of tenderness. Plain films of the left knee, tibia, and fibula are similarly unremarkable. What is the most likely diagnosis?

(A) Acute compartment syndrome
(B) Exertional compartment syndrome
(C) Left knee osteoarthritis
(D) Left-sided patellofemoral pain syndrome
(E) Left tibial stress fracture

13. A 23-year-old man with new-onset back and buttock pain presents to his primary care physician for evaluation. He states that he has morn-

ing stiffness in his back that resolves over the course of the day. Further testing is negative for rheumatoid factor and positive for human leukocyte antigen (HLA)-B27 surface antigen. For which of the following conditions is the patient at greatest risk?

(A) Aortitis
(B) Splenomegaly
(C) Thrombocytopenia
(D) Uveitis
(E) Xerostomia

14. A 55-year-old white man presents to the ED complaining of diffuse, constant bone pain for the past 3 months. He is a schoolteacher, and denies any recent history of trauma or infection. He does note that his favorite fitted baseball hat no longer fits. His temperature is 37.6°C (99.7°F), blood pressure is 120/75 mm Hg, pulse is 85/min, and respiratory rate is 22/min. Physical examination reveals no focal points of tenderness. Mild frontal bossing and bilateral tibial bowing are noted. A skull film is shown in the image. What is the most likely diagnosis?

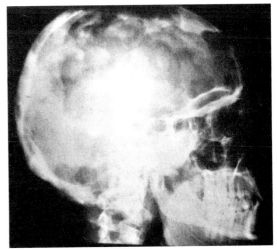

Reproduced, with permission, from Kasper DL, Braunwald E, Fauci AS, Hauser SL, Longo DL, Jameson LJ, Isselbacher KJ, eds. *Harrison's Online.* New York: McGraw-Hill, 2005: 2280.

(A) Ankylosing spondylitis
(B) Paget's disease
(C) Pituitary adenoma
(D) Rickets
(E) Scurvy

15. A 45-year-old woman presents to her primary care physician complaining of difficulty sleeping and extreme fatigue with minimal exertion. These symptoms have been persistent over the past 3 months. She describes her pain as a stiff ache throughout her back and shoulders. Although the stiffness typically improves over the course of the day, any major form of exertion leaves her muscles aching. She denies any recent history of trauma or infection. Physical examination reveals points of increased tenderness over the medial aspect of the upper border of the trapezius muscle bilaterally and above the medial border of the scapular spine. X-rays of the shoulder are normal. What is the most likely diagnosis?

(A) Fibromyalgia
(B) Frozen shoulder syndrome
(C) Malingering
(D) Osteoarthritis
(E) Rheumatoid arthritis

16. A 35-year-old woman presents to her primary care physician with complaints of progressive weakness over the past month. She states that she has noticed an increasing amount of difficulty associated with getting out of chairs, climbing stairs, brushing her hair, and lifting her 3-year-old son out of his playpen, an activity that she was able to do without difficulty prior to the onset of her weakness. She admits to missing 3 days of work approximately 6 weeks ago due to "a bad cold." Physical examination is remarkable for symmetric proximal muscle weakness. Several tests are ordered to establish a diagnosis. Which of the following most strongly supports a diagnosis of polymyositis?

(A) β-Amyloid deposits noted on muscle biopsy
(B) Increased creatine kinase levels
(C) Normal creatine kinase levels
(D) Perifascicular atrophy noted on muscle biopsy
(E) Positive rheumatoid factor

17. A 75-year-old white man presents to his primary care physician complaining of lower back and leg pain. The pain is brought on by walking, has been steadily worsening over the past few years, and is not relieved by non-steroidal anti-inflammatory drugs. In the past the pain was confined only to his lower back and upper leg/thigh, but in recent months it has started to shoot past his knees. He states that the pain is worst with walking, and he denies any recent trauma or illness. On physical examination, his lower extremities are neurovascularly intact, with full 5/5 strength, intact sensation, and 2+ dorsalis pedis and posterior tibial pulses. Which is the most appropriate next step in the diagnosis of this patient?

(A) CT of the spine
(B) Electromyography of the lower extremities
(C) Lumbar spine plain films
(D) MRI of the lower back
(E) Whole body positron emission tomographic scan

18. A 55-year-old woman presents to her primary care physician complaining of fever, headache, and general malaise over the past 2 weeks. For the past month, she has had recurrent headaches of increasing frequency. On further questioning, the patient indicates that she has felt feverish and generally "not well" for the past 2 weeks. She denies any recent trauma, increase in stress, or known exposure to infection. Her temperature is 38.2°C (100.8°F), heart rate is 92/min, and blood pressure is 114/85 mm Hg. On physical examination, the patient has marked tenderness over her temples. The physician orders a stat erythrocyte sedimentation rate level, and finds it to be markedly increased at 109 mm/h. What is the most likely diagnosis in this case?

(A) Cluster headaches
(B) Migraine headaches
(C) Temporal arteritis
(D) Tension headaches
(E) Trigeminal neuralgia

19. A 75-year-old man presents to his family physician with a 3-day history of joint pain. The patient has had various "aches and pains" in his joints over the years, but in the past 3 days, he has noticed that his first metatarsophalangeal (MTP) joint in his left foot has become very painful. He describes the pain as a dull, constant ache at a 7 of 10 on the pain scale. He

denies any recent trauma or exposure to infectious agents. The remainder of his musculoskeletal examination is within normal limits, with full range of motion and no focal tenderness in any of his other joints. On physical examination, the first MTP in the left foot is warm, erythematous, and extremely tender to the touch. Synovial fluid was clear with no WBCs or RBCs and negative Gram stain. Results of tissue biopsy are shown in the image. What is the most likely diagnosis?

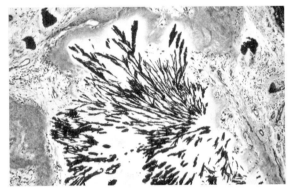

Reprinted, with permission, from PEIR Digital Library (http://peir.net).

(A) Acute gout
(B) Osteoarthritis
(C) Rheumatoid arthritis
(D) Septic arthritis
(E) Systemic lupus erythematosus

20. A 26-year-old woman was hit by a car and brought to the trauma bay with a blood pressure of 62/40 mm Hg. On examination, she was unresponsive, her pupils were equally round and reactive, her distal pulses were weak, and her extremities were cold. X-ray of the chest was taken and was normal. Peritoneal lavage showed no blood in the abdomen. After receiving 2 L of lactated Ringer's solution, her blood pressure was 71/46 mm Hg. The pelvis was unstable with compression, and an anteroposterior x-ray of the pelvis confirmed a pelvic fracture. What is the next best step in management?

(A) Application of an external fixation device
(B) Exploratory laparotomy with packing of the pelvis

(C) Open reduction and internal fixation of the fracture
(D) Pelvic CT with contrast
(E) Surgical exploration of pelvic hematoma

21. A 28-year-old woman presents to her primary care physician complaining of a rash and hair loss. She says that while on a cruise last month, she got a bad sunburn on her cheeks and nose, but the redness has not subsided. She also notes that she has been losing large clumps of hair in the shower for the past several weeks. On further review of systems, she notes feeling very fatigued for the past few months and has lost 4.5 kg (10 lb). She has a temperature of 38.3°C (100.9°F), a heart rate of 92/min, and a blood pressure of 110/72 mm Hg. Her muscles are diffusely tender and her shoulders, knees, and ankles have decreased passive range of motion secondary to pain and stiffness. She has 1+ pitting edema in her legs up to the mid-calf bilaterally. Laboratory workup reveals positive antinuclear antibody and positive anti–double-stranded DNA antibody. Which of the following additional laboratory findings might be found in this patient?

(A) Anticentromere antibodies
(B) Antineutrophil cytoplasmic antibodies
(C) Leukopenia
(D) Macrocytic anemia
(E) Thrombocytosis

22. A 26-year-old patient was diagnosed with rheumatoid arthritis (RA) 1 month ago. She returns to her primary care physician for a follow-up visit and is interested in learning how RA might affect her, other than the joint destruction it can cause. The patient is most likely to develop which of the following?

(A) Myocarditis
(B) Nodules
(C) Pericarditis
(D) Renal failure
(E) Splenomegaly

23. A 9-year-old girl presents to her pediatrician with a 3-week history of spiking fevers at night up to 39.4°C (102.9°F). The fevers usually subside with acetaminophen or ibuprofen but eventually return. She has also been complaining of pain in her legs. The mother is very concerned because her daughter has developed a salmon-colored rash on her chest and arms that flares every time she has a fever spike. Her temperature is 38.3°C (100.9°F), heart rate is 96/min, and blood pressure is 104/56 mm Hg. Bilateral anterior cervical and axillary lymphadenopathy is present. Cardiac examination reveals a regular rate and rhythm with no murmurs or rubs. The abdomen is soft and nontender, and her liver is palpable 3 cm below the costal margin. Her right knee and left ankle are swollen and warm, with decreased range of motion. What is the most likely diagnosis in this patient?

    (A) Acute rheumatic fever
    (B) Juvenile rheumatoid arthritis
    (C) Parvovirus B19 infection
    (D) Reiter's syndrome
    (E) Septic arthritis

24. A man presents to his primary care physician with a chief complaint of lower back pain. He is not particularly concerned about the pain, as it is not causing him significant distress. However, he works at a factory and he would like a letter to be sent to his boss, stating that he needs some time off to recuperate. Before agreeing to write the letter, the physician takes a more detailed history. Which of the following findings would be most reassuring to the physician?

    (A) Age of 60 years
    (B) Duration of symptoms >1 month
    (C) History of prostate cancer
    (D) History of recurrent urinary tract infection
    (E) Relief of pain with nonsteroidal anti-inflammatory drugs
    (F) Unexplained weight loss

25. A 74-year-old woman presents to her primary care physician with a 1-month history of temporal headaches, fevers, and general malaise. The headaches are described as a throbbing pain, especially localized to her temporal regions bilaterally. She denies any recent trauma or exposure to infectious agents. Her temperature is 38.0°C (100.4°F), heart rate is 82/min, and blood pressure is 119/96 mm Hg. On physical examination, the patient is extremely tender over her temples, and abnormally thickened temporal arteries are palpable bilaterally. Laboratory tests demonstrate an erythrocyte sedimentation rate of 31 mm/h. What is the most appropriate initial step in treatment for this patient?

    (A) Acetazolamide
    (B) Atenolol
    (C) Methotrexate
    (D) Nifedipine
    (E) Oral prednisone

EXTENDED MATCHING

Questions 26 and 27

For each of the following patients with joint complaints, identify the type of arthritis.

    (A) Ankylosing spondylitis
    (B) Fibromyalgia
    (C) Gonococcal arthritis
    (D) Gout
    (E) Osteoarthritis
    (F) Polymyalgia rheumatica
    (G) Psoriatic arthritis
    (H) Reactive arthritis
    (I) Reiter's syndrome
    (J) Rheumatoid arthritis
    (K) Systemic lupus erythematosus

26. A 65-year-old man presents to the ED with 10 of 10 pain in his right first toe. The pain started suddenly last night with no precipitating trauma. His toe is extremely tender to the touch, and is very warm and swollen.

27. A 58-year-old woman has pain and stiffness in her hands that increases throughout the day. Physical examination shows bony enlargement of the distal interphalangeal joints. X-rays of the hands show joint space narrowing with subchondral sclerosis.

Questions 28–30

Match each of the following clinical scenarios with the one most appropriate diagnosis.

(A) Behçet's syndrome
(B) Churg-Strauss vasculitis
(C) Disseminated intravascular coagulation
(D) Giant cell arteritis
(E) Hemolytic-uremic syndrome
(F) Henoch-Schönlein purpura
(G) Idiopathic thrombocytopenic purpura
(H) Kawasaki disease
(I) Microscopic polyangiitis
(J) Polyarteritis nodosa
(K) Takayasu's arteritis
(L) Thromboangiitis obliterans
(M) Thrombotic thrombocytopenic purpura
(N) Wegener's granulomatosis

28. A 27-year-old man presents to the clinic with several weeks of malaise, fatigue, and low-grade fever. He mentions that he has had some testicular and abdominal pain after eating. He also states that he has been "tripping over his feet," and a neurologic examination demonstrates a right foot drop. His history is significant for hepatitis B.

29. A 52-year-old woman with recurrent sinusitis and a chronic cough develops hemoptysis. A urinalysis shows microhematuria, and a kidney biopsy demonstrates granulomatous inflammation within the arterial walls.

30. A 36-year-old man with asthma and chronic allergies presents to his physician with mononeuropathy of his ulnar nerve and mild pleuritic chest pain. His differential demonstrates 11.7% eosinophils. An x-ray of the chest shows a right-sided pulmonary infiltrate.

1. **The correct answer is A.** This patient has symptoms and signs suggestive of systemic sclerosis, or scleroderma. The swollen, indurated fingers and hands are a classic finding in cutaneous systemic sclerosis. The fact that the skin findings are limited to the hands and do not extend proximally indicates that this woman has limited cutaneous systemic sclerosis (LCSS), as opposed to diffuse disease. LCSS is typically associated with the **CREST** syndrome: **C**alcinosis, **R**aynaud's phenomenon, **E**sophageal dysmotility, **S**clerodactyly, and **T**elangiectasias. This patient demonstrates many of the components of CREST, including nodules in the finger pads, which represent calcific deposits in the subcutaneous tissue. She also has Raynaud's phenomenon, or episodic vasoconstriction of the small arteries in the fingers, causing pallor and cyanosis when patients are exposed to cold temperatures or emotional stress, and rubor on rewarming. She also has a history of reflux and dysphagia, which are signs of esophageal dysmotility. LCSS is typically associated with elevated levels of anti-centromere and/or anti-nucleolar autoantibodies.

Answer B is incorrect. Antineutrophil cytoplasmic autoantibody (ANCA) is typically found in patients with Wegener's granulomatosis, a vasculitis that affects medium- and small-sized vessels. Wegener's classically affects the lungs and kidneys. Pulmonary symptoms include cough, dyspnea, and hemoptysis. Renal involvement is usually a pauci-immune glomerulonephritis. ANCA may also be positive in microscopic polyangiitis, Churg-Strauss syndrome, and several other vasculitides, but it is not associated with systemic sclerosis.

Answer C is incorrect. Anti-Scl-70 is frequently elevated in patients with diffuse cutaneous systemic sclerosis (DCSS). These patients will have skin findings extending proximally past the wrists. They will also lack other signs of CREST syndrome that are seen in this patient. Patients with DCSS are at increased risk of pulmonary fibrosis, the leading cause of death in patients with scleroderma.

Patients with DCSS may also have cardiac abnormalities and renal disease.

Answer D is incorrect. Anti-Smith autoantibodies are elevated in patients with systemic lupus erythematosus (SLE). SLE is an autoimmune disorder that most commonly affects young women. It can cause widespread systemic disease including renal failure, central nervous system disturbances, and pulmonary disease. There is a wide range of clinical manifestations of SLE, but common presenting symptoms include fever, fatigue, weight loss, malar rash, photosensitivity, alopecia, arthritis, myalgias, pleuritic chest pain, and neurologic changes. Patients with SLE may also have elevated anti–double-stranded DNA autoantibodies.

Answer E is incorrect. Anti-SSA is elevated in patients with Sjögren's syndrome, which is characterized by dry eyes, dry mouth, and enlarged salivary glands. It may also be elevated in patients with systemic lupus erythematosus, but is not associated with systemic sclerosis.

2. **The correct answer is D.** This patient is presenting with a lupus-like syndrome. He has malar rash, fevers, and arthritis, all signs that are seen in patients with lupus. Patients with drug-induced lupus usually have positive antinuclear antibodies, but tend to have a less severe presentation compared to patients with systemic lupus erythematosus. The syndrome usually resolves several weeks after discontinuing the medication. Procainamide is a class IA antiarrhythmic drug that is used in some patients with Wolff-Parkinson-White syndrome to prevent atrial fibrillation, and can cause a drug-induced lupus-like syndrome. Other drugs that cause it include hydralazine, isoniazid, minocycline, propylthiouracil, lithium, carbamazepine, and phenytoin.

Answer A is incorrect. Amiodarone is a class III antiarrhythmic agent that is sometimes used to treat patients with Wolff-Parkinson-White syndrome. Its major use is to prevent orthodromic atrioventricular reentrant tachycardia. Amiodarone can be a very toxic medication, but it is not typically associated with a drug-induced lupus-like syndrome. Side effects of amiodarone include pulmonary toxicity, thyroid dysfunction, liver toxicity, ocular disease, and gastrointestinal upset.

Answer B is incorrect. Hydralazine is an antihypertensive medication that is frequently associated with an increased risk of developing drug-induced lupus. However, it is not a drug that is used to manage arrhythmias in Wolff-Parkinson-White syndrome.

Answer C is incorrect. Isoniazid is an antibiotic that is also associated with causing a drug-induced lupus-like syndrome. However, it is not used to treat Wolff-Parkinson-White syndrome. Isoniazid is most commonly used in the treatment and prophylaxis of tuberculosis.

Answer E is incorrect. Sotalol is a class III antiarrhythmic agent that may be used to treat patients with Wolff-Parkinson-White syndrome; however, it does not cause a lupus-like syndrome. The most common adverse effect of sotalol is cardiac toxicity, including bradycardia and arrhythmias.

3. **The correct answer is E.** This patient is presenting with signs and symptoms suggestive of Duchenne's muscular dystrophy (DMD). DMD is present at birth, but typically does not begin to manifest until age 3–5 years. DMD classically affects the proximal musculature, so patients will have difficulty climbing stairs. This patient is displaying a positive Gower's sign. However, patients with proximal muscle weakness will roll to the prone position and use their arms to climb up their legs, as opposed to using truncal muscles to get into a sitting position and then thigh muscles to rise to standing. Patients with DMD develop hyperlordosis and scoliosis because of weakness of truncal muscles. The chest deformity, along with muscle weakness, impairs respiratory function, and patients often require tracheostomy. Calves are enlarged due to pseudohypertrophy. Creatine kinase is elevated, indicating a primary muscle disorder as opposed to a neurologic disorder. Death occurs in the third decade due to respiratory failure or cardiomyopathy. DMD is inherited in an X-linked recessive fashion. Clues in the family

history include a maternal uncle who died of respiratory failure in his 20s, and normal, unaffected females

Answer A is incorrect. In autosomal dominant disorders, the disease will affect any individual carrying a single mutation. Unless this boy has a new, spontaneous mutation, his mother must be a carrier of the mutation. Therefore, she would also be expected to have the disease. Autosomal dominant disorders include Huntington's disease and neurofibromatosis.

Answer B is incorrect. Although this family history might suggest an autosomal recessive pattern of inheritance, Duchenne's muscular dystrophy is always inherited as an X-linked recessive condition. Common autosomal recessive disorders include cystic fibrosis and sickle cell disease.

Answer C is incorrect. Autosomal trisomies include trisomies 13, 18, and 21. These disorders present with many congenital anomalies at birth, including cardiac defects, limb abnormalities, and craniofacial dysmorphia.

Answer D is incorrect. Mitochondrial disorders are inherited from the mother. The mitochondrial myopathies can also affect muscle strength, but the mother and sister would also be affected, because all offspring of affected females show signs of disease.

4. **The correct answer is E.** This patient's clinical presentation suggests rhabdomyolysis. A history of trauma followed by an extended period of inactivity is a classic cause of rhabdomyolysis. Urine positive for blood by dipstick but negative for RBCs by microscopic examination suggests the presence of myoglobin secondary to rhabdomyolysis. The widespread muscle cell damage that occurs in rhabdomyolysis leads to the release of intracellular components into the systemic circulation. Among these, elevations of potassium, phosphate, uric acid, and structural proteins such as myoglobin can lead to serious problems such as acute renal failure (ARF). Myoglobin accumulation in the kidney can lead to myoglobinuria and ARF, as evidenced by a sharp rise in creatinine levels (out of proportion to

increases in blood urea nitrogen). An elevation of serum phosphate drives calcium concentration down as the two ions complex with each other.

Answer A is incorrect. In rhabdomyolysis, the potassium, phosphate, uric acid, and creatinine would increase, not decrease, and the complexing of phosphate to calcium would cause serum calcium levels to decrease.

Answer B is incorrect. Potassium, phosphate, and creatinine would be increased, not decreased. Serum calcium should decrease, not increase.

Answer C is incorrect. Potassium and uric acid levels would be increased, not normal. In addition, serum calcium would be decreased.

Answer D is incorrect. Uric acid would also increase along with potassium, phosphate, and creatinine.

5. **The correct answer is C.** This patient has a clinical presentation suggestive of polymyalgia rheumatica (PMR). PMR is a disorder that is linked to temporal (giant cell) arteritis, and almost exclusively occurs in patients > 50 years old. PMR typically presents as subacute or chronic onset of symmetrical pain and morning stiffness in large proximal joints including the shoulder, hip girdle, and neck. Patients may report trouble getting dressed because of stiffness in these joints. Patients may also have systemic symptoms including weight loss and fatigue. When present, the pain of PMR is due to synovitis and bursitis of the joints, rather than actual muscle tenderness as the name implies. The classic laboratory finding in both PMR and temporal arteritis is elevated erythrocyte sedimentation rate, usually > 40 mm/h and sometimes exceeding 100 mm/h. The rapid response to prednisone further confirms the diagnosis, as both PMR and temporal arteritis typically have a dramatic response to even low-dose steroid.

Answer A is incorrect. Patients with fibromyalgia tend to be < 50 years old and complain of diffuse musculoskeletal pain. Physical examination typically reveals muscle tenderness. Laboratory workup is unremarkable, including a normal erythrocyte sedimentation rate. Fibromyalgia would not rapidly resolve after a short course of steroids.

Answer B is incorrect. Osteoarthritis (OA) is a very common cause of joint pain in older patients. OA commonly involves the hips, knees, spine, and hands. The pain associated with OA tends to worsen throughout the day with increasing activity, as opposed to inflammatory pain, which is most severe in the morning, after an extended period of inactivity. Patients with OA would not be expected to have an elevated erythrocyte sedimentation rate or rapid response to steroids.

Answer D is incorrect. Polymyositis is another rheumatologic disorder that typically presents with proximal muscle weakness. Patients may also complain of difficulty getting dressed, but this is due to actual muscle weakness as opposed to joint stiffness, as seen in polymyalgia rheumatica. Patients with polymyositis typically do not complain of pain in the hip girdle. On examination, they will have muscle tenderness and diminished muscle strength, but should have full range of motion of all joints including the shoulders. Laboratory findings include elevated muscle enzymes such as creatine kinase.

Answer E is incorrect. Rheumatoid arthritis (RA) may present with similar symptoms as polymyalgia rheumatica (PMR), including symmetric polyarthritis and morning stiffness. However, RA tends to involve more joints than PMR, and also involves smaller joints including the hands and feet, which are typically spared in PMR. In addition, RA is usually a difficult disease to manage and requires high-dose steroids or other disease-modifying antirheumatic drugs, so this patient's rapid response to low-dose steroids is unlikely to be seen in a patient with RA.

6. **The correct answer is E.** The scaphoid is the most commonly fractured carpal bone. It articulates with the distal radius, trapezium, and capitate, and is restricted from motion during radial deviation and dorsiflexion (outstretched arm). Thus any forceful stress exerted on the scaphoid in this position results in fracture. Tenderness, swelling, or bruising in the anatomic snuffbox, a triangular depression on

the dorsal aspect of the hand bordered by the extensor and abductors of the thumb, can be highly indicative of a scaphoid fracture. Initial plain film radiographs do not always detect scaphoid fractures, especially in nondisplaced fractures. Thus, as a general rule, a patient with a clinically suspected scaphoid fracture but negative initial x-ray is treated with a short arm thumb spica splint and reevaluated in 2 weeks. Repeat x-ray films are important to detect fractures of the proximal third of the scaphoid, which are associated with avascular necrosis. Failure to accurately diagnose and treat a scaphoid fracture may result in a variety of adverse outcomes including nonunion, delayed union, decreased grip strength, decreased range of motion, and osteoarthritis of the radiocarpal joint.

Answer A is incorrect. Surgery is not indicated at this time since the initial x-ray film did not reveal a fracture. Open reduction is indicated for displaced fractures and nonunions.

Answer B is incorrect. A plaster splint is made from various crinoline-type material strips impregnated with plaster that crystallizes or sets when water is added. It provides temporary immobilization to improve pain and discomfort, minimize blood loss, decrease the risk of fat emboli, and prevent further neurovascular injury associated with fractures. However, in this case a fracture should be assumed and full-time immobilization applied until a scaphoid fracture can be ruled out weeks later.

Answer C is incorrect. Soft-tissue injuries not associated with bony fractures include sprains, strains, contusions, tendinitis, and bursitis. Traumatic injury or repeated overuse can lead to this type of injury. Treatment for most soft-tissue injuries includes rest for a certain time period, ice therapy, and nonsteroidal anti-inflammatory drugs (NSAIDs). The patient's mechanism of injury and physical examination findings are highly suspicious for a scaphoid fracture and thus warrant splint immobilization. Ice and NSAIDs can be used as adjunctive therapy.

Answer D is incorrect. A short arm cast is applied below the elbow to the hand and does not adequately immobilize the scaphoid. It is

primarily indicated for forearm or wrist fractures, or to immobilize the forearm or wrist muscles and tendons in place following surgery. In addition, repeat x-ray films are needed sooner than 4 weeks to determine whether there is a scaphoid fracture, so that appropriate measures can be undertaken in a timely fashion to prevent complications arising from this type of injury.

7. **The correct answer is E.** This patient is presenting with the signs and symptoms of classic Reiter's syndrome. Classic Reiter's syndrome is one of the spondyloarthropathies. Classic Reiter's syndrome is characterized by a triad of uveitis, urethritis, and arthritis ("can't see, can't pee, can't climb a tree"). This patient's complaints are consistent with uveitis (blurred vision, photophobia, and pain) and peripheral inflammatory arthritis (symmetric, of the large joints of the lower limbs). The mucosal ulceration seen at the urethral meatus is characteristic of circinate balanitis, a lesion caused by *Chlamydia trachomatis*, the organism implicated in the pathogenesis of Reiter's syndrome. Although some patients may report a history of penile discharge, the infection can also be asymptomatic, especially in circumcised males, who may not notice the nontender lesion. Females may have asymptomatic chlamydial infection that precedes the onset of Reiter's syndrome.

Answer A is incorrect. Rheumatoid factor is a marker found in many patients with RA, as well as several other rheumatologic conditions. Although rheumatoid arthritis can present with morning stiffness, the arthritis is typically symmetric and affects many joints. Typically it involves small joints of the hands as opposed to a single large joint of the lower extremity. Also, RA typically does not cause back pain or limited movement of the spine. The combination of findings in this patient is much more suggestive of Reiter's syndrome than RA.

Answer B is incorrect. The Venereal Disease Research Laboratory test is used to test for syphilis. Primary syphilis can cause a painless ulceration on the genitalia called a chancroid. However, early syphilis is not associated with the other findings seen in this patient, such as uveitis, sacroiliitis, and peripheral arthritis.

Answer C is incorrect. Reactive arthritis presents similarly to classic Reiter's syndrome, with inflammatory back pain and asymmetric oligoarthritis affecting the large joints. Common pathogens implicated in reactive arthritis include *Shigella*, *Campylobacter*, *Yersinia*, and *Salmonella*. However, the lack of diarrhea and the presence of a genital ulcer and uveitis are more suggestive of Reiter's syndrome due to chlamydial infection.

Answer D is incorrect. Gonococcal infection can also cause urethritis and arthritis. The arthritis caused by gonococcus involve large joints. However, gonococcus does not typically cause inflammatory back pain, and the genital lesion seen on this patient is more consistent with chlamydial infection. Gonococcus is more likely to cause a purulent urethritis.

8. **The correct answer is D.** This patient is presenting with classic signs and symptoms of rheumatoid arthritis. The combination of rheumatoid arthritis with dyspnea and crackles is suggestive of rheumatoid arthritis–associated interstitial lung disease (RA-ILD), the most common manifestation of rheumatoid lung disease. Patients with RA-ILD present with a clinical picture similar to idiopathic pulmonary fibrosis, including dyspnea, nonproductive cough, crackles, and clubbing in late disease. Lung disease is most common in patients 50–60 years old and is more common in men. Interstitial lung disease causes a restrictive pattern on pulmonary function testing. Total lung capacity, functional residual capacity, and residual volume are all decreased. FEV_1 and FVC are also decreased, but these reductions are in relation to a decreased total lung capacity, so the ratio of FEV_1:FVC is either normal or slightly increased. The carbon monoxide diffusion capacity is reduced due to inflammation and scarring of the lung tissue.

Answer A is incorrect. Decreased ratio of FEV_1:FVC is found in patients with obstructive lung disease, most commonly due to chronic obstructive pulmonary disease. Although there are a variety of obstructive lung diseases associated with rheumatoid arthritis, rheumatoid arthritis-associated interstitial lung disease is much more common. Although pa-

tients with chronic obstructive pulmonary disease may present with cough and dyspnea, this diagnosis is less likely in a patient who has never smoked.

Answer B is incorrect. Patients with restrictive lung disease have decreased residual volumes.

Answer C is incorrect. Patients with interstitial lung disease have a decreased, not increased, total lung capacity.

Answer E is incorrect. Normal or increased ratio of FEV_1:FVC with a normal carbon monoxide diffusion capacity can be seen in patients with restrictive lung disease due to extrinsic disorders. Disorders of the chest wall or pleura, or neuromuscular disorders, can decrease total lung capacity (TLC). As with intrinsic lung disorders that cause a restrictive pattern, the FEV_1:FVC in patients with extrinsic disorders will be normal to increased. This is because both FEV_1 and FVC are reduced in relation to an overall decreased TLC. However, the diffusion capacity will be normal, because the lung tissue itself is not involved in the pathology.

9. **The correct answer is C.** This patient is presenting with acute gouty arthritis. In the absence of contraindications, the initial drug of choice in a patient with acute gouty arthritis of < 24 hours' duration is a potent nonsteroidal anti-inflammatory drug (NSAID) such as indomethacin. Indomethacin can rapidly improve pain and swelling and prevent progressive inflammation. Another anti-inflammatory agent that can be used is oral colchicine, but it is sometimes reserved for patients who are intolerant of NSAIDs or those who have had prior success with colchicine, because the drug has many adverse effects, including diarrhea, at therapeutic levels. Other options include intra-articular steroid injections or oral prednisone, but patients may have rebound inflammation after withdrawal of oral steroids.

Answer A is incorrect. Acetaminophen is not used in treating acute gouty arthritis because it does not decrease inflammation.

Answer B is incorrect. Allopurinol decreases the production of uric acid by inhibiting the enzyme xanthine oxidase. It is very effective in decreasing uric acid levels in patients who have hyperuricemia secondary to overproduction. However, allopurinol should never be started during an acute gouty attack. Initiation of therapy with uric acid-lowering drugs during an acute attack can lead to a more intense and prolonged episode. Allopurinol should not be started until a few weeks after the acute attack resolves, and it should be given with colchicine to prevent recurrence.

Answer D is incorrect. Intravenous colchicine can be very effective in treating acute gouty arthritis. However, there is a high rate of toxicity including gastrointestinal upset, myopathy, agranulocytosis, and even sudden death. Its use is limited to hospitalized patients with polyarticular gout who cannot tolerate nonsteroidal anti-inflammatory drugs or oral medications. It is contraindicated in patients with leukopenia, hepatic disease, or renal insufficiency. It is not first-line therapy.

Answer E is incorrect. Probenecid is a drug that decreases serum uric acid by inhibiting urate reabsorption in the kidney. Probenecid may be used for long-term prophylaxis in patients with hyperuricemia due to decreased excretion. Like allopurinol, probenecid should not be started during an acute attack because it can intensify and prolong the episode.

10. **The correct answer is B.** This patient has signs suggestive of systemic sclerosis, or scleroderma. Pulmonary disease occurs in up to 70% of patients with scleroderma, and it is the leading cause of mortality in these patients. Pulmonary hypertension is a more rare complication of scleroderma, but patients with it may present with dyspnea, and x-ray evidence of an enlarged pulmonary artery, as in this patient (at the arrow). She most likely has limited cutaneous systemic sclerosis, which is limited to sclerosis distal to the wrists, and is often associated with **CREST** syndrome (consisting of Calcinosis, Raynaud's phenomenon, Esophageal dysmotility, Sclerodactyly, and Telangiectasias) and anticentromere antibodies.

Answer A is incorrect. Diffuse cutaneous systemic sclerosis (DCSS) is differentiated from limited cutaneous systemic sclerosis, based on extension of the sclerosis proximal to the wrists. It is commonly associated with pulmonary disease but typically causes interstitial pulmonary fibrosis. Patients may also present with exertional dyspnea, but x-ray of the chest will show symmetric basilar reticulonodular infiltrates. In addition, patients with DCSS typically have elevated antitopoisomerase or anti-Scl-70 autoantibodies, not anticentromere antibodies.

Answer C is incorrect. RA can also cause pulmonary disease that presents with dyspnea. The most common manifestation of RA lung disease is interstitial pulmonary fibrosis, but patients may also have pleural disease, lung nodules, and vasculitis. Patients with RA present with painful swelling of the joints and morning stiffness that classically affects the metacarpophalangeal and proximal interphalangeal joints of the hands. Patients with RA do not have shiny, firm skin. In addition, anticentromere antibody is not typically elevated in patients with RA.

Answer D is incorrect. Patients with SLE can have a wide range of pulmonary manifestations, including pulmonary hypertension, interstitial fibrosis, pneumonitis, pleurisy, and alveolar hemorrhage. SLE typically affects young women and can cause widespread systemic disease, including fever, fatigue, weight loss, malar rash, photosensitivity, alopecia, arthritis, myalgias, neurologic changes, and renal failure. This patient does not have any other clinical signs suggestive of SLE. In addition, patients with SLE have elevated antinuclear, anti–double-stranded DNA, and/or anti-Smith autoantibodies, not anticentromere antibody.

Answer E is incorrect. Wegener's granulomatosis is a systemic vasculitis of medium- and small-size vessels that classically affects the lungs and kidneys. Pulmonary symptoms include cough, dyspnea, and hemoptysis. X-ray of the chest may show cavitating nodules, alveolar infiltrates, and diffuse hazy opacities. Patients with Wegener's do not typically have pulmonary hypertension. Wegener's is associated with elevated levels of antineutrophil cytoplasmic antibody.

11. **The correct answer is B.** Specificity is defined as the proportion of disease-free persons appropriately classified by the screening test as negative. A test with high specificity is useful in confirming a diagnosis because a highly specific test will have few results that are false-positive. In this case, the joint fluid evaluation is used to confirm the physician's clinical suspicion and decrease the likelihood that a patient without gouty arthritis will mistakenly receive that diagnosis.

Answer A is incorrect. False negatives are diseased persons who are misclassified as negative. This parameter does not decrease with a highly specific test. High sensitivity, however, would by definition reduce the proportion of false negatives.

Answer C is incorrect. Specificity of a test is a property of the screening test and is not associated with the prevalence of the disease in a population.

Answer D is incorrect. True negatives are healthy persons who are correctly classified as being without disease. This parameter would increase with a highly specific test.

Answer E is incorrect. True positives are diseased persons who are correctly classified as positive. This parameter does not decrease with a highly specific test, although it would increase with a highly sensitive test.

12. **The correct answer is B.** Exertional compartment syndrome is a condition in which the patient experiences pain over the anterior lower leg caused by a pressure buildup within the muscles of the leg. Patients typically complain of pain after a period of activity or exercise, and it is quickly relieved by rest. As blood flow to the muscle increases with activity, the muscle swells and becomes constricted by the encompassing fascia. Pain results from the ensuing ischemia. There may also be associated numbness in the dorsum of the foot or weakness on dorsiflexion at the ankle. The diagnosis is made by measuring pressures within the leg at rest followed by a reading after some exercise. Treatment consists of a surgical fasciotomy, which involves release of the tight fascia.

Answer A is incorrect. Acute compartment syndrome differs from exercise-induced or chronic compartment syndrome in that the former occurs secondary to a traumatic injury such as a fracture of one of the long bones or a crush injury. The patient would present with severe pain and clinically tight compartments at the time of examination with associated paresthesias. Treatment involves immediate fasciotomy to prevent cell death.

Answer C is incorrect. Pain associated with knee osteoarthritis would not likely resolve within a half hour of cessation of exercise. Patients typically experience pain, soreness, and swelling with activity that does not necessarily resolve immediately after rest. Treatment includes ice, nonsteroidal anti-inflammatory drugs, and limited activity. In addition, the patient's age and lack of x-ray findings make this diagnosis unlikely.

Answer D is incorrect. Patellofemoral knee pain most commonly arises from an imbalance or irregularity of patellar movement or tracking. Conditions that predispose to these abnormalities include an imbalance in quadriceps strength, patella alta, recurrent patellar subluxation, direct trauma to the patella, and meniscal injuries. Patients suffering from any of the patellofemoral knee pain syndromes usually complain of anterior knee pain, and do not present in the manner described in the stem.

Answer E is incorrect. Stress fractures are tiny cracks in bone that result from overuse. Fatigued muscles and increasing the amount or intensity of an activity too rapidly may cause these cracks. Most stress fractures occur in the weight-bearing bones of the lower leg and the foot. Treatment consists of ice, nonsteroidal anti-inflammatory drugs, and rest for 6–8 weeks which allows ample time for healing. Evidence of fracture may never appear on plain radiographs or may not appear for 2–10 weeks after symptom onset, although triple-phase nuclear bone scans are more sensitive in the detection of stress fractures early in the clinical course. A patient with a tibial stress fracture would not be pain-free within 30 minutes of cessation of activity, nor would the patient likely experience a temporary loss of sensation over the dorsum of the foot.

13. The correct answer is D. The patient's demographic information, presentation, and study results are most consistent with a diagnosis of ankylosing spondylitis (AS). AS is a chronic inflammation of the sacroiliac joints and the spine, which can eventually lead to fusion of the vertebrae. Patients experience back pain and morning stiffness. Systemic findings are associated with the disease, including uveitis in approximately 30% of affected patients. Other associated conditions include cataracts, secondary glaucoma, aortic insufficiency, and prostatitis in men. Patients are generally managed with nonsteroidal anti-inflammatory drugs and specific exercise regimens, and may require hip replacements or spinal surgery later in the disease.

Answer A is incorrect. Aortitis, or inflammation of the aorta, can be infectious or autoimmune. It is associated with ankylosing spondylitis but affects < 5% of patients with the disease. Affected patients are at risk for a variety of complications of diminished aortic flow, including central hypertension from renal artery stenosis, vision changes, neurologic deficits, and claudication.

Answer B is incorrect. Splenomegaly occurs in about 10% of patients with systemic lupus erythematosus but is not commonly found in patients with ankylosing spondylitis. In lupus patients, it is associated with nausea, diarrhea, and vague abdominal pain.

Answer C is incorrect. Thrombocytopenia is associated with a wide variety of systemic illnesses but is not commonly associated with AS. Autoimmune etiologies for thrombocytopenia exist but are not associated with AS.

Answer E is incorrect. Xerostomia (dry mouth) is commonly associated with Sjögren's syndrome, not ankylosing spondylitis. Patients with Sjögren's have sicca symptoms: dryness of the oral mucosa, eyes, and other mucosal surfaces of the body (e.g., skin, nose, and vagina). However, they generally do not experience progressive back pain and stiffness.

14. The correct answer is B. Paget's disease is characterized by an increased rate of bone turnover, causing both excessive resorption as well as excessive formation. The history of diffuse bone pain and increasing head size in conjunction with the physical examination findings of frontal bossing and tibial bowing are suspicious for Paget's disease. The skull x-rays reveal the classic "cotton wool" appearance found in patients with Paget's disease. Additionally, these patients will have an elevated alkaline phosphatase with normal calcium and phosphate. A majority of those with Paget's disease are asymptomatic and do not require treatment. Treatment may be indicated in order to treat symptoms or to prevent complications. Treatment includes calcitonin and bisphosphonates to slow bone resorption.

Answer A is incorrect. This disorder is associated with ankylosis/fusion of joints, and does not fit well with the description and findings above. Ankylosing spondylitis typically presents in the late teens and early 20s with hip pain and lower back pain that is worst in the morning and improves with activity.

Answer C is incorrect. Hormone imbalances associated with pituitary adenomas may manifest in a number of ways including acromegalic bony changes. However, the history and findings (including the bilateral bowing of the tibias) above are most consistent with Paget's disease.

Answer D is incorrect. Rickets, or osteomalacia, is the weakening and softening of bones that is frequently associated with decreased vitamin D or calcium intake. Though it can occur in adults, it occurs most frequently in early childhood. This is particularly common in developing countries as a result of famine and malnourishment.

Answer E is incorrect. Scurvy is a disorder of collagen synthesis typically associated with vitamin C deficiency. Common manifestations of scurvy include perifollicular hemorrhages, perifollicular hyperkeratotic papules, petechiae and purpura, splinter hemorrhages, bleeding gums, hemarthroses, and subperiosteal hemorrhages.

15. The correct answer is A. This patient has a classic presentation of fibromyalgia. Patients often present with generalized musculoskeletal aching, with stiffness and fatigue that improves over the course of the day. Pain and tightness in the neck and upper back, along with areas of point tenderness, are common symptoms. Patients may complain of muscle pain and fatigue after minimal exertion, poor sleep, awaking frequently over the course of the night, and having difficulty falling back to sleep. Physical examination and radiologic studies do not typically demonstrate any joint abnormalities.

Answer B is incorrect. A patient with frozen shoulder syndrome would have significant deficits in range of motion that would be exposed during physical examination. Adhesive capsulitis, or "frozen shoulder," is a progressive disorder in which patients suffer from shoulder pain and decreased range of motion without the presence of truly intrinsic shoulder disease. This disorder often follows bouts of bursitis, and is characterized by a thickened capsule, with mild inflammatory changes, leading to decreased range of motion and increased pain.

Answer C is incorrect. Patients with fibromyalgia are often dismissed as malingerers because their symptoms are often nonfocal and vague in nature. It is important not to dismiss cases of fibromyalgia as malingering. Fibromyalgia is a real medical entity with viable treatment options, including amitriptyline, fluoxetine, chlorpromazine, or cyclobenzaprine.

Answer D is incorrect. In OA, pain is usually limited to joints, and radiologic changes, including joint space narrowing, osteophytes, and subchondral cysts, are likely to be found. The lack of proper history or x-ray findings goes against the diagnosis of OA.

Answer E is incorrect. The diffuse nature of the pain (not limited to joints) and absence of radiographic findings make RA less likely. In RA, pain usually affects joints, not muscle. In addition, one might expect to find radiologic changes, including joint space narrowing in RA. Therefore, the diagnosis of RA is unlikely.

16. **The correct answer is B.** Polymyositis, dermatomyositis, and inclusion body myositis are all idiopathic inflammatory arthropathies. Although the etiology behind these disorders is largely unknown, they typically present with progressive bilateral muscle weakness. Diagnostic distinction between the three entities is made on muscle biopsy. In addition, creatine kinase levels may provide further distinction between the disorders. Polymyositis is always associated with increased creatine kinase (CK) levels. CK levels in dermatomyositis and inclusion body myositis can be normal, and therefore cannot be used to rule out these two diseases.

Answer A is incorrect. β-Amyloid deposits are a classic biopsy finding in inclusion body myositis. It is the most common acquired myopathy in patients age 50 years or older. Patients develop progressive, asymmetric weakness of both proximal and distal muscles and generally do not respond to immunosuppressive treatment.

Answer C is incorrect. CK levels are increased, not normal, in polymyositis. Patients with dermatomyositis and inclusion body myositis can have normal CK levels, so the distinction between the disease processes must be made with biopsy findings.

Answer D is incorrect. Perifascicular atrophy is a classic biopsy finding in dermatomyositis. It affects the joints, esophagus, lungs, and heart, and presents with skin findings such as heliotrope rash and Gottron papules. Patients experience proximal muscle weakness, joint swelling, and occasional muscle tenderness.

Answer E is incorrect. Positive rheumatoid factor is not associated with polymyositis, but instead with rheumatoid arthritis. Patients begin to experience fatigue, stiffness after waking up, diffuse myalgias, and weakness. Joint pain and swelling follows, particularly in the wrist, elbow, fingers, knees, and toes. Rheumatoid arthritis classically affects the proximal joints of the hand.

17. **The correct answer is D.** Patients with lumbar spinal stenosis present when the narrowed spinal canal and degenerative joint changes compress nerve roots and become symptomatic. The best diagnostic confirmation of this disorder is lumbar spine MRI, which may demonstrate bulging/protrusion of the intervertebral disks, osteophytes at the facet joints, or

hypertrophy of the ligamentum flavum. Because this patient experiences neurogenic claudication (ischemia of compressed nerves while walking), he would be a candidate for decompression surgery.

Answer A is incorrect. CT scan would not adequately image the intervertebral disks, which can play an essential role in the development of lumbar spinal stenosis. Like plain films, spine CT is best for diagnosing bony abnormalities such as fractures.

Answer B is incorrect. Electromyography (EMG) would not provide any direct imaging data, which is essential to the diagnosis of lumbar spinal stenosis. Although EMG can detect nerve compression, results are most useful in detecting motor unit pathology such as that found in myasthenia gravis or amyotrophic lateral sclerosis.

Answer C is incorrect. Plain films do not adequately image the soft tissues that may be involved with the etiology of lumbar spinal stenosis, including bulging/protrusion of the intervertebral disks, or hypertrophy of the ligamentum flavum. Plain films are useful in evaluating bony abnormalities such as osteoarthritis.

Answer E is incorrect. Positron emission tomography (PET) scan would not adequately image the soft tissues or bony structures that must be examined in this case of lumbar spinal stenosis. PET scan is useful in assessing tissue perfusion and detecting malignancy.

18. **The correct answer is C.** This patient has temporal arteritis. Temporal arteritis, also known as giant cell arteritis, is characterized by inflammation of large to medium-size arteries, especially the temporal artery. Patients often present with headaches, fever, anemia, elevated erythrocyte sedimentation rate (ESR), and marked tenderness to palpation over the temporal regions, with a palpably thickened temporal artery noted on occasion. Laboratory abnormalities associated with temporal arteritis include elevated ESR, increased serum alkaline phosphatase levels, increased serum levels of IgG, increased serum complement levels, and normochromic or slightly hypochromic

anemia. Serum creatine kinase is not elevated in this disorder.

Answer A is incorrect. Cluster headaches are usually characterized by one to three short attacks of periorbital pain per day over a 4- to 8-week period, followed by nonsymptomatic periods of up to 1 year.

Answer B is incorrect. Migraine headaches classically present with deep throbbing pain, photophobia, and antecedent aura. They are not associated with gradual onset or elevated ESR.

Answer D is incorrect. Tension headaches are characterized by a tight band of pressure and pain surrounding the head, and may be found with increases in stress/anxiety level.

Answer E is incorrect. Trigeminal neuralgia typically presents with excruciating pain in the cheeks, gums, and lips.

19. **The correct answer is A.** Gout is a disease associated with an abnormally high level of urate in the serum. This disorder often results in recurring acute monarticular arthritis, classically affecting the first MTP joint. The image shows extracellular and intracellular monosodium urate crystals. These needle- and rod-shaped, negatively birefringent crystals are pathognomonic for gout. In addition, the monarticular acute presentation without history of trauma or infection is consistent with this diagnosis.

Answer B is incorrect. OA is joint degeneration that is usually secondary to overuse or trauma. The acute onset of this patient's toe pain and lack of supporting history make OA unlikely.

Answer C is incorrect. RA is an autoimmune joint disorder that normally presents with symmetric joint degeneration and periarticular pain and stiffness. Synovial fluid in RA shows a predominance of neutrophils and high protein. In addition, the history and physical examination findings are more consistent with this diagnosis than with RA.

Answer D is incorrect. Aspiration of a septic joint would most likely yield synovial fluid with increased white cell counts and a 75% chance of visualizing the offending organism itself.

Answer E is incorrect. SLE is an autoimmune inflammatory disorder that affects a wide variety of organs. The sign and symptoms of SLE can be remembered using the mnemonic **DOPAMINE RASH** (**D**iscoid rash, **O**ral ulcers, **P**hotosensitivity, **A**rthritis, **M**alar rash, **I**mmunologic criteria, **N**eurologic symptoms, **E**levated RBC sedimentation rate, **R**enal disease, **A**NA [antinuclear antibody] positive, **S**erositis, and **H**ematologic abnormalities). The patient's findings do not correlate well with the diagnosis of SLE, but rather are more representative of an acute gout flare.

20. **The correct answer is A.** An exsanguinating hemorrhage is likely when hypotension and shock are present in the setting of a pelvic fracture. Patients with evidence of unstable fractures of the pelvis associated with hypotension should be considered for some form of external pelvic stabilization, which has been shown to decrease mortality in these patients. The exact mechanism by which early pelvic stabilization is effective in promoting hemodynamic stability in patients with unstable pelvic fractures is not completely understood. However, some believe that reducing the pelvis back to its normal configuration reduces pelvic volume, and therefore limits the amount of blood loss to the retroperitoneal pelvic hematoma. Thus keeping the pelvic volume small may promote tamponade of the bleeding sources in the pelvis.

Answer B is incorrect. Laparotomy is not warranted without evidence of gross blood in the abdomen or evidence of intestinal perforation. The diagnostic peritoneal lavage is a reliable diagnostic test for this purpose. In addition, patients with evidence of unstable pelvic fractures who warrant laparotomy should receive external pelvic stabilization prior to any incisions.

Answer C is incorrect. Internal fixation should be considered only if the patient is hemodynamically stable.

Answer D is incorrect. Patients who are hemodynamically unstable should not be sent to the CT scanner. Once stable, a patient may be taken to the scanner. Patients with evidence of arterial extravasation of intravenous contrast in the pelvis via CT should be considered for pelvic angiography and possible embolization.

Answer E is incorrect. A pelvic hematoma should never be explored due to the risk of uncontrollable bleeding.

21. **The correct answer is C.** This woman is presenting with signs and symptoms suggestive of SLE. It can cause widespread systemic disease including renal failure, central nervous system disturbances, and pulmonary disease. Antinuclear antibody is positive in almost all patients with SLE, but it is not specific. Anti–double-stranded DNA and anti-Sm antibodies are highly specific for lupus, so their presence confirms the diagnosis of SLE. Patients with SLE frequently have hematologic abnormalities. Leukopenia is a very common finding. It is usually lymphopenia as opposed to neutropenia, so patients are not at significantly increased risk of infection.

Answer A is incorrect. Anticentromere antibodies are specific for CREST syndrome, or limited cutaneous systemic sclerosis. The **CREST** syndrome consists of **C**alcinosis, **R**aynaud's phenomenon, **E**sophageal dysmotility, **S**clerodactyly, and **T**elangiectasias.

Answer B is incorrect. Antineutrophil cytoplasmic antibody (ANCA) is a common finding in patients with Wegener's granulomatosis, which is a systemic vasculitis that classically affects the lung and kidney. ANCA may also be positive in microscopic polyangiitis, Churg-Strauss syndrome, and several other vasculitides, but is not associated with systemic lupus erythematosus.

Answer D is incorrect. Anemia is a very common finding in patients with SLE, but it is typically a normochromic, normocytic anemia due to chronic disease. Rarely, patients with SLE can have a hemolytic anemia. Macrocytic anemia is typically caused by folate or vitamin B_{12} deficiency and can also be seen in patients with alcohol abuse, liver disease, and hypothyroidism.

Answer E is incorrect. Patients with SLE typically develop thrombocytopenia, not thrombocytosis. Patients may present with purpura or easy bruising and bleeding.

22. **The correct answer is B.** RA is an autoimmune disorder with potential for multiple organ system involvement. The most common presentation of RA is that of an inflammatory symmetric synovitis of the peripheral joints. The disease is also associated with several extra-articular manifestations, including nodules, splenomegaly, interstitial fibrosis, and vasculitis. Rheumatoid nodules are present in 20–35% of patients with RA and usually form on pressure points on the body.

Answer A is incorrect. Myocarditis is a possible extra-articular manifestation of RA; however, it is rare.

Answer C is incorrect. Pericarditis is a possible extra-articular manifestation of RA that occurs in < 10% of RA patients over their lifetime. However, 30% of patients may have evidence of pericardial effusions on echocardiography that are of no clinical significance.

Answer D is incorrect. Patients with RA can develop renal disease, including focal glomerulonephritis or toxicity from RA treatments, but this is very rare.

Answer E is incorrect. Splenomegaly (as part of Felty's syndrome with granulocytopenia) is a possible extra-articular manifestation of RA; however, it is uncommon.

23. **The correct answer is B.** The combination of several weeks of high-spiking fevers, arthritis, and salmon-colored rash is highly suggestive of systemic-onset juvenile rheumatoid arthritis (JRA). The salmon-colored macular rash is activated by heat and is frequently found in warm areas of the body such as the axilla and the waist. The rash is commonly triggered by a fever spike, but subsides when the temperature returns to normal. Physical examination findings in systemic-onset JRA include lymphadenopathy, hepatomegaly, and splenomegaly. There is no specific test for JRA, so the diagnosis is typically made by clinical presentation.

Answer A is incorrect. Acute rheumatic fever (ARF) is a complication of group A streptococcal pharyngitis. It is characterized by five major criteria: migratory arthritis of the large joints, carditis, rash, chorea, and subcutaneous nodules. The rash of ARF is erythema marginatum, a pink, nonpruritic rash with sharply defined borders and central clearing that predominantly occurs on the trunk. Fever is one of the minor criteria of ARF, along with arthralgias and previous rheumatic heart disease. Diagnosis of ARF by Jones' criteria requires the presence of two major, or one major and two minor, criteria in addition to evidence of a recent streptococcal infection.

Answer C is incorrect. Parvovirus can also cause fever, rash, and arthritis, and is often considered in the differential diagnosis of systemic-onset JRA. However, viral infections rarely cause the spiking fevers that are seen in patients with systemic-onset JRA. In addition, the rash of parvovirus is classically a "slapped-cheek" appearance, as opposed to the rash shown above. Viral exanthems tend to persist regardless of temperature, as opposed to the rash of JRA that fluctuates with fever.

Answer D is incorrect. Reiter's syndrome is characterized by a classic triad of uveitis, urethritis, and arthritis ("can't see, can't pee, can't climb a tree"). Reiter's is typically caused by *Chlamydia trachomatis*. It is one of the spondyloarthropathies in which patients have axial and sacroiliac inflammatory arthritis. Patients may also have asymmetric involvement of large peripheral joints, particularly of the lower limbs.

Answer E is incorrect. Septic arthritis is a common disorder in patients in this age group. However, the history of several weeks of spiking fevers and rash is less consistent with an acute bacterial infection. In addition, acute bacterial septic arthritis typically affects a single joint.

24. **The correct answer is E.** Low back pain is a very common complaint seen by the primary care physician. The most common origin of low back pain is musculoskeletal, such as strain of paraspinal muscles or injury to ligaments or fascia. However, back pain can be the presenting symptom of a more serious underlying disorder such as malignancy. In the initial work-up of a patient with back pain, a detailed history is essential in determining which patients can be managed conservatively and

which need further diagnostic evaluation. Pain relieved by nonsteroidal anti-inflammatory drugs is unlikely to be due to malignancy or infection.

Answer A is incorrect. Age > 50 years in a patient with back pain is associated with a greater risk of malignancy. More benign causes of low back pain, such as musculoskeletal pain, tend to occur in younger patients.

Answer B is incorrect. Pain that lasts < 1 month is concerning for a more serious condition such as malignancy or infection. Ninety percent of patients with low back pain will recover spontaneously within 4 weeks. As a result, symptoms lasting > 1 month are an indication for further evaluation.

Answer C is incorrect. Any patient with a history of malignancy presenting with low back pain should have further radiographic evaluation to rule out metastatic disease. A history of prostate cancer is particularly concerning, given the propensity of prostate cancer to metastasize to the lumbar spine.

Answer D is incorrect. History of recurrent urinary tract infection can be an indication that the patient has back pain due to pyelonephritis. Further workup including complete blood cell count, erythrocyte sedimentation rate, and radiographic imaging should be performed.

Answer F is incorrect. Any systemic symptoms including fever, weight loss, and night sweats should raise the suspicion that back pain is due to either malignancy or infection, and thus warrants further evaluation.

25. **The correct answer is E.** The patient suffers from temporal arteritis. Temporal arteritis, also known as giant cell arteritis, is characterized by inflammation of large to medium-size arteries, especially the temporal artery. Patients often present with headaches, fever, anemia, elevated ESR, and marked tenderness to palpation over the temporal regions. Occasionally, a palpably thickened temporal artery is noted. This disorder generally responds well to steroid therapy. Current guidelines dictate that initial treatment of temporal arteritis should be 40–60 mg of oral prednisone per day for approxi-

mately 1 month, followed by a gradual taper. This decreases the risk of the long-term sequelae of the disease, namely, visual loss, aortic aneurysm, and aortic dissection.

Answer A is incorrect. Acetazolamide is a carbonic anhydrase inhibitor and does not play a role in the initial treatment of temporal arteritis.

Answer B is incorrect. Atenolol is a β-blocker and does not play a role in the initial treatment of temporal arteritis.

Answer C is incorrect. Methotrexate is an immunosuppressive agent (like prednisone); however, it is not indicated for use in the treatment of temporal arteritis because studies examining its effects have been inconclusive.

Answer D is incorrect. Nifedipine is a calcium channel blocker and does not play a role in the initial treatment of temporal arteritis.

Questions 26 and 27

26. **The correct answer is D.** Acute gouty arthritis is typically monarticular, presenting with severe pain, redness, swelling, and warmth of the affected joint. A classic location of acute gouty arthritis is the first metatarsophalangeal joint, a condition known as podagra. Gout most commonly occurs in middle-aged to elderly men and is caused by hyperuricemia. Acute gouty arthritis typically has a sudden onset, often at night, and tends to last for 3–10 days.

27. **The correct answer is E.** This patient has a clinical presentation suggesting OA. The dull, aching pain caused by OA worsens with activity and may resolve with rest. Patients may also complain of stiffness and limited mobility. Multiple joints are typically involved. In the hand, the proximal and distal interphalangeal joints are classically affected, while the metacarpophalangeal joints are spared. Enlargement of the distal interphalangeal and proximal interphalangeal joints results in Heberden's and Bouchard's nodes, respectively. The major radiographic signs of osteoarthritis include joint space narrowing, subchondral sclerosis, osteophytes, and subchondral cysts.

Answer A is incorrect. Ankylosing spondylitis is a spondyloarthropathy that typically affects young men. It primarily causes inflammatory back pain and sacroiliitis. Other manifestations include anterior uveitis, aortic regurgitation, bowel ulcerations, and IgA nephropathy.

Answer B is incorrect. Patients with fibromyalgia fulfill two criteria: (1) chronic pain for at least 3 months in all four quadrants of the body and along the axial skeleton and (2) tenderness in 11 of 18 specific anatomic points. They often have multiple associated conditions, such as irritable bowel syndrome, tension headaches or migraines, anxiety disorders, thyroid dysfunction, sleep disorders, depression, and dysmenorrhea.

Answer C is incorrect. Gonococcal arthritis typically causes monarticular arthritis, tenosynovitis, and dermatitis. Patients usually have an acute onset of arthritis, often accompanied by systemic symptoms such as fever and chills. Patients may have pain in the right upper quadrant due to perihepatitis, a condition known as Fitz-Hugh–Curtis syndrome.

Answer F is incorrect. Polymyalgia rheumatica is a rheumatic syndrome that consists of aching pain in the neck, shoulders, and pelvis. Pain is most severe in the proximal muscles. There are no signs of atrophy, but patients do have a reduced range of motion because of their pain.

Answer G is incorrect. Psoriatic arthritis is a spondyloarthropathy that causes inflammatory back pain and oligoarthritis of large peripheral joints. The pain is usually insidious in onset and is worst in the morning or after a long period of inactivity. Patients must have cutaneous signs of psoriasis to be diagnosed with psoriatic arthritis.

Answer H is incorrect. Reactive arthritis is another spondyloarthropathy that typically follows a gastrointestinal infection. Common pathogens implicated in reactive arthritis include *Shigella*, *Campylobacter*, *Yersinia*, and *Salmonella*.

Answer I is incorrect. Classic Reiter's syndrome is also a spondyloarthropathy that typically occurs after infection with *Chlamydia trachomatis*. The classic triad of findings includes uveitis, urethritis, and arthritis ("can't see, can't pee, can't climb a tree"). Other findings may include circinate balanitis and keratoderma blennorrhagicum.

Answer J is incorrect. RA causes symmetric polyarticular inflammation that commonly affects the hands, feet, knees, and ankles. Pain is classically most severe in the morning and improves throughout the day. Patients also complain of morning stiffness that prevents them from getting out of bed. In contrast to OA, patients with RA typically have inflammation of the metacarpophalangeal and proximal interphalangeal joints, with sparing of the distal interphalangeal joints.

Answer K is incorrect. SLE is an autoimmune disorder defined by the presence of antinuclear antibodies. The arthritis of lupus is typically a symmetric polyarthritis that is nondeforming and nonerosive. It generally affects the metacarpophalangeal and proximal interphalangeal joints of the hands, wrists, and knees.

Questions 28–30

28. **The correct answer is J.** Polyarteritis nodosa is a vasculitis of small or medium-size arteries that can cause aneurysms secondary to infiltration and destruction of the blood vessel wall by neutrophils. The most common manifestations are constitutional symptoms, myalgias, and arthralgias, but it may also involve the central nervous system, gastrointestinal tract, and kidneys. This patient's foot drop is secondary to infiltration of the artery supplying the common peroneal nerve, and his postprandial pain is secondary to "intestinal angina" of one of the mesenteric vessels. Treatment is with corticosteroids and cyclophosphamide if refractory.

29. **The correct answer is N.** Wegener's granulomatosis is caused by inflammatory infiltration of small and medium-size arteries. The disease tends to affect the sinuses, upper and lower airways, and kidneys. Symptoms may include cough, hemoptysis, pleuritis, and dyspnea. Although only a minority of patients present with glomerulonephritis early on, approximately

three-fourths of patients eventually develop the complication. Most patients with Wegener's granulomatosis are circulating antineutrophilic cytoplasmic antibody–positive. Initial treatment is with cyclophosphamide.

30. **The correct answer is B.** Churg-Strauss vasculitis is a vasculitis affecting small and medium-size arteries (but typically smaller arteries than those affected by Wegener's granulomatosis). The vasculitis is seen in the setting of asthma and allergic rhinitis. Asthma usually precedes evidence of vasculitis by up to 20 years. The criteria for diagnosis include the presence of asthma, eosinophilia, mono- or polyneuropathy, pulmonary infiltrates, paranasal sinus abnormalities, and extravascular eosinophils.

Answer A is incorrect. Behçet's disease is a systemic vasculitis that affects arteries and veins of all sizes. Clinical manifestations include recurrent oral aphthous and genital ulcers, eye lesions, skin lesions, and a positive pathergy test (a pinprick that turns into a pustule).

Answer C is incorrect. Disseminated intravascular coagulation is seen in many different clinical scenarios, including sepsis, postdelivery (eg, with amniotic embolus), and trauma, as well as in the setting of neoplasia. It is characterized by diffuse bleeding from venipuncture sites, mucosal bleeding, and hypotension. Prothrombin time and partial thromboplastin time are both increased, as is bleeding time. A positive D-dimer and increased fibrin split products with decreased circulating fibrinogen are indicative of a diffuse coagulation process.

Answer D is incorrect. Giant cell arteritis is a vasculitis that typically affects the cranial branches of the aortic arch. Patients can present with headache, scalp pain, constitutional symptoms, or absent temporal artery pulsations. It is associated with polymyalgia rheumatica (pain and weakness of the shoulder and pelvic girdle). Disease activity is associated with an elevated ESR. Temporal artery biopsy demonstrates mononuclear cell or granulomatous inflammation, usually with multinucleated giant cells.

Answer E is incorrect. Hemolytic-uremic syndrome is associated with a mild viral illness or gastroenteritis with *Escherichia coli* O157:H7. The characteristic presentation involves anemia, thrombocytopenia, and acute renal failure.

Answer F is incorrect. Henoch-Schönlein purpura occurs most frequently in children and causes palpable purpura unrelated to thrombocytopenia along with arthritis, abdominal pain, and glomerulonephritis. The disease typically follows an upper respiratory tract infection and is diagnosed by demonstrating IgA deposition in the cutaneous blood vessel wall.

Answer G is incorrect. Idiopathic thrombocytopenic purpura (ITP) is characterized by petechiae, purpura, ecchymoses, and mucosal bleeding. A complete blood count shows very low platelets, and a peripheral blood smear demonstrates large platelets with the absence of schistocytes. ITP can resolve spontaneously, but treatment in adults usually includes corticosteroids; intravenous immunoglobulin and anti-Rh$_o$(D) are reserved for uncontrollable hemorrhage or extremely low platelet counts.

Answer H is incorrect. Kawasaki's disease is a vasculitis of childhood affecting small and medium-size muscular arteries (especially the coronary arteries). Diagnosis requires a fever for at least 5 days and four of the following: rash, conjunctival injection, erythematous mucous membranes, cervical lymphadenopathy, and changes in the hands or feet (e.g., desquamation).

Answer I is incorrect. Microscopic polyangiitis is a vasculitis of small and medium-size arteries and veins that can cause mononeuritis multiplex, necrotizing glomerulonephritis, and pulmonary capillaritis, leading to alveolar hemorrhage and hemoptysis. In contrast to polyarteritis nodosa, it tends to involve the lung. It differs from Wegener's granulomatosis in that patients with microscopic polyangiitis do not exhibit granulomatous inflammation. Patients tend to be perinuclear antineutrophilic cytoplasmic antibody–positive.

Answer K is incorrect. Takayasu's arteritis, also known as "pulseless disease," is a vasculitis that affects young women and demonstrates vasculitis of the aorta and its branches. Patients can present with constitutional findings and claudication of the extremities. Clinical findings include an absent or decreased brachial artery pulse, subclavian bruit, pain along the vessels, and unequal pulses.

Answer L is incorrect. Thromboangiitis obliterans (also known as Buerger's disease) is an inflammatory disease of the small and medium-size arteries, veins, and nerves of the distal extremities. Biopsy demonstrates a highly cellular and inflammatory thrombus that spares the vessel wall. Clinical findings typi-cally involve ischemia of the digits. There are no specific laboratory anomalies for the disease. The typical patient is a young (i.e., < 45 years) male smoker.

Answer M is incorrect. Thrombotic thrombo-cytopenic purpura is a microangiopathic hemolytic anemia characterized by fever, anemia, acute renal failure, thrombocytopenia, and neurologic abnormalities. A peripheral blood smear demonstrates thrombocytopenia and the presence of schistocytes. Indirect bilirubin and lactate dehydrogenase will be high secondary to hemolysis.

CHAPTER 10

Neurology

1. A 4-year-old boy is discovered to have an IQ of 60 and is referred to a pediatrician. His mother reports that he was born 5 weeks premature by spontaneous vaginal delivery after an uncomplicated pregnancy. His developmental history is notable for initially sitting at 9 months, saying his first word at 16 months, walking at 19 months, and climbing up stairs at 3.5 years. He plays cooperatively with the other children. On physical examination, he is cooperative with the examiner, responding in three-word sentences. He walks on his tiptoes with a scissored gait. His legs are hypertonic bilaterally with brisk patellar reflexes; he has ankle clonus and upgoing toes bilaterally. What is the most likely diagnosis?

   (A) Autism
   (B) Cerebral palsy
   (C) Down's syndrome
   (D) Duchenne's muscular dystrophy
   (E) Fragile X syndrome

2. A 42-year-old man presents to urgent care with back pain for 2 days that began while he was moving furniture during home remodeling. The pain is sharp, travels down his left leg, and feels "like an electric shock." It is relieved with rest and aggravated with walking. His temperature is 36.9°C (98.5°F), blood pressure is 122/70 mm Hg, heart rate is 68/min, and respiratory rate is 12/min. The patient appears uncomfortable, and when asked to describe the location of the pain, places his entire hand flat on the lumbar region to the left of the spine. Straight leg raise on the left is positive for replication of the pain. Reflexes are decreased in the left lower extremity. Which of the following is the most appropriate next step in the care of this patient?

   (A) CT of the spine
   (B) Lumbar series x-ray
   (C) MRI of the spine
   (D) Neurosurgical consultation
   (E) Rest and nonsteroidal anti-inflammatory drugs

3. The parents of a 6-month-old child bring him to a pediatrician because they are concerned

he might be having seizures. They describe the events as "convulsions" lasting under a minute and occurring in clusters of increasing frequency and severity. They also report that the child can no longer sit on his own. On examination the child initially seems healthy and is afebrile, but experiences a series of five extensor-type spasms of the neck and trunk. Which of the following tests can confirm the diagnosis of West's syndrome?

   (A) CT scan of the head
   (B) Electrocardiogram
   (C) Electroencephalogram
   (D) Electromyography
   (E) Lumbar puncture

4. A 21-year-old woman presents to her obstetrician for urinary problems. She states that she has been stressed because she is working hard to do well on her finals at college. Over the last 2 weeks she finds herself continually rushing to the bathroom, "because I feel like I need to go, but I can't." This has never happened to her before, and she has begun wearing pads "just in case." She denies fevers and dysuria. She is otherwise healthy, exercises regularly, and takes a multivitamin daily. Her physical examination is normal, as is her urinalysis. Cystometry is performed, and her detrusor contraction to bethanechol chloride is greatly exaggerated. What is the most likely etiology of this woman's urinary urgency?

   (A) Acute cystitis
   (B) Chronic bladder distention
   (C) Detrusor muscle inflammation
   (D) Multiple sclerosis
   (E) Pelvic floor damage

5. A 2.5-month-old African-American boy is brought to the emergency department (ED) for evaluation of fever. Two days prior to admission, the patient developed a fever to 39.1°C (102.3°F) and became irritable with nasal discharge and decreased oral intake. His birth history is unremarkable. He lives at home with his mother and 6-year-old brother who attends elementary school where several kids have been absent for illness. His heart rate is

137/min, blood pressure is 72/48 mm Hg, respiratory rate is 35/min, and temperature is 39.3°C (102.7°F), rectal. Neurologic examination is remarkable for a lethargic-appearing child who is responsive to stimulation. His anterior fontanelle is open and bulging. The resident caring for the patient is certain that he has acute bacterial meningitis and orders a lumbar puncture. According to the table, which of the following cerebrospinal fluid results from the lumbar puncture would be most consistent with acute bacterial meningitis?

(A) A
(B) B
(C) C
(D) D
(E) E

6. A 55-year-old man reported experiencing a headache while lifting heavy boxes. The headache was acute in onset, but gradually worsened over several hours. It was associated with nausea. No over-the-counter analgesics alleviated the symptoms. His past medical history is significant for a recent diagnosis of adult polycystic kidney disease. The man was brought to the ED by his wife. By the time he arrived in the ED he had a decrease in level of consciousness. Which of the following should be performed first in order to confirm a diagnosis?

(A) Comprehensive metabolic panel and complete blood count
(B) Electroencephalogram
(C) Lumbar puncture
(D) Neuroimaging with CT
(E) Neuroimaging with MRI
(F) Positron emission tomography scan

7. A 16-year-old boy is brought to the ED by paramedics while seizing. The neighbors who called 911 report that he has a long-standing seizure disorder and add that they believe he often abuses cocaine; they are unaware of how long he was seizing before they found him 20 minutes ago. On arrival to the ED the patient's pulse is 125/min, blood pressure is 160/100 mm Hg, temperature is 38.9°C (102°F), and respiratory rate is 22/min. On examination the patient has his arms extended rigidly at his side and is arching his back rhythmically and appears to be aspirating. Nasopharyngeal intubation is successful on the second attempt by the ED resident on call; intravenous access is obtained. Which of the following is the most appropriate next step in management?

(A) Intravenous glucose, thiamine, and naloxone, and oxygen via face mask
(B) Intravenous lorazepam and phenytoin
(C) Intravenous phenobarbital
(D) Neuromuscular blockade
(E) Placement of electroencephalographic monitor

CHOICE	PRESSURE (mm H$_2$O)	WBC COUNT (mm^3) [PREDOMINANT CELLS]	PROTEIN (mg/dL)	GLUCOSE (mg/dL)
A	60	2 [lymphocytes]	30	70
B	228	3780 [polymorphonuclear leukocytes]	327	36
C	115	980 [mononuclear cells]	123	62
D	123	300 [mononuclear cells]	194	42
E	97	415 [lymphocytes]	138	69

8. An 80-year-old white man is brought to clinic by his son who is concerned that his father has become more forgetful over the past year, cannot follow instructions, is unable to drive his car or manage his checkbook, and has had a decline in being able to manage activities of daily living. He has no significant medical history other than diabetes, and has no past psychiatric history. His Mini Mental State Examination score is 17. Which of the following criteria would help establish a diagnosis of Alzheimer's disease?

(A) A high level of protein 14-3-3 in the cerebrospinal fluid
(B) Focal neurologic findings and evidence of prior strokes
(C) Gait dysfunction and urinary incontinence
(D) Gradual onset of symptoms and continued cognitive decline
(E) Lewy bodies in the brain stem on autopsy

9. A 79-year-old man who was diagnosed with late onset bipolar disorder is hospitalized after sustaining a fracture. During admission, he is alert and fully oriented, and receives pain medication. Two days after surgery to reduce the fracture, the patient was verbally unresponsive, disoriented, displayed a clouding of consciousness, and could only utter short phrases. A Mini Mental State Examination (MMSE) was administered at that time, and his score was 10 of 30. A day later, the patient displayed good eye contact and normal psychomotor activity. His score on the MMSE was 24 of 30. What is the most appropriate approach to this patient's disorder?

(A) Chlordiazepoxide, thiamine, folic acid, and a multivitamin
(B) Discontinue unnecessary medications, pan-culture, and check for electrolyte abnormalities
(C) Donepezil
(D) Lithium and a sedative drug
(E) Watchful waiting

10. A 36-year-old woman who received no prenatal care gave birth to a full-term 3200-g (7.1-lb) girl. The infant's physical examination is notable for a flat nasal bridge, upslanting palpebral fissures, prominent epicanthal folds, and a pansystolic murmur. A karyotype is sent, and is found to be abnormal. In utero, the infant's condition could have been predicted by which of the following results on a triple marker screen?

CHOICE	MATERNAL SERUM α-FETOPROTEIN	ESTRADIOL	β-HUMAN CHORIONIC GONADOTROPIN
A	↓	↓	↓
B	↓	↓	↑
C	↓	↑	↑
D	↑	↓	↓
E	↑	↓	↑

(A) A
(B) B
(C) C
(D) D
(E) E

11. An 80-year-old man with long-standing Parkinson's disease has been chronically treated with L-dopa in order to alleviate the movement symptoms associated with the disease. Which of the following medications is synergistic with L-dopa and augments its action?

(A) Amantadine
(B) Benztropine
(C) Bromocriptine
(D) Carbidopa
(E) Selegiline

12. A 67-year-old man is found on the floor in his home unresponsive and unarousable. On physical examination the patient is breathing spontaneously and has bounding radial pulses bilaterally. He does not open his eyes, makes no sounds, and withdraws to sternal rub. What is the next step in the management of this patient's condition?

(A) Administer naloxone, thiamine, and dextrose
(B) Check brain stem reflexes
(C) Check serum electrolytes

(D) Intubate

(E) Undress the patient

13. A homeless man is brought to the ED in a confused state following a seizure in public. Witnesses report the seizure as occurring suddenly and lasting at least 2 or 3 minutes. A first responder on the scene says "he swung his arms and his entire body shook." On examination, the patient's tongue is unharmed, although his pants are covered in fresh urine. He is oriented to person but not place or time and has no recollection of what happened, but is aware he has "some sort" of seizure disorder for which he "occasionally" takes an unnamed medication that he is not carrying. More indepth questioning reveals that he has been using increasing amounts of cocaine and heroin since he was kicked out of a group home and rarely takes his seizure medication as a result. An electroencephalogram of this patient during the episode would most likely show which of the following?

(A) A 3-Hz spike-and-wave pattern

(B) A triphasic discharge pattern in sporadic fashion

(C) Generalized seizure activity affecting one hemisphere

(D) Seizure activity involving both hemispheres

(E) Seizure activity localized to a discrete portion of one hemisphere

14. A 30-year-old patient presents with a gradually increasing headache, which she describes as being a "dull aching feeling" at the top of her head. Despite having no previous history, she describes having suffered uncontrollable jerking movements yesterday, subsiding only after 30 seconds. She states that the worst aspect of the headache is the fact that it reaches a crescendo in the morning, making it difficult for her to get to work on time. What is the likely diagnosis?

(A) Brain tumor

(B) Cluster headache

(C) Epidural hemorrhage

(D) Migraine headache

(E) Subdural hemorrhage

(F) Tension headache

15. A 16-month-old toddler is brought to the clinic for worsening coordination. The parents state that the patient was developing well until the age of 5 months. Prior to then, the patient had an appropriate social smile, recognized caregivers, and cooed. At the age of 11 months, she could say a few words, but over the past 3 months has not learned any new words and is not speaking her first words anymore. She was walking with assistance at 12 months, but now has lost coordination and cannot walk. Her parents note that she has developed a peculiar behavior of wringing her hands for long periods of time. This disorder is almost exclusively found in which of the following populations?

(A) Ashkenazi Jews

(B) Females

(C) Fragile X syndrome

(D) Males

(E) Southeast Asians

(F) Trisomy 21 genotype

16. A 38-year-old man with prior head trauma from a motor vehicle accident and no significant past medical history presents with episodes of dizziness induced by rolling over to one side while lying down in bed, that last < 1 minute, and are associated with intense nausea. These episodes have occurred periodically for the past 2–3 months. Nothing alleviates the symptoms. What is the first step in diagnosing the patient's symptoms?

(A) Brain stem evoked audiometry

(B) Dix-Hallpike maneuver

(C) Electronystagmography

(D) Lumbar puncture

(E) Neuroimaging

17. A 13-year-old boy with a previous history of seizures is brought to the physician's office by his parents for staring spells that occur in the morning. His parents report that his epilepsy has been well controlled, and it has been several years since his last seizure. However, they say that he has trouble with spastic movements of his arms and legs almost every morning. An electroencephalogram taken during one of these events would be likely to show which of the following?

(A) A 3-Hz spike-and-wave pattern
(B) "Beta buzz" evolving into diffuse poly-spikes
(C) Generalized seizure activity affecting one hemisphere
(D) Seizure activity involving both hemi-spheres
(E) Seizure activity localized to a discrete por-tion of one hemisphere

18. During a routine eye examination in a 31-year-old patient, an ophthalmologist notices pig-mented hamartomas of the iris. Not knowing what to make of this, the doctor does a full physical examination which is unremarkable, with the exception of the skin findings shown in the image. The patient notes a family his-tory of similar skin findings. Which of the fol-lowing is the most likely diagnosis?

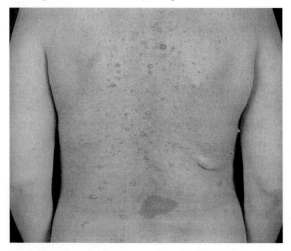

Reproduced, with permission, from Wolff K, Johnson RA, Surmond D. *Fitzpatrick's Color Atlas & Synopsis of Clinical Dermatology*, 5th ed. New York: McGraw-Hill, 2005: Figure 15-29.

(A) Multiple neuroendocrine neoplasia type I
(B) Neurofibromatosis type I
(C) Neurofibromatosis type II
(D) Tuberous sclerosis
(E) Von Hippel–Lindau syndrome

19. A 45-year-old patient with a newly diagnosed brain tumor presents with a speech impedi-ment. He is not able to repeat anything that is said to him or name objects. However, he has preserved fluency of speech and good compre-hension of spoken and written language. He has no other symptoms or neurologic deficits, and his neurologic examination is otherwise unremarkable. What is the most likely diagno-sis?

(A) Broca's aphasia
(B) Conduction aphasia
(C) Global aphasia
(D) Transcortical sensory aphasia
(E) Wernicke's aphasia

20. A 48-year-old auto mechanic presents to the clinic with complaints of many years of "pins and needles" in his left hand that initially oc-curred only while working but have worsened substantially. He claims the pain wakes him al-most every night. On examination, marked weakness and wasting of the left hand muscles are evident. What is the patient's most likely diagnosis?

(A) Amyotrophic lateral sclerosis
(B) Angina
(C) Carpal tunnel syndrome
(D) Multiple sclerosis
(E) Myasthenia gravis

21. A 56-year-old white man is diagnosed with sub-arachnoid hemorrhage following rupture of a cerebral aneurysm in the anterior circulation. The hemorrhage is confirmed on CT of the head, but the decision is made for the patient to undergo endovascular coiling rather than surgical clipping. Roughly 1 week after the original bleed, the patient suffers an acute de-cline in his mental status, with a confirmed new infarct on MRI. Based on the history and time course, what was the likely etiology of the new infarct?

(A) Atherosclerosis
(B) Cardiogenic thromboembolism
(C) Hydrocephalus
(D) Vasospasm

22. A 65-year-old African-American man presents with new-onset aphasia and left-sided homonymous hemianopsia. Results of a CT scan of the head are shown in the image. This patient's stroke involves which vascular territory?

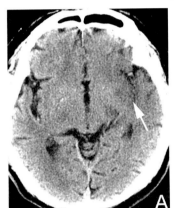

Reproduced, with permission, from Kasper DL, Braunwald E, Fauci AS, Hauser SL, Longo DL, Jameson LJ, Isselbacher KJ, eds. *Harrison's Online.* New York: McGraw-Hill, 2005: Figure 349-12.

(A) Anterior cerebral artery
(B) Basilar artery
(C) Lacunar territories
(D) Middle cerebral artery
(E) Posterior cerebral artery

23. A 72-year-old woman presents complaining of poor sleep and decreased appetite. She is a retired high school teacher who lives with her husband. Their children live in the neighborhood and visit on a regular basis. The patient has no history of psychiatric disorders or major medical illnesses aside from hypertension well controlled on a diuretic. For the past month, the patient has been less interested in many activities that she previously enjoyed. In particular, she no longer reads books and has become reluctant to garden or play with her grandchildren. During the past 3 weeks, her husband has taken over most of the household chores.

When the physician begins the examination, the patient becomes tearful and reluctant to answer questions, frequently saying, "I don't know." Her Mini Mental State Examination score is 24/30, losing points for short-term recall. She also performs poorly on simple executive tasks. Which of the following is the most likely diagnosis?

(A) Alzheimer's dementia
(B) Delirium
(C) Normal aging
(D) Pseudodementia
(E) Vascular dementia

24. A 24-year-old woman with Graves' disease presents complaining of blurry vision during her afternoon commute driving home from work. Administration of edrophonium leads to transient resolution of her clinical symptoms. The physician diagnoses her with myasthenia gravis. In discussing the patient's treatment options with her, which of the following can the physician describe as potentially curative?

(A) Intravenous immune globulin
(B) Neostigmine
(C) Plasmapheresis
(D) Prednisone
(E) Thymectomy

25. A 50-year-old man suffers from headaches. They occur in periodic cycles, only several months out of the year, with one to two headache attacks per day. The headaches are severe; located behind the right eye; and are associated with a red, tearing, right eye and nasal stuffiness on the same side. What is the first step in management of this patient's condition?

(A) Anticonvulsants
(B) Avoiding factors that precipitate these headaches (e.g., alcohol or physical stress)
(C) β-Blockers
(D) Nonsteroidal antiinflammatory drugs
(E) Tricyclic antidepressants

26. A 54-year-old white man presents to the local emergency department with altered mental status and largely unintelligible speech. On further examination, he has considerable gait difficulties and eye movement abnormalities. During the few moments that he is somewhat lucid, he cannot recall where he lives, where he was born, or what he does for a living. The patient's past history includes alcoholism, and his current glucose level is 50 mg/dL. Which of the following should be given to the patient immediately?

(A) Folate
(B) Glucose
(C) Thiamine
(D) Vitamin B_6
(E) Vitamin B_{12}

27. A 64-year-old African-American woman with a history of hypertension and a recent myocardial infarction is brought to the ED by ambulance after developing paralysis of one side of her body and having trouble talking. Her vital signs are stable, but her blood pressure is 190/90 mm Hg. Brain imaging identifies a large ischemic area in the right anterior and middle cerebral artery distribution. Bedside carotid duplex shows complete occlusion of the right internal carotid just distal to the bifurcation. Laboratory values show a platelet count of 250,000/mm³, blood glucose of 110 mg/dL, and normal coagulation times. She has no known drug allergies and is fecal occult blood test negative. Administering which of the following drugs would constitute emergent, evidence-based therapy in this patient?

(A) Aspirin
(B) β-Blocker
(C) Intravenous nitroprusside
(D) Tissue plasminogen activator
(E) Urokinase

28. A 15-year-old boy suffers a blow to the right side of his head during a football game, and loses consciousness. Following a return of consciousness for roughly 5 minutes, he begins to show signs of altered mental status, nausea, and vomiting. CT of the head shows acute blood in the intracranial compartment. What structure likely was injured?

(A) Basilar artery
(B) Dural venous sinus
(C) Middle meningeal artery
(D) Superior sagittal sinus
(E) Vertebral artery

29. A 3-day-old boy presents to the ED after his mother found him rhythmically shaking his extremities for 1 minute. He was born at term via spontaneous vaginal delivery after an uncomplicated pregnancy. His Apgar scores were 8 and 9 at 1 and 5 minutes, respectively. His birth weight is 3100 g (6.8 lb). His family history is notable for a brother who died at age 6 years from mycobacterial pneumonia. His temperature is 36.5°C (97.7°F), blood pressure is 70/50 mm Hg, respiratory rate is 30/min, and heart rate is 110/min. He has a squared nose, cleft palate, and a harsh systolic ejection murmur along the sternal border. Laboratory tests show:

WBC count	6200/mm³
Hemoglobin	15 g/dL
Platelet count	190,000/mm³
Serum calcium	6.2 mg/dL
25-Hydroxyvitamin D	50 ng/mL
Phosphorus	4 mg/dL
Magnesium	2 mg/dL

Which of the following is the most likely diagnosis?

(A) Beckwith-Wiedemann syndrome
(B) Chronic granulomatous disease
(C) DiGeorge's syndrome
(D) Multiple endocrine neoplasia type I
(E) Niemann-Pick disease

30. A 76-year-old man with chronic hypertension presents to the emergency department with altered mental status and elevated blood pressure in the 230/140 mm Hg range as a result of noncompliance with blood pressure medication. ED doctors suspect a bleed based on CT of the head. Where do bleeds typically occur in this patient population?

(A) Basal ganglia/thalamus
(B) Brain stem
(C) Epidural space
(D) Ventricles

31. The parents of a 6-year-old boy bring their child to the physician for episodes "too numerous to count" of the child staring off "into space" while fluttering his eyes. His attention returns after 5–10 seconds, and he is never aware of the lapses in his attention. Which antiepileptic is the first-line agent for children with this disorder?

    (A) Carbamazepine
    (B) Gabapentin
    (C) Ethosuximide
    (D) Tiagabine
    (E) Valproate

32. A young girl hops and skips her way into her pediatrician's office. She takes a seat beside her mother and is able to copy crosses in the workbook the nurse hands her but is not able to print her name. She then counts to 10 and begins to sing a song she was taught by her older sister. How old is she?

    (A) 2 years old
    (B) 3 years old
    (C) 4 years old
    (D) 5 years old
    (E) 6 years old

33. A 4-year-old boy is brought to the local ED by his mother because he is "not acting right." His mother, who is pregnant, reports that he seemed well last night, but this morning he was uncharacteristically groggy and appeared "flushed." He fell over twice while walking around the house and "passed out" for 20 seconds while eating breakfast. Although he did not hit his head, he did complain of a headache. On the way to the hospital, he vomited once; it was nonbloody and nonbilious. There are no sick contacts in the household, but his father awoke with an unusually severe headache this morning. The family is vacationing at a nearby mountain resort noted for its "rustic log cabins with wood-burning fireplaces." His temperature is 37°C (98.6°F), blood pressure is 90/50 mm Hg, pulse is 130/min, and respiratory rate is 26/min. The patient is minimally cooperative; he refuses to walk, preferring to nap in his mother's arms. There is no evidence of head trauma and his physical examination is otherwise unremarkable. Further testing would likely reveal which of the following abnormalities?

    (A) Blood glucose of 60 mg/dL
    (B) Low partial pressure of arterial oxygen measured in arterial blood gas testing
    (C) Metabolic acidosis with increased anion gap
    (D) Pulmonary effusion on x-ray of the chest
    (E) Pulse oximetry of 89%

34. A 75-year-old man with a history of carotid stenosis presents with acute left-sided hemiparesis and aphasia. He was brought to the ED from his nursing home by an ambulance, which was held up in traffic for at least half an hour. He remains somewhat responsive with stable vital signs but his neurologic deficits are unchanged. The physician also notes that his clothing is soiled with urine and feces, although he is known to be continent at baseline. Which of the following is the most appropriate initial imaging study for this patient?

    (A) Carotid ultrasound
    (B) Cerebral angiography
    (C) Conventional radiography
    (D) CT of the head without contrast
    (E) MRI of the brain

35. A 36-year-old woman presents to the ED after experiencing a seizure in her apartment 3 hours earlier. She has no known prior medical problems, and takes only aspirin for some recent headaches. She is currently lethargic but responsive and coherent. Her temperature is 37.2°C (98.9°F), blood pressure is 117/68 mm Hg with no orthostatic changes, and pulse is 70/min. Physical examination reveals anicteric sclerae with reactive pupils and moist mucous membranes. Laboratory tests show:

Na+	124 mEq/L
Ca2+	9.8 mg/dL
Cl−	100 mEq/L
HCO3−	19 mEq/L
Blood urea nitrogen	9.2 mg/dL
Creatinine	0.9 mg/dL
Glucose	110 mg/dL

Liver function tests, amylase, lipase, and bilirubin are normal. Urine electrolytes reveal an elevated urine sodium. Which of the following is the most likely cause of this patient's hyponatremia?

(A) Bartter's syndrome
(B) Brain tumor
(C) Hyperglycemic crisis
(D) Primary biliary cirrhosis
(E) Subarachnoid hemorrhage

36. A 58-year-old African-American man with a history of hypertension and diabetes presents to the ophthalmology clinic for a routine examination. The patient has no visual complaints. Visual acuity is 20/20 in both eyes. Funduscopic examination reveals enlarged optic nerve head cupping with significant rim pallor in both eyes. Gonioscopy reveals open angles, and applanation tonometry reveals borderline intraocular pressures. Given his diagnosis, what agent could be used to treat this patient's condition?

(A) Corticosteroids
(B) Intravenous mannitol
(C) Isoproterenol
(D) Phenoxybenzamine
(E) Pilocarpine

37. A 50-year-old man presents to the ED with a headache that began suddenly in the middle of the night. He says that the pain is severe and is located behind his right eye. When the pain started, he began to see double. The patient notes a history of poorly controlled hypertension and mitral valve prolapse. One year prior to presentation, an ultrasound of the right upper quadrant to evaluate for gallstones showed several small hepatic cysts. He was told to follow-up but never did. The patient has a blood pressure of 165/90 mm Hg, heart rate of 62/min, temperature of 36.6°C (97.8°F), and respiratory rate of 20/min. Physical examination shows his body habitus is normal, and he looks uncomfortable. On neurologic examination, he has a blown right pupil that does not respond to light in the ipsilateral or contralateral side. The left pupil is both directly and consensually responsive to light. The patient is unable to elevate, depress, or adduct the right eye. The double vision is only present when both eyes are open and is worse in right lateral gaze. The rest of his cranial nerves are intact, and no other neurologic abnormalities are noted. On abdominal examination, there are bilateral, easily palpable large kidneys, the left one greater than the right. No hepatosplenomegaly is appreciated. Laboratory tests show:

Na+	140 mEq/L
K+	3.8 mEq/L
Cl−	126 mEq/L
HCO3−	9 mEq/L
Blood urea nitrogen	10 mg/dL
Creatinine	1.5 mg/dL
Total bilirubin	0.8 mg/dL
Aspartate transaminase	12 U/L
Alkaline phosphatase	55 U/L

What disease would explain this man's presentation?

(A) Budd-Chiari syndrome
(B) Caroli's disease
(C) Marfan's syndrome
(D) Metastatic renal cell carcinoma
(E) Multiple sclerosis
(F) Polycystic kidney disease

38. A 20-year-old college student was brought to the ED after she was hit on the head by a stray baseball. The patient was conscious when the first responders arrived at the scene, but she began complaining of a severe headache and

then lost consciousness en route to the hospital. Initial CT scan showed a large epidural hematoma that would require emergent evacuation. The patient had not regained consciousness, and the ED clerk had not yet found her emergency contact information. Which of the following is the most appropriate next step in the patient's care?

(A) Ask the patient's dormitory housemaster to sign a consent form for emergency treatment
(B) Infuse mannitol to decrease intracranial pressure while waiting for the patient's parents to arrive
(C) Perform emergent evacuation of epidural hematoma
(D) Perform serial neurologic examinations while waiting for the clerk to obtain the information about the patient's emergency contact
(E) Wait for the parents to arrive before proceeding with any treatment

39. A middle-aged man is brought to the ED by ambulance after developing acute-onset hemiparesis and aphasia while at work. Brain imaging identifies a large ischemic area in the right anterior cerebral artery/middle cerebral artery distribution. Bedside carotid duplex shows complete occlusion of the right internal carotid artery just distal to the bifurcation. Laboratory tests show a platelet count of 250,000/mm³, blood glucose of 110 mg/dL, and normal coagulation times. His blood pressure is 140/85 mm Hg and he is afebrile. Due to confusion and aphasia, it is almost impossible to obtain a history from the patient. The physician is planning on administering thrombolytics, but needs certain key information beforehand. Suddenly, the patient's wife arrives in the ED. Which of the following items in the patient's recent medical history is a contraindication to thrombolytic therapy?

(A) Bruise on the leg
(B) Documented carotid stenosis
(C) Myocardial infarction 10 years ago
(D) Peptic ulcer at the age of 16, treated
(E) Stroke 2 months ago

40. A 6-month-old boy of Ashkenazi Jewish descent presents to his pediatrician's office. His mother is concerned that "he isn't developing right." At 2 months, he was following objects as they moved across the midline and lifting his head. However, for the past month, he has been less alert, startles more easily, and has not been lifting his head. Physical examination is unremarkable, except the ophthalmologic examination shown a bright red macula surrounded by a whitish ring. What is this patient's clinical prognosis?

(A) Death by age 4–5 years
(B) Future organomegaly and easy bruising
(C) Hyperactivity if left untreated
(D) Opisthotonos
(E) Spasticity and rigidity in type A of this condition

41. A 64-year-old smoker presents to the clinic with gradual-onset distortion of straight lines, blurring of small objects, and disturbances in color vision. He has decreased visual acuity in the central visual fields of both eyes. Funduscopy shows drusen accompanied by a choroidal neovascular membrane, subretinal hemorrhages, subretinal fibrosis, and retinal hemorrhage. What would be the next most appropriate step in management of the patient?

(A) Atropine
(B) Laser photocoagulation
(C) Timolol
(D) Topical steroids
(E) Trabeculectomy

42. A 22-year-old previously healthy woman presents to the ED complaining of the worst headache of her life, which started suddenly 3 hours ago. She denies photo- or phonophobia, but complains of blurry vision associated with the onset of the headache. CT scan of the head without contrast reveals a Fisher grade III subarachnoid hemorrhage. The patient is transported back to the trauma bay, at which time she loses consciousness and seizes. What is the first step in management of this patient after the seizure?

    (A) Antiepileptic and mannitol
    (B) Cervical spine evaluation/immobilization
    (C) Intubate the patient
    (D) Start oxygen by nasal cannula
    (E) Trauma survey

43. A 58-year-old woman has been suffering from daily headaches for months. They are not associated with an aura, nausea, vomiting, or photophobia. They last for 6 hours per day and occur about half the month. Her medical history is significant only for arthritis, for which she has been taking high doses of nonsteroidal anti-inflammatory drugs and acetaminophen-based analgesics daily for the past several months. She has been gradually escalating her analgesic dose to manage her condition. Her physical examination is within normal limits. Which of the following is most likely to be effective in preventing her daily headaches?

    (A) Behavioral modification therapies
    (B) Controlling her analgesic use
    (C) Prophylactic treatment with β-blockers
    (D) Treatment with selective serotonin reuptake inhibitors
    (E) Treatment with tricyclic antidepressants

44. A 34-year-old woman is seen by a neurologist complaining of a 3-month history of headaches. The neurologist promptly orders an MRI of the brain which reveals a tumor that has a large central lesion in the posterior parietal lobe, along with multiple, smaller satellite lesions around it. Following surgical resection, the pathologic specimen seen in the image is obtained. What tumor type does the MRI and pathology results most likely indicate?

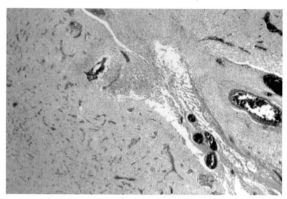

Reproduced, with permission, from PEIR Digital Library (http://peir.net).

    (A) Acoustic schwannoma
    (B) Cavernous malformation
    (C) Glioblastoma multiforme
    (D) Medulloblastoma
    (E) Meningioma

45. After a sailing accident in which a man falls overboard, he arrives at the ED with a temperature of 25°C (77.0°F), no spontaneous respirations or cardiac activity, and a depressed skull fracture. Rewarming is begun, the man is intubated and mechanically ventilated, and cardiotropic medications are administered, resulting in a faint, palpable, pulse. The "doll's-eyes" reflex is absent. There is no deviation of the eyes in response to irrigation of the ear canal with ice water. His Glasgow Coma Scale score is 3/15. Body temperature after CT is 28.1°C (82.5°F). Which of the following characteristics would prevent brain death from being declared in this patient at this time?

    (A) Artificial ventilation
    (B) Body temperature
    (C) Cardiac activity
    (D) Glasgow Coma Scale score 3/15
    (E) Skull fracture

46. An 8-year-old girl is brought to the ED for evaluation of a "seizure." She first complained of stomach pain and soon afterward smacked her lips for 10 minutes. During that time she was unresponsive, and she does not remember the event. There is no history of head trauma or a history of seizures. Her mother had seizures that resolved in puberty and is distraught about her daughter's seizure. On examination, her

temperature is 37.8°C (100.0°F), blood pressure is 90/60 mm Hg, heart rate is 70/min, and respiratory rate is 22/min. She is drowsy but is able to be aroused. Her neck is supple, and the remainder of the neurologic examination is normal. A complete metabolic panel, complete blood cell count, and liver function tests are normal. A prolactin level is slightly elevated. A CT scan of the head with contrast is negative. An electroencephalogram shows slow waves throughout, with sharp waves over the left temporal region. What is the most appropriate therapy for this child?

(A) Acetaminophen
(B) Aspirin
(C) Cefotaxime and vancomycin
(D) Ethosuximide
(E) Phenobarbital

47. A 65-year-old woman is brought to the physician by her son because he is concerned about her memory loss over the past year. Yesterday, after going for a walk, she could not remember her way back, even though she was only two blocks away from the house. Although the patient denies any major problems, her son says she is forgetful and becomes confused. There is a family history of dementia. She has no history of drug or alcohol abuse. Her vital signs are within normal limits. She is oriented to person, place, and time. She can recall past events quite well but her recent memory is impaired. She has difficulty recalling the names of common objects. Her physical examination, laboratory test results, and thyroid tests indicate no abnormalities. Which is the most appropriate step in management?

(A) Bupropion
(B) Donepezil
(C) Doxepin
(D) Gingko biloba
(E) Thiamine
(F) Vitamin E

48. A 12-month-old boy is brought to his pediatrician by his parents. He had had a normal, healthy childhood until 1 month ago. His parents complain that over the past month he has been vomiting frequently, and also appears to be increasingly irritable. He is now taking more naps during the day and is playing less than usual. His parents also think there is a problem with his sight, as he often does not appear to see toys and furniture that are directly in his line of vision. On physical examination, the patient has lost 3.6 kg (8 lb) since his last visit 6 weeks ago. He is afebrile, has a pulse of 140/min, a blood pressure of 90/56 mm Hg, and a respiratory rate of 24/min. An image from an ophthalmologic examination is shown. Which of the following is the most appropriate next step in managing this patient?

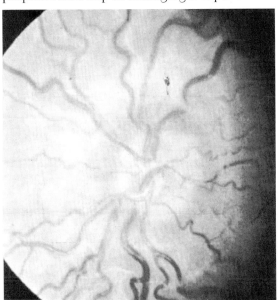

Reproduced, with permission, from Ropper AH, Brown RH. *Adams and Victor's Principles of Neurology*, 8th ed. New York: McGraw-Hill, 2005: Figure 13-9.

(A) Administer mannitol
(B) Administer timolol
(C) CT scan of the head without contrast
(D) Lumbar puncture
(E) MRI scan of the brain

HIGH-YIELD SYSTEMS

Neurology

49. A 79-year-old woman is in the early stages of Alzheimer's disease. She has some mild recent memory loss and difficulty with everyday motor tasks, which has been progressive over 2 years. She has no living will and has not designated a durable power of attorney in the event that she becomes incapacitated. Which of the following is true regarding advance directives in patients with early Alzheimer's disease?

(A) Family members should be allowed to decide on future treatment plans
(B) It is impossible for these patients to make decisions regarding their health care due to loss of self-identity
(C) Patients generally do not have a sufficient level of executive function to designate a health care proxy
(D) Substituted judgment should be applied to determine the patient's proxy
(E) The physician should discuss the course and prognosis of the disease with the patient

50. A 50-year-old man presents to his primary care physician with difficulty achieving an erection. He states that he has noticed a decrease in his sex drive during the past 2–3 months. The man has a history of diet-controlled hypertension and had a left total knee replacement 1 year ago. He states that he is in a monogamous relationship with his wife and has been for 22 years. The patient's blood pressure is 130/90 mm Hg, temperature is 37.2°C (98.9°F), and heart rate is 86/min. On examination, his confrontational visual fields reveal a small bitemporal superior visual field loss. The rest of the man's cranial nerves are normal. His abdominal, genital, and prostate examinations are unremarkable. Laboratory tests show:

WBC count	5600/mm^3
Hematocrit	40%
Platelet count	156,000/mm^3
Aspartate aminotransferase	20 U/L
Alkaline phosphatase	50 U/L
Blood urea nitrogen	18 mg/dL
Creatinine	0.9 mg/dL
Cortisol (fasting)	11 μg/dL
Prolactin	38 ng/mL
Thyroid-stimulating hormone	2.8 μU/mL
Total testosterone	190 ng/mL
Free testosterone	40 pg/L

Which of the following diagnostic tests is most appropriate to perform?

(A) Brain MRI
(B) β-Human chorionic gonadotropin
(C) Mammogram
(D) No tests are necessary
(E) Scrotal ultrasound

1. **The correct answer is B.** This child has cerebral palsy (CP), which is the most prevalent nonprogressive motor disorder in children. The most common type of CP is pyramidal, accounting for 75% of the cases. Mental retardation is present in 90% of cases of pyramidal CP. Pyramidal CP is nonprogressive and characterized by spasticity, hyperreflexia, slow effortful voluntary movements, and impaired fine motor function. Delayed developmental milestones, persistence of infantile reflexes (e.g., Babinski's reflex), contractures, and weakness or underdevelopment of affected limbs are common. Children typically walk on their toes and have a scissor gait. The cause of CP is usually not clearly defined; however, risk factors include prematurity, perinatal asphyxia, intrauterine growth restriction, infection, trauma, brain malformation, and hemorrhage.

Answer A is incorrect. Autism is characterized by poor verbal and nonverbal communication skills, repetitive stereotyped behaviors, mental retardation, abnormal responses to the environment, and poor social skills. These symptoms are present before the age of 3 years. Spasticity, hyperreflexia, voluntary movement disorders, and impaired fine motor function are not typically part of this condition, so autism is an unlikely diagnosis in this patient.

Answer C is incorrect. Down's syndrome is the most common cause of mental retardation. It is characterized by abnormal facies (flat facial profile and prominent epicanthal folds), a simian crease, and cardiac malformations. However, Down's syndrome does not cause spasticity, hyperreflexia, or other movement complaints described in this patient, so this answer is incorrect.

Answer D is incorrect. Duchenne's muscular dystrophy (DMD) is the most common hereditary neuromuscular disease and is sometimes associated with mental retardation. There is a progressive loss of muscle strength. The classic sign is a Gowers' maneuver, in which a child pushes off the floor and walks his hands up his legs to assume a standing position. DMD typi-cally affects the limb girdle muscles initially and is progressive, which makes this diagnosis incorrect in this patient.

Answer E is incorrect. Fragile X syndrome is the most common cause of mental retardation in male patients. It is characterized by abnormal facies (macrocephaly, elongated face, and prominent ears), macro-orchidism, and stereotyped behavior rather than movement problems; therefore, this answer is not the most likely diagnosis.

2. **The correct answer is E.** The patient's symptoms are consistent with a herniated nucleus pulposus. Spontaneous improvement is the rule; > 90% of patients have resolution within 6 weeks of pain onset. Conservative treatment involves rest: 1–2 days of bedrest (longer is counterproductive, as deconditioning begins) followed by 2–3 weeks of activity limitation (reduce lifting and twisting) with reassessment prior to lifting activity restriction. Nonsteroidal anti-inflammatory drugs, moist heat, and gentle exercise to promote joint mobility are all typically helpful.

Answer A is incorrect. Imaging is reserved for patients with systemic symptoms (fever and weight loss) when cancer or infection is high on the differential, in patients with trauma (e.g., motor vehicle accident), and in patients who do not improve with more conservative measures.

Answer B is incorrect. Imaging is reserved for patients with systemic symptoms (fever and weight loss) when cancer or infection is high on the differential, in patients with trauma (e.g., motor vehicle accident), and in patients who do not improve with more conservative measures.

Answer C is incorrect. Imaging is reserved for patients with systemic symptoms (fever and weight loss) when cancer or infection is high on the differential, in patients with trauma (e.g., motor vehicle accident), and in patients who do not improve with more conservative measures.

Answer D is incorrect. Surgical decompression of the nerve root would be reserved for cases intractable to more conservative measures.

3. **The correct answer is C.** The child has a classic clinical presentation of West's syndrome, which is characterized by infantile spasms, arrest of psychomotor development and a hypsarrhythmia pattern on electroencephalogram.

Answer A is incorrect. Although inferior to MRI, CT would be useful if one suspected seizures secondary to a central nervous system neoplasm.

Answer B is incorrect. ECG would not be useful in this context, but is easily confused with electroencephalogram.

Answer D is incorrect. Electromyography would not be useful in this context, but is often confused with electroencephalogram and is useful in the diagnosis of many neurodegenerative syndromes in adults.

Answer E is incorrect. Lumbar puncture (LP) would be more helpful in diagnosing infectious causes of meningitis. On rare occasion, LP might reveal a metabolic cause of West's syndrome such as nonketotic hypoglycinemia.

4. **The correct answer is D.** Bethanechol chloride is a parasympathomimetic drug that is used during cystometry to aid in diagnosis. Lack of a contraction to bethanechol chloride suggests detrusor muscle damage and an increased response suggests upper motor neuron dysfunction. Multiple sclerosis is an autoimmune disease that is the result of central nervous system demyelination. It most commonly affects young women and can be exacerbated by stress. Bladder spasticity and urinary retention can be the presenting symptoms.

Answer A is incorrect. Although acute cystitis is common in young women, it is often accompanied by dysuria and RBCs, WBCs, and bacteria in the urine. The response to bethanechol chloride should not be influenced by cystitis.

Answer B is incorrect. Chronic bladder distention, often secondary to outflow obstruction, presents with overflow incontinence, not spasticity, and would not be expected to lead to an increased response to bethanechol chloride.

Answer C is incorrect. The response to bethanechol chloride should be decreased in cases of detrusor dysfunction due to muscle damage.

Answer E is incorrect. Pelvic floor damage, often secondary to trauma such as childbirth, leads to sphincteric insufficiency and stress, or in severe cases, total incontinence. Spasticity would be an unlikely presentation. Furthermore, the response to bethanechol chloride would not be expected to be increased.

5. **The correct answer is B.** Acute bacterial meningitis in an infant often manifests with signs and symptoms similar to those in the vignette (i.e., fever, increased irritability or lethargy, decreased oral intake, papilledema, and a bulging fontanelle). Laboratory evaluation of cerebrospinal fluid obtained from a lumbar puncture will demonstrate an elevated opening pressure (usually 100–300 mm H_2O) with 100–10,000 WBCs, most of which will be polymorphonuclear leukocytes. Protein levels are elevated (100–500 mg/dL), and glucose is decreased to < 50% of serum glucose levels. Acute bacterial meningitis is a life-threatening condition that must be rapidly diagnosed and treated in affected patients to reduce morbidity and mortality.

Answer A is incorrect. This is typical of cerebrospinal fluid (CSF) findings in a normal individual. Normal opening pressure is 50–80 mm H_2O, and generally < 5 WBCs are present with ≥ 75% lymphocytes. Normal protein levels are 20–45 mg/dL and normal CSF glucose levels are > 50 mg/dL, or approximately 75% serum glucose.

Answer C is incorrect. These cerebrospinal fluid findings are typical of viral meningitis. In such patients, pressure is normal or slightly elevated (80–150 mm H_2O), and there are rarely ≥ 1000 cells present. Polymorphonuclear leukocytes predominate early in the course of the illness, and mononuclear cells (monocyte + lymphocyte) predominate throughout the illness. Protein is often elevated to 50–200 mg/dL and glucose levels are often normal but may be decreased, depending on the viral pathogen.

Answer D is incorrect. This is representative of fungal meningitis. Pressure is often elevated, and 5–500 WBCs are present, with polymorphonuclear leukocytes predominating early in the course, and mononuclear cells predominate throughout the majority of the illness. Protein levels are often 25–500 mg/dL and glucose levels are generally < 50 mg/dL.

Answer E is incorrect. Acute syphilis and leptospirosis will provide cerebrospinal fluid findings as seen in this option. Pressure is elevated at 50–500 mm H_2O and WBCs are predominantly present, 50–200 mg/dL of protein is found, and glucose levels are usually normal.

6. **The correct answer is D.** Neuroimaging with CT is the first essential step in confirming a diagnosis of cerebral hemorrhage, which is suspected given the patient's history of presentation and the acuity of the symptoms. Patients with adult polycystic kidney disease are at increased risk for developing berry aneurysms.

Answer A is incorrect. Testing the patient's blood has no immediate role in the establishment of a diagnosis of cerebral hemorrhage.

Answer B is incorrect. EEG, while useful for diagnosing seizure disorders, has no utility in diagnosing acute cerebral hemorrhage.

Answer C is incorrect. Although a lumbar puncture may have diagnostic value in order to assess the presence of RBCs or the presence of xanthochromia, it should not be performed without having had a prior CT/MRI, because surrounding edema may cause shifts in brain content, and brain herniation into the spinal canal can occur, leading to death.

Answer E is incorrect. Although MRI can be helpful to determine the presence of blood or other abnormalities, scanning may take up to an hour. This patient has a possible acute bleed and needs to be assessed quickly.

Answer F is incorrect. A positron emission tomography scan has no role in the acute diagnosis of a cerebral hemorrhage.

7. **The correct answer is B.** Status epilepticus (SE) refers to a continuous state of seizure activity or a series of seizures during which there is no return to consciousness in the inter-ictal period. The minimal duration of seizure activity in SE has traditionally been cited as 15–30 minutes. Practically speaking, anyone who is brought to an emergency department who has been seizing for > 5 minutes will be treated as having SE. SE is a medical emergency with a wide range of potentially lethal complications and 20% mortality. Following a basic primary survey (**ABCs**; **A**irway, **B**reathing, and **C**irculation) the next step in management is the administration of a benzodiazepine and a loading dose of phenytoin.

Answer A is incorrect. At many centers intravenous glucose, thiamine, naloxone, and oxygen via face mask are given presumptively to all unconscious patients that arrive in the emergency department. While these therapies have little risk and may be appropriate in this patient, the next logical step in a patient with presumed status epilepticus would be the administration of medication capable of ending seizure activity.

Answer C is incorrect. If intravenous (IV) benzodiazepines and phenytoin are ineffective, phenobarbital may be given IV, but it is not a first-line agent.

Answer D is incorrect. Brief neuromuscular blockade may become necessary if rapid sequence induction intubation is required to secure the patient's airway. However, in this patient with a secure airway, further blockade is unnecessary unless the patient develops respiratory distress and requires paralysis and mechanical ventilation or rhabdomyolysis.

Answer E is incorrect. Complex studies such as electroencephalographic monitoring and brain imaging, although they may be useful in establishing the diagnosis, are best deferred until the patient has been stabilized.

8. **The correct answer is D.** Gradual onset of symptoms and continued cognitive decline are criteria for diagnosing Alzheimer's disease (AD) according to the *Diagnostic and Statistical Manual of Mental Disorders, Fourth Edition, Text Revision*. Other criteria include impairment of recent memory (inability to learn new information) and at least one of the following: disturbance of language; inability to

execute skilled motor activities in the absence of weakness; disturbances of visual processing; or disturbances of executive function (including abstract reasoning and concentration). Behavioral problems are common in patients with AD; personality changes (ranging from progressive passivity to open hostility) may precede the cognitive impairments. AD is the most common form of dementia in the elderly, accounting for 60–80% of cases. The brains of individuals with AD are characterized by extracellular deposition of amyloid-β protein, intracellular neurofibrillary tangles, and loss of neurons.

Answer A is incorrect. A high level of protein 14-3-3 in the cerebrospinal fluid (CSF) is associated with Creutzfeldt-Jakob disease (CJD). CJD is the most frequent of the human prion diseases. Rapidly progressive mental deterioration and myoclonus are the two cardinal clinical manifestations of CJD. Myoclonus, especially provoked by startle, is present in > 90% of patients at some point during the illness. The gold standard of diagnosis involves brain biopsy. The etiology of CJD can be familial or iatrogenic (from corneal transplantation or dural grafts). There is no effective treatment for CJD which is uniformly fatal.

Answer B is incorrect. Focal neurologic findings and evidence on physical examination consistent with prior strokes is associated with vascular dementia. Vascular dementia would also be suggested if a patient has an abrupt onset of symptoms followed by stepwise deterioration, and has infarcts on cerebral imaging. Although diabetes is associated with vascular disease and the risk factors of stroke, there are no focal neurologic deficits or a prior history of strokes.

Answer C is incorrect. A triad of gait dysfunction, urinary incontinence, and cognitive dysfunction help establish a diagnosis of normal pressure hydrocephalus (NPH). This patient does not have these symptoms. Furthermore, CT scan of the head may show dilated cerebral ventricles. NPH occurs in elderly patients and is due to an increased subarachnoid space volume that does not accompany increased ventricular volume. Some believe that the initial event is diminished absorption of cerebrospinal

fluid at the arachnoid villi. Clinical symptoms result from distortion of the central portion of the corona radiata by the distended ventricles. Dementia results from distortion of the periventricular limbic system.

Answer E is incorrect. Lewy bodies in the brain stem on autopsy are seen in dementia with Lewy bodies (DLB) associated with Parkinson's disease. DLB is the second most common form of neurodegenerative dementia after Alzheimer's disease. The core clinical features of DLB are a gradually progressive dementia; fluctuations in cognitive function; persistent, well-formed visual hallucinations; and spontaneous motor features of parkinsonism. Supportive features of DLB include repeated falls, syncope, sensitivity to neuroleptic medications, delusions, hallucinations in nonvisual senses, rapid eye movement sleep behavior disorders, and depression. The diagnosis is based on history and clinical features.

9. **The correct answer is B.** This patient meets the diagnostic criteria for delirium. Characteristics of delirium include rapid onset, a fluctuating and cloudy level of consciousness, impaired orientation, disordered thinking, and usually complete reversibility of the condition (as with this patient who returned to normal functioning a day later). Postoperative delirium is common in patients who are elderly, regardless of preexisting psychopathology. The proper approach is to identify and correct underlying causes such as dehydration, electrolyte imbalance, infection, and polypharmacy.

Answer A is incorrect. The combination of chlordiazepoxide (Librium), thiamine, folic acid, and a multivitamin is used to treat alcohol withdrawal. There is no mention of alcohol use and dependence in this patient.

Answer C is incorrect. Donepezil is the treatment of choice for patients with Alzheimer's disease (dementia). The patient's condition can be clinically differentiated from dementia on the basis that dementia is a chronic disease, has an insidious onset, and is chronically progressive. Level of consciousness and orientation is intact initially, but the majority of case.

Answer D is incorrect. Lithium and a sedative drug are used in cases of acute manic episodes. Although the patient in this case has a previous diagnosis of bipolar disorder, there is no evidence that he is having an acute manic episode that would involve an expansive or irritable mood lasting at least 1 week, grandiosity, pressured speech, or flight of ideas.

Answer E is incorrect. Delirium is a medical urgency, and its cause must be identified as soon as possible.

10. **The correct answer is B.** The infant has Down's syndrome; classic physical findings include flat facial profile, prominent epicanthal folds, upslanting palpebral fissure, clinodactyly, simian crease, and congenital heart disease. At 15–18 weeks of gestation a triple marker screen can be performed. This is the classic profile seen in trisomy 21. An amniocentesis is offered to women who have abnormal triple screens or those who will be > 35 years old at the time of delivery. Karyotyping is performed on amniotic fluid and allows a definitive diagnosis to be made. The infant was at increased risk of having Down's syndrome because her mother is > 35 years old.

Answer A is incorrect. These results are classically seen in fetuses with trisomy 18. Trisomy 18, Edward's syndrome, classically presents with rocker-bottom feet, low-set ears, micrognathia, prominent occiput, clenched hands, and congenital heart disease.

Answer C is incorrect. These results are abnormal but are not specific for any particular condition. The α-fetoprotein and β-human chorionic gonadotropin suggest Down's syndrome; however, the estradiol is trended in the wrong direction.

Answer D is incorrect. These results are abnormal but are not specific for any particular condition. Although an elevated α-fetoprotein is seen in neural tube defects, β-human chorionic gonadotropin and estradiol are not markers for this condition.

Answer E is incorrect. These results are abnormal but are not specific for any particular condition. Although the estradiol and β-human chorionic gonadotropin levels suggest Down's syndrome, the α-fetoprotein is trended in the wrong direction.

11. **The correct answer is D.** Parkinson's disease is a degenerative disorder of the central nervous system characterized by muscle rigidity, tremor, bradykinesia, and in extreme cases, akinesia. The primary symptoms are the results of excessive muscle contraction secondary to insufficient formation and action of dopamine. Carbidopa augments the action of L-dopa by increasing L-dopa's entry into the brain. This effect is accomplished by preventing its peripheral conversion to dopamine, with the added benefit of preventing side effects of L-dopa.

Answer A is incorrect. Amantadine is a dopamine reuptake inhibitor that has also been used as an independent treatment of Parkinson's disease.

Answer B is incorrect. Benztropine is an antimuscarinic that reduces parkinsonian tremor and rigidity.

Answer C is incorrect. Bromocriptine directly activates the dopamine receptor and is independently used to treat Parkinson's disease.

Answer E is incorrect. Selegiline is a selective monoamine oxidase-B inhibitor that increases dopamine levels in the brain.

12. **The correct answer is D.** The first step in the diagnosis and clinical assessment of a patient with altered consciousness is to perform a primary survey that provides rapid identification of potentially fatal conditions. This patient was "found down" and his provider should have a high degree of suspicion for injury. The primary survey can be remembered as **ABCDE**— **A**irway, **B**reathing, **C**irculation, **D**isability, and **E**xposure. This patient is breathing, but this does not mean the airway is clear! The breathing could be labored or difficult due to impending airway compromise or obstruction. Thus the first step in management would be establishing a definite airway by intubation. Once the ABCs have been examined, disability should be ascertained by using the Glasgow Coma Scale (GCS). This patient has a GCS score of 6. Any patient with a GCS score of < 8 should be intubated to establish a definitive

airway. (Notice that we did not need the patient's GCS in order to arrive at our first management step, but the GCS confirmed our decision.)

Answer A is incorrect. A patient may experience obtundation secondary to a number of factors, including pharmaceutical sedation or comorbid disease processes. Although reversing common reversible causes with naloxone, thiamine, and dextrose is a reasonable step, the first priority is the primary survey, which can be remembered as **ABCDE**—**A**irway, **B**reathing, **C**irculation, **D**isability, and **E**xposure.

Answer B is incorrect. Checking brain stem reflexes is an important part of the neurologic examination of a patient with altered mental status; however, this should occur after airway, breathing, and circulation are properly maintained.

Answer C is incorrect. A patient can have an altered mental status secondary to electrolyte imbalances and comorbid disease processes; although a serum electrolyte panel should be examined, diagnostic testing belongs in the secondary survey. The first step in clinical assessment is to complete the primary survey, which can be remembered as **ABCDE**—**A**irway, **B**reathing, **C**irculation, **D**isability, and **E**xposure.

Answer E is incorrect. Exposure of the patient is the last step in the primary survey. Removal of clothing from the patient aids the primary survey and is necessary to complete the secondary survey. It should be performed after the **ABC**s are managed (**A**irway, **B**reathing, and **C**irculation), and the patient's disability level has been determined, but before the secondary survey is started.

13. **The correct answer is D.** This patient with an underlying seizure disorder has most likely suffered a grand mal (tonic-clonic) seizure involving both cerebral hemispheres and resulting in complete loss of consciousness. These types of seizures begin suddenly with tonic extension of the back and extremities and typically last for several minutes. Patients often experience incontinence and/or tongue biting during the seizure. The post-ictal period is marked by

confusion as the patient slowly returns to consciousness. In this patient the most likely underlying cause is low serum antiepileptic levels secondary to medication noncompliance.

Answer A is incorrect. Absence seizures have a characteristic 3-Hz spike-and-wave pattern. These are typically very brief, lasting only a few seconds, and occur many times per day in affected children. Focal seizures, whether simple or complex, do not result in loss of consciousness and typically involve a discrete region in one cerebral hemisphere. While it is possible for a focal seizure to generalize into a grand mal seizure, there is no evidence that this occurred in this patient.

Answer B is incorrect. This electroencephalogram pattern is typical for Creutzfeldt-Jakob disease.

Answer C is incorrect. Partial seizures cause activity in only one hemisphere as opposed to both hemispheres. In this case, symptoms may not be bilateral.

Answer E is incorrect. Focal seizures cause activity located to a discrete portion of one hemisphere and may not cause tonic-clonic reactions.

14. **The correct answer is A.** Brain tumors often present with a headache that is <u>worse in the morning</u> and gets better with vomiting. This is because lying down all evening while asleep causes increased intracranial pressure (ICP), which when further exacerbated by a mass lesion causes a headache in the morning that is relieved with vomiting. In addition, other presenting features can include seizures, focal neurologic deficits, and signs and symptoms of increased ICP.

Answer B is incorrect. The patient's headache does not show ipsilateral conjunctival injection and tearing, as would be expected in cluster headaches.

Answer C is incorrect. Some history of traumatic head injury would be expected to cause an epidural hemorrhage. Epidural hematomas present with a lucid interval prior to a precipitous decline in level of consciousness, although this only occurs in 10–30% of cases.

Other symptoms include focal neurologic signs, seizures, nausea and vomiting, and headache.

Answer D is incorrect. The lack of a family history, the lack of an aura, and the age of onset point away from migraines.

Answer E is incorrect. Some history of traumatic head injury would be expected to cause a subdural hemorrhage. Any focal neurologic signs following blunt head trauma or a Glasgow Coma Scale score < 15 after head trauma warrants investigation for subdural or epidural hematoma.

Answer F is incorrect. Tension headache is a diagnosis of exclusion; here, the focal neurologic signs clearly point away from this diagnosis.

15. **The correct answer is B.** Rett's syndrome is a genetic neurodegenerative disease found almost exclusively in females. Patients have normal physical, mental, and social development until about the age of 5 months and then begin to regress in development. Language and coordination are the most common functions that are adversely affected.

Answer A is incorrect. Rett's syndrome has not been shown to have an increased prevalence in Ashkenazi Jews.

Answer C is incorrect. Fragile X is a syndrome in males and is associated with mental retardation.

Answer D is incorrect. This disorder occurs very rarely in males. The *MECP2* gene responsible for Rett's syndrome is located on the X chromosome. The mutation is often sporadic but has been found to more often occur in the paternally derived X chromosome, which combined with the often lethal phenotype seen in males might explain the extreme female predominance. However, the exact mechanism for the gender predominance remains unknown.

Answer E is incorrect. Rett's syndrome has not been associated with any ethnic or racial group.

Answer F is incorrect. Trisomy 21 or Down's syndrome is characterized by mental retarda-tion, but the patients do not have a normal phase of development as seen in Rett's patients.

16. **The correct answer is B.** The patient's symptoms and clinical history indicate the presence of positional vertigo, of which the most common form is benign paroxysmal positional vertigo (BPPV). The first step in diagnosis, before more complex tests are undertaken, is to perform a thorough neurologic examination, including the Dix-Hallpike maneuver. With the patient sitting, the neck is extended and turned to one side. The patient is then placed supine rapidly, so that the head hangs over the edge of the bed, and is observed for nystagmus. The patient is then returned to upright, observed for another 30 seconds for nystagmus, and the maneuver is repeated with the head turned to the other side. If the patient has BPPV, the Dix-Hallpike maneuver will provoke upward beating torsional nystagmus, with the upper poles of the eye beating toward the floor, usually lasting 30 seconds or less.

Answer A is incorrect. Brain stem evoked audiometry is often used to diagnose sensorineural hearing loss and entails measuring responses in brain waves that are stimulated by a clicking sound to check the central auditory pathways of the brain stem. The test is about 90% sensitive for diagnosing acoustic neuromas.

Answer C is incorrect. With typical benign paroxysmal positional vertigo, further testing is not necessary. Electronystagmography is indicated only if there is preexisting vestibular disease.

Answer D is incorrect. There is no indication for a lumbar puncture for diagnosing a patient with classic symptoms of benign paroxysmal positional vertigo.

Answer E is incorrect. Neuroimaging is necessary when the nystagmus is incongruent with the classic posterior canal presentation of benign paroxysmal positional vertigo.

17. **The correct answer is D.** This patient suffers from myoclonic seizures as a result of juvenile myoclonic epilepsy (JME). Myoclonic seizures

involve both cerebral hemispheres but rarely cause a loss of consciousness or post-ictal confusion. JME typically occurs in adolescents with a history of generalized seizures and responds well to anticonvulsant medications

Answer A is incorrect. Absence seizures have a characteristic 3-Hz spike-and-wave pattern on electroencephalogram and are brief, 2- to 3-second seizures that may occur many times per day in affected children. However, absence seizures typically present between 4 and 8 years of age and are not associated with a loss of postural muscle tone. This patient is not suffering from absence seizures.

Answer B is incorrect. Tonic seizures consist of sudden-onset tonic extension or flexion of the head, trunk, and/or extremities for several seconds. They typically occur in relation to drowsiness and are often associated with other neurologic abnormalities. Electroencephalogram shows an electrodecremental response, which is a high-frequency electrographic discharge in the β frequency ("beta buzz") with relatively low amplitude compared to the background rhythm. The pattern can evolve into slow spike-and-wave complexes or diffuse polyspikes.

Answer C is incorrect. The definition of a generalized seizure is one that involves both cerebral hemispheres. Involvement of only one hemisphere would by definition not be a generalized seizure.

Answer E is incorrect. Focal seizures involve seizure activity localized to a discrete portion of one hemisphere. Whether simple (awareness unaffected) or complex (behavior, memory, or awareness modified), focal seizures do not result in loss of consciousness. Although it is possible for a focal seizure to generalize into a grand mal seizure, there is no evidence that this occurred in this patient.

18. **The correct answer is B.** The skin findings in the image are café-au-lait spots, and the eye finding is an accurate description of a Lisch nodule, all consistent with neurofibromatosis type I (an autosomal dominant disease caused by a gene found on chromosome 17).

Answer A is incorrect. Neither Lisch nodules nor café-au-lait spots are found in multiple

neuroendocrine neoplasia (MEN) type I. MEN type I is typified by the "**3 P's**": **P**ituitary (usually prolactinoma), **P**arathyroid (hypercalcemia), and **P**ancreatoma (gastrinoma). MEN type I is autosomal dominant and tends to present in middle age.

Answer C is incorrect. Lisch nodules are consistent with neurofibromatosis (NF) type I, not NF type II. NF type II is associated with acoustic neuromas, as well as multiple intracranial meningiomas. The gene for type II NF is located on chromosome 22.

Answer D is incorrect. Neither Lisch nodules nor café-au-lait spots are found in tuberous sclerosis. Tuberous sclerosis is associated with hypopigmented macules (ash leaf spots), shagreen spots (leathery cutaneous thickening of the skin), facial hamartomas, seizures, and mental retardation. Tuberous sclerosis is inherited in an autosomal dominant fashion, and it presents in childhood as mental retardation, epilepsy, and facial hamartoma.

Answer E is incorrect. Neither Lisch nodules nor café-au-lait spots are found in von Hippel–Lindau syndrome (VHL). VHL presents with several hemangiomas in many organs. It is associated with a renal cell cancer and polycythemia (due to increased erythropoietin).

19. **The correct answer is B.** The patient suffers from conduction aphasia, which is characterized by problems with repeating what is said and naming, but preserved fluency and comprehension. Anatomically the lesion occurs at the arcuate fasciculus between Broca's and Wernicke's area.

Answer A is incorrect. Broca's aphasia is characterized by preserved comprehension, but problems with language production. These patients speak nonfluently, haltingly, and without much intonation. Naming and repetition are also impaired. They are aware of their problem and may often become depressed. Interestingly, some patients can maintain fluency when singing. Broca's area includes the posterior part of the inferior frontal gyrus and a surrounding rim of prefrontal heteromodal cortex.

Answer C is incorrect. This is caused by a large lesion in the dominant hemisphere, leading to problems with language production, comprehension, and repetition. It can be conceptualized as a combination of Broca's and Wernicke's aphasia.

Answer D is incorrect. This type of aphasia is characterized by impaired comprehension of language, but preserved repetition and fluency.

Answer E is incorrect. Wernicke's aphasia represents a problem with language comprehension, which affects both language output and input. Language output is paraphasic and circumlocutious. Repetition, naming, reading, and writing are also impaired although certain axial tasks such as opening one's eyes may be preserved. Wernicke's area includes the posterior third of the superior temporal gyrus and a surrounding rim of inferior parietal and midtemporal cortex.

20. **The correct answer is C.** The mechanic has signs and symptoms of carpal tunnel syndrome, which is entrapment of the median nerve characterized by pain and paresthesias in the medial portion of the palm that may radiate proximally down the forearm. Carpal tunnel syndrome often presents as a work-related illness in persons whose jobs require prolonged use of the hand and wrist. If left uncorrected, carpal tunnel syndrome can lead to severe neuropathy and muscle wasting distal to the point of median nerve entrapment.

Answer A is incorrect. Amyotrophic lateral sclerosis (ALS) is an idiopathic disease that results in chronic, progressive degeneration of neurons in the spinal cord, brain stem, and motor cortex. In ALS, both upper and lower motor neuron signs and involvement of more than one extremity are expected to be seen.

Answer B is incorrect. Angina is typically described as acute, localized squeezing/burning chest pain that may radiate to the arm, neck, jaw, or abdomen. Angina is typically transient and is worse on exertion; it is improved by rest or vasodilators such as nitroglycerine. This patient's symptoms seem more neuropathic and are confined to an extremity with clear signs of neuropathy, making angina a much less likely cause.

Answer D is incorrect. Currently believed to have an autoimmune etiology, multiple sclero-

sis (MS) is a chronic progressive neurologic disease that results in demyelinating lesions of various portions of the central nervous system. MS is twice as common in females. To be diagnosed with MS, a patient must present with multiple neurologic complaints distinct in "time and space." To the physician's knowledge, this patient only has one chronic neurologic complaint.

Answer E is incorrect. Myasthenia gravis is an autoimmune disease caused by antibodies against the acetylcholine receptors of the postsynaptic cleft. It is most common in young women, although elderly men can be affected. It typically presents with double vision that is worse as the day progresses and/or difficulty swallowing and proximal muscle weakness. Unilateral muscle wasting is not characteristic of myasthenia gravis.

21. **The correct answer is D.** Vasospasm typically occurs 3–14 days after rupture of an aneurysm and has a mortality rate approaching 12%. Roughly 70–90% of all patients will experience vasospasm after an aneurysmal rupture, and about one-half will result in an ischemic stroke. Given such high odds, this is the most likely etiology of a stroke in this patient.

Answer A is incorrect. Atherosclerosis can induce blood clots and lead to ischemic events. The most common locations in the brain for thrombotic events include the intracerebral arches, the branches of the circle of Willis, and the posterior circulation. Again, the history of recent aneurysmal rupture leads one to suspect vasospasm over other causes.

Answer B is incorrect. Twenty percent to 30% of all ischemic strokes occur due to a cardiogenic thromboembolism and may be caused by a number of pathogenic factors. Common causes include stasis due to atrial fibrillation or myocardial infarction and endothelial abnormalities due to valvular diseases. In this case, however, the recent history of aneurysmal rupture leads one to suspect vasospasm.

Answer C is incorrect. Although hydrocephalus is a common complication of subarachnoid hemorrhage (SAH), the time course makes this unlikely to be the cause of a new infarct. After SAH, roughly 20% of patients can expect to develop hydrocephalus.

22. **The correct answer is D.** Middle cerebral artery (MCA) strokes typically present with aphasia (dominant hemisphere), neglect (non-dominant hemisphere), contralateral hemiparesis, gaze preference, or homonymous hemianopsia. The CT scan demonstrates ischemic stroke of the MCA territories with ensuing edema.

Answer A is incorrect. Anterior cerebral artery strokes present with leg paresis, amnesia, personality changes, foot drop, gait dysfunction, or cognitive changes.

Answer B is incorrect. Basilar strokes present with coma, cranial nerve palsies, apnea, visual symptoms, drop attacks, or dysphagia.

Answer C is incorrect. Lacunar strokes are caused by the occlusion of single deep penetrating arteries resulting in small subcortical infarcts < 15 mm that appear as small lesions (the word lacune derives from their lake-like radiologic appearance) on CT or MRI. They account for some 15–25% of strokes in the United States and typically present with pure motor or sensory deficits, dysarthria, or ataxic hemiparesis.

Answer E is incorrect. Posterior cerebral artery strokes present with homonymous hemianopsia, memory deficits, or dyslexia/alexia.

23. **The correct answer is D.** Pseudodementia is a condition by which depression in persons who are elderly may present as symptoms of cognitive impairment. Pseudodementia can be differentiated from other causes of dementia by the time of onset, its tendency to occur for days to weeks, cognitive changes, personality changes, past medical history positive for mood disorder, and patient awareness and distress of the cognitive changes.

Answer A is incorrect. Alzheimer's dementia typically has a vague onset. The patient is often unaware or unconcerned with their cognitive deficits. Additionally, patients tend to exhibit prominent cognitive impairment, and CT results may be abnormal.

Answer B is incorrect. Delirium is mainly differentiated from dementia based on the patient's level of consciousness and orientation. Patients with delirium who reveal a fluctuating level of consciousness and orientation may be impaired in comparison to patients with dementia. Other factors include rapid onset, duration, psychomotor retardation, and reversibility.

Answer C is incorrect. Normal aging is associated with a decreased ability to learn new material and slowing of cognitive processes.

Answer E is incorrect. Vascular dementia is the second most common cause of dementia. Patients with vascular dementia usually have a medical history of hypertension and/or stroke. Also, vascular dementia usually progresses in a stepwise fashion with each recurrent infarct.

24. **The correct answer is E.** Myasthenia gravis is an autoimmune disease caused by antibodies against postsynaptic acetylcholine receptors at the neuromuscular junction. Thirty to fifty percent of patients with thymoma have myasthenia gravis. If a thymoma is present, surgical resection can often be curative.

Answer A is incorrect. Intravenous immune globulin (IVIG) is a pooled product of human gamma-globulin. In severe cases, IVIG can be used to provide temporary relief, such as during a myasthenic crisis when patients are at risk of respiratory failure. The exact mechanism of how IVIG works in myasthenia gravis is not understood. Although this therapy may provide some symptomatic relief, it is not curative. Infusions are required every few weeks, take multiple hours to administer, and are quite expensive.

Answer B is incorrect. Neostigmine is an acetylcholinesterase inhibitor used to increase the concentration of acetylcholine at the neuromuscular junction in patients with myasthenia. Although this therapy may provide some symptomatic relief, it is not curative. The medicine must be administered for life to prevent recurrence of symptoms.

Answer C is incorrect. Plasmapheresis involves exchanging the patient's plasma for fresh frozen plasma. It is often used in preparation for surgery, as short-term management of an exacerbation, or to provide temporary relief during a crisis when the patient is at risk of respiratory failure. Weakness improves within days, but the improvement is not curative. It only lasts 6–8 weeks.

Answer D is incorrect. Prednisone is used to downregulate the immune system in patients with myasthenia. Although this therapy provides temporary relief, it is not curative, and the disease will continue without further steroid treatment.

25. **The correct answer is B.** This patient is suffering from cluster headaches. Treatment is primarily focused on avoiding factors that exacerbate these headaches, particularly alcohol and/or strenuous physical exercise. This should be the first step in management before pharmacotherapy is initiated. If therapy is indicated, patients will typically require both prophylactic and abortive therapy for relief of their symptoms. Abortive therapy includes oxygen administration and the use of triptans. Prophylactic therapy includes the use of prednisone, lithium, and calcium channel blockers.

Answer A is incorrect. Anticonvulsants such as valproate are good prophylactic medications against migraine headaches, less so for cluster headaches.

Answer C is incorrect. β-Blockers are good prophylactic medications for migraine headaches. Their role in cluster headaches is less well defined.

Answer D is incorrect. Nonsteroidal antiinflammatory drugs are helpful in stopping a headache once it has begun. However, it has a greater abortive role in migraine and tension-type headaches.

Answer E is incorrect. Tricyclic antidepressants are good prophylactic medications against migraine headaches and have been used in tension headaches, but their role in cluster headaches is less well defined.

26. **The correct answer is C.** The patient's presentation corresponds to the classic presentation of thiamine deficiency, with the patient perhaps suffering from permanent Korsakoff's syndrome as evidenced by amnesia. However, thiamine should be administered in the hope that the patient simply has reversible Wernicke's encephalopathy. Both disorders are caused by the same pathophysiology of thiamine deficiency. Wernicke's encephalopathy refers to an acute presentation of the symptoms described in the question. Korsakoff's or Wernicke-Korsakoff syndrome refers to the persistence of these symptoms, particularly amnesia, and may be warded off by proper treatment of Wernicke's syndrome.

Answer A is incorrect. Folate deficiency does not produce neurologic deficits, with the exception of some memory loss and personality changes. Most commonly, folate deficiency presents with gastrointestinal symptoms, such as a swollen and red tongue, nausea, emesis, diarrhea, and abdominal pain after meals.

Answer B is incorrect. Glucose should not be given in a patient with suspected thiamine deficiency because high-dose glucose administration can precipitate symptoms of thiamine deficiency. This is because even more substrate is given for biochemical pathways that do not have proper substrates.

Answer D is incorrect. Vitamin B_6 deficiency would not present in this manner. Such deficiency usually presents with bilateral distal extremity numbness, weakness, sideroblastic anemia, and skin changes, such as erythematous itching and burning, blisters, and hyperpigmentation with thickening.

Answer E is incorrect. The patient does not have sensory and motor deficits consistent with vitamin B_{12} deficiency. The classic triad of vitamin B_{12} deficiency includes weakness, sore tongue, and paresthesias. However, the chief symptoms are usually weight loss and anorexia, malaise, and neurologic symptoms such as paresthesias and gait abnormalities.

27. **The correct answer is A.** Aspirin has been shown to reduce morbidity and mortality in acute ischemic stroke when administered within 48 hours. This assumes that there is no aspirin allergy, no gastrointestinal bleeding, and no tissue plasminogen activator use, all of

which are reasonable assumptions in this patient with no known drug allergies and a negative fecal occult blood test, and in whom thrombolytics are contraindicated.

Answer B is incorrect. β-Blockers are useful when given following acute myocardial infarction in the absence of bradycardia, hypotension, or pulmonary edema, but they have not been shown to improve outcomes following acute stroke.

Answer C is incorrect. Although this patient is hypertensive, it would be advisable to allow her pressure to increase to 200/100 mm Hg following a stroke to maintain cerebral perfusion. Administering intravenous nitroprusside in this patient at this time could potentially lower her pressure enough to compromise her cerebral perfusion.

Answer D is incorrect. Thrombolytic therapy is contraindicated in this patient because her systolic pressure is > 185 mm Hg and she has suffered a recent myocardial infarction. Other contraindications to thrombolytics include diastolic blood pressure > 100 mm Hg, glucose < 50 mg/dL or > 500 mg/dL, age > 18 years, International Normalized Ratio > 1.7, use of heparin in the past 48 hours with prolonged partial thromboplastin time, platelet count < 100,000/mm³, stroke or head trauma within the past 3 months, prior intracranial hemorrhage or major surgery in the past 14 days, gastrointestinal or urinary bleeding in the past 21 days, and seizures present at the onset of stroke.

Answer E is incorrect. Urokinase is also thrombolytic therapy, and because the patient has suffered a recent myocardial infarction and has a systolic blood pressure > 185 mm Hg, urokinase is contraindicated.

28. **The correct answer is C.** The patient, with his characteristic lucid interval, has suffered an epidural hematoma, which is characteristically caused by damage to the middle meningeal artery.

Answer A is incorrect. Damage to the basilar artery would likely produce intraparenchymal bleeding, not an epidural hematoma. The basilar artery arises from the confluence of the two

vertebral arteries at the level of the medulla oblongata. It ascends in the central gutter (sulcus basilaris) inferior to the pons and divides into the two posterior cerebral arteries.

Answer B is incorrect. The dural venous sinus would not be injured in this type of injury. Damage to the venous sinus typically presents with thrombosis.

Answer D is incorrect. The superior sagittal sinus is not typically affected by this mechanism. Damage to the venous sinus typically presents with thrombosis.

Answer E is incorrect. Damage to the vertebral artery would likely produce intraparenchymal bleeding, not an epidural hematoma.

29. **The correct answer is C.** This child has DiGeorge's syndrome, a disease caused by a deletion of chromosome 22q11. This chromosomal anomaly causes abnormal development of the third and fourth pharyngeal pouches, resulting in midline defects. Abnormal facies, cleft palate, congenital heart defects, thymic aplasia, and parathyroid hypoplasia characterize DiGeorge's syndrome. Patients often present in the neonatal period with tetany or seizures secondary to hypocalcemia. Hypocalcemia can be detected on physical examination by positive Trousseau's and Chvostek's signs. These children are also susceptible to infection due to thymic aplasia and a decreased number of T lymphocytes.

Answer A is incorrect. Beckwith-Wiedemann syndrome is characterized by perinatal growth acceleration, hemihypertrophy, macroglossia, linear ear creases, abdominal wall defects, exophthalmos, and transient neonatal hypoglycemia. Patients with Beckwith-Wiedemann syndrome are at increased risk of developing Wilms' tumor.

Answer B is incorrect. Chronic granulomatous disease (CGD) is characterized by recurrent mucous membrane infections, abscesses, and poor wound healing. This disease is a result of a defect in neutrophil-mediated phagocytosis due to a lack of reduced nicotinamide adenine dinucleotide phosphate activity. CGD is usually diagnosed between 3 and 8 years of age after multiple infections. It is not associated with hypocalcemia, abnormal facies, or cardiac defects.

Answer D is incorrect. Multiple endocrine neoplasia type I causes a predisposition to developing tumors of the parathyroid, pituitary, and pancreas. Parathyroid tumors cause hyperparathyroidism and consequently hypercalcemia. They are not associated with hypocalcemia, abnormal facies, cardiac defects, or predisposition to infections.

Answer E is incorrect. Niemann-Pick disease results from deficiency of sphingomyelinase, leading to buildup of sphingomyelin and cholesterol. The infantile form presents with hepatosplenomegaly, failure to thrive, and rapidly progressive neurodevelopmental regression. It is not associated with cardiac malformations or immunodeficiency and does not cause hypocalcemia.

30. **The correct answer is A.** The basal ganglia and thalamus are the classic sites of a hypertensive bleed. This is because the small perforator arteries come directly off much larger vessels. This results in higher blood pressures than are usual in arteries of that size, and they are thus more prone to hypertensive bleeding.

Answer B is incorrect. Bleeding in the brain stem is generally due to a hemorrhagic stroke. This can be caused by chronic hypertension, but bleeding is more likely to occur in the basal ganglia and thalamus during an acute hypertensive event. The prognosis for brain stem bleeds depends on the size of the hemorrhage but is generally poor because the brain stem is one of the eloquent areas of the brain.

Answer C is incorrect. Bleeding in the epidural space is most likely to be an epidural hematoma. This is usually the result of trauma. Prognosis is good if treated appropriately and early.

Answer D is incorrect. Bleeding in the ventricles is typically due to subarachnoid hemorrhage in adults. Aneurysmal bleeding has an extremely poor prognosis if not caught in time, leading to an almost 40% mortality rate.

31. **The correct answer is C.** Ethosuximide is the first-line agent and is effectively only against absence seizures. Seizures will eventually resolve spontaneously, but ethosuximide is potentially useful in minimizing symptoms and associated learning deficits and behavioral problems during childhood.

Answer A is incorrect. Carbamazepine has been reported to exacerbate absence seizures and is contraindicated in such patients.

Answer B is incorrect. Gabapentin has been reported to exacerbate absence seizures and is contraindicated in such patients.

Answer D is incorrect. Tiagabine has been reported to exacerbate absence seizures and is contraindicated in such patients.

Answer E is incorrect. Valproate can be useful for absence patients but is normally used as second-line therapy in those who have had inadequate relief of symptoms from ethosuximide. Other useful second-line agents include lamotrigine, topiramate, and zonisamide.

32. **The correct answer is C.** A 4-year-old child is able to hop and skip, draw crosses, count to 10, and sing songs or recite poems from memory.

Answer A is incorrect. A 2-year-old child can walk up and down stairs, build a six-cube tower, and use two-word sentences, but he or she will not have achieved the milestones listed for 3-, 4-, and 5-year-old children.

Answer B is incorrect. A 3-year-old child can ride a tricycle, draw a circle, and use three-word sentences, but he or she will not have achieved the milestones listed for 4- and 5-year-old children.

Answer D is incorrect. A 5-year-old child will be able to do these tasks, as well as jump over some obstacles, tie shoelaces, copy a square, and print his or her name.

Answer E is incorrect. A 6-year-old child can ride a bicycle, knows his or her left hand from his or her right, can carry on a telephone conversation, enjoys constructive and creative play, and can read and write some words.

33. **The correct answer is C.** Carbon monoxide poisoning should be considered in any case of headache with altered mental status. The

father's headaches may be a coincidence, but should increase the index of suspicion for carbon monoxide exposure. Children are at especially high risk of carbon monoxide poisoning due to their increased respiratory rate and minute volume. Prolonged exposure to even low levels of carbon monoxide may produce moderate to severe poisoning. Mild exposure may result in headaches, somnolence, dizziness, and nausea. Symptoms of moderate to severe toxicity may include chest pain, dyspnea, headache, ataxia, confusion, seizures, coma, and eventually death. In severe poisoning, tissue hypoxia may cause an increased anion gap metabolic acidosis secondary to increased lactic acid production. His symptoms (loss of consciousness and difficulty walking) are concerning for more severe poisoning, and an acidosis may be present.

Answer A is incorrect. Blood sugar is not affected by bloodstream carbon monoxide levels. Hypoglycemia might cause headaches and confusion, but symptoms would not persist after a meal, as occurred in this case.

Answer B is incorrect. Carbon monoxide (CO) does not affect the concentration of dissolved oxygen in serum. Since partial arterial oxygen pressure (PaO_2) measures dissolved oxygen only, PaO_2 is normal in cases of CO poisoning.

Answer D is incorrect. Abnormalities may be seen on x-ray of the chest in cases of CO toxicity and usually include pulmonary edema or infiltrates secondary to aspiration pneumonitis. However, in most cases of CO poisoning, x-ray of the chest is normal.

Answer E is incorrect. Conventional pulse oximeters, which use two wavelengths of light, can only differentiate oxyhemoglobin from deoxyhemoglobin. Carboxyhemoglobin and methemoglobin are misinterpreted as oxygenated hemoglobin; therefore pulse oximetry will most likely appear normal even in the presence of severe hypoxia. Methemoglobinemia may be due to inherited defects in oxidative stress reduction pathways (such as glucose-6-phosphate dehydrogenase deficiency or pyruvate kinase deficiency), certain medications, or environmental exposures (particularly nitrites or nitrates).

34. The correct answer is D. CT without contrast is the imaging study of choice in this patient, chiefly because of its speed, safety, and efficacy in distinguishing between the most common causes of neurologic injury. When stroke is suspected, the scan is performed without contrast in order to aid in distinguishing between hemorrhagic and ischemic stroke. An infused CT is contraindicated as an initial study because of the risk of further damage to the brain parenchyma from extravasated contrast dye if the stroke is hemorrhagic.

Answer A is incorrect. If this patient's stroke is in fact related to his carotid disease, then a duplex ultrasound may indeed help identify the underlying cause and direct subsequent therapy (e.g., emergent carotid endarterectomy). While this would be an appropriate test following a CT scan of the head showing a stroke in the anterior circulation, it would be inappropriate as an initial diagnostic study.

Answer B is incorrect. Cerebral angiography is traditionally regarded as the gold standard for identifying vascular pathology (e.g., aneurysms or occlusion). However, because it is invasive and carries the risk of substantial complications, it is rarely used.

Answer C is incorrect. Conventional radiography has no role in the evaluation of patients with acute neurologic injury unless cervical spine injury is suspected, in which case an odontoid view and a lateral cervical spine film should be obtained. In this instance, it will offer no information as to whether or not the patient has suffered a stroke.

Answer E is incorrect. A properly performed MRI of the brain has anatomic resolution that is superior to CT of the head in many ways. MRI is more sensitive in detecting early ischemic changes, imaging the brain stem/posterior fossa, and determining the date of injury. However, because the image acquisition times are considerably longer for MRI, obtaining high-quality images is dependent on the patient's ability to sit still. Due to this current limitation, MRI is typically reserved for the subacute setting and is often used to follow-up CT findings in stroke victims.

35. The correct answer is B. This patient has a normal blood pressure and heart rate, moist mucous membranes, and gives no history of recent fluid losses. She demonstrates euvolemic hyponatremia without symptoms of acute water intoxication such as confusion, anorexia, nausea, vomiting, or coma. Common causes of euvolemic hyponatremia include the syndrome of inappropriate secretion of antidiuretic hormone (SIADH), a reset osmostat, and isotonic salt losses with free water repletion. In this case, the patient has experienced recent onset of headaches and now a seizure, raising the possibility of a slowly progressing intracranial process. A hyponatremic seizure at a sodium concentration of 124 mEq/L is unlikely given the clinical scenario of a chronic disorder. The history of recent-onset headaches and seizure should raise concern for intracranial malignancy, which is often associated with inappropriate ADH secretion from the pituitary gland. This is confirmed by elevated urine sodium levels in the setting of clinically normal volume status. Nonsteroidal anti-inflammatory drugs potentiate the action of ADH and are also associated with development of SIADH.

Answer A is incorrect. Bartter's syndrome is a defect in sodium transport at the loop of Henle leading to hypokalemia, metabolic alkalosis, and hypercalciuria. It presents early in life and is associated with growth defects, low blood pressure, and mental retardation. It is not associated with hyponatremia.

Answer C is incorrect. Hyperglycemia in the setting of diabetes (diabetic ketoacidosis or hyperosmolar hyponatremic nonketosis) can lead to hyperosmotic hyponatremia. High plasma glucose pulls water out of cells and results in a dilutional hyponatremia. At the same time, the increased osmotic pressure leads to an osmotic diuresis. The resultant hypovolemic, hyperosmolar hyponatremia must be corrected by volume replacement and insulin. Adjusted plasma sodium levels (2 mEq/L for every 100 mg/dL of glucose > 200 mg/dL) may actually show hypernatremia in these cases.

Answer D is incorrect. Cirrhosis-induced hypoalbuminemia combined with peripheral vasodilation leads to free water retention and hyponatremia. In early stages of cirrhosis, transaminases and bilirubin are usually elevated, but in late-stage liver disease, as the number of normal hepatic cells dwindles, transaminases may drop to near-normal levels. These patients are hypervolemic, demonstrating edema and ascites, but are intravascularly volume depleted, with water losses caused by decreased oncotic pressures and subsequent loss across the capillary membranes.

Answer E is incorrect. Other intracranial processes (subarachnoid hemorrhage) are associated with a process known as cerebral salt wasting, thought to be due to increased levels of brain natriuretic peptide and concurrent aldosterone suppression. Despite hyponatremia and high plasma antidiuretic hormone, cerebral salt wasting can be differentiated from the syndrome of inappropriate secretion of antidiuretic hormone by signs and symptoms of hypovolemia.

36. The correct answer is E. This patient has chronic (open-angle) glaucoma. This condition is diagnosed by an increased intraocular pressure, abnormal optic disk findings, and typical visual field loss. The eye is not red or painful, the pupil and cornea appear normal, and it commonly affects both eyes. Open-angle glaucoma can be treated with a variety of medications. Pilocarpine is a muscarinic agonist that produces rapid miosis and contraction of the ciliary muscles. This can be used in the acute treatment of closed- or open-angle glaucoma to open the trabecular meshwork around Schlemm's canal, increasing drainage of aqueous humor and decreasing intraocular pressure. Other agents that increase aqueous humor secretion include prostaglandins (latanoprost) and epinephrine. Open-angle glaucoma can also be treated with agents that decrease secretion, including β-blockers (timolol), carbonic anhydrase inhibitors, and α_2-agonists (brimonidine).

Answer A is incorrect. Corticosteroids are the treatment of choice for a number of ophthalmic conditions including uveitis, retrobulbar neuritis, optic neuritis, and allergic conjunctivitis. However, steroids are not indicated for the treatment of glaucoma.

blockage of aqueous outflow
pain
conj injection halos

Answer B is incorrect. Unlike open-angle glaucoma, narrow-angle glaucoma is caused by the blockage of the aqueous outflow passageway. Dilation of the pupils may precipitate an attack since the iris bunches up and narrows the angle. This condition presents with intense pain and conjunctival injection. The patient may see halos around lights, may have decreased vision, and may present with nausea and vomiting. Treatment includes pilocarpine to constrict the pupil, topical β-blockers, carbonic anhydrase inhibitors, and α$_2$-agonists. Patients should also be treated with intravenous mannitol, an osmotic agent that draws water out of the eye and reduces pressure. Intravenous mannitol is not used for the treatment of chronic glaucoma.

Answer C is incorrect. Isoproterenol is a β-agonist. It has no use in the ophthalmic treatment of glaucoma. Glaucoma is treated with topical β-blockers.

Answer D is incorrect. Phenoxybenzamine is a nonselective α-blocker. It has no use in the ophthalmic treatment of glaucoma. Glaucoma is treated with α$_2$-agonists.

37. **The correct answer is F.** The acute problem is an abrupt enlarging of an aneurysm that is causing a third nerve palsy. This is a rare "prodrome" before the rupture of a berry aneurysm, and the growing aneurysm is likely at the junction of the internal carotid and posterior communicating arteries. Polycystic kidney disease would relate the cerebral berry aneurysm with the patient's other diagnoses of mitral valve prolapse, hepatic cysts, large palpable kidneys, hypertension, and an elevated creatinine. This autosomal dominant disease is usually asymptomatic until patients are > 30 years old.

Answer A is incorrect. The Budd-Chiari syndrome is a decrease in the normal outflow of hepatic blood due to occlusion of the hepatic vein. The process is typically secondary to a hypercoagulable state. Budd-Chiari typically presents with sudden onset of massive ascites. The neurologic symptoms could have been associated with a vascular event secondary to a hypercoagulable state, but this would not explain

the patient's other clinical manifestations accompanied by normal liver function tests.

Answer B is incorrect. Caroli's disease is characterized by large intrahepatic bile ducts that are segmentally dilatated. The disease is associated with autosomal recessive (juvenile) polycystic kidney disease. Normal liver function tests essentially rule out this diagnosis.

Answer C is incorrect. Marfan's syndrome is an inherited disorder of connective tissue. The incidence is about 1 in 10,000, making it one of the most common connective tissue disorders. Mitral valve prolapse and aneurysms are found in this disorder. Marfan's is not known to be associated with renal cysts, and no mention of a marfanoid body habitus is made in relation to this patient.

Answer D is incorrect. Renal cell carcinomas can metastasize to the liver and the brain. The chance, however, that the hepatic cysts represent metastatic cancer 1 year prior to presentation without a history of weight loss or abnormal liver function test is unlikely.

Answer E is incorrect. Multiple sclerosis is not likely in this situation. The disease is usually found in women who are of childbearing age from northern latitudes. The disease can cause central nervous system lesions that lead to cranial nerve abnormalities; however, this patient has other findings such as palpable kidneys that make polycystic kidney disease a more parsimonious diagnosis.

38. **The correct answer is C.** Emergency treatments in life-threatening situations do not require consent; consent is implied. Therefore, the most appropriate next step is to perform emergency evacuation of the hematoma before further neurologic deficits develop. Should all relevant parties be present, consent authority would serially fall upon (1) the patient's spouse; (2) an adult child of the patient who has the waiver and consent of all other qualified adult children of the patient to act as the sole decision maker; (3) a majority of the patient's reasonably available adult children; (4) the patient's parents; or (5) the individual clearly identified to act for the patient before the patient became incapacitated, the patient's

nearest living relative, or a member of the clergy.

Answer A is incorrect. In the case of a life-threatening condition, consent to treatment is implied.

Answer B is incorrect. While medical management to decrease intracranial pressure may be appropriate in other types of intracranial hemorrhage, a progressing epidural hematoma must be surgically evacuated to relieve the pressure.

Answer D is incorrect. Serial neurologic examinations are appropriate for conscious patients while waiting for a neurosurgery consult, but the patient in the case was already unconscious, and the operation must be performed immediately.

Answer E is incorrect. Consent to treatment is implied when emergency treatment for a life-threatening condition is required. This applies whether or not the patient is a minor.

39. **The correct answer is E.** Thrombolytic therapy is contraindicated in any patient with: stroke or head trauma in the past 3 months, recent myocardial infarction, prior intracranial hemorrhage, or major surgery in the past 14 days. Other contraindications in the patient's history include gastrointestinal or urinary bleeding in the past 21 days, or seizures present at the onset of a stroke.

Answer A is incorrect. A bruise is not a contraindication, assuming the platelet count, prothrombin time, and activated partial thromboplastin time are normal.

Answer B is incorrect. While carotid stenosis can increase the risk of an ischemic stroke, it is not a contraindication to the administration of tissue plasminogen activator because it does not increase the risk of bleeding.

Answer C is incorrect. A myocardial infarction (MI) 10 years ago is not a contraindication. It must be a recent MI.

Answer D is incorrect. Only recent peptic ulcers are a contraindication (within the last 21 days).

40. **The correct answer is A.** The "cherry-red" retinal lesion is characteristic of infantile Tay-Sachs disease. Absence of hexosaminidase A in WBCs is diagnostic for Tay-Sachs disease. Tay-Sachs has an autosomal recessive inheritance. It is most prevalent among Ashkenazi Jews (1:25–30 are carriers). Infantile Tay-Sachs presents at 4–5 months of age with loss of motor skills, increased startle reaction to noise, and retinal cherry-red spots. Seizures develop by 2 years of age, and children typically do not survive past age 4–5 years.

Answer B is incorrect. Deficiency of β-glucocerebroside leads to accumulation of glucocerebroside in the reticuloendothelial system. Gaucher's disease is diagnosed by the presence of Gaucher cells in the bone marrow. Gaucher cells have a characteristic "crinkled paper" appearance. Patients typically present in adolescence with bone pain, hepatosplenomegaly, and anemia. Thrombocytopenia often causes easy bleeding and bruising. On x-ray, an Erlenmeyer flask deformity of the distal femur is commonly noted.

Answer C is incorrect. Presence of phenylketones in the urine is diagnostic for phenylketonuria (PKU). PKU presents with fair skin, eczema, and musty body odor. As the child ages, mental retardation, hyperactivity with purposeless movements, rhythmic rocking, and athetosis will become evident if left untreated.

Answer D is incorrect. Krabbe's disease results from the absence of β-galactosidase and leads to accumulation of galactocerebroside. This disease presents during the first year of life with optic atrophy, seizures, and spasticity. Opisthotonos, or abnormal posturing characterized by rigidity and arching of the back with the neck hyperextended, occurs, and the child usually dies by age 3 years.

Answer E is incorrect. Niemann-Pick disease results from deficiency of sphingomyelinase, leading to a build-up of sphingomyelin and cholesterol. Type A presents with hepatosplenomegaly, failure to thrive, and rapidly progressive neurodevelopmental regression leading to spasticity and rigidity in later stages. Type B has a more variable course and pulmonary involvement.

41. **The correct answer is B.** Age-related macular degeneration (ARMD) is a degenerative disease of the macula (central portion of the retina) that results in the loss of central vision. ARMD is classified as wet (neovascular or exudative) or dry (atrophic) type. Risk increases as patients age, with smoking being a major modifiable risk factor in this disease process. Laser photocoagulation can reduce the risk of severe visual loss in patients with treatable exudative ARMD, typically with drusen accompanied by a choroidal neovascular membrane. The laser photocoagulation should be applied within 72 hours of the fluorescein angiography.

Answer A is incorrect. Atropine is an antimuscarinic agent that results in mydriasis and is not an acceptable form of treatment for age-related macular degeneration.

Answer C is incorrect. Timolol is a nonselective β-antagonist that reduces the production of aqueous humor in the eye. It can be used topically in treatment of open-angle glaucoma.

Answer D is incorrect. Topical steroids are not indicated for treatment of exudative age-related macular degeneration.

Answer E is incorrect. Although trabeculectomy can provide curative treatment for glaucoma, this patient has exudative age-related macular degeneration. Trabeculectomy is not indicated in this situation.

42. **The correct answer is C.** Intubation is the most important first step in cases in whom the patient is not conscious, including apnea, decreased mental status, impending airway compromise (e.g., burn injury or maxillofacial trauma), closed head injuries, and failed bag ventilation. Intubation is also indicated in patients with a Glasgow Coma Scale (GCS) score < 8. (Remember, the GCS is a neurologic scale that affords one a reliable, objective way of assessing the level of consciousness of a person, for initial as well as continuing assessment. It has value in predicting ultimate outcome.)

Answer A is incorrect. Antiepileptics and mannitol for volume status are indicated, but the patient's airway should be secured first.

Answer B is incorrect. Cervical spine evaluation is indicated in a patient who presents as a trauma victim, but unless this patient sustained an injury during the seizure there is no indication for cervical spine management in this patient.

Answer D is incorrect. Most post-ictal patients breathe spontaneously, even if they remain unconscious. However, delaying intubation would not be advisable in a patient with a massive intracranial hemorrhage, since respiratory control could rapidly become compromised.

Answer E is incorrect. While a full trauma survey would be appropriate if the patient came into the emergency department seizing, airway management is the first step in this instance. Once the patient's airway is secure and she is not actively seizing, additional components of the trauma survey can be conducted as pertinent to the case.

43. **The correct answer is B.** The patient most likely suffers from chronic daily headaches induced by analgesic medication overuse (e.g., acetaminophen), also known as analgesic rebound headaches. They typically last at least 4 hours per day and occur 15 days per month and are seen most commonly in women in their fifties. The first step in prevention would be to withdraw the patient from the offending medication. If there is another underlying headache syndrome, this will then reveal itself. Another analgesic can be used instead, or the same one can be later reintroduced, but with the instruction to consume it less often and in lower doses.

Answer A is incorrect. Although behavioral therapies such as relaxation therapy and biofeedback can be successful in the management of headaches, it would not be the first-line or sole preventive measure for medication-induced headaches.

Answer C is incorrect. β-Blockers have a greater impact for prophylactic treatment of migraine headaches than for headaches due to chronic analgesic use.

Answer D is incorrect. Selective serotonin reuptake inhibitors are a newer addition to the prophylactic treatment of headaches. Although useful, the first step in management of medication overuse headaches is to control the offending medication rather than start a new drug treatment.

Answer E is incorrect. Tricyclic antidepressants such as amitriptyline and nortriptyline are useful prophylactic agents in the long-term treatment and prevention of migraines and tension headaches. However, the first step in management of medication overuse headaches is to control the offending medication, rather than start a new drug.

44. **The correct answer is C.** Astrocytomas are the most common tumor type, and of these, glioblastoma multiforme (GBM) is the most common primary brain tumor. Imaging can reveal a tumor mass that often crosses the corpus callosum into the contralateral cerebral hemisphere, or a multicentric appearance with satellite lesions. GBM is a low-grade lesion, with extensive necrosis and hemorrhage within the tumor. Such lesions have a poor prognosis, with mean survival often < 1 year. Histopathology shows poorly differentiated, pleomorphic astrocytic cells with nuclear atypia. Necrosis along with microvascular proliferation are often seen.

[handwritten margin note: crosses corpus callosum, multicentric w/ satellite lesions, necrosis & hem. w/in tumor]

Answer A is incorrect. Schwannomas arise from the superior division of cranial nerve VIII, are pathologically characterized by an Antoni A or B pattern, and present with such symptoms as hearing loss and dizziness.

Answer B is incorrect. Cavernous malformations are one of a group of vascular malformations, and would not be characterized by neoplastic tissue.

Answer D is incorrect. Medulloblastomas are tumors of childhood, and would not be seen in this age group. Histopathology characteristically shows small round blue cells.

Answer E is incorrect. Meningiomas are the most common low-grade intracranial tumors, most often appearing in middle-aged women and often presenting on the cerebral convexities. Histopathology characteristically shows plump pink cells with small amounts of hemosiderin. Psammoma bodies may be seen.

45. **The correct answer is B.** A diagnosis of brain death requires a core body temperature of at least 32.2°C (90.0°F). Lower temperatures exhibit a neuroprotective effect via enzyme inhibition, and patients have been successfully resuscitated with neurologic recovery even after long periods of cardiac arrest, if the patient's core body temperature was low at the time of arrest. Other requirements include the absence of intoxication or poisoning, the absence of metabolic or endocrine derangements, evidence of a catastrophic cerebral event, and the absence of brain stem reflexes, such as the "doll's-eyes" (oculocephalic) reflex and the vestibulo-ocular reflex (response to caloric stimulation).

Answer A is incorrect. The presence of artificial ventilation does not hamper a diagnosis of brain death.

Answer C is incorrect. Historically, cardiac arrest was used to define death. A brain death definition is now used, and a heartbeat does not preclude brain death.

Answer D is incorrect. Because one point for each category defines the bottom of the Glasgow Coma Scale, it is not possible to score lower than 3. A patient scoring 3/15 is profoundly comatose, and coma and/or absence of cerebral motor responses is required to diagnose brain death.

Answer E is incorrect. Evidence of a devastating neurologic event is required to diagnose brain death; the presence of a skull fracture does not prevent this diagnosis.

46. **The correct answer is E.** The event described in this case is a classic complex partial seizure. This patient is too old to have a febrile seizure, which is defined as a seizure in a child < 4 years associated with a temperature > 100.4°F (38°C) in the absence of a systemic infectious, inflammatory, or metabolic underlying condition. Abnormalities seen on electroencephalogram (EEG) are an indication to treat a first nonfebrile seizure if the family so chooses. When there is an abnormal EEG, the risk of another seizure during the next year increases from 15% to 41%. A family history of epilepsy increases the risk of recurrent seizures. Pheno-

barbital is the first-line anticonvulsant for children with partial seizures.

Answer A is incorrect. Acetaminophen will control fever. Antipyretic therapy is appropriate therapy for a febrile seizure. However, this child is too old to have febrile seizures, which occur in children between 6 months and 6 years of age.

Answer B is incorrect. It is important to control the fever in febrile seizures. However, aspirin should not be used because it can lead to Reye's syndrome. Reye's syndrome results in encephalopathy and fatty degeneration of the liver. Most significantly, this child is not having a febrile seizure, and an anticonvulsant is more appropriate for her.

Answer C is incorrect. This antibiotic combination would be appropriate if the child was suspected of having meningitis. A lumbar puncture (LP) should be performed on children who have focal neurologic signs, nuchal rigidity, or are < 6 months to evaluate for meningitis in the absence of contraindications. Some experts recommend that all children < 1 year have an LP if they have any focal neurologic signs. This child is old enough to exhibit the classic signs if meningitis were present and, therefore, her low-grade temperature does not warrant an LP.

Answer D is incorrect. Ethosuximide is the first-line treatment for absence seizures. Absence seizures appear as staring spells lasting 5–10 seconds. On EEG, they show classic three-per-second spike-and-wave discharges. Ethosuximide is inappropriate therapy for partial seizures.

47. **The correct answer is B.** Confusion, getting lost, and intact long-term memory in the presence of difficulties with recent memories are all suggestive of Alzheimer's disease. Donepezil, rivastigmine, galantamine, and tacrine are cholinesterase inhibitors that are FDA-approved treatments for dementia of the Alzheimer's type. While these drugs do not alter the underlying disease process, they can retard the cognitive decline in some patients with mild to moderate Alzheimer's disease. Of the three drugs, donepezil has the most favorable adverse-effect profile.

Answer A is incorrect. Bupropion is a nonseratonergic antidepressant.

Answer C is incorrect. Doxepin is a psychotropic drug with antidepressant and anxiolytic effects.

Answer D is incorrect. Gingko biloba has been studied as a supplement to cholinesterase inhibitors, but is not proven effective as a stand-alone drug.

Answer E is incorrect. Thiamine (vitamin B_{12}) is used for thiamine deficiency which causes apathy, irritability, depression, and severe memory impairment if deficiency is prolonged. Thiamine deficiency may be secondary to familial poverty or caused by chronic alcohol abuse.

Answer F is incorrect. Vitamin E has been studied as a supplement to cholinesterase inhibitors, but is not proven effective as a stand-alone drug.

48. **The correct answer is C.** This patient exhibits symptoms of elevated intracranial pressure (ICP). Possible physical examination findings include papilledema; a dilated ipsilateral pupil; cranial nerve palsies of the third (most common), fourth, and sixth nerves; and nuchal rigidity. Hemiparesis, hypertonia, hyperreflexia, or Cushing's triad (systemic hypertension, bradycardia, and respiratory depression) are late signs. In a case of suspected elevated ICP, the patient should be stabilized and a CT scan of the head without contrast should be performed. A midline shift or effacement of the sulci or basilar cisterns are possible findings on CT scan of the head that confirm the diagnosis of elevated ICP. The etiology of the elevated ICP, such as a mass or hemorrhage, may also be evident on CT scan. Other possible causes of elevated ICP are hydrocephalus, vasculitis, infarcts, and central nervous system infection.

Answer A is incorrect. Mannitol is an osmotic agent that establishes a gradient between plasma and parenchyma, causing a diuresis and reduction in brain water content. It can be used to decrease intracranial pressure. In this patient, CT scan of the head and other studies should be carried out to establish intracranial hypertension before mannitol is considered.

Answer B is incorrect. Primary infantile glaucoma is a rare disease that begins within the first 3 years of life. It is caused by an anomaly of the trabecular meshwork, leading to impaired drainage of aqueous fluid. It classically presents with tearing, photophobia, and eyelid squeezing, and is treated with surgery. A β-blocker such as timolol can be used postoperatively to decrease aqueous production and prevent or postpone the need for a second surgery.

Answer D is incorrect. An LP can trigger herniation in the setting of elevated intracranial pressure due to a mass. Therefore, CT scan of the head should be obtained to rule out a mass before an LP is performed. If central nervous system infection is strongly suspected, antibiotic therapy should be initiated, even if the LP must be delayed.

Answer E is incorrect. A CT scan of the head without contrast is the initial imaging study of choice in children with suspected intracranial hypertension. If the initial CT scan is normal or if findings such as a neoplasm, hemorrhage, or unexplained hydrocephalus are noted, an MRI of the brain can be considered for further evaluation.

49. **The correct answer is E.** Due to the relentlessly progressive nature of Alzheimer's disease, it is important for patients to have a living will or durable power of attorney. However, this does not need to occur before the onset of disease because the majority of patients still have the capacity for self-determination at the time of diagnosis. Treatment decisions are likely to be more in line with the patient's desires if the patient is involved early in deciding who should serve as a proxy. The physician should have a discussion with the patient regarding disease course and prognosis as soon as possible.

Answer A is incorrect. Family members should be involved in the discussion about future care, but the patient should decide who will ultimately make treatment decisions.

Answer B is incorrect. Patients with early Alzheimer's disease still retain executive function and self-identity, and should be allowed to make health care decisions and select a proxy.

Answer C is incorrect. Patients with early Alzheimer's disease still retain executive function and self-identity, and should be allowed to make health decisions and select a proxy.

Answer D is incorrect. Substituted judgment comes into play when a health care proxy is faced with a decision for an incompetent patient when that patient did not make any specific requests pertaining to the situation. Substituted judgment cannot be used to choose a health care proxy.

50. **The correct answer is A.** The presentation and laboratory findings suggest that the man needs to be evaluated for a prolactinoma. Headache and visual field defects, classically bitemporal hemianopsia, are characteristic of a prolactinoma. As a result, central imaging is warranted. In fact, any elevation of prolactin that cannot be attributed to another cause (e.g., neuroleptic medication) warrants central nervous system imaging to evaluate for the presence of a macroadenoma, microadenoma, or other central lesion.

Answer B is incorrect. β-Human chorionic gonadotropin (β-hCG) is elevated in patients with choriocarcinoma (100%), embryonal carcinoma (40–60%), and seminoma (5–10%), so it is often included in the initial screening panel for testicular cancer. Testicular cancer is most common in men from puberty to age 35, and clinical presentation can include a neck mass (supraclavicular node), dyspnea (pulmonary metastases), back/bone pain (spinal/skeletal metastases), central nervous system/peripheral nervous system signs, leg swelling (inferior vena cava involvement), or gynecomastia (systemic endocrine effects). Isolated erectile dysfunction is less common. β-hCG is also a test that is used to determine pregnancy status. In a woman with hyperprolactinemia, pregnancy must be considered as a cause of elevated hormone levels.

Answer C is incorrect. Mammography is not needed for this patient. Patients with prolactinoma can present with gynecomastia, and even in rare cases, galactorrhea. However, neither are mentioned in the stem.

Answer D is incorrect. Accepted management of elevated prolactin levels requires imaging regardless of the degree of prolactin elevation. Higher levels would suggest that the lesion was indeed a macroadenoma.

Answer E is incorrect. Scrotal ultrasound is used in the evaluation of scrotal masses, and has no utility here. The man is not noted to have any masses in his testicles or any testicular pain.

CHAPTER 11

Obstetrics

1. A 14-year-old G1P0 woman who is 29 weeks pregnant with twins presents to the emergency department (ED) following a seizure. She was watching television and stood up to go to the bathroom when she "fell down and started shaking." The patient has no history of seizures and is otherwise healthy. She missed her last obstetrician's appointment, and her aunt states that her niece has had a lot of headaches and swelling over the past 2 days. On examination, she is somnolent and difficult to arouse, and has edema of her hands and face. Her vitals are blood pressure 205/120 mm Hg, pulse 80/min, and respiratory rate 16/min; the fetal heart rate is 130/min. Which is the most correct advice for the patient's aunt?

(A) Your niece has a life-threatening condition called eclampsia, and needs to be put on strict bed rest and monitored until the baby can be delivered at term

(B) Your niece has a life-threatening condition called eclampsia, and the baby needs to be delivered as soon as possible

(C) Your niece has a life-threatening condition called eclampsia, but this can be managed with anti-seizure medications until the baby can be delivered at term

(D) Your niece has a life-threatening condition called preeclampsia, and needs to be put on strict bed rest and monitored until the baby can be delivered at term

(E) Your niece has a life-threatening condition called preeclampsia, and the baby needs to be delivered as soon as possible

2. A 19-year-old woman at 32 weeks' gestation is the driver in a front-end motor vehicle crash. The air bags did not inflate, and the patient sustained blunt trauma to the abdomen. The patient is taken to a nearby ED in stable condition, where she notes a small amount of bright red blood on her underwear. Maternal vital signs are significant for a heart rate of 110/min and a blood pressure of 110/55 mm Hg. What is next most appropriate step in management?

(A) Administration of $Rh_o(D)$ immune globulin

(B) Disseminated intravascular coagulation panel

(C) External fetal heart rate and uterine monitoring

(D) Immediate cesarean delivery

(E) Immediate vaginal delivery

(F) Internal fetal heart rate and uterine monitoring

3. A 19-year-old G1P0 woman presents to the ED in active labor and delivers a full-term male infant. The infant appears healthy with the exception of jaundice (bilirubin 10 mg/dL, > 95th percentile). The mother does not speak any English, but a cousin states that she has seen the mother taking pills prescribed by her doctor, although she does not know the reason she was taking medication. Based on the newborn's jaundice, which drug was she most likely taking?

(A) Angiotensin-converting enzyme inhibitor

(B) Lithium

(C) Phenytoin

(D) Tretinoin

(E) Trimethoprim-sulfamethoxazole

4. A 16-year-old girl presents to the ED complaining of fever, chills, abdominal pain, and vaginal bleeding. She gives a history of unprotected sexual activity with her 17-year-old boyfriend over the past several months. Her last menstrual period was 8 weeks ago. She reports having a dilatation and curettage procedure at an unlicensed abortion clinic recently to try to abort her pregnancy. Vital signs are significant for a fever of 38.7°C (101.7°F), a heart rate of 120/min, and a blood pressure of 100/70 mm Hg. Pelvic examination reveals cervical motion tenderness, tissue in the internal os, and foul-smelling vaginal discharge. Urine β-human chorionic gonadotropin is positive. What is the most likely diagnosis?

(A) Ectopic pregnancy

(B) Pelvic abscess

(C) Septic abortion

(D) Threatened abortion

(E) Vaginal laceration

5. A 24-year-old woman presents to her primary care physician with a complaint of 1 week of increased vaginal discharge with an unpleasant odor. She is sexually active with one partner and uses oral contraception for birth control. A pregnancy test is negative. Gynecologic examination reveals a pink cervix and a thin white discharge. The discharge has a positive amine "whiff" test and a pH of 6; results of wet saline mount microscopy are shown in the image. Which of the following is the most likely diagnosis?

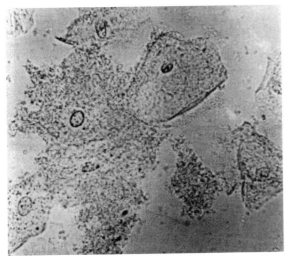

Reproduced, with permission, from Tintinalli JE, Kelen GD, Stapczynski S, Ma OJ, Cline DM. *Tintinalli's Emergency Medicine: A Comprehensive Study Guide*, 6th ed. New York: McGraw-Hill, 2004: 691.

(A) Bacterial vaginosis
(B) *Neisseria gonorrhoeae* cervicitis
(C) *Trichomonas vaginalis*
(D) Vaginal candidiasis
(E) Vulvar candidiasis

6. A 30-year-old obese G3P2 woman with no significant past medical history is in active labor at 41 weeks' gestation. She had an uncomplicated pregnancy with appropriate prenatal evaluation. The patient ruptured membranes spontaneously 30 minutes ago. Contractions occur regularly every 2–3 minutes. Early decelerations are noted on the fetal heart rate monitor with each of the past five contractions. Which is the most appropriate next step in management?

(A) Change the maternal position
(B) No further management is required
(C) Place a fetal scalp probe
(D) Prepare for emergent cesarean delivery
(E) Start an amnioinfusion of saline

7. A 25-year-old G2P1 woman who is 36 weeks pregnant presents to her obstetrician complaining of restlessness and weakness for the past month. She states that her boyfriend recently left her and their 2-year-old son, and she feels overwhelmed with this pregnancy. She denies feeling depressed but does report that she has trouble sleeping. She had an upper respiratory infection last month, "caught from my son," and states that she still has a sore throat. Her blood is drawn, and laboratory tests show:

WBC count	80,000/mm^3
Hemoglobin	11.0 g/dL
Hematocrit	40%
Platelet count	250,000/mm^3
Thyroid-stimulating hormone	0.5 µU/mL
Free thyroxine	4.0 ng/dL

Which of the following is the next step in management?

(A) Levothyroxine
(B) Partial thyroidectomy
(C) Postpartum thyroid hormone levels
(D) Propylthiouracil treatment
(E) Radioiodine treatment

8. A 19-year-old G0 woman presents to her family physician complaining of dysmenorrhea for the past year. She reports severe right-sided pain that coincides with days 1–5 of her menstrual cycle. Her menses occur regularly every 28 days, and she requires three to four pads per day for the first two days of her bleeding and one to two pads per day for the remainder. She has never had surgery. She is not sexually active and does not smoke. Her last menstrual period was 1 week ago. Vital signs are temperature 36.7°C (98.1°F), blood pressure 121/74 mm Hg, heart rate 80/min, and respiratory rate 14/min. Physical examination reveals a thin, healthy-appearing young female. Pelvic examination reveals a normal sized uterus and no cervical motion tenderness. What is the most likely diagnosis?

(A) Ectopic pregnancy
(B) Endometriosis
(C) Leiomyoma
(D) Pelvic inflammatory disease
(E) Polycystic ovary syndrome

9. A 36-year-old G1P0 woman pregnant with twins presents to her obstetrician for her routine 32-week appointment. She has gained 5.4 kg (12 lb) in the past 2 weeks. When questioned about her weight gain, she states that she has had headaches and some blurred vision for the past 2 weeks, which she thinks is secondary to dehydration. To circumvent this she has been drinking a lot of water, which she claims "is not really working, and is making me swell, even my hands!" She also has had some epigastric pain for the past 2 weeks, which she attributes to "all the water I've been drinking." Her vitals are blood pressure 142/90 mm Hg, pulse 105/min, and respiratory rate 18/min. Her urine reveals 1+ glucosuria and 4+ proteinuria. What is the next best step in management?

(A) Administer magnesium sulfate only
(B) Expectant management
(C) Magnesium sulfate therapy, steroids, and induction of labor
(D) Oral antihypertensive therapy
(E) Platelet transfusion

10. A 24-year-old woman with chronic hypothyroidism presents to her gynecologist for her annual examination. She recently got married, and she and her husband would like to conceive. Her hypothyroidism is well controlled and stable on thyroxine, and she has no other medical conditions. She is healthy and does not smoke or drink alcohol. She would like to know if she should keep taking her thyroxine. Which is the most correct advice to give this patient?

(A) No, thyroxine is generally accepted as safe during pregnancy, but if you are not comfortable taking it, there is no evidence that being hypothyroid will affect your baby
(B) No, thyroxine is not safe when taken during pregnancy; it is better for both you and your baby for you to be hypothyroid
(C) No, but we would want to keep you euthyroid for the sake of your baby, so you would be switched to methimazole
(D) Yes, but we would likely be able to decrease your thyroxine during pregnancy because pregnancy is accompanied by mild physiologic hyperthyroidism
(E) Yes, in fact we would likely need to increase your thyroxine during pregnancy to avoid hypothyroidism, which may adversely affect your baby

11. A 24-year-old G1P0 woman at 31 weeks' gestation presents to the ED with a 4-hour history of abdominal cramping and contractions. The contractions have been regularly spaced at 10 minutes, but seem to be increasing in intensity. She has had a small amount of vaginal discharge, but is unable to definitively say whether or not her water has broken. She has not had any vaginal bleeding. Her temperature is 36.8°C (98.3°F), her blood pressure is 137/84 mm Hg, her pulse is 87/min, and her respiratory rate is 12/min. Physical examination reveals a nontender abdomen with palpable contractions every 8 minutes. Which is the next step in the management of this patient?

(A) Cervical culture for Group B streptococci
(B) Digital cervical examination and assessment of dilation and effacement
(C) Quantification of strength and timing of contractions with an external tocometer

(D) Speculum examination to rule out rupture of membranes and visually assess cervical dilation and effacement

(E) Ultrasound examination of the fetus

12. A 32-year-old G3P3 woman is postoperative day 5 after an emergent cesarean section due to fetal distress. The patient progressed rapidly through passive labor without incident, but after the patient's membranes were ruptured manually, a fetal scalp probe was placed in the active phase secondary to several runs of mid-late decelerations. Cesarean section was ultimately performed after 2 hours of active labor secondary to fetal distress. The patient presents now with a fever to 38.7°C (101.7°F) and uterine tenderness. Laboratory values reveal a WBC count of 14,000/mm³, with 70% neutrophils and 4% bands. Which of the following is the most appropriate antibiotic(s)?

(A) Ampicillin and gentamicin
(B) Cefotaxime and levofloxacin
(C) Clindamycin and gentamicin
(D) Imipenem
(E) Metronidazole and doxycycline

13. A 32-year-old G3P3 woman presents to her obstetrician for help conceiving. She states that her cycles have not been regular since the birth of her third child 3 years ago. Furthermore, despite the fact that she readily became pregnant with her other three children, she has failed to become pregnant despite trying over the past 2 years. She has no significant past medical history and takes only prenatal vitamins. Although she says that she has not been ill lately, she reports feeling "tired and cold all the time." She also reports that she has had trouble sleeping over the last several months. Her physical examination is normal. Laboratory tests show:

WBC count	9000/mm³
Hemoglobin	8.0 g/dL
Platelet count	300,000/mm³
Hematocrit	40%
Thyroid-stimulating hormone	0.5 μU/mL
Free thyroxine	2.0 ng/dL
Luteinizing hormone	0.5 mU/mL
Follicle-stimulating hormone	0.5 mU/mL

Which of the following will this woman likely need to take to conceive?

(A) Clomiphene
(B) Levothyroxine
(C) Prednisone
(D) Progesterone
(E) Propylthiouracil

14. A 22-year-old G1P0 woman who is 10 weeks pregnant with twins presents to the ED for vomiting and dizziness. She has had "morning sickness" for the past month, when she would vomit once or twice a day. However, over the past week she has been vomiting multiple times a day, and she has been unsuccessful at "keeping anything down" for the past 2 days. She denies fever or change in her bowel movements; her last bowel movement had been that morning and was well formed. She has otherwise been healthy. Physical examination reveals a tired-appearing, pale woman with poor skin turgor. Otherwise, her examination is unremarkable. Her blood pressure is 110/75 mm Hg lying down and 90/45 mm Hg sitting up. Her pulse is 80/min lying down and 115/min sitting up. Her respiratory rate is 24/min, and her temperature is 37.2°C (99.0°F). Laboratory tests show:

WBC count	14,000/mm³
Platelet count	350,000/mm³
Na⁺	150 mEq/L
K⁺	4 mEq/L
Cl⁻	88 mEq/L
HCO₃⁻	26 mEq/L
Hemoglobin	15 g/dL
Hematocrit	40%
Aspartate aminotransferase	80 U/L
Alanine aminotransferase	85 U/L

What is this woman's most likely diagnosis?

(A) Acute viral hepatitis A
(B) Hyperemesis gravidarum
(C) Preeclampsia
(D) *Salmonella* food poisoning
(E) Viral gastroenteritis

15. A 21-year-old woman presents to the clinic in tears. She states that she recently found out she was pregnant at 10 weeks' gestation. She is a recovering alcoholic but recently relapsed, consuming several drinks a day. She is nervous about the effects of her drinking on her fetus. The physician should tell her that her child is at greatest risk for which of the following?

(A) Eclampsia
(B) Hypoplastic lung
(C) Macrosomia
(D) Microcephaly
(E) Polyhydramnios

16. A 28-year-old G1P0 woman at 12 weeks' gestation presents for routine follow-up with her obstetrician. She complains of mild nausea and occasional vomiting, but otherwise is doing well and reports no other symptoms or complications. Her physical examination is unremarkable and fetal ultrasound is normal for gestational age. Laboratory tests show:

Free triiodothyronine	180 ng/dL
Free thyroxine	2.2 ng/dL
Total thyroxine	12 µg/dL
Thyroid-stimulating hormone	0.1 µU/mL

Results of a thyroid-stimulating hormone–receptor antibody test are negative. Which of the following explains these findings?

(A) Acute infectious thyroiditis
(B) Graves' disease
(C) Hashimoto's thyroiditis
(D) High serum estrogen concentration
(E) High serum β-human chorionic gonadotropin concentration

17. A 23-year-old G1P0 woman is seen in the antepartum care unit. She presents at 37 weeks' gestation with regular contractions and is two fingerbreadths dilated on sterile pelvic examination. Results of electronic fetal heart monitoring are shown in the image. What mechanism best explains the findings on this tracing?

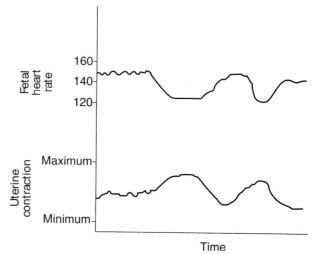

Reproduced, with permission, from USMLERx.com.

(A) Artifact from strong uterine contractions
(B) Compression of the umbilical cord by uterine contractions
(C) Fetal arrhythmia
(D) Pressure on the fetal head coincident with uterine contraction
(E) Reflex response to fetal hypoxia from fetal anemia

18. A 27-year-old G1P0 woman at 27 weeks' gestation presents to the emergency department following a motor vehicle accident. The patient specifically denies any abdominal pain or cramping, contractions, or vaginal bleeding. Examination reveals a gravid, nontender abdomen and a closed, noneffaced cervix with no evidence of vaginal bleeding. Fetal heart monitoring shows a fetal heart rate of 145/min, with variable accelerations and no decelerations. The patient is Rh-negative with no history of blood transfusion, while the father is of unknown Rh status and unavailable. The results of the Kleihauer-Betke test, in which maternal blood is exposed to acid, shows a combination of pale and stained RBCs. What is the next appropriate step in management?

(A) Administer an appropriate dose of intramuscular $Rh_0(D)$ immune globulin
(B) Amniocentesis to measure the amniotic fluid bilirubin level
(C) Emergent cesarean section
(D) Induction of vaginal labor with prostaglandins and oxytocin
(E) Treatment with betamethasone

19. A 27-year-old G1 woman is 20 weeks pregnant. She is currently in her third year of a family practice residency and would like to travel to Africa and Asia as part of an outreach mission with her program. She has received all of her childhood immunizations. She presents to the obstetric clinic inquiring about the safety of immunizations during pregnancy. Which of the following vaccines is contraindicated in pregnancy?

(A) Hepatitis A
(B) Hepatitis B
(C) Influenza
(D) Tetanus
(E) Typhoid
(F) Varicella

20. A 28-year-old G0 woman presents to the clinic complaining of inability to conceive and amenorrhea. She has been taking a low-dose oral contraceptive pill for the past 6 years, which she discontinued 3 months ago when she and her husband decided they wanted to have children. They have been sexually active with each other two to three times per week over the past 3 months, but the patient has not become pregnant. The patient denies a history of sexually transmitted disease and states that until recently she has always had regular menstrual cycles. She has not had a period since discontinuation of the oral contraceptive. What is the next most appropriate step?

(A) Administer a progesterone challenge
(B) Check follicle-stimulating hormone and luteinizing hormone levels
(C) Observation
(D) Perform a hysterosalpingogram
(E) Perform a pelvic ultrasound

21. A 31-year-old G3P2 woman at 37 weeks' gestation presents to the labor and delivery floor after 2 hours of contractions of increasing frequency and intensity. An epidural anesthetic is requested on admission and placed. The patient continues to have contractions for the next 15 hours, during which time her membranes rupture spontaneously. Vaginal examination at that time reveals a cervix which is soft, 3 cm dilated, in an anterior position, and 80% effaced. The fetal head is at the −1 station. Fetal heart tracings reveal a baseline heart rate of 156/min, with variable accelerations and no significant decelerations. What would be the next appropriate step in management?

(A) Apply intravaginal prostaglandin E_2
(B) Attempt forceps-facilitated delivery
(C) Begin an infusion of oxytocin
(D) Increase the rate of intravenous fluids to hydrate the patient
(E) Proceed to cesarean section

22. A 24-year-old G2P2 woman presents to the ED complaining of vaginal bleeding and abdominal cramping. She is sexually active in a monogamous relationship with her husband. Her last menstrual period was 6 weeks ago. The patient is afebrile, and vital signs are within normal limits. Pelvic examination is notable for a dilated cervix, fetal tissue in the vaginal vault, and no cervical motion tenderness. What is the most likely cause of this patient's abortion?

(A) Acute maternal infection
(B) Chromosomal abnormality
(C) Maternal exposure to environmental chemicals
(D) Maternal smoking
(E) Trauma

23. A 30-year-old G0 woman with a past medical history significant only for dysmenorrhea presents to an infertility clinic with her husband for a follow-up visit. The couple has been trying to get pregnant for the past 3 years with no success. Their infertility workup thus far has included a semen analysis, hysterosalpingogram, and estrogen, progesterone, and follicle-stimulating hormone blood levels, all of which were normal. Currently the woman feels well; her only complaint is frustration regarding her inability to conceive. A pelvic ultrasound done last week demonstrated a 3-cm well-circumscribed mass on the patient's left ovary. Her last menstrual period was 3 weeks ago. The mass most likely represents which of the following?

    (A) Corpus luteum cyst
    (B) Ectopic pregnancy
    (C) Endometrioma
    (D) Leiomyoma
    (E) Tubo-ovarian abscess

24. A 37-year-old G2P1 woman at 38 weeks' gestation, with regular prenatal care, presents to the labor and delivery floor after several hours of increasingly frequent and strong contractions and her amniotic membranes are ruptured. On examination her cervix is soft, anterior, and completely effaced and dilated. Labor continues for another 3 hours, at which time the fetus has still not been delivered. The fetal mean heart rate is 146/min, with variable accelerations and no appreciable decelerations. Evaluation of the fetus and maternal pelvis indicate that anatomic factors are adequate for vaginal delivery. Which of the following is an indication for forceps-assisted delivery?

    (A) Fetal distress during the active stage of labor
    (B) Labor complicated by shoulder dystocia
    (C) Prolonged active stage of labor due to inadequate contraction strength
    (D) Prolonged latent stage of labor due to inadequate contraction strength
    (E) Prolonged second stage of labor due to inadequate contraction strength

25. A 30-year-old G3P2 woman at 25 weeks' gestation has a history of gestational diabetes in her previous pregnancy. Her fasting blood glucose level at her initial 10-week screening visit was 110 mg/dL and urinalysis was negative for glucose in the urine. The patient has not been taking her own blood sugars at home, but she has been adhering to a low-carbohydrate diet. Over the past several weeks, she has noticed increased fatigue and polyuria. What is the next appropriate step?

    (A) Administer a 3-hour glucose tolerance test
    (B) Administer a 50-g 1-hour glucose tolerance test
    (C) Begin insulin therapy
    (D) Check a urinalysis and start insulin if urinalysis reveals glucose in the urine
    (E) Prescribe metformin to be taken daily

26. A 47-year-old G1P0 woman at 38 weeks' gestation presents to the obstetrics clinic for a prenatal visit. The patient had difficulty becoming pregnant but was successful after using in vitro fertilization assistance. She has a history of recurrent herpes outbreaks, and currently complains of pain and tingling in the area where she normally breaks out. Routine rectovaginal culture at 36 weeks was positive for Group B streptococci. Which of the following would be a clear indication for delivering the child by cesarean section?

    (A) Active maternal herpes virus infection
    (B) Advanced maternal age
    (C) In vitro fertilization
    (D) Macrosomia
    (E) Maternal colonization with Group B streptococci

27. A 31-year-old woman with systemic lupus erythematous (SLE) is 4 weeks pregnant, and presents to her obstetrician for her first prenatal visit. She is very concerned that the lupus will affect her baby. She was diagnosed with SLE 5 years ago and her symptoms have been well controlled on low-dose prednisone. She has baseline renal insufficiency, with a creatinine of 1.3 mg/dL, which has been stable for the past 6 months. This is her first pregnancy. For which of the following is the baby at increased risk?

(A) Acute renal failure
(B) Chorioretinitis
(C) Complete heart block
(D) Ebstein's anomaly
(E) Rash

28. A 28-year-old G2P1 woman with a past medical history significant for hypertension is in active labor at 42 weeks' gestation. She had an uncomplicated pregnancy and ruptured membranes spontaneously 2 hours ago. Fetal heart tracings are reassuring, contractions occur regularly every 2–3 minutes, and the patient's blood pressure is 110/75 mm Hg. The on-call physician is suddenly called into the patient's room by the nurse because of the findings on the fetal heart monitor, as shown in the image. Which of the following is the most likely cause?

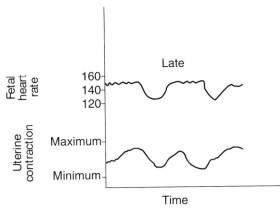

Reproduced, with permission, from USMLERx.com.

(A) Fetal head compression
(B) Fetal myocardial depression
(C) Fetal vagal stimulation
(D) Placental abruption
(E) Placenta previa

29. A 34-year-old G1P0 woman at 29 weeks' gestation with placenta previa diagnosed by ultrasound presents to the ED complaining of 2 hours of vaginal bleeding which has now stopped. She denies any abdominal pain, cramping, or contractions associated with the bleeding. Her temperature is 36.8°C (98.2°F), blood pressure is 118/72 mm Hg, pulse is

75/min, and respiratory rate is 13/min. She reports that she is Rh-positive, her hemoglobin is 11.1 g/dL, and coagulation tests, fibrinogen, and D-dimer levels are all normal. On examination her gravid abdomen is nontender. Fetal heart monitoring is reassuring, with a heart rate of 155/min, variable accelerations, and no decelerations. Two large-bore peripheral intravenous lines are inserted and two units of blood are typed and crossed. What is the most appropriate next step in management of this patient?

(A) Admit to the antenatal unit for bed rest and betamethasone
(B) Admit to the antenatal unit for bed rest and blood transfusion
(C) Admit to the antenatal unit for bed rest and treatment with $Rh_o(D)$ immune globulin
(D) Emergent cesarean section
(E) Outpatient expectant management

30. A 32-year-old G3P2 woman at 35 weeks' gestation has a past medical history significant for hypertension. She was well controlled on hydrochlorothiazide and lisinopril as an outpatient, but these drugs were discontinued when she found out that she was pregnant. Her blood pressure has been relatively well controlled in the 120s systolic off medication, and urinalysis has consistently been negative for proteinuria at each of her prenatal visits. She presents now to the obstetric clinic with a blood pressure of 142/84 mm Hg. A 24-hour urine specimen yields 0.35 g of proteinuria. Which of the following is the next most appropriate step?

(A) Administer oral furosemide
(B) Prepare for emergent delivery
(C) Restart the patient's prepregnancy antihypertensive regimen
(D) Restricted activity and close monitoring as an outpatient following initial inpatient evaluation
(E) Start hydralazine

31. A 32-year-old G2P1 woman at 35 weeks' gestation presents to her obstetrician for a routine prenatal checkup. The mother has been previously diagnosed with mild preeclampsia, which the obstetrician has chosen to manage expectantly. During the visit, a biophysical profile (BPP) is performed and the amniotic fluid index is found to be less than 5 cm, indicating the development of oligohydramnios. The BPP is otherwise normal, with a total score of 8/10 and reassuring fetal heart tracings. How should oligohydramnios be managed in this patient?

   (A) Administration of betamethasone, then cesarean section in 24 hours
   (B) Amnioinfusion with normal saline solution
   (C) Biweekly fetal biophysical profiles
   (D) Emergent cesarean section
   (E) No change in management is necessary

32. At 38 weeks' gestation, a 4030-g (8.9-lb) boy is delivered by spontaneous vaginal delivery. During the first minute of life, he is limp, cyanotic, lacks respiratory effort, has a heart rate of 110/min, flexes his extremities, and grimaces to nasal suctioning. By 5 minutes, he continues to grimace to nasal suctioning, has a weak cry, is well perfused with a heart rate of 160/min, and is kicking both legs. Using the chart below to determine his Apgar scores, will the child need to be resuscitated?

Factor	0	1	2
Heart rate	None	< 100/min	> 100/min
Color	All blue	Body pink and extremities blue	All pink
Muscle tone	Limp	Flexion of extremities	Active motion
Respiratory effort	None	Slow/irregular	Cry
Reflex irritability	No response	Grimace	Cough or sneeze

   (A) Indicated at 1 and 5 minutes
   (B) Indicated at 1 minute and not at 5 minutes
   (C) Indicated at 5 minutes and not at 1 minute
   (D) Not indicated at 1 or 5 minutes
   (E) Not enough information to determine

33. A 23-year-old G1P0 woman presents to her obstetrician for a prenatal examination at 28 weeks' gestation. She has received poor prenatal care up to this point, but is confident about dating the pregnancy. She denies use of alcohol and illicit drugs but has continued to smoke during the pregnancy. The mother has gained only 9 kg (20 lb) during the course of the pregnancy. The mother's temperature is 36.8°C (98.2°F), pulse is 94/min, blood pressure is 138/84 mm Hg, and respiratory rate is 12/min. The fundal height is only 23 cm above the pubic symphysis. Further examination with ultrasound reveals that the fetus is < 10% of the expected weight for the gestational age with symmetric growth anomalies. What is the most likely cause for the intrauterine growth restriction of this fetus?

   (A) Inadequate maternal weight gain during pregnancy
   (B) In utero infection
   (C) Maternal hypertension
   (D) Maternal smoking
   (E) Singleton pregnancy

34. A 22-year-old obese woman presents to the obstetrics-gynecology clinic complaining of mild abdominal pain and vaginal bleeding. The patient states that she is sexually active with her boyfriend and uses condoms "basically all the time." She states that her last menstrual period was 7 weeks ago and insists that her periods have always been irregular, occurring every 3–4 months. She denies any past medical history but states that she used to have a problem with excess facial hair prior to starting low-dose oral contraceptive pills. What is the first step in the diagnostic evaluation of this patient?

   (A) Endometrial biopsy
   (B) Progesterone challenge
   (C) Prothrombin time/partial thromboplastin time
   (D) Thyroid-stimulating hormone
   (E) Ultrasound of the ovaries
   (F) Urine β-human chorionic gonadotropin

35. A full-term 2200-g (4.9-lb) boy was born to a 30-year-old G4P2 woman whose pregnancy was complicated by a seizure disorder for which she inconsistently took carbamazepine. The pregnancy was also notable for an abnormal triple screen for which an amniocentesis was declined. His Apgar scores are 7 and 9 at 1 and 5 minutes, respectively. On examination, his temperature is 37.0°C (98.6°F), blood pressure is 65/45 mm Hg, heart rate is 110/min, and respiratory rate is 30/min. His head circumference is below the fifth percentile. There is a small fleshy sac protruding from the sacral spine. His reflexes are 2+ throughout, and his strength is 5 of 5 in all extremities. His fingernails are very small. What is the most likely diagnosis?

(A) Anoxia due to maternal seizing
(B) Fetal alcohol syndrome
(C) Perinatal exposure to carbamazepine
(D) Trisomy 18
(E) Trisomy 21

36. A 23-year-old primigravid woman at 36 weeks' gestational age has an uncomplicated pregnancy and presents to the labor and delivery unit with intense cramping that began several hours ago. Leopold maneuvers reveal a fetus appropriate in size for gestational age in vertex presentation. Tocometry reveals four irregular contractions lasting more than 30 seconds over 30 minutes. The fetal heart tracing is reassuring. She is one fingerbreadth dilated on sterile vaginal examination. After 6 hours, she is 1 cm dilated. A prostaglandin gel is administered, and 2 hours later she is 2 cm dilated. At this time, oxytocin infusion is begun, and the cervix begins to dilate and become effaced more rapidly. Tocometry reveals powerful and regular contractions. After 4 hours of oxytocin

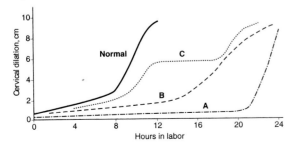

Reproduced, with permission, from USMLERx.com.

infusion, she fails to progress. Based on the image what curve best represents the labor curve of this patient, and what is the possible etiology?

(A) Curve A; inadequate cervical ripening
(B) Curve A; primigravid patient
(C) Curve B; inadequate force of uterine contractions
(D) Curve B; inadequate maternal sedation
(E) Curve C; cephalopelvic disproportion
(F) Curve C; occiput anterior

37. A 28-year-old woman and her husband present to her obstetrician's office. They have been married for 7 years and have been trying to become pregnant for the past 2 years. Prior to this the woman had an intrauterine device, which she had in place for 5 years. Both are healthy without any medical problems, and both deny a history of sexually transmitted diseases. The woman states that her cycles have always been regular (every 28 days, lasting for 5 days) since she was 14 years old. She also denies menorrhagia and dysmenorrhea. What is the most likely cause of this couple's infertility?

(A) Endometriosis
(B) Low sperm concentration
(C) Pelvic inflammatory disease
(D) Premature ovarian failure
(E) Prior placement of an intrauterine device

EXTENDED MATCHING

Questions 38–40

For each patient with vaginal bleeding, select the most appropriate diagnosis.

(A) Abruptio placentae
(B) Ectopic pregnancy
(C) Breakthrough bleeding
(D) Cervical carcinoma
(E) Endometrial cancer
(F) Foreign body
(G) Normal menses
(H) Placenta previa
(I) Preterm labor
(J) Threatened abortion
(K) Vulvar carcinoma

38. A 27-year-old G3P2 woman at 30 weeks' gestation presents to the emergency obstetrics clinic following a 35-mph rear-end collision with another car. She has no previous medical history and her pregnancy has been uncomplicated. She is anxious and complains of sudden onset of severe abdominal pain, dark vaginal bleeding, and uterine contractions. She is hemodynamically stable but tachycardic. On examination there is hypertonicity of the uterus and a nonreassuring fetal heart tracing.

39. A 32-year-old G6P5 woman at 29 weeks' gestation with a history of four previous cesarean sections presents to the emergency obstetrics clinic with painless vaginal bleeding that began this morning and ceased shortly thereafter. She reports normal fetal movement and denies vaginal loss of fluid or uterine contractions. Her vital signs are normal and on examination her uterine fundus is nontender and appropriately enlarged for gestational age. There is no active bleeding from the vaginal canal. Fetal heart tracing is normal and transvaginal sonography reveals a viable fetus and a low-lying placenta with its posterior edge 1 cm from the internal cervical os.

40. An 18-year-old G1P0 woman at 35 weeks' gestation presents to the emergency antepartum clinic for evaluation. She reports a gushing loss of fluid from her vagina this morning with back pain, abdominal cramping, and vaginal spotting for the past several hours. The woman has normal, stable vital signs and fetal heart tracing detects a fetal heart rate of 140/min without decelerations, and a tocometer detects uterine contractions every 10 minutes lasting 30 seconds each. Sterile vaginal examination reveals a cervical os that is dilated at two fingerbreadths.

1. **The correct answer is B.** This patient's seizure, hypertension, headache, and facial edema are consistent with a diagnosis of eclampsia. Eclampsia is defined as seizure activity or coma in an obstetric patient with preeclampsia. Delivery is an immediate necessity once the patient is stabilized to prevent maternal and fetal mortality.

Answer A is incorrect. Delaying delivery once a seizure has occurred is contraindicated because eclampsia is life threatening and will lead to multiorgan system failure.

Answer C is incorrect. Preventing seizures is critical in eclampsia but will not prevent the multiorgan system failure that will occur if delivery is postponed.

Answer D is incorrect. Preeclampsia develops after 20 weeks' gestation and is defined by a blood pressure > 140/90 mm Hg in a previously normotensive patient, plus proteinuria. Hypertension, headache, and edema are also symptoms of preeclampsia; however, once a patient has a seizure, she is classified as having eclampsia.

Answer E is incorrect. Preeclampsia does not require immediate delivery. Mild preeclampsia can be handled as an outpatient. Severe preeclampsia can be monitored in an intensive care unit setting. Immediate delivery for severe preeclampsia is only indicated for fetal age > 30 weeks or fetal distress.

2. **The correct answer is C.** Abruptio placentae refers to premature separation of a normally implanted placenta after 20 weeks of gestation, but prior to delivery of the infant. Since the detached portion of the placenta is unable to exchange gases and nutrients, the fetus can become compromised if the area of separation is large. This patient is at risk for placental abruption secondary to compression-decompression and acceleration-deceleration stresses of a motor vehicle crash. Vaginal bleeding in this setting is concerning, as bleeding is one of the first signs of abruption. It is unlikely that a complete abruption has oc-

curred, as the patient is not frankly hypotensive and her bleeding was minimal. All women > 24 weeks of gestation subjected to abdominal trauma should have continuous fetal and uterine monitoring with an external fetal heart rate to assess for preterm labor and/or an abruption. Signs of fetal compromise are associated with moderate to severe abruption and would necessitate immediate delivery.

Answer A is incorrect. Administration of $Rh_o(D)$ immune globulin is appropriate in an unsensitized Rh-negative female. This patient's blood type would need to be established prior to administration of this drug.

Answer B is incorrect. While patients with placental abruptions are at risk for developing disseminated intravascular coagulation (DIC), this patient does not exhibit signs of a coagulopathy. A DIC panel should be included in routine laboratory blood work on this patient; however, it is an inappropriate first step prior to the establishment of external fetal and uterine monitoring.

Answer D is incorrect. Although cesarean section is the appropriate method of delivery in a patient with a placental abruption, delivery is only warranted when there are signs of fetal or maternal compromise. This patient is at risk for fetal distress due to uteroplacental insufficiency, although further evaluation of the fetus is necessary prior to delivery.

Answer E is incorrect. Vaginal delivery is an inappropriate treatment for a patient with a placental abruption. Patients with abruptions who demonstrate signs of maternal or fetal distress and thus require emergent delivery should be delivered by cesarean section.

Answer F is incorrect. Internal monitoring requires the rupture of membranes, which would be inappropriate management of this patient prior to delivery.

3. **The correct answer is E.** Sulfonamides, used to treat urinary tract infections, can displace bilirubin from albumin, leading to toxicity. Newborns with hyperbilirubinemia are at risk

for neurotoxicity. At extremely elevated levels (i.e., > 25–30 mg/dL) these babies are at risk for development of kernicterus. When to start phototherapy is controversial, though many physicians would start phototherapy at bilirubin levels from 10–15 mg/dL.

Answer A is incorrect. Angiotensin-converting enzyme (ACE) inhibitors have been associated with fetal renal defects, renal dysgenesis/dysplasia, renal failure, oligohydramnios, persistent anuria following delivery, hypotension, pulmonary hypoplasia, limb contractures secondary to oligohydramnios, and stillbirth. ACE inhibitors should be avoided during pregnancy, particularly in the second and third trimesters. ACE inhibitors have not been associated with fetal jaundice.

Answer B is incorrect. Lithium can cause cardiac abnormalities, but has not been associated with fetal jaundice.

Answer C is incorrect. Several antiseizure medications are teratogenic: phenytoin can cause fetal hydantoin syndrome (growth retardation, underdeveloped nails, and mental deficiency); carbamazepine is associated with neural tube defects and other major malformations; valproate is associated with neural tube defects; and phenobarbital can cause cardiac defects and hemorrhagic disease of the newborn due to vitamin K depletion. However, these medications have not been associated with jaundice.

Answer D is incorrect. Tretinoin (retinoic acid) is a treatment for acne, and can cause severe fetal abnormalities and/or spontaneous abortion, but has not been associated with jaundice.

4. **The correct answer is C.** This patient most likely has a septic abortion. Common presenting symptoms include fever, malaise, chills, abdominal or pelvic pain, and vaginal bleeding with or without retained products of conception. Septic abortions do not commonly complicate spontaneous abortions, but can occur as complications of illegally performed induced abortions, foreign bodies, invasive gynecologic procedures, or incomplete spontaneous abortions.

Answer A is incorrect. While ectopic pregnancy may present with vaginal bleeding and abdominal or pelvic pain, the internal cervical os would be closed in an ectopic pregnancy, which contrasts with the patient's presentation. Also, an ectopic pregnancy rarely presents with fevers and chills, symptoms more consistent with septic abortion.

Answer B is incorrect. A pelvic abscess is a complication of pelvic inflammatory disease or other upper genital tract infection. While a pelvic abscess would produce high fevers and abdominal pain, it is unlikely to produce vaginal bleeding. Additionally, the internal os would be closed.

Answer D is incorrect. A threatened abortion presents as pregnancy with painless vaginal bleeding. The internal os is closed. Some of these women will ultimately lose the pregnancy, while a majority will continue to carry the pregnancy successfully to full term.

Answer E is incorrect. While ectopic pregnancy may present with vaginal bleeding and abdominal or pelvic pain, the internal cervical os would be closed in an ectopic pregnancy, which contrasts with the patient's presentation. Also, an ectopic pregnancy rarely presents with fevers and chills, symptoms more consistent with septic abortion.

5. **The correct answer is A.** Bacterial vaginosis is caused by an imbalance in vaginal flora, with reduced numbers of lactobacilli and increased proportions of bacteria such as *Gardnerella*, *Mobiluncus*, or *Peptostreptococcus* species. Signs of bacterial vaginosis include a thin white vaginal discharge, vaginal pH > 4.5, fishy odor on 10% potassium hydroxide "whiff" test, and clue cells on saline mount microscopy (as seen in the image). This diagnosis is established if three of these four criteria are met.

Answer B is incorrect. Patients suffering from *Neisseria gonorrhoeae* cervicitis often complain of vaginal pruritus and discharge. However, up to 50% of patients may not manifest any symptoms at all. Diagnosis is established by identification of *N. gonorrhoeae* on chocolate agar culture or by DNA probe testing. The potassium hydroxide "whiff" test would be negative and no clue cells would be expected.

Answer C is incorrect. Similarly to bacterial vaginosis, *Trichomonas vaginalis* may present with malodorous vaginal discharge and elevated vaginal pH. However, *Trichomonas* is distinguished from bacterial vaginosis by the often yellow-green color of the vaginal discharge, and the visualization of the mobile protozoan with multiple flagella on microscopy.

Answer D is incorrect. Patients with candidiasis often complain of a thick vaginal discharge, vaginal pruritus, and/or dysuria. Signs of candidiasis include vaginal pH in the range of 4–5, and budding hyphae or spores when examined on a slide treated with 10% potassium hydroxide preparation, which lyses the cells in the sample and makes the yeast easier to visualize. Clue cells are not seen in candidiasis.

Answer E is incorrect. Vulvar candidiasis presents with pruritus and redness of the external genitalia. Vaginal discharge would not be expected, vaginal pH would remain normal, and clue cells would not be visualized on wet mount.

6. **The correct answer is B.** Early decelerations are shallow, symmetric decelerations in which the nadir of the deceleration is coincident with the peak of the uterine contraction. They are mediated by vagal stimulation due to fetal head compression from the contracting uterus and thus indicate a normally functioning fetal autonomic nervous system. They are not associated with fetal hypoxia, acidosis, or poor neonatal outcome. No further management is necessary.

Answer A is incorrect. Altering the mother's position (from back to side or side to back) is indicated to relieve cord compression. Variable decelerations, not early decelerations, are a sign of cord compression and thus a change in this patient's position is not necessary.

Answer C is incorrect. A fetal scalp probe is an invasive procedure in which an electrode is inserted transcervically into the fetus's scalp. It is indicated when external fetal heart rate monitoring is inadequate. Internal monitoring provides an accurate beat-to-beat and

baseline measurement of the fetal heart rate variability.

Answer D is incorrect. Cesarean section is appropriate in cases of fetal distress. Early decelerations are not a sign of fetal distress and thus normal labor and delivery should be allowed to continue.

Answer E is incorrect. An amnioinfusion is used to prevent or relieve umbilical cord compression during labor. Cord compression, which is manifested by repetitive variable decelerations, can compromise fetal blood flow and oxygenation.

7. **The correct answer is D.** This woman is exhibiting signs of subacute thyroiditis, consistent with a low thyroid-stimulating hormone and high thyroxine. This commonly follows a viral upper respiratory infection, and pain from the thyroid can be referred to the throat. Thyroid disorders are common during pregnancy (0.5–2% of pregnant women develop hyperthyroidism) and may be subtle and/or present in the context of normal or near normal thyroid hormone levels. Medical management is the treatment of choice in pregnant patients or in those with mild hyperthyroidism.

Answer A is incorrect. Levothyroxine is used to treat hypothyroidism. Symptoms of hypothyroidism are weakness, fatigue, cold intolerance, constipation, weight gain, depression, menstrual irregularities, and hoarseness. On examination, these patients will have dry, cold, puffy skin; edema; thin eyebrows; bradycardia, and delayed relaxation of deep tendon reflexes.

Answer B is incorrect. Surgery is indicated for pregnant women who cannot tolerate thioamides (e.g., propylthiouracil) or for those with severe hyperthyroidism, such as those with goiters large enough to obstruct the airway or esophagus, or those with a nonfunctional thyroid nodule that may be thyroid cancer. This patient's symptoms are mild, and given the potential risks associated with surgery, medical management is preferred.

Answer C is incorrect. Although postpartum thyroid hormone levels will have to be obtained, leaving this woman untreated puts her fetus at risk for growth restriction, craniosynostosis, and death.

Answer E is incorrect. Radioiodine treatment leads to radioactive destruction of the majority of the thyroid gland secondary to thyroid cells taking up the radioactive iodine. Although commonly used for hyperthyroidism, radioisotope treatment is contraindicated during pregnancy due to the potential hazard to the fetus.

8. **The correct answer is B.** Endometriosis is characterized by the presence of endometrial glandular and stromal tissue outside of the uterine cavity or musculature. Although endometriosis can be asymptomatic, patients commonly experience chronic pelvic pain that is often more severe during menses, dysmenorrhea, dyspareunia, abnormal menstrual bleeding, and infertility. A definitive diagnosis is made by direct visualization of the ectopic endometrial tissue via laparoscopy or laparotomy, although patients are often treated empirically with oral contraceptives to avoid a surgical procedure.

Answer A is incorrect. An ectopic pregnancy is a pregnancy that has implanted at a site other than the endometrium of the uterine cavity. Pregnancy should always be considered in a woman of reproductive age complaining of pelvic pain or vaginal bleeding. This patient, however, is not sexually active and reports a last menstrual period of 1 week ago.

Answer C is incorrect. Leiomyomata are benign neoplasms of smooth muscle origin that commonly occur in the uterus, but can form in the broad ligament. They typically occur in middle-aged women and cause menorrhagia, often with resulting iron deficiency anemia, and infertility. They are generally not associated with pelvic pain or dysmenorrhea.

Answer D is incorrect. Pelvic inflammatory disease occurs as a result of an ascending infection of the female genital tract. It commonly occurs in young women and is caused by anaerobic and sexually transmitted microorganisms. Clinical features include fever, chills, unilateral pelvic pain, and cervical motion tenderness. This patient reports none of these symptoms.

Answer E is incorrect. Polycystic ovary syndrome (PCOS) is a constellation of symptoms characterized by multiple ovarian cysts, amenorrhea and infertility secondary to anovulation, hirsutism, and obesity. While the ovarian cysts can often cause unilateral pelvic pain, this patient does not exhibit other classic signs of PCOS.

9. **The correct answer is C.** This woman presents with preeclampsia, which is characterized by hypertension ($\geq$ 140/90 mm Hg) and proteinuria. Nondependent edema, such as facial or hand edema, is usually present as well but is not a necessary criterion. Proteinuria is defined as excretion of $\geq$ 300 mg of protein in 24 hours. The patient is experiencing both subjective as well as objective signs of severe disease, as evidenced by her headaches, visual changes, epigastric pain, and a urine dipstick > 3. A dipstick of 1+ to 2+ is more consistent with mild disease. The underlying pathophysiology of preeclampsia is vasospasm and leaky vessels, but its origin is unclear. Vasospasm and endothelial leakage cause local hypoxemia of tissue, which can lead to hemolysis, necrosis, and end-organ damage. It is cured only by termination of pregnancy and almost always resolves after delivery. Thus, the management of the disease will depend on the gestational age of the fetus, together with the severity of the disease. If the pregnancy is at term, then delivery is indicated. If the pregnancy is preterm, then severity of disease is assessed. If severe preeclampsia is present, then delivery is usually indicated regardless of gestational age. Administration of magnesium sulfate serves as anticonvulsant therapy and should be given during labor to prevent eclampsia.

Answer A is incorrect. Magnesium sulfate alone is not the proper course of action here given the severity of preeclamptic disease. This anticonvulsant is administered as an adjunct to labor, in which it is used to prevent seizures in the setting of severe preeclampsia. However, it will not treat the underlying disease, which will progress and may result in life-threatening complications if delivery is prolonged. Since magnesium sulfate is excreted via the kidneys, it is vital to monitor renal function through urine output, in addition to other potential side effects or signs of toxicity such as respiratory depression, dyspnea secondary to pulmonary edema, and abolition of the deep tendon reflexes.

Answer B is incorrect. Expectant management is an option in premature pregnancies with mild disease. These patients can then be monitored for worsening disease while prolonging the pregnancy to as close to term as possible to allow for fetal lung maturity.

Answer D is incorrect. Antihypertensive medication is indicated in preeclampsia to treat the hypertension, but it will not treat preeclamptic symptoms or prevent any feared complications such as seizures.

Answer E is incorrect. Although complications of preeclampsia include placental abruption, eclampsia, coagulopathies, hepatic subscapular hematoma, hepatic rupture, renal failure, and uteroplacental insufficiency, there are no indications present to warrant the administration of a platelet transfusion. **HELLP** syndrome (**H**emolysis, **E**levated **L**iver enzymes, and **L**ow **P**latelets) is a feared complication of severe preeclampsia and may warrant a platelet transfusion in addition to other therapies, of which delivery is again the best treatment.

10. **The correct answer is E.** During pregnancy there is an increase in circulating thyroid-binding globulin as a result of estrogen stimulation of hepatic enzymes. As a result, pregnant women will often need to increase thyroxine supplementation during their pregnancy. Maternal thyroid hormones are important for fetal neuron development and studies have shown that children whose mothers had hypothyroidism during pregnancy had lower IQs and other developmental problems. Therefore, it is important that hypothyroidism be well controlled during pregnancy.

Answer A is incorrect. Maternal thyroid hormones are important for fetal neuron development. Therefore, it is important that hypothyroidism be well controlled during pregnancy.

Answer B is incorrect. Thyroxine is considered safe during pregnancy. Maternal thyroid hormones are important for fetal neuron de-

velopment. Therefore, it is important that hypothyroidism be well controlled during pregnancy.

Answer C is incorrect. Methimazole is used in treating hyperthyroidism and is not considered safe in pregnancy, as it causes fetal aplasia cutis congenita.

Answer D is incorrect. Although pregnancy is accompanied by a pseudohyperthyroidism (an increase in thyroid-binding globulin results in an elevated total triiodothyronine and thyroxine [T_4]), individuals who take T_4 tend to need higher levels of thyroxine during pregnancy.

11. **The correct answer is D.** Serial assessment of the cervix for changes in dilation and effacement is an important aid in the diagnosis of preterm labor. Examination may be accomplished by either gentle digital examination or by visual inspection with the aid of a speculum. Digital examination is contraindicated in preterm patients whose water has broken as a preventive measure against chorioamnionitis. In a patient who is unsure of the status of her membranes at the time of presentation, it would be prudent to perform a speculum examination of the cervix.

Answer A is incorrect. Group B streptococcal (GBS) colonization is associated with preterm labor, and may complicate the neonatal course of children delivered to colonized mothers. GBS cultures are often taken from women who are in preterm labor, and antibiotic treatment is often initiated until cultures are determined to be negative. However, a GBS test is not diagnostic for preterm labor since patients may be in false labor even if they are colonized with GBS.

Answer B is incorrect. Digital examination is contraindicated in preterm patients whose water has broken as a preventive measure against chorioamnionitis. In a patient who is unsure of the status of her membranes at the time of presentation, it would be prudent to perform a speculum examination of the cervix.

Answer C is incorrect. External tocometers are useful for determining timing and duration of contractions, but are unable to measure the strength of uterine contractions. Therefore, they are of limited use in the diagnosis of preterm labor.

Answer E is incorrect. Ultrasound examination can determine fetal viability and gestational age, and amniotic fluid volume. It may also be used to monitor patients for intrauterine bleeding. However, fetal ultrasound is rarely useful as a diagnostic examination for preterm labor.

12. **The correct answer is C.** This patient is suffering from postpartum endometritis, with risk factors including nonspontaneous rupture of membranes, internal fetal monitoring, and cesarean section. Postpartum endometritis is usually a polymicrobial infection caused by anaerobes and aerobes from the genital tract. Endometrial cultures are generally not helpful in identifying organisms, as infection may result from organisms that typically colonize the genital tract, such as Group B streptococci, as well as from organisms introduced via instrumentation. Management of these patients involves sending blood cultures and subsequently treating with parenteral broad-spectrum antibiotics, including coverage for β-lactamase–producing microbes. The gold standard treatment is intravenous clindamycin and gentamicin.

Answer A is incorrect. This combination does not provide adequate coverage for β-lactamase-producing organisms. Ampicillin may be combined with sulbactam and used as an alternative to the clindamycin/gentamicin combination.

Answer B is incorrect. This combination does not provide adequate anaerobic coverage or coverage of β-lactamase–producing organisms.

Answer D is incorrect. Imipenem is active against aerobes, anaerobes, and β-lactamase-producing organisms. However, it is not the appropriate first-line drug for such an infection, but may be used if the patient does not respond clinically to less potent antibiotics. Additionally, imipenem enters breast milk and thus must be used with caution in breast-feeding mothers.

Answer E is incorrect. Metronidazole may be used with ceftriaxone or levofloxacin as an alternate therapy; however, it provides inappropriate coverage when combined with doxycycline. Furthermore, doxycycline is contraindicated in nursing mothers because it causes tooth discoloration and enamel hypoplasia during tooth formation in infants.

13. **The correct answer is A.** This patient is likely suffering from postpartum pituitary necrosis (Sheehan's syndrome), which is believed to be a consequence of reduced blood flow to the pituitary during delivery or the postpartum period. This woman is exhibiting signs of hypothyroidism (low thyroid-stimulating hormone and thyroxine) and will likely need levothyroxine treatment. However, she is likely not ovulating secondary to her pituitary dysfunction (low follicle-stimulating hormone and luteinizing hormone). In cases such as these, ovulation often needs to be induced with an agent such as clomiphene.

Answer B is incorrect. Levothyroxine should be part of this woman's prescriptive regimen to combat her hypothyroidism. However, she will likely need direct ovulation stimulation to become pregnant.

Answer C is incorrect. Prednisone in addition to the levothyroxine would be used to treat this woman's hypothyroidism during pregnancy, but it would not help her conceive.

Answer D is incorrect. Progesterone is used as an exogenously administered hormone to maintain the corpus luteum and induce the secretory phase of the endometrium for implantation, but it would not lead to conception in a woman who is not ovulating.

Answer E is incorrect. Propylthiouracil is used to medically manage hyperthyroidism, not hypothyroidism.

14. **The correct answer is B.** Hyperemesis gravidarum is defined as persistent severe vomiting during pregnancy and is principally a diagnosis of exclusion. It can lead to severe dehydration, hypochloremic acidosis, hypokalemia, and a transient elevation in liver enzymes. It is more common in multiple pregnancies, as in this scenario, and is believed to be due to increasing β-human chorionic gonadotropin levels.

Answer A is incorrect. Although viral hepatitis A does cause nausea and vomiting and an increase in liver enzymes, it is also associated with malaise, fatigue, low-grade fevers, and jaundice. Given this woman's history of a multiple gestation pregnancy with accompanying morning sickness in the absence of any other signs or symptoms, the most likely diagnosis is hyperemesis gravidarum.

Answer C is incorrect. Although preeclampsia is more common in multiple gestations, it is rare before 20 weeks' gestation. In addition, patients with preeclampsia rarely have isolated acute nausea and vomiting. Other signs and symptoms such as severe hypertension, edema, proteinuria, sudden weight gain, headache, and vision changes usually accompany the gastrointestinal distress.

Answer D is incorrect. *Salmonella* food poisoning usually causes vomiting in the context of diarrhea and fever.

Answer E is incorrect. Viral gastroenteritis can cause nausea and vomiting, but given a lack of bowel changes or other symptoms, this woman's history is more consistent with hyperemesis gravidarum.

15. **The correct answer is D.** The prevalence of fetal alcohol syndrome (FAS) among moderate to heavy drinkers and alcoholics is 10–50%. The diagnosis is based upon three criteria: growth retardation (confirmed pre- or postnatal weight or height ≤ 10th percentile), facial dysmorphia (smooth philtrum, thin vermilion border, short palpebral fissures, hypoplastic midface, and microcephaly), and central nervous system abnormalities (structural or functional abnormalities, including mental retardation). FAS patients also have an increased risk of cardiac defects.

Answer A is incorrect. Preeclampsia is defined as new-onset hypertension, proteinuria, and/or nondependent edema occurring at > 20 weeks' gestation. Eclampsia is seizures in a patient with preeclampsia. Risk factors include nulliparity, black race, extremes of age, multiple gestation, molar pregnancy, renal disease, family history of preeclampsia, and chronic hypertension. Preeclampsia is not associated with fetal alcohol syndrome.

Answer B is incorrect. Pulmonary hypoplasia occurs secondary to severe reduction in amniotic fluid and is often related to kidney dysgenesis or dysfunction, not fetal alcohol syndrome.

Answer C is incorrect. Macrosomia is defined as fetal weight > 4.0 kg, or birth weight above the 90th percentile for gestational age. Maternal gestational diabetes mellitus is a risk factor for macrosomia. It is thought that the fetal pancreas produces excess insulin as a result of increased maternal blood glucose. This results in large fat deposits which cause the fetus to grow excessively large. Patients with fetal alcohol syndrome experience intrauterine growth restriction.

Answer E is incorrect. Excess amniotic fluid may be a result of fetal anomalies including duodenal atresia, tracheoesophageal fistula, or anencephaly. These anomalies prevent the fetus from ingesting amniotic fluid. The fetal alcohol syndrome does not include these anomalies.

16. **The correct answer is E.** The two most important factors that affect thyroid physiology in the pregnant patient are estrogen and β-human chorionic gonadotropin. Early in pregnancy, when β-human chorionic gonadotropin (β-hCG) levels peak at 10–12 weeks, patients can have subclinical hyperthyroidism because β-hCG is a weak stimulator of the thyroid-stimulating hormone (TSH)-receptor and this stimulation causes excess production of thyroid hormones and a subsequent decline in TSH due to negative feedback on the pituitary, as is seen in this patient. This transient subclinical hyperthyroidism occurs in 10–20% of patients and usually does not require therapy. Rarely, high levels of β-hCG can contribute to hyperemesis gravidarum, a syndrome consisting of nausea, vomiting, and weight loss. In addition, patients with hydatidiform mole or choriocarcinoma can have severe hyperthyroidism.

Answer A is incorrect. Acute infectious thyroiditis presents with fever, chills, and acute onset of extreme pain in the thyroid. Many patients will have a unilateral neck mass, which may be fluctuant. Thyroid function is typically normal in patients with acute infectious thyroiditis.

Answer B is incorrect. Graves' disease is the most common cause of hyperthyroidism in pregnant as well as nonpregnant patients. Patients will present with signs and symptoms of hyperthyroidism including fatigue, heat intolerance, anxiety, diarrhea, and palpitations. Patients will typically have TSH levels < 0.01 μU/mL and the serum will be positive for TSH-receptor antibodies.

Answer C is incorrect. Hashimoto's disease is a common cause of hypothyroidism. These patients will have decreased levels of free triiodothyronine and thyroxine and elevated thyroid-stimulating hormone. Hypothyroidism is rare in pregnant patients because it can cause anovulation. In addition, hypothyroidism can cause spontaneous abortion in the first trimester.

Answer D is incorrect. Elevated serum estrogen levels also cause a major change in thyroid function. Estrogen increases production as well as decreases clearance of thyroid-binding globulin. This causes an increase in total thyroxine (T_4), but the free triiodothyronine (T_3) and T_4 remain normal. The patient is clinically euthyroid and the TSH is normal. These abnormalities will typically be found in pregnant patients. However, this patient's findings of high free T_3 and T_4 as well as decreased TSH suggest a subclinical hyperthyroidism due to the effects of β-human chorionic gonadotropin.

17. **The correct answer is D.** A deceleration is a slowing of the fetal heart rate, usually lasting 10–15 seconds. Early decelerations begin and end with contractions. They are a reassuring finding and reflect an increase in vagal tone as a result of uterine contractions exerting pressure on the fetal head as it descends into the vaginal canal.

Answer A is incorrect. Fetal hypoxia from fetal anemia can result in a regular and smooth-appearing sinusoidal wave pattern. This tracing is ominous and associated with high fetal morbidity and mortality.

Answer B is incorrect. Compression of the umbilical cord leads to variable decelerations and constitutes a nonreassuring tracing. This

tracing would show a sharp fall in fetal heart rate followed by a variable recovery time. They do not display the consistent association with contractions that are seen in the "early decelerations" seen in the case above.

Answer C is incorrect. Fetal arrhythmia is not associated with early decelerations.

Answer E is incorrect. Fetal hypoxia from fetal anemia can result in a regular and smooth-appearing sinusoidal wave pattern. This tracing is ominous and associated with high fetal morbidity and mortality.

18. **The correct answer is A.** The mother has been exposed to fetal blood cells, as evidenced by the Kleihauer-Betke test. This test uses the increased resistance of fetal hemoglobin to elution by acid as compared to adult hemoglobin. Because the Rh antigen is inherited in an autosomal dominant fashion, the fetus would be Rh-negative if the father were also Rh-negative. However, because the father is unavailable for testing, it is prudent to proceed as if the fetus were Rh-positive. Thus, the mother should receive $Rh_o(D)$ immune globulin to prevent possible isoimmunization to the Rh antigen.

Answer B is incorrect. Amniocentesis to measure bilirubin levels is a method of measuring the degree to which an Rh-positive fetus, carried by an Rh-sensitized mother, is affected by hemolysis. Because the mother is not sensitized, any risk of isoimmunization would be to subsequent pregnancies, not the current one. Therefore, amniocentesis to ascertain the amniotic fluid bilirubin level is not indicated.

Answer C is incorrect. Both the mother and fetus are stable after the accident. At only 27 weeks, the fetus is still several weeks away from achieving full lung maturity, and an emergent cesarean section would put the infant at significant risk for respiratory distress syndrome. In the absence of any maternal or fetal distress, emergent cesarean section is not indicated at this time.

Answer D is incorrect. There are no signs of maternal or fetal distress that would warrant premature delivery of this infant. Thus, expectant management for a term delivery with emphasis on prevention of Rh isoimmunization of the mother is a more prudent course in this clinical situation.

Answer E is incorrect. Both the mother and the fetus appear to be stable after the automobile accident, and there are no signs of impending labor. Thus, the mother can be expectantly managed for a delivery at term. There is no need to administer betamethasone to accelerate maturation of the fetal lungs at this time.

19. **The correct answer is F.** Varicella vaccine is a live attenuated vaccine. Women who have not contracted chickenpox as children should be vaccinated prior to considering pregnancy.

    Answer A is incorrect. Two inactivated forms of the hepatitis A vaccine are available. Although limited data exist on the safety of these vaccines during pregnancy, the vaccine is presumed to be safe like other inactivated vaccines. Nonetheless, it should only be administered to high-risk women, such as those traveling to areas in which hepatitis A is endemic.

    Answer B is incorrect. Hepatitis B vaccine is a recombinant vaccine and has not been shown to be harmful to the fetus or newborn. Hepatitis B vaccine is indicated in pregnant women who are completing an immunization series that had begun prior to conception and to nonimmunized women who are at high risk of contracting hepatitis B.

    Answer C is incorrect. The influenza virus vaccine is an inactivated vaccine and should be administered to all pregnant women in October to mid-November (prior to influenza season) regardless of gestational age of the fetus.

    Answer D is incorrect. The tetanus vaccine is a modified bacterial toxoid; thus the toxoid is rendered inactive. It is safe during pregnancy and is indicated in any woman who has not completed her three-dose primary immunization or has not had a booster dose in 10 years.

    Answer E is incorrect. The typhoid vaccine is a capsular polysaccharide vaccine that must be administered parenterally. It is not a commonly administered vaccine but can be given to patients traveling to endemic areas.

20. **The correct answer is C.** Amenorrhea for 3–5 months following the discontinuation of oral contraceptive pills (OCPs) is common and should not cause concern. Patients whose menses do not return more than 5 months after discontinuation of the pill, particularly if they were taking low-dose OCPs, require a standard evaluation for amenorrhea.

    Answer A is incorrect. A progesterone challenge is given to women with amenorrhea to evaluate for ovarian estradiol production and the presence of a normal outflow tract. This patient may require such a challenge if she does not get her period within the next few months, but it is inappropriate at this point.

    Answer B is incorrect. Follicle-stimulating hormone (FSH) and luteinizing hormone (LH) levels are checked as part of the evaluation of a woman with amenorrhea. High FSH and LH levels indicate a lack of steroid hormone synthesis or anatomic abnormality of the ovarian tissue, whereas low FSH and LH levels suggest pituitary dysfunction. If this patient is still amenorrheic after two more months, she will require a complete evaluation for amenorrhea. At this time, however, she does not.

    Answer D is incorrect. A hysterosalpingogram (HSG) is performed to determine the patency of the fallopian tubes in a woman experiencing infertility. Women at high risk for tubal scarring include women with a history of sexually transmitted diseases (STDs), particularly prior chlamydial infection. This patient does not need an HSG at this time, as she does not meet the criteria for infertility (failure to conceive after 12 months of frequent intercourse without contraception) and she denies a history of STDs.

    Answer E is incorrect. A pelvic ultrasound is useful in patients who are or may be pregnant, or where there is concern for uterine or ovarian pathology (i.e., cysts or masses). It is not indicated in this patient.

21. **The correct answer is C.** This patient is experiencing a prolonged latent phase of labor. Options for managing a prolonged latent phase include rest or augmentation of labor. Augmentation of labor is often effected with oxy-

tocin intravenous infusions and artificial rupture of membranes if they have not already spontaneously ruptured. In this case of prolonged labor in which the mother has a cervix favorable for delivery and has had spontaneous rupture of membranes, an oxytocin infusion is a reasonable next step.

Answer A is incorrect. Intravaginal prostaglandin E_2 is used to induce labor when the patient has a cervix that is unfavorable for oxytocin induction. Prostaglandin E_2 is not used once labor is in progress, and carries a risk of uterine hyperstimulation, placental insufficiency, and uterine rupture.

Answer B is incorrect. Forceps delivery may be used to facilitate delivery in cases in which the power of uterine contractions alone is insufficient to deliver the infant. However, prerequisites for forceps delivery include a fully dilated cervix and fully engaged fetal head. For most forceps delivery techniques the fetal head station must be at least +2. This patient, who is still in the latent first stage of labor, has not yet progressed to a point where forceps are likely to facilitate delivery of the infant.

Answer D is incorrect. Hydration is often used to forestall premature labor. Antidiuretic hormone is manufactured in the hypothalamus along with oxytocin, and is hypothesized to exhibit some cross-reactivity with oxytocin. Decrease of ADH levels by hydration leads to lower levels of stimulation of oxytocin receptors, and thus may decrease the strength of contractions. Therefore hydration would not facilitate delivery, and may decrease the strength of uterine contractions, prolonging the labor process.

Answer E is incorrect. While the progression to active labor has been prolonged, the fetal heart rate is reassuring of the fetus' well-being. Thus, vaginal delivery may be allowed to proceed. If at any point the fetal heart rate pattern becomes nonreassuring and vaginal delivery is not imminent, a cesarean section would be indicated.

22. **The correct answer is B.** Chromosomal abnormalities, most commonly aneuploidy, account for approximately 50% of all miscarriages, particularly those occurring prior to 12 weeks' gestation.

Answer A is incorrect. Acute maternal infection, particularly toxoplasmosis, herpes simplex, or rubella, can increase the chances of early pregnancy loss. However, it is not the most common cause of miscarriage.

Answer C is incorrect. Exposure to certain environmental chemicals can also increase the chances of pregnancy loss. However, this is not the most common etiology.

Answer D is incorrect. Heavy maternal smoking is associated with an increase in pregnancy loss; however, the rate of increase of spontaneous abortions associated with smoking (~ 24%) is much less significant than the number of spontaneous abortions associated with chromosomal abnormalities (~ > 50%). Therefore, smoking is a possible cause of the abortion, but it is not the most likely cause.

Answer E is incorrect. The uterus at an early gestational age is protected from blunt trauma due to its small size. However, trauma from a gynecologic or obstetric procedure can induce a miscarriage. This patient does not report any such history.

23. **The correct answer is C.** The patient's infertility and dysmenorrhea are most likely secondary to endometriosis, and the pelvic mass is most likely an endometrioma, or "chocolate cyst." Patients with endometriosis often experience chronic pelvic pain that is more severe during menses, dysmenorrhea, dyspareunia, abnormal menstrual bleeding, and infertility. The optimal method of diagnosis is direct visualization via laparoscopy or laparotomy, following initial imaging with ultrasound. On ultrasound, an endometrioma appears as a complex mass, with varying areas of hypodense and hyperdense lesions.

Answer A is incorrect. A corpus luteum cyst is a functional ovarian cyst that occurs after an egg has been released from a follicle. Usually, the follicle (now the corpus luteum) breaks down if no pregnancy occurs, but it can become filled with blood or fluid, remaining in the ovary. This patient's adnexal mass is unlikely to be a corpus luteum cyst, as the ultrasound was performed at week two of her menstrual cycle, around the time of ovulation. Corpus luteum cysts tend to appear toward the end of the menstrual cycle.

Answer B is incorrect. This patient does not describe typical symptoms of ectopic pregnancy, namely unilateral pelvic pain, vaginal spotting, and amenorrhea. She also does not report risk factors for ectopic pregnancy, such as a history of sexually transmitted diseases, prior pelvic surgery, or previous ectopic pregnancy.

Answer D is incorrect. Leiomyomata are benign neoplasms of smooth muscle origin that commonly occur in the uterus, but can also form in the broad ligament. They generally occur in women aged 30–40 and are a common cause of infertility. They tend not to cause pelvic pain or dysmenorrhea. While this patient could have a leiomyoma, given her history, her symptoms are more likely due to endometriosis.

Answer E is incorrect. A tubo-ovarian abscess (TOA) is part of the spectrum of pelvic inflammatory disease and occurs as a result of an ascending infection of the female genital tract. The most likely causes of TOA are anaerobic and sexually transmitted microorganisms. Clinical features include fever, chills, unilateral pelvic pain, and cervical motion tenderness. This patient reports none of these symptoms.

24. **The correct answer is E.** Forceps-assisted delivery is used when the combination of uterine contractions and voluntary pushing by the mother generate insufficient force to deliver the infant. This technique is employed during the second stage of labor, at which point the membranes have ruptured, the cervix is fully dilated, and the fetal head is engaged. It is important to exclude cephalopelvic disproportion as the cause of prolonged labor before forceps delivery is attempted.

Answer A is incorrect. During the active stage of labor, delivery of the infant may still require several hours to accomplish. In cases of fetal distress, vaginal delivery should only be allowed to proceed if delivery is imminent. Cesarean section is the indicated course of action for fetal distress during active labor.

Answer B is incorrect. Forceps delivery is primarily a method of increasing the force of traction expelling the fetus from the birth canal. In shoulder dystocia, the difficulty of passage of the infant arises not from insufficient force, but rather from an anatomic obstruction of the shoulder by the pubic symphysis. Maneuvers used in shoulder dystocia include flexion of the maternal hips, suprapubic pressure, and pressure applied to the anterior or posterior shoulder of the fetus.

Answer C is incorrect. Prolonged active phase of labor can be a result of cephalopelvic disproportion or insufficient strength of uterine contractions. If disproportion is excluded, oxytocin may be used to increase the strength of uterine contractions. Amniotomy is recommended if the membranes are intact and there is prolonged active labor.

Answer D is incorrect. The causes of a prolonged latent phase of labor are numerous and include inadequate contractions, cephalopelvic disproportion, and infrequent contractions. Options for treatment of prolonged latent phase of labor include rest or augmentation of contractions with oxytocin, as well as amniotomy if the membranes are intact. Use of forceps to effect delivery at this time would be excessively morbid for both the mother and fetus.

25. **The correct answer is B.** This woman has an increased risk of developing gestational diabetes in this pregnancy, given her history of gestational diabetes in a previous pregnancy. All women with increased risk should be screened at 24–28 weeks' gestation with a random 1-hour 50-g oral glucose challenge. If positive, screening should follow with a 100-g 3-hour glucose tolerance test. If this test is positive, the woman is diagnosed with gestational diabetes. Treatment should initially begin with a trial of diet modification. If the patient fails to meet target blood sugar levels, insulin therapy should be started.

Answer A is incorrect. A 3-hour glucose tolerance test is indicated only after an initial 1-hour 50-g oral glucose challenge.

Answer C is incorrect. Insulin therapy is not appropriate at this point. This patient does not yet have a diagnosis of gestational diabetes.

Answer D is incorrect. While patients with gestational diabetes will have glycosuria, initiation of insulin therapy is not determined by the presence or absence of glucose in the urine. Insulin therapy is initiated in a patient with gestational diabetes who fails to meet target blood glucose levels with diet and exercise alone.

Answer E is incorrect. All of the oral hypoglycemic agents, including metformin, are contraindicated in pregnancy, as they can cause fetal hypoglycemia. Only insulin therapy should be administered to women with diabetes during pregnancy.

26. **The correct answer is A.** Active maternal herpes lesion or prodromal symptoms near the time of delivery are an indication to perform a cesarean section. This is because 85% of neonatal herpes infections are due to transmission near delivery. Although the majority of infants with neonatal herpes simplex virus are born to asymptomatic women, cesarean delivery is warranted in the setting of herpetic symptoms because of the significant consequences of neonatal herpes infection, which include localized infections, central nervous system involvement and disseminated disease.

Answer B is incorrect. Advanced maternal age is not a recognized indication for cesarean section.

Answer C is incorrect. In vitro fertilization increases the rate of multiple gestations up to 20%, and multiple gestations increase the rate of prematurity, intrauterine growth restriction, and nonvertex presentations. In twins, if the second twin's estimated fetal weight is less than 2000 g or external version fails to correct nonvertex presentation, cesarean delivery should be performed. However, in vitro fertilization itself is not an absolute indication for cesarean section.

Answer D is incorrect. Macrosomia is associated with a twofold increase in the likelihood of cesarean section but is not itself a clear indication for an operative delivery.

Answer E is incorrect. Maternal colonization with Group B streptococci is not an indication for cesarean section, although it increases the risk for chorioamnionitis and neonatal sepsis. Indicated treatment is a course of antibiotic therapy with intravenous penicillin during labor.

27. **The correct answer is C.** Neonatal lupus is caused by passive transfer of anti-Ro/SSA and/or anti-La/SSB antibodies. The disorder can occur in babies born to mothers with lupus, Sjögren's syndrome, or in women with no prior history of autoimmune disease. Not all women with systemic lupus erythematosus have these autoantibodies, so screening should be done at the beginning of prenatal care to determine the risk of neonatal lupus and the need for monitoring. The most serious complication of neonatal lupus is complete heart block. Neonatal lupus is the most common cause of congenital complete heart block. Fetuses at risk of neonatal lupus should have regular Doppler echocardiography to screen for the development of heart block.

Answer A is incorrect. Babies born to mothers with lupus are not at increased risk of developing renal abnormalities or acute renal failure. However, women with baseline lupus nephritis are at increased risk of developing progressive renal disease during pregnancy due to an increased burden placed on maternal kidneys.

Answer B is incorrect. Chorioretinitis is typically seen in babies with congenital infections such as toxoplasmosis and cytomegalovirus (CMV). Toxoplasmosis also presents with hydrocephalus and intracranial calcifications. CMV presents with microcephaly, hepatosplenomegaly, respiratory distress, and seizures.

Answer D is incorrect. Ebstein's anomaly is a congenital cardiac defect consisting of malformation of the tricuspid valve and right ventricle. It occurs more frequently in infants born to mothers who took lithium during pregnancy. It is not associated with maternal systemic lupus erythematosus.

Answer E is incorrect. Most babies with neonatal lupus have a rash, usually consisting of erythematous annular lesions on the scalp and periorbital area. However, the rash is typically mild and resolves by 6–8 months of age.

28. **The correct answer is D.** Mild late decelerations are due to a central nervous system reflex response to fetal hypoxia. Hypoxia generally results from uteroplacental insufficiency, which is commonly a sign of placental abruption or hypotension. Placental abruption tends to present with painful, dark vaginal bleeding that does not cease spontaneously. In this case, with a history of maternal hypertension, the patient is likely having a placental abruption and may require emergent cesarean section.

Answer A is incorrect. Fetal head compression is associated with early decelerations, which begin and end at approximately the same time as the maternal contraction. The tracing above shows late decelerations.

Answer B is incorrect. Fetal myocardial depression is manifested by severe late decelerations, and usually with absent variability. Myocardial depression is associated with severe acidosis and perinatal morbidity and mortality. The patient in this question is not exhibiting signs of severe fetal compromise.

Answer C is incorrect. Early, not late, decelerations are secondary to vagal stimulation due to fetal head compression. In early decelerations, the nadir of the heart rate deceleration occurs simultaneously with the peak of the uterine contraction.

Answer E is incorrect. Placenta previa predisposes a patient to peripartum hemorrhage and placental abruption, both of which may contribute to maternal hypotension and fetal hypoxia. In the absence of these clinical findings, placenta previa in and of itself does not cause late decelerations or fetal distress. Placenta previa presents with painless, bright red bleeding that often ceases in 1–2 hours.

29. **The correct answer is A.** Patients with placenta previa are often managed expectantly unless there is fetal distress, persistent labor, or life-threatening hemorrhage. However, up to 70% of patients experience a recurrence of bleeding and require delivery before fetal lung maturity has been achieved. Thus, preparation for preterm delivery with betamethasone to promote fetal lung maturity is indicated. The child should be delivered by cesarean section at 36 weeks, or earlier if life-threatening hemorrhage occurs.

Answer B is incorrect. At this time the bleeding from the placenta previa has ceased, the mother has a hemoglobin level of 11.1 g/dL, and the fetus has a reassuring heart tone. In this patient blood transfusion is not indicated at this time.

Answer C is incorrect. The mother is Rh-positive. $Rh_o(D)$ immune globulin is administered in the case of an Rh-negative mother and known or suspected Rh-positive fetus to prevent isoimmunization and its complications such as fetal anemia and high-output cardiac failure. Since the mother is Rh-positive, isoimmunization cannot occur.

Answer D is incorrect. Delivery in the case of placenta previa should be by cesarean section. However, most sentinel bleeds resulting from placenta previa will cease spontaneously, and thus are managed expectantly to allow for administration of betamethasone and further fetal development.

Answer E is incorrect. Rebleeding occurs in up to 70% of patients with placenta previa after the sentinel bleed. Thus, the patient should be hospitalized on bed rest and preparations should be taken for life-threatening hemorrhage and emergent cesarean section.

30. **The correct answer is D.** Preeclampsia refers to the new onset of hypertension and proteinuria (> 0.3 g in a 24-hour urine specimen) after 20 weeks' gestation in a previously normotensive female. Eclampsia refers to the occurrence of one or more generalized convulsions and/or coma in the setting of preeclampsia. In mild preeclampsia, patients do not have any features of severe disease, such as central nervous system symptoms, thrombocytopenia, or pulmonary edema. Many newly diagnosed patients need close maternal monitoring to establish disease severity and rate of progression, and to monitor for progression to eclampsia, hypertensive crisis, abruptio placentae, or **HELLP** syndrome (Hemolysis, Elevated Liver

enzymes, and **L**ow **P**latelets). However, these complications are uncommon in women beyond 32 weeks' gestation with mild hypertension (< 150/100 mm Hg), minimal proteinuria (e.g., < 1 g in 24 hours), and no other abnormalities. Therefore, patients with these findings may be managed on an ambulatory basis after initial inpatient evaluation, with frequent maternal and fetal evaluations. Restricted activity is typically recommended; there is no evidence that complete bed rest has any benefit. Antihypertensive medications are only recommended in patients with a systolic blood pressure > 150 mm Hg or a diastolic blood pressure > 100 mm Hg.

Answer A is incorrect. Diuretics are not recommended during pregnancy due to their possible teratogenic effects. Furthermore, furosemide is an ineffective antihypertensive agent in patients who are not volume overloaded.

Answer B is incorrect. Delivery of the fetus is indicated in a woman with severe preeclampsia or eclampsia.

Answer C is incorrect. Angiotensin-converting enzyme inhibitors are contraindicated in pregnancy. They cause oligohydramnios and renal damage to the fetus.

Answer E is incorrect. Hydralazine and labetalol are the two antihypertensive medications recommended in pregnancy. Medical therapy, however, is not indicated in patients with systolic blood pressures < 150 mm Hg or diastolic blood pressures < 100 mm Hg, as is the case with this patient.

31. **The correct answer is C.** Oligohydramnios in this patient is most likely a reflection of the uteroplacental insufficiency caused by the mild preeclampsia. While oligohydramnios itself poses some risk to the fetus through an increase in prevalence of cord compression, it does not require immediate delivery if there is no fetal or maternal distress. A prudent course of action would include regular monitoring with biophysical profile testing to ensure fetal well-being and induction of labor when fetal lung maturity has been achieved.

Answer A is incorrect. In cases of oligohydramnios without fetal distress, a trial of labor

once fetal maturity has been achieved is not contraindicated. While planned cesarean section in this case would be much preferable to an emergent cesarean section, there is no need to forego a trial of labor in this case.

Answer B is incorrect. Amnioinfusion is often used to treat fetuses that are experiencing severe, repeated variable heart rate decelerations indicative of cord compression during labor. It is also used as a dilutional method in labors that are complicated by thick meconium-stained amniotic fluid. It is not currently used in cases of oligohydramnios when there is no evidence of fetal distress.

Answer D is incorrect. Oligohydramnios is often caused by uteroplacental insufficiency, placental abruption or infarction, congenital abnormalities, growth restriction, fetal demise, or ruptured membranes. While oligohydramnios may be indicative of some underlying pathology, the oligohydramnios itself does not warrant emergent surgical delivery.

Answer E is incorrect. Since oligohydramnios in the third trimester is often associated with uteroplacental insufficiency, it is prudent to monitor the fetus at regular intervals for signs of distress. Biweekly biophysical profile testing is a prudent addition to this patient's care.

32. **The correct answer is B.** His Apgar scores are 3 and 8 at 1 and 5 minutes, respectively. Apgar scoring is a standardized method of summarizing an infant's overall condition at birth and predicting which infants are going to require resuscitation. Apgar scores of 0–3 indicate the need for immediate resuscitation, either bag-mask ventilation or intubation. Apgar scores of 8–10 indicate good cardiopulmonary adaptation. Apgar scores of 4–7 indicate possible need for resuscitation.

Answer A is incorrect. An Apgar score of 8 does not indicate a need for resuscitation.

Answer C is incorrect. An Apgar score of 8 does not indicate a need for resuscitation; however, a score of 3 indicates the need for immediate resuscitation.

Answer D is incorrect. An Apgar score of 3 indicates the need for immediate resuscitation.

Answer E is incorrect. The information necessary to determine Apgar scores and the need for resuscitation are provided. The Apgar system is a standardized method that incorporates the criteria known to impact survival in neonates.

33. **The correct answer is B.** Causes of symmetric intrauterine growth restriction (IUGR) include in-utero infection, multiple pregnancies, and maternal disease. Asymmetric IUGR is due to uteroplacental insufficiency from maternal hypertension, smoking, and poor nutrition. Since this fetus demonstrates symmetric growth restriction, the most likely cause of the IUGR is an early in-utero infection.

    Answer A is incorrect. Inadequate weight gain also inhibits growth by cellular hyperplasia, and causes asymmetric growth retardation. However, because nutritional deficiency only affects cellular hyperplasia rather than division, it is more amenable to reversal if the nutritional deficit is corrected.

    Answer C is incorrect. Maternal hypertension, like smoking, causes IUGR through uteroplacental insufficiency. This is likely to cause asymmetric IUGR rather than the symmetric IUGR demonstrated in this child.

    Answer D is incorrect. Maternal smoking affects fetal growth by causing a relative uteroplacental insufficiency. The fetal nutritional requirements exceed the placenta's ability to provide nutrients, especially later in pregnancy. Thus, smoking is more likely to cause asymmetric IUGR rather than symmetric IUGR.

    Answer E is incorrect. Singleton pregnancy has not been shown to be a risk factor for IUGR. Rather, multiple gestations can lead to IUGR through decreased relative amount of nutrients available to each fetus.

34. **The correct answer is F.** Pregnancy (intrauterine or ectopic) must always be ruled out in a woman of childbearing age with abnormal uterine bleeding. Ectopic pregnancy is a diagnosis that cannot be missed because it can result in maternal death, with shock secondary to tubal rupture. Although some patients with ec-

topic pregnancy present with hemodynamic instability, more than 50% of patients are asymptomatic before tubal rupture and do not have an identifiable risk factor for ectopic pregnancy. Patients may simply present with abnormal vaginal bleeding and abdominal pain.

Answer A is incorrect. Endometrial biopsy should be performed in all women older than 35 years who have abnormal uterine bleeding. Although not a common cause of abnormal uterine bleeding, endometrial carcinoma must always be ruled out in that age group. This patient is at a much lower risk for endometrial cancer given her age, and therefore an endometrial biopsy is inappropriate at this point.

Answer B is incorrect. The most common cause of vaginal bleeding in this patient's age group is anovulatory bleeding. The administration of a progesterone challenge is important in determining the etiology of anovulatory bleeding because a negative result indicates insufficient estrogen production, whereas a positive result indicates adequate endogenous estrogen production. However, urine or serum β-human chorionic gonadotropin is the first step in evaluating this patient to rule out pregnancy.

Answer C is incorrect. Coagulopathies are not a common cause of uterine bleeding but can be considered after other more frequent possibilities have been ruled out.

Answer D is incorrect. Hypothyroidism can cause heavy uterine bleeding and can be part of the workup; however, it is not the first step in the diagnostic evaluation of this patient.

Answer E is incorrect. Given the history of obesity, hirsutism, and irregular menses, polycystic ovary disease is high on the differential diagnosis. An ultrasound of the ovaries is therefore appropriate to evaluate for ovarian cysts; however, it is not the first step in evaluation of this patient because pregnancy should be ruled out first.

35. **The correct answer is C.** Carbamazepine is teratogenic, causing neural tube defects, fingernail hypoplasia, microcephaly, and intrauterine growth restriction. The presentation of neural tube defects (spina bifida and anen-

cephaly) varies based on the extent and location of the lesion. This child's lesion is consistent with a sacral meningocele. <u>Neural tube defects cause an elevated α-fetoprotein on triple screen.</u>

Answer A is incorrect. Anoxia secondary to maternal seizure is not teratogenic but may result in fetal demise, growth retardation, and brain damage.

Answer B is incorrect. Symptoms of fetal alcohol syndrome are facial abnormalities (macrognathia, thin upper lip, short palpebral fissure, epicanthal fold, and thin upper lip), poor growth (small head circumference, short length, and low weight), cardiac defects, minor joint and limb abnormalities, and developmental delay/mental retardation.

Answer D is incorrect. Trisomy 18, Edward's syndrome, classically presents with rocker-bottom feet, low-set ears, micrognathia, prominent occiput, clenched hands, and congenital heart disease. This syndrome causes a low maternal serum α-fetoprotein, low estriol, and low β-human chorionic gonadotropin on triple screen.

Answer E is incorrect. Trisomy 21, Down's syndrome, classically presents with a flat facial profile, prominent epicanthal folds, upslanting palpebral fissures, clinodactyly, simian crease, and congenital heart disease. On the triple screen, maternal serum (α-fetoprotein and estriol are low, while β-human chorionic gonadotropin is high.

36. **The correct answer is E.** Curve C represents an arrest of active phase that best fits the case presented here. It is defined as arrest of cervical dilation when a patient has entered the active phase of labor and is depicted as a flattening of the labor curve. Common causes include maternal factors (inadequate uterine contractions, small pelvic diameter, or abnormally shaped pelvis) and fetal factors (malposition and macrosomia).

Answer A is incorrect. Curve A represents a prolonged latent phase. An unripe cervix is not as easily softened and effaced. Thus, the presenting head may not progress despite adequate uterine contractions.

Answer B is incorrect. Curve A represents a prolonged latent phase. A primigravid patient is more likely to have a longer latent phase (average 6.4 hours, > 20 hours abnormal) than a multiparous woman (average 4.8 hours, > 14 hours abnormal).

Answer C is incorrect. Curve B represents a prolonged active phase. Inadequate uterine contraction is a common cause of a prolonged active phase, but in the case presented, there is an arrest, rather than a prolongation, of the active phase.

Answer D is incorrect. Curve B represents a prolonged active phase. A common cause of a prolonged active phase is excessive maternal sedation, not inadequate sedation.

Answer F is incorrect. Curve C represents an arrest of active phase. Occiput anterior is the ideal position of the fetus in vertex presentation and would not be a cause of arrest of the active phase.

37. **The correct answer is B.** Infertility can be caused by male or female factors. One-third of cases are exclusively due to female factors, 20% are exclusively due to male factors, and another 20% are due to a combination of female and male factors. Given this wife's unremarkable past medical history, female factors are less likely to be the cause of the couple's infertility. She has no symptoms of endometriosis, no history of pelvic inflammatory disease or sexually transmitted diseases, and appears to have properly functioning ovaries. Of the choices listed, a male factor is the most likely cause of this couple's infertility. The most common male factors include low semen volume, low sperm concentration, decreased sperm motility, and atypical sperm morphology.

Answer A is incorrect. Endometriosis is a common cause of female infertility, as a result of the pelvic adhesions that form from the ectopic endometrial tissue. However, this patient has none of the classic symptoms, such as severe dysmenorrhea and chronic pelvic pain that result from the adhesions. Hence, endometriosis is unlikely to be the cause of this couple's infertility.

Answer C is incorrect. Pelvic inflammatory disease (PID) is caused by ascending infection of the female genital tract, and is commonly associated with *Chlamydia trachomatis* and *Neisseria gonorrhoeae*. It is a common cause of female infertility secondary to tubal occlusion. However, this patient has neither a history of sexually transmitted diseases nor symptoms such as lower abdominal pain, vaginal discharge, low back pain, fever, nausea, and vomiting. As a result, PID is an unlikely cause of this couple's infertility.

Answer D is incorrect. A patient with premature ovarian failure would present with early amenorrhea (usually in her 30s) and premature symptoms of menopause. Given the regularity of this woman's cycles, premature ovarian failure is unlikely.

Answer E is incorrect. Intrauterine devices (IUDs) are associated with an increased risk of STDs, but there is no indication of prior STDs in this woman. IUDs are not associated with subsequent infertility in the absence of prior STD infection. This patient has no prior history of STDs or current symptoms, such as pelvic pain and abnormal vaginal discharge. STDs can lead to infertility as a result of tubal occlusion.

Questions 38–40

38. **The correct answer is A.** This is a classic presentation for abruptio placentae, which refers to the premature separation of an implanted placenta from the myometrium. Trauma commonly causes abruptio placentae, as rapid acceleration-deceleration can lead to shear stress between the placenta and uterus. There is a disruption of maternal vessels at the decidua basalis that leads to rapid accumulation of blood. The expanding hematoma causes dissection in a plane between the placenta and the uterus. Classic presentation includes painful dark vaginal bleeding, uterine contractions, and a nonreassuring fetal heart tracing.

39. **The correct answer is H.** Placenta previa refers to an abnormal location of placental implantation that lies either directly over or adjacent to the internal os of the cervix. Risk fac-

tors include grand multiparity and multiple previous cesarean sections. The classic presentation is painless vaginal bleeding beyond 24 weeks' gestation. Uterine contractions are typically absent. The bleeding typically stops and unless there is hemodynamic instability, the well being of the fetus will not be compromised. Transvaginal sonography is the gold standard for diagnosing placenta previa.

40. **The correct answer is I.** Onset of labor between 20 and 37 weeks' gestation is known as preterm labor. A diagnosis is made when there are regular contractions ($\geq$ 3 contractions every 30 minutes lasting 30 seconds each) with an associated cervical change assessed by sterile speculum examination. Patients typically present with abdominal, pelvic, and/or back discomfort; menstrual-like cramps; and a change in vaginal discharge or bleeding.

Answer B is incorrect. Ectopic pregnancy refers to implantation of a fertilized ovum in an area other than the endometrial lining of the uterus, most commonly the ampulla. It is highly unlikely that an ectopic pregnancy would survive and go unrecognized into the third trimester. All of the cases above are in the third trimester.

Answer C is incorrect. Breakthrough bleeding is not a relevant term to describe any of the situations above. This term is generally used to describe non-menses bleeding that occurs mid-cycle in a nonpregnant woman on oral contraceptive pills.

Answer D is incorrect. Though it is possible for women of these ages to have cervical carcinoma, it would not be a likely cause of the vaginal bleeding in the above cases.

Answer E is incorrect. Endometrial cancer would be a concern in a postmenopausal woman complaining of vaginal bleeding. It would not be a primary concern in a pregnant woman complaining of bleeding.

Answer F is incorrect. None of the cases reports any history of possible injury from a foreign body.

Answer G is incorrect. Normal menses is an incorrect answer in all of the above because all three women have confirmed pregnancies and therefore should not be menstruating.

Answer J is incorrect. Threatened abortion refers to vaginal bleeding with a closed os in pre-viable pregnancies. All of the above cases are at viability. At viability, what was once a "threatened abortion" now becomes "preterm labor."

Answer K is incorrect. Vulvar carcinoma is highly unlikely in the cases above. Vulvar carcinoma can generally be spotted on physical examination and no vulvar abnormalities were noted above. In addition, vulvar carcinoma in most commonly seen in postmenopausal women in their 50s and 60s.

CHAPTER 12

Gynecology

1. A woman brings her 15-year-old daughter to her pediatrician for concerns about hair growth. The child has always had a lot of body hair, and has been shaving her legs since she was 12, but recently the mother reports she has been noticing more hair, especially along the upper lip and on the chest and abdomen. The child is clearly distressed about her appearance. Further questioning reveals that although the young girl had her first menses at 11, her menstrual cycles are irregular, sometimes skipping cycles for months at a time. Physical examination reveals a young heavy-set olive-skinned teenager with moderate acne and dark hair growth along her upper lip, across her chest, and over her lower abdomen. What is the most appropriate treatment for this child's hirsutism?

(A) Danazol
(B) Insulin
(C) Levothyroxine
(D) Oral contraceptives
(E) Pergolide

2. An 18-year-old college student presents to the student health clinic with a complaint of copious yellow vaginal discharge. She has been sexually active with a new partner for the past month, but she is unsure if her partner is monogamous. A speculum examination reveals petechiae in the upper vagina and malodorous, yellow-green discharge. A potassium hydroxide preparation reveals no organisms, and a saline preparation reveals a motile protozoan. What is the most appropriate treatment?

(A) Treat her and her partner with oral fluconazole and test for other sexually transmitted diseases
(B) Treat her and her partner with oral metronidazole and test for other sexually transmitted diseases
(C) Treat her with oral fluconazole and test for other sexually transmitted diseases
(D) Treat her with oral metronidazole and test for other sexually transmitted diseases
(E) Treat her with vaginal fluconazole and test for other sexually transmitted diseases
(F) Treat her with vaginal metronidazole and test for other sexually transmitted diseases

3. A 28-year-old teacher presents to a primary care clinic complaining of 5 months of polyuria, polydipsia, and weight loss. Additionally, her menses, which have always been irregular and variable in amount, have stopped altogether. She is concerned because both her mother and maternal aunt suffer from non-insulin-dependent diabetes, and they told her they had similar symptoms before they were diagnosed. Upon questioning, she reveals that she is in a committed relationship, and has no desire to have children, so she uses barrier protection during intercourse. Physical examination reveals an obese woman, in no acute distress, with male-pattern hair distribution. Testing for β-human chorionic gonadotropin level, random blood sugar level, cholesterol panel, and a luteinizing hormone:follicle-stimulating hormone ratio suggests the patient has polycystic ovary syndrome. Although no one in her family has had cancer, she is concerned that her symptoms are a harbinger of cancer, or that she might be likely to suffer from cancer in the future. This diagnosis would most raise her risk for which kind of cancer?

(A) Cervical cancer
(B) Colon cancer
(C) Endometrial cancer
(D) Lung cancer
(E) Ovarian cancer

4. A 28-year-old G1A1 woman presents to a gynecology clinic with a chief complaint of reduced menstrual flow for the past 6 months, especially last month. She denies any pain with menstruation or irregularity in her cycle. She says that she had an elective termination by dilation and curettage approximately 9 months ago. She is sexually active with one partner and always uses condoms. Review of her records indicates a past history of abnormal Pap smears, but she has not been followed recently. She denies any history of irregular menses, and says that age of menarche was 13 years. She takes no medications. Physical examination reveals a normally developed 68-kg (150-lb) woman who is 183 cm (6 ft) tall. She is in no acute distress. A β-human chorionic gonadotropin test from her original

visit 1 week ago is negative. What is the most likely diagnosis?

(A) Asherman's syndrome
(B) Cervical stenosis
(C) Endometrial cancer
(D) Hypogonadotropic hypogonadism
(E) Pregnancy

5. A 38-year-old, G2P0, Spanish-speaking woman at 36 weeks' gestation is seen in the antepartum evaluation center with contractions and concerns that her water broke. Her nephew reports that roughly 20 years ago, while living in Nicaragua, she required an emergency cesarean section for unknown reasons. On examination, she appears in no acute distress. Her heart rate is 80/min, and her blood pressure is 110/60 mm Hg. Tocometry reveals uterine contractions lasting 30 seconds. An abdominal sonogram reveals a fetus that is of appropriate size for gestational age and is in vertex position. Fetal heart tracing is reassuring. What is the best next step in management?

(A) Administer tocolysis
(B) Augment with oxytocin
(C) Cesarean section
(D) Emergent cesarean section
(E) Manage expectantly and anticipate spontaneous vaginal delivery

6. A 42-year-old postmenopausal woman presents to the clinic complaining of vague abdominal pain, early satiety, and a 9-kg (20-lb) unintended weight loss. She has a history of normal Papanicolaou (Pap) smears. On physical examination, her abdomen is firm, with evidence of ascites with a firm, irregular, and fixed left adnexal mass palpated on vaginal examination. A CT scan of the abdomen and pelvis confirms the presence of an ovarian mass that has features that are highly suspicious for cancer. What is the best means to correctly diagnose and stage this mass?

(A) Cancer antigen-125 level
(B) α-Fetoprotein, β-human chorionic gonadotropin, and lactate dehydrogenase levels
(C) MRI of the abdomen and pelvis
(D) Percutaneous needle biopsy of the tumor for histopathologic staining

(E) Surgical exploration with tumor debulking and nodal sampling

7. A 42-year-old G1P0 woman at 18 weeks' gestation presents to the emergency obstetric evaluation center. She had an amniocentesis for genetic workup of the fetus 2 days ago without complication. She had noted loss of scant amounts of clear vaginal fluid since the procedure, but this morning she has noticed an increase in the amount of fluid leakage per vagina. She denies vaginal spotting or abdominal cramping or pressure. On examination, the patient is anxious; her temperature is 37.6°C (99.7°F), her heart rate is 90/min, and her blood pressure is 115/70 mm Hg. Sterile vaginal examination reveals clear fluid with alkaline pH leaking from the cervical os that increases with Valsalva maneuver and is pooling at the posterior fornix. She is nontender to palpation over the fundus and ultrasonography of the fetus is within normal limits. Which of the following should be tested for to prevent chorioamnionitis?

(A) *Escherichia coli*
(B) Group B streptococci
(C) *Helicobacter pylori*
(D) *Proteus mirabilis*
(E) *Staphylococcus aureus*

8. A 57-year-old G3P3 woman presents to her gynecologist with complaints of vaginal pruritus and increased vaginal discharge. The patient has no history of gynecologic surgery or sexually transmitted diseases; she is not currently sexually active. A bimanual examination and Pap smear are performed. The Pap smear is positive for malignant squamous cells. Follow-up colposcopy shows no cervical lesions, but a small lesion is noted on the lower vagina. Biopsy of this lesion confirms the diagnosis of vaginal squamous cell cancer, while cross-sectional imaging excludes invasion of surrounding tissues. What is the most appropriate course of treatment in this patient?

(A) Chemotherapy
(B) Radiation therapy
(C) Surgical excision
(D) Surgical excision and chemotherapy
(E) Surgical excision and radiation therapy

9. A 33-year-old G1P1 woman presents to her gynecologist for a Pap smear. It has been several years since a physician has last seen her. She is not currently sexually active, but takes oral contraceptives. Her vaginal examination is normal, but her Pap smear shows moderate-grade cervical intraepithelial neoplasia (CIN II), a precursor of cervical cancer. The patient undergoes colposcopy and biopsies taken at that time are confirmatory for CIN II. What is the appropriate management of this patient?

(A) Continued annual Pap smears
(B) Loop electrosurgical excision procedure
(C) Radiation therapy
(D) Serial colposcopies every 3–4 months
(E) Total abdominal hysterectomy

10. A 25-year-old G2P1 woman at 36 weeks' gestation presents to her obstetrician for a standard prenatal visit. She is experiencing occasional low back pain and fatigue. The low back pain is constant in nature, and does not feel like contractions. On physical examination, she is in no acute distress and is afebrile, with a pulse of 76/min, blood pressure of 120/80 mm Hg, and respiratory rate of 22/min. Fundal height is 34 cm. Pelvic examination reveals fluid in the vaginal canal. The patient comments that she noticed it, but wasn't worried because it wasn't bloody. She says she really is not sure if the fluid has any odor or not. She also denies any vaginal irritation. In addition to standard 32–36 week testing (chlamydia and gonorrhea cultures, repeat hematocrit, and Group B streptococcal screening), a nitrazine blue test is performed; results are positive. What conclusions may be drawn from this test?

(A) This patient has candidiasis
(B) This patient has placenta previa
(C) This patient has normal vaginal secretions
(D) This patient is in premature labor
(E) This patient may have premature rupture of membranes or bacterial vaginosis
(F) This patient's partner should be treated with antibiotics

11. A 48-year-old woman presents to her gynecologist for vaginal bleeding. She states that after a year of hot flashes and irregular cycles, she finally stopped menstruating 4 months ago. Two days ago, she began having some vaginal bleeding that was very similar to her prior menses. She is concerned because she heard that the first sign of endometrial cancer in postmenopausal women is vaginal bleeding. She is an otherwise healthy woman with no medical problems. She exercises three times a week and takes multivitamins. She had three children when she was between the ages of 29 and 35. She used oral contraceptive pills for contraception from the time she was 18 until she got married at the age of 28. What is the most appropriate next step in managing this woman's vaginal bleeding?

(A) Abdominal ultrasound
(B) Endometrial biopsy
(C) Follow-up examination in 6 months
(D) Luteinizing hormone and follicle-stimulating hormone serum levels
(E) Prescription of testosterone cream

12. A 19-year-old patient presents to her primary care physician with complaints of multiple fleshy growths around her vulva and vagina. She states that the growths are painless, and have developed within the past several months. She is not currently sexually active, but had been until 10 months ago with her previous boyfriend. She denies any vaginal pruritus or discharge, abdominal pain, fevers, dysuria, or vaginal bleeding. Physical examination of her genitalia reveals the lesions seen in the image. Which of the following is the most likely cause of these lesions?

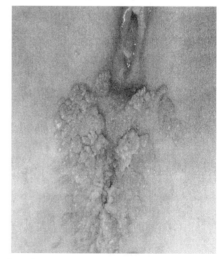

Reproduced, with permission, from Kasper DL, Braunwald E, Fauci AS, Hauser SL, Longo DL, Jameson LJ, Isselbacher KJ, eds. *Harrison's Online*. New York: McGraw-Hill, 2005: 1057.

(A) *Haemophilus ducreyi*
(B) Herpes simplex virus
(C) HIV
(D) Human papillomavirus
(E) *Treponema pallidum*

13. A 35-year-old G4P4 obese woman is referred to her gynecology clinic by her primary care physician for heavy menstruation and irregular cycles. She has noticed these symptoms for several months. She reports being a "late bloomer," with onset of menses at age 13 years. She is sexually active and monogamous with her partner of 2 years. She is on oral contraceptive pills and has a 5-year smoking history. An endometrial biopsy is read as "endometrial hyperplasia, cannot rule out intraepithelial carcinoma." Serum β-human chorionic gonadotropin is negative. Which of the following factors may have contributed to this abnormality?

(A) Body habitus
(B) Late menarche
(C) Multiparity
(D) Sexual activity
(E) Smoking history
(F) Use of oral contraceptive pills

14. A 25-year-old presents to her gynecologist complaining of irregular menstrual cycles. She states that they are irregular in length and frequency, and sometimes she misses cycles entirely. Her first menses was at age 11, but she has never had regular cycles. She has been married for 2 years and has been trying to become pregnant. Which is most likely to be used to diagnose polycystic ovary syndrome?

(A) An endometrial biopsy
(B) An exploratory laparotomy
(C) A transvaginal ultrasound
(D) Luteinizing hormone, follicle-stimulating hormone, and dehydroepiandrosterone levels
(E) Oral glucose tolerance test

15. A 65-year-old G2P2 postmenopausal woman presents to a gynecologist for the first time in many years complaining of symptoms of vaginal bleeding, pelvic pain, and increased urinary frequency. She reports that she is sexually active with her husband. After an appropriate work-up, a diagnosis of locally invasive squamous cell carcinoma of the cervix is made. The tumor has extended approximately 9 mm into the cervical stroma, grading the cancer as stage IB. The patient is informed of the diagnosis and wishes to undergo definitive therapy. What is the definitive therapy for this patient's disease?

(A) Chemotherapy
(B) Cold knife cone excision
(C) Loop electrosurgical excision procedure
(D) Radical hysterectomy
(E) Uterine artery embolization

16. A 35-year-old woman presents to the ED with nausea, vomiting, and abdominal distention. She has a history of pelvic inflammatory disease and is currently sexually active with her partner of the past 2 months. Her last menstrual period was 2 weeks ago. On examination she is febrile at 38.3°C (101.0°F), her heart rate is 110/min, and her blood pressure is 110/60 mm Hg. Abdominal examination reveals guarding and diffuse tenderness to palpation. Her abdomen is also tympanic to percussion in all four quadrants. Urine β-human chorionic gonadotropin is negative. An x-ray of the abdomen is taken and reveals large dilated and air-filled loops of small bowel with absence of air in the colon. Given the history and physical examination findings, what is the most likely etiology?

(A) Appendicitis
(B) Endometriosis
(C) Malignancy
(D) Peritonitis from ascending gynecologic infection
(E) Small bowel obstruction from adhesions

17. A 23-year-old, G0P0, African-American woman presents to her gynecologist for her annual examination. She has no significant gynecologic history, but her mother has a history of endometrial cancer. She is currently in a monogamous relationship with her boyfriend of 3 years. She denies any history of pregnancy, pelvic pain, sexually transmitted diseases, or excessive vaginal bleeding. On examination, her physician feels a firm, irregular mass. The gynecologist suspects that the patient has a uterine fibroid and confirms this diagnosis by transabdominal ultrasound. What is the underlying etiology of this uterine fibroid?

(A) Benign neoplastic growth of uterine endometrial cells
(B) Benign neoplastic growth of uterine myocytes
(C) Invasion of endometrial glandular cells into the myometrium
(D) Malignant neoplastic growth of uterine endometrial cells
(E) Malignant neoplastic growth of uterine myocytes

18. In an outpatient clinic, 500 patients suspected of human papillomavirus (HPV) infection are screened. One hundred patients are later proven to have the disease, while 400 patients are proven to be HPV-negative. The initial screening test is positive in 95 of the 100 HPV-infected patients and is negative in 380 of the 400 HPV-negative patients. What is the specificity of the screening test?

(A) 20%
(B) 83%
(C) 95%
(D) 99%
(E) 100%

19. A 52-year-old postmenopausal woman who was diagnosed with advanced ovarian cancer presents to the clinic to discuss her treatment options. She has had a CT of the abdomino-pelvic region that showed extensive disease extending from her left ovary and involving her uterus along with large pelvic nodes. What is the best treatment option for this disease?

(A) Chemotherapy and radiation therapy to the pelvis followed by surgery
(B) Extensive surgical tumor debulking followed by three to six courses of paclitaxel combined with cisplatin chemotherapy
(C) Radiation therapy to the abdomen and pelvis
(D) Three to six courses of paclitaxel combined with cisplatin and a repeat CT of the abdominopelvic region
(E) Tumor debulking only

20. A 55-year-old woman is brought to the emergency department (ED) by fire and rescue personnel because of intractable back and thigh pain for the past 3 hours. Upon presentation she says that the pain is 9 of 10 in severity and localized to her lower back. She lives with her sister, and she has no primary care physician. She denies any complaints aside from fatigue, which she attributes to her multiple jobs and caring for her sister's children. She has a pulse of 110/min, blood pressure of 140/88 mm Hg, respiratory rate of 20/min, and temperature of 37.8°C (100.1°F). On physical examination she is exquisitely tender over the L2–3 area of the spine. She also has point tenderness over the anterior right thigh. Sensation is intact over the lower extremities bilaterally and she has 5/5 strength in the lower extremities bilaterally. Breast examination shows a retracted nipple and dimpling of the right breast. What will likely represent the mainstay of treatment for this patient's symptoms?

(A) Bone marrow transplant
(B) Chemotherapy
(C) Hormone replacement therapy
(D) Radiation therapy
(E) Surgery

21. An 18-year-old college student presents to student health services with a complaint of a burning sensation while urinating and abdominal pain. She denies urinary urgency or increased frequency. She has no significant past medical history. She is currently sexually active with a new partner. She does not use barrier contraception. She denies any previous history of sexually transmitted diseases. On examina-

tion, she is afebrile, her heart rate is 70/min, and her blood pressure is 120/60 mm Hg. Examination reveals no peritoneal signs but there is tenderness to palpation over the suprapubic region. On pelvic examination, the cervix appears edematous and friable with a small amount of discharge from the os. A urine sample reveals numerous WBCs but no organisms on Gram stain. A cervical swab is sent for Gram stain and culture. What is the most likely explanation for these findings?

(A) *Chlamydia trachomatis* infection
(B) *Escherichia coli* infection
(C) Interstitial cystitis
(D) *Neisseria gonorrhoeae* infection
(E) *Proteus mirabilis* infection

22. A 25-year-old woman who is "about 5 months" pregnant with her first child presents for the first time to an obstetrician's office. She has had no prenatal care. When asked about her medical history, she states that she sometimes takes medicine for "depression," and she produces a prescription bottle with lithium tablets in it. She is otherwise healthy, and her pregnancy has been uncomplicated to date. The fundus of her uterus is 22 cm from the pubic symphysis, fetal movement is felt, and fetal heart tones are present at 130/min. Which of the following tests should be advised given the patient's lithium ingestion?

(A) Chorionic villus sampling
(B) Fetal echocardiography
(C) Fetal renal ultrasound
(D) α-Fetoprotein, β-human chorionic gonadotropin, and estriol levels
(E) Maternal oral glucose tolerance test

23. A 67-year-old postmenopausal woman presents to the clinic complaining of recurrent episodes of vaginal bleeding and pelvic discomfort. She denies a history of abnormal Pap smears. A diagnostic workup for this complaint reveals a moderately differentiated endometrial carcinoma invading more than one-half of the myometrium. Which of the following is the most important risk factor for developing endometrial cancer?

(A) Combined estrogen and progesterone therapy
(B) Human papillomavirus infection
(C) Hypothyroidism
(D) Multiparity
(E) Obesity

24. A 20-year-old woman presents to her gynecologist's office complaining of several days of vaginal itching and increased vaginal secretions that have an unpleasant odor. She denies any recent fever, back pain, hematuria, or vaginal bleeding. She has been sexually active with multiple sexual partners and rarely uses protection. On examination she has a moderate amount of frothy green discharge. Amine "whiff" test of the discharge is negative, and the pH of the discharge is 6. Multiflagellated organisms are seen on microscopy. What is the most likely diagnosis in this patient?

(A) Bacterial vaginosis
(B) *Neisseria gonorrhoeae* infection
(C) Syphilis
(D) Trichomoniasis vaginitis
(E) Vaginal candidiasis

25. A 24-year-old G0 woman presents to the ED of a local hospital stating that she was sexually assaulted. The patient is alone, and she is sobbing and is clearly anxious. She states that her last menstrual period was 3.5 weeks ago and asks the physician to please help her prevent a possible pregnancy from the assault. Physical examination is significant for bruised external labia and a .5-cm laceration in the vaginal vault. There is no vaginal discharge or cervical motion tenderness. After the appropriate psychological support is provided and a social worker is consulted, she is given one dose of 600 mg of mifepristone. Mifepristone contains which of the following?

(A) Estrogen and progestin
(B) High-dose estrogen only
(C) Progestin only
(D) Progesterone antagonist
(E) Prostaglandin

26. A 45-year-old African-American woman who had been diagnosed with polycystic ovary syndrome (PCOS) in her early 20s presents to her gynecologist for her annual visit. One of her close friends has recently been diagnosed with ovarian cancer, so she is concerned about her own cancer risk. Menarche was at age 14, and she has yet to go through menopause. She has a healthy 19-year-old daughter. She has no family history of cancer. She does not smoke or drink and exercises regularly. Aside from a diagnosis of PCOS, she is otherwise in good health. Given her health history, which of the following is true?

(A) She should have annual mammograms, although her risk of breast cancer is not changed relative to women without PCOS

(B) She should have annual mammograms because she has an increased risk of developing breast cancer relative to women without PCOS

(C) She should have annual Pap smears, although she has a decreased risk of developing cervical cancer relative to women without PCOS

(D) She should have annual Pap smears because she has an increased risk of developing cervical cancer relative to women without PCOS

(E) She should have annual Pap smears because she has an increased risk of developing ovarian cancer relative to women without PCOS

27. A 19-year-old patient presents to her gynecologist complaining of a painful genital rash. The patient states that approximately 1 week ago she had unprotected sexual intercourse with a new partner. She denies any vaginal pruritus or discharge, abdominal pain, fevers, dysuria, or vaginal bleeding. Physical examination of her genitalia reveals the lesions seen in the image. In addition to local care for the lesions, what is the most appropriate treatment for this condition?

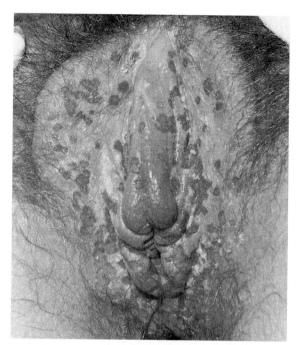

Reproduced, with permission, from Wolff K, Johnson RA, Surmond D. *Fitzpatrick's Color Atlas & Synopsis of Clinical Dermatology*, 5th ed. New York: McGraw-Hill, 2005: 900.

(A) Efavirenz
(B) Fluconazole
(C) Metronidazole
(D) Topical trichloroacetic acid
(E) Valacyclovir

EXTENDED MATCHING

Questions 28-30

For each of the following patients, select the most likely causes of urinary incontinence.

(A) Acute cystitis
(B) Acute urinary retention
(C) Neurogenic bladder
(D) Pelvic floor laxity
(E) Pyelonephritis
(F) Urethral fistulization
(G) Urethral sphincter insufficiency
(H) Urethral stricture

28. A 52-year-old woman presents to her gynecologist with a 2-month history of incontinence. She has been experiencing small amounts of urine leakage whenever her bladder is full. Urinalysis is negative for RBCs, WBCs, and bacteria. Her past medical history is significant for cervical cancer treated with surgery and radiation last year.

29. A 25-year-old female newlywed presents to the clinic with increased urgency and severe dysuria over the past day. Her physical examination is normal; blood pressure is 110/80 mm Hg, pulse is 100/min, temperature is 37.2°C (99.0°F), and respiratory rate is 16/min. Urinalysis reveals 50 WBCs/hpf, 50 RBCs/hpf, and moderate bacteriuria.

30. A 37-year-old G5P5 woman comes to her obstetrician for a routine visit. She complains about often leaking urine when she laughs or sneezes. Urinalysis is negative for RBCs and WBCs. Her past medical history is significant for breast cancer treated with radiation 3 years ago.

1. **The correct answer is D.** Given the history of irregular menses, acne, and excess weight, PCOS is the most likely cause of the patient's hirsutism. Oral contraceptive pills (OCPs) are the first-line therapy against hirsutism due to androgen excess, as seen in PCOS, as well as for unknown causes. In patients with PCOS, OCPs are also useful in establishing regular menstrual cycles.

Answer A is incorrect. Danazol is a synthetic androgen used to treat endometriosis. It would actually worsen the patient's hirsutism.

Answer B is incorrect. Many patients with PCOS are found to have high insulin levels, which are believed to stimulate androgen production in the ovaries, and are glucose intolerant. As a result, antiglycemic medications have been shown to alleviate some components of the syndrome, such as hirsutism.

Answer C is incorrect. Hypothyroidism is another cause of hirsutism. Patients would also present with weight gain, cold intolerance, and constipation. PCOS is the most likely diagnosis in this patient.

Answer E is incorrect. Hyperprolactinemia, most frequently caused by a pituitary adenoma, can present with hirsutism. Patients may also experience changes in vision, headaches, and galactorrhea. Pergolide is a dopamine agonist used to inhibit the release of prolactin. This patient's symptoms, however, are most consistent with PCOS, not a prolactinoma.

2. **The correct answer is B.** Typical signs and symptoms of *Trichomonas vaginalis* infection include a malodorous, green-yellow, frothy discharge, burning, pruritus, dysuria, frequency, dyspareunia, and punctate hemorrhages on the vagina/cervix. Metronidazole is the treatment for this infection. Oral treatment is preferred to vaginal treatment because it allows for therapeutic levels in the urethra and periurethral glands, which otherwise serve as a source for endogenous recurrence. This is a sexually transmitted disease (STD), so both she and her partner should be treated. Additionally, she

should be tested for other STDs because infection with one STD carries a higher risk of harboring another STD.

Answer A is incorrect. Oral fluconazole is used to treat fungal infections, including that of the mouth, throat, esophagus, lungs, and blood.

Answer C is incorrect. Oral fluconazole is used to treat fungal infections, including that of the mouth, throat, esophagus, lungs, and blood.

Answer D is incorrect. Treatment must also include treatment of the partner so the infection is not passed back and forth or to others.

Answer E is incorrect. Vaginal fluconazole is used to treat *Candida albicans* of the vagina, not *Trichomonas*.

Answer F is incorrect. Oral treatment is superior to vaginal treatment, so the urethra can be treated to prevent self-reinfection. Treatment must also include treatment of the partner and testing for other STDs.

3. **The correct answer is C.** Polycystic ovary syndrome (PCOS) is defined by the presence of infrequent menses and high blood levels of androgens. In addition, patients have high levels of circulating estrogens, partially due to chronic anovulation, and partially due to increased peripheral conversion of androgens to estrone due to concomitant obesity. Endometrial cancer risk is increased in the setting of unopposed estrogen exposure.

Answer A is incorrect. The risk for cervical cancer is increased for patients with multiple sexual partners, early start of sexual activity, immunocompromised status, smoking history, history of human papillomavirus infection, and history of other STDs.

Answer B is incorrect. There is no relationship between sex hormones and the development of colon cancer.

Answer D is incorrect. Lung cancer is the most common cause of cancer death in women, but it is not related to PCOS.

Answer E is incorrect. Risk factors for ovarian cancer are family history of ovarian or breast cancer, and chronic uninterrupted ovulation. The patient has no family history, and PCOS is characterized by chronic anovulation.

4. **The correct answer is A.** Asherman's syndrome is an etiology of secondary amenorrhea or hypomenorrhea characterized by the presence of intrauterine synechiae. It is usually caused by instrumentation of the uterine cavity, as is the case status–post dilation and curettage or an elective termination of pregnancy. Asherman's syndrome, although uncommon, is the most likely diagnosis given the patient's elective termination. Also, the other choices are unlikely given the patient's history. The diagnosis is confirmed by hysteroscopy.

Answer B is incorrect. Cervical stenosis is a cause of secondary amenorrhea. It may be due to congenital, inflammatory, or neoplastic causes, but the cause is usually surgical. Surgical operations such as electrocoagulation, cryotherapy, laser vaporization, conization, or cervical amputation are normally the culprits. Cervical stenosis can result in complete or partial obstruction of menstrual flow, causing amenorrhea or hypomenorrhea. It is usually diagnosed by pelvic ultrasound.

Answer C is incorrect. Endometrial cancer usually presents in older women as postmenopausal vaginal bleeding.

Answer D is incorrect. Hypogonadotropic hypogonadism is a cause of hypomenorrhea and is common in anorexic patients, athletes who train excessively, and in genetic disorders such as Kallman's syndrome. This patient's history does not suggest any of these causes.

Answer E is incorrect. Pregnancy should always be considered in cases of reduced or absent menstrual flow, but it is unlikely in the presence of a negative β-human chorionic gonadotropin test.

5. **The correct answer is C.** Vaginal birth after cesarean involving a classic, midline incision is an indication for subsequent cesarean section because the risk of uterine rupture is high. Low transverse incisions are not an indication for subsequent cesarean, and a vaginal delivery may be attempted safely. In this case, there is not enough information to proceed safely with a vaginal delivery. The cesarean section was emergent and is thus more likely to have involved a midline incision.

Answer A is incorrect. The only indication for administering tocolysis is when inhibiting uterine contractions in preterm labor will allow time for the administration of corticosteroids to promote fetal lung maturity and to decrease neonatal morbidity and mortality.

Answer B is incorrect. There is no indication for augmenting uterine contractions with oxytocin. Augmentation should only be used when there is a prolonged labor and the patient is failing to proceed through the normal stages of labor as a direct result of weak uterine contractions.

Answer D is incorrect. There are no signs of fetal or maternal distress. With no indication for emergent surgery, the preparation of the cesarean section can proceed at a normal pace.

Answer E is incorrect. Vaginal birth after cesarean is not safe if it is likely that the cesarean section involved a midline incision.

6. **The correct answer is E.** To properly stage an ovarian mass that is highly suspicious for cancer, a full exploration and inspection of all pelvic structures is required. There is no noninvasive means to consistently diagnose and stage ovarian cancer. Removal of the primary mass with histopathologic staining is required, and retroperitoneal exploration with pelvic and para-aortic nodal sampling is performed.

Answer A is incorrect. A workup for ovarian cancer should include a cancer antigen-125 (CA-125) level because certain cancers can present with an elevated level. In such instances, response to chemotherapy can be monitored by the drop in CA-125. However, cancers other than ovarian cancer may elevate the CA-125 level (e.g., endometrial cancer and certain pancreatic cancers). Benign conditions, such as endometriosis, uterine leiomyoma, and pelvic inflammatory disease, can elevate the level as well.

Answer B is incorrect. Elevated α-fetoprotein, β-human chorionic gonadotropin, and lactate dehydrogenase levels are associated with primary germ cell cancers. Measurements of these levels are performed in cases in which a firm fixed adnexal mass is palpated in a premenarchal or adolescent patient because primary germ cell cancers are more prevalent in this age group.

Answer C is incorrect. Although an MRI will show the ovarian mass and nodes that are involved, MRI images will not distinguish the type of ovarian cancer. Tissue from the mass and nodes is required to diagnose and fully stage the progression of cancer.

Answer D is incorrect. Although a needle biopsy will provide tissue to diagnose the mass, deep pelvic nodes, which are required to properly stage the spread of disease, are not reached by percutaneous needle biopsy.

7. **The correct answer is B.** Chorioamnionitis is an infection of the placental tissue and amniotic fluid. It affects about 1% of all pregnancies, increasing to 7–10% of those with preterm premature rupture of membranes, which allows ample time for vaginal organisms to move upward into the uterus. Chorioamnionitis is a potential complication of amniocentesis and can cause bacteremia in the mother and can lead to preterm birth and serious infection in the newborn. Signs of chorioamnionitis include maternal fever, fetal and maternal tachycardia, uterine tenderness, and malodorous vaginal discharge. The organisms usually responsible for chorioamnionitis are those that are normally present in the vagina, including *Escherichia coli* and Group B streptococci (GBS). GBS should be tested for and treated with antibiotics.

Answer A is incorrect. *Escherichia coli* can be a causative agent in chorioamnionitis, but is not as easily tested for since it is part of normal fecal flora.

Answer C is incorrect. *Helicobacter pylori* is the causative agent in peptic ulcer disease and plays no role in chorioamnionitis.

Answer D is incorrect. *Proteus mirabilis* is a gram-negative, facultatively anaerobic bacterium commonly implicated in urinary tract infections, not chorioamnionitis. *Proteus* infection is usually found in those with structural abnormalities of the urinary tract or those with ureteral instrumentation such as catheters, as well as nosocomial infections. *Proteus* raises urine pH and can be detected with urine Gram stain.

Answer E is incorrect. *Staphylococcus aureus* is the causative agent in toxic shock syndrome, food poisoning, and scalded skin syndrome. It is not a common pathogen causing chorioamnionitis.

8. **The correct answer is B.** Small squamous cell vaginal cancers in the upper portion of the vagina are often treated by surgical excision, which consists of radical hysterectomy, upper vaginectomy, and bilateral lymph node dissection. However, resection of malignancies in the lower portion of the vagina is difficult, and the primary treatment is radiation therapy. Early-stage cancers may be treated solely with brachytherapy, but more advanced cancers are treated with external beam radiation.

Answer A is incorrect. Several chemotherapeutic agents have been studied for use in advanced vaginal cancer, but none have been found to initiate a significant therapeutic response. Some experts advocate the use of chemotherapy in addition to radiation therapy, although randomized controlled trials investigating this issue did not find compelling evidence to support this position.

Answer C is incorrect. Surgical resection of cancer in the lower vagina is difficult, and the primary modality of treatment is radiation therapy.

Answer D is incorrect. Lower vaginal cancers are not amenable to surgical resection, and chemotherapeutic agents are of limited use in the treatment of vaginal cancer.

Answer E is incorrect. The technical difficulty of resection of lower vaginal cancers precludes surgical treatment for this disease.

9. **The correct answer is B.** Dysplastic cervical intraepithelial neoplasia (CIN II) cells most often will undergo malignant transformation if

not treated. The mean time to malignant transformation is 4 years for CIN II, but occasionally can be much quicker. While CIN I lesions can be monitored with colposcopy every 3–4 months, the standard of care for CIN II and III lesions is local excision by a loop electrosurgical excision procedure. This procedure can often be performed in the gynecologist's office.

Answer A is incorrect. Dysplastic CIN II cells most often will undergo malignant transformation if not treated, so these premalignant lesions need to be removed. Continued monitoring with annual Pap smears is insufficient management of a patient with these lesions.

Answer C is incorrect. Radiation therapy may be used to treat cervical cancer once it has invaded > 5 cm into the cervix, and is the only effective therapy for cancer that extends into the parametria. Again, radiation therapy is damaging to local tissue and is an excessively morbid treatment for a condition such as CIN II that can be sufficiently treated with local excision.

Answer D is incorrect. Serial monitoring with colposcopy every 3–4 months is appropriate treatment for mild cervical dysplasia (cervical intraepithelial neoplasia, CIN I). However, for moderate to severe dysplasia (CIN II to III), malignant transformation may occur rapidly, making local excision of the dysplastic tissue necessary.

Answer E is incorrect. Since CIN II is a premalignant lesion which has not yet spread beyond the cervical epithelium, local excision is adequate treatment. Total abdominal hysterectomy is reserved for treatment of cervical cancer that has invaded > 5 mm into the cervix, but which has not yet extended to the pelvic wall. Treatment of CIN II with hysterectomy would be excessively morbid without providing any additional benefits over treatment with loop electrosurgical excision.

10. **The correct answer is E.** This patient's presentation is consistent with both premature rupture of membranes and BV, given only the positive nitrazine paper test. Nitrazine tests nonspecifically for alkaline vaginal fluid, which may be amniotic fluid or the alkaline vaginal secretions associated with BV. At this point, no definite conclusion may be drawn. Further tests would include a wet mount in which case clue cells, or epithelial cells studded with bacteria, would be indicative of BV and evidence of ferning would suggest premature rupture of membranes. Although BV is normally associated with a foul odor, it is also notable for a lack of vaginal irritation, unlike other vaginoses.

Answer A is incorrect. Candidiasis usually presents with a white, cottage cheese–like discharge that is generally acidic in nature. Although it is common in pregnant patients, candidiasis is unlikely in the setting of no vaginal irritation.

Answer B is incorrect. Placenta previa usually presents with painless vaginal bleeding, which the patient specifically denies.

Answer C is incorrect. Vaginal secretions in pregnancy are normally thick acidic secretions.

Answer D is incorrect. Premature labor is defined as the onset of labor between 20 and 37 weeks' gestation. The diagnosis of labor requires regular uterine contractions with cervical change. This patient has no indication of cervical change on vaginal examination and a complaint of only nonspecific back pain.

Answer F is incorrect. The patient may have BV as indicated by the positive nitrazine blue test. BV is a type of vaginitis associated with an imbalance in the normal vaginal flora; however, it is not an STD. Treatment of sexual partners does not prevent recurrence of BV.

11. **The correct answer is C.** Perimenopause is the period prior to the cessation of menses; it commonly occurs up to 2 years prior to the onset of menopause. Menopause is defined as amenorrhea for 1 year's duration. This woman presents with symptoms of perimenopause (hot flashes and menstrual irregularities) of 1 year, and amenorrhea for 4 months. Because she has not had amenorrhea for a full year, she is still considered to be perimenopausal, and this episode of bleeding likely represents an anovulatory menstrual cycle. She should continue to monitor her vaginal bleeding and can be offered medications to lessen her symptoms (i.e., oral contraceptive pill).

Answer A is incorrect. An abdominal ultrasound could be used to visualize the uterine cavity and would likely reveal a thickened endometrium in a menstruating woman. It would not be helpful in ruling out endometrial cancer. This would require a biopsy.

Answer B is incorrect. Nulliparity and unopposed estrogenic states are associated with increased risk of endometrial cancer, neither of which applies to this woman. Indeed, 10 years on the oral contraceptive pill places this woman at a lower risk for endometrial cancer. However, to rule out endometrial cancer, the second most common cancer of the female genital tract, an endometrial biopsy is the standard of care if vaginal bleeding occurs more than 1 year after amenorrhea in a postmenopausal woman.

Answer D is incorrect. Because this woman is perimenopausal, luteinizing hormone and follicle-stimulating hormone levels are likely to be high and would not provide any further specific information.

Answer E is incorrect. In menopausal women, vaginal atrophy is a common cause of vaginal bleeding, which can be treated with topical estrogen or testosterone creams. However, substantial bleeding is less likely to result from vaginal atrophy than from an endometrial source.

12. **The correct answer is D.** This history and image are consistent with condyloma acuminata, commonly known as genital warts. These lesions are painless, raised, and irregular in shape. The causative organism of these lesions is the human papillomavirus (HPV), a DNA virus, a non-oncogenic strain. HPV is spread through direct skin-to-skin contact during sexual intercourse. Lesions often appear after a 6- to 12-week incubation period. Certain high-risk strains of HPV (strains 16, 18, 45, and 56) are associated with an increased incidence of cervical cancer.

Answer A is incorrect. *Haemophilus ducreyi* is the causative organism of chancroid. Chancroid lesions are irregular, erythematous lesions that have bloody or purulent secretions. These lesions arise 2–6 days after sexual con-

tact, are quite painful, and are often associated with enlarged tender lymph nodes. Treatment with a single dose of azithromycin is often curative.

Answer B is incorrect. Herpes simplex virus leads to painful vesicular lesions that often arise within days of sexual intercourse. The lesions are flat and regular, and last for 1–2 weeks. These lesions would be inconsistent with the given history and examination.

Answer C is incorrect. HIV is the organism that causes the acquired immunodeficiency syndrome. While it places a woman at a higher risk for getting HPV, it does not cause genital warts.

Answer E is incorrect. *Treponema pallidum* is the infectious agent that causes syphilis. In primary syphilis the lesion is a chancre that appears 10–60 days after disease transmission. This lesion is painless, with indurated edges and a punched out center. Six to eight weeks later secondary syphilis may develop, with constitutional symptoms and a maculopapular rash that often occurs on the hands and feet. At this time condyloma lata may form, which have a regular, round, and flat appearance that differentiates them from condyloma acuminata.

13. **The correct answer is A.** A mechanism of endometrial carcinoma and hyperplasia is abnormal proliferation of glandular elements of the endometrium under the direction of high levels of unopposed estrogen. Obesity leads to a state of high levels of estrone from the aromatization of androstenedione in peripheral fat. Other sources of estrogen include endogenous sources such as hypersecretion from the ovaries and exogenous sources such as medications.

Answer B is incorrect. Late menarche is protective while early menarche is a risk factor for endometrial hyperplasia/carcinoma, as more cycles of unopposed high estrogen increase risk.

Answer C is incorrect. Multiparity is protective, as the endometrium is not exposed to as many cycles of endometrial proliferation, while nulliparity is a risk factor.

Answer D is incorrect. Sexual activity is not known to be a risk factor for endometrial carcinoma/hyperplasia.

Answer E is incorrect. Smoking has been found to be protective in large retrospective studies. It is thought to stimulate hepatic metabolism of circulating estrogens. At the very least, it has not been found to be a risk factor.

Answer F is incorrect. Use of oral contraceptive pills has been found to be protective for endometrial carcinoma/hyperplasia due to the content of progestins in most formulations. It is proliferation of the endometrial elements under the direction of unopposed estrogen that increases risk.

14. **The correct answer is D.** A history of irregular cycles, early menarche, and infertility is highly suggestive of PCOS. It is the most common cause of anovulatory infertility in women of childbearing age. Patients have increased levels of androgens and may also present with acne, hirsutism, and weight gain. A luteinizing hormone:follicle-stimulating hormone ratio of > 3 and increased levels of dehydroepiandrosterone are consistent with a diagnosis of PCOS. Patients can be treated with adequate glucose control, and if desired, reproductive therapy.

Answer A is incorrect. An endometrial biopsy would be useful to determine if the endometrial stroma was responding to the luteal phase hormones, which can be deregulated in cases of infertility, but would not be useful in diagnosing PCOS. This is known as luteal phase defect infertility.

Answer B is incorrect. Endometriosis is the growth of uterine cells outside of the uterus. In addition to irregular bleeding or infertility, patients very commonly also present with severe pelvic pain before and during menses. An exploratory laparotomy is diagnostic for endometriosis, and therefore would not be helpful in diagnosing polycystic ovarian syndrome.

Answer C is incorrect. Although a large majority of women with PCOS do have multiple ovarian cysts, the appearance of the ovaries varies with the menstrual cycle, therefore ultrasound has a poor predictive value.

Answer E is incorrect. A significant number of women with PCOS have comorbid diabetes; however, an abnormal oral glucose tolerance test is not specific for PCOS (it is also seen in diabetes).

15. **The correct answer is D.** Patients with localized cervical cancer, such as this patient, may be treated with radical hysterectomy or radiation therapy plus chemotherapy. Both treatments have similar 5-year survival and complication rates. Patients undergoing surgery may retain ovarian function and have lower rates of vaginal stenosis. More advanced disease or bulky early disease is preferentially treated with radiation therapy and adjuvant chemotherapy.

Answer A is incorrect. Chemotherapy has been found to significantly increase the survival rate of women when used as an adjuvant to radiation therapy. Chemotherapy is also used as palliative therapy in women with recurrent or advanced disease that cannot be treated locally. However, chemotherapy alone is not used as a curative therapy for cervical cancer.

Answer B is incorrect. Cold knife cone excision is most often used to treat patients who have category II or III CIN, a precursor of cervical cancer. For this indication it has mainly been replaced by the loop electrosurgical excision procedure. It may also be used as definitive treatment for young women with malignant invasion < 3 mm into the cervix and who wish to preserve their fertility.

Answer C is incorrect. Loop electrosurgical excision procedure is used to excise CIN II or III. It is not used for resection of malignant lesions.

Answer E is incorrect. Uterine artery embolization is a procedure performed by interventional radiologists to treat uterine fibroids. These metaplastic tumors are primarily fed by the uterine artery, and embolization of their vascular supply often results in reduction of bulk symptoms and menorrhagia. It is not used to treat malignant cervical cancer.

16. **The correct answer is E.** The history, physical examination, and radiographic findings are all

highly suggestive of a bowel obstruction. In patients who experience pelvic inflammatory disease (PID), this inflammation will often lead to scar, or adhesion, formation that can affect both pelvic and abdominal processes in the future. These adhesions can lead to pelvic pain, infertility, ectopic pregnancies, and other complications. Given the history of previous PID, bowel adhesions are most likely the cause of mechanical small bowel obstruction.

Answer A is incorrect. Appendicitis does not cause small bowel obstruction.

Answer B is incorrect. Endometriosis can lead to abdominal pain occurring with menses, dysmenorrhea, abnormal uterine bleeding, dyspareunia, and infertility. Only very rarely does it cause small bowel obstruction.

Answer C is incorrect. While malignancy can cause mechanical small bowel obstruction, it is very rare in an otherwise healthy young patient.

Answer D is incorrect. Peritonitis only explains the fever and the nausea, vomiting, and abdominal tenderness. It does not explain the radiographic data.

17. **The correct answer is B.** The etiology of uterine fibroids (leiomyomas) is not fully understood, but they are believed to result from neoplastic growth of abnormal myocytes within the uterus. Leiomyomas are believed to have no malignant potential. Fibroids typically occur during childbearing age and are usually asymptomatic, requiring no treatment. However, some women suffer from heavy uterine bleeding, pain, bulk symptoms such as increased urinary frequency or pelvic pressure, and occasionally infertility.

Answer A is incorrect. Leiomyomas derive from the smooth muscle cells of the myometrium rather than the endometrium.

Answer C is incorrect. The abnormal invasion of endometrial glands into the myometrium is called adenomyosis. The surrounding myometrium undergoes hypertrophy and hyperplasia as a reaction to this invasion. Up to 60% of women who have adenomyosis also have uterine fibroids. The symptoms of

this disease include dysmenorrhea and menorrhagia, and if severe may be treated with a hysterectomy.

Answer D is incorrect. Leiomyomas derive from the smooth muscle cells of the myometrium rather than the endometrium. Additionally, leiomyomas are benign tumors.

Answer E is incorrect. Leiomyomas are benign neoplastic growths of smooth muscle myocytes from a single cell line. They are not locally invasive, do not metastasize, and are therefore not considered to be malignant.

18. **The correct answer is C.** Specificity is defined as the proportion of disease-free persons appropriately classified by the screening test as negative. To calculate specificity, the following formula is used: TN/(FP + TN). True-negative (TN) persons are disease-free persons who are correctly classified as negative, FP (false positive) refers to disease-free persons who are misclassified as positive. FP can be calculated by understanding that if 380 patients out of 400 disease-free patients were correctly classified as negative, then there were 20 false positives. Specificity can be calculated in the case given as follows: TN/(FP + TN) = 380/(20 + 380) = 95%.

Answer A is incorrect. Twenty percent would be the prevalence of the disease in this population at this time. Prevalence is number of cases disease/total population = 100/500 = 20%.

Answer B is incorrect. Eighty-three percent is the positive predictive value (PPV) of the test. PPV is calculated by the following formula: TP/(TP + FP) = 95/(95 + 20) = 83%.

Answer D is incorrect. Ninety-nine percent is the negative predictive value (NPV) of the test. NPV is calculated by the following formula: TN/(TN + FN) = 380/(380 + 5) = 99%.

Answer E is incorrect. This is the percentage of all people who were screened for HPV infection.

19. **The correct answer is B.** Tumor debulking is indicated for any stage of ovarian cancer because chemotherapy is more effective when the tumor masses are each < 1 cm in diameter.

Combined paclitaxel and cisplatin is the chemotherapy of choice for ovarian cancer.

Answer A is incorrect. Optimal treatment for advanced ovarian cancer is tumor debulking followed by chemotherapy. Although neoadjuvant chemotherapy can be used in patients in whom surgery is considered excessively risky, it is not considered standard of care. More research is needed to elucidate the optimal use of neoadjuvant chemotherapy.

Answer C is incorrect. Because advanced ovarian cancer often has peritoneal seeding and extensive volume of tumor, radiation is ineffective as the primary mode of treatment.

Answer D is incorrect. Chemotherapy is less effective when the tumors are > 1 cm in diameter, and reducing the tumor size by debulking allows for more effective chemotherapy.

Answer E is incorrect. Tumor debulking alone is not curative or effective since debulking alone will most likely leave residual disease or tumors that were too small to be visualized during intra-abdominal exploration. Some forms of early resected ovarian cancer are treated with surgery followed only by observation. However, this patient has advanced disease, and thus chemotherapy is required.

20. **The correct answer is B.** This patient likely has metastatic breast carcinoma. The finding of a retracted nipple and dimpling of the breast in a woman with no regular health care is highly suggestive of breast carcinoma. The complaint of bone pain in a patient likely to have breast cancer is an ominous one and likely represents metastases to bone. Chemotherapy is the treatment modality of choice for symptoms in metastatic disease.

Answer A is incorrect. Bone marrow transplant is not part of the standard treatment for breast cancer.

Answer C is incorrect. Hormone replacement therapy is contraindicated in patients with a diagnosis of breast cancer.

Answer D is incorrect. Radiation therapy is used as adjuvant therapy in breast cancer, either status–post local excision for large tumors or status–post lumpectomy with axillary node

dissection. This patient's tumor burden is likely to be inoperable.

Answer E is incorrect. Surgery is the mainstay of treatment for patients with small tumors.

21. **The correct answer is A.** *Chlamydia trachomatis* is an obligate intracellular organism and is one of the most common sexually transmitted organisms, causing urethritis, mucopurulent cervicitis, and late postpartum endometritis. Chlamydial infections are often asymptomatic, but may also present with signs of a urinary tract infection (nongonococcal urethritis) including dysuria and pyuria, but without any organisms visible on Gram stain of a sterile urine sample. Direct fluorescent antibody tests and DNA detection tests using polymerase chain reaction are highly sensitive and specific. Treatment consists of oral erythromycin, amoxicillin, or azithromycin. Because gonorrhea often coexists with chlamydia, therapy with an intramuscular injection of ceftriaxone is also indicated.

Answer B is incorrect. *Escherichia coli* is responsible for more than 90% of all uncomplicated urinary tract infections in women, which occur primarily via periurethral contamination during sexual intercourse or via contamination due to the proximity of the anus to the urethra. Symptoms include urinary frequency, urgency, dysuria, and low-grade fever. Gram stain reveals gram-negative bacilli.

Answer C is incorrect. Interstitial cystitis is a condition that results in recurring discomfort or pain in the bladder and the surrounding pelvic region. Symptoms are characterized by urinary urgency and increased frequency, but not commonly dysuria. Although some symptoms of interstitial cystitis resemble those of a bacterial infection, Gram stain or culture of the urine reveals no organisms. This condition is one diagnosed primarily by exclusion.

Answer D is incorrect. *Neisseria gonorrhoeae* can cause inflammation of mucous membranes including the urethra, but is more likely to be asymptomatic or minimally symptomatic. Gonococcal infection primarily manifests as male urethritis and female endocervicitis. In the female, the discharge is usually described as thin, purulent, and mildly odorous. It is an organism that would be detected on urine Gram stain, showing 5 or more WBCs per oil-immersion field with intracellular gram-negative diplococci within leukocytes.

Answer E is incorrect. *Proteus mirabilis* is a gram-negative, facultatively anaerobic bacterium commonly implicated in urinary tract infections. However, *Proteus* infection is usually found in those with structural abnormalities of the urinary tract, and those with ureteral instrumentation such as catheters, as well as those with nosocomial infections. *Proteus* raises urine pH and can be detected with urine Gram stain.

22. **The correct answer is B.** Lithium ingestion is associated with Ebstein's anomaly of the heart, which is downward displacement of the tricuspid valve resulting in tricuspid regurgitation. Fetal echocardiography can be used to visualize tricuspid regurgitation.

Answer A is incorrect. Chorionic villus sampling directly allows for evaluation of the chromosomal composition of the fetus. Lithium is not associated with fetal chromosomal abnormalities.

Answer C is incorrect. Angiotensin-converting enzyme inhibitors, not lithium, are associated with fetal renal malformations.

Answer D is incorrect. When abnormal, α-fetoprotein, β-human chorionic gonadotropin, and estriol levels, commonly known as the 'triple screen,' may be indicative of neural tube defects and chromosomal abnormalities (trisomy 13, 18, or 21) but would not be influenced by heart defects seen with lithium.

Answer E is incorrect. A maternal oral glucose tolerance test is used to test for maternal diabetes, which is not a sequela of lithium use. Testing pregnant women for diabetes is important, however, because untreated diabetes can lead to preeclampsia, macrosomia in the infant, and birth injury to both infant (brachial plexus) and mother (lacerations).

23. **The correct answer is E.** Obese patients are 3–10 times more likely to develop endometrial cancer. It is believed that the excess adipose tissue leads to increased aromatization of adrenally produced androstenedione, leading to unopposed circulating estrogen.

Answer A is incorrect. Patients on prolonged estrogen therapy with unopposed progesterone are four to eight times more likely to develop endometrial cancer. The unopposed estrogen leads to chronic endometrial proliferation and hyperplasia. This chronic hyperplasia can lead to the development of an endometrial carcinoma. The presence of progesterone prevents estrogen from inducing endometrial hyperplasia, the precursor of endometrial cancer.

Answer B is incorrect. Although HPV can predispose to genital warts and cervical cancer, it has not been linked to endometrial cancer.

Answer C is incorrect. Although hypothyroidism shows no association with endometrial cancer, patients with another endocrine disorder, diabetes, are three times more likely to develop endometrial cancer. Because diabetics are more likely to be overweight than nondiabetics, it is postulated that it is the associated obesity that leads to the increased risk for developing endometrial cancer.

Answer D is incorrect. Nulliparous, not multiparous, women are two to three times more likely to develop endometrial cancer. This is likely due to the fact that many of these women have chronic anovulation. This chronic anovulation leads to a lack of progesterone production. As a result, it is believed that there is a greater likelihood of estrogen, produced from aromatization of adrenally produced androstenedione, to be unopposed by progesterone.

24. **The correct answer is D.** *Trichomonas vaginalis* is a protozoan with multiple flagella that causes a sexually transmitted vaginitis. Most commonly occurring symptoms include increased vaginal discharge with an unpleasant odor, dysuria, and vaginal pruritus. Infection with *Trichomonas* causes an increase in vaginal pH to > 4.5 (normal vaginal pH is 3.8–4.2). Treatment with a single dose of 2 g of metronidazole is effective. The symptoms, increased vaginal pH, and flagellated organisms seen on wet mount establish the diagnosis.

Answer A is incorrect. Bacterial vaginosis (BV) is caused by an imbalance in vaginal flora, with reduced numbers of lactobacilli and increased proportions of bacteria such as *Gardnerella*, *Mobiluncus*, or *Peptostreptococcus* species. Signs of BV include a thin, white vaginal discharge, vaginal pH > 4.5, fishy odor on 10% potassium hydroxide "whiff" test, and clue cells on saline mount microscopy. Flagellated organisms would not be seen in BV.

Answer B is incorrect. Patients suffering from *Neisseria gonorrhoeae* cervicitis often complain of vaginal pruritus and discharge. However, up to 50% of patients may not manifest any symptoms at all. Diagnosis is established by identification of N. *gonorrhoeae* on chocolate agar culture or by DNA probe testing. The potassium hydroxide "whiff" test would be negative and no flagellated organisms would be seen.

Answer C is incorrect. The first manifestation of syphilis, caused by infection with *Treponema pallidum*, is a painless primary chancre sore that appears 10–60 days after the infecting sexual contact. Several weeks later, symptoms of secondary syphilis can occur, which include constitutional symptoms, a maculopapular rash on the hands and feet, and flat, broad condyloma lata. Vaginal symptoms do not result from syphilis, and flagellated organisms would not be seen. *Treponema* obtained from syphilitic lesions can be visualized with darkfield microscopy.

Answer E is incorrect. Patients with candidiasis often complain of a thick vaginal discharge, vaginal pruritus, or dysuria. Signs of candidiasis include vaginal pH in the range of 4–5, and budding hyphae or spores when examined on a slide treated with 10% potassium hydroxide preparation, which lyses the cells in the sample and makes the yeast easier to visualize. Clue cells are not seen in candidiasis.

25. **The correct answer is D.** Mifepristone is an antiprogestin that has been shown to be 100% effective at preventing pregnancy when given within 72 hours of intercourse at a one-time dose of 600 mg. Recent studies, however, have demonstrated equal efficacy of use of a 10-mg dose of this drug, intended to minimize the side-effect profile and decrease disturbances of the subsequent menstrual cycle. The high efficacy of mifepristone compared to other regimens is likely secondary to its ability to inhibit implantation as well as ovulation.

Answer A is incorrect. The Yuzpe regimen, which includes two doses of both estrogen and progestin pills taken 12 hours apart, was the first available emergency contraceptive. Due to the significant nausea and vomiting associated with their administration, these medications are disfavored. Progestin-only pills such as levonorgestrel, or antiprogestins such as mifepristone, are commonly used.

Answer B is incorrect. High-dose estrogen-only pills are equally effective when compared with the progestin-only preparation. Most clinicians, however, prefer the latter, as the progestin-only pills are administered in one day as compared with the high-dose estrogen-only pills, which require five consecutive days of medication.

Answer C is incorrect. Progestin-only pills such as levonorgestrel are given in two doses 12 hours apart, within 72 hours of unprotected intercourse. They are highly effective and have a side-effect profile that is much better tolerated than the estrogen and progestin preparations (the Yuzpe regimen). Data from multiple comparative studies show that mifepristone is as effective as levonorgestrel in preventing pregnancy.

Answer E is incorrect. Prostaglandins, particularly prostaglandin E_2, stimulate contraction of uterine smooth muscle and are thus used as abortifacients. They do not have a role in emergency contraception.

26. **The correct answer is B.** PCOS is associated with an increased risk of breast and endometrial cancer secondary to unopposed estrogen secretion. It is a syndrome, not a disease, and may present with hirsutism, menstrual abnormalities, obesity, acanthosis nigricans, and precocious puberty. It is later associated with an increased risk of infertility, metabolic syndrome, and type 2 diabetes mellitus.

Answer A is incorrect. Women with PCOS have an increased risk of breast and endometrial cancer secondary to unopposed estrogen secretion.

Answer E is incorrect. Risk factors associated with ovarian cancer include nulliparity, positive family history, early age of menarche or late age of menopause, and being of white race. Furthermore, Papanicolaou (Pap) smears do not detect ovarian cancer.

27. **The correct answer is E.** The painful vesicular nature of her lesions and the short incubation time between exposure and symptoms indicate that this patient is suffering from genital herpes. Genital herpes is most often caused by herpes simplex virus-2. Valacyclovir is an antiviral medication that is used to treat primary and recurrent episodes of genital herpes, as well as for suppression therapy to reduce the frequency of genital herpes recurrences.

Answer A is incorrect. Efavirenz is a non-nucleoside reverse transcriptase inhibitor. It prevents the reverse transcription of viral RNA into DNA. Thus it is effective treatment for a retrovirus such as HIV. However, it is not effective against a DNA virus such as herpes simplex virus that does not rely on reverse transcriptase for replication.

Answer B is incorrect. Fluconazole is an antifungal agent that inhibits fungal cell membrane synthesis, and thus is not active against the herpes simplex virus. It would not be useful in the treatment of genital herpes.

Answer C is incorrect. Metronidazole is an antibiotic that is effective in treating anaerobic bacteria and some protozoa. It is used to treat BV and Trichomonas infections, but is ineffective against viruses such as herpes simplex virus.

Answer D is incorrect. Treatment with topical trichloroacetic acid is often used to treat the condyloma acuminata lesions caused by the HPV. It is not used in the treatment of the vesicular lesions of genital herpes.

29. **The correct answer is A.** This woman presents with classic signs of acute cystitis: urgency, extreme dysuria, and lack of fever. Acute cystitis is commonly caused by coliform bacteria ascending along the urethra. It is commonly seen in young women after sexual intercourse or urethral trauma. Urinalysis is usually positive for WBCs and RBCs, and the urine may contain frank blood. Pyelonephritis also will result in urinalysis results showing WBCs, RBCs, and bacteria, but patients also usually present with high fevers, and can have costovertebral angle tenderness.

30. **The correct answer is D.** This history is one of stress incontinence (urine leakage when intra-abdominal pressure is increased during sneezing or coughing). The most likely cause of stress incontinence in a multiparous woman is sphincter insufficiency as a consequence of pelvic floor laxity. Although abdominal or pelvic radiation therapy can be associated with stricture formation and detrusor muscle damage, breast cancer radiation is unlikely to be sufficiently concentrated in the pelvis to cause such damage.

Answer B is incorrect. Patients with acute urinary retention complain about a sudden inability to urinate. All three of these women are complaining of incontinence, not retention. There are many causes of acute urinary retention including alcohol, drugs, neurologic damage, benign prostatic hyperplasia, kidney stones, and surgical complications. A catheter can usually be placed through the urethra to relieve the discomfort. The underlying cause then needs to be evaluated and appropriate steps need to be taken to prevent further complications.

Answer C is incorrect. Patients with a neurogenic bladder may complain of urinary incontinence or urinary retention. Common causes of neurogenic bladder include neuropathy, trauma, tumors of the nervous system, and autoimmune diseases leading to neurological damage.

Answer E is incorrect. Pyelonephritis is a kidney parenchymal infection most commonly caused by gram-negative aerobic bacteria such as *Escherichia coli*, the offending organism in about 80% of cases. The organisms generally spread by ascending from the lower urinary tract. The patient's symptoms are generally characterized by dysuria, urgency, frequency, costovertebral tenderness, fever, chills, nausea, and vomiting. Urinalysis will reveal pyuria and bacteriuria, including a positive culture from a clean mid-stream urine catch. Hospitalization, intravenous fluids, and parenteral antibiotics are the mainstay of treatment. Failure to treat pyelonephritis early can result in acute parenchymal injury, impaired renal tubular function, bacteremia, or sepsis leading to death.

Answer F is incorrect. A fistula refers to any abnormal connection. A urethral fistula can form between the urethra and the skin, the rectum, or a blood vessel. It is usually a complication resulting from a ureteral stent placement or other surgery in the area. Recto-urethral fistulas can also occur as a result of abnormal development in utero.

Answer G is incorrect. Urethral sphincter insufficiency generally results as a complication of surgery to the prostate or pelvic region. There are two urethral sphincters: the internal sphincter is under involuntary control and the external sphincter is under voluntary control. Neuronal or mechanical damage to the nervous supply or the sphincters themselves can lead to incontinence.

CHAPTER 13

Psychiatry

1. A 79-year-old man is admitted to the hospital for an elective total knee replacement. He lives by himself and performs all of his activities of daily living. His medical history includes degenerative joint disease, coronary heart disease, and hypertension. He has no history of psychiatric problems or alcohol and drug history. In the evening, several hours after an uneventful surgical procedure, the patient becomes diaphoretic and tachypneic. He is alert, but also agitated and confused, and cannot give full attention to the hospital staff and their questions. He does remember his name, but does not believe that he is in a hospital. Which of the following is the most likely diagnosis?

(A) Brief psychotic episode
(B) Delirium
(C) Dementia
(D) Normal aging
(E) Pseudodementia

2. A 32-year-old woman states that over the last 6 months she has felt constantly nervous. She adds that sometimes "I feel like my heart is going to burst." She also notes that her heart skips a beat from time to time, and that she is having trouble sleeping. She denies feeling depressed. The patient denies flight of ideas, pressured speech, increased goal-directed activity, hallucinations, or delusions. The patient also complains of increased bowel movements and weight loss, along with significant weakness when she attempts to climb stairs or lift heavy items. The patient's vital signs are: temperature 37.8°C (100.1°F), pulse 102/min, blood pressure 124/85 mm Hg, and respiratory rate 18/min. Neurologic examination is significant only for proximal muscle weakness and hyperactive reflexes. What would be the best treatment option for this patient?

(A) Alprazolam
(B) Investigation of surreptitious laxative abuse
(C) Methimazole
(D) Sertraline
(E) Thyroid hormone replacement

3. A 14-month-old boy is brought to the clinic by his mother because he has appeared drowsy for the past 2 days. The child is unresponsive to verbal stimuli, but on administering a sternal rub, the child flexes his arms and legs. Vital signs are blood pressure 100/60 mm Hg, pulse 60/min, respiratory rate 8/min, and temperature 35.6°C (96.0°F). On examination, the child has multiple circular scars over his forearms and a number of contusions of varying ages over his lower legs. The mother reports that he bruised his legs while walking around the house. What additional physical examination finding would support the most likely diagnosis?

(A) Bilateral retinal hemorrhages
(B) Blue sclerae
(C) Cotton wool spots
(D) Positive fecal occult blood test
(E) Seborrheic keratoses on the head

4. A 32-year-old man was apprehended by the police 2 weeks ago for running across the freeway without regard for his personal safety. The patient stated that he did this "for the heck of it." The patient appeared distracted during the initial interview, spoke rapidly, and gave long and drawn out answers. When asked about his mood, the patient said that he is feeling "okay, I'm under the weather, if you get my drift." He was admitted to the inpatient unit for observation. Since his admission, he has been saying that he will soon replace the president, that he is the next Alexander the Great, and that he was told so by voices in his head. The patient's admission laboratory values, including a drug screen for illicit substances, came back normal. What is the most likely diagnosis for this patient?

(A) Bipolar disorder without psychotic features
(B) Bipolar disorder with psychotic features
(C) Depression with psychotic features
(D) Schizophrenia, disorganized type
(E) Schizophrenia, paranoid type

5. A faculty member in physics at a major university has Asperger's disorder. He appears to stare "through" people when talking to them, as if he is talking to someone far behind them. This

professor has unusually poor social functioning. Additionally, he appears quite clumsy, constantly dropping books and materials involved in his experiments. Which of the following occurs commonly in Asperger's disorder?

(A) Delayed language function
(B) Impaired memory
(C) Intact sense of humor
(D) Low IQ
(E) Poor motor coordination

6. A 28-year-old woman visits her physician for experiencing acute attacks of headache, profuse sweating, and racing heartbeat during the past 2 months. She also had bouts of nausea, abdominal pain, and dyspnea. She is being treated with clonidine for hypertension without any response. Her blood pressure is 160/80 mm Hg and her heart rate is normal. Laboratory tests show:

Na^+	140 mEq/L
K^+	4.4 mEq/L
Cl^-	99 mEq/L
HCO_3^-	30 mEq/L
Blood urea nitrogen	10 mg/dL
Creatinine	0.4 mg/dL
Serum glucose	170 mg/dL
Total thyroxine	8 μg/dL
Thyroid-stimulating hormone	3 μU/mL

Which of the following is the most likely diagnosis?

(A) Anxiety disorder
(B) Clonidine withdrawal
(C) Hyperthyroidism
(D) Pheochromocytoma
(E) Primary hyperaldosteronism

7. A 70-year-old schizophrenic patient with a noted history of violence believes that he is the Messiah and that his doctors are Roman infidels trying to destroy him. The patient is poorly groomed, and he is currently yelling at medical personnel, saying that "in time people will worship me as a god." Which medication should be given to this patient immediately?

(A) Clozapine
(B) Electroconvulsive therapy
(C) Haloperidol

(D) Lithium
(E) Olanzapine

8. A 2-year-old boy being evaluated for an upper respiratory tract infection has very poor eye contact. The child responds to smiles with disinterest. When the physician speaks with the child, he continues to say "stick" while looking at the otoscope. The mother looks distressed, and says that this is one of the only words the child speaks. The mother states that her child has no interest in playing with other children. When the child plays with toys, he is only interested in the individual parts of the toy, such as the wheels, as opposed to the whole toy. What is the most likely diagnosis at this point?

(A) Age-appropriate behavior
(B) Asperger's disorder
(C) Autistic disorder
(D) Mental retardation
(E) Stranger anxiety

9. A 47-year-old woman is brought to the emergency department (ED) by the police after being found wandering around a local park in a nightgown. Her brother is called and he reports a worsening in impulse control in his sister over the past 2 years. During this time, she has become more sexually aggressive, fondling strangers in subways and disrobing in public. Occasionally, she laughs at unknown stimuli and cannot be redirected during these emotional outbursts. Over the last month, she has become a voracious eater and has gained 4.5 kg (10 lb). She was fired from her job as a postal worker 6 months ago for inappropriate behavior. Her blood pressure is 138/80 mm Hg; she appears older than her stated age and has a disheveled appearance. She is alert and oriented, but cannot recall why she was in the park. Physical examination reveals a mild intention tremor. Her Mini-Mental State Examination score is 27, with deficits in short-term recall. What is the most likely diagnosis?

(A) Attention deficit disorder
(B) Diffuse Lewy body dementia
(C) Histrionic personality disorder
(D) Huntington's disease
(E) Klüver-Bucy syndrome

10. A 19-year-old man is brought to the ED after having attacked his next-door neighbor with a baseball bat. The police shot the suspect twice in the leg and once in the arm while attempting to subdue him, but six police officers were still required to place him in restraints. At one point during the struggle, the patient screamed out, "I am the hand of God; you cannot beat me!" The patient's complete blood cell count and serum electrolytes are within normal limits, but laboratory studies show an elevated level of serum creatine kinase. His urine is positive for myoglobinuria as well as for an illegal substance that is known to block the ion-channel N-methyl-D-aspartate receptor complex. What is the most likely cause of this patient's presentation?

(A) Alcohol
(B) Cocaine
(C) Lysergic acid diethylamide
(D) Methamphetamine
(E) Phencyclidine

11. A 48-year-old white man complains of fatigue and weight loss. He states that over the past year he has simply lost all of his energy. The onset of these symptoms has been gradual. Despite eating high-calorie meals in an attempt to gain weight, he says he has lost 20 pounds. At times, he experiences intense nausea and vomits. On physical examination, his temperature is 36.3°C (97.3°F), heart rate 71/min, blood pressure 90/55 mm Hg, and respiratory rate 18/min. His physical examination is notable for dark pigmentation on the elbows and knees. He is slouching in his chair and appears fatigued. He endorses feelings of guilt and anhedonia. What would be the best treatment option for this patient?

(A) Fluoxetine
(B) Lithium
(C) Methimazole, a thyroid-suppressing drug
(D) Mitotane, a cortisol-suppressing drug
(E) Oral steroids

12. A 18-year-old single mother finds herself being overprotective with her child. The mother would like to go back to school and pursue her passion for writing but is unable to afford day care. She often finds herself regretting her pregnancy. The child is a product of an unplanned pregnancy. Which is the most likely defense mechanism?

(A) Idealization
(B) Projection
(C) Rationalization
(D) Reaction formation
(E) Sublimation

13. A 41-year-old man has suffered from a phobia of flying on airplanes for as long as he can remember. He avoids flying when possible and worries that the plane will inevitably crash because he is on it. His mother recently passed away, so he wants to fly back home to attend the funeral. He has no history of substance abuse and would like to try something to help him cope with the upcoming flight. What is the most appropriate management at this time?

(A) Haloperidol
(B) Lorazepam
(C) Paroxetine
(D) Phenobarbital
(E) Promethazine

14. A 15-year-old girl presents to the ED with a heart rate of 37/min. The patient's mother insisted that the girl seek medical attention because she "always seems so tired." The patient, however, denies that she is feeling very tired, and denies any other physical complaints. The patient saw a psychotherapist briefly last year for "low self-esteem." Otherwise, she has no significant psychiatric history. The patient lives with her parents and is exceptionally close with her mother. She is a straight-A student at the exclusive private high school in the neighborhood. Her temperature is 36.4°C (97.5°F), blood pressure is 90/50 mm Hg, and respiratory rate is 17/min. Her body mass index is 17 kg/m². What are the patient's physical examination and laboratory studies likely to show?

(A) Elevated amylase and lipase
(B) Multiple tattoos and piercings
(C) Orthostatic hypotension, hypothermia, and skin dryness
(D) Salivary gland hypertrophy, dental enamel erosion, and scars on the knuckles
(E) Scarring on the flexor surface of the wrist

15. An 8-year-old girl is brought to her pediatrician by her mother for odd behavior. Over the past year, the mother has noticed that her daughter's arms and legs sometimes jerk wildly for no apparent reason. Lately, one of her eyes has started to blink out of sequence with the other and she licks her lips so frequently that they are always chapped. The mother states that as a toddler her daughter exhibited strange behavior, like stacking a deck of playing cards on top of itself repeatedly for hours at a time. Additionally, the mother states that the child is very pleasant and likable, with many friends. Which of the following is the most appropriate pharmacotherapy?

(A) Buspirone
(B) Diazepam
(C) Haloperidol
(D) Sertraline
(E) Valproic acid

16. The family of a 70-year-old man believes he is depressed. According to his family, the patient "doesn't care about anything anymore." Instead, the patient sits in front of the television watching game shows all day. The family also states that the patient makes lewd comments to female visitors. On mental status examination, the patient has unkempt hair, is uncooperative, and speaks very slowly. The patient denies trouble sleeping or concentrating. The patient looks surprised when asked about guilt and suicidal ideation, and emphatically states, "Certainly not!" His affect appears constricted. The patient is oriented to person and place. He has a marked impairment in attending to external stimuli during a mental status examination. The patient has poor inhibitory functions. His language and abstraction are intact. MRI of the brain shows frontal atrophy and ventricular enlargement. What is the most likely cause of the patient's current symptoms?

(A) Alzheimer's dementia
(B) Depression
(C) Frontotemporal dementia
(D) Lewy body dementia
(E) Subcortical dementia

17. A 32-year-old woman with a history of major depressive disorder is found lying on the floor in confusion, with muscle twitching, flushing, and dilated pupils. On arrival at the ED she is found to have a widened QRS complex. On which of the following medications did she most likely overdose?

(A) Amitriptyline
(B) Bupropion
(C) Fluoxetine
(D) Lithium
(E) Phenelzine

18. The behavior of a 2-year-old is evaluated by a psychiatrist. An experiment is conducted whereby the mother leaves the playroom. The child begins to cry. When the mother returns, the child is extremely enthusiastic. Which of the following behaviors is the child exhibiting?

(A) Anxious attachment
(B) Attachment disorder
(C) Secure attachment
(D) Stranger anxiety
(E) Symbolism-based behavior

19. An 18-year-old man presents complaining of depression. He states that for most of his life he has had "a negative outlook" for reasons he cannot figure out. He says he continually makes statements to himself about how "I can't do anything" and "I'm worthless." On mental status examination he appears markedly dysphoric. His thought content is full of statements regarding his shortcomings. Which therapy is focused on changing negative thought processes?

(A) Behavioral therapy
(B) Cognitive-behavioral therapy
(C) Freudian psychoanalysis
(D) Interpersonal psychotherapy
(E) Jungian psychotherapy

20. A 62-year-old man complains that he is feeling "depressed." He says that over the last 2 years, he has begun to have a vague feeling of sadness. In addition, he notes that he is extremely fatigued during the day, frequently nodding off to sleep at work. Before going to work, he frequently takes ibuprofen to relieve nearly daily morning headaches. When asked about changes in his life over the last 2 years, he reports that he has gained a significant amount of weight due to "job stress." Further questioning reveals that he does not feel guilty, has no suicidal ideation, and still enjoys his favorite pastime of reading mystery novels and holding a biweekly book club with friends. The patient's body mass index is 42 kg/m². Physical examination of the patient is within normal limits. Which of the following treatment options is appropriate for this patient?

(A) Methylphenidate
(B) Modafinil
(C) Sertraline
(D) Thyroid hormone replacement
(E) Weight loss and continuous positive airway pressure

21. A 4-year-old child is brought to his pediatrician by his mother and father. They are worried that their baby-sitter may be hurting their child. They left the child with a baby-sitter for the first time 2 days ago. When the parents returned, the child was crying, and pleaded for them to "never leave again!" When the pediatrician questions the child alone, he denies any poor treatment by the baby-sitter or parents. He simply says "Mommy and Daddy could get sick and die when they are gone." The child's baby-sitter, when questioned by phone, states that the child "won't stop crying when his parents leave." When asked how he feels while his parents are away, the child says, "It makes me feel sick when they are gone." The child denies discomfort when he is with his parents. On physical examination, the child has no stigmata of abuse, such as scars, bruises, burns, or genital lesions. His abdomen is soft, nontender, and nondistended. The child does not complain of bone pain. What is the most appropriate next step?

(A) Call child protective services
(B) Diagnose a likely separation anxiety disorder

(C) Diagnose the patient with a generalized anxiety disorder
(D) Image the child's bones
(E) Recommend upper endoscopy

22. A 63-year-old white woman presents to the ED complaining of "palpitations." An ECG shows a long QT interval. The patient states she takes the following medications: donepezil, amitriptyline, propranolol, and warfarin. She states that she recently started a new diet consisting only of grapefruit juice and tofu. Which of the following medication effects can account for the patient's QT prolongation?

(A) Decreased metabolism of amitriptyline due to grapefruit juice
(B) Decreased metabolism of propranolol due to grapefruit juice
(C) Drug interaction between donepezil and amitriptyline
(D) Drug interaction between warfarin and amitriptyline
(E) Drug interaction between warfarin and donepezil

23. A 42-year-old woman presents to an outpatient psychiatry clinic. She has a 9-year history of depression and a 15-year history of substance abuse, including cocaine, amphetamines, and opioids. She states that she has been feeling suicidal due to a "greater depression than ever before." She also admits to feeling fatigued and having a ravenous appetite. When asked about recent substance abuse, she gives vague answers and states, "I can't really remember now. I don't want to talk about it." On mental status examination, she displays severe psychomotor retardation. Which of the following is the most likely cause of the patient's symptoms?

(A) Cocaine intoxication
(B) Cocaine withdrawal
(C) Opioid intoxication
(D) Opioid withdrawal
(E) Typical depression

24. A 6-year-old girl is brought to the outpatient clinic for a checkup. She reached all developmental milestones until the age of 24 months. Since then, she has become more distant and less socially engaging. She rarely initiates so-

cial interactions and has a short temper. Verbal language consists mostly of grunting and loud nonverbal yelling, a severe decline from her toddler years when she could speak in three- to four-word sentences. She has never been completely toilet trained and has difficulty following verbal commands from her caregivers. What is the most likely disorder in this child?

(A) Asperger's syndrome
(B) Autism
(C) Childhood disintegrative disorder
(D) Fragile X syndrome
(E) Rett's disorder

25. A 3-year-old girl is brought to the ED from her day care center. Over the course of the day, she has had four episodes of nonbloody nonbilious emesis. She has also been extremely lethargic and difficult to arouse. The day care center tried to reach her mother at work but was unsuccessful. She was born vaginally at 39 weeks' gestation after a normal uncomplicated pregnancy and delivery. She is the youngest of seven children and her father has been incarcerated for the past 2 years. Her heart rate is 60/min. Her anterior fontanelle is full and her pupils are poorly reactive to light bilaterally. Cardiac examination is normal. Her lungs are clear to auscultation bilaterally with shallow breath sounds. She has bruising and tenderness over her posterior lower ribs. X-ray of the chest is shown in the image. Which of the following is the most likely diagnosis?

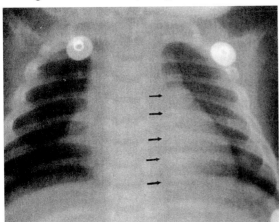

Reproduced, with permission, from Chen MYM, Pope TL, Ott DJ. *Basic Radiology.* New York: McGraw-Hill, 2004: Figure 6-9.

(A) Coagulation disorder
(B) Glutaric aciduria type 1
(C) Intracranial aneurysm
(D) Meningitis
(E) Shaken baby syndrome

26. A 29-year-old man presents to the psychiatrist at the request of his wife. The patient has received psychiatric care throughout his life, due to his repeated fights at school, bullying, taunting, and aggressive disrespect for others throughout his childhood and adolescence. The patient relates a history of lying to his wife and to other therapists, of which he seems quite proud. He has cheated on his wife many times but appears to experience little remorse about his actions. His wife demanded that he seek therapy after she learned of one of his affairs. What was the patient's most likely diagnosis as a child?

(A) Antisocial personality disorder
(B) Bipolar disorder
(C) Conduct disorder
(D) Depression
(E) Substance abuse

27. A 54-year-old man is brought to the ED in an altered mental state. He is exhibiting ataxia, nystagmus, and dysarthria and appears very somnolent. After several hours, he returns to his normal state of health. When questioned about his presentation, he replies that he "just had a few too many to drink." Which of the following would support the theory that this patient has alcohol dependence?

(A) One or more attempts to stop drinking over the last 6 months
(B) The fact that he has been arrested twice in the past 6 months on a "drunk and disorderly" charge
(C) The fact that he has been fired from three jobs in the past year for coming to work drunk
(D) The fact that his girlfriend has been threatening to leave him because of his drinking
(E) The recurrent use of alcohol while driving in the past 6 months

28. A 29-year-old woman is referred to a psychiatrist by a primary care physician. The physician informs the psychiatrist that he believes the patient is exhibiting a somatization disorder. Which of the following behaviors and symptoms will the psychiatrist note if this is the correct diagnosis?

    (A) A variety of complaints, including at least two abdominal and one neurologic
    (B) "La belle indifférence"
    (C) Physical symptoms that precisely mimic a "textbook" medical disorder
    (D) Pleasure and satisfaction on the part of the patient if she is offered admission to the hospital medical service
    (E) Relief on the part of the patient when she is informed that her problem is psychological in nature

29. A 15-year-old boy is brought to the pediatrician by his father because he has been "acting like a girl." When questioned alone, the patient states that he is uncomfortable with his life. He states that he has always had more feminine interests than most of his same-gender friends. He tries to fit in, but he simply feels more comfortable when he is hanging out with females and playing with dolls. The patient confesses that he has, for most of his life, believed that he should have been born as a girl. What is the best initial treatment option for this patient?

    (A) Alprazolam
    (B) Hormonal therapy
    (C) Paroxetine
    (D) Psychological therapy to help the patient adjust to his biological gender
    (E) Sex reassignment surgery

30. An 18-year-old woman is brought to the ED by her sister after she was found lying asleep in bed, next to an empty bottle of acetaminophen. The sister knew that "something was up" with the patient's boyfriend because she had returned home the previous night horribly upset and in tears. When asked how many acetaminophen she believed were in the bottle, the sister responded that the bottle was nearly empty, and she could not have taken any more than six pills. Which of the following questions is the most helpful during this interview?

    (A) "Do you ever hear voices or see things that other people can't see?"
    (B) "Have you ever been hospitalized for psychiatric reasons before?"
    (C) "Tell me more about your plan to commit suicide."
    (D) There is no reason to elicit more information; every suicidal patient should be hospitalized
    (E) "What recreational drugs do you use?"

31. A 12-year-old boy presented to a physician's office because of polyuria, polydipsia, nocturia, and decreased appetite for 2 months. The patient was diagnosed with attention deficit/hyperactivity disorder when he was 6 years old and is being treated with a stimulant; 9 months ago he was diagnosed with bipolar disorder and began treatment with valproic acid and olanzapine. Family history is significant for bipolar disorder and diabetes mellitus. His temperature is 36.6°C (97.9°F), pulse is 76/min, respiratory rate is 18/min, and blood pressure is 110/70 mm Hg. The patient has no abdominal pain, nausea, or vomiting. Serum glucose is reported as 300 mg/dL, and urine ketones are found in trace amounts. What is the most appropriate next step in management?

    (A) Discontinue olanzapine
    (B) Discontinue valproic acid
    (C) Monitor blood sugar for the next 6 months
    (D) Recommend diet and exercise
    (E) Start oral hypoglycemics

32. A 24-year-old psychiatry patient is extremely interested in everything the physician says, exclaiming, "Wow, doctor, you really understand me, you're the best!" She tells the physician about the verbal abuse that she suffered during her childhood from a mother who gave her notably inconsistent parenting. She says that she currently feels empty inside, like she has no direction. She discusses the large number of tumultuous relationships that she has had throughout her life, giving vague reasons as to why they have not worked out. When the physician asks her to describe herself further, she states that she is "impulsive." When the physician suggests that her personality structure may be to blame, she screams, "You're just like the rest of them!" and runs out. What is the most likely diagnosis?

(A) Antisocial personality disorder
(B) Avoidant personality disorder
(C) Borderline personality disorder
(D) Histrionic personality disorder
(E) Narcissistic personality disorder

33. A 17-year-old high school student is brought to the pediatrician by her mother for fatigue and dizziness. She has no known medical problems. Her weight is within the normal range for her height. Her respiratory rate is 10/min, heart rate is 58/min, and blood pressure lying down is 116/72 mm Hg and standing is 94/56 mmHg. Her oxygen saturation is 99% on room air. On physical examination, her skin is dry and doughy, and her capillary refill time is 3.5 seconds. Her cheeks are swollen, her oropharynx is clear, and she has erosion of the enamel on her front teeth. She has calluses over the first and second metacarpophalangeal joints of her right hand. The remainder of her physical examination is within normal limits. Laboratory studies show:

Complete blood cell count	Normal
HCO_3^-	32 mEq/L
Blood urea nitrogen	44 mg/dL
Creatinine	0.6 mg/dL
Serum amylase	142 U/L
Lipase	Normal

Which of the following is the most likely explanation of these laboratory values?

(A) Acute pancreatitis
(B) Acute renal failure
(C) Cardiac arrhythmia
(D) Respiratory acidosis
(E) Self-induced vomiting

34. A man attends three sessions per week with his psychiatrist. During each session, he begins to talk, saying whatever comes to his mind. Occasionally, the patient relates dreams that he remembers from the previous night. The psychiatrist remains silent for the majority of the session, asking only about details to clarify what the patient says. This is an example of which of the following types of therapy?

(A) Behavioral therapy
(B) Cognitive therapy

(C) Interpersonal psychotherapy
(D) Psychoanalysis
(E) Supportive psychotherapy

35. A 63-year-old white woman with a 15-year history of schizophrenia is admitted to the inpatient psychiatric ward after she was found inside a department store wearing clothing that did not belong to her. On mental status examination, the patient is sitting motionless in a chair. Her responses to questioning exhibit paucity of content. The patient also displays echopraxia while answering questions. On examination, the patient displays increased tone in the arms and legs that is proportional to the amount of force used during the examination. The patient also seems to leave her arms and legs in strange positions for extended periods of time. Vital signs are temperature 36.8°C (98.2°F), heart rate 86/min, blood pressure 123/76 mm Hg, and respiratory rate 16/min. Significant medications include haloperidol 15 mg once daily. What is the most likely diagnosis at this point?

(A) Catatonia
(B) Dystonia
(C) Mental retardation
(D) Neuroleptic malignant syndrome
(E) Serotonin syndrome

36. A 12-year-old boy is referred by a teacher to the school psychologist for his disruptive behavior. The teacher states that he has been disturbing the class during the past 8 months by talking back to her and repeatedly calling out during class without obeying the rules. His mother notes that he has been increasingly resentful and angry with her over mundane tasks, such as cleaning his room. He has been caught sneaking out through his window at night and was found smoking with his friends at a neighbor's house. What is the most likely diagnosis?

(A) Antisocial personality disorder
(B) Attention deficit disorder
(C) Conduct disorder
(D) Normal preadolescent development
(E) Oppositional defiant disorder

37. Lithium has multiple adverse effects, including neurologic effects, thyroid enlargement, and acne. Up to 20% of patients taking therapeutic doses of lithium experience polyuria and polydipsia as adverse effects of the medication. What is the mechanism of this toxicity?

    (A) Central diabetes insipidus secondary to decreased ADH release
    (B) Destruction of ADH-releasing cells in hypothalamic nuclei
    (C) Increased ADH catabolism by vasopressinase
    (D) Increased density of ADH receptors
    (E) Nephrogenic diabetes insipidus secondary to ADH antagonism

38. A 34-year-old man who was previously employed as a nurse presents to the ED with dizziness and weakness. He states that for the past few weeks he has experienced a number of episodes of fainting spells, weakness, and stomach aches. After a fingerstick test reveals a serum glucose level of 24 mg/dL, the patient is admitted to the medical service, where his glucose level is stabilized. Subsequent laboratory studies show a low C-peptide level, a high serum insulin level, and positive titers for insulin antibodies. Which of the following is the next step in the management of this patient?

    (A) CT scan of the abdomen
    (B) Endoscopy
    (C) Initiation of dialysis
    (D) Institution of insulin therapy
    (E) Psychiatric consultation

EXTENDED MATCHING

Questions 39–41

For each of the following scenarios, choose the correct antidote or treatment.

    (A) Activated charcoal
    (B) Atropine
    (C) Benzodiazepines
    (D) Deferoxamine
    (E) Dialysis
    (F) Dimercaprol
    (G) Flumazenil
    (H) Glucagon
    (I) Haloperidol
    (J) Hyperbaric oxygen
    (K) N-acetylcysteine
    (L) Naloxone
    (M) Vitamin K

39. A 23-year-old woman is brought to the ED by a group of friends, who leave immediately after dropping her off. The woman is unresponsive, with tightly constricted pupils and a respiratory rate of 6/min.

40. A 35-year-old businessman is brought to the ED by paramedics, who were summoned by the police during a routine traffic stop. The patient is jittery and exuberant. He is talking rapidly and is difficult to examine, but his pupils are noted to be large, and he is sweating. Further examination reveals his heart rate to be 120/min and his blood pressure 150/100 mm Hg. While in the ED he becomes very agitated, struggling with the nurses and stating that the doctors are "out to get me."

41. A 67-year-old homeless man presents to the ED with hypertension, diaphoresis, tachycardia, and tremor. He is agitated and confused, stating that he can feel rats crawling all over him. Physical examination reveals that he has ascites and a liver edge that is palpable 6 cm below the costal margin.

Questions 42–44

Match each of the following adverse effects with the drug with which it is most closely associated.

    (A) Amitriptyline
    (B) Buspirone
    (C) Clonazepam
    (D) Clonidine
    (E) Clozapine
    (F) Fluoxetine
    (G) Haloperidol
    (H) Lamotrigine
    (I) Lithium
    (J) Olanzapine
    (K) Reserpine
    (L) Risperidone
    (M) Sertraline
    (N) Topiramate
    (O) Valproic acid
    (P) Venlafaxine

42. Requires weekly complete blood count monitoring for a dangerous adverse effect in 1–2% of patients.

43. Is most associated with the metabolic syndrome of dyslipidemia, hyperglycemia, and weight gain.

44. Is most associated with potentially life-threatening skin eruptions.

Questions 45–47

Match each vignette with the most likely psychiatric disorder.

   (A) Antisocial personality disorder
   (B) Brief psychotic disorder
   (C) Conversion disorder
   (D) Cyclothymia
   (E) Generalized anxiety disorder
   (F) Narcolepsy
   (G) Obsessive-compulsive disorder
   (H) Oppositional defiant disorder
   (I) Panic disorder
   (J) Posttraumatic stress disorder
   (K) Rett's syndrome
   (L) Schizoaffective disorder
   (M) Schizophrenia, paranoid subtype
   (N) Social phobia
   (O) Tourette's disorder

45. A 34-year-old man begins to sweat profusely every time he has to give a presentation at the office. The sweating causes such marked anxiety at each presentation that he soon develops palpitations, dizziness, and difficulty breathing. He finds that if he has several alcoholic drinks before the presentation, he feels "calmer" and can complete the talk.

46. Two days after her husband was killed in a car crash, a 37-year-old woman becomes severely agitated, yelling and screaming, using expletives, and threatening one of her children with a knife. Her son called emergency medical services, and she was taken to the nearest ED, where she responded to intramuscular haloperidol and was eventually admitted. Four days later, her agitation had ceased, she was sincerely apologetic for her behavior, and she

returned to her premorbid level of functioning.

47. The husband of a 26-year-old woman consults his lawyer for a divorce. For the past several months, he "doesn't know whom he'll come home to." His wife is either extremely irritable and starting fights or she is in bed "depressed." She was fired from her job 3 weeks ago for inconsistent performance.

Questions 48–50

Match the following clinical scenarios with the most appropriate description.

   (A) Agoraphobia
   (B) Akathisia
   (C) Anhedonia
   (D) Ataxia
   (E) Catatonia
   (F) Compulsion
   (G) Echolalia
   (H) Delirium
   (I) Delusion
   (J) Dyskinesia
   (K) Dysthymia
   (L) Flight of ideas
   (M) Grandiosity
   (N) Hypochondriasis
   (O) Obsession
   (P) Somatization

48. Several weeks after starting a new medication, a woman with a history of schizoaffective disorder returns to her psychiatrist complaining that she "just can't sit still" and fidgets constantly.

49. Any time a young woman is aboard a bus or subway, stands in line in a crowded supermarket, or crosses a bridge, she develops a rapid heartbeat, difficulty breathing, sweating, nausea, and dizziness. She soon stops leaving the house for fear of developing the symptoms.

50. A 27-year-old man has been hospitalized eight times for acute schizophrenic episodes. When seen by his physician, he refuses to answer any questions, merely repeating whatever has been said to him.

ANSWERS

1. **The correct answer is B.** The most likely diagnosis for this patient is delirium. Clinical features typical of delirium as opposed to dementia include a relatively rapid onset, a fluctuating and cloudy level of consciousness, impaired orientation, disordered thinking, impairment of recent memory only, and reversibility of the condition.

   Answer A is incorrect. A brief psychotic episode is characterized by schizophrenia-like symptoms that last less than a month. The patient must experience delusions, hallucinations, or disorganized speech in order to be diagnosed with this condition. In some cases of delirium the patient may experience hallucinations (especially visual); however, in contrast to a brief psychotic episode, delirium is usually traceable to an underlying medical condition.

   Answer C is incorrect. In contrast to delirium, dementia is a chronic disease with an insidious onset and a progressive course. The patient's level of consciousness is generally not affected, orientation is initially intact, recent and remote memory are impaired, and the majority of cases of dementia are not reversible.

   Answer D is incorrect. Age-related cognitive decline (normal aging) involves a decreased ability to learn new information. It does not include clouding of consciousness, change of mental status, or problems with orientation.

   Answer E is incorrect. Pseudodementia is the term given to patients that experience cognitive slippage in relation to depression. The patient in this case does not show evidence of depression.

2. **The correct answer is C.** In considering anxiety disorders, one must first always rule out hyperthyroidism. Typical physical manifestations of hyperthyroidism include weight loss with preserved appetite, heat intolerance, proximal muscle weakness, and increased frequency of bowel movements. Other general signs include hyperactivity, tachycardia, palpitations, and hyperreflexia. Psychiatric manifestations include anxiety and insomnia. Methimazole, a thyroid inhibitor, is appropriate therapy in this case.

   Answer A is incorrect. Anxiety disorder is certainly in the differential for this patient. Benzodiazepines such as alprazolam are the appropriate treatment for anxiety disorder. Medical causes of her anxiety, however, would have to be ruled out first before she is considered to have an anxiety disorder.

   Answer B is incorrect. The patient does complain of weight loss, but does not have any complaints consistent with metabolic abnormalities (e.g., hyperphosphatemia), making laxative use a less likely explanation. Also, her other symptoms and complaints can be explained well by the diagnosis of hyperthyroidism.

   Answer D is incorrect. The patient does not describe any significant signs of depression, such as guilt, decreased interest in pleasurable activity, or decreased concentration. Thus, an antidepressant is not indicated.

   Answer E is incorrect. Hypothyroidism more often presents as depression than as anxiety. Other signs of hypothyroidism include deepening of the voice, lack of energy, constipation, abnormal sensitivity to cold temperatures, weight gain (often in spite of a poor appetite), and dry skin and hair.

3. **The correct answer is A.** Based on the inconsistency between the mother's explanation of the child's symptoms and the observed physical findings, the scenario is highly worrisome for child abuse. Given the child's altered mental status, it is likely that this toddler has also suffered diffuse brain injury. An ophthalmologic examination would likely reveal retinal hemorrhages if this child sustained intracranial trauma. Other indications of head trauma might include subdural hemorrhage(s) and/or white matter changes visible on brain imaging studies. All suspected cases of child abuse and neglect must be reported to the authorities.

   Answer B is incorrect. Blue sclerae is a finding in patients with osteogenesis imperfecta. This disease can be mistaken for child abuse because the patient's bones are frail and present with recurrent fractures at a young age. This patient has no evidence of fractures and has an altered mental status consistent with head injury.

Answer C is incorrect. Cotton wool spots are found in patients with a long-standing history of hypertension and are generally not observed in otherwise healthy toddlers.

Answer D is incorrect. A positive fecal occult blood test is a nonspecific test that would not specify a single diagnosis. Nevertheless, in cases of child abuse, a positive fecal occult blood test may signal that the child has sustained intra-abdominal trauma and should prompt further medical evaluation.

Answer E is incorrect. Seborrheic dermatitis is a common finding in infants and tends to be self-limited over time. The rash occurs in a "cradle cap" distribution on the scalp and presents with a characteristic flaky, scaly dermatitis with a "stuck-on" appearance. It is not indicative of child abuse or neglect.

4. **The correct answer is B.** The patient exhibits grandiosity, pressured speech, distractibility, and an increase in risk-taking behavior, all of which comprise a manic episode because they have lasted longer than 1 week. Thus, the diagnosis is bipolar disorder. Although schizophrenic patients may also engage in inappropriate actions such as running across the freeway, they often relate poorly to the staff, given their more bizarre delusions. Often, patients with schizophrenia also have flattened affect, paucity of speech, and other "negative" symptoms later in their illness, which decreases their ability to relate to staff. Because the patient is hearing voices, he certainly has psychotic features. Up to 50% of patients with bipolar disorder have psychotic features.

Answer A is incorrect. Hearing voices is a psychotic feature.

Answer C is incorrect. The patient states that his mood is okay, although he throws in some nonsensical pieces of speech after this. Additionally, most psychotic content in depression is of a negative nature.

Answer D is incorrect. This patient lacks the "negative" symptoms of schizophrenia, such as

poor motivation, self-neglect, reduced emotion, poor attention, constricted affect, and paucity of speech. Moreover, in the disorganized schizophrenic patient, the thought process would be far more difficult to understand due to loose associations. The patient is delusional, but his thought process can be understood.

Answer E is incorrect. Although this patient has psychotic features that are seen in schizophrenia, he is not experiencing paranoid thoughts. His grandiosity and pressured speech make him more likely to be suffering from bipolar disorder.

5. **The correct answer is E.** Core features of Asperger's syndrome include a lack of eye contact, a paucity of facial and gestural expressions, and a flat and emotionless tone of voice. Other characteristics of Asperger's include pronounced likes and dislikes, repetitive routines or rituals, peculiarities in speech and language, the inability to interact successfully with peers, absent sense of humor, problems with nonverbal communication, and clumsy and uncoordinated motor movements. There may, however, be special abilities (rote memory) interwoven with disabilities and unusual interest in natural sciences, complex calculations, or calendar calculating.

Answer A is incorrect. Patients with Asperger's syndrome often have excellent language function, although they have an impaired ability to appreciate the meaning of the words they are using.

Answer B is incorrect. Patients with Asperger's syndrome often have tremendous rote memories.

Answer C is incorrect. Patients with Asperger's syndrome often have little or no sense of humor.

Answer D is incorrect. Patients with Asperger's syndrome often have normal to high IQs.

6. **The correct answer is D.** Pheochromocytoma should be suspected in cases of difficult-to-control hypertension accompanied by various adrenergic symptoms such as tachycardia, sweating, nervousness, and orthostasis. These

symptoms are caused by excessive levels of nor-epinephrine or neuropeptide Y. Patients have a tumor located in either or both adrenals or anywhere along the sympathetic nervous chain. Additionally, patients may experience attacks of nausea, abdominal pain, weakness, tremor, visual disturbance, chest pain, and dyspnea. Also, mild hyperglycemia is common in cases of pheochromocytoma.

Answer A is incorrect. Pheochromocytoma may be mistaken for an anxiety disorder such as a panic attack given common physical symptoms of racing heart, sweating and nervousness, headache, muscle tension, chest pain, and abdominal distress. However, patients with pheochromocytoma more often than not present with hypertension (90%), which may be sustained or paroxysmal in nature.

Answer B is incorrect. Clonidine withdrawal syndrome can result from the abrupt withdrawal or tapering of clonidine causing a hyperadrenergic state that mimics pheochromocytoma. The syndrome consists of nausea, palpitation, anxiety, sweating, and headache, along with an elevation in blood pressure. In this clinical scenario, the patient has remained on clonidine despite a poor response.

Answer C is incorrect. Tachycardia, heat intolerance, weight loss, and anxiety are also features of hyperthyroidism. However, in this clinical scenario, serum thyroxine and thyroid-stimulating hormone levels are within the normal range and therefore rule out the diagnosis of hyperthyroidism.

Answer E is incorrect. Patients with primary hyperaldosteronism typically have other physical and biochemical findings such as hypokalemia (the patient in this clinical scenario has normal potassium) and alkalosis.

7. **The correct answer is C.** Once medical causes have been excluded, the determination of safety is important in treating psychiatric illness. It is necessary to maintain a controlled environment for the safety of both the patient and staff. Initial management of this patient includes an antipsychotic, such as haloperidol, for psychosis and agitation. Therapy with typi-cal neuroleptics, such as haloperidol and chlorpromazine, is frequently successful in amelioration of "positive" symptoms such as hallucinations, delusions, and agitation. These typical neuroleptics have little effect on negative symptoms. It is important to note that much of the aggression which occurs in schizophrenia is due to the patient's poor understanding of reality, as opposed to a premeditated, instrumental aggression which occurs in psychopathy.

Answer A is incorrect. Atypical neuroleptics, including clozapine, are thought to be effective for both positive and negative symptoms of schizophrenia. The use of clozapine is limited to refractive cases of schizophrenia due to the risk of agranulocytosis.

Answer B is incorrect. Electroconvulsive therapy (ECT) plays an important role in the therapy of treatment-resistant schizophrenia. ECT should be considered after 3–4 drug trials, and is likely most effective in patients with affective symptoms.

Answer D is incorrect. Lithium is a mood-stabilizing agent that is first-line treatment for bipolar disorder. Approximately 80% of manic patients also respond to this treatment; however, a measurable response typically takes 1–2 weeks. As such, it is not able to control psychosis and agitation in the initial period of treatment, but may be co-administered with another antipsychotic medication. Lithium is also recommended for the treatment of schizophrenic patients who have not achieved a significant response to neuroleptics alone. Lithium may be an effective adjunctive treatment for patients with significant affective symptoms.

Answer E is incorrect. Olanzapine is another atypical antipsychotic that can be very effective for treating patients with negative symptoms. It would not be the treatment of choice for this patient, as he exhibits positive symptoms.

8. **The correct answer is C.** Patients with autism have impairment in three major areas. The first area is impairment in social interaction. The child will make little eye contact, has few peer interactions, and will not engage in ap-

propriate interest-sharing activities, such as showing parents toys they are interested in. The patient also has difficulty with communication, learning and using few words. Words that are used are stereotyped and used incorrectly. Finally, patients display restricted repetitive and stereotyped patterns of behavior, interests, and activities, and interest in parts of objects. The disorder is often conceptualized as "missing the forest for the trees." Communication and social interaction may require a certain integrative function that autistic children lack. The pathogenesis of the disorder, however, remains a mystery.

Answer A is incorrect. The fact that the patient does not respond to social cues such as smiles is not normal at any age. Moreover, only using one word at age 3 years is not age-appropriate behavior. By age 3, children should be putting together three-word sentences, along with riding a tricycle and playing with other children.

Answer B is incorrect. Differentiating Asperger's disorder from autism can be difficult. Children with Asperger's disorder often display similar poor social interaction and stereotyped interests. What differentiates the two is that in Asperger's, social communication is intact. In fact, speech in Asperger's patients often develops early. The speech of Asperger's patients often has no prosody in it. These patients are often called "little professors" for their poor social interaction, narrowed interests, and excellent (but aprosic) speech.

Answer D is incorrect. Mental retardation is defined as an IQ < 70 with concurrent dysfunction in adaptive behavior as expressed in conceptual (e.g., reading, writing, and money concepts), social (e.g., self-esteem and gullibility), and practical adaptive skills (e.g., personal activities of daily living). This disorder can cause difficulty in social and communication functions. The patient's poor eye contact and social relatedness point toward autism. It is often very difficult to tell these two disorders apart.

Answer E is incorrect. Peak stranger anxiety occurs at 8–10 months of age. The child has integrated the idea that he or she is separate from mother and is separate from the rest of the world. The child feels comfortable with the mother, but is not comfortable with strangers in the world. This fear, which occurs between 6 months and 2 years of age, would not account for the behavior described in the stem.

9. **The correct answer is E.** Klüver-Bucy syndrome is classified as a syndrome within the frontal lobe dementias. Classic symptoms include hyperorality, hypersexuality, and perseverative speech or behavior. Other symptoms include apathy, personality changes, and amotivation.

Answer A is incorrect. Attention deficit disorder may present in adults, but it is characterized by inability to focus on tasks, and difficulty attending to details.

Answer B is incorrect. Diffuse Lewy body disease has prominent psychiatric signs such as personality changes, depression, and hallucinations. Patients often have weight loss, rather than weight gain. Fluctuating mental status and cognitive impairments are common. This patient, however, fits the classic presentation of Kl_ver-Bucy syndrome.

Answer C is incorrect. Histrionic personality disorder is a persistent pattern of behaviors present throughout a patient's life. Prominent signs include inappropriate sexual behavior and unstable relationships.

Answer D is incorrect. Huntington's disease is a familial dementia with anticipatory expression. It is caused by a triplet repeat and successive generations tend to express the mutation earlier in age. Symptoms of the disease include difficulty in speaking and swallowing, involuntary movements, cognitive impairment, and depression. Uncommonly, patients can present with delusions, hallucinations, and obsessive-compulsive disorders. It is uniformly fatal.

10. **The correct answer is E.** This patient is suffering from a phencyclidine (PCP)-induced psychosis. PCP is a dissociative drug that causes users to feel detached from their bodies and from their surroundings. Users generally feel numb and may have a sense of invulnera-

bility, rendering them highly dangerous both to themselves and to others. PCP noncompetitively binds to the N-methyl-D-aspartate receptor complex and inactivates the channel, resulting in a blockade of the excitatory central nervous system amino acids glutamate and aspartate. The drug is excreted in the urine and can be screened for in suspected patients who present with psychotic symptoms. Treatment consists mainly of benzodiazepines for sedation. Psychosis can be treated with an antipsychotic with low anticholinergic activity (PCP is an anticholinergic). For patients who ingest the drug, gastric lavage or charcoal can reduce the absorption of the drug via the gastrointestinal tract.

Answer A is incorrect. Alcohol is a central nervous system depressant that typically presents with disinhibition, emotional lability, slurred speech, ataxia, and somnolence. Frank psychosis is seen in the context of alcohol withdrawal, but only rarely is it seen with alcohol intoxication.

Answer B is incorrect. Cocaine can also cause substance-related psychosis with hallucinations and delusions. However, cocaine acts by preventing the reuptake of dopamine molecules released in the synaptic clefts of nerves.

Answer C is incorrect. This patient's presentation is unlikely to be due to lysergic acid diethylamide (LSD), which typically causes powerful sensory disturbances such as the movement of shapes, light, and colors. LSD usually does not produce hallucinations in the strict sense, but rather illusions and vivid daydream-like scenes. The drug acts on numerous receptors in the central nervous system, including dopamine receptors, adrenoreceptors, and serotonin receptors. However, LSD does not block N-methyl-D-aspartate receptors.

Answer D is incorrect. Amphetamines such as methamphetamine are also stimulants that can cause psychosis. However, amphetamines work by activating the release of norepinephrine and dopamine at nerve endings.

11. **The correct answer is E.** The patient is likely suffering from adrenal insufficiency and would thus need steroid replacement therapy. Significant symptoms include weight loss, anorexia,

and muscle weakness, along with fatigue, low blood pressure, and hyperpigmentation (dark skin tanning of both external and unexposed skin areas, most noticeable on skin folds, elbows, knees, knuckles, toes, lips, and mucous membranes). Patients are often noticeably sick, with nausea and vomiting. Psychiatric symptoms include apathy, irritability, and depression.

Answer A is incorrect. The patient might have major depressive disorder. However, with this patient's physical symptoms, it is more likely that a medical condition is causing the mood change. Therefore, an antidepressant would not be recommended at this point.

Answer B is incorrect. There is no evidence to indicate that the patient has a history of manic episodes, a requisite for the consideration of bipolar disorder. Thus, a mood stabilizer is not indicated.

Answer C is incorrect. The patient might be weak and have a change in mood due to hyperthyroidism. However, although the patient has lost weight, he does not have any signs of increased anxiety, palpitations, or inability to tolerate hot temperatures characteristic of hyperthyroidism. Moreover, the low blood pressure and the hyperpigmentation make adrenal insufficiency a more likely diagnosis. Thus, methimazole would not be indicated.

Answer D is incorrect. Cushing's disease, which overloads the body with cortisol, can present with depression. The patient, however, would have weight gain instead of weight loss. He would also have high blood pressure instead of low blood pressure. Other indications of Cushing's disease include stretch marks on the torso and buffalo hump due to neck adipose deposits.

12. **The correct answer is D.** With reaction formation the individual deals with intra-psychic conflict by behaviors, thoughts, or feelings that are the opposite of her own, consciously unacceptable thoughts. In this case, a mother subconsciously wishes she did not have to care for her child instead of pursuing a career. She reacts against these feelings by acting in an overprotective manner.

Answer A is incorrect. In idealization, the individual deals with emotional conflict and distress by attributing overly positive qualities to others.

Answer B is incorrect. When a person is projecting they falsely attribute their own unacceptable feelings, impulses, or thoughts onto another.

Answer C is incorrect. The process of rationalization involves the elaboration of one's own thoughts, actions, and feelings by way of reassuring explanations that conceal their true meaning.

Answer E is incorrect. Sublimation involves channeling potentially threatening and maladaptive feelings and impulses into socially acceptable outlets.

13. **The correct answer is B.** Lorazepam is a benzodiazepine (GABAergic) anxiolytic used to help patients cope with their phobias on a short-term basis. When time is a factor in developing a treatment plan, benzodiazepines are appropriate first-line agents to produce an immediate reduction in symptoms of anxiety.

Answer A is incorrect. Haloperidol is a typical antipsychotic that may be sedating, but it would not be used in this case. Rather, it is used to control psychotic symptoms such as hallucinations and delusions.

Answer C is incorrect. Paroxetine is an antidepressant in the selective serotonin reuptake inhibitor (SSRI) family. It is effective in treating specific phobias and might be helpful in long-term therapy, but because SSRIs typically require 4–6 weeks to exert therapeutic effects, a benzodiazepine would produce a much more immediate response suitable for this particular situation.

Answer D is incorrect. Phenobarbital is a barbiturate that has anticonvulsant and sedative properties. It is not indicated to treat phobias.

Answer E is incorrect. Promethazine is an antipsychotic that is effective in treating paranoia and hallucinations; however, it is not indicated for the treatment of specific phobias.

14. **The correct answer is C.** The patient likely is suffering from anorexia nervosa. *Diagnostic and Statistical Manual of Mental Disorders, Fourth Edition*, Text Revision, criteria for anorexia include a refusal to maintain body weight within a normal weight for age and height (> 15% below ideal body weight). Psychological characteristics of anorexics include a very close relationship with the significant same-sex parent and perfectionist attitudes. Anorectics also exhibit intense fear of gaining weight and a severely distorted body image. Patients who are suffering from severe malnutrition due to self-starvation often have bradycardia, hypotension, hypothermia, skin dryness, and lanugo (downy hair seen on the trunk and extremities).

Answer A is incorrect. Most laboratory values tend to remain normal in patients with eating disorders until late in their disorder following severe dietary restriction. Elevated lipase and amylase are more likely indicators of pancreatitis than a sign of a specific eating disorder.

Answer B is incorrect. Tattoos and piercings used to be a weak clinical indicator of antisocial personality disorder. In today's world, they indicate almost nothing about the person. They certainly are not an indicator of anorexia nervosa.

Answer D is incorrect. Salivary gland hypertrophy, dental enamel erosion, and Russell's sign (scars and calluses on the back of the hand) are signs that the patient purges food to stay thin. Not all anorectics engage in this behavior. These signs would be a stronger clinical indicator of bulimia.

Answer E is incorrect. Scars on the wrists, which might indicate self-injurious behavior or suicidal behavior, might be seen in anorexia. However, they are not specific for the disorder.

15. **The correct answer is C.** The girl has Tourette's syndrome, which is characterized by motor and vocal tics. Tourette's is also associated with obsessive-compulsive symptoms such as stacking a deck of cards repeatedly. In terms of pharmacotherapy, the drugs of choice for Tourette's syndrome are haloperidol, pimozide, and clonidine; haloperidol has the most benign adverse-effect profile of the three.

Answer A is incorrect. Buspirone is used to treat anxiety disorders, not Tourette's syndrome.

Answer B is incorrect. Diazepam is a benzodiazepine, which is not used for medical management of Tourette's syndrome.

Answer D is incorrect. Sertraline is an SSRI used to treat depressive disorders, not Tourette's syndrome.

Answer E is incorrect. Valproic acid can be used for many disorders such as seizure disorders and bipolar disorder. However, it is not indicated for the treatment of Tourette's syndrome.

16. **The correct answer is C.** Core features of frontal lobe dementias include insidious onset, gradual progression, and an early decline in social and interpersonal conduct. Emotional blunting and apathy also occur early without insight. There is a marked decline in personal hygiene, as well as significant distractibility and motor impersistence (failure to maintain a motor activity). In the types of frontal dementia associated with aphasia, language is affected more significantly than personality. Frontal lobe dementias may also cause patients to be apathetic when medial frontal damage occurs and disinhibited when basal-frontal dysfunction predominates. Social withdrawal and behavioral disinhibition may precede the onset of dementia by several years. In patients whose frontal lobe dementia primarily affects frontal language, loss of spontaneity of speech is often the first noticeable symptom.

Answer A is incorrect. In Alzheimer's dementia, a subjective sense of memory loss appears first, followed by loss of memory detail and temporal relationships. All areas of memory function deteriorate, including encoding, retrieval, and consolidation. Patients forget landmarks in their lives less often than other events. Agnosia (failure to recognize or identify objects), aphasia (language disturbance), and apraxia occur later; however, a mild amnestic aphasia may be an early finding. Later, patients with Alzheimer's disease become passive, coarse, and less spontaneous. The patient does not seem to have memory problems as a signif-

icant aspect of his presentation, making this diagnosis less likely.

Answer B is incorrect. It is often difficult to differentiate between the anhedonia seen in depression and the apathy seen with degeneration of the frontal lobe. Clues to the diagnosis of frontotemporal dementia are lack of depressive symptoms such as guilt and suicidal ideation. Additionally, the patient's signs of disinhibition make the diagnosis of frontotemporal dementia more likely.

Answer D is incorrect. Patients with Lewy body disease present similarly to those with Alzheimer's, but with more of a fluctuating cognitive impairment that affects memory and higher cortical functions. These patients may present with unexplained delirium. Associated features include visual or auditory hallucinations, mild extrapyramidal signs, or repeated and unexplained falls.

Answer E is incorrect. Patients with subcortical dementias have a diagnosed disorder of deeper brain structures in the presence of a relatively unaffected cerebral cortex. The principal features of subcortical dementias include slowed mentation, impairment of executive function, recall abnormalities, and visuospatial disturbances. Subcortical dementias may occur in Parkinson's disease, Huntington's disease, and progressive supranuclear palsy, and in inflammatory, infectious, vascular, and demyelinating illness. This patient does not have any of the prerequisite disorders for subcortical dementia.

17. **The correct answer is A.** Amitriptyline is a tricyclic antidepressant used to treat major depression as well as in the treatment of neuropathic pain. It is associated with primarily anticholinergic adverse effects, sedation, sexual dysfunction, and arrhythmias. It can be lethal in overdose, causing coma, convulsions, and cardiac arrhythmias. Overdose is treated with intravenous fluids for hypotension, sodium bicarbonate if the QRS interval is > 100 msec for cardioprotection, and α-adrenergic vasopressors if refractory.

Answer B is incorrect. Bupropion is a heterocyclic antidepressant used in treatment of depression as well as for smoking cessation. Its most typical adverse effects include headache, dry mouth, insomnia, and dizziness, but it can also cause stimulant effects, aggravation of psychosis, and seizures. The medication is contraindicated in patients with known seizure disorder or in those with anorexia nervosa or bulimia nervosa (due to increase in seizures).

Answer C is incorrect. Fluoxetine is an SSRI used in the treatment of depression, obsessive-compulsive disorder, bulimia nervosa, panic disorder without agoraphobia, and premenstrual dysphoric disorder. Adverse effects include decreased libido, insomnia, headache, anxiety, nervousness, nausea, diarrhea, anorexia, dry mouth, weakness, and tremor. It is relatively safe in overdose, but when used in conjunction with monoamine oxidase inhibitors can cause serotonin syndrome (fever, myoclonus, cardiovascular collapse, and mental status changes).

Answer D is incorrect. Lithium is used in the therapy of bipolar disorder, particularly treatment and prophylaxis of bipolar disorder. Adverse effects include electrolyte abnormalities, diabetes insipidus, leukocytosis secondary to demargination, and hypothyroidism. It has a narrow therapeutic range, so levels are checked often. In overdose, patients may have confusion and seizures.

Answer E is incorrect. Phenelzine is a monoamine oxidase inhibitor used in the treatment of depression, especially atypical depression. Common adverse effects include orthostasis and sexual dysfunction, but when combined with tyramine-containing foods (in addition to some over-the-counter cold medications), can cause hypertensive crisis. When used in conjunction with other antidepressant medications (e.g., SSRIs), it can cause the serotonin syndrome, which includes symptoms of confusion, tremor, myoclonus, hyperthermia, sinus tachycardia (not a widened QRS complex), and dilated pupils.

18. **The correct answer is C.** This child is showing secure attachment style. The child's behavior, especially toward the parent upon reunion, is indicative of the quality of the overall parent-child attachment. Children who are distressed when the mother leaves and happy at her return are showing secure attachment.

Answer A is incorrect. Children with anxious attachment are extremely depressed when their mother departs. The child will be ambivalent when she returns, seeking to remain close to the mother but resentful, and resistant when the mother initiates attention.

Answer B is incorrect. Attachment disorder occurs in children who fail to develop secure attachment to loving, protective caregivers. These children are left without an important foundation for healthy development and may develop emotional, behavioral, social, and developmental problems. This child is displaying normal secure attachment; therefore, the child's behavior does not suggest an attachment disorder.

Answer D is incorrect. Stranger anxiety occurs between 6 months and 2 years of age, and it is a normal part of development. It reflects preferential attachment to the mother over other possible attachment figures. Stranger anxiety would be reflected if the child began crying when being handled by strangers and if he or she was then soothed by the mother. This anxiety is not what is demonstrated.

Answer E is incorrect. Symbolism-based behavior occurs during Piaget's preoperational stage of cognitive development. Examples of this behavior include using a transitional object, such as a blanket, to represent a parent. The preoperational stage lasts from about 2 to 7 years of age. The symbolic thinking permits more flexibility and planning in parent-child problem solving during this stage.

19. **The correct answer is B.** Cognitive-behavioral psychotherapy holds that the best way to treat mental illness is to focus on the cognitions that lead to negative emotions. The prototypical example is a patient who is depressed because of negative cognitions, such as feeling "I'm worthless." Cognitive-behavioral therapy states that one should attempt to consciously rephrase those statements, saying, "Wait, why would I be more worthless than anyone else? I may feel that, but it just isn't true." Then the patient rephrases the statement as "I'm as wor-

thy as anyone else." Though the patient may not believe it at first, the thoughts will begin to reinforce themselves.

Answer A is incorrect. Behavioral therapy uses the principles of classical conditioning or operant conditioning to address change at the behavioral level. It does not focus on thoughts.

Answer C is incorrect. Freudian psychotherapy holds that there is a personal unconscious that motivates our behavior. Research has demonstrated that emotional memory is formed through the amygdala pathway during the first 3 years of life, even though our hippocampus (our conscious memory) is not working during those 3 years. Thus, there is an unconscious (emotional memory) of which we are not aware. Freudian psychotherapy attempts to uncover the patterns and assumptions we make about other people based on these early emotional memories.

Answer D is incorrect. Interpersonal psychotherapy focuses on a person's individual life events and transitions. Its major foci include interpersonal disputes, role transitions, grief, and interpersonal deficits. It attempts to examine interpersonal disputes to see how intractable they really are, to examine old and new roles, to examine the relationship between the deceased and the patient during times of grief, and to look at the components of interpersonal deficits. Communication and thought processes are only considered in the context of the aforementioned foci of interpersonal therapy.

Answer E is incorrect. Jungian psychotherapy differs from freudian psychoanalysis in stating that in addition to the personal unconscious, there is a collective unconscious. This collective unconscious is inherent in all human beings. It is a genetic model for how we perceive things, such as our parents and our loved ones. Jungian psychotherapy holds that these collective symbols are expressed in myth and religion. Jung felt that the best way to get in touch with our collective unconscious is through dreams and art. Thus his therapy had a creative focus.

20. The correct answer is E. Sleep apnea is characterized by interrupted breathing of 20 sec-

onds or more during sleep, and it may be classified as central, obstructive, or mixed. The most common of these is obstructive sleep apnea, in which the patient has an intermittent upper airway obstruction. Often this airway obstruction is from the accumulation of fat on the sides of the upper airway, which causes the airway to become narrow and predisposed to closure when the muscles relax. Obese patients are more prone to this phenomenon. Patients may complain of snoring, morning headaches, dry mouth on awakening, or gasping during sleep. They may also have depressed mood, impaired concentration, impotence, and personality changes. Patients suffering from obstructive sleep apnea are at increased risk of pulmonary hypertension, right-sided heart failure, stroke, myocardial infarction, and sudden death. Primary treatment for patients with sleep apnea is weight loss and nasal continuous positive airway pressure.

Answer A is incorrect. Narcolepsy, which may be treated with methylphenidate, is classically associated with uncontrollable sleep attacks in which the patient abruptly falls asleep in inappropriate, embarrassing, and even dangerous situations. Examples include falling asleep while eating, driving, and having intercourse. Most narcoleptics experience related symptoms, including cataplexy (sudden loss of muscle tone), hypnagogic hallucinations (dream-like experiences while falling asleep but not yet asleep), and sleep paralysis (brief paralysis associated with the onset of sleep or wakefulness). However, only 10–15% of narcoleptic patients will have all four classic symptoms.

Answer B is incorrect. Modafinil, a non-amphetamine stimulant, is also used to treat narcolepsy. It would not be recommended in sleep apnea.

Answer C is incorrect. Although the patient does complain of vague depressive symptoms, he states that he is not feeling guilty, is not having suicidal ideation, and is still able to enjoy his favorite hobby. Moreover, a patient with depression can present with insomnia or hypersomnia, but this patient reports neither symptom. Rather, he is having difficulty staying awake during the day. This patient would not meet the *Diagnostic and Statistical Manual of Mental Disorders*, Fourth Edition, Text Revision, criteria for depression, which requires at least five of the following symptoms to be present in any 2-week period: depressed mood, anhedonia, change in appetite, insomnia or hypersomnia, psychomotor agitation or retardation, fatigue, feelings of worthlessness, diminished ability to think or concentrate, or recurrent thoughts of death/suicidal ideation. Thus, an antidepressant would not be the first treatment option.

Answer D is incorrect. Hypothyroidism can certainly cause weight gain and fatigue, along with depressed mood. Morning headache, however, is more characteristic of obstructive sleep apnea. Moreover, the patient does not have other manifestations of hypothyroidism such as muscle weakness, change in skin or hair, muscle cramps, or constipation.

21. **The correct answer is B.** The child most likely has separation anxiety disorder, which is developmentally inappropriate and excessive anxiety concerning separation from home or from those to whom the individual is attached. This can take the form of recurrent distress when separated, excessive worry about harm befalling attachment figures, and repeated nightmares with themes of separation.

    Answer A is incorrect. There is no evidence that the baby-sitter is abusing this child. However, a high index of suspicion is always necessary. Police data suggest that roughly 7000 to 8000 baby-sitter offenses—the majority of which are sex crimes—are reported to police over the course of a year.

    Answer C is incorrect. Generalized anxiety disorder in children involves excessive anxiety and worry about a number of events or activities such as school performance, social relations, or clothes, which causes significant impairment or distress. It is manifested by somatic symptoms, self-consciousness, and social inhibition. In this child, the distress seems to revolve around separation, as opposed to other aspects of life.

    Answer D is incorrect. In 2001, child protective service agencies investigated more than 3.25 million reports of child abuse and neglect in the United States. This is an increase of 2% from the previous year. Teachers, law enforcement officers, social service workers, and physicians made 56% of the reports. In this case, however, there is no evidence that the child has been abused. Thus, further studies, such as bone imaging, to ascertain abuse are not necessary.

    Answer E is incorrect. The child is likely experiencing symptoms of nausea caused by the significant distress of physical separation, which is common in separation anxiety. This conclusion can be drawn from the fact that the patient has no physical complaints when the child is with his parents, and the child has no abdominal tenderness. If this child had physical symptoms, a more complete gastrointestinal physical workup would be indicated.

22. **The correct answer is A.** Grapefruit juice is a potent inhibitor of the cytochrome P450 (CYP450) isoenzyme system, which metabolizes many tricyclic antidepressants. This inhibition likely increased the effective dose of the patient's amitriptyline. Other substrates of this system include clozapine, propranolol, warfarin, theophylline, and tacrine. Other inhibitors of the CYP450 system include fluvoxamine and quinolones. Inducers of CYP450 enzymes include omeprazole, phenobarbital, phenytoin, nicotine, and charcoal-broiled meat.

    Answer B is incorrect. Decreased metabolism of propranolol might result from consumption of grapefruit juice, which leads to decreased metabolism of propranolol. Decreased levels of propranolol would likely lead to increased heart rates and/or blood pressure, as opposed to QT prolongation.

    Answer C is incorrect. Donepezil does not interact to any appreciable degree with the cytochrome P450 system.

    Answer D is incorrect. Both warfarin and amitriptyline are metabolized by the cytochrome P450 system, but neither inhibits the system.

    Answer E is incorrect. There is presently no known drug interaction between donepezil and warfarin.

23. **The correct answer is B.** In humans, discontinuation of cocaine leads to dysphoria (a so-called crash). Hypersomnolence and anergia are also common, along with increased appetite.

Answer A is incorrect. Cocaine's physiologic action is a blockade of norepinephrine and dopamine reuptake in the brain. Due to the noradrenergic blockade, patients intoxicated with cocaine will likely have tachycardia, hypertension, dilated pupils, and hyperthermia. The dopaminergic reuptake blockade is responsible for hallucinations, particularly formication (the feeling of insects crawling under the skin), and increased sexual arousal. The increased dopamine in the nigrostriatal pathway may also cause stereotyped movements and an increase in motor activity.

Answer C is incorrect. The characteristic pharmacologic action of opioids is analgesia. Opioids, at lower doses, may have a behaviorally disinhibiting effect, which presents as impaired judgment and social functioning. They are, however, sedating at higher dosages due to factors such as respiratory depression. Other major features of intoxication are feelings of euphoria or dysphoria, facial flushing, and pupil constriction.

Answer D is incorrect. Opioid withdrawal may cause depression; however, it also causes many other prominent symptoms that are not present in this case. Autonomic symptoms are typically characteristic of opioid withdrawal. These include goose flesh, tachycardia, and increased blood pressure. Musculoskeletal symptoms, such as joint and muscle aches, are also extremely characteristic of opioid withdrawal.

Answer E is incorrect. Typical depression is usually characterized by a decrease in both appetite and sleep. Atypical depression, however, may be characterized by an increase in these neurovegetative functions, as opposed to a decrease.

24. **The correct answer is C.** Childhood disintegrative disorder is a disorder of early childhood and usually presents prior to age 10 years. Patients generally have normal psychosocial development during the first 2 years of their lives and then begin to regress. Areas of dysfunction can include language, social play, bowel or bladder control, and motor skills.

Answer A is incorrect. Asperger's syndrome is characterized by impaired social functioning, although it is not usually as severe as in autism. Patients can have stereotyped behaviors and may persevere in an activity for hours on end.

Answer B is incorrect. Autism is characterized by marked impairment in communication and social interactions. Patients may also exhibit repetitive or stereotyped behavior, hobbies, or interests. Many patients also have mental retardation. Patients do not have a normal phase of development, as shown in this history.

Answer D is incorrect. Fragile X is a syndrome that occurs in male patients and is associated with mental retardation, macroorchidism, and large ears.

Answer E is incorrect. Rett's disorder, which the patient does not have, is a genetic neurodegenerative disease found only in female patients. Patients have normal physical, mental, and social development until about the age of 5 months and then begin to regress in development. Language and coordination are the most common functions that are adversely affected.

25. **The correct answer is E.** X-ray of the chest demonstrates numerous fractures of the ribs, as indicated by the arrows. Shaken baby syndrome is a group of findings secondary to violent shaking in children which occurs most commonly in infants, but may occur in children as old as 4 years. These findings include subdural hematoma and possible subarachnoid bleeding (not as common), occult fractures (21–53%, especially posterior rib or long bone fractures), and retinal hemorrhages (50–100%). Other signs may include vomiting, anorexia, irritability, seizures, and lethargy. On physical examination, apnea, bradycardia, hypothermia, bulging fontanelles, bruises, nystagmus, and decreased reactivity of the pupils may be present secondary to head trauma.

Answer A is incorrect. Intracranial hemorrhage may occur with coagulation disorders. Other manifestations including ecchymoses, hematomas, or hemarthroses are usually present. Retinal hemorrhages are rare and if present, are usually at the posterior pole.

Answer B is incorrect. Glutaric aciduria is a metabolic condition caused by a deficiency in riboflavin-dependent glutaryl-CoA dehydrogenase, resulting in an increase in glutaric acid and 3-hydroxyglutaric acid in urine. In contrast to shaken baby syndrome victims, skeletal abnormalities are not observed in patients with glutaric aciduria type 1, but macrocephaly and acute encephalopathic crises are observed.

Answer C is incorrect. Intracranial aneurysms are often asymptomatic until they rupture, resulting in subarachnoid hemorrhage. Less commonly, intracranial aneurysms may manifest with headache, loss of visual acuity, facial pain, and cranial nerve palsies. If the intracranial aneurysm ruptures, a severe headache results. Loss of consciousness, seizure, nausea, and nuchal rigidity may also occur.

Answer D is incorrect. Meningitis results from intracranial infection that causes inflammation of the meninges. It typically presents with fever, headache, nuchal rigidity, photophobia, nausea, and/or seizures.

26. **The correct answer is C.** The patient has antisocial personality disorder, which is characterized by deceitfulness, aggressiveness, and irritability, as exhibited by repeated physical fights, impulsiveness, and a reckless disregard for his own and others' safety. However, to be diagnosed with antisocial personality disorder, the patient also has to have had conduct disorder, which is the childhood precursor to antisocial personality disorder that occurs before age 15 years. Criteria for conduct disorder include cruelty to people and animals, destruction of property, deceitfulness or theft, and serious violation of parental rules.

Answer A is incorrect. The patient currently has antisocial personality disorder, but he would not have been diagnosed with this as a child because it is only diagnosed in adults. In many cases, children with conduct disorder go on to develop antisocial personality disorder.

Answer B is incorrect. The patient is impulsive, which could indicate manic episodes. However, the patient has a significant history of repeated fighting as a child and adult, making conduct disorder and subsequent antisocial personality disorder a more likely diagnosis.

Answer D is incorrect. Although children with depression may often be agitated and unhappy, leading to an increased incidence of school fights, his current antisocial behavior makes childhood depression a less likely diagnosis.

Answer E is incorrect. Children with conduct disorder often abuse substances. However, there is no evidence that this is the case.

27. **The correct answer is A.** The *Diagnostic and Statistical Manual of Mental Disorders*, Fourth Edition, Text Revision, defines dependence as a maladaptive pattern of substance use leading to clinically significant impairment or distress, as manifested by three or more of the following occurring at any time in the same 12-month period: tolerance; withdrawal; taking the substance in larger amounts or over a longer period than was intended; persistent but unsuccessful efforts to cut down; spending a great deal of time in obtaining, using, or recovering from the substance; stopping of important activities because of substance use; or continuing the use despite knowledge of the problem. In this case, the presence of several attempts to stop would be indicative of dependence.

Answer B is incorrect. The use of alcohol in the face of legal ramifications indicates alcohol abuse, not dependence.

Answer C is incorrect. The failure to fulfill role obligations at work indicates alcohol abuse, not dependence.

Answer D is incorrect. The presence of social/interpersonal problems indicates alcohol abuse, not dependence.

Answer E is incorrect. The *Diagnostic and Statistical Manual of Mental Disorders* defines alcohol abuse as a maladaptive pattern of substance use leading to clinically significant impairment or distress, as manifested by one (or more) of the following, occurring within a 12-month period: recurrent substance use resulting in failure to fulfill major role obligations;

recurrent substance use in situations in which it is physically hazardous; recurrent substance-related legal problems; and/or continued substance use despite having persistent or recurrent social or interpersonal problems. In this case, the recurrent use of alcohol while driving indicates abuse, not dependence.

28. **The correct answer is A.** Somatization disorder is a chronic psychiatric condition that typically presents with a long-standing history of unsubstantiated medical complaints of pain in at least four sites, including two gastrointestinal symptoms, one sexual symptom, and one neurologic symptom. Patients with somatization disorder do not produce their symptoms intentionally and do not realize any gain from them. Referral to a psychiatrist is an important component of treatment, since behavioral and cognitive techniques can help such patients express their emotional needs in a more constructive way. Once the disorder is identified, it is important for the medical team to minimize inappropriate medical interventions. This patient exhibits some classic symptoms of narcolepsy, including cataplexy and sleep paralysis. Methylphenidate is an amphetamine derivative that is used to treat attention-deficit/hyperactivity disorder and narcolepsy.

    Answer B is incorrect. "La belle indifférence" refers to the lack of concern that many patients with conversion disorder exhibit with regard to their condition. Conversion disorder is characterized by the sudden loss of an aspect of physical functioning, often secondary to acute psychological distress. It is monosymptomatic and almost always involves a single motor or sensory symptom.

    Answer C is incorrect. A "textbook presentation" points more to a factitious disorder than to a somatization disorder, as the latter is often characterized by vague and indistinct complaints. Patients with factitious disorders consciously feign symptoms to be in the "sick role." Although they consciously fake symptoms, their motivation is unconscious. In factitious disorder, there is no obvious secondary gain such as money, drugs, or avoidance of work. Patients with malingering are seeking secondary gains.

    Answer D is incorrect. Pleasure and satisfaction derived from an offer of a medical hospitalization points more toward a factitious disorder than to a somatization disorder. Factitious disorders result when a patient feigns or induces a medical condition in order to receive some form of secondary gain.

    Answer E is incorrect. Patients with somatization disorder often lack insight and are highly offended if it is implied that their symptoms are psychological in nature.

29. **The correct answer is D.** This patient has gender identity disorder. Early psychological therapy to help the person focus on his or her biological gender role can result in less transsexual behavior in the future. However, adults with persistent gender identity disorder may seek sex change surgery.

    Answer A is incorrect. Alprazolam is a benzodiazepine. Medication is not a recommended part of the treatment for gender identity disorder. However, it may be used to treat comorbid anxiety and depression.

    Answer B is incorrect. Hormone therapy would be useful if the patient were going to have gender reassignment. It would not be appropriate while a young patient is receiving psychotherapy.

    Answer C is incorrect. Paroxetine is a SSRI. Medication is not a recommended part of the treatment for gender identity disorder. However, it may be used to treat comorbid anxiety and depression.

    Answer E is incorrect. Gender reassignment may be appropriate later in life for persistent gender identity disorder. It would not be appropriate until psychotherapeutic prevention has been attempted.

30. **The correct answer is C.** One of the most important things to remember when interviewing a suicidal patient is that patients may tend to minimize their own symptoms, expressing a denial of what they were really hoping to accomplish. However, all aspects of the patient's suicide attempt, any previous suicide attempts, and the meaning behind the current crisis must all be explored. These questions will en-

able the interviewer to learn more about the patient, her feelings, and what is currently happening in her life that led to this event.

Answer A is incorrect. If the patient is psychotic, then appropriate medications should be initiated; however, the details of her suicide attempt must be elicited first.

Answer B is incorrect. Although a good psychiatric history is important, in the acute setting it is more important to address the sincerity of the patient's suicide attempt, and evaluate whether she is still a danger to herself.

Answer D is incorrect. Any patient who is a danger to herself should be hospitalized, but to do so without an understanding of her actions would not be appropriate.

Answer E is incorrect. Although it is important to address substance abuse as a contributor to any suicide attempt, the details of the suicide and plan are more important in the acute setting.

31. **The correct answer is A.** The patient presents with symptoms of diabetes mellitus after treatment with an atypical antipsychotic (olanzapine). Hyperglycemia, diabetes mellitus, and acute-onset diabetic ketoacidosis have been reported with atypical antipsychotics, especially olanzapine and clozapine. The most appropriate next step in management of this patient would be to discontinue olanzapine.

Answer B is incorrect. Valproic acid has many adverse effects including gastrointestinal effects, tremors, weight gain, and hepatotoxicity. Diabetes has not been associated with valproic acid (although rare cases of pancreatitis have).

Answer C is incorrect. Olanzapine has been linked with acute-onset ketoacidosis, therefore immediate attention is required and monitoring blood sugars would not be an appropriate next step in management of this patient.

Answer D is incorrect. Olanzapine has been linked with acute-onset ketoacidosis, therefore immediate attention is required and diet and exercise alone would not be appropriate.

Answer E is incorrect. In this clinical scenario, the onset of diabetes is correlated with use of an atypical antipsychotic medication and therefore discontinuation of the offending agent altogether will most likely stop symptoms of diabetes. Oral hypoglycemics would be indicated for long-term therapy of non-drug associated type 2 diabetes.

32. **The correct answer is C.** The patient displays many of the characteristics and feelings that are seen in borderline personality disorder. These patients often have childhoods that are characterized by inconsistent parenting and often a significant amount of abuse. The parents may not reinforce the validity of the patient's inner feelings. The patients tend to divide people into all good or all bad categories, a well-known phenomenon termed splitting. They often have chronic feelings of emptiness and have many relationships that are labile in nature. Borderline patients have severe trouble regulating their emotions, as seen when the patient could not control her own anger at the therapist, and are therefore very impulsive.

Answer A is incorrect. The patient does not show a consistent disregard for the rules of society and the rights of others, which is characteristic of antisocial personality disorder.

Answer B is incorrect. The patient does not discuss being extremely afraid of situations that may result in interpersonal rejection, a key characteristic of avoidant personality disorder.

Answer D is incorrect. Although the patient displays shallow emotions, a characteristic of histrionic personality disorder, she also displays splitting, impulsivity, and volatile characteristics more indicative of a borderline personality disorder. Histrionic personality disorder is characterized by a pervasive pattern of excessive emotionality and attention seeking.

Answer E is incorrect. The patient does not exhibit grandiosity in her self-perception, making narcissistic personality disorder less likely.

33. **The correct answer is E.** This patient is exhibiting many signs of self-induced vomiting. The bicarbonate level is high, consistent with a metabolic alkalosis. She has parotid gland swelling, dental pitting, and Russell's sign (the metacarpophalangeal calluses caused by teeth

rubbing against the joint during vomiting). She is orthostatic, and her blood urea nitrogen and creatinine levels are indicative of hypovolemia. Increased serum amylase can be seen with prolonged vomiting. Her fatigue and dizziness are most likely secondary to dehydration and the possible electrolyte abnormalities (e.g., low potassium) associated with chronic vomiting. The mother is not aware of any abnormal eating patterns or chronic vomiting, consistent with the patient concealing her behaviors, which is often seen in bulimia nervosa.

Answer A is incorrect. Acute pancreatitis is characterized by the abrupt onset of pain in the epigastric region radiating to the back, usually caused by alcoholism or gallstones. This patient does not have any abdominal pain, thereby reducing the likelihood of pancreatitis. She does have an elevated amylase, but the lipase is normal; this abnormality is most likely secondary to chronic vomiting, not pancreatitis.

Answer B is incorrect. Acute renal failure is defined as an abrupt decrease in renal function leading to the retention of creatinine and blood urea nitrogen (BUN). Acute renal failure can be caused by prerenal causes such as hypovolemia. Although the BUN in this case is elevated, the creatinine is normal. Thus, the etiology of these laboratory abnormalities is not acute renal failure.

Answer C is incorrect. Although sustained vomiting can lead to electrolyte abnormalities such as hypokalemia, which can lead to arrhythmias, this patient's dizziness is much more attributable to volume loss. It would not, however, be unreasonable to obtain an ECG to evaluate her cardiac function.

Answer D is incorrect. Respiratory acidosis can be caused by carbon dioxide retention secondary to airway obstruction or chronic obstructive pulmonary disease. This woman has an increased bicarbonate, which could be due to renal compensation for a respiratory acidosis. However, based on her normal respiratory/pulmonary examination and normal oxygen saturation, there does not seem to be any primary pulmonary process. The increased bi-

carbonate level is most likely due to a primary metabolic alkalosis.

34. **The correct answer is D.** There are many different types of psychotherapy, each of which has its unique advantages and disadvantages. This therapy is psychoanalysis, in which the psychiatrist plays a neutral role, listening for any connections in what the patient says. The patient speaks freely, a technique called "free association," in which whatever is on the patient's mind is of psychoanalytic interest. Dreams, and their subsequent analysis, can also play a large role in psychoanalysis, which may give the therapist more clues to valuable connections in the patient's life. Clarification, confrontation, and interpretation are also used in this modality.

Answer A is incorrect. Behavioral therapy, sometimes closely linked to cognitive therapy in cognitive-behavior therapy, is based on the hypothesis that all human behavior grows out of conditioned reactions from childhood and that all psychopathology is the result of inappropriate conditioning from childhood. Behavior therapy is best suited for patients with a circumscribed disorder, such as anxiety, and not disorders that are long term or chronic. The focus of therapy is to lessen the anxiety associated with a particular situation or behavior and to gradually teach relaxation techniques when faced with the problematic environment.

Answer B is incorrect. Cognitive therapy, developed for mild to moderate depression and dysthymia, relies on the theory that there is a close link between a person's habits or patterns of conscious thought and that person's moods, and that certain thoughts can cause and/or maintain a person's depressed mood. The goal of therapy is to have the patient actively identify his or her negative thoughts and then change the content of those thoughts to reflect a more positive view of him- or herself.

Answer C is incorrect. Interpersonal therapy was developed in response to the theory that depression is a defect in interpersonal relations. The patient describes in detail his or her relationships to other people in his or her life, and deficiencies in relationships are examined. The patient is encouraged to become more aware of his or her own feelings toward others, and he or she becomes more able to express feelings and communicate freely.

Answer E is incorrect. The goal of supportive therapy is to support the patient at his or her highest level of functioning. The therapist provides a warm, empathetic environment that should be seen as a reliable source of support and help. Supportive therapy is used in response to an acute event ("crisis intervention"), in the case of a patient with long-term chronic medical problems, or for chronic psychiatric patients (e.g., with schizophrenia) that cannot make use of other types of therapies.

35. **The correct answer is A.** Catatonia is an alteration in neuromuscular tone that occurs as part of many psychiatric disorders, including schizophrenia, mania, depression, and anxiety, and as part of certain neurologic disorders. Symptoms include negativism (resistance to following directions), mutism (paucity of speech), echopraxia (repetition of movements made by another person), waxy flexibility (when the patient can be moved and molded into strange body positions that he or she will maintain), paratonia (involuntary resistance to passive movement), and stereotyped mannerisms.

Answer B is incorrect. Dystonias are involuntary movements of the agonist/antagonist muscles in a given area of the body. Examples include neck muscle dystonia (retrocollis/torticollis) and extraocular muscles (oculogyric crisis). These movement disorders result from dopamine antagonism in the nigrostriatal dopamine pathways of the basal ganglia. Dystonia is a known adverse effect of typical neuroleptics such as haloperidol. Although the patient is taking haloperidol, she does not exhibit dystonic symptoms.

Answer C is incorrect. Mental retardation might include cognitive symptoms such as echolalia, but would not be likely to include the motor component mentioned.

Answer D is incorrect. Neuroleptic malignant syndrome is a rare, idiosyncratic but life-threatening reaction to antipsychotics that causes lead pipe rigidity; autonomic symptoms,

including diaphoresis, high fever, hypertension, and increased heart rate; and neurologic dysfunction.

Answer E is incorrect. Serotonin syndrome occurs from hyperstimulation of 5-HT$_{1a}$ receptors, often as a result of interaction between monoamine oxidase inhibitors or typical neuroleptics and SSRIs. The classic triad of symptoms that characterizes serotonin syndrome includes altered mental status with significant restlessness, autonomic dysfunction, and neuromuscular abnormalities. Autonomic symptoms include nausea, vomiting, and hyperthermia, while neuromuscular abnormalities include myoclonus, nystagmus, hyperreflexia, and lower extremity rigidity.

36. **The correct answer is E.** Oppositional defiant disorder (ODD) is a persistent pattern of hostile, defiant behavior toward authorities that persists for more than 6 months. Symptoms are seen in multiple settings, such as home and school. To diagnose ODD, the behavior must be frequent and consistent when compared with other children of the same age and development status, and when the disruptive nature of the behavior causes a significant degree of impaired social and school functioning.

Answer A is incorrect. Antisocial personality disorder is a persistent pattern of behavior with a central theme of disrespect for the rights of others. Patients may exhibit milder signs and/or be diagnosed with conduct disorder during adolescence but are diagnosed with this disorder only after the age of 18.

Answer B is incorrect. Attention deficit disorder is a disorder of inattention and impaired ability to focus on given tasks. Patients can be hyperactive and become easily bored because they are frustrated by their limitations. But this patient is predominantly negative and hostile toward authority figures.

Answer C is incorrect. Conduct disorder may have a similar presentation to oppositional defiant disorder; however, conduct disorder is characterized by violence and a consistent disregard for the property and well-being of others. Patients may have engaged in theft, assault, and injury of animals or small children.

Answer D is incorrect. Normal adolescents are prone to confrontation and arguments while trying to assert their independence. This patient's behavior, however, is impairing his school and home functioning. He appears to have a disregard for authority and an intentional defiance of all rules and regulations

37. **The correct answer is E.** Lithium is typically used to treat bipolar disorders. Chronic lithium use can cause nephrogenic diabetes insipidus by increasing resistance to ADH. The drug accumulates in the collecting tubule cells and interferes with ADH function. The other answer choices are mechanisms of central diabetes insipidus.

Answer A is incorrect. Decreased ADH release causes central diabetes insipidus and occurs in a variety of disorders. It may be a complication following neurosurgery or trauma but is not the cause of lithium-related diabetes insipidus.

Answer B is incorrect. Destruction of ADH-releasing cells occurs in idiopathic central diabetes, most likely through an autoimmune mechanism.

Answer C is incorrect. Increased ADH catabolism is the mechanism of central diabetes insipidus that can occur in pregnancy.

Answer D is incorrect. This would lead to the exact opposite effect, as well as decreased thirst and urine volume. Lithium toxicity is believed to cause a decrease in density of ADH receptors.

38. **The correct answer is E.** It would appear that this patient is suffering from factitious disorder. The serologic profile of a patient injecting exogenous insulin is characterized by low C-peptide levels because the production of the endogenous insulin is suppressed along with C-peptide by-product levels. Antibodies are also produced against the exogenous insulin. Given that this patient has prior medical knowledge, it must be assumed that he administered the medication to himself-a behavior that is consistent with factitious disorder. Patients with factitious disorder simulate physical or psychiatric illness in order to gain attention from medical personnel and often have an extensive history of prior surgeries and hospitalizations. A psychiatric consultation should be called before any other medical interventions are initiated.

Answer A is incorrect. This patient has a psychiatric condition that warrants evaluation. However, a CT scan would be helpful if an insulinoma was suspected. An insulinoma would cause low blood glucose levels, but C-peptide would be high, as it is a by-product of endogenous insulin.

Answer B is incorrect. Endoscopy is used to visualize the gastrointestinal tract in order to evaluate for pathology within the gastrointestinal system, including malignancy, ulcers, or inflammatory conditions. This patient's low blood sugar is better explained by a psychiatric condition, and thus psychiatric evaluation is the most appropriate step in management at this time.

Answer C is incorrect. Dialysis would be indicated if this patient's low sugar was due to a metabolic abnormality such as acidosis (pH < 7.1), abnormal electrolytes (K^+ > 6.5 mEq/L or rapidly rising), intoxication (e.g., lithium or aspirin), volume overload, or uremia with related pericarditis, neuropathy, or unexplained decline in mental status.

Answer D is incorrect. Insulin therapy would be appropriate in a patient with diabetes and high blood sugar levels. However, this patient already has dangerously low blood sugar due to inappropriate use of insulin.

Questions 39–41

39. **The correct answer is L.** This patient is exhibiting classic signs of opiate overdose, which include depressed respiration, constricted pupils, somnolence, and eventually coma. Treatment is with naloxone, an opiate antagonist.

40. **The correct answer is I.** This patient is exhibiting signs of cocaine intoxication, as shown by his sympathetic arousal and exuberant mood. Haloperidol is the appropriate treatment for an agitated or psychotic substance-abusing patient. It should be noted that while

the same symptoms can be seen in amphetamine intoxication, the treatment would be the same for any severe agitation.

41. **The correct answer is C.** This patient is experiencing delirium tremens (DT), a consequence of alcohol withdrawal that usually appears 2–7 days after a patient stops drinking. DT is characterized by tachycardia, hypertension, diaphoresis, confusion, hallucinations (especially tactile), and tremors. The main treatment is with benzodiazepines.

Answer A is incorrect. Activated charcoal is a nonspecific binding substance that is used to clear the gastrointestinal tract of substances that have not yet been absorbed. It would be used in the setting of ingestion of salicylates, barbiturates, theophylline, and the like.

Answer B is incorrect. Atropine is the antidote for anticholinesterases and organophosphates such as pesticides.

Answer D is incorrect. Deferoxamine is the treatment for an iron overdose.

Answer E is incorrect. Dialysis is used to clear the blood of substances for which no other remedy is known (e.g., salicylates and barbiturates) and is used only as a last-line therapy.

Answer F is incorrect. Dimercaprol is used to treat overdoses of heavy metals such as lead, arsenic, mercury, and gold.

Answer G is incorrect. Flumazenil is used to treat an overdose of benzodiazepines.

Answer H is incorrect. Glucagon is used to treat an overdose of β-blockers.

Answer J is incorrect. Hyperbaric oxygen treatment is used for carbon monoxide exposure.

Answer K is incorrect. N-acetylcysteine is the antidote for acetaminophen overdose.

Answer M is incorrect. Vitamin K is used to reverse the effects of a warfarin overdose.

Questions 42–44

42. **The correct answer is E.** Clozapine is an antipsychotic medication that improves the negative symptoms of schizophrenia but can cause agranulocytosis in 1–2% of patients taking it. As a result, patients must agree to a weekly blood draw to check WBC count throughout therapy and for 4 weeks after stopping the drug. Agranulocytosis is an absolute contraindication for continuing the drug.

43. **The correct answer is J.** Olanzapine is an atypical antipsychotic associated with increased triglycerides, somnolence, hyperglycemia, and weight gain. The drug itself is particularly effective for negative symptoms of schizophrenia and for agitation.

44. **The correct answer is H.** In approximately 10% of patients, lamotrigine causes a skin rash. Development of this potentially life-threatening rash is associated with rapid increase in the drug dosage. Development of any type of rash is an absolute contraindication for continuation of lamotrigine.

Answer A is incorrect. Amitriptyline is a tricyclic antidepressant used to treat major depression and in the treatment of neuropathic pain. It is associated with primarily anticholinergic adverse effects, sedation, sexual dysfunction, and arrhythmias. It can be lethal in overdose, causing coma, convulsions, and cardiac arrhythmias.

Answer B is incorrect. Buspirone is an effective anxiolytic that does not promote dependence or tolerance. Its most common adverse effect is dizziness.

Answer C is incorrect. Clonazepam is a benzodiazepine used in the treatment of anxiety (especially for the immediate relief of anxiety symptoms) and panic disorder, and as an adjunct treatment of some seizures. Its adverse effects include ataxia, confusion, memory disturbances, drowsiness, and somnolence.

Answer D is incorrect. Clonidine is a centrally acting adrenergic agonist that inhibits the sympathetic nervous system via central α_2-adrenergic receptors. In psychiatry, it can be used in the treatment of attention deficit/hyperactivity disorder, and in targeting anxiety and hyperarousal in posttraumatic stress disorder.

Answer F is incorrect. Fluoxetine is a SSRI used in the treatment of depression, obsessive-compulsive disorder, bulimia nervosa, panic disorder without agoraphobia, and premenstrual dysphoric disorder. Adverse effects include decreased libido, insomnia, headache, anxiety, nervousness, nausea, diarrhea, anorexia, dry mouth, weakness, and tremor.

Answer G is incorrect. Haloperidol is a high-potency typical antipsychotic medication that is associated with more extrapyramidal symptoms (EPS) than the low-potency agents (e.g., chlorpromazine). Typical antipsychotics in general can cause EPS, hyperprolactinemia, anticholinergic effects, and sedation, and are more associated with neuroleptic malignant syndrome than are atypical antipsychotics.

Answer I is incorrect. Lithium is used in the therapy of bipolar disorder, particularly treatment and prophylaxis of bipolar disorder. Adverse effects include electrolyte abnormalities, diabetes insipidus, leukocytosis secondary to demargination, and hypothyroidism.

Answer K is incorrect. Reserpine is an antihypertensive medication that is also used in the treatment of agitated psychotic states (eg, schizophrenia) and in management of tardive dyskinesia. It acts by depletion of sympathetic biogenic amines (e.g., norepinephrine and dopamine). Adverse effects include sedation and dizziness.

Answer L is incorrect. Risperidone is an atypical antipsychotic medication. Adverse effects include extrapyramidal adverse effects, insomnia, agitation, anxiety, headache, and weight gain.

Answer M is incorrect. Sertraline is an SSRI used in treating major depressive disorder. Adverse effects include insomnia/somnolence, dizziness, headache, dry mouth, and sexual adverse effects (e.g., ejaculatory disturbances).

Answer N is incorrect. Topiramate is an anticonvulsant and mood stabilizer. Adverse effects include weight loss, anorexia, psychomotor slowing, memory difficulties, difficulty concentrating, nausea, drop in serum bicarbonate, and paresthesias.

Answer O is incorrect. Valproic acid is a mood stabilizer that can cause thrombocytopenia and bleeding, in addition to hepatic failure, pancreatitis, and hyperammonemia; it is also considered a teratogen.

Answer P is incorrect. Venlafaxine is a serotonin norepinephrine reuptake inhibitor. Its adverse effects include central nervous system effects (headache, insomnia/somnolence, dizziness, and nervousness), gastrointestinal effects (nausea, dry mouth, constipation, and anorexia), genitourinary effects (abnormal ejaculation or orgasm), weakness, and diaphoresis and hypertension.

Questions 45–47

45. **The correct answer is N.** Social phobia results in a disabling sense of anxiety in situations in which the patient is expected to perform or will be scrutinized by others, as in this scenario. It can severely impact the life of the patient, from office presentations to talking to unfamiliar people. It can be treated with antidepressants and benzodiazepines; some patients respond to a presituational β-blocker aimed at minimizing somatic complaints.

46. **The correct answer is B.** Brief psychotic disorder is the development of psychotic symptoms (usually auditory hallucinations) occurring in the setting of a psychosocial stressor (e.g., the loss of a loved one). For the diagnosis to apply, it must resolve within 1 month. In comparison to the other psychotic diagnoses, it has a much better prognosis.

47. **The correct answer is D.** Patients with cyclothymia alternate between hypomania and dysthymia. The mood swings are much more frequent than in bipolar disorder, but the "highs" (hypomanic episodes) are not as pronounced and the "lows" (dysthymic episodes) are less debilitating. Many patients are aware of feeling chronically depressed, without recognizing their own hypomanic episodes.

Answer A is incorrect. Patients with antisocial personality disorder have been termed *sociopaths*; they violate the rights of others, the law, and social norms. They are impulsive, and they lack remorse for their behavior.

Answer C is incorrect. Usually related to some psychosocial trauma, conversion disorder presents with a motor or sensory dysfunction (blindness, paralysis, or seizure) that is incompatible with any known medical diagnosis.

Answer E is incorrect. The diagnosis of generalized anxiety disorder (GAD) depends on duration of symptoms for more than 6 months and at least three somatic symptoms for the same time period. It is not uncommon to see patients with GAD self-medicate with benzodiazepines or alcohol. The treatment for GAD is usually with a SSRI or other anxiolytic (e.g., buspirone).

Answer F is incorrect. Narcolepsy is a disease in which the patient falls asleep suddenly; these sleeping episodes (both normal and narcoleptic) begin with rapid eye movement sleep. Treatment is usually with stimulants (e.g., amphetamines).

Answer G is incorrect. The diagnosis of obsessive-compulsive disorder requires the presence of both obsessions and compulsions. The treatment of obsessive-compulsive disorder is usually a combination of cognitive-behavioral therapy or psychodynamic therapy and either clomipramine or an SSRI such as fluoxetine.

Answer H is incorrect. Oppositional defiant disorder is a pattern of negativistic, defiant, disobedient, and hostile behavior toward authority figures for more than 6 months that is mostly diagnosed in adolescence (before age 18). However, the patient does not violate social norms or the rights of others (as in antisocial personality disorder). The treatment involves both individual and family therapy.

Answer I is incorrect. Patients with panic disorder experience abrupt onset "attacks," consisting of several somatic symptoms and a feeling of impending doom. These attacks can be brought on by particular environments (e.g., agoraphobia).

Answer J is incorrect. Posttraumatic stress disorder (PTSD) is characterized by symptoms resulting from an extremely traumatic stressor (assault, active combat, or witnessing a violent event). The patient relives the event via nightmares and flashbacks, experiences a state of increased arousal (hypervigilance and exaggerated startle), and tends to avoid stimuli associated with the event. The syndrome is also marked by psychic numbing (detachment, social withdrawal, and anhedonia). In addition to supportive and cognitive-behavioral therapy, SSRIs can be helpful in the treatment of PTSD.

Answer K is incorrect. Rett's syndrome is a genetic neurodegenerative disorder of women with progressive developmental impairment after approximately 5 months of normal development.

Answer L is incorrect. The most important feature of schizoaffective disorder is the presence of mood symptoms (depression, mania, or mixed) in conjunction with psychotic symptoms. However, the psychotic symptoms must then continue for at least 2 weeks after the resolution of the mood symptoms.

Answer M is incorrect. Patients with schizophrenia must have two or more of the following for at least 6 months: hallucinations, delusions, disorganized speech, affective flattening, alogia, and avolition. To be classified in the paranoid subtype, patients must have delusions or hallucinations, but cognitive function and affect are relatively preserved. Of all the subtypes of schizophrenia, this one has the best prognosis.

Answer O is incorrect. Tourette's disorder is characterized by multiple vocal and motor tics occurring many times per day. It is more common in men, is known to have a genetic predisposition, and usually begins in the teenage years. Treatment is usually with haloperidol, pimozide, or clonidine, and psychological counseling can help with social adjustment.

Questions 48–50

48. **The correct answer is B.** Akathisia is a feeling of restlessness (either subjective or objective), or "not being able to sit still." It is considered an extrapyramidal adverse effect and is associated with the use of many antipsychotic medications, especially the typical antipsychotics. It can be treated with β-blockade and by decreasing the dosage of the antipsychotic med-

ication. Benzodiazepines and anticholinergics (as in the treatment of other extrapyramidal symptoms) may also help.

49. **The correct answer is A.** Agoraphobia is defined by the *Diagnostic and Statistical Manual of Mental Disorders*, Fourth Edition, Text Revision, as "anxiety about being in places or situations from which escape might be difficult (or embarrassing) or in which help may not be available in the event of having an unexpected or situationally predisposed panic attack or panic-like symptoms." This young woman's symptoms are consistent with panic disorder with agoraphobia, which occurs in 30–50% of all patients with panic disorder.

50. **The correct answer is G.** Echolalia is the immediate and involuntary repetition of words or phrases just spoken by others. It can be seen in autism and many forms of schizophrenia.

Answer C is incorrect. Anhedonia is the complete loss of pleasure in activities, people, or things that were previously pleasurable. For example, a person with major depression may no longer enjoy baseball games, which he or she had once followed religiously.

Answer D is incorrect. Ataxia is loss of coordination, most commonly due to disturbance in the cerebellum or neuronal pathways leading into and out of the cerebellum.

Answer E is incorrect. Catatonic schizophrenia is marked by at least two of the following: excessive motor activity, immobility, extreme negativism, mutism, waxy flexibility, echolalia (repeating another's words), or echopraxia (mimicking another's movements). Although the patient in the second vignette displays echolalia, he only has one symptom of catatonia and therefore could not be diagnosed with catatonic schizophrenia based on this presentation.

Answer F is incorrect. Compulsions are conscious, repeated acts or behaviors that are uncontrollable. In obsessive-compulsive disorder, compulsions are done to neutralize the anxiety invoked by an obsession.

Answer H is incorrect. Delirium is defined as a disturbance of consciousness or a waxing and waning of normal levels of consciousness. It can be experienced as confusion, disorientation, cognitive impairment, or inability to concentrate. Delirium can be due to many different etiologies, including structural damage to the brain, infection, metabolic disorders, drugs, neoplasms, and autoimmune conditions.

Answer I is incorrect. Delusions are disorders of thought content. Subtypes of delusions include paranoid, persecutory, bizarre, somatic, grandiose, or referential. They are based on incorrect perceptions that do not stem from a social or cultural belief system (e.g., religious beliefs).

Answer J is incorrect. Dyskinesia is also known as pseudoparkinsonism, or the shuffling gait and cogwheel rigidity seen in both parkinsonism and as an adverse effect of many antipsychotic medications (especially the typical antipsychotics). It can be remedied with anticholinergics (e.g., benztropine) or dopamine agonists (e.g., amantadine).

Answer K is incorrect. Dysthymia is a milder form of major depression, consisting of at least 2 years of depressed mood with effects on eating, sleeping, energy level, self-esteem, difficulty concentrating, or feelings of hopelessness.

Answer L is incorrect. Flight of ideas is a rapid flow of thought, manifested by accelerated speech with abrupt changes from topic to topic, often a characteristic of the thought pattern of patients with mania.

Answer M is incorrect. Grandiosity is an inflated self-esteem and feeling of entitlement that may be seen in mania. A person with bipolar disorder may believe that nothing can stop him or her from getting what he or she wants, and the person may become extremely agitated or irritated if obstructed.

Answer N is incorrect. Hypochondriasis is the preoccupation with or fear of having a serious medical illness despite adequate medical reassurance.

Answer O is incorrect. Obsessions are persistent, intrusive ideas, thoughts, impulses, or images that cause anxiety or stress. Common obsessions are contamination and fear of harm to oneself. The patient experiences obsessions as inappropriate thoughts or impulses from his or her own mind (as opposed to thought insertion, which is experienced as coming from the outside). In obsessive-compulsive disorder, obsessions are neutralized or prevented by compulsions.

Answer P is incorrect. *Somatization* is the term applied to the experience of multiple, unexplainable somatic symptoms that are not due to any medical condition or to the effects of a drug. The symptoms are not produced intentionally, and the patients are unaware of having any psychiatric problems. Symptoms are often related to pain at many different anatomic sites (most commonly, the back, the joints, and the abdomen).

CHAPTER 14

Pulmonary

1. A 78-year-old man is seen in the doctor's office for a nonproductive cough, 9-kg (20-lb) unintentional weight loss, and bilateral breast enlargement, all occurring within the past 6 months. He has smoked two packs per day for the past 40 years. His past medical history is otherwise unremarkable, and he takes no medications. His temperature is 36.7°C (98.1°F), blood pressure is 125/85 mm Hg, pulse is 68/min and regular, respiratory rate is 15/min, and oxygen saturation is 99% on room air. There are crackles at the left lower lung field and a ridge of symmetric glandular tissue (1 cm in diameter) around the nipple-areolar complexes of both breasts. Complete blood cell count shows a WBC count of 6000/mm³ hemoglobin of 14.7 g/dL, and platelet count of 210,000/mm³. All other laboratory results are normal. X-ray of the chest shows a focal 5-cm mass lesion in the left lower lung corroborated by CT scan. Which of the following is most likely histologic type of lung cancer present in this patient?

(A) Adenocarcinoma
(B) Bronchoalveolar cell carcinoma
(C) Large cell carcinoma
(D) Small cell carcinoma
(E) Squamous cell carcinoma

2. A 30-year-old patient with a history of mild persistent asthma (baseline peak expiratory flow rate of 85%) presents to the emergency department (ED) with shortness of breath and wheezing not relieved by her albuterol inhaler for the past 12 hours. She was able to tolerate pulmonary function tests and a set was performed. Which of the following is the most likely test result?

(A) Decreased FEV_1, normal/increased FVC, decreased FEV_1:FVC ratio, with post-bronchodilator FEV_1 increased by 13%
(B) Decreased residual volume and total lung capacity
(C) Increased FEV_1, increased FVC, normal FEV_1:FVC ratio

(D) Increased residual volume, increased total lung capacity, increased FEV_1
(E) Normal FEV_1, decreased FVC, increased FEV_1:FVC ratio

3. A 3-year-old boy presents to the ED with a fever and difficulty breathing. He is the product of a normal pregnancy. He has been healthy since birth, and his immunizations are up to date. This morning he appeared to be in his usual state of health and was dropped off at day care by his father. Later on, his teacher noticed that he had suddenly become fussy and flushed, and could not be consoled with toys, rocking, or hearing a story. He also felt warm to the touch and was drooling more than usual. When she took his temperature, it was 39°C (102.2°F). His parents were contacted immediately, and the patient was brought to the ED. He appears toxic and anxious, and has loud labored breathing. He is sitting upright, bracing himself on his arms, with his neck hyperextended and mouth open. His temperature is 40°C (104°F), respiratory rate is 50/min, pulse is 140/min, and blood pressure is 102/62 mm Hg. Oxygen saturation is 100% on room air. Lateral x-ray of the neck is shown in the image. Laryngoscopy reveals a large cherry-red epiglottitis. What is the most appropriate next step in management?

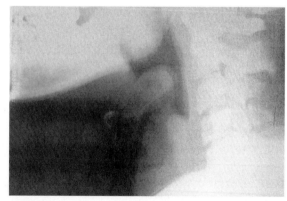

Reproduced, with permission, from Stone CK, Humphries RL. *Current Emergency Diagnosis & Treatment.* New York: McGraw-Hill, 2004: Figure 48-4.

(A) Antibiotic therapy
(B) Corticosteroids
(C) Nasotracheal intubation
(D) Observation
(E) Tracheostomy

4. A 27-year-old woman is 7 months pregnant with her first child. Her pregnancy has been uncomplicated to date. She presents to the ED complaining of sudden-onset, right-sided chest pain that is exacerbated with deep breathing, and shortness of breath, which began 1 hour ago. She denies leg pain, and says the swelling that is apparent has been unchanged since the sixth month of her pregnancy. Her temperature is 37.9°C (100.3°F), blood pressure is 130/87 mm Hg, pulse is 107/min and regular, respiratory rate is 24/min, and oxygen saturation is 90% on room air, increasing to 98% with 4 L oxygen via nasal cannula. Physical examination is significant for crackles at the lower right lung field and a negative Homans' sign bilaterally. X-ray of the chest appears normal, D-dimer is elevated, and ECG shows sinus tachycardia, right-axis deviation, S wave in lead I, Q wave in lead III, and an inverted T wave in lead III. Which of the following is the most appropriate next step in diagnosis?

(A) Arterial blood gas analysis
(B) Lower extremity Doppler ultrasound
(C) MRI
(D) Pulmonary angiography
(E) Ventilation/perfusion scan

5. A 65-year-old smoker previously diagnosed with chronic obstructive pulmonary disease presents to the ED complaining of worsening cough and sputum production. She reports feeling breathless when climbing the stairs to her first floor walk-up apartment, and has moderate difficulty in providing her history in complete sentences. In the ED, x-ray of the chest shows hyperinflated lungs with flattened diaphragms, attenuated vascular markings, and a narrow mediastinum. What agent(s) will provide the greatest relief of symptoms in the ED?

(A) Antibiotics
(B) Magnesium sulfate
(C) N-acetylcysteine
(D) Salmeterol and ipratropium bromide
(E) Theophylline

6. After an uncomplicated pregnancy and cesarean section for breech presentation, twins are born at 32 weeks' gestation to a 24-year-old primigravida mother. Twin A weighs 1610 g (3.5 lb) and has Apgar scores of 8 and 9 at 1 and 5 minutes, respectively. Twin B weighs 1600 g (3.5 lb) and has Apgar scores of 7 and 8 at 1 and 5 minutes, respectively. Within minutes of birth, twin B becomes mildly cyanotic and tachypneic with subcostal retractions, expiratory grunting, and nasal flaring. Twin B's blood pressure is 58/39 mm Hg, heart rate is 130/min, respiratory rate is 100/min, and temperature is 37.0°C (98.6°F). Twin B is intubated and given 70% fraction of inspired oxygen. Compared to twin A, what is twin B at greater risk of developing?

(A) Apnea of prematurity
(B) Gastroesophageal reflux disease
(C) Hyperbilirubinemia
(D) No difference because they are both premature
(E) Retinopathy of prematurity

7. A 32-year-old white man with HIV and a recent CD4+ count of 400/mm³ presents to the ED with a 3-day history of fever, anorexia, cough, and night sweats. He recently returned from a camping vacation in Arizona, approximately 1 month prior to presentation. He also describes diffuse joint pains. On physical examination, his temperature is 38.9°C (102°F), his oxygen saturation is 99% on room air, and there is a rash on his arms and hands. There is dullness to percussion at the right lung base. X-ray of the chest reveals a small right-sided infiltrate and hilar lymphadenopathy. Sputum analysis does not reveal any organisms. He reportedly had a negative purified protein derivative test 2 months ago. Which is the most likely diagnosis?

(A) Coccidioidomycosis
(B) Histoplasmosis
(C) Lung carcinoma
(D) Pneumocystis jiroveci (formerly carinii) pneumonia
(E) Sarcoidosis
(F) Tuberculosis

8. A 55-year-old man was admitted to the hospital 2 weeks ago for rapid onset of cough, fatigue, and pleuritic chest pain. He has worked as a sandblaster for the past year. When first seen in the hospital, he denied hemoptysis and smoking. Currently, the patient is intubated and on assist-control ventilation. His temperature is 36.7°C (98°F), pulse is 96/min, blood pressure is 138/85 mm Hg, and respiratory rate is 18/min. A recent arterial blood gas study showed a pH of 7.42, partial pressure of arterial carbon dioxide of 36 mm Hg, and partial pressure of arterial oxygen of 110 mm Hg while on 100% fraction of inspired oxygen. Physical examination is significant for diffuse crackles throughout both lung fields, a loud pulmonic component of the second heart sound, and jugular venous distention of 9 cm with a prominent A wave, a left parasternal heave, and symmetric 3+ lower extremity pitting edema. Which of the following is the correct diagnosis?

(A) Asbestosis
(B) Berylliosis
(C) Byssinosis
(D) Coal worker's pneumoconiosis
(E) Silicosis

9. A 45-year-old Haitian immigrant presents to the ED with a chief complaint of productive, blood-tinged cough for 2 months. He has been in the United States for 1 month. His temperature is 40.1°C (104.2°F), and his heart rate is 105/min. On physical examination, he appears cachectic, and pulmonary rales are heard throughout his lung fields. X-ray of the chest reveals multiple bilateral upper lobe cavitary lesions with associated intrathoracic adenopathy. Sputum culture is pending. Which of the following tuberculosis medications can potentially cause optic neuritis?

(A) Ethambutol
(B) Isoniazid
(C) Levofloxacin
(D) Pyrazinamide
(E) Rifampin
(F) Streptomycin

10. A 30-year-old man has episodes of wheezing and shortness of breath two to three times per week. Approximately every 2 weeks he awakens at night due to cough and difficulties breathing. He reports having similar symptoms since he was a child, but believes that they are worsening somewhat now. His symptoms are worsened by cold air and exercise and are improved by rest. What is the most appropriate treatment for this patient?

(A) Daily high-dose inhaled corticosteroid and β-agonist when needed
(B) Daily high-dose inhaled corticosteroid with oral steroids for exacerbations and short-acting β-agonist when needed
(C) Daily low-dose inhaled corticosteroid and short-acting β-agonist when needed
(D) Daily oral steroids and long-acting β-agonist
(E) Short-acting β-agonist when needed

11. A 38-year-old man is being seen in his physician's office after being involved in a car accident. He now has a vague pain along his right sternal border, where he crashed into the steering wheel. On examination, his temperature is 36.6°C (97.8°F), pulse is 80/min, blood pressure is 123/75 mm Hg, respiratory rate is 14/min, and oxygen saturation is 99% on room air. Physical examination is significant for point tenderness over the right sternal border. An x-ray of the chest shows no broken ribs but a single, well-circumscribed pulmonary nodule, 1.5 cm in diameter, located in the left lower lung field. A search through the patient's electronic medical file reveals that he had an x-ray of the chest taken 2 years ago. The radiology report from that time reveals that the nodule was only 0.75 cm in diameter. To characterize the lesion, a CT scan of the chest is performed and shows "popcorn" calcification within the lesion. Which of the following risk factors most increases the chances of malignancy?

(A) Discrete border
(B) Doubling time
(C) Nodule diameter of 1.5 cm
(D) Patient age
(E) "Popcorn" calcification

12. A 27-year-old white woman comes to the ED with a 2-week history of shortness of breath,

nonproductive cough, fever, and chills. Her past medical history is significant for intravenous drug abuse, with her last use 6 years ago. She also gets frequent vaginal yeast infections, which persist despite treatment with over-the-counter metronidazole. The patient denies sick contacts, tobacco use or exposure to other irritants, and recent travel. On physical examination, the patient is a sick-appearing young woman with tachypnea and an oxygen saturation of 91% on 3 L of oxygen by nasal cannula. X-ray of the chest is shown in the image. What does this patient's x-ray of the chest show?

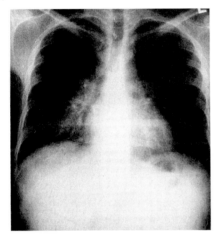

Reproduced, with permission, from Hall JB, Schmidt GA, Wood LDH. *Principles of Critical Care*, 3rd edition. New York: McGraw-Hill, 2005: Figure 48-1.

(A) Bilateral enlarged hilar lymphadenopathy
(B) Diffuse ground-glass infiltrates
(C) Hyperinflation
(D) Localized air-fluid level in 2-cm left upper lobe lesion
(E) Normal x-ray of the chest

13. A 30-year-old woman presents to her physician's office with 3 months of nonproductive cough, exertional dyspnea, fatigue, malaise, and blurred vision. She denies weight loss, fever, chills, sweats, recent travel, or sick contacts. She works on the assembly line of an electronics plant. Vital signs are unremarkable. Physical examination reveals she has tender red papules over her shins. The patient said she first noticed the bumps when she changed oral contraceptive pills (her only medication), but assumed they would disappear. X-ray of the chest shows bilateral hilar lymphadenopathy with pulmonary infiltrates. Laboratory tests show:

WBC count	5600/mm^3
Hemoglobin	14.3 g/dL
Platelet count	300,000/mm^3
Na$^+$	140 mEq/L
K$^+$	4.2 mEq/L
Cl$^-$	108 mEq/L
Ca^{2+}	16 mg/dL
CO$_2$	24 mmol/L
Blood urea nitrogen	10 mg/dL
Creatinine	1.0 mg/dL

Culture of bronchoalveloar lavage fluid is negative. Which of the following is the most likely diagnosis?

(A) Berylliosis
(B) Fungal infection
(C) Lymphoma
(D) Sarcoidosis
(E) Tuberculosis

14. A 30-year-old man presents to the resuscitation bay with gunshot wounds in the anterior and posterior left chest. Although in distress and dyspneic, the patient is cooperative. He has a patent airway and is moving all extremities. His pulse is 120/min, blood pressure is 120/90 mm Hg, and respiratory rate is 30/min. He has bounding distal pulses, and no other injuries are identified on secondary examination. X-ray of the chest reveals fluid in the pleural space, and a left chest tube thoracostomy yields 600 mL of bright red fluid. Over the next hour, 750 mL of blood is collected. What is the most appropriate next step in management?

(A) Autotransfuse with the collected blood and continue to observe closely
(B) Insert another chest tube
(C) Left thoracotomy
(D) Remove the chest tube and suture the incision closed
(E) Thoracentesis

15. A 25-year-old man is recovering in the hospital from an open repair of his broken femur, which he suffered during an automobile accident. On postoperative day 3, he develops sudden-onset shortness of breath and vague chest discomfort. His temperature is 37.6°C (99.6°F), heart rate is 108/min, blood pressure is 95/62 mm Hg, respiratory rate is 42/min, and oxygen saturation is 89% on room air. Physical examination is significant for jugular venous distention to 9 cm and an accentuated pulmonic component of the second heart sound. A quantitative plasma D-dimer enzyme-linked immunosorbent assay is elevated at 900 ng/mL. A pulmonary angiogram is shown in the image. Which of the following is most likely to be decreased?

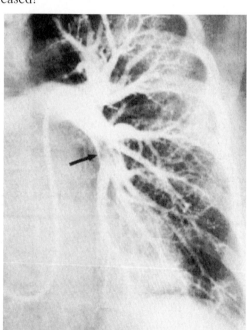

Reprinted, with permission, from Brunicardi FC, Andersen DK, Billiar TR, Dunn DL, Hunter JG, Matthews JB, Pollock RE, Schwartz SI. *Schwartz's Principles of Surgery,* 8th edition. New York: McGraw-Hill, 2005: Figure 23-9.

(A) Airway resistance
(B) Alveolar dead space
(C) Alveolar ventilation
(D) Pulmonary compliance
(E) Pulmonary vascular resistance

16. A 5-year old girl is brought to the ED in December by her mother who complains that her daughter seems confused. The mother reports that her daughter has complained of intermittent headaches since the two of them moved into the first floor of an older apartment building 6 months ago. The mother has been at home with the daughter for the past 24 hours and the girl appears lethargic and is complaining of joint aches, nausea, and a headache. Her pulse is 120/min, blood pressure is 130/85 mm Hg, and respiratory rate is 25/min with an oxygen saturation of 100% by pulse oximeter. The girl's mother also notes having a slight headache that started this past day. Which of the following diagnostics should be most rapidly pursued?

(A) Arterial blood gas
(B) CT scan of the head
(C) Direct laryngoscopy
(D) ECG
(E) Toxicology screen

17. A 33-year-old African-American homeless man presents to the ED with a chief complaint of fever, cough, and malaise. His past medical history is significant for being HIV-positive from previous intravenous drug abuse but records indicate that he has been lost to follow-up for several years. He says he has lost significant weight over the past month. X-ray of the chest reveals intrathoracic lymphadenopathy, right middle lobe consolidation, and a right-sided pleural effusion. Cultures of blood, sputum, and urine are pending. A smear of sputum is positive for acid-fast organisms, but a purified protein derivative test shows no reaction. Laboratory tests show:

WBC count	4200/mm³
Hematocrit	37%
Platelet count	220,000/mm³
CD4+ count	158/mm³
HIV viral load	112,000 copies/mL

Which of the following is the most likely diagnosis?

(A) Cytomegalovirus pneumonitis
(B) *Nocardia* infection
(C) *Mycobacterium avium* complex infection
(D) *Mycobacterium tuberculosis* infection
(E) *Pneumocystis jiroveci* (formerly *carinii*) pneumonia
(F) Pulmonary aspergillosis

18. A 1-year-old child with cerebral palsy secondary to perinatal asphyxia presents to her general pediatrician for a well-child visit. She was delivered at 37 weeks' gestation by emergency cesarean section for a tight nuchal chord. The patient has severe spastic quadriparesis that is limiting her movements. She also has mental retardation and is unable to speak. She has received physical and occupational therapy since early infancy; however, her parents are concerned by her lack of improvement. Which of the following is the best choice for treatment of spasticity in this child?

(A) Baclofen
(B) Botulinum toxin
(C) Carbamazepine
(D) Discontinue physical therapy
(E) Hyperbaric oxygen

19. A 58-year-old man presents to the ED complaining of fever and chills. The fever started last night and has not subsided, even though he took acetaminophen. He had a successful appendectomy 3 days ago and was discharged from the hospital 2 days ago. His only medication is ibuprofen, which is adequately controlling his pain. He is a 30 pack-year smoker with a chronic cough productive of white sputum. He has noticed increased sputum production, which has become yellowish-green. He denies dysuria, urgency, or frequency. His temperature is 38.4°C (101.1°F), heart rate is 88/min, respiratory rate is 16/min, and blood pressure is 126/74 mm Hg. On examination, he appears to be tired but not in acute distress. Pulmonary examination is limited secondary to deep inhalation, causing coughing and slight abdominal pain. There is no tactile fremitus or dullness to percussion. Abdominal examination is significant for a slightly erythematous, appropriately tender healing incision in the right

lower quadrant without exudates and normal active bowel sounds. Extremities are warm and well perfused without erythema or edema. Pulses are intact. Which of the following most likely could have prevented this condition?

(A) Aggressive incentive spirometry
(B) Early removal of the Foley catheter
(C) Early removal of the intravenous catheter
(D) Pre- and postoperative antibiotic prophylaxis
(E) Use of compression stockings and subcutaneous heparin

20. A 20-year-old woman with a history of well-controlled asthma presents to her physician with a 4-week history of shortness of breath, chest tightness, wheezing, and irritating cough. She started working at the local cotton mill at about the same time the symptoms developed. On further questioning, the patient reveals that the symptoms are worse when she first enters the mill, especially after being away over the weekend. Although the symptoms do persist throughout the week, they are not as severe as they are on Mondays. She denies fever, chills, sweats, or exposure to sick persons. She also does not smoke. Her only medication is an albuterol inhaler, which she used sparingly until the development of her current symptoms. Her temperature is 36.7°C (98°F), heart rate is 85/min, blood pressure is 120/80 mm Hg, respiratory rate is 14/min, and oxygen saturation is 99% on room air. Physical examination is unremarkable. X-ray of the chest is normal. Which of the following is the most likely diagnosis?

(A) Byssinosis
(B) Community-acquired pneumonia
(C) Exposure to grain dust
(D) Farmer's lung
(E) Influenza

21. A 35-year-old HIV-positive man (CD4+ count 150/mm^3) is seen in the ED with right-sided chest pain. The patient has become progressively dyspneic over the past few days. Suddenly, 30 minutes ago he noticed a sharp pain in his chest associated with shortness of breath. His temperature is 37.7° (99.9°F), blood pressure is 128/84 mm Hg, pulse is 102/min and regular, respiratory rate is 25/min, and oxygen saturation is 90% on room air. Physical examination reveals diminished right-sided breath sounds and hyperresonance. Jugular venous distention is 5 cm and there is no tracheal deviation. ECG shows sinus tachycardia. X-ray of the chest shows a right-sided pneumothorax occupying approximately 10% of the right thoracic cavity. Which of the following etiologies most likely caused this patient's presentation?

(A) Intravenous drug use
(B) Kaposi's sarcoma
(C) *Mycobacterium tuberculosis*
(D) *Pneumocystis jiroveci* (formerly *carinii*) pneumonia
(E) Toxoplasmosis

22. A 75-year-old man develops increased ventilatory requirements several days after requiring intubation for respiratory failure. X-ray of the chest shows bilateral infiltrates, and based on his ventilatory settings, the ratio of the partial pressure of arterial oxygen to the fraction of inspired oxygen is 190. What is the most common underlying etiology of acute respiratory distress syndrome?

(A) Aspiration of gastric contents
(B) Drug overdose
(C) Lung or bone marrow transplantation
(D) Massive blood transfusion
(E) Near-drowning
(F) Sepsis

23. A 31-year-old G4P3 woman gave birth via repeat cesarean section to a full-term, 3700-gm (8.2-lb) baby girl. There were no complications during the pregnancy or delivery. Two hours after the birth the resident is called to evaluate the baby girl. She is afebrile, but is breathing rapidly with mild subcostal retractions. Breath sounds are equal and clear bilaterally. S1 and S2 are normal and the point of maximal intensity is not displaced. X-ray of the chest reveals a flattened diaphragm, prominent vascular markings, and fluid lines in the fissures. Which of the following is the most likely diagnosis?

(A) Diaphragmatic hernia
(B) Neonatal respiratory distress syndrome
(C) Pulmonary hemorrhage
(D) Pulmonary interstitial emphysema
(E) Transient tachypnea of the newborn

24. A 67-year-old man presents to his primary care physician with complaints of dyspnea on exertion over the past 6 months that has progressively worsened to dyspnea at rest. He denies cough and wheezing and has had no fevers, night sweats, or unintentional weight loss. The physician takes a detailed social history and learns that the man has never smoked and worked as a shipbuilder for over 30 years. Which of the following radiographic findings on x-ray of the chest would confirm the most likely diagnosis?

(A) Bilateral diffuse infiltrates
(B) Bilateral hilar adenopathy
(C) Consolidation of lung tissue
(D) Focal mass with air bronchograms
(E) Multiple pleural plaques with patchy parenchymal opacities

25. A 23-year-old man is seen in the ED for sudden-onset, right-sided pleuritic chest pain that developed 30 minutes ago while he was watching television. The patient also complains of difficulty breathing. He has no prior medical history, denies smoking and intravenous drug use, and does not take any medications. His temperature is 37.3°C (99.1°F), blood pressure is 130/82 mm Hg, pulse is 92/min and regular, respiratory rate is 20/min and shallow, and oxygen saturation is 98% on room air. He is 196 cm (6 ft 5 in) tall with a body mass index of 18 kg/m^2. Diminished breath sounds, hyperresonance, and decreased tactile fremitus are prominent in the right lung field. The trachea is midline. X-ray of the chest shows a 10% pneumothorax on the right. Which of the following is the most appropriate initial management?

(A) Observation with supplemental oxygen
(B) Open thoracotomy with oversewing of the pleural blebs and scarification of the pleura
(C) Needle decompression
(D) Thoracoscopy with stapling of blebs
(E) Tube thoracostomy with doxycycline pleurodesis

26. A 53-year-old man presents to the clinic with complaints of increasing shortness of breath, a nagging cough, and weight loss over several months. He reports no history of cigarette smoking but has worked underground in the New York City subway system for the past 20 years. Spirometry tests are ordered that demonstrate a forced expiratory volume in 1 second:forced vital capacity ratio ($FEV_1:FVC$) of 0.7, and an FEV_1 value that is 60% of expected. The FEV_1 improves to 70% of expected with bronchodilator treatment. Which of the following is the most likely diagnosis?

(A) Asthma
(B) Chronic aspiration
(C) Chronic obstructive pulmonary disease
(D) Histoplasmosis
(E) Tuberculosis

27. A 22-year-old woman with a history of mild persistent asthma comes to the primary care clinic after an ED visit 2 days ago for an acute asthma exacerbation. She notes an increase in frequency of wheezing and shortness of breath for the past 4 months, with daily symptoms, and has been symptomatic for at least 2 nights per week. She has also had three ED visits during the same period. Her current asthma medications include montelukast (leukotriene inhibitor) daily and an albuterol inhaler as needed. The patient's peak flow in the ED is 75% of predicted. What is the next most appropriate step in management of this patient?

(A) Add an inhaled β-adrenergic agonist and low-dose inhaled steroid to the regimen
(B) Add systemic steroids to the regimen
(C) Admit to the hospital for further pulmonary workup

(D) Discontinue the leukotriene inhibitor and change the regimen to daily low-dose inhaled steroids
(E) Start cromolyn sodium

28. A 78-year-old woman is seen in the ED for difficulty breathing and cough over the past 4 hours. She has a history of congestive heart failure for which she takes hydrochlorothiazide, metoprolol, and enalapril. Her oxygen saturation is 92% on room air. On examination there is a high-pitched systolic crescendo-decrescendo murmur best heard at the right upper sternal border with radiation to the carotids, and rales are present in both lung fields on inspiration. There is 2+ symmetrical pitting edema bilaterally in the lower extremities. X-ray of the chest shows an enlarged heart and prominent pulmonary vasculature. Which of the following is the most likely cause of the patient's pulmonary edema?

(A) Decreased capillary fluid oncotic pressure
(B) Decreased interstitial fluid hydrostatic pressure
(C) Increased capillary fluid hydrostatic pressure
(D) Increased capillary permeability
(E) Increased interstitial fluid oncotic pressure

29. A 55-year-old man presents to his physician's office with increasing dyspnea on exertion. He denies chest pain, diaphoresis, nausea, or vomiting. He has been involved in eight motor vehicle accidents in the past 3 years. Past medical history is significant for hypertension, for which he takes a diuretic. His temperature is 37.2°C (99.0°F), blood pressure is 121/82 mm Hg, pulse is 85/min, respiratory rate is 14/min, and oxygen saturation is 99% on room air. Physical examination is significant for diffuse and laterally displaced point of maximal intensity and an S_3 gallop. Which of the following is the most appropriate next step in diagnosis?

(A) Cardiac catheterization
(B) Echocardiogram
(C) Exercise tolerance test
(D) Polysomnography
(E) X-ray of the chest

30. A 74-year-old man presents to his primary care physician complaining of dyspnea and cough with blood-tinged sputum for the past several weeks. He has diabetes and elevated cholesterol. Medications include a sulfonylurea and a statin. The patient has a 50 pack-year smoking history and a family history of hypertension. On examination, vital signs are within normal limits; abdominal striae and moon facies are noted, along with a trucal fat distribution. X-ray of the chest reveals a single central nodule, and follow-up CT again demonstrates the nodule and multiple solid hepatic masses. Which of the following is the most likely diagnosis?

(A) Adenocarcinoma of the lung
(B) Carcinoma metastatic to the lung
(C) Large cell carcinoma of the lung
(D) Small cell carcinoma of the lung
(E) Squamous cell carcinoma of the lung

31. A 21-year-old nonsmoking college student is brought into the local ED with a cough, weight loss, and low-grade fever. Occasionally, his sputum is tinged with blood. X-ray of the chest is shown in the image. He reports traveling to Haiti on a "medical mission" trip several years ago. Which of the following is the most likely diagnosis?

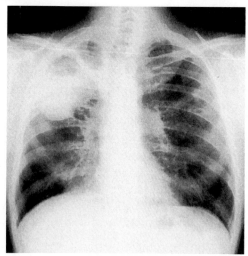

Reproduced, with permission, from Doherty GM, Way LW. *Current Surgical Diagnosis and Treatment*, 12th edition. New York: McGraw-Hill, 2006: Figure 18-19.

(A) Aspergillosis
(B) *Klebsiella* infection
(C) Lung cancer
(D) Sarcoidosis
(E) Tuberculosis

32. A 5-month-old infant has failed to gain weight despite a good appetite. The child's mother reports that the baby has up to eight bulky, foul-smelling, oily stools per day. A sweat chloride test reveals a chloride of 78 mEq/L. Which of the following sequelae is most likely to occur as a result of this patient's disease?

(A) Cirrhosis and subsequent hepatic failure
(B) Dehydration, electrolyte abnormalities, and acute hypotension
(C) Esophageal ulceration or strictures and upper gastrointestinal bleeding
(D) Purple lines on the gums, red-brown discoloration of the urine, and renal tubular acidosis
(E) Recurrent airway disease with eventual respiratory insufficiency associated with bronchiectasis

EXTENDED MATCHING

Questions 33 and 34

For each of the following patients, select the microorganism that is most likely responsible for the infection.

(A) *Actinomyces israelii*
(B) *Aspergillus flavus*
(C) *Blastomyces dermatitidis*
(D) *Candida albicans*
(E) *Cryptococcus neoformans*
(F) *Histoplasma capsulatum*
(G) *Mycobacterium tuberculosis*
(H) *Nocardia asteroides*
(I) *Sporothrix schenckii*

33. A 32-year-old farmer from Mississippi presents with fever and cough. His symptoms are mild and developed gradually. X-ray of the chest shows pulmonary infiltrates. Fungal culture on Sabouraud agar at 25°C yielded nonencapsulated mycelial forms and spores. Blood agar at 37°C yielded yeast forms.

34. A 32-year-old Hispanic immigrant presents to the ED with a nonproductive cough, fevers, night sweats, and anorexia. X-ray of the chest shows cavitary pneumonia and healed granulomas.

Questions 35–37

For each patient with pulmonary edema, select the most likely cause.

  (A) Acute aortic insufficiency
  (B) Acute mitral regurgitation
  (C) Acute respiratory distress syndrome
  (D) Aspiration pneumonia
  (E) Cardiac arrhythmia
  (F) Epidural hemorrhage
  (G) Epileptic seizures
  (H) Myocardial infarction
  (I) Rheumatic heart disease
  (J) Subarachnoid hemorrhage
  (K) Subdural hemorrhage
  (L) Viral meningoencephalitis

35. A 55-year-old man with a history of polycystic kidney disease is on a plane from New York to Los Angeles when he develops a sudden-onset, intensely painful headache, neck stiffness, tactile fever, nausea, and vomiting. After the plane lands the patient is rushed to the local ED, where he complains of shortness of breath in addition to his persistent headache. On examination there is no photophobia, Brudzinski's and Kerning's signs are both negative, and rales are auscultated on inspiration. X-ray of the chest shows a "bat-wing" appearance of the hilar shadows.

36. A 35-year-old woman presents to the ED complaining of shortness of breath that began 3 hours ago while walking to the store and has still not subsided. She reports that she had "a severe bout of some throat infection" as a child, for which she was not treated. She denies a history of asthma or smoking. Her vital signs are normal. On examination there is a low-pitched diastolic rumble audible at the apex and an opening snap.

37. A 22-year-old unresponsive man is transported to the intensive care unit (ICU) after being involved in a motor vehicle accident. The pa-

tient was unrestrained, and his car crashed head-first into a brick wall. He is on assist-control ventilation with a fraction of inspired oxygen of 0.85, partial pressure of oxygen of 90 mm Hg, and oxygen saturation of 94%. Vital signs are otherwise normal. X-ray of the chest taken in the ICU shows interstitial pulmonary edema and bilateral perihilar alveolar edema, producing a characteristic "butterfly" pattern. Noncontrast CT of the head does not reveal intracranial hemorrhage.

Questions 38–40

For each patient with a solitary pulmonary nodule, select the most likely etiology.

  (A) Adenocarcinoma
  (B) Aspergilloma
  (C) Bronchogenic cyst
  (D) Carcinoid lung tumor
  (E) Cavitating abscess
  (F) Coccidioidomycosis
  (G) Hamartoma
  (H) Histoplasmosis
  (I) Lipoma
  (J) *Mycobacterium tuberculosis* infection
  (K) Neurilemmoma
  (L) Pulmonary arteriovenous malformation
  (M) Rheumatoid nodule
  (N) Sarcoidosis
  (O) Squamous cell carcinoma
  (P) Thymoma

38. A 55-year-old unrestrained driver in a motor vehicle collision presents with complaints of tenderness over the right side of his chest. He has no prior medical history and denies a history of smoking. On examination, there is bruising and tenderness over the 8th, 9th, and 10th ribs on the right. Imaging studies are negative for fracture but do reveal a single 1.8-cm pulmonary nodule with a "popcorn" pattern of calcification in the apex of his right lung, within 8 mm of the superior lobar bronchus.

39. A 43-year-old man from the central United States presents with 6 months of productive cough, intermittent night sweats, and 6.8-kg (15-lb) weight loss. He denies a history of smoking or recent travel outside the United States. The patient's last CD4+ count 2 weeks

ago was 900/mm^3. His temperature is 37.8°C (100.0°F); other vital signs and physical examination are unremarkable. X-ray of the chest shows a 2.7-cm lesion in the right upper lung field. Stain and cultures are negative for acid-fast bacilli.

40. A 72-year-old man is seen in the doctor's office for a nonproductive cough and 9-kg (20-lb) unintentional weight loss over the past 4 months. The patient has no past medical history, takes no medications, and denies smoking. His temperature is 36.7°C (98.1°F), blood pressure is 131/84 mm Hg, pulse is 75/min and regular, and respiratory rate is 16/min. Examination is significant for finger clubbing. X-ray of the chest shows a focal 1.8-cm peripheral nodule in the left lower lobe. A CT scan confirms the presence of the 1.8-cm lesion in the left lower lobe that does not invade the visceral pleura or lobar bronchus.

1. **The correct answer is C.** Primary lung cancer is the leading cause of cancer death. The most significant risk factor is smoking because it raises the lifetime relative risk of lung cancer 10- to 30-fold when compared with the lifetime risk of nonsmokers. Patients with lung cancer can present with cough, hemoptysis, chest pain, and unintentional weight loss. Physical examination may reveal crackles or atelectasis. Lung cancer is usually first noted as a nodule on x-ray of the chest but is best defined on CT. Fine-needle aspiration under CT guidance or bronchoscopy with biopsy or brushings can usually establish the histologic diagnosis. Gynecomastia, defined as the benign proliferation of glandular tissue in the male breast and seen clinically as a firm mass extending concentrically from the nipple-areolar complex, is a feature of large cell carcinoma. Large cell carcinoma behaves similarly to poorly differentiated non-small cell lung cancer and may produce β-human chorionic gonadotropin (β-hCG), resulting in gynecomastia, milky nipple discharge, and elevated serum concentrations of plasma β-hCG. Large cell carcinoma of the lung carries a poor prognosis (mean survival time of 7–19 months) and has often metastasized at time of diagnosis.

Answer A is incorrect. Digital clubbing and hypertrophic pulmonary osteoarthropathy can occur with any histologic subtype of lung cancer, but they are most often associated with adenocarcinoma of the lung. Thrombophlebitis and nonbacterial verrucous endocarditis are cardiovascular complications of adenocarcinoma.

Answer B is incorrect. Bronchoalveolar cell carcinoma is a subtype of adenocarcinoma. It is most often associated with multiple nodules on imaging studies, interstitial infiltration, and prolific sputum production.

Answer D is incorrect. A variety of syndromes associated with ectopic hormone production are seen with small cell carcinoma, the subtype of lung cancer highly associated with smoking. These include the syndrome of inappropriate secretion of antidiuretic hormone and the syndrome of ectopic ACTH production.

Answer E is incorrect. The paraneoplastic syndrome associated with squamous cell carcinoma is hypercalcemia, due to the ectopic production of parathyroid hormone–related peptide (PTHrP). Pathologic fractures and kidney stones are also commonly seen as a result of PTHrP production.

2. **The correct answer is A.** Pulmonary function tests measure several different lung volumes that can differentiate obstructive and restrictive lung diseases, including FEV_1 (forced expiratory volume; the amount forcibly exhaled in 1 second), FVC (forced vital capacity; the total volume that can be forcibly exhaled), RV (residual volume; the amount left in the lungs after forced exhalation), and TLC (total lung capacity; the total volume of the lungs after inhalation). In obstructive lung diseases like asthma, lung volumes (TLC and RV) are typically increased, while in restrictive lung diseases like sarcoidosis lung volumes are less than normal. In both obstructive and restrictive disease FEV_1 and FVC are reduced, but in obstructive disease FEV_1 is more dramatically reduced, resulting in a decreased FEV_1:FVC ratio. In hyperresponsive airway obstruction like that seen in asthma, The FEV_1 will improve with bronchodilators.

Answer B is incorrect. RV and TLC are typically normal or increased in asthma due to airway obstruction that leads to air trapping and hyperinflated lungs.

Answer C is incorrect. The forced expiratory volume in 1 second always decreases in asthma exacerbation.

Answer D is incorrect. While increased residual volume and total lung capacity are characteristic of asthma, increased forced expiratory volume in 1 second is not.

Answer E is incorrect. The forced expiratory volume in 1 second always decreases in asthma exacerbation.

3. The correct answer is C. Epiglottitis is a potentially fatal condition that is characterized by high fever, pharyngitis, dyspnea, and rapidly progressing respiratory obstruction. *Staphylococcus aureus*, group A streptococci, *Streptococcus pneumoniae*, *Haemophilus influenzae* type A and nontypeable strains, and *Haemophilus parainfluenzae* are the most common pathogens. *Haemophilus influenzae* type b (Hib) is a less common cause of epiglottitis due to immunization with Hib vaccines. Epiglottitis is a pediatric emergency that often occurs in 2- to 7-year-old children. It typically manifests in a healthy child who has an abrupt onset of fever and sore throat, and then appears toxic with labored breathing and difficulty swallowing within several hours. The child usually drools and keeps his or her neck hyperextended in an attempt to maintain a patent airway. Diagnosis requires visualization of a cherry-red swollen epiglottis by laryngoscopy. Lateral radiographs of the upper airway show the thumb sign with a swollen epiglottis. An artificial airway is created by nasotracheal intubation.

Answer A is incorrect. Appropriate antibiotic therapy should be started that provides coverage against *Staphylococcus aureus*, group A streptococci, *Streptococcus pneumoniae*, and *Haemophilus influenzae*. However, it is more important to secure the patient's airway first.

Answer B is incorrect. Corticosteroids are not indicated in the management of epiglottitis.

Answer D is incorrect. Epiglottitis is a true pediatric emergency. The airway should be secured immediately if epiglottitis is suspected, regardless of the degree of respiratory distress, because 6% of affected children without an artificial airway die.

Answer E is incorrect. Tracheostomy is reserved for cases in which severe epiglottic edema prevents intubation via the nasopharyngeal airway.

4. The correct answer is E. Pregnancy is an independent risk factor for the development of venous thromboembolism (VTE). Studies have shown that the incidence of VTE during pregnancy is approximately 1 in 1500, with the majority of events occurring in the postpartum period, and equal distribution of the remaining VTE events among the three trimesters. The clinical diagnosis of VTE during pregnancy is insensitive and nonspecific because of normal physiologic changes associated with pregnancy. For example, lower extremity swelling and tachypnea are common in normal pregnancies and in pulmonary embolism (PE). Furthermore, tests for D-dimer are of limited diagnostic utility in pregnancy because of the normal elevation of D-dimer in uncomplicated pregnancy. X-ray of the chest may be normal initially but may later show Westermark sign (dilatation of pulmonary vessels and a sharp cutoff), atelectasis, small pleural effusion, and elevated diaphragm. The ECG findings described here are collectively nicknamed the "S1Q3T3 pattern," which is a nonspecific finding encountered in any case of acute cor pulmonale (tension pneumothorax, bronchospasm, or PE). An S1Q3T3 pattern alone is not sufficient for diagnosis of PE. A definitive diagnostic strategy is necessary in pregnant patients suspected of VTE. Ventilation/perfusion lung scanning is currently considered the diagnostic modality of choice in the pregnant population.

Answer A is incorrect. Arterial blood gases are neither sensitive nor specific with regard to the diagnosis of PE. If an arterial blood gas were performed, respiratory alkalosis would be a common finding because it is a feature of both pregnancy and PE. Similar to the nonpregnant population, a normal partial pressure of carbon dioxide, partial pressure of oxygen, and arterial-alveolar gradient are common with PE.

Answer B is incorrect. If the patient is stable and has a nondiagnostic ventilation/perfusion scan, lower extremity Doppler ultrasound is a reasonable test to document deep vein thrombosis (DVT). Because treatments for DVT and submassive PE are the same, identification of DVT is sufficient to terminate the workup of PE.

Answer C is incorrect. MRI is a modality that can detect thigh and pelvic DVT in the nonpregnant population with a sensitivity approaching 100%. Comparable studies have not been performed in the pregnant population. Furthermore, although no birth defects have been attributed to MRI, studies of safety have not been adequate to date. CT and ventilation/perfusion scanning are superior to MRI in the evaluation of lung vasculature in cases of suspected pulmonary embolism.

Answer D is incorrect. Pulmonary angiography is the most specific examination employed to diagnose pulmonary embolism (PE), and may be used in patients with a high clinical pretest probability of PE, but a low- or intermediate-probability ventilation/perfusion scan and negative lower extremity ultrasound. Thus, pulmonary angiography should only be used after these tests have been tried. It can detect emboli as small as 1–2 mm.

5. **The correct answer is D.** This patient has chronic obstructive pulmonary disease (COPD). Exacerbations of COPD are often treated with an anticholinergic agent (ipratropium bromide) plus a β-agonist (a short-acting one such as albuterol or a long-acting β-agonist such as salmeterol if administration of the short-acting agent is required too frequently). While asthma is a possible diagnosis, this patient's age, history of smoking, and previous diagnosis of COPD make COPD exacerbation more likely. In asthma exacerbations, intravenous steroids are first-line therapy, whereas in COPD exacerbations, anticholinergic agents are first-line therapy.

Answer A is incorrect. Infections are responsible for > 50% of exacerbations, whether they be viral or bacterial, and in the setting of a history of a change or increase in sputum, it is recommended to treat empirically for bronchitis/pneumonia even without an infiltrate on x-ray of the chest. However, in the emergency department setting, a β-agonist, an anticholinergic agent, and supplemental oxygen would provide faster symptomatic relief.

Answer B is incorrect. Magnesium sulfate has a bronchodilating effect that may be of benefit in asthma. Its use should be reserved for life-threatening bronchospasm that is refractory to all other interventions.

Answer C is incorrect. N-acetylcysteine may be used for its mucolytic/antioxidant properties, but again, in the acute setting, a combination of a β-agonist, an anticholinergic agent,

and supplemental oxygen would provide faster symptomatic relief.

Answer E is incorrect. A methylxanthine like theophylline may be added in addition to the β-agonist and anticholinergic agent to produce modest improvements in expiratory flow rates, vital capacity, and arterial oxygen and carbon dioxide levels in patients with moderate to severe COPD. However, it would not be used alone as a first-line agent in an acute COPD exacerbation. In addition, serum levels should be monitored in an attempt to minimize toxicity. Nausea, tachycardia, and tremor are reported side effects.

6. **The correct answer is E.** Given both the symptoms and time course, twin B has developed respiratory distress syndrome (RDS). RDS and treatment with oxygen exposure and mechanical ventilation predispose to retinopathy of prematurity. RDS and its treatment also predispose to bronchopulmonary dysplasia (also referred to as chronic lung disease), persistent patent ductus arteriosus, interventricular hemorrhage, and necrotizing enterocolitis.

Answer A is incorrect. Both twins are equally likely to develop apnea of prematurity because they are equally premature.

Answer B is incorrect. Both twins are at slightly increased risk of developing gastroesophageal reflux disease because they are premature.

Answer C is incorrect. Both twins are at risk of hyperbilirubinemia because they are premature.

Answer D is incorrect. The development of RDS places the affected infant at a much higher risk for developing certain complications specifically associated with RDS and its treatments.

7. **The correct answer is A.** Coccidioidomycosis, which is caused by a soil-dwelling fungus, is a pulmonary infection endemic to the southwestern United States. The incubation period can be from 1–4 weeks after exposure, but it typically presents 10–14 days after exposure. Patients with lymphoma or AIDS, patients of Filipino, Native American, Mexican, or African-

American descent, and pregnant women can often progress to the disseminated form which can be fatal. Skin rashes can be part of the presentation, including toxic erythema, erythema nodosum, and erythema multiforme, which appear to be part of a hypersensitivity reaction. Amphotericin B, ketoconazole, fluconazole, and itraconazole can all be used as therapies.

Answer B is incorrect. Histoplasmosis is linked to bat exposure and bird droppings and is especially common in the Ohio and Mississippi river valleys. Patients are usually asymptomatic unless they are immunocompromised. If disseminated histoplasmosis is suspected, the diagnosis is made by culturing the affected organ, or by a urine polysaccharide antigen screen.

Answer C is incorrect. Lung cancer is not likely in this young patient, even one who is immunocompromised. Also, the onset is fairly acute to be a malignancy.

Answer D is incorrect. Although this patient has risk factors for an opportunistic infection, *Pneumocystis jiroveci* pneumonia usually presents with a decreased oxygen saturation and a history of shortness of breath, classically with diffuse ground-glass infiltrates on x-ray. Furthermore, *P. jiroveci* pneumonia is not commonly seen until the CD4+ count falls below 200/mm³.

Answer E is incorrect. Sarcoidosis is a disease that is diagnosed by the findings on x-ray of the chest of bilateral hilar lymphadenopathy and reticular opacities. Fifty percent of patients are asymptomatic and the findings on x-ray of the chest are incidental. In those patients that are symptomatic, the traditional restrictive lung disease symptoms of cough, dyspnea, and chest pain are the most common complaints. In the patient described above, the onset of symptoms is unusually acute for sarcoidosis and the temporal association with travel to a region endemic for coccidioidomycosis makes that the more likely cause.

Answer F is incorrect. Tuberculosis (TB) is not likely, as he had a negative purified protein derivative (PPD) test, so this option is less likely than coccidioidomycosis. However,

patients with end-stage HIV (CD4+ count < 200/mm³) can also have a falsely negative PPD. Extrapulmonary TB is often seen in HIV patients with lymphadenitis and/or miliary disease. A person with TB usually presents with slowly progressive malaise, anorexia, weight loss, fever, and night sweats. Furthermore, acid-fast bacteria can be seen on sputum examination, although this is not 100% sensitive for finding the bacteria.

8. **The correct answer is E.** Acute silicosis develops in persons exposed to exceptionally high concentrations of silica. Silicosis can occur in mining, quarrying, or construction that involves drilling, cutting, grinding, blasting, or crushing the earth's crust. Acute silicosis symptoms develop suddenly and include weight loss, fatigue, chest pain, and cough. On examination, patients have diffuse crackles, signs of cyanosis and cor pulmonale, and respiratory failure. Signs of cor pulmonale in this patient include the loud pulmonic component of the second heart sound, which indicates pulmonary artery hypertension, and the prominent A wave and left parasternal heave, which both indicate right ventricular hypertrophy. X-ray of the chest usually shows silicoproteinosis, the hallmark of acute silicosis. There is a characteristic basilar alveolar pattern, without rounded opacities or calcifications. For patients with acute silicosis, survival beyond 4 years after the onset of symptoms is rare. Patients are encouraged to avoid further exposure and to quit smoking; however, no specific treatment cures or alters the course of the disease.

Answer A is incorrect. Asbestosis is most commonly encountered by workers involved in the mining, milling, and manufacturing of asbestos products, as well as those involved in the building trades of pipe fitting and boiler making. The major health effects of asbestos, such as pulmonary fibrosis, lung cancer, and mesothelioma, do not present acutely.

Answer B is incorrect. Berylliosis most commonly produces a chronic interstitial pneumonitis. Berylliosis is encountered in high technology industries, such as aerospace, nuclear, and electronics plants, ceramics plants, plating facilities, and dental material and dye manufacturing.

Answer C is incorrect. Byssinosis is caused by inhalation of organic dust, specifically cotton dust. After exposure for 10 years, workers with recurrent symptoms such as chest tightness or a decrease in FEV_1 may develop an obstructive pattern on pulmonary function testing.

Answer D is incorrect. Coal worker's pneumoconiosis (CWP) has important medical significance in nations where the coal mining industry is important. CWP can cause the development of chronic bronchitis and obstructive lung disease. Furthermore, the chest radiography of CWP is starkly different than that seen in acute silicosis. In simple CWP, radiographic abnormalities consist of small (1- to 5-mm diameter), irregular opacities. In complicated CWP, nodules range in size from 1 cm to involvement of an entire lobe and are generally confined to the upper lung zones.

9. **The correct answer is A.** Combination therapy with isoniazid, rifampin, ethambutol, and pyrazinamide is the standard first-line therapy for tuberculosis. They are all available in single daily oral doses. The important adverse effect of ethambutol is optic neuritis, which is rare at usual therapeutic doses.

Answer B is incorrect. Hepatotoxicity is the main concern with isoniazid.

Answer C is incorrect. Of the antituberculosis drugs listed, levofloxacin is the only one that is not considered to be first-line therapy but may be a reasonable choice as a second-line drug in the setting of resistance or toxicity to other medications. Note that it is not approved by the U.S. Food and Drug Administration for this use.

Answer D is incorrect. As with isoniazid and rifampin, hepatotoxicity of pyrazinamide is an important concern. Gastrointestinal intolerance is common.

Answer E is incorrect. Rifampin may cause an orange discoloration to bodily fluids, including tears, sweat, and urine. A major adverse effect is the induction of hepatic enzymes, which may decrease the efficacy of other medications.

Answer F is incorrect. Streptomycin must be given parenterally, thus limiting its use. It may still be used in the first-line treatment of tuberculosis. Ototoxicity is the major concern with this drug.

10. **The correct answer is C.** This patient has mild persistent asthma, defined as daytime symptoms two or more times per week and nighttime symptoms as often as once every 2 weeks. The most appropriate treatment choice for mild persistent asthma is a daily inhaled corticosteroid with a short-acting β_2-agonist as needed, although recent studies show that the inhaled corticosteroid may be equally effective if taken only in relation to symptoms.

Answer A is incorrect. This answer is an appropriate treatment regimen for moderate persistent asthma, depending on the degree of severity of symptoms. Moderate persistent asthma is defined as daytime symptoms daily and nighttime symptoms at least once each week in the absence of treatment. There are asthma attacks at least two times weekly.

Answer B is incorrect. This answer is an appropriate treatment regimen for moderate persistent asthma, depending on the degree of severity of symptoms. Moderate persistent asthma is defined as daytime symptoms daily and nighttime symptoms at least once each week in the absence of treatment. There are asthma attacks at least two times weekly.

Answer D is incorrect. This is a treatment option for severe persistent asthma, which typically requires multiple adjunctive treatment strategies. Severe asthma is defined as symptoms constantly throughout the day in the absence of treatment, and frequent day and nighttime attacks.

Answer E is incorrect. This is the most appropriate treatment for mild intermittent asthma, defined as daytime symptoms no more than two times per week, and nighttime symptoms no more than two times per month, which requires no daily treatment.

11. **The correct answer is B.** A solitary pulmonary nodule is defined as a lung nodule, < 3 cm in size, that is discovered on x-ray or CT scan of the chest. Solitary pulmonary nodules have a

40% chance of being malignant. Review of old x-rays is crucial because they can give an indication of the nodule's doubling time. A doubling time between 20 and 400 days is more concerning for malignancy. For example, small cell cancer doubles every 30 days, adenocarcinoma doubles every 180 days, and well-differentiated cancers have an even longer doubling time. Benign processes generally have doubling times that are < 20 days (infection) or > 450 days (old granulomas). The doubling time for this patient is not 2 years. On x-ray of the chest, a pulmonary nodule appears as a coin-shaped lesion, when in actuality it is best approximated as a three-dimensional sphere. Thus, if a calculation is performed for the volume of the nodule/sphere, we observe close to an eightfold increase in size. Thus, the lesion doubled in size three times during the 2-year period, meaning that the doubling time was 2 years divided by 3, or every two-thirds of a year (243.5 days).

Answer A is incorrect. Benign nodules tend to have a smooth, discrete border, while malignant lesions have an irregular border.

Answer C is incorrect. Nodule size is directly related to the likelihood of malignancy. Generally, a nodule > 3 cm diameter significantly increases the likelihood of malignancy. In one study, 80% of nodules > 3 cm were malignant compared with 20% in nodules < 2 cm.

Answer D is incorrect. The likelihood of malignancy increases with age. In one study, the chances of a nodule being malignant as a function of age were 3% (ages 35–39 years), 15% (ages 40–49 years), 43% (ages 50–59 years), and 50% in patients > 60 years old. In another study, nodules in patients > 50 years old had a 65% likelihood of malignancy, whereas those in patients < 50 years old had a 33% likelihood of being malignant. Given the patient's young age (38 years), doubling time is a much more likely risk factor for malignancy.

Answer E is incorrect. The presence of certain patterns of calcification (best seen on CT) favors the lesion being benign. Such patterns include "popcorn" calcification, diffuse/homogenous calcification, central calcification, and laminated/concentric calcification. However, the existence of areas of calcification is not associated with a benign lesion. An eccentric lesion having an asymmetric area of calcification should raise concern of malignancy.

12. **The correct answer is B.** Diffuse ground-glass infiltrates are seen in *Pneumocystis jiroveci* (formerly *carinii*) pneumonia, characterized by shortness of breath, nonproductive cough, and extremely decreased oxygen saturation. This is most common in patients with HIV with CD4+ counts < 200/mm^3, but it can also occur in non-HIV patients. The patient's history of intravenous drug use puts her at increased risk for HIV.

Answer A is incorrect. Sarcoidosis is often detected by radiographic abnormalities showing bilateral hilar lymphadenopathy. Pulmonary symptoms of cough, dyspnea, and chest pain are common symptoms in sarcoidosis. Patients may also have fever, fatigue, malaise, and weight loss. Sarcoidosis is more common among African-American women. This patient's demographics make sarcoidosis less likely, and her x-ray of the chest argues against this diagnosis.

Answer C is incorrect. This finding would be likely in the case of asthma or emphysema. Asthma manifests as intermittent dyspnea, wheezing, and cough. In patients with asthma without an additional concomitant pulmonary process, x-ray of the chest is commonly normal or shows some hyperinflation. Our patient has no previous history of asthma or smoking and presents with acute symptoms, including fever, that are more suggestive of an infectious etiology.

Answer D is incorrect. A lung abscess would be unlikely to present with this clinical picture. Lung abscesses typically occur with aspiration pneumonia. Patients with lung abscesses present with indolent symptoms (cough, fever, and night sweats) that develop over weeks to months. Patients typically have putrid sputum. X-ray of the chest can be used to visualize pulmonary lesions, but CT scan is preferred for diagnosis. In this patient without aspiration, a lung abscess is unlikely.

Answer E is incorrect. This is possible, but with the patient's significant hypoxia and fever suggesting an infectious process, it is unlikely that the patient would have a negative x-ray of the chest.

13. **The correct answer is D.** The combination of constitutional symptoms, respiratory complaints, erythema nodosum, blurred vision, and bilateral hilar lymphadenopathy in a young adult strongly suggests the diagnosis of sarcoidosis; however, a biopsy of the pulmonary lymphadenopathy, which showed noncaseating granulomas, would be necessary to make a definitive diagnosis. Bilateral hilar lymphadenopathy on x-ray of the chest is pathognomonic for sarcoidosis, but a similar pattern can be seen in lymphoma, tuberculosis, fungal infection, and brucellosis. Elevated serum angiotensin-converting enzyme levels and hypercalcemia are other findings characteristic of sarcoidosis. The Kveim-Siltzbach skin test, which entails an intradermal sarcoid protein injection and is positive in 70–80% of patients, is now less commonly used with the advent of transbronchial biopsy of lung parenchyma.

Answer A is incorrect. Workers in high-technology fields, such as aerospace, nuclear, and electronics plants, ceramics industries, plating facilities, dental material sites, and dye manufacturing, can develop an interstitial lung disease called berylliosis. In berylliosis, x-ray of the chest shows bilateral hilar lymphadenopathy with interstitial infiltrates, and a biopsy of the lesion shows noncaseating granulomas. Both findings are similar to sarcoidosis. Distinction can be made between sarcoidosis and berylliosis by measuring tissue levels of beryllium. While the patient does work in an electronics plant and may have a component of berylliosis, the overall clinical picture is more consistent with sarcoidosis.

Answer B is incorrect. The distinction between pulmonary fungal infection and sarcoidosis is important. After all, starting a patient on systemic steroids for sarcoidosis can be disastrous if the patient actually has a fungal infection. However, the clinical picture is more consistent with sarcoidosis, and the negative bronchoalveolar lavage culture argues against a fungal infection.

Answer C is incorrect. The x-ray of the chest may be consistent with lymphoma, either Hodgkin's or non-Hodgkin's. However, the patient lacks the symptoms and signs typically present in lymphoma patients: fever (temperature > 38.5°C [101.3°F]), night sweats, 10% weight loss over the preceding 6 months, and hepatosplenomegaly.

Answer E is incorrect. While the x-ray of the chest can also be indicative of pulmonary tuberculosis (TB), it is difficult to explain the other findings present in the case by this diagnosis. TB does not cause hypercalcemia or erythema nodosum. Rather, findings sometimes seen in TB, but not present in this patient, are hyponatremia from the syndrome of inappropriate secretion of antidiuretic hormone, leukocytosis, fever, and chest pain.

14. **The correct answer is C.** Patients with a hemothorax that is bleeding at a rate > 200 mL/h require an urgent thoracotomy to control the hemorrhage. It is likely that the internal thoracic and/or intercostal arteries are lacerated.

Answer A is incorrect. Hemothoraces that are less severe (< 200 mL/h) can be treated with autotransfusion of the collected blood.

Answer B is incorrect. Inserting another chest tube will not help control the bleeding, which is the priority.

Answer D is incorrect. Removing the chest tube will not correct the source of bleeding, and the patient is at risk for exsanguinating.

Answer E is incorrect. Thoracentesis is used for diagnosis when the etiology of pleural fluid is uncertain. In the setting of a gunshot wound and bright red fluid in the pleural space, hemothorax is highly suspected, and urgent attention is needed due to the extent of bleeding.

15. **The correct answer is D.** The patient's presentation (history of stasis, tachypnea, dyspnea, tachycardia, hypotension, low-grade fever, elevated jugular venous distension, and accentuated pulmonic component of the second heart sound) in combination with an elevated D-dimer on enzyme-linked immunosorbent assay and findings on CT angiogram are diagnostic for a large pulmonary embolus (see arrow in

image). Pulmonary embolism has many effects on pulmonary physiology. The compliance of the lungs, which is defined as the volume change per unit pressure change, decreases. The decrease occurs for a number of reasons, such as lung edema, lung hemorrhage, and loss of surfactant.

Answer A is incorrect. Airway resistance increases, rather than decreases, as a result of a pulmonary embolus. The increase in airway resistance is due to bronchoconstriction of unused/underperfused portions of lung.

Answer B is incorrect. Alveolar dead space is defined as an area of the lung that is ventilated but not perfused. Anatomically, this usually represents the area at the top of the lung. In pulmonary embolus, alveolar dead space increases, rather than decreases, due to vascular obstruction.

Answer C is incorrect. In pulmonary embolus (PE), alveolar ventilation increases, rather than decreases, due to stimulation of irritant receptors. Alveolar ventilation is defined as the volume of fresh air reaching the alveoli per minute. Mathematically it is expressed as $V_A =$ (tidal volume − anatomic dead space) × respiratory rate. In PE, the increase in respiratory rate causes an increase in alveolar ventilation.

Answer E is incorrect. Pulmonary vascular resistance (PVR) is derived from Ohm's law and is defined as PVR + (input pressure − output pressure)/blood flow. If an embolus blocks one or several lobes of the lung, pulmonary vascular resistance rises. This rise, however, is less than what might be expected because pulmonary arterial pressure rises, causing PVR of nonembolized lung to decrease.

16. **The correct answer is A.** It is critical to obtain an arterial blood gas (ABG) analysis, including measurements of carboxyhemoglobin and methemoglobin (which must be specifically requested), to establish a diagnosis and assess hypoxemia in a patient who presents with a history and symptoms suggestive of carbon monoxide (CO) poisoning or toxic ingestion. Common symptoms include dyspnea, headache, lethargy, and depressed mental status. Pulse oximetry cannot be used to rule out hypoxemia in the setting of CO poisoning, since

the saturation recorded is the sum of oxygen- and CO-bound hemoglobin; however, a low saturation by pulse oximetry is an especially ominous sign. An ABG is also important to assess for metabolic acidosis, which could be secondary to hypoxia.

Answer B is incorrect. This is an important part of the workup of carbon monoxide poisoning and other causes of mental status change in a child, but assessment for hypoxemia is most urgent.

Answer C is incorrect. Laryngoscopy and bronchoscopy are important if smoke inhalation is suspected; look for singed nose hairs, facial burns, hoarseness, wheezing, and carbonaceous sputum. These patients require early intubation since upper airway edema can quickly become complete obstruction.

Answer D is incorrect. An ECG would be especially important in the assessment of carbon monoxide (CO) poisoning in elderly patients and other patients with a history of cardiac disease to evaluate the extent of ischemic damage secondary to the carbon monoxide ingestion. The diagnosis of CO poisoning and degree of hypoxemia should be obtained first in this case.

Answer E is incorrect. A toxicology screen is an important part of the differential diagnosis in this scenario, but is not the most urgent diagnostic, given the high suspicion of carbon monoxide poisoning based on the history and the need to assess for hypoxemia.

17. **The correct answer is D.** There is a wide differential diagnosis in the AIDS patient with pulmonary complaints. Tuberculosis is an important consideration. X-ray of the chest may be atypical in the setting of a low CD4+ count. The pleural effusion likely represents tuberculosis pleuritis. Purified protein derivative reactivity is useful to diagnose tuberculosis infection only among HIV-infected individuals with CD4+ counts ≥ 500 cells/mm³. Among individuals with lower counts, lowering cutoff levels or using an anergy panel does not permit comparable reactivity to that observed among HIV-uninfected individuals.

Answer A is incorrect. While evidence of cytomegalovirus (CMV) infection on autopsy is prevalent among HIV-positive individuals, CMV as a sole cause of pulmonary complaints is not common. Nevertheless, the presence of CMV by bronchoalveolar lavage culture or histology (not seen in this case) is indicative of a poor prognosis.

Answer B is incorrect. *Nocardia* is an opportunistic bacterial infection that often appears in immunocompromised hosts as partially acid-fast filamentous branching rods on smear of the sputum. The pulmonary symptoms of *Nocardia* infection are relatively nonspecific and overlap with those of tuberculosis (fever, chills, anorexia, weight loss, and hemoptysis). However, tuberculosis in this setting is far more common.

Answer C is incorrect. *Mycobacterium avium* complex infections in HIV-positive individuals are most common with CD4+ counts < 50/mm^3. The presentation is usually that of disseminated disease and is seldom localized to the lungs. The organism would appear as acid-fact bacteria.

Answer E is incorrect. This patient's clinical presentation should immediately raise concern for *Pneumocystis jiroveci* pneumonia. While the radiograph may be normal, the typical presentation is usually bilateral alveolar infiltrates. The acid-fast bacillus–positive smear makes tuberculosis more likely.

Answer F is incorrect. Pulmonary aspergillosis is a relatively uncommon disease, even in HIV patients. The disease is characterized by fever and cough accompanied by cavitary or focal alveolar infiltrates that may be bilateral. Diagnosis is made through a positive bronchoalveolar lavage and culture.

18. **The correct answer is A.** Cerebral palsy (CP) is a group of clinical syndromes characterized by motor and postural dysfunction due to disorders of early brain development. CP ranges in severity and can result from ischemic, metabolic, genetic, infectious, developmental, and acquired etiologies. CP is often associated with epilepsy and visual, speech, and intellectual abnormalities. Some patients may exhibit spasticity, or strong sustained contractions and hyperreflexivity. Baclofen is a muscle relaxant that reduces the involuntary, abnormal movements and posturing affecting these patients by inhibiting reflex pathways in the spinal cord.

Answer B is incorrect. Botulinum toxin is being studied for the treatment of spasticity in specific muscle groups. It is not recommended for children under 18 years of age and is used primarily in calf muscles. However, it may be considered for focal aspects of generalized spasticity.

Answer C is incorrect. Carbamazepine is an antiepileptic that has been used in children who have cerebral palsy with dystonia. Dystonia is the involuntary and sometimes painful contractions of muscle tissue leading to jerking and twisting movements of body parts.

Answer D is incorrect. Physical therapy is an established component of the management of cerebral palsy. It is started and continued at home by the parents, with the intention of reducing muscle tone.

Answer E is incorrect. Hyperbaric oxygen does not improve spasticity in children with cerebral palsy.

19. **The correct answer is A.** The most likely cause of this patient's fever is pneumonia. The mnemonic for postoperative fever is the "6 W's": **W**ind (pneumonia and atelectasis), **W**ater (urinary tract infection [UTI]), **W**ound, **W**onder drugs (i.e., erythromycin, isoniazid, penicillin, captopril, aspirin, allopurinol, and heparin), **W**alking (deep vein thrombosis), and "**W**hat happened" (medical interventions such as blood transfusions or intravenous lines). Immediately (approximately within the first 24 hours), the most common causes are postoperative inflammation, streptococcal or clostridial wound infections, or transfusion reaction. In the acute postoperative period (approximately 3–7 days), the most common cause of fever is pneumonia, which is often associated with intraoperative ventilator use, or previously acquired infections. Other causes at this time include UTI, intravenous site infection/thrombosis, or noninfectious wound complication, such as hematoma or foreign body reaction. Incentive spirometry encourages air movement and clearance of secretions, and has

been shown to decrease the occurrence of postoperative pneumonia. In a patient with underlying lung disease, the risk of acquiring a respiratory infection following surgery is increased.

Answer B is incorrect. Although a urinary tract infection (UTI) is in the differential diagnosis, it is much less likely. There are no urinary symptoms, and there is no history of prolonged catheterization. The risk of acquiring a UTI postoperatively increases with duration of catheterization.

Answer C is incorrect. Findings suggestive of catheter infection, such as localized erythema, tenderness, and swelling, are not seen in this case.

Answer D is incorrect. A wound infection (nonclostridial) is the most common cause of fever in the subacute postoperative period (approximately 1 week to 1 month). The timing (3 days post-surgery) and benign surgical site described in the case make this diagnosis less likely.

Answer E is incorrect. Deep vein thrombosis typically presents in 4–6 days; however, no risk factors (e.g., prolonged immobilization or hypercoagulable state) are mentioned, and the patient is not exhibiting symptoms of calf tenderness or leg swelling to suggest this diagnosis.

20. **The correct answer is A.** This presentation is classic for cotton dust exposure, or byssinosis, a type of hypersensitivity pneumonitis. Byssinosis affects workers who are exposed to the processing of cotton, flax, and hemp to make cotton cloth, linen, and rope. Clinically it is divided into two stages, an occasional (early) and a regular (late) stage of chest tightness that occurs toward the end of the first day of the work week. Those with asthma and chronic bronchitis tend to be susceptible to byssinosis. Eighty percent of workers exposed to cotton dust may show a significant drop in their FEV_1 over the course of a Monday shift (hence the term *Monday chest tightness*). Removal from exposure to the inciting antigen results in subsiding of symptoms within 12 hours to several days and complete resolution of clinical and radiographic findings within several weeks.

The disease may recur with re-exposure. When exposure reaches 10 years, workers are more likely to have an obstructive pattern on pulmonary function testing. The level of disability is related to quantity and duration of exposure. Cigarette smoking has an additive effect on the patient's level of disability, such that the patients most debilitated by byssinosis are smokers. X-ray of the chest in early byssinosis typically shows no active disease.

Answer B is incorrect. Community-acquired pneumonia would be expected to cause fever, chills, pleuritic pain, and sputum production, all of which this patient denies. Also, pneumonia would not be expected to have the fluctuating course that is seen in byssinosis.

Answer C is incorrect. The findings in workers exposed to grain dust are identical to those in cigarette smokers: persistent cough, mucus secretion, wheezing, dyspnea on exertion, reduced FEV_1, and reduced FEV_1:FVC.

Answer D is incorrect. Farmer's lung occurs when a person is exposed to moldy hay containing spores of actinomycetes. The inhalation of the spores results in a hypersensitivity pneumonitis. The patient with farmer's lung typically presents 4–8 hours after exposure, complaining of fever, chills, malaise, cough, and dyspnea with wheezes. To differentiate this condition from influenza or pneumonia, an adequate history documenting exposure to moldy hay is crucial. Nevertheless, the patient's lack of fever, chills, or sweats, and the cyclical nature of the patient's symptoms, makes byssinosis the most likely diagnosis.

Answer E is incorrect. Patients with influenza characteristically present with fever, chills, myalgia, cough, fatigue, and headache. This patient denies these symptoms and exposure to sick persons, thus influenza is unlikely.

21. **The correct answer is D.** Pneumothorax is an uncommon but potentially fatal complication of HIV believed to occur in 2–6% of HIV patients at some point during their infection. More than 80% of the cases of pneumothorax in HIV patients occur in conjunction with *Pneumocystis jiroveci* pneumonia. Extensive tissue invasion within the alveolar interstitium is common in severe *P. jiroveci* pneumonia,

and may be an important factor in causing necrosis and subsequent pneumothorax. Patients with pneumothorax present with the sudden onset of unilateral pleuritic chest pain and dyspnea. Physical examination can reveal decreased or absent breath sounds, hyperresonance, and decreased tactile fremitus on the affected side.

Answer A is incorrect. Pneumothorax may result from unsuccessful attempts to inject drugs into the central circulation via the subclavian and jugular veins ("pocket shots"). However, there is no evidence that this patient uses injection drugs.

Answer B is incorrect. Kaposi's sarcoma is a vascular tumor arising from infection with human herpesvirus 8. Kaposi's sarcoma is the most common tumor arising in patients with AIDS and is 20,000 times more common in AIDS patients than in the general population. While Kaposi's sarcoma does occur in conjunction with pneumothorax in HIV patients, it is not as frequent as *Pneumocystis jiroveci* pneumonia.

Answer C is incorrect. *Mycobacterium tuberculosis* is a mycobacterial opportunistic infection encountered in AIDS. *Mycobacterium tuberculosis* has no association with pneumothorax in HIV patients.

Answer E is incorrect. Toxoplasmosis is a protozoan opportunistic infection encountered in AIDS. Toxoplasmosis has no association with pneumothorax in HIV patients.

22. **The correct answer is F.** Acute respiratory distress syndrome (ARDS) is the presence of pulmonary edema in the absence of volume overload or depressed left ventricular function. Early disease may manifest with only mild tachypnea. Sepsis accounts for the majority of cases of ARDS and is an especially important cause of ARDS in patients with a history of alcoholism. the ratio of the partial pressure of arterial oxygen to the fraction of inspired oxygen ($PaO_2:FiO_2$) is used to assess respiratory status. Values < 300 in the setting of bilateral x-ray of the chest infiltrates and a pulmonary capillary wedge pressure of < 18 mm Hg define acute lung injury (ALI), a pulmonary syndrome

characterized by noncardiogenic pulmonary edema. ARDS is a more severe form of ALI with a $PaO_2:FiO_2 < 200$.

Answer A is incorrect. Aspiration of gastric contents is a less common cause of acute respiratory distress syndrome.

Answer B is incorrect. Drug overdose of medications such as aspirin, opioids, tricyclic antidepressants, and cocaine may result in acute respiratory distress syndrome, but it is not the most common cause.

Answer C is incorrect. Lung or bone marrow transplantation is a cause of acute respiratory distress syndrome but is a much less common etiology than sepsis in causing this clinical syndrome.

Answer D is incorrect. Massive blood transfusion is a less common cause of acute respiratory distress syndrome.

Answer E is incorrect. Near-drowning is a less common cause of acute respiratory distress syndrome.

23. **The correct answer is E.** X-ray of the chest demonstrated fluid in the fissures, prominent pulmonary vascular markings, and overexpansion (as evidenced by flattening of the diaphragm). The history and imaging findings are consistent with transient tachypnea of the newborn (TTN). TTN is caused by a temporary pulmonary edema that results from delayed clearance of fetal lung fluid. TTN typically presents with mild to moderate respiratory distress within the first 6 hours of life, manifested by tachypnea, cyanosis, subcostal retractions, nasal flaring, and grunting. In mild TTN, respiratory distress persists for 12–24 hours, but can last up to 48–72 hours in more severe cases. Breath sounds are usually clear but can be coarse. Risk factors for TTN include premature birth, precipitous birth, and cesarean section. These are thought to contribute to impaired clearance of fetal lung fluid due to the absence of the "thoracic squeeze" the baby normally experiences during passage through the birth canal. However, regardless of gestational age and method of delivery, all infants are at risk for developing TTN.

Answer A is incorrect. X-ray of the chest in an infant with a diaphragmatic hernia would reveal air-filled bowel in the chest. The physical exam of this patient is not consistent with a diaphragmatic hernia, in which one would expect absent or decreased breath sounds on the side of the hernia and heart sounds displaced to the opposite side of the thorax. Clinically, patients with diaphragmatic hernias are usually in severe respiratory distress.

Answer B is incorrect. In neonatal respiratory distress syndrome (NRDS), x-ray of the chest reveals a fine reticular granular pattern and air bronchograms. Although this neonate's history is consistent with NRDS, more acute respiratory distress would be expected. Also, this infant is at low risk of developing NRDS because she is full-term.

Answer C is incorrect. On x-ray of the chest, diffuse opacification of one or both lungs and air bronchograms would be seen in a case of pulmonary hemorrhage.

Answer D is incorrect. On x-ray of the chest, pulmonary interstitial emphysema (PIE) appears as linear lucencies radiating from the hilum or as large cyst-like blebs. This neonate's time course is consistent with PIE, in which infants develop respiratory distress within 48 hours of birth. However, neonates with PIE are typically more ill and have hypotension, bradycardia, and hypoxia. PIE usually affects extremely preterm infants with neonatal respiratory distress syndrome NRDS or sepsis.

24. **The correct answer is E.** This patient most likely suffers from asbestosis, a condition typically found in shipyard and textile workers. X-ray of the chest often demonstrates small bilateral parenchymal opacities, and 50% of patients with asbestosis will have multiple pleural plaques.

Answer A is incorrect. Bilateral diffuse infiltrates are seen in several conditions, including atypical pneumonia. A patient might present with nonproductive cough, dyspnea, and fever.

Answer B is incorrect. Bilateral hilar adenopathy is characteristic of sarcoidosis. Sarcoidosis occurs most often in African-American women and causes non-caseating granulomas in various organ systems.

Answer C is incorrect. Consolidation of lung tissue suggests a bacterial pneumonia. Look for a patient with an acute onset of fever, productive cough, and decreased breath sounds over the consolidation.

Answer D is incorrect. A focal mass would suggest primary lung carcinoma, but this patient has no smoking history and no constitutional symptoms, making this a much less likely diagnosis. Patients with lung carcinoma might present with chronic cough, dyspnea, weight loss, hemoptysis, and paraneoplastic syndromes.

25. **The correct answer is A.** Primary spontaneous pneumothorax is most commonly due to a rupture of subpleural apical blebs, which usually occurs in tall, thin young men. The history and physical examination presented are classic for pneumothorax: sudden-onset unilateral pleuritic chest pain and dyspnea. X-ray of the chest is the diagnostic modality of choice because it shows a visceral pleural line and/or lung retraction from the chest wall when pneumothorax is present. Observation with supplemental oxygen is the best approach for pneumothoraces occupying < 15% of the hemithorax because these often resolve spontaneously. The rate of reabsorption is 1.25% of the volume of the hemithorax per 24 hours. The rate is increased with the administration of supplemental oxygen.

Answer B is incorrect. Open thoracotomy has been largely replaced by video-assisted thoracoscopy because hospitalization time is shorter and postoperative pain is less. Currently, thoracotomy is indicated after thoracoscopy has failed or if thoracoscopy is unavailable. If thoracotomy is undertaken, the pleural blebs are oversewn and the pleura scarred.

Answer C is incorrect. The initial treatment for patients with pneumothoraces occupying > 15% of the hemithorax is aspiration of the pleural space. Usually an 8F catheter is threaded over an 18-gauge needle. Once in proper position, the needle is removed and the air in the pleural space is manually evacuated.

However, if the patient is unstable, then aspiration should be bypassed in favor of tube thoracostomy.

Answer D is incorrect. An alternative to tube thoracostomy is video-assisted thoracoscopy. With this procedure, the bullae are treated with wedge resection via an endoscopic stapler. The indications for thoracoscopy include failure of aspiration treatment, failure of lung reexpansion after 3 days of tube thoracostomy, persistence of bronchopleural fistula after 3 days, and recurrent pneumothorax after pleurodesis. Video-assisted thoracostomy is a safe and effective management option for the treatment and prevention of pneumothorax.

Answer E is incorrect. A patient with a primary spontaneous pneumothorax that fails aspiration should be treated with tube thoracostomy. For a patient being managed with a chest tube, the tube can be clamped when no air has been seen emanating from the thoracic cavity for 12 hours. The chest tube may be removed after there has been no evidence (radiographic or clinical) of pneumothorax for 24 hours. Instillation of a pleurodesis agent such as doxycycline decreases the recurrence rate of pneumothorax.

26. **The correct answer is C.** This man's age, symptoms, and history suggest a diagnosis of chronic obstructive pulmonary disease (COPD). The diagnosis is supported by a decreased forced expiratory volume in 1 second:forced vital capacity ratio (FEV_1:FVC) of 0.7 and a FEV_1 value that is 60% of expected. Although the obstructed airways are not completely reversible, which differentiates it from asthma, it is common to see up to a 15% improvement in FEV_1 after bronchodilator therapy, even in patients with COPD.

Answer A is incorrect. Asthma is largely due to hyperreactive airways, which become inflamed and constrict in response to a variety of triggers (cold, infection, exercise, or allergens). The airway constriction, however, is largely reversible with bronchodilator treatment.

Answer B is incorrect. Chronic aspiration typically occurs in one of two settings. First, in the setting of neurologic impairment due to de-

mentia or following a stroke, aspiration may be secondary to a loss of cough and swallow reflexes. Second, a pharyngeal or esophageal disorder, such as laryngopharyngeal or gastroesophageal reflux, cricopharyngeal spasm, strictures, Zenker's diverticulum, achalasia, or changes post-radiation or post-surgery for neoplastic processes, may also result in aspiration. There is no history that indicates that any of these risk factors are present.

Answer D is incorrect. Chronic histoplasmosis would be associated with a restrictive lung disease pattern, which would result in normal or increased forced expiratory volume in 1 second:forced vital capacity ratio. Also, the subway worker does not directly work with soil, where the histoplasmosis fungus resides. In addition, histoplasmosis is most often found in the midwestern and southeastern states and along the Ohio and Mississippi river valleys.

Answer E is incorrect. No history of prior positive purified protein derivative test, immunocompromised status, travel history, or sick contacts are present that would suggest a diagnosis of tuberculosis. Also no history of chills or sweats is given and the spirometry results indicate that a minimally reversible obstructive lung process is at work.

27. **The correct answer is A.** This patient now has moderate persistent asthma, with daily symptoms and more than one night per week of symptoms, along with worsening end-expiratory flow rate. The recommended treatment for moderate persistent asthma is low- to medium-dose inhaled steroids along with a long-acting bronchodilator, either a β-adrenergic agonist or theophylline.

Answer B is incorrect. This is appropriate for a severe asthma exacerbation requiring hospitalization, not as a control treatment for moderate persistent asthma. Signs of respiratory distress indicating that hospitalization is needed include dyspnea at rest, retractions, paradoxical breathing, and use of accessory muscles of respiration.

Answer C is incorrect. The patient's symptoms have resolved with treatment in the emergency department and she does not require hospitalization at this point.

Answer D is incorrect. This is appropriate for mild persistent asthma (> 2 episodes per week but < 1 per day).

Answer E is incorrect. Cromolyn sodium is more useful in the pediatric population or patients with mild persistent asthma. Cromolyn is an inhaled nonsteroidal anti-inflammatory drug used for asthma prophylaxis. The drug stabilizes mast cells, leading to decreased pulmonary inflammation.

28. **The correct answer is C.** The patient is suffering from aortic stenosis (AS) which is causing pulmonary edema. The classic triad of symptoms of AS includes congestive heart failure, syncope, and angina. Aortic stenosis causes cardiogenic pulmonary edema by making it harder for the left ventricle to move blood forward, resulting in increased filling pressures in the pulmonary capillaries. Patients with pulmonary edema complain of dyspnea, orthopnea, and paroxysmal nocturnal dyspnea, and rales will classically be heard with auscultation. X-ray of the chest often shows an enlarged heart and prominent pulmonary vasculature. The primary pathogenic mechanism in cardiogenic pulmonary edema is an increase in the capillary fluid hydraulic pressure due to left ventricular systolic or diastolic dysfunction.

Answer A is incorrect. Decreased capillary fluid oncotic pressure, which occurs in states of hypoalbuminemia, could precipitate pulmonary edema.

Answer B is incorrect. Decreased capillary interstitial pressure causes pulmonary edema. This condition arises from the rapid removal of pleural effusion.

Answer D is incorrect. Increased capillary permeability can cause pulmonary edema. Sepsis, radiation, oxygen toxicity, and the acute respiratory distress syndrome are possible causes of increased capillary permeability.

Answer E is incorrect. Pulmonary edema can be caused by an increase in interstitial oncotic pressure, which would drive fluid from the capillaries into the interstitium. The interstitial oncotic pressure is derived from filtered plasma proteins and proteoglycans in the interstitium. Aortic stenosis,

29. **The correct answer is D.** The patient's history and physical examination are highly suspicious for sleep apnea. Obstructive sleep apnea (OSA) is most prevalent in men ages 30–60 years, who present with a history of snoring, excessive daytime sleepiness, nocturnal choking or gasping, witnessed apneic episodes, moderate obesity, and hypertension. The patient's dyspnea on exertion, diffuse and laterally displaced point of maximal intensity, and S3 gallop are all signs and symptoms of left heart failure, a manifestation of OSA. It is believed that left heart failure arises from repetitive episodes of nocturnal asphyxia and concomitant negative intrathoracic pressure. The negative intrathoracic pressure increases cardiac afterload, which manifests over time as left heart failure. The definitive diagnostic modality for OSA is a sleep study (polysomnography). Polysomnography documents arousals, obstructions, episodes of hypoxemia, and the various stages of sleep. A sleep study would be useful in this case because it would confirm the diagnosis and establish the need for therapeutic intervention with continuous positive airway pressure.

Answer A is incorrect. Cardiac catheterization would not be useful in the diagnosis of OSA.

Answer B is incorrect. Echocardiography may be helpful in detecting wall motion abnormalities and roughly gauging cardiac function, but it would also not help confirm the diagnosis of OSA.

Answer C is incorrect. Exercise tolerance testing is used to diagnose coronary artery disease (CAD), evaluate patients with known CAD, localize ischemia, and risk-stratify patients after acute coronary syndrome. At this time, however, the patient lacks symptoms that would suggest CAD, namely substernal chest pain provoked by exertion and relieved by rest or nitroglycerin. Furthermore, an exercise tolerance test would not be expected to help confirm the diagnosis of OSA.

Answer E is incorrect. An x-ray of the chest may show an enlarged heart, but it would not be expected to help confirm the diagnosis of OSA.

30. **The correct answer is D.** Key features include the central location, history of smoking (small cell carcinomas are closely associated with a history of smoking), and the presence of a paraneoplastic syndrome, in this case Cushing's syndrome from tumor elaboration of ACTH outside hypothalamic-pituitary-adrenal axis regulation. The syndrome of inappropriate ADH secretion and Eaton-Lambert syndrome are other paraneoplastic syndromes associated with small cell lung carcinoma. Metastases are commonly present at the time of diagnosis. Favored sites are brain, liver, and bone.

Answer A is incorrect. Adenocarcinoma is incorrect because it typically presents peripherally and is not associated with Cushing's syndrome.

Answer B is incorrect. Cancer metastatic to the lung is incorrect. In this instance, there is a single lesion in the lung and multiple lesions in the liver. The site of multiple solid masses is more likely the destination of the metastasis, while the solitary nodule in the lung is likely to be the primary.

Answer C is incorrect. Large cell carcinoma is incorrect because they typically present on the periphery, are not associated with Cushing's syndrome, and are the least frequent type of lung cancer.

Answer E is incorrect. Squamous cell carcinoma is incorrect. Although squamous cell lung carcinoma presents centrally and is clearly linked to smoking, a paraneoplastic syndrome marked by excess ACTH would not be expected. Excess parathyroid hormone and resultant hypercalcemia, however, is associated with squamous cell cancers.

31. **The correct answer is E.** The classic symptoms of cough, low-grade fevers, and wasting should raise the suspicion of pulmonary tuberculosis (TB), given the patient's age, clinical presentation, and history of previous travel to an area with a high incidence of TB. The addition of abscesses and fluid levels on x-ray demonstrate that the pneumonia is cavitary. TB is one of the more prominent cavitary pneumonias. Blood streaking of the sputum is frequently documented as in this patient. Some other risk factors for TB include HIV-positivity, imprisonment, homelessness, and malnourishment. A purified protein derivative test can be used to screen for a latent infection, but will tell you nothing in a patient with active TB. The first-line treatment for TB is a combination of four drugs: isoniazid, rifampin, ethambutol, and pyrazinamide for a minimum of 6 months.

Answer A is incorrect. *Aspergillus* infection in the lung can cause invasive aspergillosis, aspergilloma, chronic necrotizing *Aspergillus* pneumonia, and allergic bronchopulmonary aspergillosis, none of which will offer a more appropriate diagnosis than TB. *Aspergillus* is often seen in neutropenic patients and is seen as a "fungus ball" with cavitation on x-ray of the chest. The treatment for *Aspergillus* infection is amphotericin B or itraconazole.

Answer B is incorrect. *Klebsiella* produces lobar pneumonias that more classically involves "currant jelly" sputum. *Klebsiella* pneumonia is often seen in alcoholics and diabetics, and is often antibiotic-resistant.

Answer C is incorrect. Lung cancer can cause wasting, low-grade fevers, cough, and night sweats. It is certainly a possible cause of pulmonary nodules; however, while it may be hard to immediately discount the possibility of its occurrence, the constellation of symptoms, including the lack of a smoking history, and history of international travel should make one lean more heavily toward TB.

Answer D is incorrect. Sarcoidosis is an idiopathic disorder that typically presents in African-Americans in their 20s to 30s. About 50% of patients realize that they have sarcoidosis by an x-ray of the chest, which reveals bilateral mediastinal adenopathy. Sarcoidosis can mimic TB, but is a diagnosis of exclusion, and TB should be ruled out before this diagnosis is entertained.

32. **The correct answer is E.** This patient has cystic fibrosis (CF), which may be diagnosed in childhood with failure to thrive and failure to gain weight despite a good appetite. Children often have bulky, foul-smelling stools as a result of pancreatic insufficiency. CF disease in the lung accounts for most of the morbidity

and mortality from this disease. Bacteria in the lungs of CF patients, typically *Pseudomonas* or *Burkholderia cepacia*, infect the bronchial tree, provoking an intense inflammatory response. Infection stimulates mucus production, and damage to the wall of the airway with resultant bronchiectasis ensues.

Answer A is incorrect. Cirrhosis and hepatic failure are possible complications of hepatitis.

Answer B is incorrect. The salt-wasting forms of congenital adrenal hyperplasia, a disorder of defective steroidogenic pathways, are associated with these complications.

Answer C is incorrect. Esophageal ulceration or strictures and upper gastrointestinal bleeding are possible complications of gastroesophageal reflux disease.

Answer D is incorrect. This answer describes possible sequelae of lead poisoning.

Questions 33 and 34

33. **The correct answer is F.** This patient's fungal culture is typical for *Histoplasma capsulatum*. Pulmonary histoplasmosis should always be included in the differential diagnosis if sarcoidosis, tuberculosis, or malignancy is suspected. Cases are most common in the Ohio and Mississippi river valleys after exposure to bird or bat droppings. In immunocompetent patients, more than 95% will have asymptomatic disease, but severe illness can occur. The vast majority of cases are self-limiting and do not require treatment, but itraconazole or amphotericin B can be given in severe cases.

34. **The correct answer is G.** This patient's symptoms and x-ray of the chest are concerning for reactivation TB. Definitive diagnosis can be made by identification of acid-fast bacilli on sputum smear or culture of *Mycobacterium tuberculosis* from sputum. Skin testing is often done when TB is expected, but is neither sensitive nor specific for identifying active TB. Multidrug resistance (to isoniazid and rifampin) has resulted in the use of a four-drug regimen with directly observed therapy in endemic areas. Patients can be treated with isoniazid, rifampin, an aminoglycoside (e.g., strep-

tomycin or amikacin), and a quinolone (e.g., levofloxacin or moxifloxacin).

Answer A is incorrect. *Actinomyces israelii* are anaerobic gram-positive bacteria of the family Actinomycetaceae and typically manifests clinically as patients with draining sinus tracts. Involvement of the lungs is rare. *Actinomyces* are constituents of normal oral flora and humans are the only reservoir. The typical patient is a male (male-to-female ratio 2:1) with poor oral hygiene. *Actinomyces* is best grown on brain-heart infusion broth at 37°C with 6–10% carbon dioxide. *Actinomyces* is characterized by "sulfur granules" in pus (not actually sulfur, but they appear yellow). Treatment is with penicillins or tetracyclines.

Answer B is incorrect. *Aspergillus* can manifest as pulmonary disease as either allergic bronchopulmonary aspergillosis (ABPA) or as aspergilloma. ABPA most often occurs in patients with cystic fibrosis or asthma who present with bronchial obstruction, fever, malaise, and expectoration of brownish mucus plugs. X-ray of the chest would show upper lobe infiltrates and atelectasis from mucoid impaction. ABPA is diagnosed by skin test reactivity as well as serum IgG and IgE to *Aspergillus*. Aspergillomas usually arise in previous lung cavities due to TB, sarcoidosis, or other fungal infections. Pulmonary infection can be asymptomatic or manifest as hemoptysis. Diagnosis is usually by x-ray of the chest showing a solid mass surrounded by a radiolucent crescent. Culture from sputum (without radiologic findings) cannot be used in diagnosis due to colonization of *Aspergillus* in patients with any type of lung disease. Medical treatment is rarely helpful. Patients are treated by surgical resection of the aspergilloma or lobectomy.

Answer C is incorrect. *Blastomyces* is endemic to the Ohio and Mississippi river basins (similar to histoplasmosis) as well as the Midwest and along the Great Lakes, and occurs most often in those with significant exposure to soil. Blastomycosis can be asymptomatic or manifest as acute or chronic pneumonia. Hematogenous spread to extrapulmonary sites is common. Blastomyces can be identified by fungal culture growth at 37°C revealing broad-based budding yeast. Unlike histoplasmosis, blastomycosis should be treated with amphotericin B or an azole (ketoconazole or fluconazole) if there is extrapulmonary disease. The one exception is mild disease in an immunocompetent host, which can be followed by observation.

Answer D is incorrect. Pneumonia due to *Candida* is rare unless it is part of systemic illness in immunocompromised hosts. It is difficult to identify candidal pneumonia since positive cultures cannot distinguish between oropharyngeal contamination (normal colonization) or a pathologic state. Fungal culture reveals yeast and pseudohyphae. Unless there is involvement of other organs, treatment is not indicated. When other organs are involved, treatment with amphotericin B and fluconazole is initiated.

Answer E is incorrect. Most people have been exposed to *Cryptococcus* and are asymptomatic. However, some immunocompetent people can still develop symptomatic disease characterized by cough, chest pain, fever, weight loss, or hemoptysis. Diagnosis is made by culturing the organism from sputum (characteristic encapsulated yeast forms). The most common finding on x-ray of the chest is non-calcified pulmonary nodules; cavitation is rare. Patients with symptoms can be treated with fluconazole or amphotericin B.

Answer H is incorrect. *Nocardia* is an uncommon aerobic gram-positive bacteria of the family Nocardiaceae and typically is responsible for opportunistic infections, but infection can occur in the immunocompromised. *Nocardia* are endemic to soil and aquatic environments and are acquired by inhalation. *Nocardia* infection most commonly occurs in patients who use steroids (e.g., asthma, chronic obstructive pulmonary disease, and transplant recipients) or patients with solid or hematologic malignancies, but it rarely occurs in AIDS patients due to their prophylaxis with trimethoprim-sulfamethoxazole. Isolation of *Nocardia* from sputum indicates infection. *Nocardia* appear as filamentous gram-positive branching rods on Gram stain and are differentiated from *Actinomyces* by acid-fast staining. Culture should be grown on buffered charcoal yeast extract (the same as that used for *Legionella*) or Thayer-Martin agar. A brain MRI should be obtained due to its propensity for central nervous system involvement. Treatment has not been studied in formal trials, but sulfonamides are typically given.

Answer I is incorrect. *Sporothrix* is not highly virulent and disease is limited to cutaneous and lymphatic structures. Expect *Sporothrix* infection in a rose gardener who has pricked her fingers with a thorn. Involvement of the respiratory system is rare but can occur with inhalation of conidia in patients with chronic obstructive pulmonary disease, AIDS, or alcoholism. The typical patient with pulmonary disease is a middle-aged male alcoholic who presents with symptoms and an x-ray of the chest that is concerning for TB. In this question, immigration from an endemic area for TB and no mention of alcohol abuse makes TB a more likely option. Growth of *Sporothrix* on Sabouraud agar at 25–27°C reveals thin, septate hyphae with branching and stranding; conidia arrange themselves around the hyphae in a bouquet-like fashion. Pulmonary infection is deadly if untreated and should be treated with amphotericin B or itraconazole.

Questions 35–37

35. **The correct answer is J.** The patient shows symptoms classic for a subarachnoid hemorrhage (SAH). SAH is typically caused by a ruptured aneurysm, arteriovenous malformation, or trauma to the circle of Willis. Berry aneurysms are associated with polycystic kidney disease and coarctation of the aorta. Patients with an SAH experience a sudden-onset intensely painful headache, neck stiffness, tactile fever, nausea and vomiting, and a fluctuating level of consciousness. Subarachnoid hemorrhage is a known cause of pulmonary edema and is believed to be due to massive sympathetic discharge following SAH. Other causes of neurogenic pulmonary edema include epileptic seizure and head injury. Subdural and epidural hematomas are not known to cause pulmonary edema.

36. **The correct answer is I.** Rheumatic heart disease can cause a variety of valvular disorders:

aortic stenosis, aortic insufficiency, mitral regurgitation, and mitral stenosis. Pulmonary edema and dyspnea are clinical manifestations of mitral stenosis. The edema and dyspnea can be precipitated by tachycardia (as during exercise), volume overload, and atrial fibrillation. Recurrent bronchitis (seen in this patient) is a frequent pulmonary symptom of mitral stenosis due to congestion. Classically, physical examination of mitral stenosis reveals a low-pitched diastolic rumble audible at the apex and an opening snap.

37. **The correct answer is C.** The patient is suffering from acute respiratory distress syndrome (ARDS), which is defined by noncardiogenic pulmonary edema. There are many direct and indirect etiologies of ARDS. Direct causes include aspiration, pneumonia, inhalation injury, and pulmonary contusion. Indirect causes include sepsis, shock, disseminated intravascular coagulation, and pancreatitis. Four criteria define ARDS without biopsy, all of which are present in this patient. The four criteria include acute onset, bilateral patchy airspace disease, pulmonary capillary wedge pressure < 18 mm Hg, and a partial pressure of oxygen to fraction of inspired oxygen ratio of < 200.

Answer A is incorrect. Acute aortic insufficiency (regurgitation) is a serious disease with high mortality. It is characterized by acute cardiovascular collapse and may present as severe dyspnea, hypotension, or angina. Causes include trauma, aortic dissection, and infections (rheumatic fever or endocarditis).

Answer B is incorrect. Acute mitral regurgitation is a life-threatening complication of papillary muscle rupture following myocardial infarction. It leads to massive pulmonary congestion, and frequently, death.

Answer D is incorrect. Aspiration pneumonia occurs when a patient inhales material from the oropharynx that is colonized by upper airway flora. It is common in people with impaired consciousness or impaired ability to swallow (i.e., intubated patients or the comatose). In most cases, the organisms isolated include *Staphylococcus aureus*, *Streptococcus pneumoniae*, Enterobacteriaceae, and *Hae-mophilus influenzae*. In alcoholics, *Klebsiella* is classic. Intubated patients are at risk of *Pseudomonas aeruginosa* infection.

Answer E is incorrect. Cardiac arrhythmias may be life threatening if they lead to ventricular fibrillation. The patients listed here do not have stories suggestive of arrhythmia.

Answer F is incorrect. Epidural hematoma is usually the result of blunt trauma to the cranium and frequently involves laceration of branches of the middle meningeal artery. It is a high pressure bleed that produces a biconvex (lens-shaped) hyperdensity on CT scan of the head. Epidural hematomas have the unique property of being limited by suture lines (because the dura is attached firmly to the skull at the suture lines).

Answer G is incorrect. Epilepsy is characterized by a pattern of recurrent seizures. The seizures may be either partial (focal) or generalized. Treatment is often lifelong and aimed at improving quality of life.

Answer H is incorrect. Patients with myocardial infarction classically present with substernal chest pain that radiates to the left arm/shoulder. Patients are often diaphoretic and tend to describe their discomfort as intense pressure: "It feels like there is an elephant sitting on my chest."

Answer K is incorrect. Subdural hemorrhage is commonly due to tearing of the bridging veins that extend from the cortex into the venous sinuses. It is typically a low pressure bleed and appears on a noncontrast CT scan of the head as a hyperdense crescentic mass along the cerebral convexity.

Answer L is incorrect. Inflammation of the leptomeninges (pia and arachnoid mater) is one of the most common manifestations of viral infections of the central nervous system. The term meningitis implies lack of cerebral (encephalitis) and spinal cord (myelitis) involvement, but some pathogens may cause a combination of signs and symptoms consistent with meningoencephalitis or encephalomyelitis. The term "aseptic" is often used to indicate viral etiology.

Questions 38–40

38. **The correct answer is G.** Hamartomas are the most common cause of benign tumors of the lung. The lesions are composed of cartilage surrounded by connective tissue and fat. In the United States, hamartomas represent 5–8% of all solitary pulmonary nodules and 0.25% of all autopsy cases. Most pulmonary hamartomas are asymptomatic and first noticed as an incidental finding on x-ray of the chest. The typical appearance on x-ray of the chest is a solitary pulmonary nodule with a "popcorn" calcification. The rib pain in this case is due to bruising and not fractures or the hamartoma.

39. **The correct answer is H.** Histoplasmosis is endemic in the central United States, specifically around the Mississippi River Valley. Risk factors include AIDS, spelunking, and exposure to bat or bird excrement. Chronic infection is associated with low-grade fever, anorexia, weight loss, night sweats, and productive cough. X-ray of the chest may reveal hilar or mediastinal adenopathy, in addition to a solitary pulmonary nodule or a focal infiltrate. Complement fixation antibody titers of 1:16 or 1:32 are presumptive for a diagnosis of histoplasmosis. Identifying organisms by silver stain on biopsy (bone marrow, lymph node, or liver) or bronchoalveolar lavage is diagnostic. TB and fungi (both histoplasmosis and coccidioidomycosis) are the most frequent causes of infectious granulomas that present as solitary pulmonary nodules. TB is less likely given the negative smear and culture (which can take weeks to complete). Coccidioidomycosis should be suspected, rather than histoplasmosis, if the patient is in the southwestern United States.

40. **The correct answer is A.** Patients with lung cancer typically present with a history of cough, hemoptysis, weight loss, and chest pain. Adenocarcinoma is the most common non-small-cell type of lung cancer, representing 35–40% of all lung cancers. Adenocarcinoma is most often located peripherally and is the subtype most commonly associated with nonsmoking patients. Furthermore, digital clubbing can occur with any type of lung cancer but is most frequently associated with adenocarcinoma. Although all subtypes of lung cancer can present

as a solitary pulmonary nodule, this presentation is most frequently associated with adenocarcinoma and large cell carcinoma.

Answer B is incorrect. Aspergilloma may manifest as an asymptomatic radiographic abnormality in a patient with preexisting cavitary lung disease due to sarcoidosis, tuberculosis, or other necrotizing pulmonary processes. It is caused by the fungus *Aspergillus* and is far more prevalent in immunocompromised hosts. It is unlikely here due to the lack of history of preexisting cavitary disease.

Answer C is incorrect. Bronchogenic cysts are rare, congenital lesions that are often identified secondary to infection. More than half of all patients with bronchogenic cysts are asymptomatic. The most common symptoms are chest pain and dysphagia due to compression of mediastinal structures. This diagnosis is unlikely due to its extremely low incidence.

Answer D is incorrect. One to six percent of all lung tumors are carcinoid tumors. Although these neoplasms are capable of producing a variety of substances, including biologically active peptides and hormones, most are inactive. Carcinoids developing within large airway structures grow slowly; can become quite large; and can cause persistent atelectasis, recurrent pneumonia, pulmonary abscess, and bronchiectasis. Although peripheral carcinoid lung tumors are in the differential for a solitary pulmonary nodule, they are relatively rare.

Answer E is incorrect. Cavitating abscesses on x-ray of the chest may appear as an area of thick pneumonic consolidation, depending on the stage of the abscess and preceding the emergence of the typical cavitary air-fluid form. However, this does not correspond to the appearance of these x-rays.

Answer F is incorrect. Coccidioidomycosis would be suspected, rather than histoplasmosis, if the patient were in or had recent travel history to the southwestern United States, Mexico, or Central and South America. It is caused by breathing in spores of a fungus found in desert regions.

Answer I is incorrect. A pulmonary lipoma occurs in the pulmonary parenchyma. Lipomas are asymptomatic and are usually first observed on x-ray or CT scan of the chest. Unlike hamartomas, lipomas have a uniform fatty density with soft tissue strands due to their fibrous stroma.

Answer J is incorrect. TB and fungi (both histoplasmosis and coccidioidomycosis) are the most frequent causes of infectious granulomas that present as solitary pulmonary nodules. TB is less likely given the negative smear and culture.

Answer K is incorrect. Neurilemmoma is a neurogenic tumor that arises from the cells of the nerve sheath and the paraganglionic and autonomic ganglia. They comprise approximately 21% of all adult mediastinal tumors and are believed to be Schwann cells derived from the neural crest. These masses usually arise from the side of a nerve, are well encapsulated, and have a unique histologic pattern. The benign lesion essentially manifests with cosmetic deformity, a palpable mass, and/or symptoms similar to a compressive neuropathy. Neurologic symptoms tend to present late. Symptoms can be vague, with an average interval of up to 5 years before the diagnosis is established. Neurilemmoma is the most common neurogenic tumor.

Answer L is incorrect. The clinical presentation of pulmonary arteriovenous malformation (PAVM) may vary from no symptoms to severe illness. Symptoms generally develop between the fourth and the fifth decades of life. The most common complaints are epistaxis, dyspnea, platypnea, and hemoptysis. A PAVM may be suspected in the case of the incidental finding of a solitary pulmonary nodule on x-ray of the chest; however, the extremely low incidence of PAVMs (approximately 1:40,000) makes it unlikely.

Answer M is incorrect. Extra-articular manifestations of rheumatoid arthritis (RA) are more likely to be present in patients with severe RA. The absence of RA in this patient makes a rheumatoid nodule an unlikely diagnosis. In fact, pleural effusion is the most common manifestation of RA in the chest. Nodules are relatively rare, usually multiple, located at the bases, subpleural in location, and can appear with cavitation.

Answer N is incorrect. A solitary lung mass is a rare thoracic presentation of sarcoidosis, making this diagnosis unlikely. Also, it is usually asymptomatic, although it can be accompanied by a dry cough that persists, excessive tearing, or skin rash. A diagnosis of pulmonary sarcoidosis can only be confirmed after other diagnoses have been ruled out and when there is histologic evidence of noncaseating granuloma from a thoracic biopsy. The cause of sarcoidosis is unknown, and it can appear and disappear suddenly.

Answer O is incorrect. Squamous cell carcinoma accounts for 25–30% of all lung cancers. The classic manifestation is a cavitary lesion in a proximal bronchus. It has a distinct dose-response relationship to tobacco smoking. It is more likely to be associated with hypercalcemia due to parathyroid-like hormone production. The typical location and associated hypercalcemia make this diagnosis unlikely.

Answer P is incorrect. Thymoma is the most common neoplasm of the anterior mediastinum and accounts for 50% of anterior mediastinal masses. Peak incidence is in the fourth to fifth decade of life. Presenting symptoms include cough, chest pain, superior vena cava syndrome, dysphagia, and hoarseness, and do not typically include night sweats, phlegm production, or weight loss. On x-ray of the chest, the lesion typically appears as a smooth mass in the upper half of the chest, overlying the superior portion of the cardiac shadow near the junction of the heart and great vessels. This location does not correspond to the x-ray of the chest in question.

CHAPTER 15

Renal/Genitourinary

1. A 65-year-old man with chronic obstructive pulmonary disease requiring home oxygen at night and cor pulmonale presents to the emergency department (ED) with worsening shortness of breath. On examination, the man's respiratory rate is 22/min and he has a heart rate of 104/min. He has distant breath sounds and is using accessory muscles of breathing. In addition to his baseline chronic respiratory acidosis, the man is found to have a metabolic acidosis on arterial blood gas analysis. Laboratory tests show:

Na^+	*AG = 7.6*	138 mEq/L
K^+		3.6 mEq/L
Cl^-		118 mmol/L
HCO_3^-		16 mEq/L
Phosphate		2.0 mg/dL
Glucose		98 mg/dL
Blood urea nitrogen		10 mg/dL
Creatinine		0.8 mg/dL

Urinalysis is positive for glucose. Which of the following diagnoses explains this patient's laboratory findings?

(A) Right heart failure
(B) Steroid-induced glucosuria
(C) Type I renal tubular acidosis
(D) Type II renal tubular acidosis
(E) Type IV renal tubular acidosis

2. A 37-year-old man presents to the ED complaining of swelling of his legs, hands, and face for 4 days. On examination he is afebrile with generalized edema of his upper and lower extremities as well as his face. His examination is otherwise notable only for scars in a linear pattern on his middle to lower arms bilaterally. Basic metabolic panel and complete blood cell count are normal, but liver function tests show total protein of 5.4 mg/dL and albumin of 2.8 mg/dL. Urinalysis shows 3+ protein without significant red or white blood cells. What is the most likely etiology of this patient's disease?

(A) Antibody deposition
(B) Cardiomyopathy

(C) Cocaine abuse
(D) Heroin abuse
(E) Hyperglycemia
(F) Streptococcal infection

3. A 75-year-old man with chronic obstructive pulmonary disease and coronary artery disease presents to the ED complaining of blood in his urine for the past several days. He denies any difficulty passing his urine or any frequency, urgency, or flank pain. He smokes about a pack of cigarettes a day and has done so for the past 50 years. The patient has a temperature of 36.6°C (97.9°F), heart rate of 60/min, and blood pressure of 128/85 mm Hg. Digital rectal examination reveals a normal prostate with no nodules. Urinalysis shows < 10 RBCs/hpf and 4 WBCs/hpf. There are no casts or crystals. His hemoglobin is 12 g/dL and WBC count is 9800/mm^3. What is the most likely diagnosis?

(A) Acute bacterial prostatitis
(B) Adenocarcinoma of the bladder
(C) Adenocarcinoma of the prostate
(D) Benign prostatic hyperplasia
(E) Interstitial cystitis
(F) Transitional cell carcinoma of the bladder

4. An 83-year-old woman who lives alone is admitted for confusion. She is accompanied to the hospital by her neighbor, who states that as recently as 3 months ago, the patient was able to perform basic and independent activities of daily living, and enjoyed gardening in her yard. However, after her husband's death 6 weeks ago, the patient has not been seen outside her home. When the neighbor went to check on the patient today, she found her to be awake and alert but confused. Her house was uncharacteristically unkempt, and a few empty TV dinners were strewn around the living room. Her blood pressure is 106/66 mm Hg, heart rate is 68/min, and temperature is 37.3°C (98.1°F). The remainder of her examination is unremarkable, except for marked temporal wasting. Laboratory studies show:

Na$^+$	137 mEq/L
K$^+$	3.5 mEq/L
Total Ca^{2+}	6.9 mg/dL
Mg^{2+}	1.5 mEq/L
Blood urea nitrogen	8 mg/dL
Creatinine	0.5 mg/dL
Inorganic phosphate	3.1 mg/dL
Albumin	1.5 g/dL

What is the next step in managing this patient's low calcium levels?

(A) This patient has low blood urea nitrogen levels; therefore, her hypocalcemia likely does not represent a decrease in active calcium; she does not need calcium repletion at this time

(B) This patient has low creatinine levels; therefore, her hypocalcemia likely does not represent a decrease in active calcium; she does not need calcium repletion at this time

(C) This patient has low creatinine levels; therefore, her hypocalcemia is likely more severe than measured; she needs aggressive calcium repletion

(D) This patient is hypoalbuminemic; therefore, her hypocalcemia likely does not represent a decrease in active calcium; she does not need calcium repletion at this time

(E) This patient is hypoalbuminemic; therefore, her hypocalcemia is likely more severe than measured; she needs aggressive calcium repletion

5. A 64-year-old man with a history of diabetes and colon polyps is admitted for episodic chest pain. The pain started 2 days ago and is sharp, nonradiating, and intermittent. It is worse with recumbency and with deep inspiration. His blood pressure is 118/68 mm Hg and drops to 116/64 mm Hg with inspiration, pulse is 80/min, and temperature is 37.3°C (99.2°F). On physical examination the patient is in significant distress. Further examination reveals the absence of jugular venous distention, cardiac friction rub, and normal pulmonary examination. Extremities are warm and well perfused. An ECG is obtained, as shown in the image. Laboratory tests show:

Blood urea nitrogen	73 mg/dL
Creatinine	6.3 mg/dL
Glucose	150 mg/dL
Creatine kinase-myocardial bound	1 IU/L
Troponin-I	< 0.3 IU/L

Which of the following is the most appropriate next step in the management of this patient?

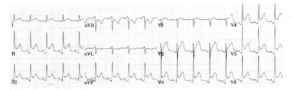

Reproduced, with permission, from Fuster V, Alexander RW, O'Rourke RA, eds. *Hurst's The Heart*, 11th edition. New York: McGraw-Hill, 2004: Figure 13-12.

(A) Hemodialysis
(B) Intravenous pyelogram
(C) 2 L normal saline at 225 mL/h
(D) Percutaneous angioplasty
(E) Pericardiocentesis

6. A 47-year-old man presents to his primary care physician complaining of urinary frequency, urgency, and pain with urination for the past 2 days. On further questioning, the patient reports feeling feverish and having a vague backache. He has no past medical history but has a brother who was diagnosed with prostate cancer 2 years ago at age 60 years. The patient has a temperature of 38.5°C (101.2°F) and blood pressure of 128/80 mm Hg. Digital rectal examination reveals an enlarged prostate that is tender with irregular contour. Urinalysis reveals 5–10 WBCs/hpf and 3–5 RBCs/hpf. A complete blood count is notable only for a WBC count of 15,000/mm^3. Prostate-specific antigen level was tested at the patient's request and was elevated at 4.8 ng/dL. What additional test would best confirm the patient's diagnosis?

(A) Blood culture
(B) Serial serum prostate-specific antigen
(C) Transrectal ultrasound
(D) Transrectal ultrasound and transrectal prostate biop
(E) Urine culture (± prostate massage)

7. A 35-year-old man with appendiceal carcinoma presents to the urgent care clinic 1 week after receiving chemotherapy with oxaliplatin, 5-fluorouracil, and leucovorin. He complains of severe fatigue progressively worsening over the past 4 days, with decreased oral intake of food and liquids. Review of systems reveals back pain that he has had for several months. Physical examination shows a lethargic, ill-appearing man with normal vital signs. He has a draining enterocutaneous fistula with an ostomy bag but no other abnormalities. Complete blood count shows mild anemia and leukocytosis. Electrolyte panel shows normal sodium and potassium with blood urea nitrogen of 76 mg/dL and creatinine of 3.3 mg/dL. Urinalysis is essentially normal. He has been taking aspirin for the pain. What is the most likely cause of renal failure in this patient?

(A) Acute interstitial nephritis secondary to aspirin
(B) Direct renal toxicity of oxaliplatin
(C) Hypovolemia secondary to chemotherapy and inadequate oral intake of fluids
(D) Nephrolithiasis
(E) Obstruction of the ureter by the tumor

8. A 50-year-old man complains to his physician of difficulty with erections. Over the past several months, his erections have been very painful. He denies any genital pain when his penis is not erect. His penis has also acquired a prominent curve when it is erect. The patient has a blood pressure of 130/78 mm Hg and a heart rate of 79/min. Genital examination reveals his penis is atraumatic and has a palpable dense plaque on the dorsal aspect of the shaft. There is no discharge from the meatus. What is the next step in managing the condition that is causing the patient's erectile dysfunction?

(A) Ascorbic acid
(B) Immediate decompression of the corpora cavernosa
(C) Observation and emotional support
(D) Penile prosthesis
(E) Surgical treatment

9. A 23-year-old woman clinic patient has recently been diagnosed with systemic lupus erythematosus. At the time of diagnosis, she had an elevated RBC sedimentation rate and markedly elevated anti-double-stranded DNA titers. At her rheumatologist's office, it was discovered that she had traces of blood in her urine and proteinuria. Renal biopsy was scheduled, and she was started on a 2-month course of prednisone. Over the course of her therapy, which medication adverse effect is this patient most likely to experience?

(A) Hair loss
(B) Hypertension
(C) Hypoglycemia
(D) Leukopenia
(E) Weight loss

10. A 3-year-old girl who has a past history of recurrent cystitis is brought to the ED. Her father has noticed 24 hours of decreased oral intake and an oral temperature of 38.8°C (101.9°F). On physical examination, the child has a blood pressure of 80/40 mm Hg, a heart rate of 120/min, and a respiratory rate of 28/min. The child appears well developed with marked costovertebral angle tenderness on the left. The child does not have a sacral tuft of hair or sacral dimple. Her urine culture grows > 100,000 colony-forming units of *Escherichia coli*. An ultrasound is done that does not show any hydronephrosis, but does show a small wedge-shaped area of scarring on the left upper pole of the kidney and blunted calyces on the left kidney. Following administration of intravenous antibiotics and resolution of her acute illness, what test is the most appropriate?

(A) CT scan without contrast
(B) Cystoscopy
(C) Intravenous pyelogram
(D) Spine MRI
(E) Voiding cystourethrogram

11. A 43-year-old woman with familial cystinuria seeks evaluation for intermittent flank pain. She has a history of kidney stones but has been episode free since undertaking a strategy of pharmacologic management and aggressive hydration 2 years ago. She admits to "getting lazy" with her fluid intake over the past several months but insists she is continuing her medication, although she cannot remember its name. Initial x-ray of the abdomen reveals a

small opacity within the proximal right ureter. Urinalysis demonstrates a urine pH of 7.8 and no trace of cystine crystals. Urinary calcium is elevated at 325 mg/24 h. Which of the following medications taken for prevention of cystine stones most likely contributed to this stone formation?

(A) Allopurinol
(B) Enalapril
(C) Furosemide
(D) Hydrochlorothiazide
(E) Potassium bicarbonate

12. A 60-year-old man with celiac sprue is in relatively good health and presents to the doctor for an annual check-up. He has a family history of coronary artery disease and a brother that had a myocardial infarction at age 55 years. He has a blood pressure of 128/78 mm Hg and a heart rate of 70/min. He mentions that his friend has just been diagnosed with prostate cancer and wants to know what screening test would be appropriate. What is the recommended screening test for prostate cancer in this patient?

(A) Cystoscopy
(B) Digital rectal examination and prostate-specific antigen
(C) Prostate-specific antigen alone
(D) Transrectal needle biopsy
(E) Yearly history and physical examination

13. A 5-year-old girl with acute lymphoid leukemia has been hospitalized on the pediatric hematology-oncology service for more than 2 months. A physician has been assigned to take care of her on his first day. During this time, the young patient has had many infections, including *Candida* septicemia. For the past 2 weeks, her main problem has been persistent hypokalemia, despite daily repletion. What laboratory value should the physician check on this patient, and is it expected to be high or low?

(A) Ca^{2+}, high
(B) Ca^{2+}, low
(C) Mg^{2+}, high
(D) Mg^{2+}, low
(E) Na^+, high
(F) Na^+, low

14. A 62-year-old police officer is brought to the ED after having a seizure that began spontaneously while he was sitting at his desk. He has no history of seizures or neurologic disorders. On physical examination, the patient has a temperature of 37.3°C (99.2°F), blood pressure of 110/90 mm Hg, and heart rate of 100/min. He localizes pain on deep palpation of the nail beds and sternal rub but is still in a state of altered consciousness. Laboratory tests show:

Glucose	88 mg/dL
Na^+	120 mEq/L
K^+	4.5 mEq/L
Cl^-	94 mmol/L
CO_2	24 mmol/L
Blood urea nitrogen	20 mg/dL
Creatinine	1.0 mg/dL

A urine specimen from a Foley catheter shows a urine osmolality of 300 mOsm/kg and urine Na^+ of 40 mEq/L. After treatment of the acute hyponatremia with slow administration of hypertonic saline, an extensive workup reveals a neoplasm. What is the most likely neoplasm based on the patient's hyponatremia?

(A) Insulinoma
(B) Multiple myeloma
(C) Small cell lung cancer
(D) Testicular embryonal tumor
(E) Thymic carcinoid

15. A 48-year-old man is brought to the ED confused and disoriented. He reports recent onset of nausea and has had several episodes of emesis in the past 4 days. On further questioning he also notes a metallic taste in his mouth, frequent hiccups, and pruritus. On physical examination there is a rough, Velcro-like sound heard across his precordium. Based on this patient's symptoms, which of the following is the most likely diagnosis?

(A) Addisonian crisis
(B) Fulminant hepatic failure
(C) Heroin withdrawal
(D) Renal insufficiency
(E) Vitamin B_{12} deficiency

16. A 60-year-old man presents to the urologist complaining of difficulty urinating. He states that he frequently gets out of bed in the middle of the night to go to the bathroom. Once he gets to the bathroom he can't urinate and must "bear down" to do so. He denies any history of sexually transmitted disease, trauma to the genitourinary tract, or prior genitourinary instrumentation. On rectal examination, the patient has an enlarged prostate and one 1-cm area of induration that is located on the middle posterior aspect of the prostate. He has a prostate-specific antigen level of 6 ng/mL (normal: 0–4 ng/mL), a blood urea nitrogen of 20 mg/L, and a creatinine of 1.6 mg/L. The patient undergoes a transrectal prostate biopsy, and no dysplasia or atypia is present. Given the clinical scenario and pathologic findings, what is the most appropriate treatment?

(A) Brachytherapy
(B) Finasteride
(C) Radical retropubic prostatectomy
(D) Transurethral resection of the prostate
(E) Watchful waiting

17. A 45-year-old woman presents to her physician complaining of lower extremity edema. Her temperature is 36.7°C (98.1°F), blood pressure is 150/90 mm Hg, heart rate is 80/min, and respiratory rate is 14/min. In addition to the finding of 1+ pitting edema of her ankles bilaterally, she has diffuse crackles on pulmonary examination. She denies shortness of breath, chest pain, or orthopnea. Initial laboratory evaluation reveals an albumin of 1.8 g/dL (normal: 3.5–5.5 g/dL), a total cholesterol of 200 mg/dL, and a protein C level of 2.1 μg/mL (normal: > 4 μg/mL). Urinalysis reveals heavy proteinuria. Which of the following disorders is most often associated with this presentation?

(A) Alcohol consumption
(B) Asthma
(C) Diabetes mellitus
(D) Hypertension
(E) Minimal change disease

18. A 23-year-old construction worker is admitted after his right leg became trapped under a concrete block at his construction site. After removal of the block, there were visible signs of crush injury to his thigh, and he was airlifted to a local hospital. In transit, he received several bags of intravenous fluids and analgesics. He is alert and oriented on arrival at the hospital. His blood pressure is 140/80 mm Hg, pulse is 70/min, and respiratory rate is 12/min. Physical examination is significant for multiple contusions and abrasions on the anterior portion of his right thigh. Distal pulses are palpable, and sensation in the affected extremity is normal. Laboratory studies show:

K+	6.1 mg/dL
Phosphorus	8.2 mg/dL
Ca^{2+}	6.3 mg/dL
Uric acid	20 mg/dL

What additional laboratory finding is most consistent with his likely diagnosis?

(A) Creatine kinase levels < 1000 IU/L
(B) Decreased serum lactic acid dehydrogenase
(C) Elevated homocysteine levels
(D) Elevated troponin I levels
(E) Positive urine dipstick for blood without red cells on microscopic examination

19. A 20-year-old man with no past medical history presents to a urologist after 2 years of unsuccessful attempts at conceiving a child. The man states that his wife is 24 years old and has no medical problems. She was evaluated for infertility by a gynecologist, and no abnormalities were found. The man has no history of sexually transmitted disease or urologic diseases. Physical examination reveals a tall man with long legs who appears younger than his stated age. He has minimal facial hair and a slight fullness to his breasts bilaterally (see image). The patient's testicles are 2.2 cm long and firm. A semen sample is obtained, which shows no sperm. For what disease is this man at increased risk?

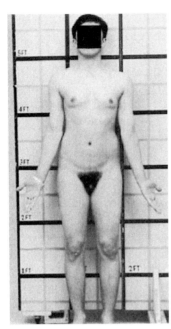

Reproduced, with permission, from Gardner DG, Shoback D. *Greenspan's Basic and Clinical Endocrinology*, 8th ed. New York: McGraw-Hill, 2007: Figure 13-7.

(A) Germ cell tumor
(B) Paraphimosis
(C) Peyronie's disease
(D) Renal cell carcinoma
(E) Transitional cell carcinoma

20. A 42-year-old woman with a family history of adult polycystic kidney disease presents to the ED complaining of gross blood in her urine, 3 days of fever, and right-sided abdominal pain. A review of systems reveals that she has had dysuria and urinary frequency as well. She has had similar symptoms twice in the past year and was treated for a urinary tract infection. Her temperature is 38.6°C (101.4°F), pulse is 82/min, respiratory rate is 18/min, and blood pressure is 160/100 mm Hg. Urinalysis shows many white and red blood cells as well as 1+ protein and positive leukocyte esterase. Which of the following is most likely to be iatrogenic in this patient?

(A) Ampicillin
(B) Angiotensin-converting enzyme inhibitor
(C) Gentamicin
(D) Low-protein diet
(E) Percutaneous cyst drainage

21. A 37-year-old man with a history of alcoholism and ulcerative colitis is being evaluated for an elevated blood urea nitrogen (BUN) level. He was first admitted after complaining of weakness and lightheadedness several weeks ago following an episode of bloody diarrhea. Initial work-up revealed heme-positive stool and hemoglobin of 7.1 mg/dL. A colonoscopy was performed revealing severe colitis. He was transfused with 2 U of packed RBCs. Ten days later, he began to complain of abdominal pain and was febrile. Currently, his blood pressure is 100/60 mm Hg and pulse is 110/min. Physical examination shows abdominal tenseness with rebound and pale extremities. Emergent colectomy is performed, and broad-spectrum antibiotics are started. In recovery, laboratory values demonstrated an elevation in his BUN to 82 mg/dL. Urinalysis was heme negative and did not reveal any casts. What is most likely to have contributed to this patient's azotemia?

(A) Alcoholism
(B) Blood transfusion
(C) Broad-spectrum antibiotics
(D) Gastrointestinal bleeding
(E) Glomerulonephritis

22. A 67-year-old woman with type 2 diabetes mellitus, asthma, coronary artery disease, and atrial fibrillation was admitted to the hospital for fluid repletion 3 days ago after a 1-week history of diarrhea. Laboratory studies show:

Serum glucose	400 mg/dL
Na$^+$	156 mEq/L
Blood urea nitrogen	30 mg/dL
Creatinine	0.9 mg/dL

Examination revealed dry mucous membranes and tenting of the skin on her hands. She was given insulin and promptly started on 0.45% saline at 200 mL/h. On her second hospital day, her glucose had normalized, she produced 100 mL/h of urine, and her sodium was within normal limits. Later in the day, she began to complain of fatigue and weakness. By hospital day 3, she had difficulty moving her limbs and was complaining of severe constipation. An ECG from her second hospital day is shown in the image. Which of the following would have prevented her most recent symptoms?

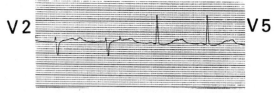

Reproduced, with permission, from Fuster V, Alexander RW, O'Rourke RA, eds. *Hurst's The Heart*, 11th ed. New York: McGraw-Hill, 2004: Figure 13-34.

(A) Administration of 20 mEq/h of potassium chloride
(B) Continuation of her home dose of albuterol
(C) Epinephrine bolus
(D) Phosphate repletion
(E) Using 1.8% saline instead of 0.45% saline for fluid replacement

23. A 50-year-old man presents to his primary care physician with the chief complaint of inability to achieve an erection. The patient has type 2 diabetes mellitus that is well controlled with diet and exercise, atrial fibrillation, and seasonal allergies, and a past surgical history of a bilateral varicocelectomy. He currently takes warfarin and intranasal steroids. The man states that his problem with achieving an erec-

tion has been going on for the past 3 weeks. He admits to having masturbated about a week ago. He did this because he noticed that he was able to have a normal erection when the woman with whom he is having an affair left for the morning. He states that it took him about 3 minutes to reach climax and ejaculate. He denies any curvature of the penis with erection or when flaccid. The man is afebrile, has a heart rate of 110/min that is regularly irregular, and a blood pressure of 130/85 mm Hg. Physical examination reveals his abdomen is soft, with no palpable masses. The man has an uncircumcised penis that is normally developed and two testicles that are normal in size and texture. What is the most likely cause of the man's erectile dysfunction?

(A) Diabetes mellitus
(B) Medication
(C) Peyronie's disease
(D) Prior genitourinary surgery
(E) Psychogenic

24. A 38-year-old man was thrown from his motorcycle and brought to the ED by emergency medical services. The paramedics report his initial vital signs were blood pressure 83/52 mm Hg, pulse 128/min, and respiratory rate 33/min. He was given 2 L of lactated Ringer's solution en route, and medical antishock trousers were applied. His vital signs on arrival to the trauma bay were blood pressure 108/76 mm Hg, pulse 105/min, and respiratory rate 28/min. On examination, pelvic compression elicits severe pain, and blood is noted at the urethral meatus. Which of the following is the most appropriate next step in evaluation of blood at the urethral meatus?

(A) Abdominal ultrasound
(B) Digital rectal examination
(C) Foley catheter insertion and urinalysis
(D) Intravenous pyelogram
(E) Retrograde urethrogram

25. A 40-year-old woman presents to the urologist for the evaluation of a renal mass discovered incidentally on CT scan of the abdomen. The mass on CT scan was 5 cm in diameter, originating from the upper pole of the right kidney. The center of the mass contains an area of cal-

cification. The patient has a distant history of acute pancreatitis secondary to a scorpion bite and a 20 pack-year smoking history. She does not drink alcohol. The decision was made to proceed with surgical removal of the mass, and a partial nephrectomy was performed. The patient did well postoperatively, and her Foley catheter was removed on postoperative day 2. That evening, she had substantial output into a Jackson-Pratt drain that the surgeons left in place. The output of the drain has been 30 mL/h for the past few hours, and the fluid is light pink to clear. The patient is examined and states that she is not in pain. She has a temperature of 37.7°C (99.8°F), heart rate of 80/min, and blood pressure of 110/70 mm Hg. What test or procedure would be appropriate to confirm the suspected diagnosis?

(A) Exploratory laparotomy
(B) Jackson-Pratt amylase
(C) Jackson-Pratt creatinine
(D) Serum amylase
(E) Serum hemoglobin

26. A 70-year-old woman with a history of renal artery stenosis presents to the ED with decreased urine output. She was recently started on a new medication by a physician, and a few days later noticed that she was producing less urine. Otherwise, she feels well and has no complaints. She is afebrile and her blood pressure is 156/88 mm Hg. Laboratory tests show:

Na$^+$	139 mEq/L
K$^+$	4.1 mEq/L
HCO$_3$$^-$	24 mEq/L
Blood urea nitrogen	41 mg/dL
Creatinine	1.8 mg/dL
Urine Na$^+$	6 mEq/L
Urine creatinine	11 mg/dL

Which of the following medications did she likely start recently?

(A) Amikacin
(B) Benztropine
(C) Cimetidine
(D) Enalapril
(E) Hydroxyurea

27. A 52-year-old man is recovering from a total colectomy for colorectal adenocarcinoma 1 day ago in the surgical intensive care unit. He is currently being maintained on a patient-controlled analgesia pump, half of a normal saline drip, and intravenous cefazolin. Additionally, he takes nothing by mouth. He has no complaints, appears well, and is conversational. Relevant laboratory findings are a serum sodium level of 110 mEq/L; his sodium level was 137 mEq/L 1 day earlier. What is the next step in the management of this patient?

(A) Discontinue cefazolin
(B) Discontinue patient-controlled analgesia pump
(C) Draw blood for laboratory tests from the other arm
(D) Restrict fluid intake
(E) Switch to hypertonic saline infusion

28. A 4-month-old boy born at 29 weeks' gestation is brought to the pediatrician for a well-baby examination. During the pregnancy, an amniocentesis was performed out of concern for advanced maternal age (40 years). Results were normal, and the karyotype was normal, 46,XY. The child has been feeding well, and interacts with his mother and father by tracking their faces and vocalizing when excited. On physical examination, the patient has a temperature of 36.4°C (97.5°F) and heart rate of 120/min. The genitourinary examination shows a well-formed penis with no evidence of hypospadias or epispadias and a well-formed scrotum with no palpable testes. On abdominal examination, there is a mass palpable in the left lower quadrant. The mass is 1 cm in diameter and found midway between the pubic symphysis and the anterior superior iliac crest. This mass does not move on gentle manipulation. What is the likely diagnosis?

(A) Bilateral anorchia
(B) Congenital adrenal hyperplasia
(C) Cryptorchidism
(D) Retractile testis (pseudocryptorchidism)
(E) Strangulated inguinal hernia

29. A 65-year-old patient with a history of bipolar disorder, well-controlled with lithium, is being evaluated for hypernatremia. Her only complaint is 4 months of polyuria and thirst. Her blood pressure is 106/68 mm Hg and pulse is 102/min. Physical examination reveals her mucous membranes are dry, and skin turgor is normal. The remainder of the physical examination is unremarkable. Laboratory studies show:

Na^+	147 mEq/L
K^+	4.7 mEq/L
Cl^-	110 mEq/L
HCO_3^-	24 mEq/L
Blood urea nitrogen	12 mg/dL
Creatinine	1.1 mg/dL
Plasma osmolality	305 mOsm/kg
Urine osmolality	200 mOsm/kg

Which of the following is most likely to resolve this patient's electrolyte imbalance?

(A) Exogenous ADH
(B) Fluid restriction
(C) Intravenous fluids
(D) Salt restriction
(E) Thiazide diuretic

30. A 47-year-old woman comes to the ED with the chief complaint of "cold fingers." She has had intermittent episodes of this condition for several years, but today the pain was unbearable. On review of systems she mentions chronic symptoms of reflux and progressive difficulty moving her fingers. When the physician examines her, he notes the appearance of her fingers (as seen in the image), and he also sees multiple telangiectasias on her skin and hard nodules on the extensor surfaces of her forearms. If the associated electrolyte abnormality is found, what is the first step that should be taken in correcting it?

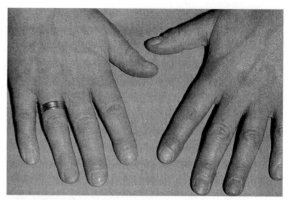

Reproduced, with permission, from Wolff K, Johnson RA, Surmond D. *Fitzpatrick's Color Atlas & Synopsis of Clinical Dermatology*, 5th ed. New York: McGraw-Hill, 2005: Figure 14-32.

(A) Insulin and bicarbonate
(B) Intravenous calcium gluconate
(C) Intravenous glucose
(D) Intravenous normal saline
(E) Oral calcium channel blocker

31. A 43-year-old man with hypertension and acute myelogenous leukemia is admitted to the hospital for fever and chills. He is currently receiving chemotherapy, but he does not know which kind. On admission the man is febrile to 38.5°C (101.3°F) and has a respiratory rate of 12/min. His blood work is notable for a WBC count of 10,000/mm³ and an absolute neutrophil count of 900/mm³ . The patient undergoes blood cultures, urine cultures, sputum cultures, and a chest x-ray, all of which are negative. He is started on empiric broad-spectrum antibiotics. The patient continues to spike temperatures to 38.5°C (101.0°F). The decision is made to start the patient on empiric antifungal therapy with amphotericin B, given that fungi can be difficult to isolate and the man continues to show signs of infection. For which of the following does amphotericin put the patient at greatest risk?

(A) Leukocytoclastic vasculitis
(B) Nephrogenic diabetes insipidus
(C) Type I distal renal tubular acidosis
(D) Type II proximal renal tubular acidosis
(E) Type IV distal renal tubular acidosis

32. The radiograph below was taken in a 36-year-old man who presented to the ED with severe left flank pain and one episode of hematuria. Which of the following measures could cause another episode of this pathology?

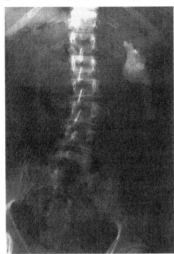

Reproduced, with permission, from Tanagho EA, McAninch JW. *Smith's General Urology*, 16th edition. New York: McGraw-Hill, 2004: Figure 15-16.

(A) Calcium restriction
(B) Increased fluid intake (> 2 L/d)
(C) Protein restriction
(D) Sodium restriction
(E) Thiazide diuretic

33. A pediatrician notes bilateral abdominal masses in a 4-month-old girl. The girl's mother reports that the child has been very irritable and is not interested in eating, and has noticeably decreased formula intake. The patient has a temperature of 36.6°C (97.8°F), blood pressure of 140/90 mm Hg, respiratory rate of 30/min, and heart rate of 120/min. Abdominal examination reveals marked upper abdominal fullness and irregularly contoured bilateral masses, but no apparent tenderness to palpation. There are increased tortuous makings surrounding the child's umbilicus. Normal bowel sounds are heard. Relevant laboratory findings are shown below.

WBC count	6000/mm^3
Creatinine	1.0 mg/dL
Aspartate aminotransferase	8 IU/L
Alanine aminotransferase	12 IU/L

A CT scan with intravenous contrast is performed, and the kidneys are 10 cm in the vertical dimension (10–12 cm is normal size in full-grown adults) with cortical cystic lesions, and exhibit poor uptake of the contrast. What is the most likely diagnosis?

(A) Autosomal dominant polycystic kidney disease
(B) Autosomal recessive polycystic kidney disease
(C) Bilateral megaureters
(D) Chronic viral hepatitis
(E) Medullary cystic disease

34. A 56-year-old man presents to the ED for severe pain in his right ankle. The pain began 4 days ago, and he denies any history of trauma. His only medical problem is recent diagnosis of hypertension, for which he takes a mild antihypertensive. His temperature is 37.2°C (98.9°F), blood pressure is 138/68 mm Hg, pulse is 80/min, and respiratory rate is 14/min. On examination his ankle is swollen, red, and diffusely tender. Joint fluid aspirate reveals needle-shaped negatively birefringent crystals under polarized light microscopy. What medication is likely responsible for this condition?

(A) Atenolol
(B) Diltiazem
(C) Enalapril
(D) Hydralazine
(E) Hydrochlorothiazide

35. A 55-year-old man with a past medical history significant for diabetes presents with fever, malaise, and dysuria. On physical examination he has costovertebral angle tenderness, and has a temperature of 37.6°C (99.6°F). The remainder of the physical examination is unremarkable. He also has a past medical history significant for untreated benign prostatic hyperplasia. What intervention is most likely to prevent the recurrence of these symptoms?

(A) Increase fluid intake
(B) Lithotripsy
(C) Surgical intervention to remove an obstructing renal calculus
(D) Treatment for benign prostatic hyperplasia
(E) Treatment with antibiotics

36. A 33-year-old African-American man presents to a rural clinic with a 2-day history of painful genital sores. The man admits to sexual contact with multiple partners and has never been tested for sexually transmitted diseases, including HIV. On physical examination, there are two tender sores with sharp edges and a yellowish exudate on his penis. Tender unilateral inguinal adenopathy is also noted. Which of the following is most likely to confirm the diagnosis?

(A) Fluorescent treponemal antibody absorption test
(B) HIV viral load
(C) Polymerase chain reaction for *Haemophilus ducreyi*
(D) Serology for L1, L2, and L3 serotypes of *Chlamydia trachomatis*
(E) Tissue biopsy
(F) Tzanck smear

37. A 78-year-old man is admitted to the medical intensive care unit (ICU) with aspiration pneumonia and sepsis. Before his ICU stay, he had been treated at his nursing home with sulfamethoxazole-trimethoprim for a urinary tract infection. In the ICU, he is treated with additional antibiotics for pneumonia and large volumes of fluid. He becomes hemodynamically stable with treatment, but his fever persists, and he develops a maculopapular rash on his chest, abdomen, and thighs. A complete blood count shows a WBC count of $12,000/mm^3$ (66% neutrophils, 23% lymphocytes, and 9% eosinophils). Urinalysis reveals blood urea nitrogen of 34 mg/dL and a creatinine level of 2.1 mg/dL. Cultures are negative. Which of the following is the most likely diagnosis?

(A) Acute interstitial nephritis
(B) Glomerulonephritis
(C) Hypovolemic renal failure
(D) Nephrolithiasis
(E) Pyelonephritis

EXTENDED MATCHING

Questions 38–40

For each patient with renal failure, select the most likely etiology.

(A) Alport's syndrome
(B) Diabetic nephropathy
(C) Focal segmental glomerulosclerosis
(D) Goodpasture's syndrome
(E) IgA nephropathy
(F) Lupus nephritis
(G) Membranoproliferative nephropathy
(H) Membranous nephropathy
(I) Minimal change disease
(J) Poststreptococcal glomerulonephritis
(K) Renal amyloidosis
(L) Wegener's granulomatosis

38. A 10-year-old boy is brought to his pediatrician because his mother notices that his legs and arms have looked "puffy" for the past 3 days. The pediatrician notices that he just saw this child in the clinic 2 weeks earlier with the chief complaint of a sore throat and prescribed antibiotics. On examination, the boy has diffuse upper and lower extremity edema, and his blood pressure is 168/110 mm Hg. Urinalysis shows microscopic hematuria and 1+ proteinuria.

39. A 23-year-old man calls his primary care physician in a panic because he noticed that the toilet was full of bright red blood after urinating. A review of systems is positive for a recent "bad cold." Based on a urinalysis showing gross hematuria and 1+ protein, the physician recommends a renal biopsy, which shows diffuse mesangial IgA deposits.

40. An 8-year-old girl is brought to her pediatrician after complaining to her father that her ballet outfit, purchased 1 month earlier, feels too tight. In the review of systems, her father notes that she has not been to her biweekly ballet class very often recently because she has been sick repeatedly with mild colds. On examination, she has 2+ edema to the knees and elbows bilaterally. Laboratory testing shows albumin level of 2.4 g/dL and total protein of 5.3 g/dL, and urinalysis shows 4+ protein. Her symptoms and laboratory studies improve dramatically after 4 weeks of prednisone.

ANSWERS

*[handwritten: FANCONIS
1. Nor AG MA
2. Hypopho
3. Glycosuri]*

1. **The correct answer is D.** The clinical scenario is consistent with a generalized proximal renal tubular dysfunction known as Fanconi's syndrome. The patient's Fanconi's syndrome is manifest as evidence of a nongap metabolic acidosis accompanied by hypophosphatemia and glycosuria (with normal blood glucose levels).

   Answer A is incorrect. Right heart failure is also known as cor pulmonale. This classically occurs secondary to the hypoxia and pulmonary hypertension that result from chronic obstructive pulmonary disease. This is not related to the laboratory findings.

   Answer B is incorrect. Steroids may cause hyperglycemia. However, the glycosuria that is seen with steroids should be accompanied by hyperglycemia, not a blood glucose of 98 mg/dL.

   Answer C is incorrect. Type I renal tubular acidosis (RTA) is a distal process. It occurs from a renal distal tubular insult, which causes a defect in urinary ammonium production and urine acidification. A type I RTA would not cause urine phosphate and glucose wasting, which are more indicative of proximal tubule dysfunction.

   Answer E is incorrect. The most common type of renal tubular acidosis is type IV. This type is characterized by hyperkalemic, hyperchloremic metabolic acidosis.

2. **The correct answer is D.** This patient presents with generalized edema, hypoalbuminemia, and marked proteinuria, findings strongly suggestive of a nephrotic syndrome. The track marks on his arms are highly suggestive of drug abuse. Putting this picture together, one can deduce that the patient has focal segmental glomerulosclerosis (FSG), a nonspecific nephrotic syndrome that may be secondary to heroin abuse. Other causes of secondary FSG include lithium and malignancy, particularly lymphoma.

   Answer A is incorrect. Antibody deposition in the glomerular basement membrane is seen in Goodpasture's syndrome, a type of nephritic syndrome that presents with hemoptysis and respiratory symptoms in addition to renal findings.

   Answer B is incorrect. Cocaine abusers can develop dilated cardiomyopathy, which can lead to congestive heart failure. Heart failure can cause edema, but the edema would likely be confined to the lower extremities, and other findings on examination would include gallops or murmurs, elevated jugular venous pressure, and signs of pulmonary vascular congestion.

   Answer C is incorrect. Cocaine may be injected and leave marks such as those seen on the arms of this patient. Also, cocaine may cause acute renal failure secondary to rhabdomyolysis, but red urine and myoglobulinemia would also be seen.

   Answer E is incorrect. Diabetic patients with diabetic nephropathy can present with proteinuria in the nephrotic range. Diabetic nephropathy is particularly common in diabetics with poor glycemic control. However, there is no evidence that this patient has diabetes; he does not complain of polyuria or polydipsia and he has no glucose or ketones reported in his urine.

   Answer F is incorrect. Streptococcal infection can cause postinfectious glomerulonephritis, a type of nephritic syndrome that presents with hypertension, hematuria, and mild proteinuria, usually several weeks after an upper respiratory infection. The patient presented here has a nephrotic, not nephritic, picture.

3. **The correct answer is F.** The patient has transitional cell carcinoma (TCC). Most bladder cancers are TCCs. The disease is more common in men (2.7:1 male-to-female ratio), and the mean age of diagnosis is 65 years. Smoking and exposure to industrial solvents and dyes such as aniline are other risk factors for TCC. Painless hematuria is the presenting symptom in about 90% of bladder carcinomas. Irritative voiding symptoms can also occur, depending on the location and size of the lesion.

Answer A is incorrect. Acute bacterial prostatitis usually presents with perineal, suprapubic, or sacral pain. Patients may complain of irritative voiding symptoms. Depending on the severity, pain, fever, and urinary obstruction with retention can occur. Prostate examination would be contraindicated in such men because it may result in sepsis.

Answer B is incorrect. Primary adenocarcinomas of the bladder are rare. Adenocarcinoma accounts for approximately 2% of bladder tumors in the United States. Transitional cell carcinoma constitutes the vast majority of bladder neoplasms.

Answer C is incorrect. Prostate cancer may present as a focal nodule within the prostate during digital rectal examination. Many prostate cancers are only detected by biopsy prompted by an elevated prostate-specific antigen.

Answer D is incorrect. The patient is not presenting with obstructive symptoms that would be consistent with benign prostatic hyperplasia (BPH). BPH may also result in an enlarged prostate on digital rectal examination.

Answer E is incorrect. Interstitial cystitis presents with pain during periods of bladder distention. This pain is often relieved by voiding. Frequency, urgency, and nocturia are also common. The diagnosis is often one of exclusion, although cystoscopy can aid in the diagnosis.

4. **The correct answer is D.** This patient is undernourished and in a neglected state of health. Often, the only manifestation of poor nutrition in an elderly patient is subtle changes in routine laboratory values including creatinine, a reflection of decreased muscle mass; albumin, a reflection of poor protein intake; and calcium. Because active, ionized calcium is only a fraction (45%) of what is measured in total calcium, there are some settings in which a low total calcium measurement does not reflect overall calcium depletion. Specifically, when circulating albumin levels are decreased, the 40% of total calcium that is normally bound to albumin is also low, and calcium measurements will be demonstrably low. In-

deed, for each 1 g/dL reduction in albumin levels, the total calcium concentration will be lowered by 0.8 mg/dL. This reduction does **not** represent a reduction in ionized calcium, and thus will not cause clinical hypocalcemia.

Answer A is incorrect. Blood urea nitrogen (BUN) levels correlate to dietary intake and hydration status. In an undernourished elderly woman, it is not surprising that as protein intake decreased, BUN dropped slightly. BUN, however, plays no role in the measurement of total or ionized calcium levels.

Answer B is incorrect. Creatinine levels correlate to lean muscle mass levels. In an undernourished and elderly woman, it is not surprising that creatinine levels are subnormal. Creatinine levels, however, play no role in the measurement of total or ionized calcium levels.

Answer C is incorrect. Because creatinine plays no role in determining calcium levels, this answer is incorrect.

Answer E is incorrect. Decreased serum albumin levels lead to an underestimation of clinically important calcium levels. Aggressive calcium repletion is not warranted.

5. **The correct answer is A.** With significant azotemia, friction rub, and presentation typical of pericardial irritation, this patient is likely suffering from uremic pericarditis. In addition, his ECG shows ST segment elevations, which are characteristic of the early stages of pericarditis. His stable blood pressure, with absent pulsus paradoxus, and general appearance suggest pericarditis without tamponade physiology. This is an important distinction to make because it greatly influences the initial management of uremic pericarditis. In the presence of tamponade, drainage of the effusion is of paramount importance before other measures are undertaken to reverse the cause of the disease. Because this patient likely does not have tamponade, initial management consists of emergent hemodialysis. As uremic patients are coagulopathic, heparin should not be used in the extracorporeal circuit during hemodialysis.

Answer B is incorrect. Intravenous pyelogram (IVP) is a diagnostic study that allows for examination of both the upper and the lower urinary tract. It is employed in renal failure patients to evaluate for reversible causes of renal failure such as pyelonephritis, renal calculi, or obstruction. IVP cannot reverse this patient's uremic pericarditis.

Answer C is incorrect. This patient is likely suffering from chronic or acute chronic renal failure and subsequent uremia. These patients are likely to be volume overloaded because decreased renal function leads to accumulation of ingested fluids. Administration of intravenous fluids without instituting hemodialysis will not address the pericardial process and may put additional strain on the heart.

Answer D is incorrect. Heart catheterization is an unnecessary procedure for this patient because his process is not ischemic in nature.

Answer E is incorrect. Pericardial fluid drainage should take precedence over dialysis only if tamponade physiology is present.

6. **The correct answer is E.** The diagnosis is acute bacterial prostatitis. Acute bacterial prostatitis is the most commonly diagnosed urologic disorder in men younger than 50 years. If prostatitis is suspected, the clinician should send a urine culture, and some clinicians suggest doing this after gentle prostatic massage. The prostatic expressate can also be cultured and/or analyzed microscopically. Although prostatic massage is the most complete way to document the diagnosis, care should be taken during the manipulation of the prostate. If the patient does have acute bacterial prostatitis, vigorous massaging can lead to bacteremia. In addition, this maneuver can be extremely painful for the patient. The diagnosis is generally a clinical one in combination with a positive urine culture. The presentation of urgency, frequency, and/or retention in addition to systemic signs such as fever would be enough to make the presumptive diagnosis. Furthermore, if the patient is in retention and the clinician is suspicious of prostatitis, the placement of a suprapubic tube would be safer than risking sepsis by placing a conventional Foley catheter.

Answer A is incorrect. A blood culture is unnecessary. A source of infection is apparent, and urine culture will likely identify the organism. Urosepsis is not suspected because the patient appears well with normal blood pressure.

Answer B is incorrect. In prostatitis, elevated levels of prostate-specific antigen (PSA) are often observed. Serially, measuring the PSA is not useful in the diagnosis or treatment of prostatitis. PSA is used in the screening of prostate cancer. A physician should, however, wait until the prostatitis has resolved before carrying out such screening. In patients with prostate cancer, PSA levels can be used postoperatively to assess for completeness of the proctectomy and disease recurrence.

Answer C is incorrect. Transrectal ultrasound is not necessary for the diagnosis of prostatitis. Transrectal ultrasound would only be indicated if the patient did not respond to conventional antibiotic therapy or if prostatic abscess was suspected. In addition, ultrasound of the bladder and kidneys to assess for substantial postvoid residual or hydronephrosis from urinary obstruction may also be indicated. CT scan may also be useful if an abscess was suspected.

Answer D is incorrect. Transrectal ultrasound with transrectal prostate biopsy is used in evaluating men suspected of having prostatic cancer. The elevated prostate-specific antigen in this case can be explained by the patient's probable infection, and thus no testing for prostate cancer is necessary at this point.

7. **The correct answer is C.** This patient presents with prerenal failure, as evidenced by the blood urea nitrogen:creatinine ratio > 20:1. His fatigue and malaise is likely secondary to renal failure. Oxaliplatin is associated with dehydration in some patients, and patients are encouraged to keep up their oral fluid intake after treatment. This patient also has a potentially high-output fistula, which can contribute to hypovolemia if he fails to keep up his oral fluid intake.

Answer A is incorrect. Nonsteroidal anti-inflammatory drug–induced acute interstitial nephritis would present with an intrinsic renal failure picture, with blood urea nitrogen:creatinine ratio < 20:1 and WBCs with casts on urinalysis.

Answer B is incorrect. Oxaliplatin may increase serum creatinine but does not have acute renal failure as a major adverse effect. Additionally, drug-induced acute renal failure would be expected to show an intrinsic renal failure picture, with blood urea nitrogen:creatinine ratio < 20:1. This patient has a prerenal failure profile.

Answer D is incorrect. The patient does complain of back pain, which might suggest nephrolithiasis. Nephrolithiasis may cause ureteral obstruction, but it would be highly unlikely to have bilateral obstruction causing postrenal failure. Kidney stones may also be associated with acute tubular necrosis, but this would present with an intrinsic renal failure, including blood urea nitrogen:creatinine < 20:1 and granular or renal tubular casts on urinalysis.

Answer E is incorrect. Obstruction distal to the kidneys can cause postrenal azotemia, which would present with a similar clinical picture. However, bilateral ureteral obstruction is highly unlikely in this patient, and his tumor is likely too superior to cause urethral obstruction.

8. **The correct answer is C.** Peyronie's disease is a clinical problem affecting middle-aged and older men that is caused by the development of a fibrous plaque involving the tunica albuginea. Patients present with a curvature of the penis, pain with erection, and poor erection distal to the area of induration. In about 50% of cases, the induration spontaneously resolves. Because often no medical treatment is needed, observation and emotional support are advised as the first line of therapy. If the induration does not resolve, medical treatment can be attempted. Medical treatment includes vitamin E, calcium channel blockers, and locally injected steroids to aid in the breakdown of connective tissue. Surgical treatment involves excision of the plaque and skin graft. Complications of surgery include loss of sexual function and damage to the urethra. Medical treatment has limited success, but should be attempted prior to surgical correction.

Answer A is incorrect. Ascorbic acid or vitamin C is not used in the treatment of Peyronie's disease. However, there is some support for treating this disorder with vitamin E and aminobenzoic acid, which are thought to break down the fibrous connective tissue of the plaque.

Answer B is incorrect. Priapism, or prolonged painful erection, is treated with decompression of the corpora cavernosa.

Answer D is incorrect. After failed medical therapy, if the patient remains impotent, a penile prosthesis can be inserted as an alternative to surgical management.

Answer E is incorrect. The Nesbit procedure is successfully used in patients with Peyronie's disease that can achieve an erection but have failed conservative management. The procedure involves making an incision in the tunica albuginea and placing a plicating stitch on the convex side of the penis across from the point of greatest curvature, thus straightening the penis. Plaque removal and grafting have also been utilized.

9. **The correct answer is B.** Corticosteroids are a very commonly used class of medication. In this case, steroids are used to control the renal manifestations of her systemic lupus erythematosus. However, they can lead to multiple local and systemic adverse effects that a clinician must be able to recognize. Commonly, these include acne, hirsutism, hypertrichosis, and weight gain. Corticosteroid use is less commonly associated with diabetes, hypertension, arrhythmias, and osteoporosis. Other important adverse effects include reduced defense against infection and several psychiatric disturbances, including euphoria, psychosis, and depression.

Answer A is incorrect. Patients taking corticosteroids are likely to experience hypertrichosis, not hair loss.

Answer C is incorrect. Corticosteroids typically cause hyperglycemia, not hypoglycemia, by increasing hepatic gluconeogenesis and by inhibiting peripheral utilization and glucose uptake.

Answer D is incorrect. Corticosteroids produce a leukocytosis, not leukopenia, by causing an increase in absolute neutrophil counts, or neutrophilia. This is caused by decreased neutrophil adhesion and increased release of stores of the bone marrow.

Answer E is incorrect. Patients taking corticosteroids are likely to experience weight gain, not weight loss.

10. **The correct answer is E.** The girl has pyelonephritis and a scar from a previous insult. A voiding cystourethrogram, carried out after the acute infection is resolved, will help determine if the patient has vesicoureteral reflux (VUR), a condition that results from an abnormal connection of the ureters and bladder and is associated with urinary tract infections (UTIs) and renal damage. VUR is diagnosed if radiopaque contrast material fills the bladder and ascends into the ureters while the child is voiding. Reflux should be sought in children with unexplained failure of renal growth, those with renal scarring, or in children with febrile UTI.

Answer A is incorrect. A CT scan without contrast is helpful in the evaluation of stones. This patient does not exhibit symptoms of renal colic, so stones are unlikely, and thus a noncontrast CT has little utility.

Answer B is incorrect. Cystoscopy allows direct visualization of the bladder. This modality can help define some pediatric urologic issues such as ureteroceles, foreign objects, tumors, posterior urethral valves in boys, and vesicoenteric fistula, but does not allow investigation of the upper tract. The patient does not seem to have any indication for cystoscopy.

Answer C is incorrect. An intravenous pyelogram is a very useful test to assess structural or anatomic defects within the genitourinary tract. The contrast dye is injected intravenously and its excretion into the collecting system is captured with x-ray imaging. This modality can identify reflux in some cases. However, the test does not necessarily capture images of the patient voiding. The voiding process produces pressure that might cause the urine (or contrast) to reflux into the upper tract, which would not be recognized if the bladder was not contracting.

Answer D is incorrect. An MRI of the spine is a useful test to evaluate children suspected of having spinal cord abnormalities. The physical examination findings of a tuft of hair or a sacral dimple might suggest that this test is the appropriate imaging modality. In the absence of this finding or other neurologic deficits, MRI is not the most appropriate imaging study at this time.

11. **The correct answer is E.** Cystinuria is typically caused by a genetic defect in the tubular amino acid transport system. This disorder is difficult to adequately treat. There are no medications that can reverse the defect in cystine transport, and thus most therapies target increasing the solubility of the molecule in urine. As with calcium stones, increasing the urine volume and thus decreasing the cystine concentration by adequate hydration helps prevent crystallization. Urine alkalization with potassium bicarbonate also helps increase the solubility of cystine. However, elevation of the urine pH can increase the risk of calcium phosphate stone formation, especially in the setting of low urine volume. The patient's new stone is likely to be a calcium stone because it is radiopaque and urinary calcium is elevated.

Answer A is incorrect. Allopurinol is a xanthine oxidase inhibitor used for the treatment of hyperuricemia and uric acid stones associated with gout. It effectively lowers urinary uric acid levels and is helpful in preventing gouty flares. It plays no role in the treatment of stones due to cystinuria.

Answer B is incorrect. Enalapril is an angiotensin-converting enzyme inhibitor that works to decrease the glomerular hydrostatic pressure and relieve hypertension. It plays no role in the treatment of cystine stone formation. Captopril, another drug in the same class as enalapril, has been used in patients with cystine stones, with limited success. Its mechanism relies on the binding of a sulfhydryl group on the drug to cystine residues.

Answer C is incorrect. Loop diuretics increase the level of calcium in the urine and thus can contribute to the formation of calcium stones. There is no role, however, for loop diuretics in the treatment of cystinuria.

Answer D is incorrect. Thiazide diuretics decrease the level of calcium in the urine and are often given to patients with recurrent calcium nephrolithiasis. There is no role, however, for thiazides in the treatment of stone disease from cystinuria.

12. **The correct answer is B.** The most sensitive method for screening men for prostate cancer employs both prostate-specific antigen (PSA) and digital rectal examination (DRE). The use of PSA helps detect cancer earlier, and its use is likely responsible for the increase in detection of prostate cancer. DRE will help identify cancer in men that might not have a PSA elevation. Screening beginning at age 50 years is considered appropriate for most men. However, risk factors such as having a first-degree relative with prostate cancer or being African-American may necessitate earlier screening beginning at age 40.

Answer A is incorrect. Cystoscopy is used in surveillance of bladder cancer and may be a part of a hematuria workup. It does not have a role in the screening or management of prostate cancer.

Answer C is incorrect. If the practitioner had only one test to screen for prostate cancer, PSA would be the first choice. PSA has relatively low specificity, as it can be elevated in settings other than prostate cancer. However, a combination of PSA and digital rectal examination provides a more thorough screening program.

Answer D is incorrect. Biopsy is the only way to confirm prostate cancer, but is not an appropriate screening test. Biopsy of the prostate should be undertaken if the PSA is > 4.0 ng/mL, if there is a significant rise in the PSA, or the digital rectal examination is abnormal.

Answer E is incorrect. A yearly history and physical examination would not be sufficient for the screening of prostate cancer. The man should, however, have a yearly history and physical as part of his regular health maintenance.

13. **The correct answer is D.** When repleting a patient's potassium, always remember to replace his or her magnesium as well. Hypomagnesemia can prevent correction of hypokalemia, even if the potassium is repleted appropriately. The other electrolytes may also be abnormal in this very ill child, but they are not the most pertinent to make note of when treating hypokalemia.

Answer A is incorrect. Hypercalcemia will not prevent the correction of hypokalemia.

Answer B is incorrect. Hypocalcemia will not prevent the correction of hypokalemia.

Answer C is incorrect. Hypermagnesemia will not prevent the correction of hypocalcemia.

Answer E is incorrect. Hypernatremia will not prevent the correction of hypokalemia.

Answer F is incorrect. Hyponatremia will not prevent the correction of hypokalemia.

14. **The correct answer is C.** The syndrome of inappropriate secretion of antidiuretic hormone (ADH) occurs in about 50% of patients with small cell lung cancer (SCLC). This inappropriate production of vasopressin does not always cause the overt symptoms of hyponatremia that this scenario depicts. The patient may compensate for the hyponatremia by decreasing water intake, and thus increasing production of atrial natriuretic peptide. Tumors that secrete ADH include those with neuroendocrine features. These can be varied and include carcinoids, non-SCLC, central nervous system neoplasms, and cancers of the head and neck and genitourinary and gastrointestinal tract.

Answer A is incorrect. Insulinomas need to be considered when working up hypoglycemia. The hypoglycemia often occurs during fasting. The patient's normal glucose makes this unlikely. Insulinomas are unrelated to hyponatremia.

Answer B is incorrect. Multiple myeloma (MM) is an aberrant proliferation of plasma cells in the bone marrow, resulting in the clonal production of a monoclonal immunoglobulin. Invasion of the bone can lead to osteolytic lesions, osteopenia, and pathologic fractures. MM is frequently accompanied with anemia, hypercalcemia, and renal insufficiency. This patient does not have any of these findings. Furthermore, MM is not associated with inappropriate ADH secretion or hyponatremia.

Answer D is incorrect. Testicular embryonal tumors can cause a paraneoplastic syndrome. However, they do not cause the syndrome of inappropriate secretion of ADH. These tumors can be a source of intact human chorionic gonadotropin (hCG), which can lead to elevated steroidogenesis and aromatase activity. Elevated hCG levels can lead to gynecomastia in men, while women are usually asymptomatic.

Answer E is incorrect. Thymic carcinoma is not frequently associated with the syndrome of inappropriate ADH secretion but is the second most common cause of ectopic ACTH production. Fifteen percent of cases of ectopic ACTH production are attributed to thymic carcinoma, while > 50% of cases are attributed to small cell lung cancer.

15. **The correct answer is D.** Perhaps because of the crucial role of kidneys in filtering toxins from the plasma, renal dysfunction often presents with a wide range of signs and symptoms. As uremic toxins increase, patients will complain of pruritus, nausea and vomiting, hiccups, and a metallic taste in the mouth. Other signs include altered sensorium, malaise, asterixis, and pericardial friction rub in cases of uremic pericarditis (the sound heard on physical examination in this case). Signs and symptoms of altered volume status may also be present, as renal failure can be caused by hypovolemia (prerenal disease) or can cause hypervolemic states (oliguria or anuria).

Answer A is incorrect. The most common manifestation of acute adrenal insufficiency is shock, but nonspecific symptoms may predominate in the initial manifestations of the syndrome. These include nausea and vomiting, weakness, and abdominal pain. Changes in arousal may also occur, ranging from fatigue and lethargy to coma.

Answer B is incorrect. Symptoms of hepatic failure include nausea, anorexia, jaundice, and abdominal pain. Hepatic encephalopathy, if present, can lead to asterixis, confusion, and even coma.

Answer C is incorrect. Signs and symptoms of opiate withdrawal are opposite to the effects often associated with opiate use and abuse. These include anxiety, tremor, and flulike symptoms such as rhinorrhea, sneezing, nausea, and vomiting. Other common symptoms include papillary dilation, lacrimation, yawning, and diarrhea.

Answer E is incorrect. Vitamin B_{12} deficiency is most often due to pernicious anemia, which causes macrocytic anemia. Vitamin B_{12} deficiency may also lead to signs and symptoms discernible on examination. Classically, mental sluggishness, a shiny tongue, and a shuffling, broad-based gait are associated with pernicious anemia–induced vitamin B_{12} deficiency. Patients may also exhibit personality changes and memory impairment. Other nonspecific neurologic findings due to damage to the posterior and lateral spinal columns include loss of dexterity, paresthesias, and weakness.

16. **The correct answer is D.** The patient has benign prostatic hyperplasia. The biopsy revealed a prostate that has undergone regular proliferation. This disease can cause elevated levels of PSA, as can prostate cancer. The nodule was suspicious enough to warrant a biopsy that revealed benign disease. This disease can be managed expectantly, with medication, or with surgery, depending on the severity of symptoms and associated findings. The man presented has renal failure secondary to the obstruction and moderate to severe symptoms. Thus, transurethral resection of the prostate is the best treatment.

Answer A is incorrect. Brachytherapy would be another treatment option had the biopsy shown more dysplasia and irregularity consistent with carcinoma. Brachytherapy involves placing radioactive seeds within the tumor, allowing for localized radiation therapy.

Answer B is incorrect. Finasteride is a 5α-reductase inhibitor that can be used to treat benign prostatic hyperplasia. This is frequently used in medical treatment of this condition. The presence of renal disease (i.e., elevated creatinine) would encourage more aggressive steps to prevent further renal damage.

Answer C is incorrect. Radical retropubic prostatectomy (RRP) would be a possible choice if the biopsy had shown prostatic carcinoma. RRP is much too aggressive an approach for benign prostatic hyperplasia.

Answer E is incorrect. Watchful waiting would be acceptable if the man was less symptomatic and did not have an elevated creatinine level.

17. **The correct answer is C.** This patient exhibits pedal and pulmonary edema, hypoalbuminemia, hyperlipidemia, decreased levels of protein C, and proteinuria. This constellation of findings is typical of nephrotic syndrome. Other important abnormalities seen in this disorder include hypercoagulability (secondary to the decreased anticoagulant effect of protein C), milky-appearing serum, and frothy urine. The most common cause of nephrotic syndrome in adults is diabetes and ensuing diabetic nephropathy.

Answer A is incorrect. Acute alcohol consumption is associated with significant electrolyte disturbances such as hyponatremia and hypokalemia. Of those alcoholics that progress to cirrhosis, some can suffer from hepatic-induced renal failure (hepatorenal syndrome); however, there is no known association between alcohol consumption and nephrotic syndrome.

Answer B is incorrect. Asthma is not associated with the development of nephrotic syndrome.

Answer D is incorrect. Hypertensive nephrosclerosis is a well-known phenomenon which typically leads to progressive renal impairment and mild proteinuria. It is not associated with frank nephrotic syndrome.

Answer E is incorrect. Minimal change disease is by far the most common cause of nephrotic syndrome in children, but is actually less common in adults, in whom it is often more severe. Nephrotic syndrome is a triad of proteinuria (> 3 g/24 hours), hypoalbuminemia (< 3.0 g/dL), and peripheral edema. Hyperlipidemia and thrombotic disease are also seen frequently.

18. **The correct answer is E.** This patient has suffered rhabdomyolysis secondary to a crush injury and is at risk for pigment (myoglobin)-induced renal failure. Even without overt renal failure, myoglobinuria is common after crush injuries and is manifested by the finding of blood on urine dipstick but the absence of RBCs on microscopic examination. The dipstick assay reacts with both hemoglobin and myoglobin, and thus will indicate the presence of blood in either case. But because the glomeruli are intact, no blood passes into the urine. Intracellular contents of muscle cells leak out as circulation returns to the damaged tissue. Lactate dehydrogenase, uric acid, phosphate, and potassium levels can increase rapidly, and patients must be monitored for signs of cardiac and systemic irregularities, such as peaked T waves and/or muscle weakness. In severe cases, dialysis is employed to manage severe hyperkalemia.

Answer A is incorrect. A hallmark of rhabdomyolysis is the elevation of creatine kinase (CK) levels, which can climb to > 100,000 IU/L. In the case of severe crush injuries, high levels are all the more likely. Treatment strategies for acute rhabdomyolysis usually involve following plasma CK levels, aggressive hydration, and urine alkalinization.

Answer B is incorrect. In addition to creatine kinase, serum lactate dehydrogenase levels increase during rhabdomyolysis.

Answer C is incorrect. Homocysteine levels can increase with end-stage renal disease (ESRD), most likely secondary to decreased glomerular filtration. This poses a potential risk to ESRD patients who are already at increased risk for cardiovascular events because elevated homocysteine levels are associated with increased risk of coronary events. Although this patient may have some renal impairment, no evidence is provided that he suffers from ESRD.

Answer D is incorrect. Troponin I is specific to cardiac tissue and is unlikely to be elevated in a crush injury that does not involve direct damage to the myocardium.

19. **The correct answer is A.** The man described has Klinefelter's syndrome. The classic triad is small, firm testes, azoospermia, and gynecomastia. The syndrome (47,XXY) is associated with an increased likelihood of germ cell tumors in extragonadal sites. Breast cancer is also much more likely in these patients.

    Answer B is incorrect. Paraphimosis describes a retracted foreskin that cannot be replaced to its normal position.

    Answer C is incorrect. Peyronie's disease is a disease in which a hard plaque develops on the penis resulting in painful erection, curvature of the penis, and poor erection quality. It is not associated with Klinefelter's syndrome.

    Answer D is incorrect. Renal cell carcinoma is not associated with Klinefelter's syndrome.

    Answer E is incorrect. The risk factors for transitional cell carcinoma include exposure to dyes and smoking. There is no known relationship to Klinefelter's syndrome.

20. **The correct answer is E.** This patient most likely has acute pyelonephritis, a common complication of polycystic kidney disease. This condition must be distinguished from an infected cyst, which would present with a normal urinalysis due to lack of direct communication between the infected cyst and the urinary tract. Percutaneous cyst drainage would be useful if the patient had an infected cyst, but of no diagnostic and therapeutic value in a patient with pyelonephritis. Since this is also an invasive procedure that carries the risk of infection and bleeding, it is also the most likely to result in an iatrogenic injury.

    Answer A is incorrect. Gentamicin and ampicillin are the standard antibiotic treatments for acute pyelonephritis in polycystic kidney disease.

    Answer B is incorrect. Angiotensin-converting enzyme inhibitors are effective for treating hypertension in polycystic kidney disease and have been shown to minimize glomerular injury.

    Answer C is incorrect. Gentamicin and ampicillin are the standard antibiotic treatments for acute pyelonephritis in polycystic kidney disease.

    Answer D is incorrect. A low-protein diet may slow the progression of kidney disease in polycystic kidney disease (PCKD). Low protein can reduce intraglomerular pressure and may therefore slow the drop in glomerular filtration rate seen in patients with PCKD.

21. **The correct answer is D.** Retention of BUN, or azotemia, is a laboratory finding with multiple etiologies. Azotemia is most often a manifestation of volume status (as in the case of contraction azotemia) and prerenal failure. As blood volume or effective volume decreases, proximal tubular reabsorption of sodium is accompanied by reabsorption of urea such that the urea:creatinine ratio is often > 20:1. There are, however, several other important causes of elevation in BUN. These include processes that result in increased circulating amino acid levels such as gastrointestinal bleeding (from direct digestion of blood protein).

    Answer A is incorrect. Although alcoholism can lead to poor nutrition and hydration, leading to prerenal azotemia, the most likely cause is volume depletion due to gastrointestinal bleeding.

    Answer B is incorrect. Blood transfusion should actually act to decrease BUN by increasing intravascular volume, thus increasing the glomerular filtration rate.

    Answer C is incorrect. Broad-spectrum antibiotics do not typically lead to azotemia. Some antibiotics, such as aminoglycosides, cause nephritis.

    Answer E is incorrect. Urinalysis was heme negative and did not reveal any negative casts; therefore, the patient most likely does not have a glomerulonephropathy. With glomerulonephritis, hematuria and RBC casts are usually seen.

22. **The correct answer is A.** This patient was admitted with hyperglycemia and dehydration. This is a common presentation for diabetics with poor glycemic control, especially when

combined with poor fluid intake. Initial management of the hyperglycemia includes insulin administration and volume repletion. With insulin administration, however, most patients should receive potassium, as insulin drives potassium intracellularly. Water loss also depletes body stores of potassium because of aldosterone-mediated sodium retention (and potassium excretion). This patient is manifesting classic symptoms of moderate to severe hypokalemia. The ECG shows flattened T waves, which is commonly seen in hypokalemia (as opposed to peaked T waves in hyperkalemia). In severe cases, one would also expect to see flaccid paralysis, hypercapnia, and rhabdomyolysis.

Answer B is incorrect. In addition to insulin, β-agonists drive potassium intracellularly. Continuation of her home dose of albuterol would worsen, not lessen, her symptoms of hypokalemia.

Answer C is incorrect. Epinephrine, through its β-agonism, also drives potassium intracellularly. This would worsen, not lessen, her hypokalemic symptoms.

Answer D is incorrect. Although insulin drives phosphate intracellularly, this patient shows no signs of acute hypophosphatemia (hemolytic anemia, increased susceptibility to infection, hypercapnia, encephalopathy, and heart failure).

Answer E is incorrect. This patient is hypernatremic in addition to being hypokalemic. Volume correction with hypertonic saline is not indicated in this setting. Hypotonic saline, or in more severe cases 5% dextrose in water, are both reasonable approaches to volume replacement.

23. **The correct answer is E.** This man is likely having situational difficulty with erections. This illustrates the importance of a good doctor-patient relationship, allowing personal issues to be explored. This man is having an extramarital affair. New sexual partners, extramarital sexual relations, conflicts with a partner, questions about sexual identity, childhood abuse, and fear of disease or pregnancy are all possible contributors to the situational erectile dysfunction that this case illustrates. Psycho-

logical factors may often coexist with organic causes.

Answer A is incorrect. Diabetes is one of many diseases that can cause or contribute to difficulty with erections. Other risk factors for erectile dysfunction include coronary artery disease, alcoholism, peripheral vascular disease, neurologic disorders, smoking, hyperlipidemia, and low high-density lipoprotein cholesterol. However, this man is capable of achieving an erection, thus there is no reason to suspect diabetic neuropathy of the penis.

Answer B is incorrect. Medications are often implicated in men with erectile dysfunction. The history, however, states that the man was able to achieve an erection with self-stimulation. The difference in ability to achieve and maintain an erection in different situations is not explained by medication.

Answer C is incorrect. Peyronie's disease is the development of a fibrous area within the corpora cavernosa. This disease can contribute to or cause erectile dysfunction, and occurs most often in men aged 45–60 years. The history specifically states that the man does not notice any curvature of the penis, and physical examination does not mention a plaque, making this a very unlikely diagnosis.

Answer D is incorrect. Prior surgeries should always be considered when evaluating a man for erectile dysfunction (ED). Surgeries that may cause ED include procedures on the prostate, penis, abdomen, and pelvic vasculature. The varicocelectomy is not likely to cause ED unless there was a bilateral insult in the blood supply to the testicles, causing an anorchid state. The physical examination is not consistent with bilateral testicular atrophy.

24. **The correct answer is B.** Blood at the urethral meatus suggests urethral injury. A rectal examination can evaluate for a high-riding, ballotable prostate, which further suggests urethral injury. After digital rectal examination, a more definitive test such as a urethrogram can be performed.

Answer A is incorrect. Although an abdominal ultrasound may be used in the initial evaluation of trauma, it will not provide any information about either the pelvic fracture or the potential for urethral injury.

Answer C is incorrect. A Foley catheter should never be placed in a patient with suspected urethral damage because the catheter could increase the urethral injury.

Answer D is incorrect. An intravenous pyelogram does not adequately assess urethral injury in the setting of trauma and takes too long to obtain to be of use in emergent situations.

Answer E is incorrect. A urethrogram is the definitive study for suspected urethral injury. However, a rectal examination should be done first as part of the rapid trauma survey to assess the position of the prostate, as well as to assess rectal tone and determine the presence of gross blood.

25. **The correct answer is C.** The fluid in the Jackson-Pratt (JP) drain is urine. This is secondary to a leak in the resected kidney. A urine leak such as this should be considered when injury to the ureter, kidney, or bladder is possible (i.e., iatrogenically in obstetric/gynecologic or urologic surgery). The suspicion that fluid contains urine can be easily confirmed by sending the fluid for a creatinine level. When this level is higher than expected in the patient's blood (there is no reason to suspect an elevated serum creatinine in this patient), the suspicion is confirmed. The timing also suggests that the patient has a urine leak because the Foley catheter has just been removed. The catheter had been keeping the bladder empty so the urine had a low resistance path to follow and the JP was relatively urine free.

Answer A is incorrect. An exploratory laparotomy is not needed in this situation. Furthermore, a urine leak such as this can usually be managed expectantly. Drainage of the bladder with a catheter may aid the healing of the iatrogenic injury.

Answer B is incorrect. A Jackson-Pratt amylase would be useful if fluid of pancreatic origin was suspected. The patient does not have pancreatitis, or more specifically, a pseudocyst, making the diagnosis of pancreatic fluid unlikely. Also, given that the surgical procedure was urologic in nature, a urine leak is more likely.

Answer D is incorrect. A serum amylase test has no role here. Serum amylase is used in diagnosing pancreatitis. The patient has no epigastric pain, and there is no reason to think that an acute attack of pancreatitis would cause an increase in drain output.

Answer E is incorrect. Serum hemoglobin should be checked postoperatively if bleeding is suspected. However, the fluid is described as clear and not grossly bloody.

26. **The correct answer is D.** This woman presents with hypertension and decreased urine output several days after starting a new medication. Her elevated creatinine makes the diagnosis of acute renal failure likely. Two other factors in the stem point to a probable etiology. Her blood urea nitrogen:creatinine ratio is greater than 20:1, and her fractional excretion of sodium (FE_{Na}) is < 1%. [FE_{Na} is calculated as follows: (urine sodium × plasma creatinine)/(plasma sodium × urine creatinine) × 100.] These two indices suggest a prerenal cause of her renal failure. Of the medications listed, only enalapril is commonly associated with causing prerenal failure. It does this by acutely decreasing the glomerular filtration rate by selectively dilating the afferent arteriole. Additionally, renal artery stenosis is a relative contraindication for angiotensin-converting enzyme inhibitors, as it causes hypoperfusion of the kidney, leading to a higher sensitivity to the decrease in glomerular filtration rate that these medications cause.

Answer A is incorrect. Aminoglycosides affect tubular cell function and have a high risk of causing nephrotoxicity. Often presenting with casts and proteinuria, aminoglycosides are most often associated with acute tubular necrosis.

Answer B is incorrect. Benztropine is an anticholinergic agent used commonly to combat some of the side effects of neuroleptic medication. As an anticholinergic agent, it often causes urinary retention, and in severe cases can lead to obstructive (postrenal) uropathy.

Answer C is incorrect. Although cimetidine is commonly associated with elevations in serum creatinine because it blocks tubular secretion of creatinine, most cimetidine-related renal disease occurs because of interstitial nephritis.

Answer E is incorrect. Hydroxyurea is a uric acid derivative commonly used as maintenance chemotherapy in patients with sickle cell disease. In patients taking hydroxyurea, there is an increased risk of uric acid crystal formation in the renal tubules, leading to an intrarenal obstruction. However, this medication is not known to cause prerenal renal failure.

27. **The correct answer is C.** This patient has a dangerously low serum sodium value but no apparent symptoms of hyponatremia (confusion, stupor, or seizures). Therefore, it is likely that this value is spurious. This is a common occurrence in patients who are phlebotomized in the same arm as the intravenous infusion, proximal to the catheter site.

    Answer A is incorrect. There is no association between intravenous cefazolin and hyponatremia.

    Answer B is incorrect. Patient-controlled analgesia pumps are not a significant source of free water and are unlikely to contribute to hyponatremia.

    Answer D is incorrect. Fluid restriction is the appropriate treatment for mild, asymptomatic hyponatremia (sodium < 120 mEq/L). However, it is important to ensure the hyponatremia is real before initiating treatment.

    Answer E is incorrect. Hypertonic saline can be used for the treatment of severe, symptomatic hyponatremia. In severe cases (seizures), correction should not exceed 1.5 to 2 mEq/h, especially if hyponatremia has been long standing. Too-rapid correction of the hyponatremia can result in central pontine myelinolysis. This patient does not have true hyponatremia, so correction is not warranted.

28. **The correct answer is C.** The diagnosis is cryptorchidism. The mass that is felt is likely the testis trapped in the inguinal canal. The testes are characteristically unable to be manipulated into the scrotum, as seen in this case. This disorder is also more likely to occur

in premature infants. The testes have a good chance of descending by 1 year of age. Thus, at this point, no correction is needed. If the testes are not appreciated on physical examination, imaging with ultrasound or MRI can be useful. If MRI is not feasible, the presence of testicular tissue can be established by administering 1500 U human chorionic gonadotropin intramuscularly for 3 days. If testicular tissue is present, there should be a significant rise in testosterone.

Answer A is incorrect. Bilateral anorchia should be in the differential for nonpalpable gonads in this child. The mass that is felt, however, is likely one of the testicles. If bilateral anorchia existed, it would be manifest with decreased testosterone and increased gonadotropin.

Answer B is incorrect. Virilizing forms of congenital adrenal hyperplasia can give females the phenotypic appearance of a man due to fusion of the labial scrotal folds. The clitoris may also overdevelop, giving the appearance of a penis. The karyotype excludes this as a diagnosis because these female pseudohermaphrodites are 46,XX.

Answer D is incorrect. Retractile testis (pseudocryptorchidism) can mimic true cryptorchidism. This occurs from a hyperactive cremasteric reflex that draws the testicle into the inguinal canal. These testicles should be able to be pulled back into the scrotum. Cold room temperature, genital manipulation, and fear can cause the reflex to occur. The typical age for this to occur is older than the clinical scenario (5–6 years old).

Answer E is incorrect. Cryptorchid males are more likely to have inguinal hernias. In fact, about 90% of these cryptorchid boys have hernias on the ipsilateral side due to the persistently open processus vaginalis. The examination, however, would not be consistent with a strangulated inguinal hernia (i.e., the child is feeding well and not in any obvious distress).

29. **The correct answer is E.** This patient is suffering from lithium-induced nephrogenic diabetes insipidus (DI) and demonstrates typical elevations in plasma osmolality without com-

pensatory elevations in urine osmolality. Indeed, normal renal function would yield a urine osmolality closer to 700 mOsm/kg or higher in this situation. In the setting of prolonged lithium exposure, there is a 20% risk of permanent insensitivity to ADH. In most cases, however, normal renal function returns with cessation of lithium therapy. Appropriate treatment of lithium-induced DI includes the administration of a thiazide diuretic, which decreases the delivery of filtrate to the distal tubule and limits urine volume. Other therapeutic options include nonsteroidal anti-inflammatory drugs (to decrease filtration at the glomerulus), amiloride (to prevent accumulation of lithium in the collecting duct cells), and, in cases of known partial DI, DDAVP (synthetic ADH).

Answer A is incorrect. ADH is effective for the diagnosis and treatment of central diabetes insipidus. However, this patient has nephrogenic resistance to ADH, and thus is unlikely to respond to exogenous ADH administration.

Answer B is incorrect. Temporary fluid restriction is a useful tool in the evaluation of polyuria and hyponatremia. In the setting of elevated plasma sodium and likely volume depletion, however, fluid restriction is inappropriate and may worsen the hypernatremia.

Answer C is incorrect. Intravenous fluids are a necessary step in the resuscitation phase for the management of acute dehydration. This patient is likely to be dehydrated, but simply administering fluids will have little overall effect on her condition

Answer D is incorrect. Although this patient has an elevated sodium concentration, she is likely total body sodium depleted and thus would not benefit from salt restriction.

30. **The correct answer is D.** This patient has **CREST**, which consists of Calcinosis, Raynaud's phenomenon (presenting complaint), Esophageal dysmotility, Sclerodactyly, and Telangiectasias. CREST is a type of scleroderma that falls under the limited cutaneous systemic sclerosis designation. The prognosis is dependent on the extent of skin involvement. The initial treatment of hypercalcemia is al-

ways hydration, which can normalize the calcium level without further treatment. The empiric use of acid-reducing agents, particularly proton pump inhibitors, is generally recommended in order to prevent the development of esophageal strictures. Calcium channel blockers are useful in decreasing the frequency of attacks of Raynaud's phenomenon. The telangiectasias create a primarily cosmetic problem that can be improved with green foundation makeup or laser therapy for particularly large lesions.

Answer A is incorrect. These are treatments for hyperkalemia. Insulin promotes cellular uptake of potassium, and bicarbonate increases the pH, which also shifts potassium into the cell.

Answer B is incorrect. This is a treatment for hyperkalemia. Calcium gluconate does not correct the hyperkalemia; however, it is the most expedient method of stabilizing the myocardium.

Answer C is incorrect. Intravenous glucose ampules can be given for severe, symptomatic hypoglycemia. Also, in the case of hyperkalemia, glucose promotes insulin secretion, which subsequently promotes potassium uptake. Glucose will not have an effect on hypercalcemia.

Answer E is incorrect. Oral calcium channel blockers are used in the long-term management of Raynaud's phenomenon to prevent recurrent attacks. Oral calcium channel blockers have no role in the acute treatment of hypercalcemia in this scenario.

31. **The correct answer is C.** Amphotericin B, a broad-spectrum antifungal agent, is a drug that is infamous for numerous unpleasant adverse effects including type I (distal) renal tubular acidosis (RTA). There are newer (liposomal) preparations that are better tolerated, but these newer preparations are often very costly. The mnemonic that can be used to recall common side effects of amphotericin, fever and chills, is "shake and bake." Type I RTA is a defect in distal H^+ α-intercalated cells. Urinary pH is usually > 5.3, and serum K^+ can be high or low. Other classic causes of this disorder are collagen

vascular disease (Sjögren's syndrome), cirrhosis, and nephrocalcinosis.

Answer A is incorrect. Leukocytoclastic vasculitis is an inflammatory reaction in small vessels in such organ systems as the skin (painless, nonblanching lesions) and kidney (glomerulonephritis). Such skin physical examination findings are not mentioned in the question stem.

Answer B is incorrect. Nephrogenic diabetes insipidus is a disorder that can be caused by drugs that damage the concentrating ability of the renal collecting ducts. The usual offending agents are lithium and demeclocycline.

Answer D is incorrect. Type II renal tubular acidosis is a defect of proximal HCO_3- reabsorption. This can lead to acidemia and increased bone turnover, causing rickets and osteomalacia. The causes of this disorder include hereditary disorders (e.g., cystinosis, tyrosinemia, glycogen storage disease type 1, and Wilson's disease), Fanconi's syndrome, and treatment with carbonic anhydrase inhibitors.

Answer E is incorrect. Type IV renal tubular acidosis (RTA) is classically due to a deficiency of or resistance to aldosterone, which results in hyperkalemia and a consequent decrease in ammonium production and urine acidification. The causes of this RTA are typically hyporeninemic hypoaldosteronism with diabetes mellitus and chronic interstitial nephritis. Treatment of hyperkalemia with furosemide or potassium-binding agents will often restore ammonium production and urine acidification.

32. **The correct answer is A.** This patient has a left ureteral stone. Eighty percent of patients with renal calculi form calcium stones, most often calcium oxalate. Various forms of diet modification can help prevent calculus formation. Even though hypercalciuria is commonly found in patients who form stones, decreased calcium intake actually increases absorption and excretion of oxalate, thereby enhancing stone formation. Calcium restriction is therefore not recommended for prevention of stones.

Answer B is incorrect. Increased fluid intake increases the urine flow rate and decreases urine solute concentration, leading to decreased stone formation.

Answer C is incorrect. High protein intake causes increases in urinary calcium, uric acid, and citrate excretion. Although a low-protein diet has not been proven to prevent stone formation, a high-protein diet is a risk factor for stone formation in men.

Answer D is incorrect. Reabsorption of sodium and water in the proximal tubule creates a gradient for calcium reabsorption. Limiting sodium intake causes increased sodium reabsorption and hence increased calcium reabsorption. The resulting decrease in calcium excretion prevents stone formation.

Answer E is incorrect. Thiazide diuretics lower calcium excretion in patients with hypercalciuria, and there is some evidence that they are beneficial in patients without identified hypercalciuria as well.

33. **The correct answer is B.** This child has autosomal recessive polycystic kidney disease (ARPCKD), also referred to as infantile polycystic kidney disease. The gene responsible for this disease has been localized to chromosome 6p21, though the exact mechanism that causes this disease's clinical manifestations is unknown. The kidneys in ARPCKD are very large and have a radial spoke pattern in the cortex seen on radiography. These cysts arise from the distal tubules and collecting ducts. ARPCKD occurs in 1:20,000 births. Most cases are diagnosed in the first year of life. In addition to renal failure she also has caput medusae, a sign of the portal hypertension often caused by the disease. Of note, this patient's creatinine is 1.0 mg/dL. This might be normal in an adult, but in a patient with a smaller muscle mass such as an infant, the creatinine is abnormally high.

Answer A is incorrect. Autosomal dominant polycystic kidney disease (ADPCKD) is the more common type of polycystic kidney disease. However, patients are usually asymptomatic until the third decade of life. This child is too young for the typical presentation of the autosomal dominant form. ADPCKD disease is known to cause hypertension and renal failure, but portal hypertension is not regularly seen.

Answer C is incorrect. Bilateral megaureter would not cause the radial cystic pattern that is seen in autosomal recessive polycystic kidney disease. A megaureter is defined as a dilated ureter with or without dilation of the renal pelves and calyces. Given the poor excretion of contrast in the CT scan, the ureters are difficult to assess, but there is no indication that this is the diagnosis.

Answer D is incorrect. Chronic hepatitis can lead to scarring of the liver (cirrhosis) and eventually portal hypertension. Cirrhosis might explain the signs of portal hypertension with normal liver function tests (LFTs). At this late stage the LFTs are not elevated because the hepatocytes are damaged to the point where they cannot produce the enzymes that when present are indicative of acute cell damage. However, there is no direct relationship between chronic hepatitis and bilaterally enlarged kidneys with cysts.

Answer E is incorrect. Medullary cystic disease is an inherited disease that leads to small kidneys with medullary cysts, not large kidneys. The lesions in medullary cystic kidney disease are usually not found in the cortex, but rather appear in the medulla as the name suggests. The inheritance is in an autosomal dominant pattern. Additionally, this disease typically presents in the third or fourth decade of life. The symptoms are polyuria, anemia, and progressive renal insufficiency. There is no cure for this disease, and unfortunately patients progress to end-stage renal disease.

34. **The correct answer is E.** This patient is suffering from an acute attack of gout, characterized by an exquisitely painful joint and signs of local inflammation. Gout is caused by a precipitation of uric acid crystals, which are negatively birefringent under polarized light. In patients prone to the disease, thiazide diuretics can lead to elevations in plasma urate levels and consequent crystal precipitation in dependent joints. Hydrochlorothiazide increases plasma urate levels by blocking the secretion of urate at the distal tubule.

Answer A is incorrect. β-Blockers are associated with sexual dysfunction and bradycardia. Less commonly, they can cause hyperkalemia and increased airway reactivity. There is no association with hyperuricemia or gout.

Answer B is incorrect. Some calcium channel blockers have been associated with increased mortality when used immediately following acute myocardial infarction, although this association is controversial. More commonly, these medications are associated with headache, dizziness, and peripheral edema. There is no association with hyperuricemia or gout.

Answer C is incorrect. Angiotensin-converting enzyme inhibitors are important for the hypertensive patient. Although they are not associated with increased plasma urate levels, they can lead to hyperkalemia and angioedema.

Answer D is incorrect. Hydralazine acts on smooth muscle cyclic guanosine monophosphate to cause relaxation and vasodilatation. It has no direct action on urate.

35. **The correct answer is D.** The patient has benign prostatic hyperplasia (BPH) and diabetes which put him at an increased risk for developing complicated UTIs. BPH is a common disorder that usually occurs in men older than 50 years and manifests with increased frequency of urination, nocturia, hesitancy, urgency, and weak urinary stream. Many men with BPH are asymptomatic or have only mild symptoms, and may not require therapy. Additionally, many patients improve or stabilize without therapy. Some patients with BPH can develop acute urinary retention, UTIs due to chronic retention, hydronephrosis, and even renal failure. Medical therapy includes (-adrenergic antagonists and 5α-reductase inhibitors. Men who develop upper tract injury (e.g., hydronephrosis or renal dysfunction), or lower tract injury (e.g., urinary retention, recurrent infection, or bladder decompensation) may require invasive therapy with transurethral resection of the prostate. Untreated BPH can cause acute urinary retention, recurrent UTIs, hydronephrosis, and even renal failure.

Answer A is incorrect. Increased fluid intake is often recommended for patients with recurrent kidney stones; however, the patient has an underlying anatomic abnormality (BPH) that puts him at greater risk for recurrent kidney stones and pyelonephritis, so his BPH must be addressed in order to lower this risk.

Answer B is incorrect. Lithotripsy would be indicated if a renal calculus was indicated by the diagnostic workup. Shock wave lithotripsy employs high-energy shock waves produced by an electrical discharge. The shock waves are transmitted through water and directly focused onto a renal/ureteral stone. The change in tissue density between the soft renal tissue and the hard stone causes a release of energy at the stone's surface. This energy fragments the stone.

Answer C is incorrect. Surgical intervention to remove a renal calculus would be indicated if there was a suspicion of an obstructing stone; however, extracorporeal shock wave lithotripsy is typically the treatment of choice for stones that do not pass on their own, although other options include pyelolithotomy and percutaneous nephrolithotomy.

Answer E is incorrect. Treatment with antibiotics would treat this episode, but would not prevent future episodes from occurring.

36. **The correct answer is C.** The lesion described is consistent with chancroid caused by *Haemophilus ducreyi*, a deep painful lesion with an exudate. There are often multiple lesions and it is associated with inguinal adenopathy in about half of patients. Chancroid ranks third behind herpes simplex virus and syphilis as a cause of genital ulcers in the United States, but it should always be kept in the differential diagnosis. The diagnosis is usually made on clinical evidence, but polymerase chain reaction testing for the causative organism shows promise. Treatment is with a single 1-g dose of azithromycin given orally.

Answer A is incorrect. The primary chancre of syphilis is usually a single painless papule that appears on the genitals. Inguinal lymphadenopathy can be present but is generally bilateral and painless. The treatment of choice is penicillin.

Answer B is incorrect. While this patient is at high risk for HIV, the lesion is not consistent with this diagnosis.

Answer D is incorrect. Lymphogranuloma venereum is caused by certain serotypes of *Chlamydia trachomatis*. The primary genital lesion is a small, painless vesicle that appears from days to weeks after infection that often goes unnoticed. The lesion resolves in a few days, but most presentations include fever, chills, myalgias, and painful inguinal lymphadenopathy (two-thirds are unilateral). The Frei test is now obsolete, and a complement fixation test as well as a microimmunofluorescence test have replaced it.

Answer E is incorrect. Biopsy can be useful for the diagnosis of human papillomavirus infection when it is not clinically obvious, and also for evaluating malignancies.

Answer F is incorrect. The Tzanck smear is used to detect the presence of multinucleated giant cells indicative of herpes simplex virus (HSV) infection. HSV is the leading cause of painful genital ulcers, but the lesions are usually multiple small vesicles. Genital herpes may be associated with reactive lymphadenopathy.

37. **The correct answer is A.** This patient has intrinsic renal failure due to acute interstitial nephritis (AIN), most likely caused by the antibiotics he has received. Penicillins, cephalosporins, and sulfonamides are among the causes of AIN, and drugs account for 70% of cases of AIN. AIN is an inflammatory process of the renal tubules similar to an allergic reaction. Findings include rash, fever, and eosinophilia, as well as WBCs and WBC casts on urinalysis.

Answer B is incorrect. Glomerulonephritis can present with laboratory values consistent with intrinsic renal failure; however, the urinalysis will show hematuria and RBC casts. Glomerulonephritis is not associated with eosinophilia.

Answer C is incorrect. This patient, who was previously septic, has been adequately volume resuscitated and is hemodynamically stable, so there is no reason to suspect that he has continuing renal failure secondary to hypovolemia. Furthermore, hypovolemic renal failure would have a prerenal picture with a blood urea nitrogen:creatinine ratio > 20:1.

Answer D is incorrect. There is no evidence that this patient has urinary obstruction with postrenal failure secondary to kidney stones.

Answer E is incorrect. Pyelonephritis can present with fever, as well as WBCs and WBC casts, on urinalysis, especially in a patient with recurrent UTI. However, this patient has negative urine cultures and no left shift on complete blood count. Additionally, rash and eosinophilia would not be explained by pyelonephritis.

Questions 38–40

38. **The correct answer is J.** Postinfectious glomerulonephritis most often occurs 1–3 weeks after group A β-hemolytic streptococcal infection and presents with a nephritic picture, including edema, hypertension, and oliguria. Urinalysis shows red cells and non-nephrotic range proteinuria. Treatment is symptomatic therapy. The major goal is to control edema and blood pressure, so water and salt might be restricted. Dialysis would only be used in the event of life-threatening hyperkalemia and clinical manifestations of uremia.

39. **The correct answer is E.** IgA nephropathy is most commonly seen in young men and children, and is often associated with upper respiratory infection, gastrointestinal symptoms, or flulike illness. The presenting symptom is red- or cola-colored urine, and the characteristic biopsy, which is the standard for diagnosis, shows focal glomerulonephritis with mesangial IgA deposition. Again, aggressive treatment of blood pressure is key, often with use of an angiotensin-converting enzyme inhibitor.

40. **The correct answer is I.** Minimal change disease is a type of nephrotic syndrome seen most commonly in children, often after viral upper respiratory tract infection. Symptoms include edema and increased susceptibility to infection, and laboratory testing shows characteristic decreases in serum albumin and total protein, as well as a high degree of proteinuria. Response to steroids among children is excellent and can be diagnostic of the condition.

Answer A is incorrect. Alport's syndrome is a hereditary nephritic syndrome that presents in males 5–20 years old. It is associated with painless hematuria and nerve deafness. On electron microscopy, the glomerular basement membrane is split.

Answer B is incorrect. Diabetic nephropathy can present with either diffuse hyalinization or nodular glomerulosclerosis (Kimmelstiel-Wilson lesions). It is the result of long-standing, poorly controlled diabetes mellitus, and presents with gross proteinuria and renal failure, as well as increased mesangial matrix on light microscopy.

Answer C is incorrect. Focal segmental glomerulosclerosis causes a nephrotic syndrome that is usually idiopathic but that can be related to heroin abuse and HIV infection.

Answer D is incorrect. Goodpasture's syndrome is a nephritic disease that presents mainly in men in their mid-20s. It presents with hemoptysis and hematuria as a result of antibodies against type IV collagen in the basement membranes, which stains in a linear fashion on immunofluorescence.

Answer F is incorrect. Lupus nephritis can present with either a nephritic or a nephrotic picture in the setting of systemic lupus erythematous. Subendothelial deposits are seen on light microscopy.

Answer G is incorrect. Membranoproliferative nephropathy has a distinctive "tram-track," double-layered basement membrane. It is a slowly progressive nephritic syndrome that is usually idiopathic.

Answer H is incorrect. Membranous nephropathy is the most common cause of a nephritic syndrome. It is an immune complex disease that presents with a "spike and dome" appearance of IgG and C3 in the glomerular basement membrane. Its causes are unknown, but it has been shown to be associated with malaria, hepatitis B virus, syphilis, and gold treatment.

Answer K is incorrect. Renal amyloidosis is a disease that is secondary to the deposition of amyloid in the glomerulus. It is most frequently seen in the context of malignancy or inflammatory disease. Amyloid deposits are seen in a Congo red or apple green stain in abdominal fat, the glomerulus, and many other tissues.

Answer L is incorrect. Wegener's granulomatosis is a vasculitis that affects mainly the lungs and kidneys. It presents with hemoptysis, hematuria, a nephritic picture, and positive tests for circulating anti-neutrophilic cytoplasmic antibodies.

Full-Length Examinations

Test Block 1

1. A 60-year-old white man presents to his primary care physician for an annual examination. He has a history of hypertension that is controlled with diet and medication. He has felt well. He has, however, noticed for the past 10 months a nonresolving small bump next to his nose that occasionally bleeds when he scratches it. He is a banker and does not spend much time outdoors, but had frequent sunburns as a boy. Examination reveals a 0.6-cm flesh-colored papule with telangiectatic vessels, a rolled edge, and slight central crusting located on the cheek (see image). Which of the following is the expected progression of this lesion?

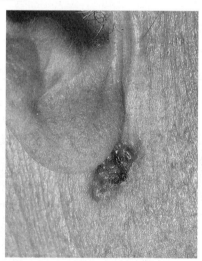

Reproduced, with permission, from Wolff K, Johnson RA, Surmond D. *Fitzpatrick's Color Atlas & Synopsis of Clinical Dermatology*, 5th ed. New York: McGraw-Hill, 2005: Figure 11-17.

(A) Good prognosis if excised early, but a propensity for lymphatogenous metastasis mandates frequent follow-up after excision
(B) Occurs exclusively within the epidermis and has no malignant potential
(C) Slow growth with destruction of local tissue that may extend along nerves to penetrate into the central nervous system
(D) Undergoes an initial radial growth phase that is followed by a vertical growth phase; prognosis is significantly related to depth of the lesion at time of excision
(E) Will remain stable for an indefinite period, and is likely to regress with residual scarring if untreated

2. A 41-year-old man presents to his physician because of recurrent suicidal thoughts. He has been depressed for over 6 months and can find no interest in life anymore. He has difficulty sleeping and constantly feels fatigued. He feels guilty about his role as a father and husband and feels "things might be better off without me around." What would be the next appropriate question to ask the patient?

(A) "Do you think you can do it?"
(B) "Everyone feels this way sometimes."
(C) "Have you ever killed anyone before?"
(D) "Have you thought of a plan, or a way to commit suicide?"
(E) "How would you feel if your wife committed suicide?"
(F) "Why do you want to die?"

3. A patient comes to the emergency department (ED) complaining of acute-onset tearing pain in his back. On x-ray of the chest, it is noted that he has a widened mediastinum. What is the most common etiology of this condition?

(A) Atherosclerosis
(B) Hypertension
(C) Protein C deficiency
(D) Rheumatic heart disease
(E) Trauma

4. A 12-year-old boy is referred to his physician for "blinking too much," which his mother thinks she first noted more than 1 year ago. The boy states that he does not notice it is occurring unless someone tells him about it. When he is nervous, it seems to worsen. He is embarrassed about it and wants to control it. What class of medications has been shown to worsen this condition?

(A) Antipsychotic
(B) Depressants
(C) Hallucinogens

(D) Selective serotonin reuptake inhibitors
(E) Stimulants

5. A 33-year-old woman presents to the ED with diffuse, cramping abdominal pain; nausea; and emesis that began this morning. The abdominal pain is diffuse throughout her entire abdomen, and the patient also describes her abdomen as looking slightly enlarged. She has a history of chronic pancreatitis, as well as a cholecystectomy and two cesarean sections. The patient states that she has had flatus but no bowel movements since the pain began. Vital signs include temperature 37.1°C (98.7°F), blood pressure 130/80 mm Hg, heart rate 96/min, and respiratory rate 15/min. On physical examination, there is diffuse abdominal tenderness with distention and high-pitched bowel sounds without rebound tenderness or guarding present. The remainder of the physical examination is not contributory. Given the clinical picture and upright x-ray of the abdomen shown in the image, which of the following is the most likely diagnosis?

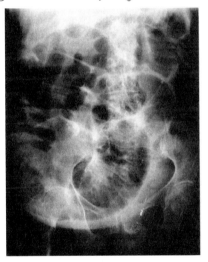

Reprinted, with permission, from Brunicardi FC, Andersen DK, Billiar TR, Dunn DL, Hunter JG, Matthews JB, Pollock RE, Schwartz SI. *Schwartz's Principles of Surgery*, 8th ed. New York: McGraw-Hill, 2005: Figure 27-14.

(A) Colon cancer
(B) Mesenteric ischemia
(C) Pancreatitis
(D) Perforated gastric ulcer
(E) Small bowel obstruction

6. A 23-year-old nursing student presents to the ED with shortness of breath, "racing heart," and a feeling that "something terrible" is happening. She states that this episode began 30 minutes earlier when she awoke from sleep drenched in sweat. She has had several similar episodes in the past, but they resolved without intervention. She states that she has been very anxious about her health lately, and has had intermittent fevers that occur in the evenings and resolve by morning for several weeks. After the patient is stabilized, what is the most appropriate next step in managing this patient's care?

(A) Bronchoscopy
(B) HIV testing
(C) PPD placement
(D) Selective serotonin reuptake inhibitor therapy
(E) X-ray of the chest

7. A 57-year-old man status post–kidney transplant 1 month ago presents to the ED with a 2-day history of fever and abdominal pain. On physical examination, he has a fever of 38.5°C (101.3°F). He complains of rebound tenderness during his abdominal examination. Which of the following is the most likely causative organism?

(A) Enterococci
(B) *Pneumocystis jiroveci* (formerly *carinii*)
(C) *Pseudomonas aeruginosa*
(D) *Staphylococcus aureus*
(E) *Streptococcus pneumoniae*

8. A 45-year-old man presents to his primary care physician asking about whether he needs to receive the influenza A vaccine. For which of the following patients is the trivalent inactivated flu vaccine specifically recommended?

(A) A 38-year-old man with a childhood history of asthma that has since resolved
(B) Healthy adults older than 45 years
(C) Healthy children older than 6 months
(D) Patients with diabetes insipidus
(E) Patients with G6PD deficiency

9. A 65-year-old man recently started taking an antihyperglycemic medication for elevated blood glucose and glycosylated hemoglobin. During his next office visit, he is back under good glycemic control but now complains of nausea since he started the medication. On further questioning, he admits to having mild abdominal pain and nausea. His blood pressure is 102/76 mm Hg, heart rate is 112/min, and respiratory rate is 24/min. Laboratory tests show:

Na^+	134 mEq/L
K^+	4.7 mEq/L
Cl^-	101 mEq/L
HCO_3^-	7.1 mmol/L
Blood urea nitrogen	16 mg/dL
Creatinine	1.4 mg/dL
Pco_2	16 mm Hg
pH	7.24

Which antihyperglycemic medication most likely caused this patient's acute presentation

(A) Acarbose
(B) Glipizide
(C) Metformin
(D) Repaglinide
(E) Rosiglitazone

10. A 17-year-old boy with a history of mild hemophilia type A presents to the ED with right lower quadrant abdominal pain. Yesterday, the patient developed periumbilical abdominal pain, nausea, vomiting, and anorexia. This morning, the pain radiated to the right lower quadrant. On physical examination, the patient has positive psoas and obturator signs. An ultrasound was performed in which a nonperforated appendix was noncompressible with a wall thickness of 5 mm. A diagnosis of acute appendicitis was made based on the clinical history and examination findings. The patient's coagulation factor VIII level is slightly lower than normal. Which of the following should this patient receive prior to undergoing an appendectomy to reduce the risk of hemorrhage?

(A) Aspirin
(B) Desmopressin
(C) Packed RBCs
(D) Platelets
(E) Whole blood

11. An 18-year-old G2P2 woman presents to her gynecologist's office complaining of several days of vaginal itching and discomfort on urination. She denies any recent fever, back pain, hematuria, or vaginal bleeding. She has been sexually active with one partner and uses barrier protection "most of the time." A urine β-human chorionic gonadotropin is negative. On examination she has a moderate amount of yellow discharge. Results of Giemsa staining of McCoy cells are shown in the image. Which of the following is the most effective oral pharmacotherapy for this disorder?

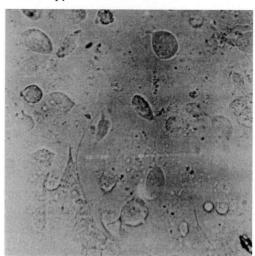

Reproduced, with permission, from Tintinalli JE, Kelen GD, Stapczynski S, Ma OJ, Cline DM. *Tintinalli's Emergency Medicine: A Comprehensive Study Guide*, 6th ed. New York: McGraw-Hill, 2004: Figure 108-3.

(A) Azithromycin
(B) Fluconazole
(C) Metronidazole
(D) Penicillin
(E) Vancomycin

12. A 55-year-old woman with a medical history significant for a prior myocardial infarction and hypertension is suffering from unilateral throbbing headaches preceded by a 10-minute visual aura. The headaches last between 10 and 24 hours and are accompanied by photophobia. She has tried nonsteroidal anti-inflammatory drugs to stop the headaches once they occur, but they are not effective. Which medication is the next logical abortive therapy to try in this patient?

(A) Acetaminophen
(B) β-Blockers
(C) Ergotamine
(D) Triptans
(E) Valproate

13. A 63-year-old man is brought into the ED by his wife after he complains of acute-onset chest pain, "like an elephant is sitting on my chest." After the patient is stabilized, his electrocardiogram is noted to have ST-segment elevations in leads II, III, and aVF. This patient is most likely suffering an acute myocardial infarction affecting which part of the heart?

(A) Anterior
(B) Indeterminate
(C) Inferior
(D) Lateral
(E) Posterior

14. A 34-year-old man with a history of Crohn's disease presents to the ED with 2 days of increasing abdominal pain. The pain is diffuse, although most intense in the periumbilical region. On questioning, he notes that he has not had a bowel movement since the onset of the pain, nor has he vomited. On initial physical examination, his abdomen is very distended and tender to palpation. His blood work is significant for bicarbonate of 24 mEq/L. Thirty minutes later, his clinical condition has worsened. Which of the following additional findings would most indicate the need for emergent surgery?

(A) Absence of bowel sounds
(B) Absence of flatus
(C) Bilious vomiting
(D) Diffuse rebound tenderness
(E) Metabolic alkalosis

15. A 30-year-old woman visits her primary care physician due to several months of dyspnea and fatigue. The physician obtains an x-ray of the chest, which demonstrates bilateral hilar adenopathy, and the patient is referred to a pulmonologist. Considering the diagnosis of sarcoidosis, the pulmonologist performs pulmonary function testing. Which of the following results of pulmonary function testing listed in the table below is characteristic of sarcoidosis?

(A) A
(B) B
(C) C
(D) D
(E) E

CHOICE	TOTAL LUNG CAPACITY	FEV$_1$	FEV$_1$:FVC RATIO	CARBON DIOXIDE DIFFUSING CAPACITY
A	↓	↓	normal	↓
B	↓	↓	normal	normal
C	↑	↓	↓	↓
D	↑	↓	↓	normal
E	↑	↓	normal	↓

16. A 77-year-old white man is brought to the clinic by his daughter, who says that her father has become more forgetful in that he has had trouble remembering important family occasions and difficulty managing his finances. These behaviors have progressively worsened in the past year, but her father denies that anything is wrong. He has no history of depression, anxiety, or head trauma. His neurologic examination is normal. His medical history is significant for type 2 diabetes diagnosed 20 years ago and atrial fibrillation. An uncle was diagnosed with Parkinson's disease at the age of 60 years. What is the most likely diagnosis?

(A) Alzheimer's disease
(B) Delirium
(C) Dementia with Lewy body
(D) Progressive supranuclear palsy
(E) Vascular dementia

17. A 56-year-old woman with a past medical history significant for type 1 diabetes mellitus presents to the ED with right-sided flank pain that radiates to the lower abdomen and groin. The patient notes chills, nausea, and one episode of vomiting this morning, as well as increased frequency of urination. On presentation, the patient's temperature is 38.8°C (101.8°F), blood pressure is 130/82 mm Hg, heart rate is 92/min, respiratory rate is 14/min, and blood glucose is 147 mg/dL. On physical examination, there is right-sided costovertebral angle tenderness. Urine analysis is notable for pyuria and bacteriuria. Which of the following is the most likely pathogen involved in this patient's diagnosis?

(A) *Enterobacter* spp.
(B) *Escherichia coli*
(C) *Klebsiella* spp.
(D) *Proteus* spp.
(E) *Pseudomonas* spp.
(F) *Staphylococcus* spp.

18. A 6-month-old girl presents with increasing frequency of stools over the last 2 weeks. Her mother describes smelly loose stools that float, and reports a history of flatulence and fussiness after feeding. Birth history is significant for failure to pass meconium in the first 24 hours. She is feeding with formula and occasional rice cereal. Physical examination is significant for weight below the fifth percentile. Stool is guaiac-negative, and cultures are negative. Which of the following tests would confirm the diagnosis?

(A) Endoscopic biopsy of the small intestine
(B) Sweat chloride test
(C) Stool qualitative fat
(D) Ultrasound of the pancreas
(E) X-ray of the abdomen and pelvis with contrast

19. A 48-year-old man presents to the ED 30 minutes after the sudden onset of an episode of diaphoresis and crushing substernal chest pain. The pain is minimally improved by nitrates. On admission, he is tachycardic and there are crackles on his lung examination. His ECG on admission reveals hyperacute T waves and ST-segment elevations in the precordial leads but with no Q waves. A representative section of his left anterior descending artery is shown in the illustration. Which of the following is the most likely diagnosis?

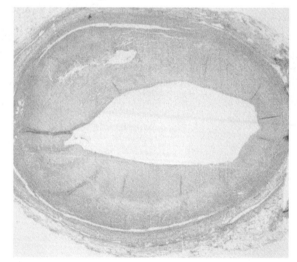

Reproduced, with permission, from PEIR Digital Library (http://peir.net).

(A) Aortic dissection involving coronary arteries
(B) Noninfarction subendocardial ischemia
(C) Noninfarction transmural ischemia
(D) Non-ST elevation (non-Q wave) myocardial infarction
(E) ST elevation (Q wave) myocardial infarction

20. Two months after undergoing a pneumonectomy for a lung nodule, a 54-year-old male smoker presents to his physician complaining of productive cough, a fever of 38.2°C (100.8°F), and chills for 2 days. A thorough review of systems reveals a 2.7-kg (6.0-lb) weight loss over the past 2 months and intermittent hip pain. Laboratory tests show:

Na$^+$	120 mEq/L
K$^+$	4.2 mEq/L
Cl$^-$	104 mEq/L
HCO$_3^-$	25 mEq/L
Blood urea nitrogen	24 mg/dL
Creatinine	0.09 mg/dL
WBC count	14,400/mm^3
Hemoglobin	35.6 g/dL
Hematocrit	14.3%
Platelet count	256,000/mm^3

What is the most likely cause of this patient's hyponatremia?

(A) Pneumonia
(B) Postsurgical atelectasis
(C) Recent head trauma
(D) Recurrence of small cell lung carcinoma
(E) Renal failure

21. A 35-year-old man who was recently diagnosed with HIV presents for his initial evaluation at an HIV clinic. The patient is afebrile, and his vital signs are within normal limits. He has no complaints, and his physical examination is unremarkable. A series of baseline laboratory studies are drawn, including a complete blood cell count, liver enzymes, and hepatitis and syphilis serologies. In addition, a purified protein derivative skin test is conducted. The patient's CD4+ count is found to be 322/mm^3. Three days later, the clinic nurse notes an area of slight induration measuring 7 mm in diameter. Which of the following is the proper course of action?

(A) Admit to the hospital in respiratory isolation; culture sputum for acid-fast bacilli
(B) Continue to monitor serial purified protein derivative tests; do not administer treatment at this time
(C) Obtain an x-ray of the chest and do not administer treatment if clear
(D) Obtain an x-ray of the chest and prescribe a 9-month course of isoniazid
(E) Start oral trimethoprim-sulfamethoxazole

22. A 75-year-old man with a history of coronary artery disease, congestive heart failure, type 2 diabetes, and chronic obstructive pulmonary disease who is status post a myocardial infarction is scheduled for thoracotomy for non-small-cell lung cancer. Before his surgery, he has a discussion with his long-time physician and his wife about the risks involved in the procedure, given his extensive comorbidities. He decides that he does not want to live with lung cancer and wants to proceed with the surgery, but he states that if the surgery is complicated and he cannot be extubated, he wants to have care withdrawn and die with dignity after a week. He signs a living will to this effect. His surgery is, in fact, complicated with major episodes of hypoxia and hypotension, and he remains intubated 1 week post surgery. At this point his wife, unwilling to let go, approaches the team and says, "I know he will pull through, please do not give up on him yet." What is the most appropriate course of action for the physicians?

(A) Call a family meeting to see what the patient's two daughters want to do; try to reach a consensus about whether to extubate
(B) Call the ethics committee to help decide how to treat the patient from this point forward
(C) Explain that there is little hope for recovery given the patient's multiple medical problems and difficult surgery; therefore, the team can decide to extubate the patient and withdraw care
(D) Explain to the wife that although they understand how difficult it is for her, her husband's wishes as stated in his living will must be respected, despite the fact that he cannot state his wishes himself at this point
(E) Extubate the patient without any further discussion

23. A 60-year-old man presents to the ED with severe headache and diaphoresis that has been occurring intermittently for the previous 24 hours. He also notes occasional palpitations. The patient's blood pressure is 220/110 mm Hg, and he has papilledema on funduscopic examination. Intravenous phentolamine is effective at improving his blood pressure. Subsequent measurement of 24-hour urinary catecholamine metabolites yields the following results:

Urine catecholamines	260 µg
Norepinephrine	225 µg
Epinephrine	1.6 µg
Metanephrine	3.0 mg
Vanillylmandelic acid	12 mg

With which of the following neoplastic diseases is this patient's cancer often associated?

(A) Insulinoma
(B) Medullary thyroid cancer
(C) Pancreatic adenocarcinoma
(D) Papillary thyroid carcinoma
(E) Pituitary adenoma

24. A 48-year-old man presents to the ED with a 4-hour history of new-onset shortness of breath, difficulty breathing while supine, and nonproductive cough. Medical history reveals he had rheumatic fever as a child. Vital signs are within normal limits, and oxygen saturation is 97% on room air. On examination there is a low-pitched diastolic rumble as well as an opening snap, both best auscultated at the apex. Rales and musical rhonchi are auscultated on inspiration in both lung fields. ECG shows an irregularly irregular rhythm. Creatine kinase–myocardial bound fraction, troponin T, and troponin I are negative 6 hours after the onset of symptoms. Testing reveals the thyroid-stimulating hormone level is normal. Which of the following is the most likely cause of the patient's pulmonary edema?

(A) Acute aortic insufficiency
(B) Acute mitral regurgitation
(C) Mitral stenosis
(D) Myocardial ischemia
(E) Thyroid disease

25. A 29-year-old man is brought into the ED by his sister, who indicates that the patient has been extremely agitated and has not moved his head for nearly an hour. She notes that he currently lives at home with her, after a month-long stay in a psychiatry facility for schizophrenia. She provides a list of his medications, which she updated this morning after his psychiatrist increased the dosage of one of his medications. Which of the following treatments should be provided?

(A) Alprazolam
(B) Diphenhydramine
(C) Haloperidol
(D) Muscle relaxants
(E) Sertraline

26. The state university's center for biological research is conducting a cross-sectional survey to determine the relationship between fruit consumption and colorectal cancer. Participants are selected randomly and contacted by telephone. Which of the following parameters can be determined from this type of study?

(A) Attributable risk
(B) Causation
(C) Incidence
(D) Prevalence
(E) Relative risk

27. A 15-year-old girl presents to a urologist for a follow-up visit. As a young child, the patient had frequent urinary tract infections (UTIs) and an episode of pyelonephritis. The subsequent workup led to the diagnosis of bilateral grade 4 vesicoureteral reflux (VUR). The patient has been on and off antibiotic prophylaxis for several years, with her last breakthrough UTI when she was 13 years old. She notes that she has not had any leaking or loss of urine during the day or at night. She has just become sexually active with her boyfriend and states that she has been using condoms. In the office, she has a temperature of 36.6°C (97.8°F) and blood pressure of 120/85 mm Hg. Physical examination reveals her abdomen is soft, and there is no tenderness to palpation. The patient is a well-developed, Tanner stage IV girl. Her blood urea nitrogen is 15 mg/dL and creatinine is 1.5 mg/dL, and are unchanged from the past two visits. Today, a voiding cystourethrogram shows left-sided grade 3

VUR and right-sided grade 4 VUR, with no residual contrast postvoid. At this point, what is the most appropriate step in management?

(A) Bilateral ureteral reimplant
(B) Continue antibiotic prophylaxis
(C) 99m-Technetium dimercaptosuccinic acid scan
(D) Repeat voiding cystourethrogram yearly
(E) Video urodynamics

28. A child is brought to his pediatrician for evaluation of a rash, as shown in the image. The child has had recurrent episodes with this skin irritation, which appears to be nonpainful and nonpruritic and has not spread to other regions of the body. The boy's mother notes that the lesions are "weepy" and ooze fluid that forms golden-colored crusts over the affected skin. The patient has mild local lymphadenopathy but no constitutional symptoms. Which is the most appropriate treatment for this patient?

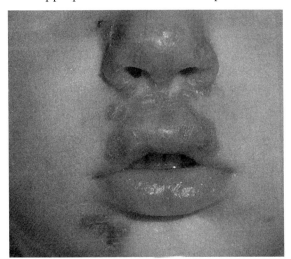

Reproduced, with permission, from Wolff K, Johnson RA, Surmond D. *Fitzpatrick's Color Atlas & Synopsis of Clinical Dermatology*, 5th ed. New York: McGraw-Hill, 2005: Figure 22-10.

(A) Acyclovir
(B) Change facial soaps
(C) Hydrocortisone cream
(D) Intravenous vancomycin
(E) Topical mupirocin
(F) Tretinoin cream

29. A 39-year-old obese African-American man presents with several episodes of weakness and tingling in his right forearm. This morning he became extremely concerned when he was unable to grip his coffee cup and could not open the car door. He is an electrician and has been unable to go to work for the past week as a result of these episodes. He notes that he has also been awakened at night with numbness and tingling in the same arm. He has a history of diabetes and has smoked for 25 years. He reports that his father also has diabetes and recently had coronary artery bypass surgery. Physical examination reveals weak grip of the right hand compared to the left with signs of thenar atrophy. Which of the following would be the most appropriate next diagnostic test in this patient?

(A) Cerebral angiogram
(B) CT scan of the head
(C) Electroencephalogram
(D) Electromyography
(E) MRI of the head

30. A 42-year-old woman complains of stomachaches and headaches nearly every day for the past 10 months, as well as occasional dry throat and palpitations. She has been feeling restless, has difficulty concentrating at work, and worries constantly about her relationships, health, and finances, despite having no significant problems in these areas. She denies drug or alcohol abuse. Her temperature is 36.9°C (98.5°F), blood pressure 132/80 mm Hg, pulse 106/min, and respiratory rate 16/min. Examination indicates an alert and oriented patient with no memory deficits and an unremarkable physical examination. Thyroid-stimulating hormone levels and urine toxicology indicate no abnormalities, and an ECG shows sinus tachycardia. Which of the following is the most likely diagnosis?

(A) Acute stress disorder
(B) Adjustment disorder with anxiety
(C) Generalized anxiety disorder
(D) Hypochondriasis
(E) Malingering

31. An unconscious 24-year-old man is brought to a rural urgent care clinic by his family. The patient is cyanotic and has clearly swollen lips and tongue. His mother states that he is extremely allergic to peanuts and the problem developed suddenly at a restaurant next door. The clinic has no supplies to intubate the patient. Which of the following medications is contraindicated for this patient?

   (A) Albuterol
   (B) Diphenhydramine
   (C) Epinephrine
   (D) Labetalol
   (E) Methylprednisolone
   (F) Ranitidine

32. A 59-year-old man presents to the clinic with a broad-based unsteady gait. He is unable to walk in a straight line and moves from side to side as he walks. His upper limb coordination is intact. He has no history of vertigo, and no nystagmus is noted on physical examination. Which of the following is the most likely cause of this patient's symptoms?

   (A) Cerebellar hemisphere infarction
   (B) Cerebellar vermis lesion
   (C) Hydrocephalus
   (D) Ménière's disease
   (E) Vestibular neuronitis

33. A 17-year-old basketball player pivots as his flexed knee is straightening. He notices instant pain in the knee but continues to play and finishes the game. The next day he is limping in practice, and he tells the coach that his knee has been catching, locking, and giving way. The athletic trainer examines the knee, finding joint effusion and medial joint line tenderness. Which of the following is the most likely diagnosis?

   (A) Chondromalacia patella
   (B) Medial collateral ligament tear
   (C) Medial meniscus tear
   (D) Pes anserine bursitis
   (E) Quadriceps tendonitis

34. A 33-year-old woman with no significant past medical history is rushed to the ED by ambulance after a gunshot wound to the left chest. Primary survey reveals that the patient is breathing, is tachycardic with a palpable pulse, has a Glasgow Coma Scale score of 7, and has a gunshot wound on the left side of her chest. The patient is intubated, connected to a positive-pressure ventilator, central and peripheral intravenous (IV) access is obtained, and IV fluids are started through peripheral IV sites. An ECG shows sinus tachycardia and electrical alternans. The patient is now found to be pulseless with no discernable blood pressure. Per advanced cardiac life support protocol, chest compressions are started, followed by administration of dobutamine, atropine, and sodium bicarbonate. A bedside echocardiogram is obtained and shows a substantial amount of fluid in the pericardium and chamber collapse. Emergent pericardiocentesis is performed and a substantial amount of blood drains from the pericardial space. Unfortunately, the patient remains pulseless and is pronounced dead after 30 minutes of further resuscitation efforts. A gross pathology specimen of the heart from the autopsy is shown in the image. Which intervention may have worsened this patient's condition and should have been avoided?

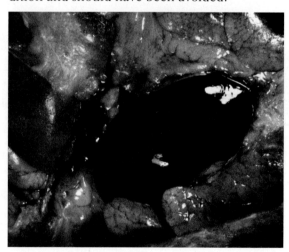

Reprinted, with permission, from PEIR Digital Library (http://peir.net).

   (A) Administration of dobutamine
   (B) Echocardiogram
   (C) Insertion of a central line
   (D) Pericardiocentesis
   (E) Positive-pressure mechanical ventilation

35. A 34-year-old patient seeks the advice of his family physician regarding colorectal cancer screening. He has asthma, for which he uses

an albuterol inhaler and inhaled cortico-steroids. He eats a high-fiber, low-fat diet and exercises regularly. The patient is concerned about his risk for colorectal cancer because his father was diagnosed with colon cancer at age 45 years and died 3 years later; his paternal grandfather was found to have colon cancer at age 57 years and died the following year. At what age should this patient's first screening colonoscopy be performed?

(A) 35 years
(B) 40 years
(C) 45 years
(D) 48 years
(E) 50 years

36. A 33-year-old woman presents to the ED complaining of intermittent palpitations, sweating, and headaches for 6 months. She has also noticed that her clothes seem looser over the past few months. She denies any psychiatric disorders or significant past medical history and is not taking any medications. The patient's pulse is 90/min, blood pressure 170/93 mm Hg, and respiratory rate 21/min. Her oxygen saturation is 100% on room air. She is a thin, diaphoretic woman, with an otherwise unremarkable physical examination. The patient is admitted to the hospital, and 24-hour urine metanephrine excretion is 2 mg/d. Other significant laboratory values include an elevated erythrocyte sedimentation rate and elevated plasma total catecholamines. Which of the following is the most appropriate pharmacotherapy?

(A) Immediately start intravenous nitroprusside and titrate to control blood pressure
(B) No pharmacotherapy is indicated, so proceed immediately to surgery
(C) Start hydrochlorothiazide 12.5 mg orally four times a day and titrate to control blood pressure
(D) Start propranolol 40 mg orally twice a day; titrate dosage to control blood pressure and symptoms
(E) Start with phenoxybenzamine 10 mg orally four times a day; titrate dosage to control blood pressure and symptoms

37. A 42-year-old white mother of two with a prior history of intermittent right upper quadrant (RUQ) abdominal pain following meals, but who never sought medical attention, presents to the ED with a more severe episode of a similar pain. She has also had nausea and vomiting. On physical examination, she is febrile to 38.2°C (100.8°F), obese, and has tenderness to palpation in the RUQ. A RUQ ultrasound reveals some stones in her gallbladder. Laboratory tests show:

WBC count	13,000/mm^3
Hematocrit	36%
Na$^+$	142 mEq/L
K$^+$	4.5 mEq/L
Cl$^-$	103 mEq/L
Ca^{2+}	9.4 mEq/L
Carbon dioxide	24 mmol/L
Blood urea nitrogen	12 mg/dL
Creatinine	0.7 mg/dL
Glucose	100 mg/dL
Total bilirubin	3.8 mg/dL
Total protein	7.7 g/dL
Albumin	4.5 g/dL
Aspartate aminotransferase	130 U/L
Alanine aminotransferase	150 U/L
Alkaline phosphatase	300 U/L
Amylase	< 30 U/L
Lipase	8 U/L

Which of the following is most likely responsible for her symptoms and laboratory values?

(A) A stone obstructing her common bile duct
(B) A stone obstructing her common hepatic duct
(C) A stone obstructing her cystic duct
(D) A stone obstructing her hepatoduodenal ampulla (of Vater)
(E) Stones in her gallbladder

38. A 24-year-old G1P0 woman at 32 weeks' gestation presents to the ED after experiencing regular contractions approximately 10 minutes apart for 3 hours. On presentation, her vital signs are temperature 37.7°C (99.8°F), blood pressure 136/87 mm Hg, pulse 95/min, and respiratory rate 18/min. While in the ED, her membranes rupture spontaneously, and she progresses through labor and delivers a premature infant 6 hours later. Which of the following could have caused premature labor and delivery?

(A) Antihypertensive treatment with nifedipine
(B) Excessive water intake
(C) Untreated *Chlamydia* cervicitis
(D) Untreated preeclampsia
(E) Use of nonsteroidal anti-inflammatory drugs

39. Which of the following medications is most associated with QT prolongation?

(A) Chlorpromazine
(B) Clozapine
(C) Haloperidol
(D) Olanzapine
(E) Quetiapine
(F) Ziprasidone

40. A boy is seen at a rural health clinic in Bolivia. He demonstrates significant mental retardation, motor spasticity, and an abnormal gait. The child is also deaf and mute. The patient is of appropriate height and sexual development, and he has no macroglossia or goiter. His mother experienced considerable fatigue and cold intolerance throughout her pregnancy. Thyroid testing is obtained and thyroxine and thyroid-stimulating hormone levels are found to be normal. What is the cause of this patient's condition?

(A) Autoimmune thyroiditis
(B) Current iodine deficiency
(C) Dyshormonogenesis
(D) Hypopituitarism
(E) Iodine deficiency late in pregnancy and after birth
(F) Maternal iodine deficiency during early pregnancy
(G) Thyroid dysgenesis

Questions 41 and 42

For each of the following patients, select the most likely diagnosis.

(A) Acute lymphocytic leukemia
(B) Acute myelocytic leukemia
(C) Burkitt's lymphoma
(D) Chronic lymphocytic leukemia, blast crisis
(E) Chronic myelogenous leukemia
(F) Ewing's sarcoma
(G) Follicular lymphoma
(H) Mantle cell lymphoma
(I) Mucosa-associated lymphoid tissue lymphoma
(J) Neuroblastoma
(K) Pheochromocytoma
(L) Primary cutaneous anaplastic large cell lymphoma
(M) Sézary syndrome

41. A 55-year-old man with a history of atopic dermatitis presents to the ED with diffusely erythematous skin, fever, and general malaise. Peripheral blood smear shows cerebriform nuclei and cells with scant cytoplasm.

42. A 5-year-old boy from Kenya is brought to the pediatrician after his mother palpates an abdominal mass while bathing him. Biopsy of the mass shows numerous pale macrophages among lymphoid cells with a high mitotic index.

Questions 43 and 44

For each of the patients with a urinary complaint, select the test that would most likely lead to the correct diagnosis.

(A) Bladder biopsy
(B) Complete blood cell count
(C) CT scan of the pelvis
(D) Cystoscopy
(E) Digital rectal examination
(F) Fasting blood glucose
(G) β-Human chorionic gonadotropin and (-fetoprotein
(H) Pap smear
(I) Prostate-specific antigen

(J) Salt-load response
(K) Urinalysis and urine culture
(L) Water deprivation test
(M) Wet prep

43. A 15-year-old boy presents to his physician complaining of polyuria and polydipsia for the past few weeks. He also admits to wetting the bed twice last week. He is sexually active and denies dysuria and urethral discharge. On physical examination, the boy is very thin, and review of medical records indicates a 6.8-kg (15-lb) weight loss over the past year. His temperature is 37.2°C (98.9°F), heart rate is 84/min, respiratory rate is 14/min, and blood pressure is 120/80 mm Hg. He has a normal abdominal examination with no palpable masses. As a young child he was part of an immunology study that did genetic testing, and he is known to be human leukocyte antigen-DR3-positive.

44. An 18-year-old girl presents to her physician complaining of urinary urgency, frequency, and slight burning and discomfort when she voids for the past 2 days. She denies fever or chills, but did note a spot of blood on the toilet paper yesterday. She has no past medical history. She takes oral contraceptives, and her last menstrual period was 9 days ago. She had intercourse for the first time 4 days ago, and wore a female condom. She has a heart rate of 80/min, respiratory rate of 12/min, and temperature of 37.2°C (98.9°F). On examination she has mild discomfort on deep palpation of the lower abdomen.

Questions 45 and 46

For each neonate with jaundice, select the most likely diagnosis.

(A) ABO incompatibility
(B) α_1-Antitrypsin deficiency
(C) Biliary atresia
(D) Breast-feeding
(E) Cephalhematoma
(F) Crigler-Najjar syndrome
(G) Gilbert's syndrome
(H) Hereditary spherocytosis
(I) Neonatal hepatitis
(J) Physiologic
(K) Rh incompatibility
(L) Sepsis
(M) Toxoplasmosis infection

45. A 29-year-old G2P1 type A Rh-positive woman delivers a 3620-g (8-lb) girl. The infant's examination is notable for frontal bossing and extreme pallor. The cord blood is Coombs' positive. At 3 hours of age, her hemoglobin is 6 mg/dL, total bilirubin is 13 mg/dL, conjugated bilirubin is 1 mg/dL, and reticulocyte count is 4/dL.

46. At 38 weeks' gestation, a 3100-g (6.8-lb) boy was born to a type B, Rh-negative 23-year-old primigravida by spontaneous vaginal delivery. He is being exclusively breast-fed but is only latching on to the breast for short periods of time. On the third day of life, he appears jaundiced. His total bilirubin is 15 mg/dL, his conjugated bilirubin is 0.8 mg/dL (normal < 2 mg/dL), and his liver function tests are normal.

1. **The correct answer is C.** This is a classic description of nodular basal cell carcinoma (BCC). BCC is usually described as a pearly, telangiectatic nodular lesion with rolled borders. As the tumor outgrows its blood supply it can develop central crusting and ulceration. BCC is the most common tumor of the skin, and is referred to as an epithelioma due to the low metastatic potential. Major risk factors are childhood sun exposure, fair skin, chronic dermatitis, and xeroderma pigmentosum. BCC is usually very slow-growing, but can result in extensive destruction of local tissues and extension into the central nervous system if untreated. Basal cell nevus syndrome, a genetic form of BCC, is associated with a mutation in the *PTCH* gene.

Answer A is incorrect. This course is typical of squamous cell carcinoma (SCC). SCC is classically a scaly, erythematous lesion that may ulcerate. Three percent of cutaneous SCCs metastasize, typically to adjacent lymph nodes. Risk factors for metastatic lesions include location in scar tissue, immunodeficiency, exposure to x-rays and ultraviolet radiation, and location on the head or neck. Prognosis is excellent if completely excised (95% cure rate), but survival is only 50% at 5 years if metastatic.

Answer B is incorrect. This course is typical of seborrheic keratosis (SK), which can mimic malignant melanoma, SCC, or BCC, but is a benign lesion. Horny cysts embedded in the surface of the lesion, when present, support this diagnosis. Abrupt eruption of multiple pruritic SKs may occur as a paraneoplastic syndrome (the sign of Leser-Trélat, most commonly seen with gastrointestinal adenocarcinomas), but this association is controversial.

Answer D is incorrect. This description characterizes malignant melanoma (MM). Though pigmented BCC can resemble MM, the lesion described here is classic nodular BCC and should not be confused with MM.

Answer E is incorrect. This describes the course of keratoacanthoma, which can mimic SCC but typically appears suddenly and grows rapidly to approximately 1–2 cm within a couple of weeks. The lesion is a dome-shaped papule that may crust, and typically remains stable for months to years before regressing. Since scarring is typical, these are usually excised.

2. **The correct answer is D.** This patient is contemplating suicide and is in great danger to himself. Questions should be nonjudgmental, yet direct. It is important to elucidate details of the plan and preparations that have been made to implement the plan.

Answer A is incorrect. A willingness to die is not helpful information in determining suicidality. Patients may feel too depressed to realistically determine whether they want to die or not.

Answer B is incorrect. Normalizing the situation may make the patient feel disregarded. Ask about specific details regarding the plan.

Answer C is incorrect. Asking about homicide does not help gather information about the current suicidality.

Answer E is incorrect. Using guilt or blame is not a useful tool when discussing suicide with a patient.

Answer F is incorrect. Patients may not have a specific reason for contemplating suicide. It is more helpful to discuss how close they are to actually attempting suicide.

3. **The correct answer is B.** Aortic dissection, especially in the ascending portion, is most commonly associated with hypertension. Acute management of this potentially life-threatening condition involves blood pressure control and prompt evaluation for surgical repair.

Answer A is incorrect. Aortic aneurysms, especially in the abdomen, are most commonly associated with atherosclerosis. Until they rupture, these generally present no distress to the patient and may be discovered incidentally. Aortic aneurysms larger than 5 cm are generally treated surgically.

Answer C is incorrect. Protein C is an anticoagulant, therefore a hereditary protein C deficiency leads to a hypercoagulable state. This is not, however, an etiology of aortic dissection.

Answer D is incorrect. Rheumatic heart disease is a childhood sequela of bacterial infection that is not commonly seen in patients who were born in the era of antibiotics. When it is seen, it commonly leads to mitral, and less frequently aortic, valvular disease. It is not, however, an etiology of aortic dissection.

Answer E is incorrect. Trauma is a possible etiology of aortic dissection, and this must be ruled out in incidents of trauma, but hypertension is still the most common etiology of aortic dissection.

4. **The correct answer is E.** Stimulants or dopamine agonists can worsen or even precipitate tics in patients. This patient likely has a motor tic disorder that can be treated with haloperidol, pimozide, or clonidine.

Answer A is incorrect. Antipsychotics can be used to lessen the severity of these involuntary movements.

Answer B is incorrect. Depressants are not known to produce or worsen tics.

Answer C is incorrect. Hallucinogens may produce bizarre behavior but not perseverative or stereotyped behaviors such as in this case.

Answer D is incorrect. Selective serotonin reuptake inhibitors have not been shown to increase the prevalence of tics in patients.

5. **The correct answer is E.** The most common causes of small bowel obstruction include peritoneal adhesions (from previous abdominal surgery), hernias, and cancer or tumors. The abdominal pain typically presents with nausea and/or vomiting, and patients may have a distended abdomen along with high-pitched bowel sounds. Supine and upright x-rays of the abdomen are useful in making the diagnosis because dilated loops of small bowel can be seen, along with air-fluid levels and lack of gas in the colon. Some patients with partial small bowel obstruction can initially be treated conservatively with close observation, intravenous

fluids, and a nasogastric tube for proximal decompression. However, patients with peritoneal signs should be taken to the operating room for surgical decompression and repair.

Answer A is incorrect. The acute onset of diffuse abdominal pain and emesis in a patient with a history of previous abdominal surgeries supports a diagnosis of small bowel obstruction more than colon cancer. Although tumors and cancers of the small bowel can cause obstruction, it is unlikely that colon cancer would produce the history, physical examination findings, and radiographic findings noted in this case.

Answer B is incorrect. Mesenteric ischemia may present with abdominal pain, nausea, and vomiting; however, the radiographic findings are not typically seen in a patient with mesenteric ischemia. In addition, the majority of cases of mesenteric ischemia occur in older patients who have cardiac abnormalities or atherosclerosis.

Answer C is incorrect. Patients with a diagnosis of pancreatitis may present with diffuse abdominal pain, nausea, and vomiting; however, the radiographic findings are not typically seen in a patient with pancreatitis

Answer D is incorrect. A patient with a perforated gastric ulcer typically presents with acute, severe abdominal pain and free intraperitoneal air. This radiograph does not show free intraperitoneal air but rather shows dilated loops of small bowel, air-fluid levels, and absence of gas in the colon. These signs/symptoms are consistent with a diagnosis of small bowel obstruction rather than a perforated gastric ulcer.

6. **The correct answer is E.** The patient is describing symptoms that are consistent with Hodgkin's disease, including night sweats and Pel-Ebstein (cyclic) fevers. Her shortness of breath may be consistent with a mediastinal mass caused by adenopathy. The patient may also be suffering from other chest pathology, including pulmonary tuberculosis, asthma, and cardiomyopathy, and an x-ray of the chest would be useful in the diagnosis or exclusion of any of these conditions.

Answer A is incorrect. A bronchoscopy may be warranted in the future but is not indicated in the absence of known lung pathology.

Answer B is incorrect. Again, HIV testing might be prudent in this patient; however, an x-ray will provide immediate answers regarding her current symptoms.

Answer C is incorrect. PPD placement might help in the diagnosis of pulmonary tuberculosis; however, this diagnosis will take 24–48 hours. An x-ray is a more appropriate next step in this patient's care.

Answer D is incorrect. Although the patient's symptoms are consistent with a panic attack, the presence of night sweats and intermittent fevers warrants further diagnostic evaluation and testing before empirically treating the patient for panic disorder with a selective serotonin reuptake inhibitor.

7. **The correct answer is C.** Patients with a recent history of kidney transplant are at an increased risk of bacterial infections. Septicemia and peritonitis in these patients is often caused by *Pseudomonas aeruginosa*. Patients with cystic fibrosis and patients with HIV can also be at an increased risk of infection with this organism.

Answer A is incorrect. Patients who have received liver transplants, not kidney transplants, are at an increased risk for infection with enterococci.

Answer B is incorrect. Patients with HIV and low CD4+ counts, as well as infants 2–8 months old, have the most increased risk for infection with *Pneumocystis jiroveci* (formerly *carinii*). Rather than peritonitis and septicemia, *P. jiroveci* usually causes pneumonia with characteristically low oxygen saturation.

Answer D is incorrect. *Staphylococcus aureus* is a common pathogen, but not one that would carry an increased risk for this patient as opposed to other immunosuppressed patients.

Answer E is incorrect. Patients who have received a bone marrow transplant or who are functionally asplenic are at an increased risk of infection with *Streptococcus pneumoniae* and other encapsulated organisms. The greatest risk of infection with these organisms in the transplant patient is in the late posttransplantation period, or more than 100 days posttransplant.

8. **The correct answer is C.** The trivalent inactivated influenza A vaccine is indicated in children older than 6 months only in the setting of asthma, cystic fibrosis, diabetes, HIV, bronchopulmonary dysplasia, sickle cell anemia, and chronic heart disease.

Answer A is incorrect. Adults who have chronic pulmonary disorders, including chronic obstructive pulmonary disease and asthma, are recommended to receive vaccination for influenza A.

Answer B is incorrect. Adults who are elderly (older than 65 years) are susceptible to life-threatening complications of influenza, such as pneumonia. Some recommend immunization beginning at age 50 years.

Answer D is incorrect. Patients with diabetes mellitus, not insipidus, have reduced immune capabilities and are recommended to receive the influenza vaccine.

Answer E is incorrect. Patients with hemoglobinopathies, not G6PD, have increased susceptibility to complications triggered by influenza infection.

9. **The correct answer is C.** This patient was started on an antihyperglycemic agent, and quickly developed gastrointestinal symptoms and an anion gap metabolic acidosis with compensatory respiratory alkalosis. This patient was likely on metformin, a biguanide that lowers blood glucose levels by decreasing hepatic glucose production and increasing insulin sensitization. Metformin is a known cause of lactic acidosis, which occurs extremely rarely in healthy individuals (5 cases per 100,000), but more commonly in patients with renal, heart, or liver disease. The mortality rate of metformin-treated patients with lactic acidosis is close to 50%. Neither arterial lactate levels nor plasma metformin concentrations are good predictors of mortality. Death more closely correlates with underlying comorbid conditions. Supportive care is given to patients with

mild to moderate lactic acidosis. For patients with profound metformin-induced lactic acidosis (pH < 7.10), use of hemodialysis or sodium bicarbonate infusion is recommended.

Answer A is incorrect. An α-glucosidase inhibitor, acarbose, inhibits intestinal absorption of carbohydrates. Because of this mechanism of action, these drugs have a high rate of unpleasant adverse effects, such as flatulence and diarrhea.

Answer B is incorrect. Sulfonylureas achieve glycemic control by increasing β-cell secretion of insulin. The main adverse effect for patients is hypoglycemia. Rarely, sulfonylureas have been known to cause nausea and photosensitivity.

Answer D is incorrect. Meglitinides act in a similar fashion to the sulfonylureas by increasing β-cell insulin secretion. The main adverse effect on patients is hypoglycemia.

Answer E is incorrect. Thiazolidinediones increase insulin sensitivity at the muscles and liver by increasing the utilization, and decreasing the production, of glucose. Because of this mechanism, the main adverse effect for patients is weight gain. Rarely, these medications can also exacerbate congestive heart failure.

10. **The correct answer is B.** Desmopressin is a vasopressin analog that promotes the release of von Willebrand's factor and factor VIII from tissue stores. Administration of desmopressin will lead to a rapid increase in a patient's factor VIII level and is therefore useful in patients with mild hemophilia type A (with a deficiency in coagulation factor VIII) to decrease bleeding during surgery. In patients with mild hemophilia, desmopressin is preferable to replacement therapy with coagulation factor VIII, which should be used for severe hemophilia A or active bleeding because it is not associated with a risk of viral transmission (HIV or hepatitis) and achieves the same ultimate goal of increasing the coagulation factor concentrations. Because of past experience with viral transmission, cryoprecipitate should not be used to treat hemophilia A.

Answer A is incorrect. Nonsteroidal anti-inflammatory drugs such as aspirin are associated with an increased risk of bleeding. These medications should not be used in patients who are prone to bleeding, including hemophiliacs or patients with von Willebrand's disease. Administration of aspirin is also contraindicated in this patient, especially prior to surgery.

Answer C is incorrect. Packed RBC transfusions do not include platelets or clotting factors. Because this patient is deficient in clotting factor VIII, there is no utility in transfusing packed RBCs to this patient preoperatively.

Answer D is incorrect. This patient has a diagnosis of hemophilia type A. This is a hereditary bleeding disorder in which there is a deficiency of coagulation factor VIII. This disorder is not associated with abnormal platelet function or quantitative platelet deficiencies. Therefore, there is no utility in transfusing platelets into this patient preoperatively.

Answer E is incorrect. Administration of whole blood will replenish RBCs and some clotting factors; however, it is deficient in platelets and clotting factors V, VIII, and XI. Because this patient is deficient in clotting factor VIII, providing whole blood to this patient preoperatively has little if any utility. In addition, whole blood transfusions are associated with a small yet quantifiable risk of transmission of viral infections (HIV and hepatitis).

11. **The correct answer is C.** The constellation of symptoms and the presence of *Trichomonas vaginalis* protozoa on Giemsa staining establish the diagnosis of trichomoniasis vaginitis. The treatment of choice for this condition is one dose of 2 g of metronidazole.

Answer A is incorrect. Azithromycin is a macrolide antibiotic that inhibits RNA synthesis by binding to the 50S ribosomal RNA subunit. It is used to treat chlamydial infections but is not therapeutic for trichomoniasis.

Answer B is incorrect. Fluconazole is an antifungal medication that inhibits cell membrane synthesis of various fungi. It is often used to treat vaginal candidiasis, but is has no antiprotozoal activity and thus is ineffective against *Trichomonas vaginalis* infections.

Answer D is incorrect. Penicillin is an antibiotic whose mechanism of action involves interruption of cell wall synthesis. Its spectrum of activity includes most gram-positive cocci, most anaerobes, and a limited number of gram-negative bacteria. It is not active against *Trichomonas vaginalis*.

Answer E is incorrect. Vancomycin is an antibiotic that is effective against numerous gram-positive organisms, including methicillin-resistant *Staphylococcus aureus*, and which is almost always administered as an intravenous infusion. The exception to this is when it is used to treat *Clostridium difficile* infections, for which vancomycin must be given orally. Vancomycin is not active against *Trichomonas vaginalis*.

12. **The correct answer is A.** If nonsteroidal anti-inflammatory drugs (NSAIDs) are not effective, other analgesics such as acetaminophen, and acetaminophen/caffeine combination medications (such as Excedrin and other over-the-counter migraine analgesics) can be used to abort a migraine attack. NSAIDs alleviate pain associated with an attack and the caffeine dilates coronary vessels and breaks the headache.

Answer B is incorrect. β-Blockers are used as prophylactic therapy for migraine headaches, preventing migraines from occurring. They do not help end a headache once it has occurred.

Answer C is incorrect. Ergotamines should be avoided in patients with coronary artery disease and hypertension because they cause coronary artery vasoconstriction and hypertension. Ergotamine is contraindicated in women who are or may become pregnant, since the drugs may cause fetal harm. Ergotamine is also contraindicated in patients with peripheral vascular disease, coronary heart disease, uncontrolled hypertension, stroke, impaired hepatic or renal function, and sepsis.

Answer D is incorrect. Triptans can be helpful, but have been linked to coronary artery constriction and should be avoided in patients with cardiovascular risk factors.

Answer E is incorrect. Valproate is an anticonvulsive medication that is most effective as

prophylactic treatment of migraine headaches because it helps prevent migraines, but is not helpful in stopping an attack once it has occurred.

13. **The correct answer is C.** In a standard 12-lead ECG, ST elevations in leads II, III, and aVF indicate an evolving myocardial infarction in the inferior portion of the heart. The posterior descending artery (usually a branch of the right coronary artery) supplies the inferior portion of the ventricle.

Answer A is incorrect. ST elevations in leads V_1, V_2, V_3, and V_4 indicate an evolving myocardial infarction in the anterior portion of the heart. The left anterior descending artery supplies the anterior portion of the left ventricle.

Answer B is incorrect. One of the primary purposes of performing an ECG is for more accurate assessment of the location of ischemic portions of the heart. Therefore, the presence of ST elevations in different leads is very helpful in determining which portions of the heart might be experiencing infarction.

Answer D is incorrect. ST elevations in leads V_5 and V_6 indicate an evolving myocardial infarction in the lateral portion of the heart. The left circumflex artery supplies the lateral portion of the left ventricle.

Answer E is incorrect. ST depressions in V_1 and V_2 would suggest ischemia in the posterior portion of the heart. The posterior descending artery supplies the posterior portion of the heart.

14. **The correct answer is D.** Diffuse rebound tenderness most likely indicates generalized peritonitis, which, combined with signs and symptoms of small bowel obstruction (SBO), most likely indicates rupture of inflamed, obstructed small bowel. This is a surgical emergency requiring an immediate operation. The other symptoms that are worrisome in a patient believed to have an SBO are tachycardia, hypotension, and metabolic acidosis.

Answer A is incorrect. Bowel sounds can be variable in small bowel obstruction, although the classic presentation is high-pitched tinkles and peristaltic rushes. Although the absence of bowel sounds indicates a progression, it does not necessarily warrant a surgical emergency.

Answer B is incorrect. The absence of flatus indicates a complete obstruction (obstipation). This is worrisome for a complete obstruction but does not warrant a surgical emergency.

Answer C is incorrect. Bilious vomiting is commonly seen in SBO, and the more proximal the obstruction, the more common is the bilious vomiting (although it will not be seen if the obstruction is proximal to the second portion of the duodenum where the common bile duct empties into the duodenum). Although SBO is an indication for surgery within 24 hours, additional diagnostics would need to be performed to confirm this diagnosis.

Answer E is incorrect. Metabolic alkalosis is commonly seen in patients with small bowel obstruction, particularly those who have experienced vomiting (this is from the loss of acidic gastric contents). Metabolic acidosis is significantly more concerning because it implies likely strangulation and necrosis of the intestines, and would require an immediate operation.

15. **The correct answer is A.** Abnormal results on pulmonary function testing (PFTs) in patients with sarcoidosis typically follow a restrictive pattern due to interstitial lung disease, as is demonstrated in this set of results. Sarcoidosis is a progressive disease characterized by non-caseating granulomas that can lead to decreased lung compliance thus leading to a restrictive pattern on the PFTs.

Answer B is incorrect. This set of results is typical of restrictive lung disease due to extrapulmonary etiology, such as obesity, pleural effusion or thickening, neuromuscular weakness, or kyphoscoliosis. It is distinguished from the correct answer by the normal carbon dioxide diffusing capacity, which suggests that oxygen exchange is still maintained in the affected areas of the lung.

Answer C is incorrect. This set of results is typical of obstructive lung disease due, for example, to emphysema.

Answer D is incorrect. This set of results is typical of obstructive lung disease due, for example, to chronic bronchitis. It is differentiated from the previous example of obstructive disease by the normal carbon dioxide diffusing capacity, which suggests that emphysematous changes have not yet begun to occur in the lung parenchyma itself.

Answer E is incorrect. This set of results is atypical of either restrictive or obstructive disease. Total lung capacity is decreased in restrictive disease, but the FEV_1:FVC ratio is decreased in obstructive disease. Neither is representative of a patient with sarcoidosis.

16. **The correct answer is A.** Alzheimer's disease is manifested by a progressive dementia, with memory loss, general cognitive dysfunction, and functional impairments. Although Alzheimer's patients can have imaging findings suggestive of increased cerebral atrophy, it is not uncommon for CT studies to be normal and age appropriate.

Answer B is incorrect. Delirium has a more acute onset of days to weeks, not months to years. Patients generally have a more clouded sensorium, with fluctuations in level of consciousness. It is usually reversible.

Answer C is incorrect. Dementia with Lewy bodies is classically seen in patients with Parkinson's disease or Parkinsonian features. The dementia is progressive, with episodes of waxing and waning of cognitive function, and is set apart from other dementia syndromes by the following key symptoms: increased daytime drowsiness and sleep, episodes of starring into space, disorganized flow of ideas, and visual hallucinations. Although this patient has a family history of Parkinson's disease, he does not show any symptoms such as tremor, bradykinesia, or cogwheel rigidity.

Answer D is incorrect. Progressive supranuclear palsy is a dementia syndrome characterized by vertical supranuclear palsy with downward gaze disturbance. There is also associated postural instability and personality changes such as apathy, anxiety, and disinhibition.

Answer E is incorrect. What differentiates vascular dementia from other types of dementia is the observed onset of cognitive symptoms immediately following a stroke, with infarcts seen on imaging and findings on physical examination consistent with a prior stroke. The onset of cognitive dysfunction is very abrupt rather than progressive, and then followed by a continued deterioration. Although atrial fibrillation increases his risk for a stroke, there is no history of a stroke and no focal neurologic deficits.

17. **The correct answer is B.** This patient has a clinical presentation most consistent with acute, uncomplicated pyelonephritis. She presents with fever, chills, nausea, vomiting, costovertebral tenderness, increased urinary frequency, and a urinalysis that is consistent with an infectious process. *Escherichia coli* is the causative pathogen most commonly seen in urinary tract infections (UTIs) (in both uncomplicated upper and lower tract infections). This organism accounts for 70–95% of UTIs. Because this patient does not have an indwelling urinary catheter in place and was not hospitalized at the time of presentation, other pathogens are even less likely to be causative in this case.

Answer A is incorrect. Although *Enterobacter* spp. may account for some cases of pyelonephritis, *Escherichia coli* is the most common uropathogen responsible for urinary tract infections (UTIs). UTIs due to *Enterobacter* are seen among hospitalized patients rather than in the ambulatory population.

Answer C is incorrect. Although *Klebsiella* spp. may account for some cases of pyelonephritis, *Escherichia coli* is the most common uropathogen responsible for urinary tract infections (UTIs). UTIs due to *Klebsiella* are seen among hospitalized patients rather than in the ambulatory population.

Answer D is incorrect. Although *Proteus* spp. may account for some cases of pyelonephritis, *Escherichia coli* is the most common uropathogen responsible for urinary tract infections (UTIs). In cases of UTIs due to *Proteus*, the alkaline urine promotes the development of a struvite stone that may form staghorn calculi in the urinary tract.

Answer E is incorrect. Although *Pseudomonas* spp. may account for some cases pyelonephri-

tis, *Escherichia coli* is the most common uropathogen responsible for urinary tract infections (UTIs). UTIs due to *Pseudomonas* are seen among hospitalized patients rather than in the ambulatory population.

Answer F is incorrect. Although staphylococci may account for 5–20% of urinary tract infections (UTIs), *Escherichia coli* has been associated with 70–95% of UTIs and therefore is more likely to be involved in the pathogenesis described. UTIs due to *Staphylococcus* infections, although relatively uncommon, occur more frequently in young, ambulatory women.

18. **The correct answer is B.** Cystic fibrosis often presents primarily with gastrointestinal symptoms in infancy, most commonly a failure to thrive and malabsorption. These effects are due to thick pancreatic secretions secondary to ineffective chloride transport, which leads to plugging of the pancreatic acini. This means that the pancreatic enzymes cannot enter the gastrointestinal tract, and the lack of pancreatic enzymes leads to malabsorption of fats. Parents will report typically foul-smelling oily stools and difficulty feeding. Seven to ten percent of patients will have a history of meconium ileus at birth. Diagnosis can be confirmed by a sweat chloride test result > 60 mEq/L.

Answer A is incorrect. A biopsy may be useful in diagnosing malabsorptive disorders due to mucosal abnormalities such as celiac disease. However, since there is nothing in her diet yet that would expose her to gluten, celiac disease is not a likely diagnosis.

Answer C is incorrect. Stool qualitative fat would only confirm a malabsorptive process, which is already suggested by the patient's presentation. It would not help in diagnosing the etiology of that process.

Answer D is incorrect. Pancreatitis may result from plugging of acini with thick secretions, leading to autodigestion of the pancreatic tissue. An ultrasound of the pancreas may show this autodigestion, but it will not make the etiology clear, and will therefore not help in diagnosis of cystic fibrosis.

Answer E is incorrect. An x-ray of the abdomen and pelvis could show anatomic abnormalities and intestinal obstruction, but has no role in diagnosing cystic fibrosis.

19. **The correct answer is E.** You should be familiar with the forms of acute coronary syndrome. Acute coronary syndrome encompasses unstable angina, non-ST-elevation myocardial infarction, and ST-elevation myocardial infarction (STEMI). A STEMI is defined as ST-segment elevation of ≥ 1 mV in concordant limb leads or ≥ 2 mV in concordant precordial leads in a patient with chest pain. Given the history and the histopathologic specimen, this is likely acute thrombosis of his left anterior descending artery, causing an ST-elevation MI. Q waves are usually preceded by hyperacute T waves and ST elevations. The next finding is T-wave inversions. Q waves are often the last finding.

Answer A is incorrect. Aortic dissection classically presents with a tearing sensation in the affected area. The specific chest pain symptoms expressed in the context of ECG and pathologic findings strongly contradict this diagnosis.

Answer B is incorrect. Noninfarction subendocardial ischemia is classical angina and is often seen on ECG as transient ST depressions. This, along with the pathologic specimen, argues against the diagnosis of angina.

Answer C is incorrect. Noninfarction transmural ischemia is seen in Prinzmetal's angina. It is manifest by transient ST-segment elevations. While the vignette does not indicate whether this is a transient process, you should assume from the large acute thrombus in the left anterior descending artery that this will result in a myocardial infarction.

Answer D is incorrect. A non-ST elevation myocardial infarction would have ST depressions or T-wave inversions without Q waves.

20. **The correct answer is D.** This patient most likely has the syndrome of inappropriate antidiuretic hormone (SIADH) secretion due to ectopic production of ADH by a bronchogenic small cell lung carcinoma. ADH acts on the collecting tubules to increase the retention of free water. SIADH, therefore, is not caused by a lack of sodium but by excess free water. How-

ever, the sodium level will be decreased in the laboratory values because of the increased water uptake. Plasma osmolality decreases due to free water retention and inability to diurese and dilute the urine. Therefore, urine electrolyte levels will be relatively elevated. Treatment is free water restriction and diuresis if the patient is stable, and infusion of isotonic saline if neurologic symptoms appear. This carcinoma is strongly correlated with smoking history and is a rapidly progressive tumor. Weight loss is typical of the presentation of this carcinoma, and hip pain suggests bony metastasis.

Answer A is incorrect. This patient most likely has a pneumonia, which can cause SIADH in some cases. Small cell lung carcinoma, however, is a more likely cause of SIADH in this patient given his smoking history, history of lung nodule, weight loss, and bone pain.

Answer B is incorrect. Postsurgical atelectasis can cause syndrome of inappropriate ADH but would not be commonly seen 2 months after surgery.

Answer C is incorrect. Head trauma can cause SIADH; however, this patient has no history of trauma.

Answer E is incorrect. Renal failure can present with hyponatremia; however, this patient has no evidence of renal failure given his normal blood urea nitrogen and creatinine.

21. **The correct answer is D.** *Mycobacterium tuberculosis* has become much more prevalent in the United States as a result of the HIV epidemic. In fact, infection with HIV may increase a patient's risk of developing active tuberculosis (TB) by a factor of more than 15. All HIV-infected individuals should be screened for latent TB infection by means of a purified protein derivative skin test. HIV-infected individuals who have a skin test reaction of more than 5 mm or who have close household contacts with persons with active TB should automatically receive prophylactic treatment for TB.

Answer A is incorrect. Although respiratory isolation in the ward would be required if this patient were detectably ill, there is no indication that he needs to be hospitalized. A 9-month course of isoniazid is indicated only because of the patient's high risk of developing active tuberculosis.

Answer B is incorrect. Monitoring serial purified protein derivative tests (PPDs) is a proper course of action for any HIV-positive individual with a PPD of < 5 mm; however, this patient has a PPD of > 5 mm and should be treated accordingly.

Answer C is incorrect. Even if x-ray of the chest is clear, current guidelines indicate that all HIV-positive patients with a PPD test of > 5 mm should receive prophylactic antituberculous therapy.

Answer E is incorrect. Trimethoprim-sulfamethoxazole is not active against *Mycobacterium tuberculosis*. The patient's CD4+ count is higher than 200/mm³, so prophylaxis against *Toxoplasma gondii* and *Pneumocystis jiroveci* (formerly *carinii*) pneumonia is therefore not indicated.

22. **The correct answer is D.** A living will specifically states the wishes of a patient and is meant to be used in lieu of a direct discussion with the patient if the patient is unable to state his wishes at any point. Because this patient made his wishes very clear, both verbally and in writing, his wife cannot override his living will now that he cannot speak for himself.

Answer A is incorrect. There is no need for a family meeting to decide whether to extubate the patient because the living will clearly states the patient's wishes.

Answer B is incorrect. Because the patient has a living will, there is no need for an ethics consult in this case to help mediate decision making between the medical team and patient's family.

Answer C is incorrect. Luckily, in this case, the patient has stated his wishes clearly before undergoing surgery, so there is no need for the team to decide how to proceed.

Answer E is incorrect. It is appropriate to address both the concerns and the needs of the patient's family, in this case his wife, before extubating the patient, even though ultimately this is the final outcome.

23. **The correct answer is B.** The patient has a pheochromocytoma, which is associated with multiple endocrine neoplasia (MEN) types 2A and 2B. MEN 2A includes medullary thyroid carcinoma, pheochromocytoma, and parathyroid hyperplasia. MEN 2B includes medullary thyroid carcinoma, pheochromocytoma, and mucosal/gastrointestinal neuromas. Other neoplastic diseases associated with pheochromocytoma include von Hippel–Lindau syndrome and neurofibromatosis.

Answer A is incorrect. Insulinoma is part of MEN type I and is not typically associated with pheochromocytoma.

Answer C is incorrect. Pancreatic adenocarcinoma is associated with Peutz-Jeghers syndrome (36% lifetime risk) and hereditary pancreatitis (40% lifetime risk). It is not typically associated with pheochromocytoma.

Answer D is incorrect. Papillary thyroid cancer typically affects women (2.5:1, male-to-female) in their 30s and 40s, contains calcified psammoma bodies, and is not typically associated with pheochromocytoma.

Answer E is incorrect. Pituitary adenoma is not typically associated with pheochromocytoma. It is part of MEN type I, along with pancreatic neuroendocrine tumors and parathyroid hyperplasia.

24. **The correct answer is C.** The history of rheumatic fever should raise suspicion of mitral stenosis, caused by the fusion of the commissures, producing the typical "fish mouth" valve. The clinical manifestations of mitral stenosis include dyspnea, pulmonary edema, and atrial fibrillation. Other findings consistent with mitral stenosis are a low-pitched diastolic rumble at the apex, an opening snap, and x-ray of the chest showing a dilated left atrium (straightening of the left heart border and elevation of the left main stem bronchus). Mitral stenosis causes an increase in the pulmonary capillary hydraulic pressure, resulting in a net increase in fluid transported into the interstitium. This patient would be treated with warfarin for his atrial fibrillation and diuretics for his pulmonary congestion.

Answer A is incorrect. Acute aortic insufficiency (AI) causes an increase in left ventricular volume, with elevation of left ventricular end-diastolic and left atrial pressure, resulting in pulmonary edema. AI, however, typically presents with a diastolic decrescendo murmur at the left upper sternal border and a wide pulse pressure (> 60 mm Hg).

Answer B is incorrect. Pulmonary edema can also arise from acute mitral insufficiency, which results from papillary muscle dysfunction or chordae tendineae rupture following myocardial infarction. With acute mitral insufficiency, the ability of the left atrium to fill the left ventricle is reduced, resulting in pulmonary edema. However, the patient's presentation and physical findings are not consistent with mitral insufficiency. While these patients do present with pulmonary edema, there is a high-pitched, blowing, holosystolic murmur at the apex, laterally displaced point of maximal intensity, and history of severe substernal chest pain (if infarction is the cause of the patient's acute mitral insufficiency).

Answer D is incorrect. Acute onset of severe myocardial ischemia can lead to a sudden loss of systolic and diastolic function, resulting in decreased cardiac output and pulmonary edema. The presentation, however, is not typical for myocardial ischemia. The patient lacks angina with or without radiation of pain to the neck, jaw, shoulders, or arms for > 30 minutes. However, 23% percent of myocardial infarctions (MIs) are atypical or silent. If this were an atypical MI, the cardiac enzymes would still be elevated. In fact, the sensitivity of creatine kinase-myocardial bound, troponin T, and troponin I > 6 hours after the onset of symptoms is 91%, 94%, and 100%, respectively.

Answer E is incorrect. In the presence of diastolic dysfunction, fever, sepsis, and anemia thyroid disease can precipitate hemodynamic decompensation and the development of pulmonary edema. A normal thyroid-stimulating hormone level, however, argues against thyroid disease.

25. **The correct answer is B.** Contraction of the neck muscles in an unnatural position is known as torticollis; in this case, the patient is experiencing an acute dystonic reaction as an adverse effect to one of his antipsychotic medications, most likely a high-potency typical antipsychotic such as haloperidol, droperidol, fluphenazine, or thiothixene. Treatment of acute dystonia is with an anticholinergic such as benztropine or with diphenhydramine; the patient will literally "loosen up" within a matter of seconds. Prophylaxis for acute dystonic reactions can be provided with benztropine.

Answer A is incorrect. Alprazolam is a short-acting benzodiazepine that is used to treat anxiety. It has no role in the treatment of acute dystonia.

Answer C is incorrect. Haloperidol and other typical antipsychotic medications are responsible for causing acute dystonias such as in this patient. Initiating haloperidol would only worsen the patient's torticollis.

Answer D is incorrect. Although it would appear that the neck muscles are in spasm, muscle relaxants are not indicated; an acute dystonic reaction warrants administration of diphenhydramine.

Answer E is incorrect. Sertraline is a selective serotonin reuptake inhibitor used primarily in the treatment of depression and anxiety disorders. It has no role in the treatment of acute dystonia.

26. **The correct answer is D.** Prevalence is the number of cases of a disease or condition in the population at a given point in time. Cross-sectional studies collect information on disease presence and on risk factors for its development simultaneously.

Answer A is incorrect. Attributable risk is calculated in cohort studies and is the difference in incidence rate between study and control groups. Cross-sectional studies do not produce the data required for this calculation.

Answer B is incorrect. Causation cannot be determined from cross-sectional studies because information on exposure to potential risk factors and information on presence or absence of disease is collected at the same point in time. Chi-square analysis may reveal significant associations based on data gathered in a cross-sectional survey, which in turn can suggest causal relationships. However, only prospective studies can actually prove causation.

Answer C is incorrect. Incidence refers to the number of new cases of a disease or condition in a population per unit of time.

Answer E is incorrect. Relative risk reflects the "strength" of association between exposure to a risk factor and development of a disease or condition. It is calculated in cohort studies.

27. **The correct answer is A.** The patient has high-grade reflux that has persisted past puberty. Although there is much debate over the management of VUR in younger patients, the situation in this case is much clearer. High-grade reflux in females that persists into adulthood with no clear secondary cause should be managed surgically. Surgical correction in this population is favored because of the increased likelihood of the complications of UTIs during pregnancy. During pregnancy, physiologic relaxation of the ureter allows for more urinary stasis and makes women with bacteriuria much more susceptible to developing pyelonephritis. Untreated upper tract infections are associated with morbidity for both the mother and the fetus, including premature labor, low birth weight, preeclampsia, and maternal anemia. This patient is also a candidate because she is already exhibiting the feared complication of untreated VUR, which is renal failure (creatinine 1.5 mg/dL).

Answer B is incorrect. Given this patient's elevated creatinine, infection despite prophylaxis, and risks associated with antibiotics, antibiotics should only be used as a temporizing therapy (i.e., until elective surgery can be performed).

Answer C is incorrect. Dimercaptosuccinic acid scans are used to assess the extent of renal scarring that can result from episodes of pyelonephritis. The test is useful in situations where reflux surgery is more questionable or where evidence of organ damage is required before proceeding to surgical management.

Answer D is incorrect. There is little utility in continuing to repeat the voiding cystourethro-

gram (VCUG) in this patient. She is already developed (Tanner stage IV) and voiding well (no residual urine on VCUG, no incontinence, and no other urinary complaints). If the patient was prepubescent or had voiding dysfunction, such as a problems with filling and emptying the bladder, yearly VCUG would be more appropriate.

Answer E is incorrect. Video urodynamics are not necessary in this case. In general, urodynamics are the study of storage and voiding function of the lower urinary tract. Video urodynamics are a way to gather data on voiding and filling pressures and a way to capture radiographic evidence of function. This test is more useful in situations where voiding dysfunction is suspected. This patient does not have difficulty voiding. The test is more often used in the peri–potty training period, or if other signs or symptoms suggest voiding abnormalities.

28. **The correct answer is E.** Impetigo is a bacterial skin infection commonly caused by either *Staphylococcus aureus* or group A *Streptococcus*. It characteristically results in crusting skin lesions that are often nonpainful and nonpruritic. The progression of the irritation is generally initiated with a tiny vesicle or pustule that rapidly develops into a honey-colored crusted plaque. The infection may be spread to other parts of the body by contact with fingers, clothing, towels, or other materials that come into contact with the impetiginous lesions. For patients with a limited number of lesions, treatment with topical antibiotic (mupirocin) is preferred; for more widespread, severe cases, oral antibiotics may be used (erythromycin, cephalexin, or dicloxacillin).

Answer A is incorrect. Acyclovir is not indicated for the treatment of bacterial skin infections. Acyclovir is commonly employed in the treatment of herpes simplex lesions, varicella zoster virus (chickenpox), or herpes zoster.

Answer B is incorrect. Changing facial soaps will not treat a bacterial skin infection. Although milder facial soaps may reduce subsequent irritation of the skin, antibiotic therapy is still required for cases of impetigo.

Answer C is incorrect. Topical steroids, such as hydrocortisone, are not routinely indicated for the treatment of bacterial skin infections. Topical steroids are more commonly employed for conditions such as contact dermatitis, seborrhea dermatitis, or atopic dermatitis (eczema).

Answer D is incorrect. Intravenous vancomycin is not indicated for the treatment of impetigo. For severe, widespread impetigo, a course of oral antibiotics is generally sufficient.

Answer F is incorrect. Tretinoin cream is not indicated for the treatment of bacterial skin infections. Tretinoin cream is typically used in the treatment of acne vulgaris.

29. **The correct answer is D.** The man has signs and symptoms of carpal tunnel syndrome, entrapment of the median nerve characterized by pain and paresthesias in the medial portion of the palm. Carpal tunnel is often a clinical diagnosis, although several objective examination findings and studies can be of use, including nerve conduction studies by electromyography.

Answer A is incorrect. Angiography is used in the setting of an acute ischemic stroke, when identifying the vascular anatomy would change medical or surgical management. This invasive maneuver is far too risky in a patient whose symptoms are not very likely to be attributable to stroke; in such a patient if stroke were more likely than carpal tunnel syndrome (the correct diagnosis), then a CT scan of the head would be a better initial study.

Answer B is incorrect. A CT scan of the head would be useful to determine if the patient's symptoms had a cerebrovascular etiology. However, the fact that he reports chronic intermittent numbness and tingling that occasionally wake him at night, and the fact that he has weakness and atrophy in the distribution of the median nerve distal to the carpal tunnel are highly suggestive of carpal tunnel syndrome. While this man clearly has risk factors for stroke, the more likely diagnosis is carpal tunnel syndrome.

Answer C is incorrect. An electroencephalogram would be useful if there were reason to suspect that the man's symptoms were due to a seizure disorder. However, there is no history of uncontrollable movements, loss of consciousness, or sensory disturbance other than the paresthesias indicative of carpal tunnel syndrome. It would be very unusual for a focal simple seizure to present in this manner, moving it far lower on the differential than carpal tunnel or stroke.

Answer E is incorrect. An MRI of the head would be one modality to look for a stroke, and is more sensitive than CT in identifying early ischemic strokes. However, there is nothing in the stem to suggest an acute pathology, and in this case the test would be a waste of resources. More importantly, the clinical diagnosis of carpal tunnel is most likely, and an MRI of the head would not be indicated.

30. **The correct answer is C.** The patient presents with typical features of generalized anxiety disorder (GAD). The diagnostic criteria for GAD include excessive anxiety and worry occurring more days than not for at least 6 months about a number of events or activities. Additionally, at least three of the following six symptoms must be present: restlessness, fatigue, difficulty concentrating, irritability, muscle tension (e.g., headaches), and sleep disturbance. The symptoms typically cause clinically significant distress or impairment in social, occupational, or other areas of functioning.

Answer A is incorrect. Acute stress disorder is characterized as excessive and persistent anxiety, nightmares, agitation, and sometimes depression following an extraordinary life event (war, natural disaster). It is similar to posttraumatic stress disorder but is less severe and involves a shorter time frame.

Answer B is incorrect. This patient has no exposure to an obvious stressor; therefore, the diagnosis of adjustment disorder with anxiety is not the most appropriate one.

Answer D is incorrect. Although the patient presents with several physical complaints (e.g., headaches, stomachaches, palpitations), her anxiety is not confined to having a serious illness, as in hypochondriasis.

Answer E is incorrect. There is no evidence that the patient is malingering. Malingering involves the voluntary production of psychological and physical symptoms to accomplish a specific goal (receive compensation, legitimize taking a sick day from work). In this situation, the patient enjoys her work and does not appear to have any ulterior motives when discussing her symptoms.

31. **The correct answer is D.** The patient is suffering from allergen-induced anaphylaxis, a type I hypersensitivity reaction due to diffuse release of vasoactive amines (i.e., histamine). A β-blocker would play no role in resuscitating this patient, and would worsen the patient's hypotension and bronchospasm. In fact, patients chronically on β-blocker therapy undergoing an anaphylactic reaction may be refractory to treatment with epinephrine, and in these patients glucagon should be administered, as it has inotropic and chronotropic effects not mediated by β-receptors.

    Answer A is incorrect. Albuterol (a β-adrenergic agonist) can assist in relaxing the airway and improving ventilation.

    Answer B is incorrect. Diphenhydramine (primarily an H_1 histamine blocker) is useful to counteract the effects of histamine.

    Answer C is incorrect. Epinephrine is the treatment of choice for severe anaphylactic shock because it reverses the severe hypotension and bronchospasm.

    Answer E is incorrect. Methylprednisolone (a potent corticosteroid) is useful to limit the inflammatory response in severe allergic reactions.

    Answer F is incorrect. Ranitidine, an antagonist of the H_2 histamine receptor, can be used to counteract the effects of histamine on myocardial and peripheral vascular tissue in patients experiencing anaphylactic shock.

32. **The correct answer is B.** The cerebellum integrates and coordinates sensory perception and motor output. Therefore, cerebellar lesions do not cause paralysis, but typically cause fine motor movement disorders, as well as deficits in equilibrium, posture and motor learning. The patient presents with gait ataxia, which is typically of a vermis lesion.

    Answer A is incorrect. A cerebellar hemisphere lesion would present with ipsilateral limb ataxia. Hemispheric lesions are characterized by decomposition of movement, dysmetria and rebound, intention tremor, or kinetic tremors (presenting in motion). Hemispheric cerebellar dysfunction is best ascertained clinically via the finger-to-nose and heel-to-knee tests.

    Answer C is incorrect. The classic triad of clinical features in normal pressure hydrocephalus includes gait disturbance, urinary incontinence, and cognitive disturbance. These features are believed to be derived from dysfunction of the periventricular white matter tracts, especially of the frontal lobe connections. A patient with hydrocephalus would more likely present with a frontal ataxia, also known as a magnetic gait or gait apraxia with impaired gait initiation. There is the appearance of the patient's feet being "stuck" to the floor, with short steps, decreased stride length and height, a broadened base, and outwardly rotated feet.

    Answer D is incorrect. Meniere's disease is associated with episodic vertigo, sensorineural hearing loss, an aura of fullness or pressure in the ear or side of the head, and tinnitus. The episodic vertigo can be followed by a period of nausea and unsteadiness for several hours.

    Answer E is incorrect. Patients with vestibular neuronitis present with rapid onset of a severe vertigo along with nausea, vomiting, and gait instability. The physical examination is significant for a spontaneous vestibular nystagmus that is unilateral, horizontal, or horizontal-torsional, and that is suppressed with visual fixation and does not change direction with gaze. The beating of the fast phase is away from the affected side. This patient does not exhibit nystagmus.

33. **The correct answer is C.** This case describes the usual mechanism of injury for a meniscal tear. Pain, catching, locking, and giving way are common symptoms of a torn meniscus. The joint line tenderness and effusion further

suggest meniscus tear as the cause of the patient's symptoms.

Answer A is incorrect. A chondromalacia patella is a chronic overuse injury with an insidious onset that causes anterior knee pain. It is related to problems with patellar tracking.

Answer B is incorrect. A medial collateral ligament injury is possible with the action described and can present with joint line tenderness. However, the mechanical symptoms of catching and locking are more consistent with meniscal injury.

Answer D is incorrect. Pes anserine bursitis can cause pain on the medial aspect of the proximal tibia. This is more likely to develop insidiously and would not cause joint line tenderness.

Answer E is incorrect. Quadriceps tendonitis can cause giving way, but not catching or locking, which implies an intra-articular pathology. It would also not be associated with joint line tenderness.

34. **The correct answer is E.** This patient had cardiac tamponade from a hemopericardium. Positive-pressure mechanical ventilation can be harmful in patients with cardiac tamponade because it increases intrathoracic pressure and leads to a further decrease in cardiac output.

Answer A is incorrect. The value of inotropic support in cardiac tamponade is unknown. Although dobutamine should theoretically improve the patient's hypotension, the patient's endogenous inotropic stimulation may be at its maximal amount in cardiac tamponade, making dobutamine have little additional effect. Although it is unknown whether the use of dobutamine in cardiac tamponade is beneficial, there is no evidence that administering inotropic drugs to patients with tamponade has a negative effect on them.

Answer B is incorrect. Echocardiography can be used to aid in diagnosing cardiac tamponade. Although the diagnosis of cardiac tamponade should have been made sooner and could have been made based on clinical signs and symptoms alone, echocardiography did not worsen the patient's condition.

Answer C is incorrect. Obtaining central access is indicated in a patient who has lost a large amount of blood and is hemodynamically unstable. This patient's hemopericardium was secondary to her gunshot wound and unrelated to insertion of the central line.

Answer D is incorrect. Pericardiocentesis is the recommended intervention for cardiac tamponade, but this procedure was not performed early enough in this patient to save her life.

35. **The correct answer is A.** For patients with a family history of colon cancer, with polyps in a first-degree relative diagnosed at younger than 60 years, or with two first-degree relatives diagnosed at any age, the American Cancer Society recommends that screening begin 10 years prior to the age at which the youngest family member to have colorectal cancer was diagnosed, or at age 40 years, whichever is earlier.

Answer B is incorrect. Screening guidelines recommend patients with a family history of colon cancer be screened at an age 10 years prior to the age at which the youngest family member was diagnosed. This patient's father was diagnosed at age 45 years; thus, the patient should have been screened at age 35 years, and so this answer is incorrect.

Answer C is incorrect. Forty-five years is the age at which the patient's father (the youngest family member to receive the diagnosis) was diagnosed; therefore, screening of the patient should have begun 10 years prior to this.

Answer D is incorrect. Forty-eight years is the age at which the patient's father died of colon cancer, which is not relevant to screening of family members.

Answer E is incorrect. Fifty years is the age at which cancer screening should begin for patients without high risk for colorectal cancer. This patient is at high risk given his family history of colorectal cancer in a first-degree relative.

36. **The correct answer is E.** This woman has a clinical picture and laboratory findings consistent with pheochromocytoma. The classic triad of symptoms in a patient with a

pheochromocytoma includes episodic headache, sweating, and tachycardia. In addition, one expects elevated urine and plasma catecholamines. Prior to surgical removal of tumor, pharmacotherapy is used to better control the patient's blood pressure. Because a pheochromocytoma secretes catecholamines, it is recommended that an α-adrenergic blocker such as phenoxybenzamine is started. After approximately 2 weeks of therapy, the patient should be ready for surgery. A β-blocker should be given only after phenoxybenzamine.

Answer A is incorrect. Nitroprusside is indicated in hypertensive emergencies. There is no indication that this woman is having a hypertensive emergency, so nitroprusside would not be our first-line treatment.

Answer B is incorrect. Although surgery to remove the tumor is indicated, it is recommended that the patient is first medically managed using an α-adrenergic blocker to control blood pressure.

Answer C is incorrect. Thiazide diuretics, such as hydrochlorothiazide (HCTZ), are a good first-line treatment in patients with essential hypertension. However, this patient has a pheochromocytoma, a cause of secondary hypertension, so HCTZ would not be the most appropriate treatment.

Answer D is incorrect. A β-blocker, such as propranolol, should never be the first antihypertensive started in patients with a suspected diagnosis of pheochromocytoma. Peripheral β-adrenergic receptors cause vasodilatation, and blocking these receptors with unopposed α-adrenergic receptor stimulation can lead to vasoconstriction, or increased blood pressure in the setting of decreased heart contractility and heart rate due to the β_1-adrenergic effects on the heart. This would essentially mean that a weaker heart would be pumping against a higher afterload. However, once an α-blocker such as phenoxybenzamine has been started, a β-blocker may be added to decrease tachycardia.

37. **The correct answer is A.** This patient is presenting with signs and symptoms that are highly suspicious for biliary colic with obstruc-

tion or inflammation of the biliary tree. Ultrasound shows stones in the gallbladder, but those stones are not necessarily responsible for her current pain. The laboratory findings can help pinpoint the site of obstruction by observing its effects. In this case, a stone appears to be obstructing the common bile duct. The elevated total bilirubin implies obstruction at this site, with consequent backup of bile into the liver, causing some hepatocellular damage (i.e., elevated aspartate aminotransferase and alanine aminotransferase). Additionally, the elevated alkaline phosphatase indicates biliary obstruction. The lack of an increase in amylase and lipase makes obstruction at the ampulla less likely (such an obstruction would cause pancreatic inflammation). A patient with choledocholithiasis should undergo extraction of stones from the common bile duct. This may be achieved endoscopically, via endoscopic retrograde cholangiopancreatography and sphincterotomy, or operatively.

Answer B is incorrect. The common hepatic duct is formed by the convergence of the right and left hepatic ducts. The cystic duct joins the common hepatic duct to form the common bile duct. Therefore, gallstones are not found in the common hepatic duct.

Answer C is incorrect. A stone obstructing her cystic duct would not result in an elevation of her total bilirubin, aspartate aminotransferase, alanine aminotransferase, or alkaline phosphatase. However, it would cause the pain of biliary colic observed in this patient. These symptomatic patients should be treated with cholecystectomy.

Answer D is incorrect. If a stone was obstructing the ampulla of Vater, some pancreatic inflammation would be expected from the concomitant obstruction of the common bile duct and the pancreatic duct, with a resulting increase in amylase and lipase. Definitive treatment includes cholecystectomy with cholangiography and removal of visualized stones from the common bile duct.

Answer E is incorrect. The stones observed in her gallbladder are not those responsible for her symptoms and laboratory values. They are not obstructing and are not causing a backup of bile from ductal obstruction. However, the stone, which is not obstructing the common bile duct, was likely formed in the gallbladder. Asymptomatic gallstones require no treatment. However, approximately 1–2% of people per year with this condition develop symptoms of gallstone disease. These symptomatic patients should be treated with cholecystectomy.

38. **The correct answer is C.** Genital tract infections have been implicated as a cause of increased rates of preterm labor. In addition, *Chlamydia* infection increases the rate of chorioamnionitis, which also causes a rise in the rate of preterm labor. It is postulated that the inflammatory response of the mother or fetus is the mechanism of preterm labor induced by infectious causes.

Answer A is incorrect. Nifedipine is also an effective tocolytic. The mechanism of action involves blockage of influx of calcium into the intracellular space through the cell membrane and sarcoplasmic reticulum.

Answer B is incorrect. Hydration is often used as a method to forestall premature labor. ADH is manufactured in the hypothalamus along with oxytocin and is hypothesized to exhibit some cross-reactivity with oxytocin receptors. Thus, hydrating a patient in preterm labor may decrease ADH levels and may delay cervical change and decrease contractions.

Answer D is incorrect. Complications of preeclampsia include fetal distress or stillbirth, intrauterine growth restriction, oligohydramnios, or progression to eclampsia. Delivery is the definitive treatment for preeclampsia, and therapeutic delivery necessitated before maturity is reached can lead to complications of prematurity in the infant. However, premature labor is not caused by preeclampsia.

Answer E is incorrect. Nonsteroidal anti-inflammatory drugs (NSAIDs) have been clinically demonstrated to be effective tocolytics with minimal maternal adverse effects. The mechanism of action is decreased production of prostaglandins, which leads to decreased intracellular levels of calcium and inhibition of uterine contractions. However, use of NSAIDs may cause multiple fetal complications, including premature closure of the ductus arteriosus and oligohydramnios.

39. **The correct answer is F.** Ziprasidone is the atypical antipsychotic that is most associated with QT prolongation.

Answer A is incorrect. Chlorpromazine is a typical antipsychotic with severe sedative adverse effects and a large likelihood of causing severe orthostatic hypotension, with a decreased risk of extrapyramidal symptoms.

Answer B is incorrect. Clozapine is an antipsychotic medication that improves the negative symptoms of schizophrenia but can cause agranulocytosis in 1–2% of patients taking it. As a result, patients must agree to a weekly blood draw to check WBC count throughout therapy and for 4 weeks after stopping the drug. Agranulocytosis is an absolute contraindication for continuing the drug.

Answer C is incorrect. Haloperidol is a high-potency typical antipsychotic medication that is associated with more extrapyramidal symptoms (EPS) than the low-potency agents (e.g., chlorpromazine). Typical antipsychotics can cause EPS, hyperprolactinemia, anticholinergic effects, and sedation, and are more associated with neuroleptic malignant syndrome than are atypical antipsychotics.

Answer D is incorrect. Olanzapine is an atypical antipsychotic associated with increased triglycerides, somnolence, hyperglycemia, and weight gain. The drug itself is particularly effective for negative symptoms of schizophrenia and for agitation.

Answer E is incorrect. The adverse effects of quetiapine include somnolence, orthostatic hypotension, and dizziness. It may increase risk of cataracts, and frequent eye examinations are recommended with its use. It also has rare adverse effect of QT prolongation, but this effect is more commonly seen with ziprasidone.

40. **The correct answer is F.** This patient most likely has neurologic endemic cretinism, caused by maternal iodine deficiency during early pregnancy and characterized by mental retardation, spasticity, abnormal gait, and deafness. Many patients have complete deafness,

and these individuals are typically mute as well. Goiter is uncommon, and patients typically are euthyroid. This disorder is most commonly found in India, China, Indonesia, Bolivia, Ecuador, and Peru.

Answer A is incorrect. Autoimmune thyroiditis is a highly uncommon cause of congenital hypothyroidism and can cause transient hypothyroidism in infants. It is the cause of Hashimoto's thyroiditis in adults.

Answer B is incorrect. While iodine deficiency is a possible cause of hypothyroidism in children, this patient would likely have an elevated thyroid-stimulating hormone, low thyroxine, a goiter, and many of the signs and symptoms of hypothyroidism (including fatigue, cold intolerance, coarse skin, and edema).

Answer C is incorrect. Congenital errors in production of thyroid hormone, thyroid-binding globulin, and iodide transport molecules account for approximately 10% of cases of congenital hypothyroidism. Patients would not be expected to have normal thyroxine and thyroid-stimulating hormone levels.

Answer D is incorrect. Hypopituitarism can cause hypothyroidism due to low levels of thyroid-stimulating hormone release. Patients often demonstrate other manifestations of hypopituitarism, such as adrenal insufficiency or diabetes insipidus.

Answer E is incorrect. Iodine deficiency late in pregnancy and after birth is considered the cause of myxedematous endemic cretinism. Both neurologic and myxedematous cretinism are part of the spectrum of endemic cretinism, which causes irreversible changes in mental development in areas of endemic hypothyroidism. Myxedematous endemic cretinism is found predominantly in the Congo region of Africa. Disorders include mental retardation, short stature, and hypothyroidism.

Answer G is incorrect. Thyroid dysgenesis is the most common cause of congenital hypothyroidism, which is in turn the most common treatable cause of mental retardation. Neonates with thyroid dysgenesis often are not affected by hypothyroidism due to maternal thyroxine that crossed the placenta. The pa-

tient in the question would be hypothyroid if this were his diagnosis.

Questions 41 and 42

41. **The correct answer is M.** This patient's presentation is consistent with Sézary's syndrome, the most advanced stage of cutaneous T-cell lymphoma (CTCL). This phase of disease usually occurs after the more localized stages (patch, plaque, and tumor) have persisted for several years. Unfortunately, these stages may go undiagnosed or be misdiagnosed as atopic dermatitis or other skin disease and may not be recognized as malignancy. *Sézary's syndrome* is a term used to describe a systemic form of CTCL, during which Sézary cells are visible in the peripheral blood and the entire skin surface is affected. Sézary cells are recognizable for their convoluted or cerebriform nuclei and scant cytoplasm.

42. **The correct answer is C.** Palpable abdominal masses may represent several forms of malignancy in children, including neuroblastoma, Wilms' tumor, and Burkitt's lymphoma. Children from Africa, where infection with Epstein-Barr virus may lead to an endemic form of Burkitt's lymphoma, are particularly prone to this disease. The numerous benign macrophages with abundant clear cytoplasm distributed among tumor cells give the tissue biopsy a "starry sky" appearance on low-power light microscopy. Burkitt's lymphoma is associated with the t(8:14) translocations of the *c-MYC* gene.

Answer A is incorrect. Although acute lymphocytic leukemia occurs primarily in children, it also accounts for 20% of adult leukemias. Patients may complain of malaise, weight loss, bone pain, and hemorrhage. Clinical examination may reveal lymphadenopathy and/or hepatosplenomegaly in half of the patients. Biopsy in L1 type would be expected to reveal small lymphoblasts with scant cytoplasm, condensed nuclear chromatin, and indistinct nuclei. Biopsy in L2 type would be expected to reveal larger lymphoblasts with a moderate amount of cytoplasm, dispersed chromatin, and multiple nucleoli. Biopsy in

L3 type would be expected to reveal lymphoblasts with deep cytoplasmic basophilia with prominent cytoplasmic vacuolation.

Answer B is incorrect. Acute myelocytic leukemia is more common in adults, presenting with fatigue, hemorrhage, bruising, lymphadenopathy, and hepatosplenomegaly. This condition is associated with leukocytosis, blasts in peripheral blood, and the presence of Auer rods.

Answer D is incorrect. The median age for presentation of chronic lymphocytic leukemia is 60 years. When symptomatic, this condition classically presents with lymphadenopathy, hepatosplenomegaly, and lymphocytosis. Lymph node biopsy would be expected to show diffusely effaced nodal architecture with occasional residual naked germinal centers. The nodal infiltrate is usually composed of mature-appearing, small lymphocytes, with an admixture of prolymphocytes and paraimmunoblasts,

Answer E is incorrect. Chronic myelogenous leukemia (CML) typically affects patients older than 50 years. CML is a myeloproliferative disorder that is often discovered on routine blood tests, where leukocytosis and thrombocytosis are discovered. When symptomatic, fatigue, weight loss, malaise, abdominal discomfort, and bleeding due to platelet dysfunction are common. The t(9;22) translocation creates the Philadelphia chromosome, which is often seen in CML. The blast crisis refers to the proliferation of blast cells. Bone marrow biopsy in the blast crisis of this condition would be expected to reveal large foci or clusters of blasts.

Answer F is incorrect. Ewing's sarcoma may develop in any bone or soft tissue but is most common in the flat and long bones. This condition is characterized by localized pain and swelling rather than abdominal or cutaneous involvement. Histology reveals monotonous sheets of small round blue cells with hyperchromatic nuclei.

Answer G is incorrect. Non-Hodgkin's lymphomas (NHLs) commonly present with hepatosplenomegaly, widespread palpable adenopathy, and abdominal masses. Follicular lymphoma is one of the more common NHLs. Because follicular lymphoma is generally slow

growing or indolent, patients tend to present with generalized disease. Follicular lymphoma typically presents in older patients. Histology of affected lymph nodes reveals relatively small, well-differentiated cells organized in a nodular pattern. The classic genetic analysis demonstrates the t(14:18) translocation with overexpression of *bcl-2*. Follicular lymphoma does not classically present with atopic dermatitis.

Answer H is incorrect. Non-Hodgkin's lymphomas (NHLs) commonly present with hepatosplenomegaly, widespread palpable adenopathy, and abdominal masses. Mantle cell lymphoma is an unusual type of NHL predominantly described in older men, presenting with generalized lymphadenopathy, splenomegaly, and peripheral blood involvement. The t(11:14) translocation is usually present involving the cyclin D1 gene (*bcl-1*). Histology would be expected to show lymphoid cells with slightly irregular or cleaved nuclei.

Answer I is incorrect. Non-Hodgkin's lymphomas commonly present with hepatosplenomegaly, widespread palpable adenopathy, and abdominal masses. Mucosal associated lymphoid tissue lymphoma most commonly involves the stomach. Histology would be expected to show dense, monotonous, lymphoid infiltrate in the lamina propria, and pale-staining cells that represent marginal zone B lymphocytes.

Answer J is incorrect. Primary neuroblastoma most commonly presents as a painless abdominal mass, hypertension, respiratory distress, Horner's syndrome, or cord compression. Often, however, neuroblastoma is not diagnosed until after it has metastasized. Low-grade fever, fatigue, and failure to thrive (which is evidenced by his small size) occur with metastatic disease. Urinary catecholamines are elevated in neuroblastoma, but definitive diagnosis requires biopsy from two separate sites, which would be expected to show neuroblasts and schwannian cells, as well as rosettes, or clumps of tumor cells with indistinct borders.

Answer K is incorrect. Pheochromocytoma is a catecholamine-secreting tumor that classically presents with the triad of episodic headache, tachycardia, and sweating. Half of patients have episodic hypertension. Biopsy should be avoided when this diagnosis is suspected because uncontrolled tumor manipulation may result in a surge of catecholamine release.

Answer L is incorrect. Anaplastic large cell lymphoma (ALCL) is divided into two types of disease: primary cutaneous and primary systemic. Primary cutaneous ALCL presents in the skin without evidence of extracutaneous disease at the time of diagnosis. Cutaneous infiltrates involve both upper and deep dermis, with small, reactive lymphocytes at the periphery of the lesions.

Questions 43 and 44

43. **The correct answer is F.** The boy should be suspected to have type 1 diabetes mellitus. The first presentation often includes urinary symptoms of polyuria and polydipsia because of osmotically active glucose that spills into the urine. Children will often complain of wetting the bed at night. Human leukocyte antigen-DR3 is associated with type 1 diabetes. The fasting blood glucose would confirm the diagnosis.

44. **The correct answer is K.** This description is classic for uncomplicated lower urinary tract infection. She is not exhibiting fevers, chills, or flank pain that would suggest an upper tract infection, namely pyelonephritis. The urinalysis will screen for the diagnosis, and the culture will confirm and give bacterial sensitivities.

Answer A is incorrect. If bladder cancer is suspected, a bladder biopsy may be part of the diagnostic evaluation; however, more appropriate initial testing includes ultrasound, CT scan, and cystoscopy for direct visualization of the mass. Gross hematuria is a presenting symptom in 80–90% of patients with bladder cancer.

Answer B is incorrect. Complete blood cell (CBC) count may reveal an increased WBC count in the case of urinary tract infection but is nonspecific for the source of infection. CBC

is not essential in a new presentation of diabetes and would not be of value in the diagnostic workup.

Answer C is incorrect. CT scan of the pelvis should be done in the case of suspected intrapelvic pathology. While both cases present with urinary complaints, both are explained by diseases better evaluated by tests other than CT. In addition, radiation should be avoided in pediatric patients when possible.

Answer D is incorrect. Cystoscopy is rarely indicated for evaluation of urinary tract infection (UTI) in women, even in patients with chronic recurrent UTIs. Women with a history of childhood UTI, stones, or painless hematuria should be evaluated with cystoscopy. Most men diagnosed with UTI without an obvious source should undergo urologic evaluation.

Answer E is incorrect. Digital rectal examination, along with prostate-specific antigen (PSA), is used as a screening tool for prostate cancer. Screening is recommended for men > 50 years old.

Answer G is incorrect. β-Human chorionic gonadotropin and α-fetoprotein are appropriate in the evaluation and diagnosis of malignant germ cell tumors. In women, germ cell tumors most often present with abdominal or pelvic pain. The girl in this case does not have such symptoms, making malignant germ cell tumor an unlikely diagnosis.

Answer H is incorrect. Pap smear is used to screen for cervical cancer and precancerous lesions. Screening should be done annually in all sexually active women or those > 21 years old.

Answer I is incorrect. PSA, along with digital rectal examination, is used as a screening tool for prostate cancer. The boy in this case is too young to be considered for a diagnosis of prostate cancer, which usually occurs in men > 50 years old.

Answer J is incorrect. Salt-load response, also known as an aldosterone suppression test, is used to diagnose primary hyperaldosteronism. Patients usually present with hypertension and may have muscle weakness secondary to hypokalemia. When a sodium load is administered, urine aldosterone is measured, and if it fails to be suppressed, primary hyperaldosteronism can be diagnosed.

Answer L is incorrect. The effect of water deprivation on urine osmolality is used to distinguish primary polydipsia from diabetes insipidus in the case of polyuria. Both of these patients have a more likely reason for increased urination and should be worked up accordingly.

Answer M is incorrect. Bacterial vaginosis often presents with increased vaginal discharge and pruritus. It is diagnosed by microscopic evaluation of a wet mount preparation of vaginal specimen, which reveals clue cells.

Questions 45 and 46

45. **The correct answer is D.** Breast-feeding jaundice is the most common cause of nonphysiologic jaundice. It occurs in neonates who are being exclusively breast-fed, usually because of poor intake. Decreased milk intake leads to increased enterohepatic circulation and abnormally high reabsorption of bilirubin normally excreted in the feces. Jaundice is usually apparent on day 3 of life.

46. **The correct answer is K.** She has jaundice secondary to Rh incompatibility. The mother was exposed to Rh antigen either via her prior pregnancy or blood transfusions, and she developed antibodies to Rh factor. Maternal Rh antibody crosses the placenta and destroys fetal RBCs. The hemolysis results in unconjugated hyperbilirubinemia, anemia, and increased hematopoiesis. The diagnosis is supported by a positive Coombs' test. Giving Rh-negative women $Rh_O(D)$ immune globulin when they are exposed to Rh-positive blood can prevent Rh isoimmune hemolytic disease of the newborn.

Answer A is incorrect. ABO incompatibility can cause a generally milder neonatal jaundice that is triggered almost exclusively in type A or B neonates born to type O mothers.

Answer B is incorrect. α_1-Antitrypsin deficiency can cause neonatal hepatitis, in addition to the pulmonary manifestations.

Answer C is incorrect. Biliary atresia is a congenital defect that causes an obstructive jaundice, resulting in acholic stools.

Answer E is incorrect. Cephalhematomas are subperiosteal collections of blood that are present in 1–2% of newborns. They can cause jaundice as they decompose.

Answer F is incorrect. Crigler-Najjar syndrome results in a severe unconjugated bilirubinemia that is accompanied by normal stool color.

Answer G is incorrect. Gilbert's syndrome is generally diagnosed in adolescents that present with mild unconjugated jaundice.

Answer H is incorrect. Hereditary spherocytosis can cause an unconjugated jaundice secondary to hemolysis.

Answer I is incorrect. Neonatal hepatitis is a cause of jaundice that is generally maternally transmitted and thus the mother should be seropositive and may have passed IgG antibodies to the neonate.

Answer J is incorrect. Physiologic jaundice generally occurs in premature infants, is mild, and can be overcome with phototherapy

Answer L is incorrect. Sepsis can cause neonatal jaundice secondary to hemolysis from marked inflammation.

Answer M is incorrect. Toxoplasmosis can cause a severe congenital infection but is not generally associated with jaundice.

Test Block 2

1. An emergency cesarean section due to persistent late decelerations is performed on an afebrile, group B streptococcus–negative, 17-year-old girl at 42 weeks' gestation. A 4600-g (10.1-lb) girl is delivered. The amniotic fluid is meconium stained. The neonate's blood pressure is 50/30 mm Hg and heart rate is 100/min, and the infant has not yet taken a breath. She is cyanotic and limp on examination. What is the most appropriate next step in management?

(A) Give ampicillin and gentamicin
(B) Obtain x-ray of the chest
(C) Provide artificial ventilation with bag-mask
(D) Provide supplemental oxygen
(E) Suction trachea

2. Pain disorder is a psychological syndrome that is considered part of the family of somatoform disorders. Which of the following true of pain disorder?

(A) It occurs more often in males than in females
(B) It often gives the patient some form of secondary gain
(C) Patient are often very in touch with their emotions
(D) Patients often have good insight into their disorder
(E) The diagnosis requires pain or dysfunction at four distinct sites, at least two of which are gastrointestinal, one is neurologic, and one is sexual

3. A 68-year-old man with no previous medical problems presents to clinic with shortness of breath and swelling of his ankles. Symptoms have progressed over the past few months. On physical examination, the patient has a regular heart rate and rhythm, an S4 is heard on cardiac auscultation, and inspiratory rales are heard throughout the lower half of the lung fields. Also, 2+ pitting edema is evident over the tibial surfaces. Echocardiography reveals an ejection fraction of 60%. Which of the following is most likely to improve this patient's condition?

(A) Amiodarone
(B) Atorvastatin
(C) Digoxin
(D) Metoprolol
(E) Nitroglycerin

4. A 37-year-old G5P5 diabetic woman is immediately postpartum from delivery of a 4.5-kg (10-lb) baby boy at 37 weeks' gestation. Time elapsed from the onset of labor to delivery of the placenta was 4.5 hours. Delivery was complicated by a second-degree perineal tear. Postpartum vital signs are within normal limits when the patient begins to hemorrhage vaginally. Estimated blood loss is 200 mL so far. Bimanual examination reveals a soft, enlarged, "boggy" uterus. What is the most appropriate first step in treatment?

(A) Bimanual uterine massage
(B) Hysterectomy
(C) Internal uterine massage
(D) Intravenous methylergonovine
(E) Intravenous oxytocin infusion
(F) Thorough speculum examination to evaluate for vaginal wall lacerations

5. A 27-year-old man requested an HIV test at his local hospital. The patient was a poor historian but complains of a mild nonproductive cough. He is breathing rapidly. HIV test is positive and his CD4+ count is 186/mm^3. An x-ray is ordered and is shown in the image. Which of the following is most appropriate diagnostic step?

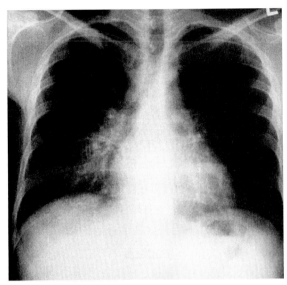

Reproduced, with permission, from Hall JB, Schmidt GA, Wood LDH. *Principles of Critical Care*, 3rd ed. New York: McGraw-Hill, 2005: Figure 48-1.

(A) Bronchoalveolar lavage and culture
(B) Bronchoalveolar lavage and serology
(C) Bronchoalveolar lavage fluid stained with methamine silver/Giemsa staining
(D) Intraoperative biopsy
(E) Intravenous blood draw and serology

6. A 46-year-old Japanese-American woman with a history of amyloidosis for which she has been repeatedly hospitalized presents to her primary care physicians with complaints of increasing shortness of breath, fatigue, chest pain, abdominal distention, and a fainting spell. Her ECG shows low-voltage QRS complexes. Her vital signs are stable, and her laboratory values are normal. What is the most appropriate next step in patient care?

(A) Cardiac enzymes
(B) CT scan of the abdomen
(C) Echocardiogram
(D) Recheck potassium
(E) X-ray of the chest

7. A 68-year-old man recently diagnosed with mild chronic obstructive pulmonary disease presents to the emergency department (ED) in the throes of a new exacerbation of symptoms. Which of the following is a reason to intubate?

(A) Forced expiratory volume in 1 second < 40% predicted
(B) Partial arterial carbon dioxide pressure > 50 mm Hg
(C) Partial arterial oxygen pressure > 50 mm Hg
(D) Respiratory rate of 25/min
(E) The patient is anxious and complains of feeling like they are "gasping for air"

8. At 39 weeks' gestation, a 3600-g (7.9-lb) boy is born to a 22-year-old primigravida by spontaneous vaginal delivery. The delivery was uncomplicated, but the pregnancy was complicated by maternal syphilis. The neonate is rapid plasma reagin–positive and is diagnosed with congenital syphilis. He becomes increasingly jaundiced; his total bilirubin at 12 hours of age is 14 mg/dL. Which of the following are most likely to be his laboratory results?

(A) Coombs' negative, elevated direct bilirubin, normal reticulocyte count
(B) Coombs' negative, normal direct bilirubin, elevated reticulocyte count
(C) Coombs' negative, normal direct bilirubin, increased number of RBCs
(D) Coombs' negative, normal direct bilirubin, normal reticulocyte count
(E) Coombs' positive, normal direct bilirubin, elevated reticulocyte count

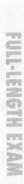

FULL-LENGTH EXAM

Test Block 2

9. An 83-year-old woman presents to the clinic with complaint of a dull lower back pain that is not affected by positional changes. It has been gradually worsening over the past several months. Her blood pressure is 161/84 mm Hg and pulse is 75/min. Cardiac examination is notable for S4. Abdominal examination reveals a pulsatile mass approximately 5.5 cm in diameter and palpable in the epigastric area. Peripheral pulses are normal. An ultrasound is shown. Which of the following is the most likely diagnosis?

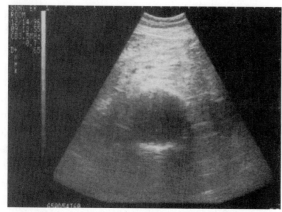

Reproduced, with permission, from Tintinalli JE, Kelen GD, Stapczynski S, Ma OJ, Cline DM. *Tintinalli's Emergency Medicine: A Comprehensive Study Guide*, 6th ed. New York: McGraw-Hill, 2004: Figure 58-2.

(A) Abdominal aortic aneurysm
(B) Colonic obstruction
(C) Intestinal arteriovenous malformation
(D) Pancreatitis with pseudocyst
(E) Peptic ulcer disease

10. A 55-year-old man with a history of diabetes, hypertension, and atrial fibrillation presents with a newly diagnosed aphasia. His word repetition ability and language comprehension are both impaired, but his fluency is preserved. Where is the lesion responsible for this kind of aphasia located?

(A) Infarct in the territory of the left posterior cerebral artery
(B) Stroke in the arcuate fasciculus
(C) Stroke in the lenticulostriate branches of the middle cerebral artery
(D) Stroke involving the inferior division of the middle cerebral artery
(E) Stroke involving the superior division of the middle cerebral artery

11. A 67-year-old man comes into the ED with a 20-minute episode of substernal chest pain. The man appears to be in moderate discomfort and indicates that the pain is in the middle of his chest. Upon questioning, the man reports that this pain is not new to him, as he has been suffering this type of pain for the past 3 years and it usually occurs after meals or at nighttime. He also complains of an acid taste in his mouth that accompanies this pain. Which of the following treatment options is appropriate for this patient?

(A) Aspirin
(B) β-Blocker
(C) Nissen fundoplication
(D) Nitroglycerin
(E) Omeprazole

12. A 26-year-old woman and her husband, her only sexual partner, present to her obstetrician seeking help after their third miscarriage in 2 years. She is healthy, and does not smoke, drink alcohol, or use recreational drugs. She is not currently on any medications and denies any history of sexually transmitted diseases. She is the oldest of seven children, and there is no record of infertility or miscarriage in her family. She has been pregnant three times, losing the pregnancies after 5, 6, or 7 weeks. What would be the most appropriate first step in determining the cause of her miscarriages?

(A) A chromosome analysis
(B) A hysterosalpingogram
(C) A 3-month trial of an oral contraceptive pill
(D) An exploratory laparotomy
(E) Vaginal and cervical cultures

13. A 24-year-old woman comes to a plastic surgeon requesting rhinoplasty. She has had five such surgeries in the past 3 years but still believes that her nose looks "hideous." She produces photographs of herself that predate her first surgery and shows them to the surgeon as proof that her nose was "monstrous." The patient's nose appears totally normal to the surgeon, both in the preoperative images and at presentation, and he states this. The patient becomes agitated and demands to have an operation, stating that she "cannot live with a de-

formed face." Which of the following is the next appropriate step in managing this patient?

(A) Perform the surgery as requested
(B) Prescribe a selective serotonin reuptake inhibitor
(C) Prescribe valium for agitation
(D) Reassure the patient that her nose is normal and gently refuse to perform the operation
(E) Refer the patient for psychotherapy

14. A 67-year-old woman is seen in the doctor's office for severe left leg pain, worse with standing and walking, starting insidiously 3 weeks ago. There has been no trauma to the area. The patient also notes that over the past 6 months, the tips of her fingers have become increasingly thick, she has lost 2.3 kg (5 lb) unintentionally, and she has been suffering from a persistent, nonproductive cough. She has a 60-pack-year smoking history and continues to smoke two packs per day. Her temperature is 36.7°C (98.1°F), blood pressure is 132/81 mm Hg, pulse is 75/min and regular, and respiratory rate is 15/min. Physical examination is significant for clubbed fingers and pain on palpation of the distal left tibia. X-ray film of the chest shows a focal 5-cm mass lesion in the left lower lung that is highly suspicious for bronchogenic carcinoma. A bronchoscopy with biopsy is pending. Based on the patient's presentation, which of the following is the most likely histologic type of lung cancer present in this patient?

(A) Adenocarcinoma
(B) Bronchoalveolar cell carcinoma
(C) Large cell carcinoma
(D) Small cell carcinoma
(E) Squamous cell carcinoma

15. A 46-year-old woman presents to the ED with acute onset of severe right upper quadrant abdominal pain that radiates to the infrascapular region. Her past medical history is significant for obesity, hypertension, obstructive sleep apnea, and gastric bypass surgery 2 years ago, after which she lost 68 kg (150 lb). The patient complains of nausea and vomiting that accompanies the pain. At presentation, her temperature is 38.9°C (101.2°F), blood pressure is 144/88 mm Hg, heart rate is 76/min, and respiratory rate is 14/min. Abdominal examination is significant for right upper quadrant tenderness along with guarding and cessation of inspired breath on deep palpation of the right upper quadrant. Which test should be ordered first to work-up this patient?

(A) Abdominal ultrasound
(B) CT scan of the abdomen
(C) Hepato-iminodiacetic acid scan
(D) MRI of the abdomen
(E) X-ray film of the abdomen

16. A 34-year-old G3P3 woman is postpartum day 14 after a vaginal delivery that was complicated by a 1500-mL hemorrhage secondary to uterine atony. The patient did not respond to oxytocin or methylergonovine and experienced an episode of profound hypotension to 60/30 mm Hg that required 2 L of normal saline and 6 U of packed RBCs. The patient was finally stabilized after emergent uterine artery embolization. Her hospital stay was further complicated by acute renal failure, presumed secondary to her hypotensive event. She is now awaiting discharge. Blood tests performed several weeks after discharge would most likely reveal which of the following?

(A) Decreased prolactin and decreased thyroid-stimulating hormone
(B) Decreased prolactin and normal thyroid-stimulating hormone
(C) Decreased prolactin and elevated thyroid-stimulating hormone
(D) Elevated prolactin and decreased thyroid-stimulating hormone
(E) Elevated prolactin and elevated thyroid-stimulating hormone

17. A 63-year-old African-American woman with osteoarthritis is seen in the ophthalmology clinic for routine examination. Her last ocular examination was 5 years ago. She reports no problems with her vision since her last examination. Her visual acuity is 20/40 in both eyes; intraocular pressure is 29 mm Hg in the right eye and 31 mm Hg in the left eye. Gonioscopic evaluation shows open anterior-chamber angle and no peripheral anterior synechiae. Results of a funduscopic examination are shown in the image. What would be the next most appropriate step in management of the patient?

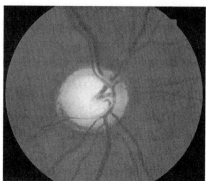

Reproduced, with permission, from Kasper DL, Braunwald E, Fauci AS, Hauser SL, Longo DL, Jameson LJ, Isselbacher KJ, eds. *Harrison's Online.* New York: McGraw-Hill, 2005: Figure 25-15.

(A) Atropine
(B) Observation with follow-up in 6 weeks
(C) Pilocarpine
(D) Timolol
(E) Trabeculectomy

18. A 5-month-old girl is rushed to the hospital by her parents because she is not moving her left side. Her mother reports that there were no problems when she was breast-fed 4 hours earlier. Prior to this she has been healthy. She was born full-term by spontaneous vaginal delivery after an uncomplicated pregnancy. Her Apgar scores were 9 at both 1 and 5 minutes. There is no family history of stroke, deep vein thrombosis, or pulmonary embolism. In the ED her temperature is 36.5°C (97.7°F), her blood pressure is 76/45 mm Hg, her respiratory rate is 26/min, and her heart rate is 96/min. Her physical examination is notable for 1/5 strength in her left arm and leg and 5/5 strength in her right arm and leg. An MRI of the head shows a right parietal infarct. In reviewing her records, it is determined that her newborn screen for inborn errors of metabolism is abnormal. Which of the following most likely led to the patient's cerebrovascular accident?

(A) Fabry's disease
(B) Homocystinuria
(C) Krabbe's disease
(D) Niemann-Pick disease
(E) Phenylketonuria

19. A 42-year-old man presents to his physician with complaints of weight gain circumferentially around his abdomen and a "hump" on his neck. Physical examination shows a rounded face and purple stretch marks on the abdomen. On CT, a solitary pituitary adenoma is noted. Unfortunately, he has contraindications to surgical resection, and alternative means of treatment must be considered. Which of the following treatment strategies is most appropriate for this patient?

(A) Glucocorticoids
(B) Insulin
(C) Ketoconazole
(D) Observation
(E) Pituitary irradiation

20. A 17-year-old G0 girl with a past medical history significant for dysmenorrhea secondary to moderate endometriosis for the past year presents with her mother to the gynecologist for follow-up. She was started on a combination oral contraceptive pill 10 months ago but experienced only mild relief of her symptoms. She returns to the gynecologist's office today to discuss the next line of therapy. What is the most appropriate next step in treating her endometriosis?

(A) Dexamethasone
(B) Electrocautery, endocoagulation, or laser resection
(C) Leuprolide
(D) Progestin only therapy
(E) Unopposed estrogens

21. A 43-year-old man develops fever, headache, and altered mental status. His past medical history is notable only for a motor vehicle acci-

dent 2 years prior, during which he sustained a splenic laceration requiring splenectomy. Which of the organisms are most likely causing this patient's symptoms?

(A) *Cryptococcus neoformans* and *Listeria monocytogenes*
(B) *Staphylococcus aureus* and *Haemophilus influenzae*
(C) *Staphylococcus aureus* and *Neisseria meningitidis*
(D) *Streptococcus pneumoniae* and *Cryptococcus neoformans*
(E) *Streptococcus pneumoniae* and *Neisseria meningitidis*

22. A 3-year-old boy presents to the pediatrician's office with 4 days of productive cough with whitish sputum and shortness of breath. His mother reports that he has had multiple episodes of upper respiratory infections in the past, and recently a few classmates at preschool were sent home because of cough and fever. She reports that her child has had no fever or rhinorrhea, no gastrointestinal symptoms, and no ear pain. On examination the boy is afebrile but tachypneic and mildly tachycardic. There is end-expiratory wheezing bilaterally. What is the most appropriate initial step in diagnosis for this child?

(A) CBC count with differential
(B) Measure peak expiratory flow rate
(C) Methacholine challenge
(D) Sputum smear
(E) X-ray of the chest

23. A 15 day-old full-term boy is brought to the clinic by his parents for shortness of breath, failure to tolerate feeding, and inadequate weight gain. On physical examination, there is no cyanosis evident on mucosal membranes. Pulmonary rales are heard bilaterally with an active precordium and a soft 2/6 holosystolic murmur most prominent at the left lower sternal border. ECG is significant for biventricular hypertrophy. X-ray of the chest shows increased pulmonary vascularity. Which of the following is the most likely etiology?

(A) Aortic stenosis
(B) Patent ductus arteriosus
(C) Tetralogy of Fallot

(D) Transposition of the great arteries
(E) Ventricular septal defect

24. A 52-year-old man develops a pruritic, scaling area on the skin of his chest. On examination an erythematous rash is noted, with plaque-like lesions measuring 5–7 cm. He is treated with a short course of oral and topical prednisone for an assumed allergic dermatitis, which brings some resolution. The patient is then lost to follow-up. He presents 7 years later with diffuse erythroderma of his entire body for 2 weeks. He states that he has been feeling run down for the past 6 months and has lost 18 pounds. On examination, he is cachectic. Complete blood cell count reveals WBC count 6000/mm^3, hemoglobin 9.5 mg/dL, and platelets 105,000/mm^3. A differential includes 21% atypical lymphocytes. A diagnosis of mycosis fungoides is made. Which of the following treatments will most likely be recommended to the patient?

(A) Conventional photon beam radiation therapy
(B) High-dose acyclovir
(C) Immediate intravenous ampicillin
(D) Topical nitrogen mustard
(E) Total skin electron beam radiation therapy

25. A 17-year-old girl was diagnosed with type 1 diabetes mellitus 7 years earlier. She recently started college and forgot to take her insulin and went to a party where she consumed several beers. She presents to the ED with rapid, deep respirations and a solvent-like odor on her breath. What treatment should be administered first?

(A) Bicarbonate repletion
(B) Glucose
(C) Intravenous fluids
(D) Potassium repletion
(E) Urinalysis

26. A 70-year-old woman was walking across her kitchen when she tripped over a throw rug and fell onto an outstretched right hand. She did not hit her head or lose consciousness. She had immediate pain and swelling in her right wrist and was brought to the ED by her daughter. X-rays were taken of the right wrist, which

revealed a dorsally displaced, dorsally angulated fracture of the distal radius with a displaced intra-articular fragment in the radiocarpal joint. There was no break in the skin. The patient is otherwise healthy, and her past medical history is significant only for a T11 compression fracture 2 years ago. What is the most appropriate treatment?

(A) Closed reduction and arm sling
(B) Closed reduction and long arm cast
(C) Ice and compressive bandage
(D) Open reduction and internal fixation
(E) Physical therapy and night splint

27. A 76-year-old man with multiple medical problems, including diabetes and coronary artery disease, is admitted to the hospital for coronary artery bypass grafting. On the second postoperative day, he develops acute shortness of breath and tachycardia, and is rushed to CT scan to rule out pulmonary embolism. That night, his nurse notices that his urine output is low despite the intravenous fluids he is receiving, and morning laboratory values show blood urea nitrogen of 45 and creatinine of 2.3. This pathology would have been resistant to which of the following prophylactic measures?

(A) Acetylcysteine administration before CT scan
(B) Aggressive intravenous saline hydration before CT scan
(C) Better chronic control of diabetes
(D) Prophylactic hemodialysis
(E) Use of MRI with gadolinium, instead of contrast CT

28. A 32-year-old G1P0 woman who is 26 weeks pregnant presents to her obstetrician for a routine prenatal visit. The pregnancy has been uncomplicated, and the patient's weight gain has been appropriate. Her blood pressure has ranged from 105/90 mm Hg to 120/85 mm Hg. Her urine has not shown any proteinuria and has been only trace positive for glucose the last two visits. During this visit, her urinalysis reveals 1+ glucosuria. The patient receives her scheduled 50-g oral glucose tolerance test, which comes back showing serum glucose of 135 mg/dL. Which of the following is the appropriate next step in managing this woman's diabetes?

(A) Dietary restrictions
(B) Exercise regimen
(C) Insulin injections
(D) Oral metformin
(E) Oral sulfonylurea

29. A 65-year-old previously healthy man with a past medical history significant for benign prostatic hyperplasia presents with fever, malaise, and dysuria. On physical examination, he has costovertebral angle tenderness and a temperature of 37.3°C (99.9°F). The remainder of the physical examination is unremarkable. What therapeutic option is indicated in this patient?

(A) 7-day outpatient course of trimethoprim-sulfamethoxazole
(B) 10-day outpatient course of ciprofloxacin
(C) 10-day outpatient course of moxifloxacin
(D) Inpatient treatment with intravenous ceftriaxone

30. At 38 weeks' gestation, a 3600-g (7.9-lb) boy is born by spontaneous vaginal delivery to a 26-year-old woman. There were no complications during pregnancy or delivery. The neonate's Apgar scores are 5 and 8 at 1 and 5 minutes, respectively. His physical examination is notable for tachypnea at 110/min, grunting, decreased breath sounds on the left side, and a sunken abdomen. He is intubated and has a nasogastric tube inserted. An x-ray film of the chest is obtained immediately and is shown in the image. What is the most appropriate treatment?

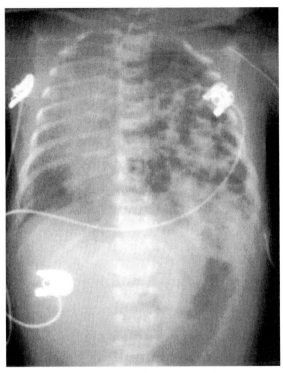

Reprinted, with permission, from Brunicardi FC, Andersen DK, Billiar TR, Dunn DL, Hunter JG, Matthews JB, Pollock RE, Schwartz SI. *Schwartz's Principles of Surgery*, 8th ed. New York: McGraw-Hill, 2005: Figure 38-3.

(A) Betamethasone
(B) Caffeine
(C) Needle decompression
(D) Surfactant
(E) Surgical correction

31. A population of 200 medical students undergoes testing for disease X. Of the 100 students with this disease, only 90 receive positive test results. Meanwhile, 25 students without disease X receive positive test results. Given this information, what is the probability that a student has disease X given that he or she tests positive for the disease?

(A) 75/(10 + 75)
(B) 75/(25 + 75)
(C) 90/(90 + 10)
(D) 90/(90 + 25)
(E) Not enough information is provided

32. A 36-year-old G2P1 woman at "about 4 months" gestation presents to her obstetrician for her first prenatal visit. She has been feeling well, but has not been to see a physician yet because of a death in the family. Her past medical history is significant for chronic hypertension, which is currently well controlled on a calcium channel blocker, and Raynaud's syndrome. Her vital signs are: blood pressure 125/85 mm Hg, heart rate 95/min, and respiratory rate 18/min. Which is the most appropriate next step in managing this patient's hypertension?

(A) Maintain the current dose of her calcium channel blocker
(B) Switch to a β-adrenergic blocker
(C) Switch to an angiotensin-converting enzyme inhibitor
(D) Switch to an angiotensin II receptor blocker
(E) Switch to hydrochlorothiazide

33. A 34-year-old woman presents to her primary care physician complaining of 2 weeks of cough and shortness of breath. A review of systems reveals that she has had two to three episodes of coughing up blood but no fever, chills, or weight loss. Her examination is notable for decreased breath sounds at both lung bases. Laboratory values include blood urea nitrogen and creatinine of 42 mg/dL and 2.3 mg/dL (previous laboratory values were within normal limits), respectively, and a urinalysis showed 2+ proteinuria, microscopic hematuria, and RBC and granular casts. X-ray of the chest shows blunting of the costodiaphragmatic angles bilaterally and a small right lower lung infiltrate. What of the following is the most likely cause of this patient's renal failure?

(A) Antibodies directed against the glomerular basement membrane
(B) Hepatitis C–associated cryoglobulinemia
(C) IgA deposition in the glomerular mesangium
(D) Postinfectious reaction
(E) Small-vessel inflammation

FULL-LENGTH EXAM

Test Block 2

34. An 18-year-old G2P2 woman presents to the ED complaining of several hours of lower abdominal cramping and a clear vaginal discharge. Her vital signs upon presentation are temperature 37.3°C (99.1°F), blood pressure 123/76 mm Hg, pulse 89/min, and respiratory rate 13/min. The patient reports that over the past several weeks she has had multiple episodes of nausea and vomiting, increasing abdominal girth, and cannot remember her last menstrual period. She reports that she has been having unprotected sex for the past several months with her boyfriend, as well as smoking, drinking alcohol, and using crack cocaine several times per week. A urine β-human chorionic gonadotropin pregnancy test is positive. Ultrasound examination shows a live fetus of approximately 24–26 weeks' gestation, and a nitrazine test of vaginal fluid is positive. Which of the following factors most likely contributed to this patient's preterm labor?

(A) Ibuprofen use
(B) Maternal obesity
(C) Multiparity
(D) Smoking and substance abuse
(E) Vaginal candidiasis

35. An 80-year-old woman presents to her primary care physician with signs of thyrotoxicosis. Blood tests reveal a low thyroid-stimulating hormone level, markedly increased triiodothyronine, and only moderately increased thyroxine. A thyroid scan shows a solitary, small "hot" nodule with complete suppression of the unaffected lobe. What is the initial treatment of choice in this patient?

(A) β-Blocker
(B) Carbimazole
(C) Propylthiouracil
(D) Radioactive iodine
(E) Thyroidectomy

36. Fine-needle aspiration biopsy has high sensitivity and moderate specificity to diagnose malignancy in a thyroid nodule. Which of the following statements is true about the use of fine-needle aspiration biopsy in this case?

(A) A positive result is a strong confirmation of disease
(B) It is a strong indicator of those who may develop the disease later on, and a moderate indicator of those who currently have the disease
(C) There is a moderately high rate of false negatives
(D) The test has a strong ability to rule out disease in healthy individuals
(E) This is a good test to use if malignancy is considered very likely in a given patient

37. A 33-year-old man comes to clinic with a rapidly expanding target-shaped rash on his shoulder in the same spot where he removed a tick 3 days ago. The physician suspects Lyme disease. Which of the following is the next step in diagnosis?

(A) Biopsy rash and culture for *Borrelia burgdorferi*
(B) Collect plasma and culture for *Borrelia burgdorferi*
(C) Collect plasma and test for Lyme antigen
(D) Collect plasma for enzyme-linked immunosorbent assay and Western blot analysis
(E) Collect urine and test for Lyme antigen

38. An 80-year-old man presents to the ED complaining of severe lower abdominal pain for 12 hours. History reveals that he has not urinated in at least 18 hours and has experienced dull back pain for about 1 week. He has not had regular medical care over the past 20 years. He is afebrile with blood pressure of 150/95 mm Hg, pulse of 88/min, and respiratory rate of 16/min. Physical examination reveals a large palpable suprapubic mass that is tender. Digital rectal examination shows an asymmetrically enlarged, firm, nodular prostate. Laboratory tests show mild anemia as well as blood urea nitrogen of 46 mg/dL and creatinine of 2.8 mg/dL. Urinalysis after suprapubic catheterization is unremarkable. Which of the following is the most likely cause of his acute renal failure?

(A) Glomerular Ig deposition
(B) Hypercalcemia
(C) Neurogenic bladder
(D) Obstructive nephropathy
(E) Renal tubular inflammation
(F) Staghorn calculus

39. A 2-year-old girl is brought to the pediatrician by her mother, who is concerned because her daughter has had difficulty walking. She had a normal birth history as well as normal development until the age of 1 year. Her mother states that her other three children all could walk by 15 months of age, and is concerned that this child continues to crawl. On physical examination, the girl appears to have an enlarged forehead as well as lateral bowing of the forearms and legs. Relevant laboratory findings include a Ca^{2+} level of 7.4 mg/dL, phosphate of 1.9 mg/dL, and parathyroid hormone of 160 pg/mL. Additionally, while the 25(OH) vitamin D level is normal, the $1,25(OH)_2$ vitamin D level is low. This patient's condition is due to an abnormality in which organ?

(A) Gut
(B) Kidney
(C) Liver
(D) Parathyroid
(E) Skin

40. A 52-year-old man with a history of major depressive episodes was admitted to an inpatient psychiatric hospital because of a suicide attempt using a kitchen knife. In the patient's words, he was trying to "release the centipedes from his blood" because they were "slowing down his brain." During the admission interview, his wife reported that he had not gone to work in more than 2 weeks, no longer showed interest in his hobbies, and refused to eat even his favorite foods. She had awakened many times over the past month to see him lying in bed and staring at the ceiling. During the mental status examination, the patient moved very slowly and deliberately, scarcely making eye contact. However, during his 3-week admission, the centipedes gradually "disappeared" from his blood, he no longer believed his mind was being slowed, and his mood improved. By the time of his discharge, his wife was thrilled to see that he had returned to his baseline. What is the most likely diagnosis?

(A) Brief psychotic episode
(B) Depression with psychotic features
(C) Schizoaffective disorder
(D) Schizophrenia
(E) Specific phobia

41. A 75-year-old man presents to the ED complaining of a rash. He states that he noticed its onset 3 days prior and that it has been worsening since then. His review of systems is notable only for feeling tired lately. He has no known allergies. Physical examination reveals erythematous lesions covering his trunk and extremities that are most severe on his legs and buttocks. He denies pruritus. The lesions do not blanch under pressure. Massive splenomegaly is observed. Complete blood count reveals WBC count 80,000/mm³, hemoglobin 8.8 g/dL, and platelets 8000/mm³. The patient's infectious workup is negative, but his bone marrow aspirate shows cells resembling mature lymphocytes packing the bone marrow. The patient is admitted to the hospital for further evaluation and supportive care. Which of the following potential therapies is the most appropriate for rapid and long-lasting correction of this patient's thrombocytopenia?

(A) High-dose corticosteroids
(B) Platelet transfusion
(C) Splenectomy
(D) Therapy with 5-fluorouracil
(E) Therapy with granulocyte colony-stimulating factor

42. The physician is consenting for a patient to be enrolled in a randomized, double-blind, placebo-controlled study. She asks about the advantage of the study being randomized. What is the form of bias reduced by randomization?

(A) Enrollment bias
(B) Lead time bias
(C) Measurement bias
(D) Observer bias
(E) Recall bias

43. A 17-year-old boy is brought to the ED by paramedics. He was found unconscious after a motor vehicle accident. Upon presentation the patient is noted to have multiple mandibular and maxillary fractures as well as an open right-sided tibial fibular fracture. The patient remains unconscious with an oxygen saturation of 78% on 2 L oxygen via face mask with a pulse of 146/min and a blood pressure of 60/20 mm Hg. What is the first step in management for this patient?

(A) Administer fluids
(B) Continue with face mask ventilation and proceed with the rest of the primary trauma survey
(C) Proceed with a cricothyroidotomy
(D) Proceed with nasopharyngeal intubation
(E) Proceed with oropharyngeal intubation

EXTENDED MATCHING

Questions 44–46

For each patient with nausea and vomiting, select the most likely diagnosis.

(A) Bulimia nervosa
(B) Digoxin toxicity
(C) Gastric outlet obstruction
(D) Gastroenteritis
(E) Gastroparesis
(F) Hepatitis
(G) Inflammatory bowel disease
(H) Intracranial hemorrhage
(I) Labyrinthitis
(J) Meningitis
(K) Migraine
(L) Myocardial infarction
(M) Pancreatic carcinoma
(N) Pancreatitis
(O) Sigmoid volvulus
(P) Small bowel obstruction

44. A 55-year-old African-American man presents with nausea and vomiting. He reports that this is the third such episode in the past week, and is accompanied by decreased appetite. He also notes that the walls and lights seem to have a yellowish-green tint. His wife complains that he has "not been acting himself," and she says he was last in the hospital for an irregular heartbeat.

45. A 85-year-old woman is brought to the ED by her daughter with vomiting, abdominal pain, distention, and constipation. Abdominal examination reveals a tympanic abdomen. X-ray of the abdomen shows an inverted U–shaped loop lacking haustration, and overlapping the liver, the dilated descending colon, and the left side of the pelvis. The ratio of air to fluid is greater than 2:1.

46. A 64-year-old woman presents with nausea and vomiting. She reports that although the vomiting can happen at any time, it usually occurs a few hours following meals. More recently she has begun lose her appetite, and notes a feeling of fullness after only a few bites of food. Her husband remarks that she has been belching a lot, and seems to have lost weight in the preceding months. Her past medical history is significant for gastroesophageal reflux disease and long-standing type 2 diabetes.

1. **The correct answer is E.** This neonate is at high risk for meconium aspiration syndrome because there is thick meconium in the amniotic fluid. To minimize this risk, the oropharynx should be suctioned as soon as the head is delivered and then again after delivery. The trachea should be suctioned through an endotracheal tube prior to respiration being initiated. This practice minimizes meconium aspiration into the smaller airways. Postterm infants are at increased risk for passing meconium in utero, likely secondary to placental insufficiency.

Answer A is incorrect. Ampicillin and gentamicin would be good treatments for group B streptococcus (GBS) but not meconium aspiration pneumonia. The history is negative for major risk factors for bacterial pneumonia because her mother is afebrile and GBS negative.

Answer B is incorrect. The infant should be stabilized before diagnostic studies are performed. Clinically, a diagnosis can be made without an x-ray of the chest. However, if one were obtained it would show patchy infiltrates, coarse streaking, and overexpansion with flattening of the diaphragm.

Answer C is incorrect. Artificial ventilation is important in patients in respiratory distress. However, in cases of meconium aspiration, the trachea should be suctioned first.

Answer D is incorrect. Supplemental oxygen is helpful when infants have respiratory depression. However, the trachea needs to be suctioned first in patients with meconium aspiration.

2. **The correct answer is B.** Patients with pain disorder often realize a secondary gain from their symptoms. This gain may take many forms, such as time off from work or sympathy from family members and friends.

Answer A is incorrect. Pain disorder is more common in females than in males.

Answer C is incorrect. Patients with pain disorder are often emotionally unsophisticated, and this is thought to be the reason they express their emotions and needs through physical means.

Answer D is incorrect. Patients with pain disorder often lack insight. They are not inventing their symptoms, and they are unaware that they are causing the pain themselves. If they were aware that this was the case, the diagnosis would be factitious disorder.

Answer E is incorrect. Pain disorder is characterized by pain at one or more sites that results in significant impairment of function and cannot be better ascribed to another source. The specific list of symptoms given here (pain or dysfunction at four distinct sites, at least two of which are gastrointestinal, one is neurologic, and one is sexual) are criteria for the diagnosis of somatization disorder, not pain disorder.

3. **The correct answer is D.** Systemic hypertension and left ventricular hypertrophy is often one of the main etiologies of diastolic dysfunction and therapy centers around aggressive treatment including β-blockers. Lowering heart rate also allows more ventricular filling time. Tachycardia should be avoided in the setting of diastolic failure.

Answer A is incorrect. In the absence of an appropriate arrhythmia, amiodarone would be unlikely to improve this patient's condition.

Answer B is incorrect. Atorvastatin is a very effective statin that can reduce cholesterol levels. There is no indication that cardiac ischemia was the cause of this patient's diastolic dysfunction.

Answer C is incorrect. Recognize that this patient has diastolic dysfunction by the normal ejection fraction in the setting of clear heart failure. In theory, digoxin is of little value in the setting of diastolic dysfunction. It may be useful in the setting of atrial fibrillation, but not in this patient's management.

Answer E is incorrect. Nitroglycerin is a potent venodilator and arterial dilator used to relieve symptoms of myocardial ischemia and reduce preload. In the setting of diastolic dysfunction, the heart relies on significant preload to maintain cardiac output. Nitroglycerin should be used judiciously to avoid potential hypotension.

4. **The correct answer is A.** In a normal postpartum uterus, continued contractions help compress the vessels and stop bleeding. This patient is experiencing postpartum hemorrhage secondary to uterine atony. Risk factors include uterine overdistention secondary to diabetes and macrosomia, and myometrial exhaustion secondary to a prolonged labor (especially third stage). The most appropriate first step in treating uterine atony is bimanual uterine massage. This technique is usually successful in controlling bleeding without the need for medication infusions.

Answer B is incorrect. Hysterectomy is appropriate in the management of postpartum hemorrhage only as a last resort when all other interventions have failed. It should never be considered an initial treatment option.

Answer C is incorrect. Uterine massage should be performed bimanually, with one hand placed over the uterus externally and one hand placed per vagina.

Answer D is incorrect. Like oxytocin, methylergonovine can be used to help control bleeding. However, it cannot be given to hypertensive patients and should only be used as a second- or third-line agent. Additionally, methylergonovine is always given intramuscularly, not intravenously.

Answer E is incorrect. Oxytocin infusion is generally used to help control bleeding secondary to uterine atony. It should, however, be administered after bimanual uterine massage has begun.

Answer F is incorrect. A thorough speculum examination, often under anesthesia, to evaluate for vaginal or cervical lacerations is an appropriate second step in management of postpartum hemorrhage. Bimanual examination in this patient strongly suggests uterine atony as the source for her blood loss and thus evaluating for and repairing vaginal or cervical lacerations is an inappropriate first step in treatment.

5. **The correct answer is C.** This patient has *Pneumocystis jiroveci* (formerly *carinii*) pneumonia. It can present with dyspnea on exertion, fever, nonproductive cough, weight loss, fatigue, and impaired oxygenation. Risk factors include impaired cellular immunity and AIDS (CD4+ count less than $200/mm^3$) as in this case. X-ray of the chest can show diffuse bilateral interstitial infiltrates with a ground glass appearance, but does not always present in that manner. Diagnosis is made based on cytology from induced sputum or silver staining of a bronchoscopy specimen.

Answer A is incorrect. While culture is important in the diagnosis of many infectious diseases, culture is not available to diagnose *Pneumocystis jiroveci* pneumonia.

Answer B is incorrect. Serology on bronchoscopy specimen is not clinically useful for *Pneumocystis jiroveci* pneumonia, but is important in the diagnosis of other opportunistic infections seen in AIDS patients, such as histoplasmosis.

Answer D is incorrect. Open lung biopsies are used when abnormalities are found on CT or x-ray of the chest and other diagnostic tests are inconclusive. It can lead to the diagnosis of cancer, benign tumors, sarcoidosis, Wegener's granulomatosis, rheumatoid lung disease, or certain infections such as aspergillosis, tuberculosis, viral pneumonia, and coccidioidomycosis.

Answer E is incorrect. Serum serology is not clinically useful for *Pneumocystis jiroveci* pneumonia, but urine and serum polysaccharide antigen testing is important in other opportunistic infections seen in AIDS patients, such as histoplasmosis.

6. **The correct answer is C.** This woman has restrictive cardiomyopathy. This condition is often brought on by infiltrative diseases, such as amyloidosis, sarcoidosis, and carcinoid syndrome, and may lead to extensive cardiac damage. Due to increased myocardial stiffness, ventricular filing is impaired, leading to the manifestations of right heart failure. To identify this condition, it is helpful to obtain an echocardiogram to distinguish it from other possible causes (valvular and other cardiomy-

opathies). A cardiac catheterization could also be done.

Answer A is incorrect. This test would be ideal if myocardial infarction was a concern. In this case, the patient's history does not fit a classic description, and she has little reason to present in an atypical fashion. If the echocardiogram did not yield any results, enzymes might help but are not necessary.

Answer B is incorrect. The abdominal distention this patient is experiencing is secondary to her right-sided heart failure, not any specific abdominal process. Therefore, this examination is unwarranted in this case.

Answer D is incorrect. Rechecking the potassium is necessary if the signs and symptoms point to potassium as being the etiology. It is most often done with laboratory error. Her ECG results do not indicate peak T waves, and the patient does not exhibit other signs or symptoms, so this test would not be pertinent at this time.

Answer E is incorrect. X-ray of the chest would not yield definitive results and therefore would not be the next best step, although it would help rule out other conditions.

7. **The correct answer is B.** Partial arterial carbon dioxide pressure > 50 mm Hg indicates severe hypercarbia in the setting of respiratory distress and is a reason to intubate.

Answer A is incorrect. Spirometry revealing a ratio of forced expiratory volume in 1 second to forced vital capacity ratio (FEV_1:FVC) < 0.7 accompanied by an FEV_1 < 40% predicted is indicative of severe chronic obstructive pulmonary disease that is GOLD (Global Initiative for Chronic Obstructive Lung Disease) stage III. An FEV_1 < 40% of predicted is not, however, used to evaluate whether a patient needs to be intubated or not.

Answer C is incorrect. Partial arterial oxygen pressure (PaO_2) < 50 mm Hg indicates severe hypoxemia in the setting of respiratory distress, and is a reason to intubate. PaO_2 > 50 mm Hg, however, is not a reason to intubate.

Answer D is incorrect. While a respiratory rate of 25/min qualifies as tachypnea, a rapid respiratory rate by itself is not a good reason to intubate. Fatigue caused by tachypnea is a valid reason to intubate.

Answer E is incorrect. Patients presenting with acute lysergic acid diethylamide intoxication will display marked anxiety or depression, delusions, visual hallucinations, flashbacks, and pupillary dilation.

8. **The correct answer is A.** Many intrauterine infections (e.g., toxoplasmosis, rubella, cytomegalovirus, herpes simplex virus, syphilis) cause a conjugated hyperbilirubinemia as a result of neonatal hepatitis. The direct Coombs' test measures the presence of antibodies attached to RBCs, while the indirect Coombs' test measures the presence of antibodies to RBCs in the blood. The test is used to evaluate for maternal antibodies against fetal hemoglobin. It involves addition of rabbit antihuman IgG to the patient's blood, which will result in aggregation of the patient's cells if the cells are coated in antibodies. Coombs' testing in this infant would only be positive if the mother had antibodies against fetal hemoglobin. The reticulocyte count is normal because there is no hemolysis.

Answer B is incorrect. Abnormal RBC morphology (e.g., hereditary spherocytosis, elliptocytosis, α-thalassemia) results in an unconjugated hyperbilirubinemia from increased destruction of RBCs. To compensate for the hemolysis, there is increased hematopoiesis reflected by an elevated reticulocyte count.

Answer C is incorrect. These laboratory values are consistent with polycythemia. An unconjugated hyperbilirubinemia occurs in polycythemia because the excess volume of RBCs results in increased RBC breakdown.

Answer D is incorrect. These laboratory values are consistent with jaundice resulting from errors in bilirubin metabolism or maternal diabetes.

Answer E is incorrect. A positive Coombs' test indicates that the mother has antibodies against fetal hemoglobin. Rh and AB incompatibility are the most common. Rh incompatibility results from prior exposure with antibody formation, which would not be present in a first pregnancy.

9. **The correct answer is A.** Abdominal aortic aneurysms (AAAs) are typically asymptomatic until rupture but can occasionally cause a dull lower back or flank pain. The aneurysms are predominantly caused by atherosclerosis, and more than 90% occur below the renal arteries. Real-time ultrasonography is the gold standard for screening for AAA because sensitivity with this imaging method approaches 100%. Routine sonographic evaluation involves measuring the longitudinal, anteroposterior, and transverse dimensions of the aorta. The normal diameter of the aorta is approximately 2 cm, and surgery is generally indicated above 4.5 cm. The finding of a pulsatile epigastric mass is highly suggestive of AAA.

Answer B is incorrect. Colonic obstruction does not fit with the gradual nature of the complaint. Colonic obstruction would present with abdominal distention and pain in a more acute fashion.

Answer C is incorrect. An intestinal arteriovenous malformation would rarely be large enough to cause somatic symptoms without also causing hemodynamic complications.

Answer D is incorrect. Although the presenting complaint could be interpreted as an episode of chronic pancreatitis, which can also present with a pseudocyst, the mass would not be pulsatile. Furthermore, one would expect pancreatitis to occur in alcoholics or patients with gallstones, neither of which is indicated in this patient.

Answer E is incorrect. Clinically significant peptic ulcer disease (PUD) would be unlikely in a patient with the finding of a pulsatile epigastric mass. Also, the pain of PUD does not characteristically localize to the back.

10. **The correct answer is D.** This patient presents with Wernicke's aphasia, featuring problems with language comprehension and impairment of both language input and output. Usually, the speech is fluent but does not make sense. Sometimes Wernicke's aphasia is accompanied by a contralateral superior homonymous quadrantanopia. The lesion is located in Wernicke's area, and is most likely caused by a stroke in the inferior division of the middle cerebral artery.

Answer A is incorrect. An infarct in the territory of the left posterior cerebral artery would render a transcortical sensory aphasia.

Answer B is incorrect. A stroke in the arcuate fasciculus would likely result in conduction aphasia, which is characterized by problems with repeating what is said, but preserved fluency and comprehension.

Answer C is incorrect. A stroke in the lenticulostriate branches of the middle cerebral artery would affect the subcortical regions of the brain, such as the internal capsule, pons, and basal ganglia, and thus would more likely present with motor and sensory symptoms instead of with aphasia, which is a manifestation of cortical damage.

Answer E is incorrect. Broca's aphasia is characterized by preserved comprehension, but problems with language production. The cause is most likely a lesion in Broca's area, usually caused by a large stroke in the territory of the superior division of the middle cerebral artery, and can present with associated right-sided hemiparesis.

11. **The correct answer is E.** The history is highly suggestive of gastroesophageal reflux disease (GERD), which presents with substernal chest pain worse after meals or when recumbent. Patients commonly also complain of an acid taste in the mouth from the reflux. Mild to moderate GERD is treated initially with lifestyle modifications including weight loss, and antacids. Pharmacologic treatment follows in patients with severe or refractory disease, with histamine-receptor antagonists (ranitidine or cimetidine) or proton pump inhibitors (omeprazole or lansoprazole). This patient has been experiencing symptoms for several years and likely has moderate to severe disease.

Answer A is incorrect. Aspirin is important in the treatment of myocardial infarction and has proven to decrease mortality in this setting. Aspirin is also indicated in the chronic treatment of stable and unstable angina, as it prevents platelet aggregation in atherosclerotic plaques.

Answer B is incorrect. A β-blocker is important in the treatment of myocardial infarction and has proven to decrease mortality in this setting. Myocardial infarction presents with crushing substernal pain, diaphoresis, nausea/vomiting, dyspnea, and bradycardia or tachycardia. There is no evidence that this patient is presenting with an acute cardiac event. β-Blockade is also indicated in the chronic treatment of stable and unstable angina, as it decreases myocardial oxygen demand.

Answer C is incorrect. This is the surgical treatment of refractory or severe gastroesophageal reflux disease. It would not be indicated as primary treatment, as pharmacologic management would be initiated first.

Answer D is incorrect. Nitroglycerin is indicated for the acute treatment of angina, as it increases oxygen delivery to the myocardium. It is also used in the treatment of myocardial infarction as a preload and afterload reducing agent.

12. **The correct answer is B.** Approximately 20% of repeated pregnancy losses are secondary to uterine pathologies. Visualizing the uterus with a hysterosalpingogram is the first step to rule out physical uterine pathology.

Answer A is incorrect. In women with an isolated spontaneous abortion prior to 11 weeks' gestation, approximately 50% are due to chromosome abnormalities. However, in women who have repeated pregnancy losses, this is not the case. Only 2–4% of these women are found to have nonviable karyotypes. As a result, chromosomal analysis is extremely low yield and often the last test to be done on these women.

Answer C is incorrect. Oral contraceptive pills (OCPs) are often used for women with endometriosis. Endometriosis is a disorder characterized by growth of endometrium outside of the uterus. OCPs can be used to minimize the growth of this ectopic endometrial stroma and thus decrease symptoms. OCPs would help to rule out uterine abnormalities as a cause for her miscarriages.

Answer D is incorrect. An exploratory laparotomy can be used to evaluate infertility, especially if endometriosis is suspected, since the procedure can help to restore fertility. However, the suspicion for endometriosis in this patient is low. In addition, exploratory laparotomy is highly invasive and should be reserved until absolutely necessary.

Answer E is incorrect. Pelvic inflammatory disease (PID) is a common cause of infertility and can lead to spontaneous miscarriage. PID is less likely to be the cause of repeated spontaneous abortions in this woman, given the frequency of her miscarriages. This test would be very low-yield in this patient.

13. **The correct answer is E.** This patient is suffering from body dysmorphic disorder, which is defined as preoccupation with some perceived physical abnormality to the point of experiencing profound distress and impairment. A referral for psychotherapy is the most appropriate next step.

Answer A is incorrect. The nature of body dysmorphic disorder is such that performing surgery is not likely to relieve the patient's suffering. Patients with this disorder are usually as certain of their abnormality after surgery as they were before. In fact, they are more likely to sue a surgeon for performing a botched procedure, since they are not able to perceive any improvement in their appearance.

Answer B is incorrect. Although selective serotonin reuptake inhibitors have been shown to be effective in treating some patients with body dysmorphic disorder, such patients should be evaluated by a psychiatrist before being placed on psychotropic medication.

Answer C is incorrect. This patient does not require sedation; she requires psychotherapy to address the underlying issues that drive her obsession.

Answer D is incorrect. While reassurance along with a refusal to perform surgery is an appropriate measure, it is not an adequate one without a referral to psychotherapy for definitive management.

14. The correct answer is A. Patients with a history of cough, unintentional weight loss, and significant smoking history should be worked up for lung cancer. Adenocarcinoma is the most common lung cancer, occurring most often peripherally. Hypertrophic pulmonary osteoarthropathy (HPOA) is common and is characterized by the proliferation of soft and osseous tissue at the distal portions of extremities. Among lung cancer patients, hypertrophic pulmonary osteoarthropathy is most frequently associated with adenocarcinoma and least frequently with small cell carcinoma. HPOA typically presents with digital clubbing, periostosis of long bones, and synovial effusions of the larger joints. Periostosis is often accompanied by pain on palpation of the affected area. When HPOA is suspected, the chest should be examined closely because lung neoplasm is the most frequent cause of acute HPOA.

Answer B is incorrect. Bronchoalveolar type of adenocarcinoma is associated with multiple nodules, interstitial infiltration, and prolific sputum production. Its appearance on x-ray of the chest mimics interstitial pneumonia. It is less predictably associated with digital clubbing or hypertrophic pulmonary osteoarthropathy.

Answer C is incorrect. Large cell carcinoma is a relatively uncommon form of bronchogenic carcinoma that may produce β-human chorionic gonadotropin (β-hCG), resulting in gynecomastia, milky nipple discharge, and elevated serum concentrations of plasma β-hCG.

Answer D is incorrect. Small cell carcinoma is strongly related to cigarette exposure and associated with Cushing's syndrome, syndrome of inappropriate antidiuretic hormone, peripheral neuropathy, subacute cerebellar degeneration, and Eaton-Lambert syndrome. Small cell carcinoma has the worst prognosis of the bronchogenic carcinomas and has metastasized at time of diagnosis in two-thirds of patients.

Answer E is incorrect. Squamous cell carcinoma is most often located centrally and associated with hypercalcemia via production of parathyroid hormone-related peptide. It is also associated with pathologic fractures and kidney stones.

15. The correct answer is A. This patient presents with acute cholecystitis. This diagnosis is supported by right upper quadrant abdominal pain that is accompanied by nausea, vomiting, fever, guarding, and a positive Murphy's sign. Although obesity increases one's risk of developing gallbladder disease, this risk is even greater following rapid weight loss (such as after gastric bypass surgery). It has even been suggested by some that patients undergoing gastric bypass or other bariatric surgery should have a prophylactic cholecystectomy A presentation suspicious for acute cholecystitis should be worked up initially with an ultrasound, as this is an inexpensive test that can be done at the bedside rapidly.

Answer B is incorrect. Although CT scan of the abdomen may show an edematous gallbladder wall with fluid surrounding the gallbladder, this test is much more expensive than an ultrasound and cannot be performed at the bedside, and therefore it is not the first test that you would order when working-up a patient with a presentation suspicious for acute cholecystitis.

Answer C is incorrect. A hepato-iminodiacetic acid (HIDA) scan may reveal a filling defect of the common bile duct, but is not useful for visualizing the gallbladder. In addition, this test is not performed at the bedside and is more expensive than an ultrasound. A HIDA scan may be useful as a second-line approach when diagnosis via ultrasound is indeterminate.

Answer D is incorrect. MRI of the abdomen is not indicated in the work-up of a patient with acute cholecystitis. This test is very expensive, cannot be performed at the bedside, and it takes longer to obtain the results when compared with abdominal ultrasound.

Answer E is incorrect. Plain abdominal films have limited utility in the diagnosis of acute cholecystitis, as they will visualize less than 15% of calculi. Right upper quadrant ultrasound has greater sensitivity and specificity than x-ray films of the abdomen in the diagnosis of acute cholecystitis.

16. The correct answer is A. This woman is at risk for Sheehan's syndrome, or postpartum pituitary necrosis, secondary to her severe obstetric hemorrhage and subsequent profound hypotension. Patients with Sheehan's syndrome have decreased levels of all hormones produced by the anterior pituitary (growth hormone, thyroid-stimulating hormone [TSH], ACTH, prolactin, luteinizing hormone, follicle-stimulating hormone), with only modest if any decrease in hormones released by the posterior pituitary (ADH, oxytocin). Therefore, blood tests will likely reveal a decrease in levels of both prolactin and TSH.

Answer B is incorrect. Both prolactin and thyroid-stimulating hormone would be decreased. Although normal levels of these hormones are possible in a patient suffering from Sheehan's syndrome, this is very unlikely. Some patients do demonstrate normal hormone levels for several months postpartum and only become aware of pituitary dysfunction when they are evaluated for amenorrhea. Sheehan's syndrome results in panhypopituitarism, as opposed to this answer's values. Most patients, however, present to their physicians within weeks of delivery, usually secondary to an inability to lactate.

Answer C is incorrect. Thyroid-stimulating hormone will be decreased, not increased.

Answer D is incorrect. Prolactin will be decreased, not increased.

Answer E is incorrect. Both prolactin and thyroid-stimulating hormone are decreased.

17. The correct answer is D. The patient has primary open-angle glaucoma, the most common type of glaucoma. The eyes undergo a progressive loss of peripheral vision and then central vision. On funduscopic examination, the optic disc's hollowed out appearance is referred to as "cupping." There are no other symptoms, which highlights the importance of measuring intraocular pressure to screen for this disease. Timolol is a nonselective β-antagonist that reduces the production of aqueous humor in the eye. It can be used topically in treatment of open-angle glaucoma. It is important to check for history of cardiac and pulmonary disease prior to prescribing.

Answer A is incorrect. Atropine is an antimuscarinic agent that results in mydriasis and is not an acceptable form of treatment for glaucoma.

Answer B is incorrect. This patient has primary open-angle glaucoma with visible cupping of the optic nerve, retinal nerve fiber layer defects, and increased intraocular pressure. It is necessary to provide the patient with a form of treatment because the pathology will likely progress without appropriate treatment. In addition, the vision loss is irreversible.

Answer C is incorrect. Pilocarpine is a muscarinic agonist that produces rapid miosis and contraction of the ciliary muscles. This can be used in the acute treatment of closed- or open-angle glaucoma to open the trabecular meshwork around Schlemm's canal, increasing drainage of aqueous humor and decreasing intraocular pressure. However, it is not typically a first-line therapy for open-angle glaucoma.

Answer E is incorrect. Although trabeculectomy can provide curative treatment of closed-angle glaucoma, it is not first-line treatment for open-angle glaucoma. A patient with closed-angle glaucoma usually presents with headache, malaise, and general distress, with loss of visual acuity as intraocular pressure increases.

18. The correct answer is B. Homocystinuria results from a defect in cystathionine or methionine synthesis, leading to accumulation of homocysteine. It can cause failure to thrive, mental retardation, osteoporosis, megaloblastic anemia, lens dislocation, and most importantly, thromboembolic events (deep vein thromboses, pulmonary emboli, and cerebrovascular accidents). Other heritable causes of hypercoagulable states include factor V Leiden mutation, protein C deficiency, protein S deficiency, antithrombin III deficiency, and defects in fibrinolysis.

Answer A is incorrect. Fabry's disease results from a deficiency of α-galactosidase A and leads to an accumulation of ceramide trihexoside. It presents with renal failure. It does not cause cerebrovascular accidents.

Answer C is incorrect. Krabbe's disease results from the absence of β-galactosidase and leads to accumulation of galactocerebroside. This disease presents during the first year of life with optic atrophy, seizures, and spasticity. It does not cause cerebrovascular accidents.

Answer D is incorrect. Niemann-Pick disease results from deficiency of sphingomyelinase, leading to a buildup of sphingomyelin and cholesterol. The infantile form presents with hepatosplenomegaly, failure to thrive, and rapidly progressive neurodevelopmental regression. It does not cause cerebrovascular accidents.

Answer E is incorrect. Phenylketonuria (PKU) results from an enzyme or cofactor deficiency that prevents phenylalanine from being converted to tyrosine. PKU classically presents with fair skin, eczema, and musty body odor. As the child ages, mental retardation will develop if left untreated. PKU does not cause cerebrovascular accidents.

19. **The correct answer is C.** Ketoconazole, an antifungal medication that can be given topically or systemically, also has the effect of decreasing adrenal steroidogenesis. Adrenal insufficiency is a possible but rare adverse effect that can be treated with steroid replacement therapy.

Answer A is incorrect. Steroid replacement therapy would exacerbate the patient's Cushing's syndrome symptoms, the opposite of the desired effect. Steroid replacement therapy may be necessary after the patient has received ketoconazole and possibly develops adrenal insufficiency.

Answer B is incorrect. One of the possible effects of Cushing's syndrome is the development of the symptoms of diabetes mellitus, secondary to glucose intolerance. Although insulin may be effective in treating those symptoms (polydipsia, polyuria, polyphagia), it will not decrease adrenal steroidogenesis.

Answer D is incorrect. The patient is symptomatic, and therefore warrants some sort of treatment, even though it will not be as effective as surgical resection. Ketoconazole would be most appropriate, given its effect of decreasing adrenal steroidogenesis.

Answer E is incorrect. Pituitary irradiation has a long lag time between treatment and remission, and remission only occurs in < 50% of patients. It is more commonly used for postoperative recurrences.

20. **The correct answer is C.** Leuprolide is a gonadotropin-releasing hormone (GnRH) analog that is commonly used to help control the symptoms of endometriosis. Release of pituitary follicle-stimulating hormone (FSH)/luteinizing hormone (LH) requires pulsatile secretion of GnRH. Constant pituitary stimulation with leuprolide, or other GnRH analogs, inhibits FSH/LH secretion, preventing normal folliculogenesis and ovulation. Impaired follicle growth and maturation causes a decreased level of circulating estrogen, which in turn decreases the proliferation of endometrial tissue and minimizes the pain associated with ectopic endometrium. Leuprolide is an appropriate medical treatment choice for endometriosis that has failed treatment of combination oral contraceptives.

Answer A is incorrect. Dexamethasone is not a treatment for endometriosis.

Answer B is incorrect. Surgical treatment is generally reserved for patients with severe disease, those who fail hormonal therapy, or the older infertile patient.

Answer D is incorrect. Progestin therapy can be used in treatment for endometriosis. However, due to its mixed results and the fact that continuous therapy can lead to breakthrough bleeding, depression, bloating, and weight gain, and is used in patients who do not desire fertility, it is not the most appropriate choice for this teenager.

Answer E is incorrect. Unopposed estrogen therapy would likely exacerbate symptoms of endometriosis. In addition, such therapy is a risk factor for acquiring endometrial cancer.

21. **The correct answer is E.** Patients who have had their spleens removed or are functionally asplenic, such as patients with sickle cell disease, can be susceptible to meningitis caused by *Streptococcus pneumoniae* and *Neisseria meningitidis*. Any encapsulated organism such

as *S. pneumoniae*, *N. meningitidis*, or *Haemophilus influenzae* may cause infection in asplenic patients, as they are unable to manufacture a new antibody immune response to these organisms after the spleen is removed. This is the reason for preoperative inoculation against these organisms in scheduled splenectomy. HIV infection and deficiency of opsonizing antibodies can also both leave the patient susceptible to meningitis caused by *S. pneumoniae*.

Answer A is incorrect. *Cryptococcus* and *Listeria* are both important causes of meningitis in patients with advanced HIV disease, but not in patients with asplenia.

Answer B is incorrect. *Staphylococcus aureus* is not more likely to cause meningitis in people with asplenia.

Answer C is incorrect. While meningococcus is an important cause of meningitis in patients with asplenia, *Staphylococcus aureus* is not likely to cause meningitis in this patient population.

Answer D is incorrect. While *Streptococcus pneumoniae* is an important cause of meningitis in asplenic patients, *Cryptococcus neoformans* is not a common cause of meningitis in this patient population. *C. neoformans* is an important cause of meningitis in patients with diseases that expose patients to high levels of corticosteroid hormones, and in patients with compromised immune systems due to HIV disease.

22. **The correct answer is B.** Peak expiratory flow rate is the maximum flow rate achieved during the forced vital capacity maneuver, beginning after full inspiration and ending at maximal expiration. This is significantly decreased during an asthmatic episode and is the simplest and fastest diagnostic step in the primary care setting.

Answer A is incorrect. Blood eosinophilia is common and may be useful if one suspects either allergy or asthma, but eosinophilia is not sensitive or specific enough to be a main diagnostic criterion for asthma. Therefore, a complete blood cell count is not indicated in the initial workup.

Answer C is incorrect. Methacholine challenge is a test for bronchial hyperresponsiveness when the patient is not acutely ill and is not specific for asthma.

Answer D is incorrect. Sputum specimen from an asthmatic may reveal Charcot-Leyden crystals and Curschmann spirals that can be diagnostic for asthma, are but not required for diagnosis.

Answer E is incorrect. In mild to moderate asthma without adventitious sounds other than wheezing, x-ray of the chest is not needed. X-ray of the chest is indicated if the patient has severe asthma and/or exacerbation requiring hospitalization. In such a case, x-ray would show barrel chest and increased lung volumes. Furthermore, subcutaneous emphysema may also be seen.

23. **The correct answer is E.** When evaluating heart defects, it is important to consider presence or absence of cyanosis, nature of any murmur, and age at presentation. Ventricular septal defects (VSDs) are the most common congenital heart defects and account for most hospital admissions for heart defects in infants 14–28 days old. The nature of symptoms is highly dependent on the size of the defect. The ECG findings and the quiet murmur in this child are consistent with a large VSD. Radiographic findings commonly include increased pulmonary vascular markings as seen in this patient. In more severe VSDs, enlargement of the left atrium and left ventricle as well as the pulmonary artery can also be seen on x-ray of the chest.

Answer A is incorrect. Aortic stenosis is usually the result of a bicuspid or single commissure valve and symptoms are largely dependent on the degree of stenosis. ECG would likely only show left ventricular hypertrophy. Most importantly, ventricular septal defects would be more common at this age.

Answer B is incorrect. Patent ductus arteriosus is often seen in premature infants and carries a female predominance. The characteristic murmur is often described as machine-like and involves both systole and diastole.

Answer C is incorrect. Tetralogy of Fallot is the second most common heart defect in infants 14–28 days old, but would likely present with cyanosis. Additionally, pulmonary blood flow would be decreased in this condition. Remember, the tetralogy includes right ventricular outflow obstruction, right ventricular hypertrophy, overriding aorta, and subaortic ventricular septal defect. Radiographic findings typically include a boot-shaped heart due to hypertrophy of the right ventricle.

Answer D is incorrect. Transposition of the great arteries is also a common heart defect, but cyanosis would likely be present from birth. Other features are variable but increased pulmonary vascular findings are typical.

24. **The correct answer is E.** The patient is presenting with end-stage mycosis fungoides, a variant of cutaneous T-lymphocyte lymphoma. This disease is generally indolent, and patients may have several years of eczematous or dermatitic skin lesions before the diagnosis is established. Skin lesions begin as patches and plaques, and may progress to tumors. In other cases, such as this one, Sézary's syndrome develops, which manifests as diffuse erythroderma and circulating tumor cells (Sézary cells). Total skin electron beam therapy is often recommended for patients with Sézary syndrome because the entire body can be treated without the morbidity that would result from conventional radiotherapy. Electron beam therapy offers the ability to treat superficial skin lesions with little penetration into deeper tissues. Unfortunately, the disease is usually not curable in late stages.

Answer A is incorrect. Conventional radiotherapy may at times be used to treat localized mycosis fungoides, particularly in the tumor stage when deeper tissue penetration may be necessary. It has little utility once the disease is present diffusely because it cannot be administered to the entire skin surface.

Answer B is incorrect. There is no indication that the patient is suffering from a viral illness that would respond to acyclovir.

Answer C is incorrect. Although the patient's condition may mimic staphylococcal scalded skin syndrome, the timing of his presentation is not as acute as it would be if he were suffering from a bacterial infection.

Answer D is incorrect. Topical nitrogen mustards are also used to treat localized disease but cannot realistically be effectively applied to the entire body.

25. **The correct answer is C.** Diabetic ketoacidosis (DKA) is one consequence of untreated diabetes mellitus (chronic high blood sugar or hyperglycemia), and is linked to an impaired glucose cycle. In a diabetic patient, DKA begins with deficiency in insulin. This is most commonly due to undiagnosed diabetes mellitus, or in patients who have been diagnosed with diabetes, failure to take prescribed insulin. DKA has a 100% mortality rate if left untreated. The treatment for diabetic ketoacidosis consists of aggressive intravenous fluids and insulin. Patients often present with significant dehydration that must be reversed as quickly as possible. Excessive alcohol intake, as in this patient, can lead to poor diabetes control (e.g., problems with medication/blood sugar balance), which can contribute to DKA. Also, while not directly causative, in some people with diabetes excess alcohol can worsen dehydration and thereby contribute to the development of DKA.

Answer A is incorrect. Bicarbonate repletion is most effective for lactic acidosis, but patients should be watched carefully for fluid overload and lactic acidosis, which can occur secondary to the amount necessary to replete. It is not indicated in diabetic ketoacidosis.

Answer B is incorrect. Glucose administration is not indicated early in the treatment of ketoacidosis, since the patient already has extremely high serum glucose levels that she cannot utilize due to her lack of insulin. Once fluids and insulin have been started, glucose could be administered to meet the child's increased metabolic needs and prevent hypoglycemia.

Answer D is incorrect. Potassium repletion is not indicated as an initial step in the treatment of diabetic ketoacidosis. Serum potassium is usually elevated in ketoacidosis secondary to hyperosmolality and insulin deficiency, which instigates potassium movement out of cells. However, with the administration of insulin there is often a rapid fall in plasma potassium concentration, which can be repleted with potassium chloride.

Answer E is incorrect. A urinalysis should be obtained to confirm the diagnosis but is not necessary to begin fluid treatment.

26. **The correct answer is D.** This patient has a Colles' fracture. In general, operative management is required if a fracture is intra-articular and/or open. Percutaneous pin fixation, open reduction and internal fixation, and external fixation are all possible ways to manage this fracture, which has a displaced intra-articular fragment.

Answer A is incorrect. Closed reduction is the treatment of choice if the fracture is displaced, closed, and extra-articular. This fracture is intra-articular. A sling would not adequately maintain the reduction and thus would not be used.

Answer B is incorrect. The fracture had a displaced intra-articular piece, so operative management is needed. A long arm cast would appropriately maintain reduction, but closed reduction cannot properly realign the joint surface.

Answer C is incorrect. Ice and compression are appropriate with isolated soft tissue injury. However, immobilization is required for fractures.

Answer E is incorrect. Although physical therapy may ultimately be needed after immobilization, initial therapy must focus on regaining proper bone and joint alignment.

27. **The correct answer is D.** This patient has contrast-induced nephropathy due to the kidneys being responsible for getting rid of the dye and it causing a renal azotemia. The patient may also have some underlying renal insufficiency due to diabetes. Of the answer choices given, prophylactic hemodialysis to remove contrast dye from the circulation is the only treatment that has not been shown to prevent acute renal failure due to contrast nephropathy.

Answer A is incorrect. Acetylcysteine may reduce the risk of contrast-induced nephropathy by an unknown mechanism.

Answer B is incorrect. Intravenous hydration with saline before and after administration of contrast has been shown to reduce the occurrence of acute renal failure, especially in patients with some underlying chronic renal insufficiency.

Answer C is incorrect. Underlying diabetic nephropathy increases the risk of contrast-induced nephropathy. Patients with better glycemic control are less likely to have underlying diabetic nephropathy and renal insufficiency.

Answer E is incorrect. Gadolinium contrast used with MRI is not associated with contrast-induced nephropathy; therefore, MRI with contrast should be considered as an alternative to CT in patients at high risk for contrast-induced nephropathy.

28. **The correct answer is A.** This woman has mild gestational diabetes (serum glucose concentration > 130 mg/dL after 50-g oral glucose tolerance test is abnormal). The first line of treatment to control blood glucose is dietary restriction. Patients are placed on the American Dietetic Association diet, which restricts calories and adheres to the conventional "food pyramid."

Answer B is incorrect. For gestational diabetes, an American Dietetic Association diet is the first line of treatment. However, diet in combination with exercise is recommended because it is more efficient than diet alone at controlling diabetes.

Answer C is incorrect. Diet control is the first line of treatment for gestational diabetes, followed by insulin injection. Therefore, this woman will only be treated with insulin if dietary restrictions alone cannot control her diabetes.

Answer D is incorrect. Oral hypoglycemic agents can cause hypoglycemia in the fetus and therefore should not be used in pregnancy.

Answer E is incorrect. Oral hypoglycemic agents can cause hypoglycemia in the fetus and therefore should not be used in pregnancy.

29. **The correct answer is B.** Acute, uncomplicated pyelonephritis is suggested by flank pain, nausea/vomiting, and fever (> 38°C [100.4°F]) with or without costovertebral tenderness, and may occur in the absence or presence of cystitis symptoms. Ciprofloxacin is an oral fluoroquinolone recommended for initial empiric treatment of infection caused by gram-negative bacilli. *Escherichia coli* accounts for 70–95% of acute, uncomplicated upper and lower urinary tract infections.

Answer A is incorrect. This treatment is inadequate because β-lactam regimens shorter than 14 days have been associated with unacceptably high failure rates.

Answer C is incorrect. Moxifloxacin, a newer fluoroquinolone, should be avoided in pyelonephritis because it may not achieve adequate concentrations in the urine to be effective.

Answer D is incorrect. This patient can receive adequate treatment as an outpatient. Indications for admission and intravenous therapy include inability to maintain oral hydration or take oral medications, uncertainty regarding the diagnosis, or severe illness with high fevers and intense pain. This patient is a relatively healthy man with no significant past medical history and a likely uncomplicated case of acute pyelonephritis.

30. **The correct answer is E.** This is a classic presentation of a congenital diaphragmatic hernia. X-ray of the chest showing bowel in the left thoracic cavity is diagnostic. The treatment for congenital diaphragmatic hernias is to support the infant's respiratory status with mechanical ventilation or extracorporeal membrane oxygenation, and then to surgically repair the defect.

Answer A is incorrect. Betamethasone is given to women who are < 35 weeks pregnant and likely to deliver in the next 7 days to increase surfactant production and prevent respiratory distress syndrome. Betamethasone does not play a role in the treatment of the tachypneic neonate.

Answer B is incorrect. Caffeine is used to treat central apnea in neonates.

Answer C is incorrect. Needle decompression treats a tension pneumothorax, which presents with respiratory distress, decreased breath sounds on the affected side, and abdominal distension. X-ray film of the chest of a tension pneumothorax shows a hyperlucent hemithorax, flattening of the diaphragm, mediastinal shift, and compression of the opposite lung. Bowel in the thoracic cavity is diagnostic of a congenital diaphragmatic hernia rather than a pneumothorax.

Answer D is incorrect. Surfactant is used to treat respiratory distress syndrome in preterm infants.

31. **The correct answer is D.** This question requires one to determine the positive predictive value (PPV) of the testing method employed. To calculate PPV, one must divide the number of true positives by the total number of people who tested positive for the disease. In this case, the number of true positives (90) is divided by the number of people who tested positive (90 + 25).

Answer A is incorrect. This fraction (true negatives/total negatives) would be used to calculate the negative predictive value of the test.

Answer B is incorrect. This fraction (true negatives/total without disease) gives the specificity of the test.

Answer C is incorrect. This fraction (true positives/total diseased) gives the sensitivity of the test.

Answer E is incorrect. This question provides us with the information necessary to calculate the positive predictive value.

32. **The correct answer is A.** Calcium channel blockers are not contraindicated during pregnancy, and are used to treat Raynaud's syndrome. Given that this woman's hypertension is controlled on a calcium channel blocker, there is no reason to switch her to a β-adrenergic blocker.

Answer B is incorrect. As this woman's hypertension is controlled on a calcium channel blocker and they are not contraindicated during pregnancy, there is no reason to switch her to a β-adrenergic blocker. Although they are generally thought to be safe in pregnancy, they are class D and may be associated with bradycardia, intrauterine growth retardation, and neonatal hypoglycemia.

Answer C is incorrect. Angiotensin-converting enzyme (ACE) inhibitors are considered teratogenic. They have been associated with renal defects, renal dysgenesis/dysplasia, renal failure, oligohydramnios, persistent anuria following delivery, hypotension, pulmonary hypoplasia, limb contractures secondary to oligohydramnios, and stillbirth. ACE inhibitors should be avoided during pregnancy, particularly in the second and third trimesters.

Answer D is incorrect. Angiotensin II receptor blockers are contraindicated during pregnancy, as they may cause renal and pulmonary complications.

Answer E is incorrect. Thiazides are pregnancy category D drugs, and have been associated with electrolyte disorders and thrombocytopenia in newborns.

33. **The correct answer is A.** This patient has Goodpasture's syndrome characterized by deposition of antibodies to the basement membrane in glomeruli and alveoli. This leads to glomerulonephritis with symptoms of renal failure, hematuria, and nephritic range proteinuria, as well as pulmonary hemorrhage causing cough and occasionally hemoptysis and bloody effusions at the lung bases. Immunofluorescence staining of a renal biopsy sample would show the pathognomonic linear deposition of the antiglomerular basement membrane antibody.

Answer B is incorrect. Cryoglobulinemia, often associated with hepatitis B or C infection, causes glomerular disease associated with necrotizing skin lesions, arthralgias, fevers, and hepatosplenomegaly.

Answer C is incorrect. IgA deposition in the glomerular mesangium is seen in IgA nephropathy, or Berger's disease. It presents with gross hematuria and nephrotic syndrome but does not cause pulmonary symptoms.

Answer D is incorrect. Postinfectious glomerulonephritis following group A streptococcal infection causes edema, oliguria, and hypertension, and does not cause concomitant pulmonary symptoms such as those seen in this patient.

Answer E is incorrect. Inflammation of small vessels, or small vessel vasculitides, such as Wegener's granulomatosis, Churg-Strauss disease, and microscopic polyangiitis, cause pauci-immune glomerulonephritis characterized by renal failure with lack of antibodies on immunofluorescence staining.

34. **The correct answer is D.** This patient is in preterm labor. The majority of preterm labor is judged to be idiopathic; however, a number of factors predispose to preterm labor. These include prior preterm deliveries, infections, an incompetent cervix, uterine or placental abnormalities, or premature rupture of membranes. Substance abuse, especially smoking, significantly increases the risk of preterm labor.

Answer A is incorrect. Prostaglandins facilitate labor by causing maturation of the cervix and increasing the strength of uterine contractions. Nonsteroidal anti-inflammatory drugs (NSAIDs) such as ibuprofen decrease the production of many prostaglandins by blocking the enzyme cyclooxygenase. NSAIDs have been shown to have tocolytic properties, delaying the progress of labor. However, they have been associated with increased rates of neonatal complications and thus are not widely used as tocolytics.

Answer B is incorrect. Maternal obesity may contribute to gestational diabetes and macrosomia, which lead to a number of prenatal and labor complications. However, maternal obesity is not a known risk factor for preterm labor.

Answer C is incorrect. Previous pregnancies complicated by preterm labor increase the likelihood that subsequent pregnancies will also be complicated by preterm labor. However, previous term labor and delivery decrease the likelihood of subsequent preterm labor. Since this patient has two prior term deliveries, her multiparity would make her less, not more, likely to experience preterm labor.

Answer E is incorrect. Genitourinary tract infections and bacterial vaginosis have been associated with preterm labor. However, vaginal *Candida* infections have not been associated with preterm labor.

35. **The correct answer is D.** Radioactive iodine is the treatment of choice in this patient, who has a solitary toxic adenoma. It will shrink her thyroid gland, and the patient will likely become euthyroid in 1–3 months. Ultimately, 80% of patients will become hypothyroid and will require thyroid hormone supplementation (levothyroxine). Thyroid lobectomy, which would remove the tumor without eliminating thyroid function, could also be considered.

Answer A is incorrect. β-Blockers are commonly given at the beginning of thiocarbamide treatment in order to avoid symptoms of thyrotoxicosis. It is not given, however, in a similar manner with radioactive iodine treatment.

Answer B is incorrect. Carbimazole, like propylthiouracil, is a member of the thiocarbamide class of drugs, and is not appropriate for toxic adenoma.

Answer C is incorrect. Propylthiouracil is a member of the thiocarbamide class of drugs, which block thyroid hormone synthesis by inhibiting thyroid peroxidase. While a good treatment for other causes of hyperthyroidism, it is not the treatment of choice for toxic adenoma.

Answer E is incorrect. Thyroidectomy could be an appropriate treatment of toxic adenoma when the nodule is large or refractory to medical management. Hot nodules (as in this patient) have a low likelihood of cancer, thus medical treatment would be the first-line treatment before surgical intervention.

36. **The correct answer is D.** Remember "SNOUT" and "SPIN:" SeNsitivity rules OUT and SPecificity rules IN. High sensitivity rules out disease in those who test negative, while high specificity confirms disease in those who test positive. A highly sensitive test is good for screening because it will not miss many individuals with disease.

Answer A is incorrect. A positive result from a test with high specificity is needed to confirm disease. In the case of high sensitivity, as in this case, a negative test rules out or confirms lack of disease.

Answer B is incorrect. Sensitivity and specificity are not predictors of who may or may not develop a disease.

Answer C is incorrect. A highly sensitive test may have a high false-negative ratio, but it will also have a low false-positive ratio. These parameters make this a good test to screen for a condition. However, this answer choice is incomplete because a high false-negative ratio on its own is not sufficient to screen effectively.

Answer E is incorrect. Because tests with high specificity are used to confirm disease, they are more appropriate in a setting where the suspicion of malignancy is already very high. In this case, fine-needle aspiration biopsy has a high sensitivity and is used to rule out disease in healthy individuals as a screening test.

37. **The correct answer is A.** This patient's rash, erythema chronicum migrans, is suggestive of Lyme disease, caused by the spirochete *Borrelia burgdorferi*, which is transmitted by the bite of *Ixodes* ticks. It is endemic in the northeastern United States. Treatment is oral doxycycline, amoxicillin, or cefuroxime axetil. Patients with certain neurologic or cardiac forms of the illness may require intravenous treatment with drugs such as ceftriaxone or penicillin. Cultures have only been shown to be useful in diagnosing Lyme disease when taken early in the course of the disease by biopsying the characteristic rash. It is less useful in the case of later disease, or when used on plasma or cerebrospinal fluid specimens.

Answer B is incorrect. Culturing plasma is less sensitive than culturing tissue taken from the erythema chronicum migrans rash characteristic of Lyme disease.

Answer C is incorrect. The Lyme antigen test was designed to be used on urine, and does not yield reliable results.

Answer D is incorrect. This early in the course of the disease, the enzyme-linked immunosorbent assay (ELISA) test and Western blot may be falsely negative, due to the delay in seroconversion after the initial exposure. Within 1 week of exposure, sensitivity of ELISA and Western blot is only 32%. After several weeks, it rises to 87%.

Answer E is incorrect. The Lyme antigen test is unreliable, and should not be used to support the diagnosis of Lyme disease.

38. **The correct answer is D.** This is an example of postrenal, or obstructive, acute renal failure. The patient most likely has prostate carcinoma given the asymmetric, firm, nodular prostate palpable on physical examination. Back pain may be evidence of bone metastases. A benign or malignant enlarged prostate can obstruct the urinary outflow tract by blocking the urethra, leading to acute urinary retention. It may present with an acute renal failure picture such as this one, in which the patient is anuric and shows laboratory evidence of renal insufficiency.

Answer A is incorrect. Glomerular Ig deposition is seen in some forms of glomerular disease, which may present with renal insufficiency. However, glomerular disease is unlikely to present with acute urinary retention, and would present with edema, proteinuria or hematuria, hypertension, and oliguria.

Answer B is incorrect. Hypercalcemia is associated with calcium phosphate renal calculi, which can cause acute ureteral obstruction but only rarely would cause bilateral obstruction leading to an acute renal failure picture. Additionally, this patient's physical examination is not consistent with nephrolithiasis, which would present with flank pain and tenderness.

Answer C is incorrect. Neurogenic bladder is a cause of urinary retention, but is more likely to present with other signs and symptoms of neurologic disease and additional focal neurologic findings on examination.

Answer E is incorrect. Renal tubular inflammation may be seen with a number of causes of renal failure, such as acute interstitial nephritis. However, such processes would not present with urinary retention, and would most likely present with casts or WBCs on urinalysis.

Answer F is incorrect. A staghorn renal calculus can cause urinary obstruction, although it is unlikely to be bilateral or to cause acute urethral obstruction and postrenal acute renal failure. Additionally, staghorn calculi are associated with chronic urinary tract infection, which is not seen in this patient's presentation.

39. **The correct answer is B.** This girl has signs consistent with rickets, a disorder of bone mineralization due to hypocalcemia or hypophosphatemia. Children may present with dental enamel hypoplasia, delay in motor milestones, and frequent infectious diseases. Clinical presentation may also include tetany, convulsions, alopecia, and skeletal abnormalities. Skeletal findings include widened growth plates, frontal bossing, enlargement of the wrists, bowing of the distal forearm, lateral bowing of the femur and tibia, and delay in closure of the fontanelles. Hypocalcemic rickets is typically due to a deficiency or resistance to vitamin D. This patient has findings that suggest vitamin D dependent rickets type I, which is caused by a mutation in the gene that encodes the 1-α-hydroxylation enzyme in the kidney. These patients will have normal or elevated levels of the precursor, $25(OH)D$, but will have significantly low levels of the active metabolite $1,25(OH)_2D$.

Answer A is incorrect. Disorders of the gut such as inflammatory bowel disease, celiac disease, cystic fibrosis, and extensive bowel surgery may cause malabsorption of vitamin D, which can lead to rickets in children or osteomalacia in adults. These patients will have hypocalcemia and hypophosphatemia, but they will have decreased levels of both $25(OH)D$ and $1,25(OH)_2D$.

Answer C is incorrect. The liver is responsible for 25-hydroxylation of vitamin D into $25(OH)D$. A deficiency in this enzyme would result in low levels of both $25(OH)D$ and $1,25(OH)_2D$. The clinical presentation would be very similar to the patient presented here.

Answer D is incorrect. Hypoparathyroidism is a cause of hypocalcemia; however, these patients will have hyper-, not hypophosphatemia. In addition, these patients will not have elevated $25(OH)D$ or decreased $1,25(OH)_2D$.

Answer E is incorrect. Vitamin D is synthesized in the skin in response to ultraviolet radiation. Elderly patients, particularly in the winter, or other people with little sun exposure may develop vitamin D deficiency. These patients will also have hypocalcemia and hypophosphatemia, but they will have decreased levels of both 25(OH)D and 1,25(OH)$_2$D.

40. **The correct answer is B.** Depression can present with additional symptoms. In this case, the patient presented with the symptoms of major depressive disorder (namely, decreased activity, anhedonia, decreased food intake, decreased sleep, and psychomotor retardation) but has additional delusions. The key to diagnosis is that the psychotic features end with the resolution of the depressive episode. Depression with psychotic features often requires special treatment with antipsychotic medications and electroconvulsive therapy.

Answer A is incorrect. In a brief psychotic episode, the psychotic behavior is present for more than 1 day but for less than 1 month (as in this case). However, the psychotic symptoms must exist in the absence of mood symptoms. Brief psychotic disorder usually carries a much better prognosis.

Answer C is incorrect. Schizoaffective disorder is a condition in which the patient's psychiatric symptoms are present during an episode of mood disorder, but then continue for at least 2 weeks after the resolution of the mood disorder. The centipedes, in this case, disappeared with the patient's depression, thereby preventing a diagnosis of schizoaffective disorder.

Answer D is incorrect. The diagnosis of schizophrenia requires there to be continuous signs and symptoms of impaired reality testing for at least 6 months in the absence of any mood symptoms. This patient's symptoms have only been present for several weeks. In addition, peak onset in men is between the ages of 18 and 25, although schizophrenia can certainly be diagnosed in older populations.

Answer E is incorrect. The *Diagnostic and Statistical Manual of Mental Disorders*, Fourth Edition, Text Revision, criteria for specific phobia include a "marked and persistent fear that is excessive and unreasonable" and not better accounted for by some other mental disease. This patient's perception of centipedes is much better included in the diagnosis of depression with psychotic features.

41. **The correct answer is C.** The patient's condition is most consistent with a diagnosis of chronic lymphocytic leukemia (CLL). Although most patients with CLL are diagnosed incidentally or with complaints of fatigue, between 10% and 20% of patients present with massive splenomegaly and resultant anemia and thrombocytopenia. This patient has symptoms of both, and his physical examination reveals classic petechiae—likely due to a platelet count of 8000/mm^3. Splenectomy in patients with CLL-induced thrombocytopenia corrects the abnormality in 70% to 85% of cases.

Answer A is incorrect. High-dose corticosteroids are used as therapy for thrombocytopenia in patients diagnosed with idiopathic thrombocytopenic purpura, an antibody-mediated illness causing marked thrombocytopenia. Corticosteroids may also be used as part of a chemotherapeutic regimen to treat acute lymphocytic leukemia. They are generally not effective in chronic leukemias and should never be used alone in these illnesses because they may produce an incomplete remission, after which the patient has a high risk of relapse with refractory disease.

Answer B is incorrect. Platelet transfusion may improve this patient's thrombocytopenia initially; however, platelets will become sequestered in the patient's spleen rapidly. This sequestration would lead to further splenomegaly and thrombocytopenia.

Answer D is incorrect. 5-Fluorouracil is a chemotherapeutic agent used to treat many types of cancer. Although the end result of its use may be normalization of blood counts as malignant cells are killed, the immediate response is a further decrease in counts from its antimetabolic action. Therefore, the initial blood work would reveal a decrease in platelet counts.

Answer E is incorrect. Granulocyte colony-stimulating factor (G-CSF) is used to stimulate the bone marrow to produce WBCs following administration of chemotherapy. It would not be effective in treating this patient's thrombocytopenia for two reasons. Platelets are not derived from granulocytes, the site of action of G-CSF. The patient's bone marrow is packed with leukemic cells; this is the reason that his platelet count is so low, and any amount of bone marrow stimulation will be ineffective in producing normal, viable cells.

42. **The correct answer is A.** Enrollment bias is the flaw that occurs when patients are assigned to different study groups in a nonrandom fashion. When a study is randomized, it ensures that there is not a bias in the way that patients were divided into the two study groups, therefore ensuring that any difference in outcome between the two groups is due to the intervention being studied, and not because of differences between the two groups.

Answer B is incorrect. Lead time bias is when a diagnosis is made earlier than it was before, but no change is made in the true survival. Lead time bias is primarily a concern for studies that seek to measure the survival benefit of disease screening programs. Because screening tests may allow for an earlier diagnosis of a disease (e.g., lung cancer) than would otherwise have occurred, patients in the screening groups may have a longer period of survival following diagnosis than those in the unscreened group, even if the course of their disease is unchanged by medical interventions. Lead time bias refers to the mistaken interpretation of these data as demonstrating a survival benefit. This is not affected by randomized design.

Answer C is incorrect. Measurement bias is when the process of collecting data affects the outcome. For example, when asked about weekly alcohol consumption, people tend to give answers that are less than the true value. Such a bias is an example of measurement bias, which is not affected by randomized design.

Answer D is incorrect. Observer bias is when an observer's evaluation of a patient's response to treatment is affected by knowing which study group the patient is in. This is avoided by

double-blind design; randomization has no effect on observer bias.

Answer E is incorrect. Recall bias can be found in retrospective trials and involves a patient's possible exaggeration of risk factors or exposures if it is known that the patient developed the disease putatively associated with them. This is not affected by randomized design.

43. **The correct answer is C.** Cricothyroidotomy is indicated in patients who cannot be intubated or who have sustained significant maxillofacial trauma, such as this patient who has multiple maxillary and mandibular fractures. Carbon dioxide retention is a common problem with cricothyroidotomies so routine arterial blood gases should be checked on these patients. Currently, cricothyroidotomy and percutaneous transtracheal ventilation are preferred over tracheostomy in most traumas because they are relatively safe and simple. However, a disadvantage of a cricothyroidotomy is the inability to use a tube larger than 6 mm because of the limited aperture of the cricothyroid space. Cricothyroidotomy is also contraindicated in patients younger than 12 years old because of the risk of damage to the cricoid cartilage and the subsequent risk of subglottic stenosis.

Answer A is incorrect. The patient is exhibiting classic signs of shock (hypotension, tachycardia, mental status changes, tachypnea, diaphoresis, and pallor) and circulation is one of the first things to evaluate in a trauma. However, an airway is always the primary concern, and in this young patient it is likely that he will maintain circulation until an airway is secured.

Answer B is incorrect. Face mask ventilation is not adequate in this patient given the oxygen saturation level and airway patency, and adequacy of ventilation should take precedence over other treatment.

Answer D is incorrect. Nasopharyngeal intubation and oropharyngeal intubation are contraindicated in patients who have sustained significant maxillofacial trauma or who have unstable facial fractures.

Answer E is incorrect. Nasopharyngeal intubation and oropharyngeal intubation are contraindicated in patients who have sustained significant maxillofacial trauma or who have unstable facial fractures.

Questions 44–46

44. The correct answer is B. Digoxin has a low therapeutic index and toxicity is common, especially in the elderly. Toxicity is often signaled by nausea, vomiting, and anorexia. Heart palpitations may also be present. Disturbances of color vision, with a tendency toward yellow-green coloring, can occur. The patient's wife's complaint that he has "not been acting himself," might be a sign of mental status changes—also a common sign of digitalis toxicity.

45. The correct answer is E. Gastroparesis, or delayed gastric emptying, describes a paralysis of the stomach. The most common cause of gastroparesis is diabetes mellitus. As in this patient, the primary symptoms are nausea and vomiting, usually following meals. Anorexia, weight loss, and early satiety are also common. Heartburn, epigastric pain, and frequent belching also support the diagnosis of gastroparesis.

46. The correct answer is O. Sigmoid volvulus is the most common form of volvulus of the gastrointestinal tract. It is particularly common in elderly persons. Patients present with abdominal pain, distention, and constipation. Nausea and vomiting may present late. Predisposing factors include chronic constipation, institutionalization, and an excessively mobile sigmoid colon. Findings on x-ray of the abdomen are usually diagnostic.

Answer A is incorrect. Bulimia may present with vomiting, but it would be induced. Patients with bulimia nervosa have episodes of binge eating followed by a compensatory activity (such as self-induced vomiting or excessive exercise).

Answer C is incorrect. Early satiety, bloating, and vomiting are common manifestations of gastric outlet obstruction. This diagnosis needs to be confirmed with gastric emptying studies, and is most commonly a complication of peptic ulcer disease (PUD); without a history of PUD it is unlikely.

Answer D is incorrect. Vomiting, diarrhea, and abdominal discomfort are all common symptoms of gastroenteritis. In gastroenteritis there is an infectious cause (bacterial or viral), and none of the stems describe contact with anyone sick or any recent travel. So gastroenteritis is a less likely diagnosis than the correct one.

Answer F is incorrect. Hepatitis (acute or chronic) can be a cause of abdominal discomfort along with fatigue and vomiting, but it will typically present with high aminotransferases and hyperbilirubinemia. Acutely, patients will often appear jaundiced and have a tender right upper quadrant, none of which were present in any of these patients.

Answer G is incorrect. Inflammatory bowel disease often has abdominal pain and diarrhea, and is a chronic condition with a waxing and waning course. Even if this was a first presentation when a history would not be as relevant, the patient would be more likely to be having diarrhea. A Crohn's disease patient may have small intestine involvement causing constipation, but this would not be the most likely diagnosis.

Answer H is incorrect. Nausea and vomiting are common with an intracranial hemorrhage, but headache is equally common, and there is often an abnormality on neurologic examination. Also, there is often an underlying reason for the hemorrhage that has not been elicited in any of these patients, such as trauma, bleeding diathesis, drug abuse, alcoholism, or hypertension. The elderly are also more likely to have an intracranial hemorrhage, but the story here is not convincing for hemorrhage.

Answer I is incorrect. Labyrinthitis, inflammation in the vestibular labyrinth, is acute in onset, and vertigo, nausea, and vomiting are usually tied to movement.

Answer J is incorrect. Meningitis can present with nausea and vomiting, but it would be unlikely to present without any neurologic symptoms, most notably headache and a stiff neck.

Answer K is incorrect. Migraine headaches can typically involve nausea and vomiting, but unilateral or bilateral headache is a prominent symptom. Migraines also often have neurologic symptoms (such as scotomas), and may have a prodrome.

Answer L is incorrect. Myocardial infarcts may atypically present (particularly in women) with nausea and vomiting. But without identifiable risk factors (smoking, hypertension, elevated low-density lipoprotein, diabetes, or family history), a myocardial infarction is not the most likely diagnosis.

Answer M is incorrect. Pancreatic carcinomas often present clinically with an obstruction, as they are clinically silent until there is a mass effect. They may obstruct the small bowel, producing nausea and vomiting, or they may obstruct the common bile duct, producing painless jaundice.

Answer N is incorrect. Pancreatitis, an acute inflammatory process of the pancreas, presents with severe abdominal pain and nausea, and investigation would reveal elevated lipase and amylase. The two most common risk factors are alcoholism and gallstones; however, there are other causes such as hypertriglyceridemia. Without an appropriate history, pancreatitis is not the most likely diagnosis in any of these patients.

Answer P is incorrect. Small bowel obstructions are common causes of abdominal pain, nausea, and vomiting. A small bowel obstruction most commonly results from postsurgical adhesions or hernias, and tumors will rarely be the underlying cause. Patients with a small bowel obstruction are surgical emergencies, as they need treatment before the development of peritoneal signs that suggest small bowel rupture. Radiographic findings would include air- and fluid-filled loops of small bowel, and eventually free air under the diaphragm if the bowel were to rupture.

Test Block 3

1. A 34-year-old woman presents to her primary care physician complaining of puffiness in her legs, arms, and face for 3 days. She often feels a little "bloated" during her menstrual period but is currently in the middle of her cycle, and states that she has not been drinking more than usual or eating too much salt. Examination reveals generalized edema but is otherwise unremarkable. Her physician draws blood for complete blood cell count, electrolytes, and thyroid function tests, and does a dipstick urinalysis in his office which shows 2+ proteinuria. He decides to hospitalize her and perform a renal biopsy to determine the etiology of her nephrotic syndrome. Biopsy shows a thickened basement membrane and immunofluorescence reveals IgG and C3 deposits in a "spike and dome" pattern in the basement membrane. Which of the following is the most likely cause of this patient's nephropathy?

(A) Anti–glomerular basement membrane antibodies
(B) Hepatitis B virus
(C) Idiopathic
(D) Penicillamine
(E) Systemic lupus erythematosus

2. A 26-year-old woman who is 38 weeks pregnant presents to the emergency department (ED) in active labor. She has felt ill for the past 2 days and has been taking acetaminophen for fevers. Last night she broke out in an itchy rash that has spread over her arms and torso. She is a day care teacher, and 2 weeks prior a parent of one of the children in her class had called and informed the day care center that her child was diagnosed with chickenpox. She says she doesn't remember if she had ever had chickenpox as a child. The patient wants to know what this means for her baby. What is the most correct advice to give this woman?

(A) "Nothing needs to be done; chickenpox in children and newborns is usually a mild, self-limiting illness"
(B) "The chance of transmitting the virus to your baby is low, so we will monitor the baby and treat if symptoms develop"

(C) "The varicella virus is teratogenic; therefore, your newborn may have some mild birth defects"
(D) "Your baby must be treated soon after birth because chickenpox is a serious illness in newborns"
(E) "Your baby will be protected because of your antibodies to the virus"

3. A 70-year-old smoker with a 50 pack-year smoking history is currently using a daily disk inhaler that delivers salmeterol and fluticasone. In addition, she has been recently discharged from the hospital for a chronic obstructive pulmonary disease (COPD) exacerbation and is being tapered off her 2-week course of oral prednisone. At one point, theophylline was added to her regimen during the inpatient stay and she was sent home with a prescription for supplemental oxygen to be delivered for 12 hours during the night. Which of the agents that this patient is currently taking has been shown to decrease overall mortality in patients with COPD?

(A) Inhaled glucocorticoids
(B) Salmeterol
(C) Supplemental oxygen
(D) Theophylline

4. A full-term girl is born to a 38-year-old white woman who received no prenatal care. The infant is pictured on the next page. Length and weight are in the 50th percentile; head circumference is less than the fifth percentile. She has a III/VI systolic ejection murmur that is loudest at the left sternal border. She has five digits on each hand and foot, but the digits of the hand are tightly clenched (see image). The karyotype for this child would most likely show which of the following?

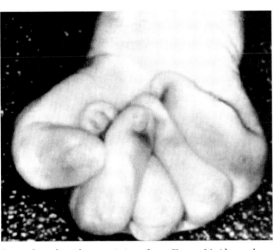

Reproduced, with permission, from Fuster V, Alexander RW, O'Rourke RA, eds. *Hurst's The Heart*, 11th ed. New York: McGraw-Hill, 2004: Figure 12-12.

(A) One X chromosome and no Y chromosome
(B) Normal 46,XY
(C) Three copies of chromosome 13
(D) Three copies of chromosome 18
(E) Three copies of chromosome 21

5. An 8-year-old boy presents to his pediatrician with recent onset of daily nosebleeds that have been occurring over the past 2 weeks. He has bruises on his legs and arms that appeared after playing on the playground at school. The patient has a history of easy bruising since early childhood. He denies painful, tender, or swollen joints. The boy's mother reports that she has a history of von Willebrand's disease. A workup for von Willebrand's disease would most likely reveal which of the following?

(A) Increased bleeding time
(B) Normal coagulation factor concentrations
(C) Prolonged prothrombin time
(D) Shortened partial thromboplastin time
(E) Thrombocytopenia

6. A 33-year-old man recently diagnosed with HIV comes to the clinic to reestablish care after not seeing a physician for more than 10 years. Which of the following immunizations is contraindicated in this patient at this time?

(A) Hepatitis A series
(B) Hepatitis B series
(C) Pneumococcal vaccine
(D) Tetanus booster
(E) Varicella vaccine

7. A 34-year-old man presents with fever and night sweats for 3 weeks and productive cough. A recent HIV test was negative. A purified protein derivative test placed on admission shows 15 mm induration. His erythrocyte sedimentation rate is 97 mm/h. His past medical history is significant for a relapse of alcoholism. Review of systems reveals generalized fatigue over the past month and a 3.2-kg (7-lb) weight loss. His temperature is 39.6°C (103.3°F), his respiratory rate is 25/min, and his oxygen saturation by pulse oximetry on room air is 86%. Bilateral pulmonary rales are noted on physical examination and moderate sternal retractions are present. X-ray of the chest reveals reticulonodular infiltrates spread evenly throughout both lung fields. Which of the following is the most likely diagnosis?

(A) Latent tuberculosis
(B) Miliary tuberculosis
(C) *Pneumocystis jiroveci* (formerly *carinii*) pneumonia
(D) Primary tuberculosis
(E) Reactivation pulmonary tuberculosis

8. A 39-year-old white man is referred to the gastrointestinal clinic for further workup of long-standing inflammatory bowel disease. He has had 1 week of worsening symptoms including frequent, loose, bloody stools and abdominal cramping. He is currently taking high-dose oral corticosteroids and cyclosporine, as his disease has been refractory to mesalamine, sulfasalazine, and lower doses of corticosteroids in the past. His laboratory tests thus far are negative for *Clostridium difficile*, ova, and parasites. Surgical resection is performed and a specimen is shown in the image. Which of the following findings is characteristic of this patient's condition?

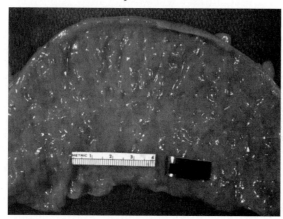

Reprinted, with permission, from PEIR Digital Library (http://peir.net).

(A) Absence of ganglion cells on full-thickness rectal biopsy
(B) An enterovesicular fistula
(C) Cobblestoning
(D) Crypt abscesses
(E) Transmural inflammation

9. A 20-year-old man presents to the clinic with a painful right testicle for the past month. The patient states that the pain has increased in intensity over the past 2 weeks. He denies any penile discharge. He is sexually active and has had several partners over the past few months. The patient has a temperature of 37.2°C (98.9°F). On examination, the testicle is swollen but no obvious mass is palpable. He is given the presumptive diagnosis of epididymitis and sent home on antibiotics. After completing the course of antibiotics, the patient returns to the clinic still complaining of swelling and a dull discomfort. What is the most appropriate imaging study at this point?

(A) CT scan of the pelvis
(B) Cystoscopy
(C) Intravenous pyelogram
(D) MRI scan of the testicles
(E) No imaging is necessary, try a second course of antibiotics
(F) Testicular ultrasound

10. A 65-year-old man in the hospital receiving spinal anesthesia for crush injuries to his lower extremities starts to notice labored breathing. He is afebrile but develops nausea and vomiting, and last had a bowel movement yesterday. His abdomen is distended and tympanic to percussion, although there are scattered bowel sounds. A plain upright abdominal film reveals a largely dilated colon extending from the cecum to the splenic flexure. Water-soluble enema fails to reveal mechanical obstruction. What is this patient's most likely diagnosis?

(A) Acute colonic pseudo-obstruction (Ogilvie's syndrome)
(B) Diverticulitis
(C) Intussusception
(D) Left-sided colonic adenocarcinoma
(E) Rectal squamous cell carcinoma

11. A patient with a history of visceral cysts and hemangioblastomas has recently been diagnosed with renal cell carcinoma at age 43. His family history is positive for a maternal grandfather and an uncle, both of whom died in their 50s from renal cell carcinoma. His mother died of a "brain tumor" shortly after giving birth to him. He has no siblings. The patient is married with three children ages 3, 5, and 9. All are healthy. Which of the following is the most appropriate next step in the management of this patient?

(A) The patient should undergo genetic testing for Osler-Weber-Rendu syndrome
(B) The patient should undergo genetic testing for tuberous sclerosis
(C) The patient should undergo genetic testing for von Hippel–Lindau disease
(D) There is no need for the patient or his children to undergo genetic testing
(E) The physician should proceed directly to testing the patient's children

12. A 26-year-old man was recently promoted to a new position in his corporation, one that requires a substantial amount of international travel. Prior to accepting the position, he had not flown in 7 years because his father was killed in an airplane crash. During his first transatlantic flight, he developed extreme anxiety, marked by palpitations, chest pain, and difficulty breathing. He was eventually demoted because of his continued refusal to attend meetings in Europe. Which of the following is this patient's most likely diagnosis?

(A) Angina pectoris
(B) Generalized anxiety disorder
(C) Hyperthyroidism
(D) Social phobia
(E) Specific phobia

13. A 68-year-old man with a history of coronary artery disease, atherosclerosis, and atrial fibrillation is brought to the ED with sudden onset of severe, crampy abdominal pain. The pain began following a massive bowel movement and was accompanied by the onset of nausea and vomiting. At presentation his temperature is 36.8°C (98.2°F), his blood pressure is 136/80 mm Hg, his heart rate is 76/min, and his respiratory rate is 14/min. On abdominal examination, the patient is writhing in pain without evidence of guarding or rebound tenderness. In addition, the patient states that his most recent bowel movement had some blood mixed in with the stool. Which test is the gold standard for the presenting condition?

(A) Angiogram
(B) Barium swallow
(C) Hepato-iminodiacetic acid scan
(D) Ultrasound of the abdomen
(E) X-ray of the abdomen

14. A 35-year-old African-American woman presents to the ED complaining of fever and cough. Her temperature is a 39.4°C (103°F), and she says that the cough is productive and the sputum looks like dark blood. On questioning she admits that she sometimes experiences shortness of breath and right-sided chest pain. She also admits binge drinking to the point of passing out several times a week. A chest radiograph is taken and shows consolidation of the upper and right middle lobe with loss of the right heart border. Which of the following is the most likely pathogen?

(A) *Klebsiella pneumoniae*
(B) *Legionella pneumophila*
(C) *Pneumocystis jiroveci* (formerly *carinii*) pneumonia
(D) *Pseudomonas aeruginosa* pneumonia
(E) *Streptococcus pneumoniae*

15. A 36-year-old woman presents to an infertility clinic with her husband. They married 1 year ago and have been trying to conceive ever since. She states that she is in good health, although she complains of irregular menses over the past year, with feelings of inadequacy, dyspareunia, difficulty sleeping, and episodes of warmth and sweating at night. Her history reveals no history of thyroid disease, no galactorrhea, and a body mass index of 30, and she uses no medications or street drugs, but notes a 15 pack-year smoking history. She has never been pregnant, nor has she ever had any sexually transmitted diseases. She has not menstruated in 4 months, but pregnancy tests have been repeatedly negative. Her husband, who is also 36, is also in good health and has two children from a previous marriage. What is the next best step in management?

(A) Obtain a hysterosalpingogram
(B) Obtain an MRI of the brain
(C) Obtain a postcoital test
(D) Obtain follicle-stimulating hormone and luteinizing hormone levels
(E) Perform a progestin challenge

16. A 40-year-old man is brought to the ED after being involved in a motor vehicle crash. He is hemodynamically stable. Primary and secondary surveys are performed, and his injuries seem to consist of a right hip dislocation and a small laceration on his forehead. His right lower extremity is shortened, flexed, adducted, and internally rotated at the hip. His right lower extremity was warm and well perfused with distal pulses intact. An orthopedic surgeon is called for a suspected closed hip dislocation. Prompt treatment will significantly reduce the incidence of which of the following complications?

(A) Avascular necrosis
(B) Femoral nerve damage
(C) Myositis ossificans
(D) Posttraumatic degenerative arthritis
(E) Recurrent dislocation

17. A 78-year-old man with a 9-year history of chronic myelogenous leukemia treated with imatinib presents with weight loss and early satiety. Splenomegaly is noted on examination, and routine laboratory evaluation reveals a WBC count of 11,000/mm–, hemoglobin of 7.5 mg/dL, and platelets of 460,000/mm–. An attempted bone marrow aspiration is unsuccessful. Bone marrow biopsy is then performed and yields the image shown. Which of the following is the most likely diagnosis?

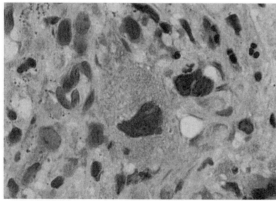

Reproduced, with permission, from Lichtman MA, Beutler E, Kipps TJ, Seligsohn U, Kaushansky K, Prchal JT. *Williams Hematology*, 7th ed. New York: McGraw-Hill, 2006: Plate XIV-11.

(A) Bernard-Soulier syndrome
(B) Idiopathic sideroblastic anemia
(C) Myelodysplastic syndrome

(D) Myelofibrosis
(E) Progression of chronic myelogenous leukemia to blast phase
(F) Second malignant neoplasm resulting from exposure to alkylating agents

18. A 71-year-old woman presents to ambulatory clinic with a chief complaint of dyspnea upon exertion. Over the past few weeks, she has had a chronic cough and shortness of breath when walking more than two city blocks. She has a long history of hypertension that has been poorly controlled in recent years. On physical examination, she has an elevated jugular venous pulse and rales are evident on lung examination. Cardiac enzymes are negative. Which modality is the most appropriate next step in distinguishing systolic from diastolic heart failure?

(A) Cardiac catheterization
(B) Clinical judgment based on physical examination
(C) CT scan of the chest
(D) Echocardiography
(E) Electrocardiogram
(F) MRI of the heart
(G) X-ray of the chest

19. A 22-month-old boy presents to the pediatrician because he has not yet begun to walk. He was able to hold his head steady at 5 months, sit unsupported at 8 months, and crawl at 12 months of age. When he crawls, he drags his legs. He takes no medications and has no known allergies. His family history is noncontributory. On examination, his legs are hypertonic bilaterally with brisk patellar reflexes; he has ankle clonus and upgoing toes bilaterally. Strength is 4 of 5 in his legs bilaterally and 5 of 5 in his arms bilaterally. What is the most appropriate therapy?

(A) ACTH and clonazepam
(B) Benztropine
(C) Diazepam and physical therapy
(D) Levodopa and carbidopa
(E) Pimozide

20. Which of the following is an appropriate choice in the management of a heroin overdose patient?

(A) Administer 4 mg of intravenous naloxone

(B) Assess the patient's kidney function

(C) Check the patient's respiratory function and establish airway access if necessary

(D) Monitor the patient for potentially life-threatening withdrawal symptoms

(E) Treat withdrawal symptoms with benzodiazepines

21. A 45-year-old HIV-positive man with a CD4+ of count 63/mm³ presents to the ED with a headache and fever. Treatment for bacterial meningitis is initiated while the physician runs additional laboratory tests. However, his symptoms fail to improve with treatment and all bacterial cultures return negative. Given the clinical scenario, which of the following laboratory tests is most likely to confirm the diagnosis?

(A) Lumbar puncture and cryptococcal antigen test

(B) Lumbar puncture and culture

(C) Lumbar puncture and India ink stain

(D) Lumbar puncture and potassium hydroxide preparation

(E) Lumbar puncture and silver stain

22. A 27-year-old G1P1 woman presents to her obstetrician 3 weeks after an uncomplicated labor and delivery of a healthy, full-term, 3.2-kg (7-lb) baby boy. The patient states that she has been nursing her son without trouble since delivery until several days ago, when she noticed that her right nipple was red, dry, and cracked. Her right breast has become increasingly sensitive, and she has continued breast-feeding her son despite the discomfort. Vital signs are notable for a temperature of 38°C (100.4°F). Physical examination reveals a warm, well-circumscribed, 5-cm erythematous patch on the right breast that is tender to light touch. No pus can be expressed from the right nipple. Which of the following is the most appropriate initial therapy?

(A) Incision and drainage

(B) Intravenous oxacillin

(C) Oral cephalexin

(D) Oral doxycycline

(E) Warm compresses

23. A 16-year-old football quarterback is in the midst of throwing a football with his shoulder in an abducted and externally rotated position. His throwing arm is suddenly hit by an oncoming defender, and he senses an immediate pop and pain in his shoulder. He is unable to move his shoulder without intense discomfort and maintains it in an adducted, externally rotated position. He states that his whole arm hurts and feels "heavy." A lump is palpated anteriorly at his shoulder, and a defect is noted below his acromioclavicular joint. The athletic trainer fears an associated nerve injury. Where should the trainer test light touch to assess the integrity of this nerve?

(A) Over the dorsum of the hand

(B) Over the medial side of the palm

(C) Over the palmar aspect of the third digit

(D) Over the palmar aspect of the thumb

(E) Over the superior lateral upper arm

24. The Framingham Heart Study began in 1950 with the intent of collecting data on risk factors and following patients over time to assess the effect of these factors on the development of disease. This is an example of which type of study design?

(A) Case-control

(B) Meta-analysis

(C) Prospective cohort

(D) Randomized controlled trial

(E) Retrospective cohort

25. A 67-year-old man is seen for increased urinary frequency. He noticed for the past year that it has been difficult for him to begin urinating. The stream has also not been as strong as it was previously. He now he has to get up two or three times a night to go to the bathroom. A physical examination showed an enlarged prostate with no nodules, induration, or asymmetry. Urinalysis showed specific gravity of 1.010 and pH of 6, and was negative for nitrites and leukoesterase. Which of the following would be the most appropriate pharmacologic management for this patient?

(A) Aspirin

(B) Bacille Calmette-Guérin

(C) Finasteride

(D) Oxybutynin

(E) Trimethoprim-sulfamethoxazole

26. A 42-year-old woman with stage IV breast cancer presents to her oncologist with a complaint of worsening chest pain over the past 2 weeks. The pain is retrosternal, worsens when she lies down, and improves when she leans forward. She carries a diagnosis of neoplastic pericarditis and has had similar symptoms in the past. She has tried nonsteroidal anti-inflammatory drugs, colchicine, and even steroids, but these medications have only given her temporary relief, and her chest pain soon returns. She has no other medical problems. She takes tamoxifen and bisphosphonates. On physical examination, she is tearful and appears to be in pain. She has a regular rate and rhythm, normal S1 and S2, and a pericardial friction rub. Her lungs are clear to auscultation bilaterally. The remainder of her physical examination is benign. Her temperature is 37.5°C (99.5°F), heart rate 80/min, blood pressure 132/78 mm Hg, and respiratory rate 16/min. Her O_2 saturation is 99%. Her ECG shows diffuse ST segment elevation. X-ray of the chest is shown in the image. Which of the following is the best way to manage this patient's chest pain?

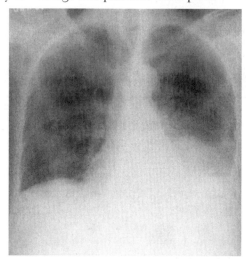

Reproduced, with permission, from Chen MYM, Pope TL, Ott DJ. *Basic Radiology.* New York: McGraw-Hill, 2004: Figure 4-52.

(A) Balloon pericardiotomy
(B) Emergent pericardiocentesis
(C) Ibuprofen 600 mg orally three times a day
(D) Morphine patient-controlled analgesia
(E) Nitroglycerin 0.3 mg sublingually as needed

27. A 21-year-old college student is brought to the ED after having attended a party at which he was offered a substance blotted on a small sheet of paper. A few minutes after placing the substance on his tongue, the student noticed that the edges of the wall had begun to look like cylindrical bars, with flashing lights alternating in bright colors alongside the bars. At one point he felt that the walls of the room were shifting horizontally and spinning. This effect lasted for about an hour and then dissipated. What is the most likely cause of this patient's presentation?

(A) Cocaine
(B) Ecstasy
(C) Heroin
(D) Lysergic acid diethylamide
(E) Marijuana

28. A 70-year-old man presents with a painless swelling of the right supraclavicular area. He states that he has lost approximately 11.3 kg (25 lb) over the past 3 months and describes generalized pruritus. On examination, he is cachectic, and his spleen is palpable 2 cm below the costal margin. A matted mass is palpable in the right supraclavicular area. X-ray of the chest reveals mediastinal lymphadenopathy. The supraclavicular mass is biopsied and reveals many Reed-Sternberg cells with few lymphocytes. The man is treated with chemotherapy and radiation therapy but shows little response. He expires from respiratory failure 6 months later. What is the most likely diagnosis?

(A) Burkitt's lymphoma
(B) Lymphocyte-depleted Hodgkin's lymphoma
(C) Lymphocyte-predominant Hodgkin's lymphoma
(D) Nodular sclerosing lymphoma
(E) Non-Hodgkin's lymphoma
(F) T-lymphocyte leukemia

29. A 15-year-old girl presents to the outpatient clinic complaining of progressive pain around her left knee that has become intractable. She states that the pain is worst at night and does not respond to nonsteroidal anti-inflammatory medications. On review of systems, she states

having intermittent fever and gradual weight loss over the past 3 months. On examination, the left thigh is swollen, tense, and tender. Laboratory results reveal hemoglobin 12.4 g/dL, WBC count 10,600/mm³, platelets 380,000/mm³, erythrocyte sedimentation rate 18 mm/h, and alkaline phosphatase 320 U/L. X-ray of the knee is shown in the image. What is the most likely diagnosis?

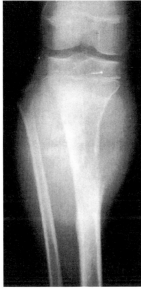

Reprinted, with permission, from Doherty GM, Way LW. *Current Surgical Diagnosis and Treatment*, 12th edition. New York: McGraw-Hill, 2006: Figure 42-49.

(A) Fibrous dysplasia
(B) Nonossifying fibroma
(C) Osteoid osteoma
(D) Osteomyelitis
(E) Osteosarcoma

30. A 45-year-old African-American diabetic man reports to his primary care physician complaining of unbearable pain in his left ear. The patient states that the pain is worse with chewing and any movement of his head or ear lobe. The primary care physician notes pus draining from the ear. There is redness around the base of the ear, and MRI shows bone involvement. The patient denies having a fever, but states that he occasionally sweats at night and has a headache. The patient's temperature is 37.9°C (100.2°F). Which of the following is the most appropriate pharmacotherapy?

(A) A fluoroquinolone plus a β-lactam
(B) Amoxicillin
(C) Amphotericin B
(D) Methicillin
(E) Topical antibiotics

31. A 72-year-old woman presents to clinic with a chief complaint of weakness and fatigue. She has had difficulty breathing over the past several weeks and now must sleep on two pillows at night to get comfortable. In addition, she reports an episode of syncope last week. Cardiac biopsy reveals amyloid deposits. Which of these findings is consistent with the biopsy results?

(A) Ejection fraction of 55% on echocardiography
(B) Harsh diastolic murmur
(C) Right lower quadrant abdominal mass
(D) Upper extremity edema
(E) U waves on ECG
(F) Wheezing on lung examination

32. A 68-year-old woman with a history of central retinal vein occlusion presents to the ophthalmology clinic for an annual examination. She has a history of cerebrovascular accident 2 years ago. She notes that for the past 3 months, she has been experiencing periorbital pain around her right eye, associated with an ipsilateral headache. She also complains of intermittent blurry vision, and "seeing halos around objects." What is the most appropriate curative treatment for this patient?

(A) Acetazolamide
(B) Atropine
(C) Laser iridotomy
(D) Pilocarpine
(E) Timolol

33. A 38-year-old African-American woman with a history of endometriosis presents to her primary care physician complaining of increasing difficulty swallowing over the last few months. It has progressively gotten worse, and she is worried because she is beginning to lose too much weight. She also reports that her skin has changed during this time period, is now more "tight," and the color has become darker, especially around her fingers and face. In addition, she reports some trouble breathing with exertion and increased fatigue. Before the physician begins the examination, the patient remembers that when she is cold, her hands hurt her and "change to all sorts of colors." Her blood pressure is 128/78 mm Hg, pulse 88/min, respiratory rate 18/min, and temperature 37.1°C (98.9°F). She denies any drug abuse or travel and has not been in contact with anyone who has been sick. On physical examination, the physician notes that her skin is indeed hyperpigmented and that it surrounds areas that are normal. The physician hears very mild rales on respiratory examination and notes telangiectasias on her face. Which of the following is the most likely diagnosis?

(A) Irritable bowel syndrome
(B) Mallory-Weiss syndrome
(C) Myasthenia gravis
(D) Primary biliary cirrhosis
(E) Scleroderma

34. A 40-year-old, G3P3 woman presents to her gynecologist for "urine leakage." She has had diabetes for many years, and it has been poorly controlled. When asked further about her urine leakage, she reports that it mainly occurs when she has a full bladder if she coughs or sneezes. Which of the following is most likely to lead to resolving this woman's incontinence?

(A) Anticholinergic medication
(B) Intermittent catheterization
(C) Sacral nerve stimulation
(D) Surgery
(E) Vaginal estrogen cream

35. A 1-week-old term girl is brought to the pediatrician for her first visit following a home birth. Her father is concerned that she sleeps too much and is only having bowel movements every 3 to 4 days. She passed meconium on the first day of life. He is worried that his daughter is sick because his wife "partied" heavily during the first 2 months of pregnancy before they realized she was pregnant. The maternal medical history is also significant for an "overactive neck gland" for which she takes medicine. On examination, the infant's height, weight, and head circumference are all in the 50th percentile. Her temperature is 35°C (95°F). She has an enlarged anterior fontanelle, enlarged tongue, poor muscle tone, and dry skin. Which of the following is the most likely etiology for the infant's condition?

(A) Inadequate nutrition from formula
(B) Maternal alcohol use during pregnancy
(C) Maternal cocaine use during pregnancy
(D) Maternal use of antithyroid medication
(E) Poorly controlled maternal diabetes

36. A 67-year-old woman was recently started on a new medication for essential hypertension. At a previous primary care visit, she had a blood pressure of 145/88 mm Hg, so she was sent home with instructions to adopt a low-salt diet. On returning to the clinic, her blood pressure was 148/90 mm Hg, and she was started on an antihypertensive. Two weeks into this course, she began to complain of muscle weakness and difficulty breathing, so she returned to her physician, who suspected a dysrhythmia and ordered an ECG (see image). Which of the following pairs of medications could have led to this adverse effect?

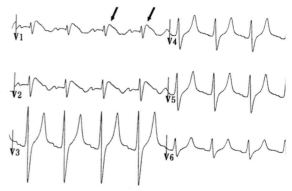

Reproduced, with permission, from Fuster V, Alexander RW, O'Rourke RA, eds. *Hurst's The Heart*, 11th ed. New York: McGraw-Hill, 2004: Figure 13-33.

(A) Acetazolamide
(B) Furosemide
(C) Hydralazine
(D) Hydrochlorothiazide
(E) Losartan

37. An otherwise healthy 25-year-old medical student presents to the ED with a 2-week history of chills, fever, and malaise. His physical examination reveals a fever of 38.3°C (101°F) and stable vital signs with no other abnormal findings. Urine, blood, and sputum cultures are taken and all are negative for growth. The patient is admitted for observation and further testing, yet after a week no explanation is found. Which of the following is the most likely cause of a fever in this patient?

(A) Collagen vascular disease
(B) Granulomatous disease
(C) Infection
(D) Neoplasm
(E) Pulmonary emboli

38. A 54-year-old man visits his physician for a regular checkup. The man has a history of diverticular disease and diabetes and has no current medical complaints. He denies tobacco use or any family history of cardiac disease. On examination, the patient is afebrile and normotensive. His lipid profile is total cholesterol 230 mg/dL, LDL cholesterol 120 mg/dL, and HDL cholesterol 47 mg/dL. In terms of managing this man's hyperlipidemia, what is the next best step?

(A) Lower LDL cholesterol to < 100 mg/dL, even as low as < 70 mg/dL
(B) Lower LDL cholesterol to < 130 mg/dL
(C) Raise HDL cholesterol to > 50 mg/dL
(D) Recommend a high-fiber and low-fat diet
(E) Recommend regular exercise

39. A 26-year-old woman, 14 weeks pregnant with her first child, presents to the ED complaining of light vaginal bleeding and mild cramping that began the previous day. Her vital signs are: blood pressure 112/80 mm Hg, heart rate 90/min, respiratory rate 16/min, and temperature 37°C (98.6°F). A pelvic examination reveals some blood in the vaginal vault without evidence of clots or tissue, and the cervical os is closed. Fetal heart tones are present at 135/min. What is the next appropriate step in management?

(A) Betamethasone administration
(B) Cervical cerclage
(C) Dilation and curettage
(D) Magnesium sulfate administration
(E) Observation

40. A 56-year-old woman is brought to the ED by her spouse for evaluation of obtundation. Earlier in the evening, the spouse reports that the patient complained of shakiness and a racing heartbeat. The patient is a type 2 diabetic and sulfonylurea pharmacotherapy was recently initiated. The patient also began taking 81 mg of aspirin at the time of her diabetes diagnosis. There is a family history of heart disease. On examination, the patient is oriented to person only, appears lethargic, and is diaphoretic. Her temperature is 36.9°C (98.4°F), blood pressure is 155/91 mm Hg, pulse is 112/min, and respiratory rate is 18/min. Laboratory studies are pending. Which of the following is most likely to be used in the management of this patient?

(A) Epinephrine
(B) Glucose
(C) Insulin
(D) Naloxone
(E) Tissue plasminogen activator

41. A 37-year-old man presents to his new primary care physician with a small, symmetric, monochromatic brown macule with regular borders that has been on his forearm "for many years." After complaining that "none of my doctors have taken me seriously," he states that he believes he is dying of melanoma. He adds that he has seen several specialists over the past year, and while all of them have assured him that his lesion is "just a mole," he is certain that this is not the case. The patient has no other complaints, no systemic symptoms, and no medical or surgical history. What is the most likely diagnosis?

(A) Basal cell carcinoma
(B) Body dysmorphic disorder
(C) Hypochondriasis
(D) Somatization disorder
(E) Squamous cell carcinoma

42. A 72-year-old woman undergoes three-vessel coronary artery bypass graft for coronary artery disease. Her postoperative course is complicated by wound infection leading to sepsis with multidrug-resistant *Klebsiella*. Her sepsis is difficult to manage, and she is on pressors, fluids, and antibiotics for several days before becoming afebrile and hemodynamically stable. Her creatinine rises postoperatively, and on postoperative day 4 electrolytes show blood urea nitrogen (BUN) of 34 mg/dL and creatinine of 2.6 mg/dL. Urine Na is 46 mEq/L, fractional excretion of sodium is calculated as 2.1%, and urine osmolarity is 310 mOsm/kg. Urinalysis shows muddy brown granular casts. Over the next week, her creatinine continues to rise despite aggressive fluid management; however, she continues to make small amounts of urine, and BUN and creatinine gradually return to normal over the next few weeks. What is the most likely pathogenesis of this woman's acute renal failure?

(A) Allergic reaction to dobutamine
(B) Autoimmune glomerular destruction
(C) Hypovolemic shock
(D) Ischemic tubular injury
(E) *Klebsiella* infection of the kidney

43. A 22-year-old G2P1 woman at 38 weeks' gestation presents to the labor and delivery suite in labor after a pregnancy with poor prenatal care. After several hours of labor, her temperature is 39.1°C (102.4°F). On examination, she has significant abdominal tenderness. A complete blood cell count shows a white count of 18,400/mm³. The child is delivered with an Apgar score of 8 but is lethargic the day after delivery, with a temperature of 34.8°C (94.6°F), respiratory rate of 24/min, heart rate of 186/min, and mean blood pressure of 32 mm Hg. For which pathogen could good prenatal care with screening and treatment have prevented these complications?

(A) *Chlamydia trachomatis*
(B) Group B streptococci
(C) HIV
(D) Toxoplasmosis
(E) *Treponema palladium*

44. On routine evaluation, a 52-year-old woman is found to have a serum calcium level of 12.2 mg/dL and an elevated serum parathyroid hormone level. On further questioning, she admits to daily muscle pain that has been increasing in intensity. The most likely cause of her condition is which one of the following?

(A) Ectopic parathyroid tissue
(B) Multiple adenoma
(C) Parathyroid carcinoma
(D) Parathyroid hyperplasia
(E) Single adenoma

EXTENDED MATCHING

Questions 45 and 46

For each patient's infection, select the most likely etiologic agent.

(A) *Bacillus cereus*
(B) *Campylobacter jejuni*
(C) *Clostridium difficile*
(D) Enteric adenovirus
(E) *Escherichia coli*
(F) *Giardia lamblia*
(G) Rotavirus
(H) *Salmonella*
(I) *Shigella*
(J) *Staphylococcus aureus*
(K) *Vibrio cholerae*
(L) *Vibrio parahaemolyticus*

45. The parents of an otherwise healthy 13-month-old boy present to the ED in the winter concerned about their son's recent diarrhea and vomiting. They report that he developed a mild fever approximately 2 days ago along with vomiting that was nonbloody and nonbilious. They took him to the pediatrician at that time, and he was diagnosed with gastroenteritis. His parents were told to monitor his fluids closely and return if his condition changed. He has now stopped vomiting but has developed watery stools that are passed approximately every 1–2 hours. His parents report that he attends day care, and recently there have been numerous children out of the program because of similar illness. His vital signs are heart rate 122/min, blood pressure 80/50 mm Hg, and

respiratory rate 28/min. His physical examination is notable for dry mucous membranes.

46. An otherwise healthy 9-year-old girl is brought to the ED after the acute development of fever (temperature 38.8°C [101.8°F]), nausea, vomiting, diarrhea, and crampy periumbilical abdominal pain. A review of her diet over the past 48 hours includes cereals, fruits, egg salad sandwiches, steamed vegetables, hamburger, grilled chicken, Christmas cookies, and homemade eggnog. At the time of evaluation, her vital signs are stable, but she has a mild fever (temperature 38.4°C [101.1°F]). She is fatigued but alert. Her abdominal examination is notable for periumbilical tenderness, but no guarding or rebound tenderness is noted, and no masses are palpated.

1. **The correct answer is C.** Nephrotic syndrome with the histology pattern of membranous nephropathy is the most common cause of nephropathy among white adults and is most frequently idiopathic. Up to one-third of patients undergo spontaneous remission, one-third continue to have proteinuria but maintain stable renal function, and the last third progress to end-stage renal failure at 5–10 years. Treatment is controversial, as corticosteroids alone as a primary therapy have not been proven to be effective and the risks of cytotoxic therapy do not justify their use when spontaneous partial to complete remission may occur in up to 40% of patients. Currently, cytotoxic therapy should only be offered to patients who are considered to be at high risk for progression based on clinical risk factors.

Answer A is incorrect. Anti-glomerular basement membrane antibodies are seen in Goodpasture's syndrome, which presents with nephritic syndrome and signs of pulmonary hemorrhage such as hemoptysis. Renal biopsy in this disorder shows linear deposits of the antibody, which is different from the histologic pattern seen in membranous glomerulonephropathies.

Answer B is incorrect. The membranous nephropathy histology may also be seen in patients with hepatitis B, but this is less common than the idiopathic form.

Answer D is incorrect. The membranous nephropathy histology may be seen in renal disease associated with the drugs penicillamine and gold, which may be used to treat rheumatoid arthritis. This patient, however, has no history of rheumatologic disease.

Answer E is incorrect. The membranous nephropathy histology may also be seen in patients with systemic lupus erythematosus, but this is less common than the idiopathic form.

2. **The correct answer is D.** Varicella is a highly contagious virus that causes a potentially life-threatening illness in newborns. The presentation is variable but can include fever, vesicular lesions, pneumonia, or meningitis. Newborns with mothers infected within 2 weeks of delivery are at greatest risk for complications, as maternal antibodies may not have been available to confer passive immunity to the infant. Patients should be treated with varicella-zoster immune globulin.

Answer A is incorrect. If untreated, chickenpox infection in newborns carries an approximately 30% mortality rate.

Answer B is incorrect. If untreated, chickenpox infection in newborns carries an approximately 30% mortality rate. Treatment with varicella-zoster immune globulin is started before symptoms develop for maximum efficacy.

Answer C is incorrect. Varicella infection during the first trimester can result in limb and digit defects, but the risk is small (approximately 1%).

Answer E is incorrect. If a woman develops symptoms from varicella virus (as this woman has), she will not have adequate antibodies against the virus in time to pass them on to the infant before delivery.

3. **The correct answer is C.** Supplemental oxygen is the only therapy demonstrated to decrease mortality in patients with chronic obstructive pulmonary disease. For patients with resting hypoxemia (resting arterial oxygen saturation < 88%, or < 90% with signs of pulmonary hypertension or right heart failure), the use of oxygen has been demonstrated to have a significant impact on mortality. The Medical Research Council Trial demonstrated that 12 hours per day was superior to no oxygen supplementation, but continuous oxygen was even better.

Answer A is incorrect. Several recent trials have failed to find a beneficial effect for the regular use of inhaled glucocorticoids on the rate of decline of lung function, as assessed by forced expiratory volume in 1 second.

Answer B is incorrect. Although chronic obstructive pulmonary disease (COPD) is characterized by airway inflammation/obstruction that is largely irreversible, salmeterol given in the acute setting can be used to improve any component of airway constriction that is reversible. No studies have shown that it affects overall mortality in COPD.

Answer D is incorrect. Theophylline has not be shown to decrease mortality in chronic obstructive pulmonary disease.

4. **The correct answer is D.** The infant pictured has microphthalmia, micrognathia, low-set/malformed ears, a short sternum, and abnormal clenched fingers, which are all signs of trisomy 18, Edwards' syndrome. Other common findings include rocker-bottom feet, a prominent occiput, and heart murmurs consistent with congenital heart disease. Risk factors include advanced maternal age, greater than 35 years.

Answer A is incorrect. Turner's syndrome, chromosomal complement XO, presents at birth with webbing of the neck and coarctation of the aorta. Often it is not detected until puberty, when these females present with primary amenorrhea secondary to ovarian dysgenesis. Short stature is another common finding in Turner's syndrome.

Answer B is incorrect. Karyotypes are useful in detecting large translocations and deletions, aneuploidy, and polyploidy. There are many congenital defects resulting from single gene disorders, microdeletions, small translocations, uniparental disomy, and environmental factors that are undetectable by karyotype analysis. Edwards' syndrome, however, is detectable by karyotype analysis.

Answer C is incorrect. Trisomy 13, Patau's syndrome, classically presents with microphthalmia, microcephaly, cleft lip and/or cleft palate, polydactyly, and congenital heart disease.

Answer E is incorrect. Trisomy 21, Down's syndrome, classically presents with flat facial profile, prominent epicanthal folds, simian creases, congenital heart disease, and mental retardation.

5. **The correct answer is A.** Von Willebrand's factor forms a bridge between platelets and ves-

sel endothelium and acts as a carrier protein for factor VIII of the coagulation pathway. Patients with von Willebrand's disease (qualitative or quantitative defects in von Willebrand's factor) therefore have defective platelet function and abnormalities in the coagulation pathway. Because bleeding time correlates with platelet function, von Willebrand's disease is associated with decreased platelet interaction with the vessel endothelium and subsequent increased bleeding time.

Answer B is incorrect. Von Willebrand's factor normally stabilizes factor VIII in the circulation. Therefore, deficiency of von Willebrand's factor may lead to factor VIII proteolysis with reduced levels of factor VIII in the circulation.

Answer C is incorrect. Because von Willebrand's factor stabilizes factor VIII of the coagulation pathway, increased partial thromboplastin time (PTT) (due to decreased factor VIII concentration) may occur in a patient with abnormal von Willebrand's factor. Factor VIII is part of the intrinsic coagulation pathway, which corresponds to PTT, not prothrombin time (PT). Therefore, decreased levels of factor VIIII will not lead to prolonged PT, only prolonged PTT.

Answer D is incorrect. Von Willebrand's factor normally stabilizes factor VIII in the circulation. Abnormalities of von Willebrand's factor, such as those seen in von Willebrand's disease, are associated with a prolonged (not shortened) partial thromboplastin time due to increased proteolysis of factor VIII and decreased factor VIII concentrations.

Answer E is incorrect. Patients with von Willebrand's disease (vWD) have normal platelet counts, but abnormal platelet function, resulting in abnormal interactions between platelets and the vessel endothelium. Because there is no indication of decreased platelet formation or increased platelet destruction in a patient with von Willebrand's disease, the patient would not have disease-related thrombocytopenia, except in the 2N variant. The 2N variant is very rare, and patients will present with hematuria, joint and soft tissue bleeding, unlike the other variants of vWD that present mostly with mucocutaneous bleeds.

6. **The correct answer is E.** Live vaccines are not recommended for immunocompromised individuals. Live attenuated viral vaccines include oral poliovirus, measles, varicella, mumps, and yellow fever vaccines.

Answer A is incorrect. The hepatitis A series is recommended for all HIV-positive patients. It can be administered with the hepatitis B vaccine.

Answer B is incorrect. The hepatitis B series is recommended for all HIV-positive patients. It can be administered with the hepatitis A vaccine.

Answer C is incorrect. The pneumococcal vaccine is recommended for all HIV-positive patients every 3–5 years.

Answer D is incorrect. A tetanus booster is recommended for all patients every 10 years.

7. **The correct answer is B.** Miliary tuberculosis (TB) refers to the hematogenous spread of *Mycobacterium tuberculosis* following reactivation of a latent infection or progressive primary infection. The clinical presentation of miliary TB varies from fever of unknown origin to multisystem organ failure. The important information here is the classic miliary pattern on x-ray of the chest indicative of hematogenous spread.

Answer A is incorrect. Latent tuberculosis would not be symptomatic, but may be accompanied by radiographic abnormalities.

Answer C is incorrect. *Pneumocystis jiroveci* (formerly *carinii*) pneumonia would be more likely in the setting of HIV, hematologic malignancy, or some other immunocompromised host.

Answer D is incorrect. While miliary tuberculosis can be a result of progressive primary infection, this is less common in the era of antibiotics. The most common symptom of primary infection is fever, with less than 25% having pulmonary complaints. The most common radiographic finding is hilar adenopathy with focal infiltrates being less common.

Answer E is incorrect. Most cases of symptomatic tuberculosis are due to reactivation of a latent infection confined to the lungs. The typical radiograph findings might reveal more discrete infiltrates or cavitary lesions involving the apical-posterior segments of the upper lobes.

8. **The correct answer is D.** Ulcerative colitis (UC) is an idiopathic autoinflammatory disorder of the colon that always involves the rectum. In fact, 40–50% of cases are limited to the rectum or rectosigmoid. Lesions may also spread proximally in a continuous manner to involve the entire colon. Findings include crypt abscesses with numerous polymorphonuclear leukocytes, friable mucosal patches that bleed easily, and pseudopolyps; the diagnosis is made on colonoscopy with biopsy showing these findings. Symptoms include bloody diarrhea and colicky abdominal pain. Ulcerative colitis is initially treated with sulfasalazine or mesalamine. Refractory disease is managed with corticosteroids and cyclosporine; however, total colectomy is curative for long-standing disease or fulminant colitis. This patient's surgical specimen shows a pan-ulcerative colitis. The mucosa has a lumpy, bumpy appearance because of areas of inflamed but intact mucosa are separated by ulcerated areas. UC carries a markedly increased risk of colorectal cancer in long-standing cases.

Answer A is incorrect. Hirschsprung's disease is caused by absence of autonomic innervation of the bowel wall, leading to inadequate relaxation and peristalsis resulting in intestinal obstruction. Patients present with abdominal distention, bilious vomiting, and failure to pass meconium in the first 24 hours of life. Diagnosis is confirmed by rectal biopsy showing an absence of ganglion cells. Treatment is via colostomy.

Answer B is incorrect. Crohn's disease involves transmural lesions that can involve the entire bowel wall thickness. As a result, these patients often develop enterovesical and enterocutaneous fistulas. Physical examination may reveal perianal fissures or fistulas.

Answer C is incorrect. Crohn's disease is an inflammatory disease of the gastrointestinal (GI) tract that may be infectious in nature. It can affect any part of the GI tract, but typically involves the ileocecal region. Symptoms include abdominal pain, watery diarrhea, fever, and weight loss. Diagnosis is based on biopsy of the affected area, showing transmural inflammation, noncaseating granulomas, cobblestone mucosal morphology, and skip lesions. Creeping fat on gross dissection is pathognomonic. Crohn's disease is managed with sulfasalazine, and then corticosteroids and immunosuppression if refractory. The newest treatment is the anti–tumor necrosis factor antibody, infliximab. Surgical resection may be necessary for perforation.

Answer E is incorrect. The inflammation seen in Crohn's disease is transmural on biopsy.

9. **The correct answer is F.** Testicular malignancy can present with testicular discomfort and swelling, which may lead a clinician to diagnose the patient with orchitis or epididymitis. The initial trial of antibiotics is reasonable, but given the persistent swelling and discomfort, an ultrasound is warranted. Despite this patient's presentation, the pathognomonic presentation for testicular cancer is a painless testicular mass.

Answer A is incorrect. A CT scan of the pelvis is a reasonable way to assess if there are large nodes or other signs of metastatic disease. The cost and exposure to radiation is not appropriate in this situation. Ultrasound is the next best step.

Answer B is incorrect. Cystoscopy is a useful tool for evaluation of the bladder. The evaluation of the testicle is not aided by cystoscopy.

Answer C is incorrect. Intravenous pyelogram is a test that helps clinicians assess the urinary tract. The test would not add any information to the evaluation of the testicle.

Answer D is incorrect. An MRI is not necessary at this point. This method of imaging would identify a lesion and its extent, but it is costly and unnecessary.

Answer E is incorrect. The persistence of symptoms should lead to imaging. Another attempt at antibiotics would probably not delay

treatment considerably, but imaging is more appropriate.

10. **The correct answer is A.** This patient has a typical presentation for Ogilvie's syndrome. Patients typically present with nausea, vomiting, constipation, diarrhea, abdominal distention, a tympanic abdomen, and positive bowel sounds, and with hypokalemia, hypocalcemia, and hypomagnesemia. X-rays show dilation of the right large intestine. Bowel distension may make breathing labored. Before making this diagnosis, mechanical obstruction must be ruled out, and toxic megacolon excluded on the basis of the clinical picture. Toxic megacolon presents with colonic dilation and fever, tachycardia, leukocytosis, and anemia. The actual etiology of Ogilvie's syndrome is unknown. Treatment includes nasogastric and rectal tube placement, frequent turning, and neostigmine to promote decompression of the colon. Serial abdominal x-rays help to monitor cecal size and determine the aggressiveness of therapy.

Answer B is incorrect. Diverticulitis would most commonly present as localized abdominal pain with possible signs of peritonitis and fever. This patient's presentation is not typical of diverticulitis.

Answer C is incorrect. Intussusception is most commonly associated with infants and a sausage-type mass felt in the left lower quadrant, as well as having "currant-jelly" stool.

Answer D is incorrect. Left-sided colonic adenocarcinoma produces colonic distention by mechanical obstruction with an "apple-core" lesion. The enema in this situation ruled out mechanical obstruction.

Answer E is incorrect. Squamous cell carcinoma of the rectum would not present with the symptoms from which this patient is suffering.

11. **The correct answer is C.** This patient has symptoms and family history suggesting von Hippel–Lindau (VHL) disease, an autosomal dominant disorder characterized by hemangioblastomas, retinal angiomas, pheochromocytoma, and renal cell carcinoma. Various manifestations of this disease have affected the

previous two generations of this patient's family, suggesting that his own symptoms are due to germline mutations. Therefore, he should undergo testing for VHL because early diagnosis would markedly improve subsequent medical care and survival rates. Individuals known to be carriers of the VHL gene should undergo annual ophthalmic and neurologic examinations, periodic imaging studies, and surveillance of renal function.

Answer A is incorrect. Osler-Weber-Rendu syndrome, also known as hereditary hemorrhagic telangiectasia, is an autosomal dominant disease in which vascular lesions (telangiectasias, arteriovenous malformations, and aneurysms) are found throughout the body, particularly in the lungs, brain, and gastrointestinal tract.

Answer B is incorrect. Tuberous sclerosis is characterized by benign tumors of the brain, eyes, skin, and kidneys that cause symptoms of mental retardation and seizures beginning in the first year of life.

Answer D is incorrect. Because early detection of von Hippel–Lindau disease and subsequent renal cell carcinoma improves survival rates in patients, it is imperative that the patient undergoes screening. If he is positive, then his children should undergo testing as well.

Answer E is incorrect. The diagnosis of von Hippel–Lindau disease in an individual who has or plans to have children is potentially important because the prognosis of patients with renal cell carcinoma, the most lethal lesion of this disease, is greatly improved with early detection. Early detection of retinal lesions may also allow for more timely laser treatment to preserve vision. The proper sequence of genetic testing is to confirm the suspected trait in the patient himself and then proceed to testing his offspring.

12. **The correct answer is E.** According to the *Diagnostic and Statistical Manual of Mental Disorders*, Fourth Edition, Text Revision, a specific fear is marked by a "persistent fear that is excessive or unreasonable, cued by the presence or anticipation of a specific object or situation." The fear may take on the qualities of a panic attack. In many cases, the feared situation may have personal meaning for the patient, as in this case. The fear is so intense that the activity (fear of flying) is avoided, resulting in functional decline. In other cases, the fear is of an object or situation that can be avoided due to limited exposure (e.g., the medical student that is afraid of snakes). The treatment of specific phobia usually involves systemic desensitization, in which the patient is progressively exposed to the activity or object that is feared, or "flooding," in which the patient is exposed directly to the feared object or activity until the symptoms of anxiety lessen.

Answer A is incorrect. Although this individual is experiencing chest pain, the story is much more consistent with one of psychiatric disease, given that the symptoms occur only in the context of flying.

Answer B is incorrect. The diagnosis of generalized anxiety disorder (GAD) depends on duration of symptoms for more than 6 months and at least three somatic symptoms for the same time period. However, because this patient's symptoms are in response to a single stimulus (flying), the diagnosis of GAD does not apply.

Answer C is incorrect. Although hyperthyroidism can produce some of the symptoms (palpitations, chest pain, and difficulty breathing), it is much more likely that the patient is experiencing a specific phobia to flying.

Answer D is incorrect. Social phobia results in a disabling sense of anxiety during situations where the patient is expected to perform or will be scrutinized by others (e.g., giving a presentation, performing in front of a large audience, or public speaking). It can severely impact the life of the patient, from office presentations to talking to unfamiliar people. It can be treated with antidepressants and benzodiazepines; some patients respond to a presituational β-blocker aimed at minimizing somatic complaints.

13. **The correct answer is A.** Embolization leading to acute mesenteric ischemia should be considered in an elderly patient that presents

with acute, intense abdominal pain that is accompanied by diarrhea, a large bowel movement, and/or nausea and vomiting. This is a diagnosis that requires immediate surgical attention and has a mortality rate of about 80%. It is very important to recognize the risk factors and examination findings so that a rapid diagnosis can be made. This condition requires emergent surgical intervention. Classically, patients with a diagnosis of acute mesenteric ischemia present with pain out of proportion to physical examination findings. The heart is the most common source of an embolus that lodges in the superior mesenteric artery, leading to acute mesenteric ischemia. An angiogram remains the gold standard for diagnosing mesenteric ischemia. If an embolus is found by angiogram, the patient must be taken to the operating room immediately.

Answer B is incorrect. Barium swallow is not indicated in the diagnosis of acute mesenteric ischemia.

Answer C is incorrect. A hepato-iminodiacetic acid (HIDA) scan is not indicated in the diagnosis of acute mesenteric ischemia. HIDA scans are a useful adjunct to ultrasound in the diagnosis of acute cholecystitis.

Answer D is incorrect. Ultrasound of the abdomen is not the gold standard for diagnosing acute mesenteric ischemia.

Answer E is incorrect. Although x-ray films of the abdomen are often ordered for patients who present with acute abdominal pain, this is not the gold standard for diagnosing acute mesenteric ischemia.

14. **The correct answer is A.** *Klebsiella pneumoniae* is a gram-negative, nonmotile, encapsulated, facultatively anaerobic, rod-shaped bacterium which is part of the normal flora of the mouth, skin, and intestines. However, it can cause urinary tract infections, wound infections, and pneumonia in certain populations. Pneumonia from this organism is typically seen in alcoholics due to aspiration of vomit. Like other aspiration pneumonias, the middle and upper lobe are often the primary areas involved, as they are the lowest points when lying down. *Klebsiella* pneumonia is characterized by a cough productive of "currant jelly" sputum.

Answer B is incorrect. *Legionella pneumophila* is a gram-negative, intracellular bacteria which can cause a pneumonia via transmission from aerosolized droplets. Common sources include hot water systems, ventilation ducts, or other areas with standing water.

Answer C is incorrect. *Pneumocystis jiroveci* (formerly *carinii*) pneumonia is an opportunistic infection seen in immunosuppressed hosts and AIDS patients. X-ray of the chest can show diffuse bilateral interstitial infiltrates with a ground-glass appearance.

Answer D is incorrect. *Pseudomonas aeruginosa* is a gram-negative, aerobic, rod-shaped bacterium which can produce a greenish color and grape-like odor in culture. It is a rare cause of community-acquired pneumonia, but rather is more associated with pneumonia of immunocompromised hosts such as those on ventilators and those with cystic fibrosis.

Answer E is incorrect. *Streptococcus pneumoniae* is a spherical, gram-positive, encapsulated, α-hemolytic bacterium responsible for causing a wide variety of infections including otitis media, cellulitis, meningitis, and pneumonia. It is the most common cause of pneumonia in adults, is lobar in nature, and often is associated with high fevers.

15. **The correct answer is D.** It is estimated that approximately 90% of normal couples should be able to conceive after 12 months of attempting to achieve pregnancy. However, approximately 10–15% of couples in the reproductive age group are affected by infertility. There are five main causes of infertility: ovulatory dysfunction, uterine and tubal disorders, male factor, cervical factor, and peritoneal factor. The patient reports a history of irregular menses in the setting of perimenopausal symptoms, including irregular cycles due to anovulatory cycles, vasomotor symptoms such as hot flashes, and vaginal dryness caused by decreased estrogen levels. Decreased estrogen levels cause a dramatic rise in follicle-stimulating hormone and luteinizing hormone levels, which are helpful in diagnosing ovarian failure.

Answer A is incorrect. A hysterosalpingogram is a radiologic study in which dye is placed into the uterine cavity via a transcervical catheter and is the initial test for intrauterine shape and tubal patency. It is best performed between days 6 and 10 of the cycle. Any uterine abnormality should be confirmed with a hysteroscopy, while tubal abnormalities are confirmed with laparoscopy, the gold standard for diagnosing tubal and/or peritoneal disease. Although uterine or tubal abnormalities can account for some barriers to conception, the patient's history is negative for congenital uterine or tubal disorders or sexually transmitted diseases, which makes a structural cause unlikely and would not explain her associated symptoms.

Answer B is incorrect. A space-occupying prolactinoma may cause secondary amenorrhea, which is defined as the absence of menstrual periods for 6 months in a woman who had previously been regular, or for 12 months in a woman who had irregular periods. Anatomic compression or high prolactin levels can inhibit proper pituitary function, resulting in hypogonadism and amenorrhea. Obtaining a serum prolactin level can help make the diagnosis. However, in the absence of galactorrhea, this diagnosis is less likely.

Answer C is incorrect. A postcoital test evaluates the cervical factor of infertility by assessing cervical mucus for motile sperm after intercourse. However, the patient related no history of a cone biopsy or cryotherapy to the cervix that may account for a negative postcoital test.

Answer E is incorrect. A progesterone challenge consists of administering this hormone to the patient for 7–10 days to see if it triggers menstruation. If a period does occur as a result of taking progestin, it means that the uterus and vagina were primed properly under the presence of estrogen, which causes the uterine lining to thicken. This confirms that estrogen is present and that the ovaries are capable of ovulating but lack proper cycling. However, if no menstruation takes place after the progestin challenge and the anatomy of the reproductive tract is found to be normal, then a lack of estrogen is the most likely cause of anovulation. Further hormone testing can then be used to make a diagnosis. This patient's presentation is most consistent with premature ovarian failure, which can be confirmed with serum follicle-stimulating hormone and luteinizing hormone levels.

16. **The correct answer is A.** Avascular necrosis is a complication of hip dislocations and occurs approximately 15% of the time. The incidence of avascular necrosis may be diminished significantly by prompt reduction of a hip dislocation. The arterial supply to the femoral head runs along the femoral neck. In a dislocated hip, the course of these vessels can be altered and blood flow hindered.

Answer B is incorrect. The femoral artery, vein, and nerve can be injured in an anterior dislocation. However, this patient suffered a posterior dislocation based on mechanism and clinical appearance.

Answer C is incorrect. Myositis ossificans can occur following hip dislocation, but it is related to muscle damage and hematoma formation rather than the timing of treatment.

Answer D is incorrect. Posttraumatic degenerative arthritis commonly develops after posterior dislocations of the hip. This complication seems to be related to the severity of the initial trauma rather than delay of treatment.

Answer E is incorrect. Although recurrent dislocation is a rare complication to traumatic hip dislocation, its incidence is not associated with time to relocation as is avascular necrosis.

17. **The correct answer is D.** Myelofibrosis refers to the conversion of bone marrow to a solid collection of fibrous tissue. It is a late manifestation of chronic myelogenous leukemia that is of unknown etiology and uniformly fatal. As the bone marrow ceases to produce RBCs, extramedullary hematopoiesis ensues, beginning in the spleen and leading to massive splenomegaly that may progress to splenic infarction. Megakaryocytes and platelets persist in the marrow, and large platelets are present peripherally. Diagnosis generally requires bone marrow biopsy because aspiration of the solid fibrous tissue is not possible.

Answer A is incorrect. Bernard-Soulier syndrome is an autosomal dominant disorder in which platelets lack the membrane glycoprotein necessary for binding von Willebrand factor to the platelet surface. It is inherited and is not related to chronic myelogenous leukemia. Patients affected by this disorder may experience spontaneous bruising, epistaxis, and petechiae. This patient's presentation is not consistent with this diagnosis.

Answer B is incorrect. Sideroblastic anemia is caused by defective iron incorporation into the heme molecule, leading to deposition of excess iron in the bone marrow and liver. Idiopathic sideroblastic anemia occurs most often in persons who are elderly and is classified as a myelodysplastic syndrome. It is characterized by macrocytic anemia and varying degrees of leukopenia and thrombocytopenia. Bone marrow aspiration demonstrates hypercellular marrow. Again, this is not consistent with the bone marrow of this patient.

Answer C is incorrect. The myelodysplastic syndromes (MDSs) are premalignant conditions in which a single clonal immature blood cell proliferates in a disordered manner, causing cytopenias, increased bone marrow cellularity, and malfunctioning peripheral cells. Although MDSs often progress to leukemias if not treated, they are not known to be *caused* by chronic myelogenous leukemia. Additionally, the bone marrow biopsy from this patient reveals decreased cellularity. In MDSs, an increase would be expected.

Answer E is incorrect. Progression to blast phase is one rapidly fatal outcome of indolent chronic myelogenous leukemia. It develops following asymptomatic disease, and results in splenomegaly, anemia, thrombocytopenia, and replacement of peripheral lymphocytes with nucleated blast cells. Bone marrow may be difficult to aspirate, but biopsy reveals hypercellularity. Although this outcome is possible for the patient in this case, the bone marrow biopsy is not consistent with this diagnosis.

Answer F is incorrect. Exposure to alkylating agents has been implicated in the pathogenesis of myelogenous leukemias. Imatinib, however, is an Abl inhibitor and is not an alkylating agent.

18. **The correct answer is D.** Systolic dysfunction and diastolic function differ in regard to their pathophysiology and management. However, they can appear similar clinically. Echocardiogram is the best (inexpensive, noninvasive, and portable) method of evaluation. It allows measurement of ejection fraction, cavity size, and wall thickness, as well as a view of any valvular abnormalities.

Answer A is incorrect. Cardiac catheterization is invasive and carries with it cost and morbidity (including contrast load). In terms of distinguishing systolic and diastolic failure, it can confirm elevated left atrial pressure, but would not be indicated unless myocardial ischemia was suspected.

Answer B is incorrect. Many of the signs and symptoms of heart failure including dyspnea, reduced exercise tolerance, edema, and the neurohormonal response are similar in both forms of heart failure. Therefore it is often difficult to distinguish the two clinically.

Answer C is incorrect. CT scan of the chest is expensive and would add little information.

Answer E is incorrect. While electrocardiogram can suggest one diagnosis over the other, it is generally unreliable.

Answer F is incorrect. MRI of the heart is very expensive and would not be very helpful.

Answer G is incorrect. X-ray of the chest in both cases may show pulmonary congestion. Systolic failure might be more associated with cardiomegaly, but this is not very reliable.

19. **The correct answer is C.** This child has spastic cerebral palsy (CP) affecting his lower limbs. CP is a general term that describes a group of disorders that appear in the first few years of life and affect a child's ability to coordinate body movements. These disorders are caused by damage to a child's brain during fetal development, birth, or the first few months after birth. CP is the most common movement disorder in children. Pyramidal CP, the most common type of CP, is characterized by spasticity, hyperreflexia, slow and effortful voluntary movements, and impaired fine motor function, and can affect all of the limbs. De-

layed developmental milestones, persistence of infantile reflexes (e.g., Babinski's reflex), contractures, and weakness or underdevelopment of affected limbs are common. Affected children classically walk on their toes and have a scissor gait. Spastic CP is treated with muscle relaxants (e.g., diazepam, dantrolene, baclofen), physical and occupational therapy, assist devices, and surgical release of contractures when necessary.

Answer A is incorrect. This is the appropriate therapy for infantile spasms (West's syndrome), which is characterized by clusters of generalized tonic-clonic seizures, very high amplitude slow waves on electroencephalogram called hypsarrhythmia, and arrest of psychomotor development at the age when the seizures began. Seizures usually begin between 3 and 12 months of age. This child is not having seizures.

Answer B is incorrect. Benztropine is an anticholinergic that treats dystonia, which occurs in Parkinson's disease and as an adverse effect associated with typical antipsychotics. This child does not have Parkinson's disease and is not taking any antipsychotic medication.

Answer D is incorrect. Levodopa and carbidopa treats Parkinson's disease, which is characterized by resting tremor, bradykinesia, rigidity, postural instability, masked facies, memory loss, and micrographia. Parkinsonism affects individuals who are in middle age and who are elderly, not children.

Answer E is incorrect. This is the appropriate therapy for infantile spasms (West's syndrome), which is characterized by clusters of generalized tonic-clonic seizures, very high amplitude slow waves on electroencephalogram called hypsarrhythmia, and arrest of psychomotor development at the age when the seizures began. Seizures usually begin between 3 and 12 months of age. This child is not having seizures.

20. **The correct answer is C.** Patients who overdose on heroin can present with respiratory compromise and may stop breathing altogether, as all opiates strongly depress respiratory drive. Therefore, any patient who presents to the ED with the hallmarks of an opioid overdose—such as pinpoint pupils, needle-track marks, and respiratory compromise—should be monitored and an emergent airway established if necessary.

Answer A is incorrect. Naloxone works as an opioid antagonist, binding strongly to the opioid receptors and reversing the effects of an opiate overdose. The reversal works immediately, and most patients recover consciousness with intravenous administration. Naloxone works so well that soon after its administration, patients may start to experience withdrawal symptoms. Administration of 0.4 mg, however, is an appropriate initial dose.

Answer B is incorrect. Once intravenous heroin users are stable, it is important to assess them for HIV, skin abscesses, and bacterial endocarditis. Kidney function, however, is not usually compromised in heroin abusers.

Answer D is incorrect. Although patients in heroin withdrawal have symptoms that are very intense and unpleasant, those symptoms are not life-threatening. Withdrawal symptoms include dysphoria, nausea, rhinorrhea, lacrimation, piloerection, muscle spasms (commonly in the legs, hence the phrase "kicking the habit"), sweating, yawning, diarrhea, fever, and insomnia.

Answer E is incorrect. To minimize withdrawal symptoms, patients can be treated with clonidine or methadone. Clonidine works to suppress the rebound hyperactivity of the sympathetic nervous system, and methadone acts as a cross-tolerant drug, since it is also an opioid but has a much longer half-life than heroin. Benzodiazepines are not used in the treatment of heroin addiction.

21. **The correct answer is A.** Cryptococcal meningitis is an opportunistic infection seen in AIDS and other immunocompromised patients. It can present as a headache, fever, and/or impaired mentation. Diagnosis is by lumbar puncture, which will show decreased glucose, increased protein, and increased leukocyte count with monocytic predominance. Cerebrospinal fluid cryptococcal antigen test is 95% sensitive in patients with the

disease and more sensitive than microscopy and culture.

Answer B is incorrect. While lumbar puncture and culture may yield a diagnosis, it often takes several days to several weeks for results and larger volumes of cerebrospinal fluid (CSF) are often required. CSF cryptococcal antigen test is much more sensitive and can be performed in a relatively short amount of time on a smaller sample size.

Answer C is incorrect. India ink stain on the cerebrospinal fluid can be used in diagnosis of cryptococcal meningitis, but is only 50% sensitive in patients with disease. The question asks for the most likely way to confirm the diagnosis of *Cryptococcus*, and therefore the more sensitive and specific test, lumbar puncture and serology, would be the better answer.

Answer D is incorrect. Potassium hydroxide preparation (KOH) is used to assess for the presence of Candida albicans, the organism responsible for thrush in immunosuppressed patients. KOH or Gram stain will show budding yeast and/or pseudohyphae if *Candida* is present.

Answer E is incorrect. Silver stain is not used in the diagnosis of cryptococcal meningitis. It can be used for diagnosis of other opportunistic infections including *Histoplasma* and *Blastomyces*.

22. **The correct answer is C.** Mastitis is a cellulitis of the periglandular breast tissue that frequently occurs within the first 3 months post partum. Mastitis results from breast-feeding–related nipple trauma and is most commonly caused by *Staphylococcus aureus*. Initial treatment consists of an oral antibiotic effective against penicillin-resistant staphylococci, such as dicloxacillin or a cephalosporin, although antibiotic coverage against oral flora from the suckling baby should be considered in a patient not responding to antistaphylococcal therapy.

Answer A is incorrect. A breast abscess can present with similar features as in mastitis, such as breast pain, systemic symptoms (e.g., fever, vomiting), and a palpable fluctuant mass. Spontaneous drainage from the mass or the nipple can also occur. Because there are no signs of pus, incision and drainage are not indicated.

Answer B is incorrect. Although intravenous (IV) oxacillin would provide adequate antistaphylococcal coverage, an IV antibiotic is generally not necessary for the treatment of mastitis. This patient is exhibiting the typical signs of a local cellulitis that can be treated with oral antibiotics. IV therapy could be considered if the infection had invaded more subcutaneous tissue or if the infection did not respond to oral antibiotics after several days of therapy.

Answer D is incorrect. Doxycycline is effective predominantly against intracellular organisms and does not have adequate antistaphylococcal coverage. Additionally, doxycycline is an absolute contraindication in actively breast-feeding mothers because tetracycline causes tooth discoloration and enamel hypoplasia in the baby's developing teeth.

Answer E is incorrect. Although warm compresses are an appropriate adjuvant to antibiotic therapy, they are not the appropriate initial treatment for mastitis.

23. **The correct answer is E.** Anterior dislocations of the shoulder can be associated with axillary artery and nerve damage. Before closed reduction and immobilization are performed, it is important to assess for neurovascular injury. The axillary nerve ends as the superior lateral cutaneous nerve supplying the area over the deltoid muscle.

Answer A is incorrect. This area is supplied by the radial nerve, which is not typically injured in an anterior shoulder dislocation. Radial nerve injury can be associated with a humeral shaft fracture and presents as a wrist drop.

Answer B is incorrect. This area is supplied by the ulnar nerve, which is not typically injured in an anterior shoulder dislocation. Ulnar nerve injury can be associated with a fracture of the medial condyle of the humerus, and these patients can present with weakness of the intrinsic muscles of the hand. They exhibit decreased ability to hold a card between the thumb and index finger, and may show "clawing" (flexion) of the fourth and fifth digits.

Answer C is incorrect. This area is supplied by the median nerve, and this area is also often used to test the C7 dermatome. Neither is typically injured in an anterior shoulder dislocation.

Answer D is incorrect. This area is supplied by the median nerve, which is not typically injured in an anterior shoulder dislocation. Median nerve injury can be associated with a supracondylar humerus fracture and presents as decreased thumb function.

24. **The correct answer is C.** This is an example of a prospective cohort study because patients were assessed for presence or absence of risk factors and followed over time for development of disease.

    Answer A is incorrect. Case-control studies assemble case groups with a disease and matched control groups without disease, and then collect retrospective data on exposure to risk factors.

    Answer B is incorrect. Meta-analysis involves a statistical combination of data from several studies, often via a literature search.

    Answer D is incorrect. Randomized controlled trials are experimental, prospective studies that are designed, for example, to test therapeutic interventions.

    Answer E is incorrect. Although the study is a cohort study, it is not retrospective. A retrospective cohort study will assemble a cohort based on history of risk factors, and examine outcomes and past exposures at the time of data collection.

25. **The correct answer is C.** This patient is suffering from benign prostatic hypertrophy, one of the most common diseases in the aging man. The patient usually develops slow and progressive urinary obstructive symptoms such as hesitancy, and irritative symptoms such as increased frequency and nocturia. Treatment is with two main classes of drugs: Finasteride, an antiandrogen that acts by inhibiting α-reductase, the

enzyme that converts testosterone to dihydrotestosterone; or terazosin/tamsulosin, selective α_1-antagonists that block the action of adrenaline on smooth muscles of the bladder and the blood vessel walls.

Answer A is incorrect. Aspirin does not have any role in treatment of benign prostatic hypertrophy.

Answer B is incorrect. Bacille Calmette-Guérin is used in the treatment of superficial bladder cancer and has no role in benign prostatic hypertrophy.

Answer D is incorrect. Oxybutynin is an anticholinergic used for the treatment of bladder spasms.

Answer E is incorrect. Trimethoprim-sulfamethoxazole is the treatment of choice for prostatitis. However, since his urinalysis shows no signs of infection, this drug would not be appropriate.

26. **The correct answer is A.** This patient has neoplastic pericarditis with pericardial effusion, which is a fluid collection in the pericardial space, as seen in the image. Pericarditis is an inflammation of the pericardial space and is a common cause of pericardial effusion. Because this patient's symptoms are bothersome, treatment is indicated. Balloon pericardiotomy, prolonged pericardial catheter drainage, surgical pericardiectomy, and intrapericardial sclerosing therapy are all appropriate methods of treatment. Balloon pericardiotomy is performed by inserting an uninflated balloon into the pericardial space, inflating the balloon, and pulling it through the pericardium to create a hole through which fluid can drain into the pleural or peritoneal space.

Answer B is incorrect. Emergent pericardiocentesis is indicated in unstable patients with cardiac tamponade. Although pericardiocentesis would relieve this patient's chest pain, the relief would only be temporary because more fluid would soon collect in the pericardial space. Therefore, pericardiocentesis would not be a good long-term solution to her pain.

Answer C is incorrect. Nonsteroidal anti-inflammatory drugs (NSAIDs) can be used in the treatment of pericarditis; however, an NSAID will only temporarily relieve this patient's symptoms and thus is not a good long-term solution.

Answer D is incorrect. A morphine patient-controlled analgesia would help control this patient's pain, but it would not treat the underlying problem of pericarditis. Thus, morphine is not a good long-term solution.

Answer E is incorrect. Nitroglycerin is used to treat chest pain in patients having angina or acute myocardial infarction. It would have little effect on pain secondary to pericarditis, as seen in this patient.

27. **The correct answer is D.** This patient's presentation is likely due to lysergic acid diethylamide (LSD), which typically causes powerful sensory disturbances such as the movement of shapes, light, and colors. LSD usually does not produce hallucinations in the strict sense, but rather illusions and vivid daydream-like scenes. The drug's action on numerous receptors, including dopamine receptors, adrenoreceptors, and serotonin receptors, may also contribute to the various physiologic reactions that users may experience, such as pupillary dilation, tachycardia, salivation, uterine contraction, and increased body temperature. Patients rarely get addicted or dependent on the drug because its rapid tolerance prevents regular use.

Answer A is incorrect. Cocaine is not the most likely cause of this patient's sensory disturbances, although it is important to note that cocaine can cause hallucinations and psychosis when taken in large amounts. Cocaine can be snorted, sniffed, injected, or smoked, but it is not usually taken orally on blotted paper.

Answer B is incorrect. Ecstasy is the street name of 3,4-methylenedioxymethamphetamine (MDMA), an illicit drug that is used recreationally. Users of ecstasy experience social disinhibition, euphoria, and heightened self-awareness; however, hallucinations are uncommon.

Answer C is incorrect. Heroin is unlikely to have caused this patient's condition, as it is usually snorted, smoked, or injected. This drug

causes an intense euphoric feeling but generally does not cause sensory disturbances. It is highly addictive, and withdrawal symptoms may develop within a day of the last heroin intake.

Answer E is incorrect. Marijuana is unlikely to be responsible for this patient's presentation, as it is usually smoked and is not known as a hallucinogenic drug. Unlike lysergic acid diethylamide, it can be abused, and users can become psychologically dependent on it.

28. **The correct answer is B.** This patient has presented with a rare form of Hodgkin's disease, the lymphocyte-depleted type. Although modern therapies have made the classic distinctions of Hodgkin's disease less important in terms of prognosis, lymphocyte-depleted disease remains quite aggressive clinically. It accounts for only 2% of Hodgkin's disease pathologies and is seen most often in older men. It is most notable for its aggressive clinical nature, and patients often present with advanced disease and significant systemic symptoms. Biopsy reveals abundant Reed-Sternberg cells with a paucity of lymphocytes compared to other forms of the disease.

Answer A is incorrect. Burkitt's lymphoma is a non-Hodgkin's lymphoma characterized by a starry sky appearance due to the ingestion of tumor cells by macrophages.

Answer C is incorrect. Lymphocyte-predominant Hodgkin's lymphoma is an uncommon form of the disease, accounting for 6% of cases. It carries an excellent prognosis. On biopsy, lymph nodes reveal diffuse lymphocytic infiltrate with few Reed-Sternberg cells. This form of the disease would not be expected to be as aggressive as this patient's illness.

Answer D is incorrect. Nodular sclerosing Hodgkin's disease is the most common form (70% of cases) and is most commonly diagnosed in young women. Histology reveals fibrosis with Reed-Sternberg and lymphoid cells. This form of the disease is less aggressive than this patient's and is uncommon in men who are elderly.

Answer E is incorrect. The Reed-Sternberg cell is pathognomonic for Hodgkin's disease, effectively ruling out non-Hodgkin's lymphoma.

Answer F is incorrect. Again, the presence of the Reed-Sternberg cell excludes a diagnosis of leukemia. In addition, leukemia would not be expected to cause such severe lymphadenopathy.

29. **The correct answer is E.** This is a classic presentation of osteosarcoma. In general, osteosarcoma will present with progressive pain that is worse at night, constitutional symptoms, and swelling/erythema over the site of the tumor. Alkaline phosphatase is elevated in more than half of all patients with osteosarcoma. The x-ray demonstrates the "sunburst" appearance of neoplastic bone formation. Of all osteosarcomas, 60% are seen in children and adolescents, with males being affected 1.5–2 times more often than females. This tumor has a tendency to affect the metaphyses of long bones, particularly the distal femur, proximal tibia, and proximal humerus. Treatment includes chemotherapy, and if possible, limb-sparing surgical resection, though amputation may be necessary in some cases. Long-term survival is 60–80%, with the best survival occurring in those patients who are responsive to chemotherapy.

Answer A is incorrect. Fibrous dysplasia also has many different appearances on x-rays and can mimic many other tumors. However, it is a benign lesion that would not present as aggressively as the lesion in this case.

Answer B is incorrect. Nonossifying fibroma is a benign lesion and so should not result in weight loss and fever. Also, it would appear radiolucent on x-rays and not radiodense as in this case.

Answer C is incorrect. The classic presentation of osteoid osteoma is night pain that responds to nonsteroidal anti-inflammatory drugs, which was not the case in this patient.

Answer D is incorrect. Infection can take on many different appearances radiographically and must always be considered with tumor. However, the normal complete blood cell count and erythrocyte sedimentation rate help to rule out this diagnostic possibility.

30. **The correct answer is A.** Otitis externa is generally treated with topical medication; however, the rarer form of it, malignant otitis externa or necrotizing otitis externa, is essentially an osteomyelitis of the temporal bone. Risk factors include diabetes and immunocompromised status. The mortality rate can be as high as 53%. Imaging studies include CT, MRI, and a combination technetium and gallium 67 scan can also be used. Aggressive parenteral antibiotic therapy aimed at *Pseudomonas* and *Staphylococcus aureus* is necessary. The excellent antipseudomonal activity of the fluoroquinolones has generally made them the treatment of choice for necrotizing otitis externa, although a combination of a β-lactam antibiotic and aminoglycoside is also effective. Treatment should also include surgical debridement of any granulation or osteitic bone.

Answer B is incorrect. Amoxicillin will not cover *Pseudomonas aeruginosa*, one of the likely infecting organisms.

Answer C is incorrect. Amphotericin B covers fungi and would be ineffective in this case.

Answer D is incorrect. Methicillin will not cover *Pseudomonas aeruginosa*, one of the likely infecting organisms.

Answer E is incorrect. Topical treatment will be insufficient to deal with this degree of infection.

31. **The correct answer is A.** The biopsy results should point to amyloidosis causing a restrictive cardiomyopathy. The hallmark of restrictive cardiomyopathies is diastolic dysfunction. This can be seen in situations in which systolic function is within normal limits and the main etiology is the inability of the ventricles to fill properly. An ejection fraction of 55% would be consistent with diastolic dysfunction.

Answer B is incorrect. A harsh diastolic murmur would not be consistent with cardiac amyloidosis. Diastolic murmurs are classified as early, mid-, or late and can be caused by a variety of pathologies. This includes aortic or pulmonary regurgitation, mitral or tricuspid stenosis, myxoma, heart block, and left-to-right shunts. None of these conditions would be definitively associated with a diagnosis of amyloid.

Answer C is incorrect. Patients with diastolic dysfunction due to restrictive cardiomyopathies will often have an enlarged, painful, and pulsatile liver. There is no relationship between a right lower quadrant mass and amyloidosis.

Answer D is incorrect. Edema is another sign of persistently elevated venous pressure and would be consistent with cardiac amyloidosis. However, this edema is generally found in the lower extremities.

Answer E is incorrect. U waves are often seen with hypokalemia.

Answer F is incorrect. Crackles upon pulmonary auscultation can be indicative of pulmonary edema due to left-sided heart failure. However, wheezing is not consistent with the biopsy results.

32. **The correct answer is C.** This patient has symptoms of subacute closed-angle glaucoma. While medical treatment can provide symptomatic relief, only laser iridotomy provides curative treatment. Laser iridotomy forms a permanent connection between the anterior and posterior chambers and prevents recurrence. In some cases, the fellow eye should undergo prophylactic laser iridotomy.

Answer A is incorrect. Acetazolamide is carbonic anhydrase inhibitor that can decrease aqueous humor secretion and reduce intraocular pressure. However, it only provides symptomatic treatment and is not curative.

Answer B is incorrect. Atropine is an antimuscarinic agent that results in mydriasis, which will further exacerbate her symptoms of closed-angle glaucoma.

Answer D is incorrect. Pilocarpine is a muscarinic agonist that produces rapid miosis and contraction of the ciliary muscles. This can be used in the acute treatment of closed- or open-angle glaucoma to open the trabecular meshwork around Schlemm's canal, increasing drainage of aqueous humor and decreasing intraocular pressure. However, it only provides symptomatic treatment and is not curative.

Answer E is incorrect. Timolol is a nonselective β-antagonist that reduces the production of aqueous humor in the eye. It can be used topically in treatment of chronic open-angle glaucoma, but does not provide curative treatment for chronic closed-angle glaucoma.

33. **The correct answer is E.** Scleroderma is a multiorgan collagen vascular disease that predominantly affects the skin and gastrointestinal system. It is caused by progressive tissue fibrosis that leads to many of the resulting symptoms. Look for sclerodactyly, dysphagia, and Raynaud's phenomenon.

Answer A is incorrect. Irritable bowel syndrome would not present with the skin and lung symptoms, and is more characterized by abdominal pain and gas than dysphagia.

Answer B is incorrect. Causing an esophageal tear secondary to vomitus, Mallory-Weiss syndrome can cause dysphagia, but the other symptoms described would not be associated.

Answer C is incorrect. Myasthenia gravis is an autoimmune disorder that can result in dysphagia but would not be characterized by the other symptoms provided in this question.

Answer D is incorrect. This condition usually presents with pruritus, fatigue, and right upper quadrant discomfort. Hyperpigmentation can be part of the manifestation of primary biliary cirrhosis, but dysphagia is not a common complaint.

34. **The correct answer is D.** This woman gives a classic history of stress incontinence, that is, urinary leak with increases in abdominal pressure (e.g., cough, sneeze, physical exertion). Her stress incontinence is likely due to pelvic floor laxity secondary to pregnancy and childbirth. Uncontrolled diabetes can lead to macrosomic infants predisposing patients to develop pelvic floor laxity. Treatment is surgical correction.

Answer A is incorrect. Anticholinergic medication such as oxybutynin can be used to treat urge incontinence.

Answer B is incorrect. Intermittent catheterization can be used to treat overflow incontinence. In patients with overflow incontinence, there is continuous leaking of small volumes of urine due to incomplete emptying of the bladder secondary to obstruction or failure of the detrusor muscle to contract. Diabetic neuropathy can also lead to overflow incontinence; however, this woman's symptoms are most consistent with stress incontinence.

Answer C is incorrect. Sacral nerve stimulation can be used to treat urge incontinence, of which this patient does not report symptoms. Urge incontinence manifests by a sudden strong desire to urinate that is difficult to suppress and may result in involuntary passing of urine if the patient does not make it to the toilet in time. It is due to detrusor instability and can be secondary to upper motor neuron lesions, infection, neoplasms, or stones.

Answer E is incorrect. Vaginal estrogen cream can be used to treat incontinence secondary to hypoestrogenism of the vaginal wall, as seen in older postmenopausal women.

35. **The correct answer is D.** The infant has transient congenital hypothyroidism, which causes lethargy, slow movement, hoarse cry, feeding problems, constipation, macroglossia, umbilical hernia, large fontanelles, hypotonia, dry skin, hypothermia, and prolonged jaundice. Congenital hypothyroidism is usually idiopathic. However, some cases may result from fetal exposure to antithyroid medications (i.e., propylthiouracil or methimazole), which can suppress the production of fetal thyroid hormone. These medications are cleared from the circulation within days, and by several weeks after delivery, most infants will become euthyroid.

Answer A is incorrect. Formula is designed to provide adequate nutrition. However, infants can be malnourished if the formula is mixed incorrectly, if an insufficient quantity is given, or under the rare circumstance that the infant is intolerant to a component of the formula. Failure to thrive, hard stools, decreased urine output, and sunken fontanelles are signs of inadequate nutrition.

Answer B is incorrect. Signs of fetal alcohol syndrome are facial abnormalities (macrognathia, thin upper lip, short palpebral fissure, and epicanthal fold), poor growth (small head circumference, short stature, and low weight), cardiac defects, minor joint and limb abnormalities, and developmental delay/mental retardation.

Answer C is incorrect. Fetal cocaine exposure can cause intrauterine growth retardation, microcephaly, and bowel atresia. It is not associated with transient congenital hypothyroidism.

Answer E is incorrect. Fetal complications of gestational diabetes mellitus (DM) include macrosomia; intrauterine growth retardation; cardiac, renal, and neural tube defects; hypocalcemia; hyperbilirubinemia; polycythemia; hypoglycemia; and respiratory distress syndrome. Gestational DM is not associated with transient congenital hypothyroidism.

36. **The correct answer is E.** This patient is manifesting classic signs of hyperkalemia, including weakness and typical ECG findings such as peaked T waves (see *arrows*) and widened electrocardiographic wave complexes. There are a few antihypertensive medications that are commonly associated with hyperkalemia. These include angiotensin-converting enzyme inhibitors, angiotensin receptor blockers (ARBs), and potassium-sparing diuretics. Losartan is an ARB. The other antihypertensives listed are either associated with hypokalemia or have no effect on potassium balance at all.

Answer A is incorrect. Carbonic anhydrase inhibitors such as acetazolamide can have a similar but less pronounced effect on potassium balance as thiazide diuretics. They can lead to increased distal sodium delivery and high aldosterone levels.

Answer B is incorrect. Loop diuretics such as furosemide and bumetanide commonly lead to hypokalemia through a similar mechanism as the thiazide diuretics.

Answer C is incorrect. Hydralazine, which upregulates cyclic guanosine monophosphate leading to smooth muscle cell relaxation, commonly leads to reflex tachycardia or drug-induced reaction. There is no association with potassium abnormalities.

Answer D is incorrect. Thiazide diuretics, such as hydrochlorothiazide, can lead to hypokalemia by increasing distal tubular delivery in the setting of high aldosterone.

37. **The correct answer is C.** Infection is the most common cause of fevers of unknown origin, defined as a fever > 38.3°C (101°F) lasting more than 3 weeks that remains undiagnosed after three outpatient visits or 3 days of hospitalization.

Answer A is incorrect. Collagen vascular disease and granulomatous diseases combined account for more than 15% of fevers of unknown origin.

Answer B is incorrect. Collagen vascular disease and granulomatous diseases combined account for more than 15% of fevers of unknown origin.

Answer D is incorrect. Neoplasm is a common cause of fever of unknown origin, but less common than either autoimmune disease or infection.

Answer E is incorrect. Pulmonary emboli are a relatively rare cause of fevers of unknown origin.

38. **The correct answer is A.** The National Cholesterol Education Program Adult Treatment Panel III has issued guidelines that recommend that any person with cardiovascular disease or diabetes mellitus achieve an LDL cholesterol level of < 100 mg/dL. However, a more recent report suggests that for patients with cardiovascular disease and diabetes (very high-risk patients), a goal of < 70 mg/dL may be a more optimal level.

Answer B is incorrect. The National Cholesterol Education Program guidelines recommend that those without cardiovascular disease and without diabetes mellitus but with at least one risk factor (including tobacco use, hypertension, high LDL, low HDL, diabetes mellitus, and obesity) achieve an LDL cholesterol goal of < 130 mg/dL. A goal of < 160 mg/dL is recommended for those without cardiovascular disease or diabetes mellitus and who have only one risk factor.

Answer C is incorrect. For those with diabetes mellitus, an HDL cholesterol level > 45 mg/dL

is desirable. This patient's HDL is over 45 mg/dL and therefore needs no intervention.

Answer D is incorrect. A high-fiber, low-fat diet is ideal, but this patient needs more immediate attention for his high LDL cholesterol level.

Answer E is incorrect. Obesity is also a risk factor, but it will not lower his hyperlipidemia as quickly as will more direct therapy to lower his LDL cholesterol level (such as drug therapy).

39. **The correct answer is E.** This patient is experiencing a threatened abortion, which is differentiated from a spontaneous abortion by the cervical os being closed. The fetus is still viable, though observation is necessary, as threatened abortions may become spontaneous abortions. Currently, there is no evidence that bed rest is helpful for preventing the opening of the os and loss of the pregnancy.

Answer A is incorrect. Betamethasone is used to mature the fetal lungs in preterm infants. At this gestational age, the fetus is not viable.

Answer B is incorrect. Cervical cerclage, or suturing the cervix closed, is a procedure that is performed if the cervix is incompetent. Patients with cervical incompetence have dilation and effacement of the cervix, usually during the second trimester. Occasionally, this will lead to loss of the fetus. There is no evidence to suggest that this woman has an incompetent cervix.

Answer C is incorrect. If the cervical os were open with bleeding at this gestational age, a spontaneous abortion would be inevitable. An emergent dilation and curettage would then be necessary to minimize the chance of retention of fetal products and subsequent infection.

Answer D is incorrect. Magnesium sulfate is a tocolytic that is used to slow down uterine contractions in preterm labor. However, this woman is only 14 weeks along. Given that she is so far from viability we would not start magnesium sulfate. It is not a long-term treatment option.

40. **The correct answer is B.** The patient is hypoglycemic, and normalization of the blood glucose level is likely to alleviate her symptoms. Sulfonylureas act primarily as insulin secretagogues, but also limit hepatic glucose production, decrease lipolysis, and decrease hepatic clearance of serum insulin. When initiating these medications, it is important to use the lowest possible dose and to increase slowly to avoid overshoot hypoglycemia.

Answer A is incorrect. Epinephrine is incorrect, as the patient already exhibits symptoms of adrenergic excess (tachycardia, tremulousness, palpitations, and diaphoresis) as would be expected with hypoglycemia.

Answer C is incorrect. Administering insulin would further decrease the blood glucose level and exacerbate the patient's symptoms.

Answer D is incorrect. Naloxone is incorrect, as it is unlikely that the patient has overdosed on opiates given her lack of respiratory depression.

Answer E is incorrect. Tissue plasminogen activator is incorrect, as it is unlikely that the patient is suffering from ischemic stroke or myocardial infarction. Although she is lethargic and obtunded, she has no focal neurologic signs. Hypotension would be expected if the cause of her mental status changes was cardiac failure. If the patient does not improve after glucose administration, further evaluation of her cardiac and neurologic status would be warranted.

41. **The correct answer is C.** This patient is exhibiting the symptoms of hypochondriasis, which involves the persistent fear and conviction that one is very ill, combined with the misinterpretation of normal bodily symptoms. The *Diagnostic and Statistical Manual of Mental Disorders*, Fourth Edition, Text Revision criteria for hypochondriasis require that the patient have at least a 6-month history of persistent and debilitating fear that is not diminished by appropriate medical evaluation and reassurance. Men and woman are equally affected, and the disorder usually presents in middle age. Treatment consists of reassurance and a referral for psychotherapy.

Answer A is incorrect. When assessing the risk of a pigmented lesion, the **ABCD** criteria apply: **A**symmetry (this lesion is symmetric), **B**order irregularity (the borders here are regular), **C**olor variegation (this lesion is monochromatic and brown), and a **D**iameter of ≥ 6 mm. Basal cell carcinoma typically presents with a slow-growing skin mass that is ulcerated, with or without pigmentation. There is a very low risk that this patient's lesion is cancerous.

Answer B is incorrect. Patients with body dysmorphic disorder are preoccupied with some perceived physical abnormality to the point of experiencing profound distress and impairment. This patient does not indicate that he feels his condition is abnormal, only that he is convinced he has a specific disorder. Hypochondriasis is thus a more likely diagnosis.

Answer D is incorrect. Somatization disorder is a chronic psychiatric condition that typically presents with a long-standing history of unsubstantiated medical complaints. The *Diagnostic and Statistical Manual of Mental Disorders*, Fourth Edition, Text Revision criteria for a somatization disorder require that the patient have a history of pain in at least four sites, including two gastrointestinal symptoms, one sexual symptom, and one neurologic symptom. This patient has only one complaint and no medical history, making somatization disorder an unlikely diagnosis.

Answer E is incorrect. When assessing the risk of a pigmented lesion, the **ABCD** criteria apply: **A**symmetry (this lesion is symmetric), **B**order irregularity (the borders here are regular), **C**olor variegation (this lesion is monochromatic and brown), and a **D**iameter of ≥ 6 mm. Squamous cell carcinoma typically presents with a raised, pigmented skin lesion that may be ulcerated, exudative, scabbed, or itchy. There is a very low risk that this patient's lesion is cancerous.

42. **The correct answer is D.** This woman most likely has acute tubular necrosis (ATN), which presents with a picture of acute renal failure, often following sepsis, hypotension, or other ischemic insult. Although prerenal failure can also result from these, it resolves more rapidly

with fluid administration, and presents with a prerenal picture, including BUN:creatinine ratio > 20:1 and $Fe_{Na} < 1\%$. ATN, in contrast, lasts longer, with creatinine elevation often persisting for several weeks, and presents with signs of renal failure such as elevated BUN and creatinine, $Fe_{Na} > 2\%$, and low urine osmolarity due to impaired urine concentrating ability despite hypovolemia. Muddy brown casts on urinalysis are characteristic of ATN.

Answer A is incorrect. Dobutamine is a commonly used pressor, which could potentially have been administered in this patient. Certain drugs such as aminoglycosides and non-steroidal anti-inflammatory drugs can cause an allergic-type renal failure called acute interstitial nephritis (AIN); however, this has not been described with dobutamine. Furthermore, in AIN, urinalysis classically shows WBCs and WBC casts, as well as eosinophils.

Answer B is incorrect. Autoimmune glomerulonephritis may be seen in conditions such as lupus and Goodpasture's syndrome. However, these causes of glomerular disease present with nephritic or nephrotic syndrome with hypertension, edema, and proteinuria, and are not consistent with this patient's presentation.

Answer C is incorrect. Hypovolemia can cause prerenal failure; however, in this condition, one would expect a higher BUN:creatinine ratio, lower Fe_{Na}, and higher urine osmolarity. Furthermore, hypovolemic renal failure should be responsive to fluids over 24–72 hours and would not take weeks to resolve.

Answer E is incorrect. Pyelonephritis does not commonly cause renal failure. Furthermore, in kidney infection, one would expect flank pain, dysuria, and WBCs or WBC casts in the urinalysis, none of which are described in this patient.

43. **The correct answer is B.** Group B streptococci (GBS) commonly colonize the gastrointestinal or genital tracts of adults. In pregnant females, colonization with GBS can lead to chorioamnionitis and sepsis. In newborn infants, group B streptococcal infection can lead to bacteremia, sepsis, and meningitis. Screening for GBS colonization is commonly done in pregnant women between 35 and 37 weeks' gestation. Women who are GBS positive then receive intravenous penicillin in labor to protect the infant from getting the infection during delivery.

Answer A is incorrect. *Chlamydia trachomatis* is a sexually transmitted disease that causes cervicitis and pelvic inflammatory disease. Infection with chlamydia during pregnancy does increase the risk of chorioamnionitis. However, conjunctivitis and pneumonia are the most common manifestations of chlamydia in newborns, not sepsis.

Answer C is incorrect. HIV may be transmitted vertically from mother to child late in pregnancy or during labor. Infection with HIV does not cause chorioamnionitis or neonatal sepsis.

Answer D is incorrect. Primary infection of a pregnant woman with toxoplasmosis can cause congenital toxoplasmosis in the newborn child. Complications of congenital toxoplasmosis include chorioretinitis, hydrocephalus, seizures, and mental retardation. The infection is often subclinical in infants with disease manifestations appearing later in life. Infection in adults is usually asymptomatic.

Answer E is incorrect. *Treponema palladium* is the causative organism in syphilis, which can cause congenital defects such as liver failure and skin lesions. However, it is not implicated in chorioamnionitis or neonatal sepsis.

44. **The correct answer is E.** Because the parathyroid hormone level and serum calcium concentration is high, the patient most likely has primary hyperparathyroidism. Single adenoma is the most frequent cause of primary hyperparathyroidism, accounting for 80% of cases.

Answer A is incorrect. Ectopic parathyroid tissue accounting for hyperparathyroidism is very rare.

Answer B is incorrect. Multiple adenomas are much less common than a single adenoma.

Answer C is incorrect. Parathyroid carcinoma is an exceedingly rare cause of primary hyperparathyroidism.

Answer D is incorrect. Parathyroid hyperplasia is the second most likely cause of primary hyperparathyroidism, accounting for 15% of cases.

Questions 45 and 46

45. **The correct answer is G.** Rotavirus is the most important cause of severe dehydrating diarrhea in early childhood. It is most commonly encountered during the winter months and is spread easily along the fecal-oral route. Child care centers and children's hospitals are common sites of encounter with the infectious agents. The virions of the rotavirus are highly contagious and shed in high concentrations in the stool before and during the clinical manifestations. Patients typically present after an incubation period of < 48 hours with low-grade to moderate-grade fever and simultaneous vomiting. Watery diarrhea is a later manifestation, often occurring for 5–7 days. Patients must be monitored closely for deteriorating clinical condition secondary to dehydration, which if left untreated can lead to eventual death. Treatment is aggressive hydration and antibiotic therapy is not recommended.

46. **The correct answer is H.** Acute enteritis is the most common manifestation of enteric salmonellosis. Patients infected with nontyphoidal *Salmonella* experience an acute onset of nausea, vomiting, and abdominal cramping, followed by mild to severe watery diarrhea that may contain blood and mucus. The incubation period for infection is typically 6–72 hours with a mean incubation period of 24 hours. The major source of nontyphoidal *Salmonella* is constituted by animals, specifically poultry and poultry products. In this case, the patient's clinical presentation is consistent with salmonellosis, and the recent inclusion of egg salad, chicken, and homemade eggnog in her diet should lead to high suspicion of the diagnosis. Therapy is aggressive hydration, and antibiotics are, in fact, detrimental and should never be prescribed.

Answer A is incorrect. *Bacillus cereus* is a gram-positive spore-forming rod that causes food poisoning when the spores land on food and germinate, creating a toxin. Ingestion of the toxin will lead to sudden onset nausea, vomiting, and diarrhea. Because the reaction is due to preformed toxins, antibiotics are not useful, and treatment is supportive.

Answer B is incorrect. *Campylobacter jejuni* is a gram-negative flagellated rod that, along with rotavirus and enterotoxigenic *Escherichia coli*, is one of the three most common causes of diarrhea in the world. Domestic animals and poultry are a reservoir for these bacteria, which are passed by the fecal-oral route and unpasteurized milk. Infection presents with a prodrome of fever, headaches, and malaise, followed by bloody, loose diarrhea. Treatment is with a fluoroquinolone and fluid resuscitation.

Answer C is incorrect. *Clostridium difficile* is the pathogen of antibiotic (usually clindamycin or ampicillin)-associated colitis. Symptoms include diarrhea, fever, and abdominal cramping. *C. difficile* toxins can be tested for in stool samples. Treatment is usually with metronidazole and discontinuation of antibiotics.

Answer D is incorrect. Enteric adenovirus is another common viral etiology of diarrhea in infants and children. However, this virus is most prevalent in the spring and summer seasons. Infection is often accompanied by fever, rhinorrhea, cough, and acute respiratory disease. No antivirals or vaccines are appropriate for the treatment of adenovirus, and aggressive hydration is the treatment of choice.

Answer E is incorrect. *Escherichia coli* bacterial colitis is caused by several subtypes of the *E. coli* bacteria. Enterotoxigenc *E. coli* causes a rice water–type stool and is often seen in travelers to third-world countries. Enterohemorrhagic *E. coli* causes a hemorrhagic colitis, and the specific subtype *E. coli* O157:H7 results in hemolytic uremic syndrome (HUS). HUS is characterized by thrombocytopenia and renal failure. Enteroinvasive *E. coli* results in colitis along with fever, and WBCs can be found in the stool. Treatment is aggressive oral hydration without antibiotic therapy.

Answer F is incorrect. *Giardia lamblia* is a flagellated protozoan that infects the duodenum and small intestine in affected patients.

Infection is often asymptomatic, but in patients manifesting symptoms, watery diarrhea is the most common presentation. Other symptoms include malaise and weakness, flatulence, abdominal distention, foul-smelling greasy stools, weight loss, and anorexia. G. lamblia has an incubation period of approximately 1–2 weeks, and diarrhea can be prolonged, lasting in some patients for several weeks.

Answer I is incorrect. *Shigella* is a nonflagellated gram-negative rod. It is found only in humans and passed by the fecal-oral route—often in communal living situations or day care. Infection presents with fever and abdominal pain, along with blood and pus-speckled diarrhea. Treatment is with fluoroquinolones and fluid resuscitation.

Answer J is incorrect. *Staphylococcus aureus* is a pathogen implicated in multiple cases of food-borne illness each year. The mechanism of infection is based on preformed toxins that are found in infected foods and are able to illicit the clinical symptoms described. The in-

cubation period for S. aureus food poisoning is within hours after ingestion, and emesis is commonly the first and most significant symptom.

Answer K is incorrect. *Vibrio cholerae* is a gram-negative flagellated rod that is passed by the fecal-oral route, usually through drinking contaminated water. It presents with sudden onset voluminous "rice water" diarrhea. Treatment is primarily with fluid resuscitation and oral rehydration as patients can lose up to 1 L of fluid in an hour, and death is commonly from dehydration. Definitive treatment is with antibiotics—either doxycycline or a fluoroquinolone.

Answer L is incorrect. *Vibrio parahaemolyticus* is a gram-negative rod that is found in marine water and is a common cause of diarrhea in Japan, where raw seafood is commonly consumed. Infection presents similarly to V. cholera with "rice water" diarrhea; however, V. parahaemolyticus typical resolves within 3 days without need for treatment.

Test Block 4

1. A 51-year-old woman presents to her primary care physician complaining of headache for the past 2 weeks. Further questioning reveals weakness over the past several months that has led to gradual impairment of physical activities. The patient has no other complaints, takes no medications other than a multivitamin, and smokes a pack of cigarettes daily. Physical examination reveals a blood pressure of 150/94 mm Hg and a respiratory rate of 8/min. Laboratory studies reveal potassium 3.1 mEq/L, and sodium 143 mEq/L. Imaging reveals bilateral adrenal hyperplasia. Which of the following medications would be most appropriate for this patient?

(A) Clonidine
(B) Hydrochlorothiazide
(C) Metoprolol
(D) Spironolactone
(E) Sumatriptan

2. The parents of a 4-week-old white boy present to the pediatric emergency department (ED) concerned about their son's feeding patterns. His mother reports he was feeding well for the first several days but developed nonbilious emesis toward the end of his second week of life. The episodes of emesis have worsened and now occur after every feeding, with some episodes being projectile in nature. Immediately after vomiting, the newborn is hungry and ready to feed again. He has a mobile, nontender epigastric mass that is olive shaped on physical examination. Heart rate is 128/min, blood pressure is 80/52 mm Hg, respiratory rate is 37/min, and temperature is 37.5°C (99.5°F). What acid-base disorder is the patient most at risk of developing?

(A) Hyperchloremic-hypokalemic metabolic acidosis
(B) Hyperchloremic-hypokalemic metabolic alkalosis
(C) Hypochloremic-hyperkalemic metabolic alkalosis
(D) Hypochloremic-hypokalemic metabolic acidosis
(E) Hypochloremic-hypokalemic metabolic alkalosis

3. A 30-year-old man is brought by ambulance to the ED after a major motor vehicle crash. He is lethargic but conscious and after the primary survey he is found to have significant hypotension and tachycardia. Secondary survey reveals an unstable pelvic girdle and what appears to be a developing pelvic hematoma. There is no blood at the urethral meatus. Anteroposterior x-ray of the pelvis is as shown in the image. Which of the following is contraindicated in this patient?

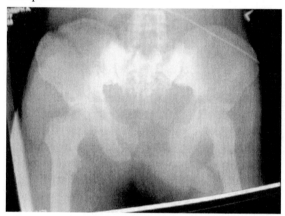

Reprinted, with permission, from Brunicardi FC, Andersen DK, Billiar TR, Dunn DL, Hunter JG, Matthews JB, Pollock RE, Schwartz SI. *Schwartz's Principles of Surgery*, 8th ed. New York: McGraw-Hill, 2005: Figure 42-41.

(A) Emergent pelvic angiography
(B) Exploration of the hematoma
(C) Manual prostate examination
(D) Orthopedic consultation for fixation
(E) Retrograde urethrogram
(F) Volume resuscitation

4. A 56-year-old man with a history of diabetes and hypertension presents to the ophthalmology clinic with a history of a blind spot in his right eye. He reports that it is painless, occurred suddenly, and is only in his right eye. On examination, he has a visual field loss in the right superior hemifield. Examination of the retina shows peripheral hemorrhages and disc congestion. What is the most likely diagnosis?

(A) Acute ophthalmic artery occlusion
(B) Branch retinal vein occlusion
(C) Central retinal vein occlusion

(D) Diabetic retinopathy
(E) Hypertensive retinopathy

5. A 25-year-old African-American woman develops a nonproductive cough and dyspnea on exertion that progressively worsens over several months. An x-ray of the chest demonstrates bilateral hilar adenopathy with interstitial infiltrates bilaterally. Biopsy of a waxy nodule on the woman's arm reveals noncaseating granuloma formation. Which of the following symptoms also occur in patients with this disease?

(A) Alopecia
(B) Ataxia and dysmetria
(C) Distal extremity weakness
(D) Keratoconjunctivitis
(E) Koilonychia

6. A 28-year-old woman presents to the ED complaining of sharp abdominal pain localized to the left lower quadrant. She reports feeling perfectly well until half an hour prior to her arrival at the ED. When asked if she could be pregnant, the patient responds that her last menstrual period was 2 weeks ago, and that she has not been sexually active during the past month. The patient's temperature is 36.9°C (98.4°F) and her blood pressure is 110/70 mm Hg. Abdominal examination elicits guarding and rebound tenderness. Pelvic examination is normal, and urine β-human chorionic gonadotropin is negative. What is the most likely etiology of this patient's abdominal pain?

(A) Acute appendicitis
(B) Acute gastritis
(C) Ectopic pregnancy
(D) Mesenteric ischemia
(E) Ruptured corpus luteum cyst

7. A 48-year-old man presents to the ED complaining of stabbing abdominal pain that increases when he tries to eat. He admits to current cocaine and alcohol use. On examination,

he is hypertensive to 162/100 mm Hg and diaphoretic. His amylase and lipase confirm that he has acute pancreatitis. He is placed on empiric antibiotics, aggressive intravenous fluids, and is made "nothing by mouth" status. His blood pressure remains elevated. What agent should the physician use to lower his blood pressure?

(A) Alprenolol
(B) Atenolol
(C) Lorazepam
(D) Metoprolol
(E) Verapamil

8. A 5-year-old boy presents with fever, pallor, and bony pain, and is diagnosed with acute lymphoid leukemia following extensive laboratory work-up and bone marrow biopsy. His laboratory studies revealed a WBC count of 240,000/mm^3, hemoglobin of 8.1 mg/dL, and platelets of 79,000/mm^3. Treatment with chemotherapy is initiated emergently. Twelve hours after his therapy is begun, he develops acute ventricular arrhythmias. Review of his bedside chart reveals anuria over the past 8 hours, despite vigorous provision of intravenous fluids. Laboratory evaluation reveals a blood urea nitrogen of 150 mg/dL and the following electrolytes: Na$^+$ 2.5 mmol/L and K$^+$ 8.9 mmol/L. Urinalysis reveals uric acid crystals in his urine. Which element of his disease and/or therapy is most likely to be accountable for his condition?

(A) Cardiac damage due to doxorubicin therapy
(B) Incorrect dosing of the anesthetic given during the bone marrow biopsy
(C) Leukemic infiltrate of the kidney leading to decreased renal function
(D) Overhydration leading to acute renal failure
(E) Rapid destruction of leukocytes by chemotherapeutic agents

9. A 58-year-old long-time alcoholic is brought to the ED after vomiting blood. After a comprehensive workup, the bleeding is determined to be due to ruptured esophageal varices. The patient has been treated for this condition several times before. He is admitted, and a management plan is determined. Four days following a new intervention, this patient becomes confused, agitated, and lethargic. On examination, he demonstrates asterixis and hyperreflexia. Given the onset of symptoms following treatment, what was the new intervention?

(A) Balloon tamponade
(B) β-Blocker therapy
(C) Endoscopic band ligation
(D) Endoscopic sclerotherapy
(E) Portosystemic shunt

10. A delirious 82-year-old man with terminal pancreatic cancer is having episodes of hypotension due to a systemic infection. The intensive care unit (ICU) team is considering use of potent intravenous antibiotics to treat the infection. Treatment is begun, despite a signed living will in the form of a "Do Not Resuscitate" (DNR). Given the signed DNR, did the ICU team make the wrong management decision?

(A) No, a DNR form should not influence action against treatable conditions
(B) No, but if a durable power of attorney was in the file, that typically supersedes an advance directive provided by the patient
(C) No, but the DNR form dictates that intravenous antibiotics should be stopped if the patient has adverse effects from the treatment
(D) Yes, a health care proxy should have been consulted before treatment was begun
(E) Yes, a signed DNR form indicates that the patient did not want to prolong his suffering, so no treatment should have been given

11. A 6-year-old boy presents with dyspnea at rest and cough productive of thick mucoid sputum over the last 5 days. He has a temperature of 39.4°C (103°F) which is only temporarily relieved by acetaminophen. He has had two episodes of pneumonia in the last 5 months, and a maternal uncle who died at an early age. On examination, he is a thin child who is breathing rapidly. Auscultation of the chest shows decreased breath sounds in both bases. X-ray of the chest shows consolidation of the left and right lower lobes. Since the patient cannot produce a good sputum sample, a bronchoscopy is performed and a lavage sample is sent. Preliminary Gram stain results are as follows:

Color: Yellow
Consistency: Thick
Neutrophils: Many
Gram stain: Numerous gram-negative rods

Which of the following causative organisms is most supportive of the presumptive diagnosis?

(A) *Klebsiella pneumoniae*
(B) *Listeria monocytogenes*
(C) *Pseudomonas aeruginosa*
(D) *Staphylococcus aureus*

12. An 82-year-old man with a history of hypertension, hypercholesterolemia, and chronic obstructive pulmonary disease presents to the ED with severe back pain. He also feels diaphoretic and nauseous. The patient states that he is usually compliant with his medications but sometimes forgets to take them all. He denies any alcohol use or illicit drug use. At presentation, his temperature is 37.1°C (98.7°F), blood pressure is 165/104 mm Hg, pulse is 112/min, and respiratory rate is 18/min. His O$_2$ saturation is 94%. On physical examination, there is no jugular venous distension, and there are diminished but equal pulses bilaterally in the lower extremities. Cardiovascular examination reveals regular rate and rhythm without murmurs, rubs, or gallops. An abdominal CT scan was obtained as seen in the image. What is the most likely diagnosis?

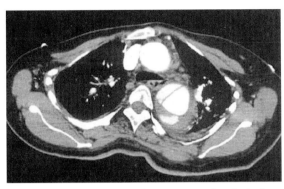

Reprinted, with permission, from Brunicardi FC, Andersen DK, Billiar TR, Dunn DL, Hunter JG, Matthews JB, Pollock RE, Schwartz SI. *Schwartz's Principles of Surgery*, 8th edition. New York: McGraw-Hill, 2005: Figure 21-12.

(A) Aortic dissection
(B) Lumbar disc herniation
(C) Pancreatic cancer
(D) Perforated peptic ulcer
(E) Ruptured aortic aneurysm

13. A 20-year-old recent immigrant presents to his primary care physician with complaints of jaundice, discoloration of his eyes, tremor, dysphagia, and depressed mood. Examination reveals jaundice, green-brown deposits in the cornea, hepatomegaly, tremor, and rigidity of the extremities. The physician suspects the patient suffers from a specific liver metabolic abnormality and wants to confirm his diagnosis with further evaluation. Which of the following would be appropriate as the next step of diagnosis?

   (A) Check the levels of serum iron, ferritin, and transferrin, and the percentage saturation of iron
   (B) Check the serum level of ceruloplasmin
   (C) Order an abdomen CT scan with contrast
   (D) Order hepatitis screening panel
   (E) Perform ultrasound-guided paracentesis

14. A 38-year-old man is brought to his doctor by his wife, who describes a distinct change in his personality over the past several weeks. Although he holds a successful job, he has not gone to work for the past week because he "doesn't feel like it." He typically sits in bed and stares blankly at the television for hours at a time. Occasionally she finds him crying for no apparent reason. He enters the examination room very slowly and refuses to make eye contact with the physician. He has lost nearly 6.8 kg (15 lb) in 1 year. When directly questioned about suicidal ideation, he indicates that he often thinks about dying and has thought about jumping out the window of his office on the 27th floor. He also states that he has never experienced anything like this before in his life. Which of the following psychiatric medications is most appropriate for this man?

(A) Amitriptyline
(B) Benztropine
(C) Citalopram
(D) Phenelzine
(E) Risperidone

15. A 58-year-old man presents to the ED with 1 day of high fever to 39.5°C (103.1°C) along with muscle aches and malaise. During the initial interview, he remembers his name but is not oriented to place or time, and he cannot recall the names of his four children. He has no known medical problems. His wife claims that he is in "perfect health" and reports that he was out playing in the yard with their grandchildren 3 days ago. They have not been out of the country in more than 2 years and have no animals at home. A peripheral blood smear demonstrates morulae within several monocytes. Additional laboratory studies are as follows:

Platelet count	84,000/mm^3
Leukocyte count	2500/mm^3
Hemoglobin	14.2 g/dL
Serum transaminases	Mildly elevated

Which of the following pathogens is most likely to have caused this patient's disease?

(A) *Babesia microti*
(B) *Borrelia burgdorferi*
(C) *Ehrlichia chaffeensis*
(D) HIV
(E) *Leishmania donovani*
(F) *Rickettsia rickettsii*
(G) *Trypanosoma brucei*

16. A 25-year-old woman presents to her primary care physician with fatigue, malaise, swollen feet, and a weight gain of > 4.5 kg (10 lb) in the past 2 weeks. She also describes a rash that is distributed primarily over her face, neck, and distal arms. On questioning, she recalls that she has also had sore knees, wrists, and ankles on and off for the past few months. Her face is quite red, exhibiting an erythematous eruption over her cheeks and the bridge of her nose, and she has small, pinpoint lesions on her buccal mucosa and hard palate. She has 2+ pitting edema up to her knees bilaterally. The remainder of her physical examination is within normal limits. Her urine dipstick shows 3+ proteinuria and microscopic hematuria. Which of the following autoantibodies would be expected to correlate with disease activity in this patient?

(A) Anticentromere antibodies
(B) Anti–double-stranded DNA antibodies
(C) Anti-Jo-1 antibodies
(D) Anti-Scl-70 antibodies
(E) La antibodies
(F) Ro antibodies

17. A 65-year-old woman with a history of coronary artery disease presents to the ED complaining of severe abdominal pain for the past 2 days, first beginning as dull pain near the umbilicus but now localized to the right lower quadrant. The patient reports that just prior to examination by the physician, she experienced a sudden decrease in intensity of pain, but she still feels very uncomfortable and must remain still on the stretcher. On examination, the patient appears in distress, and she is hypotensive with systolic blood pressure at 85 mm Hg (systolic blood pressure at triage was 110 mm Hg), and her oral temperature is 40°C (104°F). She has a diffusely tender abdomen with point tenderness in her right lower abdomen, accompanied by guarding and rebound. Laboratory values showed a leukocytosis of 20,000/mm^3 with 95% polymorphonuclear lymphocytes. Her ECG shows nonspecific ST-T changes from a baseline ECG taken 6 months ago. CT of the abdomen shows a loculated mass in the right lower quadrant. What is the most appropriate step in evaluation for further management?

(A) Blood cultures
(B) MRI of the abdomen
(C) Percutaneous drainage
(D) Ultrasound
(E) Urine culture

18. An 18-year-old woman presents to her primary care doctor for a follow-up appointment subsequent to a diagnosis of infectious mononucleosis. The patient's complete blood cell count (CBC) 1 month ago was WBC count 12,000/mm^3, hemoglobin 13.7 g/dL, and platelets 183,000/ mm^3. At follow-up, the WBC count is 7800/mm^3, hemoglobin is 14.2 g/dL, and platelet count is 78,000/mm^3. The patient denies any increased bleeding or spontaneous bleeding. Additional laboratory tests are notable for a bleeding time of 9 seconds, an activated partial thromboplastin time of 27 seconds, a prothrombin time of 12 seconds, and a normal clotting time. A diagnosis of postinfectious idiopathic thrombocytopenic purpura is made. What is the next step in management?

(A) Conservative management with follow-up and repeat complete blood count
(B) Initiate steroids
(C) Transfuse fresh frozen plasma
(D) Transfuse packed RBCs
(E) Transfuse platelets

19. A 52-year-old woman with ovarian cancer has been in the hospital for more than 4 months and is currently without decision-making capacity. On the most recent CT of the chest, abdomen, and pelvis, bulky disease was evident throughout. She has already been through two sessions of chemotherapy, the most recent of which provided minimal disease reduction. Her chosen health care proxy, in agreement with the wishes of the rest of the family, has requested a third round of chemotherapy. Her physician refuses to administer another round of chemotherapy. What is an appropriate response of the health care proxy?

(A) Because the patient chose the health care proxy when she had capacity, the physician must follow her instructions
(B) Because this treatment was partially successful the first time it was administered, the physician is ethically required to administer the chemotherapy

(C) Physician is legally and ethically required to administer the chemotherapy

(D) Physician is legally, but not ethically, required to administer the chemotherapy

(E) Physician is neither legally nor ethically required to administer the chemotherapy

20. An 11-month-old child is brought to the physician by her parents because they are concerned about "seizures" of increasing frequency and severity during which the child flails her upper extremities. Physical examination is normal except for psychomotor delay. On questioning, her parents mention that she is not speaking at all, she is not yet walking, and in fact only recently has been able to sit on her own. An EEG shows very-high-voltage, random, slow waves and spikes in all cortical areas. When her parents inquire about her prognosis, what are they told?

(A) Although her spasms will eventually regress, she is likely to be neurologically impaired

(B) Her condition is due to an infectious agent and her symptoms will most likely resolve upon treatment

(C) Her condition is entirely benign and requires no treatment

(D) She most likely has an upper respiratory tract infection that will resolve on its own

(E) The physician is obligated to contact child protective services before you can discuss her condition further

21. A 25-year-old white man presents with diarrhea, weight loss of 4.5 kg (10.0 lb) over the preceding 2 months, and RLQ pain. On examination, his temperature is 38.2°C (100.7°F), heart rate is 82/min, and blood pressure is 110/70 mm Hg. Abdominal examination reveals mild tenderness with no rebound tenderness, and a mass is palpated in the RLQ. His stool tests positive for occult blood. Subsequent colonoscopy reveals erythematous, friable mucosa with ulcerations in a longitudinal distribution. The ulcerations are segmental and interspersed with intervening normal mucosa. Colonic biopsies show a dense inflammatory infiltrate with neutrophils and mononuclear cells. The patient should be informed of which of the following?

(A) Antibiotics have been shown to benefit patients with his condition

(B) Appendectomy should be scheduled

(C) Curative proctocolectomy with ileoanal anastomoses is indicated at this time

(D) Toxic megacolon is a frequent complication of his disease

(E) Trial gluten-free diet is indicated

22. A postmenopausal 50-year-old woman with cryptogenic liver cirrhosis and coagulopathy was admitted to the hospital for severe vaginal bleeding secondary to uterine fibroids. The patient was deemed to be a poor surgical candidate because of her coagulopathy, and she was transferred to the medicine service for preoperative management, including packed red blood cells (PRBCs) and fresh frozen plasma transfusions. Although the patient initially agreed to receive transfusions, after 2 units of PRBCs she refused further transfusions, stating "I want a more definitive treatment than just receiving transfusions!" The patient's hematocrit, however, was steadily decreasing and the patient continued to experience vaginal bleeding. Although the internist thoroughly explained the nature, indications, risks, benefits, and alternatives regarding blood product transfusions, the patient still refuses to receive blood products. The patient denies feeling depressed, and is alert and oriented to time, place, and person. There are no signs of depression or suicidality. Which of the following is the most appropriate next step in patient care?

(A) Call the ethics committee and seek approval to override the patient's decision

(B) Call for psychiatry consultation to determine compete

(C) Hold transfusions and have a discussion with the gynecology consult service regarding alternatives to surgery, such as interventional radiology procedures

(D) Since the patient had given consent for earlier transfusions, the internist should continue the transfusions and reverse the coagulopathy to prepare the patient for surgery

(E) Talk to patient's husband and seek his consent for the patient's transfusions

23. A 63-year-old man presents with fatigue and frequent nosebleeds developing gradually over 4 months. He notes that he feels an abdominal fullness and becomes full easily when eating. On physical examination, he is afebrile but shows pallor of the conjunctivae and some dried blood around the nares. Splenomegaly is present, but the liver is not appreciably enlarged. The skin shows no rashes. Laboratory studies show a WBC count of 56,000/mm³ (with 59% neutrophils), a hemoglobin of 8.5 g/dL, and a platelet count of 21,000/mm³. ECG shows normal sinus rhythm with no ST-segment changes. A peripheral blood smear is shown in the image. The cells stain positively with myeloperoxidase. What is the likely diagnosis?

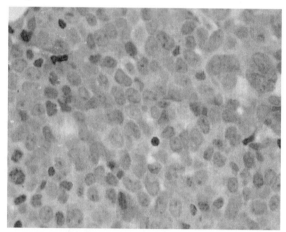

Reproduced, with permission, from Lichtman MA, Beutler E, Kipps TJ, Seligsohn U, Kaushansky K, Prchal JT. *Williams Hematology*, 7th ed. New York: McGraw-Hill, 2006: Plate XIV-9.

(A) Acute myelogenous leukemia
(B) Anemia of chronic disease
(C) Chronic myelogenous leukemia
(D) Multiple myeloma
(E) Thrombotic thrombocytopenic purpura

24. A 46-year-old man with no past medical history comes to the ED complaining of an inability to move his left leg. He takes no medications or herbal compounds and denies having any allergies. The patient currently lives with a male companion, with whom he has been monogamous for 18 months. He denies any tobacco, ethanol, or intravenous drug use and has never had an HIV test. Neurologic examination reveals no cranial nerve deficits, and strength, sensation, and tone are normal in the upper extremities. The man has substantially increased tone in both legs, left more than right, and strength is 3/5 in the right hip flexors and knee extensors and 0/5 on the left. His reflexes are increased bilaterally, left more so than the right, and four beats of clonus are detected on the left. His toes are upgoing bilaterally. Laboratory tests are remarkable for a WBC count of 3000/mm³; a lumbar puncture is unremarkable. Follow-up HIV testing is positive, and his CD4+ count is 28/mm³. An MRI of the brain shows several nonenhancing white matter lesions; no mass effect is evident. Which of the following is the likely mechanism for this patient's symptoms?

(A) Demyelination of the central nervous system
(B) Infection with *Candida albicans*
(C) Infection with JC virus
(D) Infection with herpes simplex virus type 1
(E) Infection with *Toxoplasma gondii*

25. A 55-year-old man with diabetes, hypertension, and a history of pneumonia treated as an outpatient 20 years prior presents to the clinic during early fall for a blood pressure check. He currently works as a respiratory therapist at a local hospital. The physician suggests that he receive a pneumococcus vaccination. What are his primary indications for receiving the vaccine?

(A) Age
(B) Diabetes
(C) Health care worker
(D) Hypertension
(E) Pneumonia

26. A 36-year-old African-American woman presents to the physician's office complaining of increasing dyspnea on exertion and fatigue. She has also noticed that she has been urinating more frequently, even though she has not been drinking more fluids, including caffeine. She has never traveled outside the United States. On review of systems, she also reports some blurry vision, night sweats, muscle weakness, constipation, and a 2.3-kg (5-lb) weight loss. The physician notes that the patient has some supraclavicular lymphadenopathy, so he

decides to draw blood for testing. What other laboratory abnormality would be expected?

(A) Ca²⁺: 11.3 mEq/dL.
(B) Glucose: 210 mg/dL
(C) Hemoglobin: 10.5 g/dL
(D) Na+ = 151 mEq/dL
(E) WBC count: 11,600/mm³ with 80% lymphocytes

27. A 32-year-old G2P1 woman at 32 weeks' gestation presents to the obstetrics and gynecology clinic for a follow-up visit. She complains of fatigue, polyuria, and lower back pain. Her previous pregnancy was without complications, and the child weighed 3.5 kg (7 lb 10 oz) at delivery. The patient is in no acute distress. Physical examination is notable for a fundal height of 33 cm. Extremities reveal some mild edema of the feet. A glucose loading test at 26 weeks' gestation showed a blood glucose of 145 mg/dL. Results of a subsequent glucose tolerance test are as follows:

Fasting	105 mg/dL
1 hour	210 mg/dL
2 hours	185 mg/dL
3 hours	190 mg/dL

Results of other prenatal tests have been reassuring. She denies any contractions or loss of fluid. Ultrasound reveals a fetus that is large for gestational age, with an estimated fetal weight of > 4 kg (> 8.8 lb). What is the next most appropriate prenatal test for this patient?

(A) Amniocentesis
(B) Chorionic villus sampling
(C) Cortisol level
(D) Hemoglobin A₁c level
(E) Random blood glucose

28. A 48-year-old man is rushed by ambulance to the ED after collapsing at home. According to his wife, his medical history is significant for mild asthma and recently diagnosed hypertension, for which he was prescribed 25 mg atenolol twice a day. His wife states that his blood pressure was elevated today when he checked it at the supermarket and that he had taken several additional pills to attempt to control it. His heart rate is 45/min, blood pressure 95/60 mm Hg, and respiratory rate 20/min. His O₂ saturation is 98% on 2 liters of O₂. He is obtunded. An ECG reveals complete heart block. Atropine and isoproterenol are administered. What additional intervention should be considered at this time?

(A) Amiodarone
(B) Cardiac pacing
(C) Diphenhydramine
(D) Glucagon
(E) Nebulized albuterol

29. A 60-year-old man presents to his primary care physician with the chief complaints of fatigue and unintentional weight loss over the past few months. He has noted blood in his urine, but never brought it to a physician's attention because it was never painful. Over the past 2 weeks, he has also developed a nonproductive cough. On physical examination, the man is cachectic with temporal wasting. He has a palpable, irregularly shaped mass that is located just above the pubic symphysis to the left of the midline. Digital rectal examination reveals a normal prostate and guaiac-negative stool. Urinalysis is positive for blood. CT scans of the chest, abdomen, and pelvis show a large tumor in the bladder and several suspicious-looking pelvic and cervical lymph nodes. On x-ray of the chest, four 1-cm lesions are noted in the man's left lung. He undergoes a cystoscopy and a 4-cm mass is seen on the left superior aspect of the bladder. A biopsy reveals transitional cell carcinoma. Which treatment is most appropriate for this man's disease?

(A) Intravesicular bacille Calmette-Guérin and systemic chemotherapy
(B) Pelvic exenteration and systemic chemotherapy
(C) Supportive care
(D) Systemic chemotherapy
(E) Transurethral resection of the bladder tumor, pelvic radiation, and systemic chemotherapy

30. A 32-year-old woman with long-standing schizophrenia presents with muscle cramps, nausea, and polyuria. Her lungs are clear to auscultation, and the physician does not find any signs of edema. Skin turgor appears normal. Laboratory tests show:

Na$^+$	129 mEq/L
K$^+$	3.5 mEq/L
Cl$^-$	100 mEq/L
Blood urea nitrogen	15 mg/dL
Creatinine	1.0 mg/dL
Glucose	99 mg/dL
Urine osmolality	105 mOsm/kg
Urine Na$^+$	21 mmol/L

    What is the most likely cause of her electrolyte abnormality?

    (A) Adrenal insufficiency
    (B) Dehydration
    (C) Psychogenic polydipsia
    (D) Renal failure
    (E) Syndrome of inappropriate ADH

31. A 32-year-old man previously diagnosed with myasthenia gravis presents to the ED complaining of difficulty breathing. On examination, he has marked ptosis, is dyspneic, and is having difficulty speaking and swallowing. Serial measurements of the patient's vital capacity are 700, 620, and 580 mL. X-ray of the chest reveals a right middle lobe infiltrate. Which of the following is the next best step in the management of this patient?

    (A) Albuterol nebulizer treatments
    (B) High-dose edrophonium
    (C) Inhaled racemic epinephrine
    (D) Intravenous antibiotics
    (E) Immediate endotracheal intubation and plasmapheresis

32. A 34-year-old man who lives in a homeless shelter is frequently seen by the physician who volunteers at the shelter's clinic. Over time, he builds a relationship with the physician, and the physician learns that he is homosexual, although this is not widely known. She suggests that he be tested for HIV. When he returns to the clinic for results of the test (which came back positive), she notices that he has several crusted linear wounds on his upper arms and chest. The patient tells her that he had a fight with his partner, who stabbed him several times with a kitchen knife. In which of the following circumstances will the physician be required to override patient confidentiality?

    (A) If the physician suspects abuse, she must inform the shelter
    (B) Inform the health department that the patient is HIV-positive only
    (C) Inform the patient's partner that the patient is HIV-positive only
    (D) The physician must inform both the health department and the patient's partner of his HIV status
    (E) There is no reason to break patient confidentiality

33. A 2-month-old, full-term infant is brought to his pediatrician for a rash on his scalp. The rash has been present for several days and does not seem to bother him. The mother's pregnancy and delivery were uncomplicated, and the patient has been healthy and growing well at his neonatal visits. There are no sick contacts or pets at home. On examination, the superior scalp is erythematous and slightly greasy, with a yellowish scale and plaque formation. What is the best management for this patient?

    (A) 1% Hydrocortisone cream
    (B) Oral griseofulvin therapy
    (C) Selenium sulfide shampoo
    (D) Topical emollients
    (E) Topical ketoconazole cream

34. A 64-year-old man with a history of hypertension and carcinoid tumor of the appendix presents to the ED complaining of palpitations, trouble breathing, and weakness. It has been getting worse over the past day, and this morning he nearly passed out. His blood pressure is 148/90 mm Hg, pulse is 104/min, respiratory rate is 22/min, and temperature is 37.1°C (98.9°F). Physical examination reveals an S3 gallop, a prominent S4, jugular venous distension, ascites, bipedal edema, a point of maximal impulse that is shifted down and to the left, and hepatomegaly. ECG shows QRS complexes that are low voltage, and echocardiogram establishes that left and right atria are en-

larged with a thick right ventricle. A pressure tracing shows a "dip/plateau" sign. What is the most likely diagnosis?

(A) Cerebrovascular accident
(B) Coarctation of the aorta
(C) Mitral stenosis
(D) Prinzmetal's angina
(E) Restrictive cardiomyopathy

35. A 56-year-old woman presents to the surgery clinic. A suspicious lesion was found on routine mammography 1 week earlier. The patient denies any pain at the site of the lesion, but over the past month she has experienced increased fatigue. Past gynecologic history is notable for nulliparity, onset of menarche at the age of 9 years, and age at menopause of 50 years. Her pulse is 76/min, blood pressure is 123/76 mm Hg, and temperature is 37.8°C (100.1°F). Breast examination is significant for a fixed, nontender 2-cm lump in the upper outer quadrant of the left breast. Pelvic examination is within normal limits. Mammography revealed an irregular 2-cm lump corresponding with the physical findings. A breast biopsy is performed, which shows ductal carcinoma in situ. Which aspect of this patient's history, physical examination, and laboratory findings is the most influential in determining her prognosis?

(A) Age of menarche
(B) Histology of the tumor
(C) Presence of fatigue and fever
(D) Shape of the tumor
(E) Size of the tumor

36. A 48-year-old woman with rheumatoid arthritis presents to her rheumatologist for follow-up. She was diagnosed 3 years ago, has been maintained on disease-modifying agents and nonsteroidal anti-inflammatory drugs, and has been doing well. She has no complaints at present but is concerned about her current anti-inflammatory medication and recent media reports of stroke risk demonstrated with other drugs in the same class. Recent studies examining the relationship between stroke and use of cyclooxygenase-2 inhibitors in arthritis revealed an odds ratio of 1.2. What information should the patient receive about these studies?

(A) Avoiding the use of cyclooxygenase-selective agents reduces this patient's stroke risk
(B) If a patient is exposed to a cyclooxygenase-selective agent, his or her risk of suffering a stroke is increased by a factor of 1.2
(C) Patients on cyclooxygenase-selective agents have 1.2 times as many strokes as patients not on such medications
(D) Patients with rheumatoid arthritis have 1.2 times as many strokes as patients without the disease
(E) The odds that people who suffered a stroke had previously used cyclooxygenase-2 inhibitors are 1.2 times greater than in people who did not suffer a stroke

37. A 45-year-old man presents to a psychiatrist complaining of difficulty concentrating. He states that he has had problems following conversations and watching his favorite television sitcom for the past 2 months. He also admits to feelings of guilt, fatigue, and a general lack of motivation. He says he is particularly "down" because he recently gained 4.5 kg (10 lb). His temperature is 37.1°C (98.8°F), heart rate is 76/min, and blood pressure is 142/89 mm Hg. Physical examination is notable for multiple bruises on both arms and central obesity. ACTH is 70 pg/mL (normal: 9–52 pg/mL). A CT scan of the chest indicates a bronchial tumor. Which of the following may be used to medically manage his hormonal imbalance and the underlying disease process?

(A) Fludrocortisone
(B) Fluoxetine
(C) Ketoconazole
(D) Metformin
(E) Mitotane

38. A 50-year-old woman recently diagnosed with amyotrophic lateral sclerosis presents to the office with new-onset drooling that is interfering with her ability to work. She is unmarried with no children and wishes to remain at her job. Which of the following is an acceptable solution for her problem?

(A) Baclofen, a γ-aminobutyric acid analogue muscle relaxant, 5–10 mg two to three times a day
(B) Carbamazepine, an antiepileptic, 200 mg twice daily
(C) Consult psychiatry to rule out depression
(D) Living separately from her parents
(E) Diphenhydramine, an antihistamine, 50–100 mg at night

39. A 45-year-old woman with a history of untreated gout presents to the ED complaining of severe flank pain for 1 day. A CT scan is shown in the image. Which of the following is the best way to treat this patient's condition?

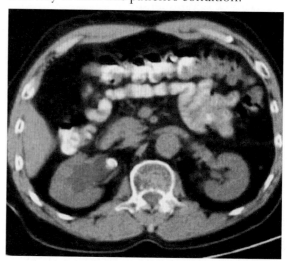

Reproduced, with permission, from Brunicardi FC, Andersen DK, Billiar TR, Dunn DL, Hunter JG, Matthews JB, Pollock RE, Schwartz SI. *Schwartz's Principles of Surgery*, 8th edition. New York: McGraw-Hill, 2005: Figure 39-7.

(A) Extracorporeal shock wave lithotripsy
(B) Hydration and alkalinization of the urine
(C) Low-sodium diet
(D) Penicillamine
(E) Thiazide diuretics

40. A 21-year-old woman presents to the ED with the complaint of severe abdominal pain for the past 6 hours. She is a college student, and her boyfriend was recently diagnosed with bacterial meningitis. After his diagnosis, the patient's boyfriend was treated with oral rifampin, and she was given prophylactic rifampin as well. The patient has a history of asthma, uses an albuterol inhaler and oral contraceptives, and has no allergies. On examination, the patient is in obvious discomfort, with pain on palpation of the lower left quadrant. Serum β-human chorionic gonadotropin is measured at 954 mg/dL, transvaginal ultrasound reveals free fluid in the cul-de-sac, and the patient undergoes laparoscopy revealing ruptured ectopic pregnancy. What is the most likely reason for the failure of the patient's oral contraceptive?

(A) Albuterol use
(B) Competition for binding sites
(C) Inactivation by a cellular pump
(D) Patient error
(E) Rifampin use

41. A 42-year-old man with recently diagnosed hypertension presents to the ED with flank pain of a few hours' duration. On physical examination the man has a blood pressure of 152/92 mm Hg, a heart rate of 78/min, and a temperature of 36.9°C (98.4°F). He has a II/VI systolic murmur at the lower sternal border with a midsystolic click, positive bowel sounds, bilateral palpable kidneys, and a liver that is 10 cm in size. No spleen tip is palpable. Urinalysis is positive for erythrocytes and leukocytes, but negative for bacteria. Relevant laboratory findings are:

WBC count   7200/mm^3
Hemoglobin   14.2 g/dL
Platelet count   250,000/mm^3
Na$^+$ 145 mEq/L
Blood urea nitrogen   20 mg/dL
Creatinine   2.2 mg/dL

On further questioning the man admits to having had several urinary tract infections over the past few months and notes that his doctor told him that he had "some sort of cardiac valve prolapse." What is the most likely diagnosis?

(A) Autosomal dominant polycystic kidney disease
(B) Autosomal recessive polycystic kidney disease
(C) Medullary cystic disease
(D) Medullary sponge kidney
(E) Nephrolithiasis
(F) Pyelonephritis

42. A 41-year-old obese woman presents to the ED with her three children. She is complaining of right upper quadrant (RUQ) pain that is worse when she eats (particularly when she eats fatty foods). On examination, she ceases inspiration on palpation of her RUQ. The physician ob-

tains an abdominal ultrasound, but the results are equivocal. What is the next appropriate test?

(A) CT of the abdomen
(B) Hepatic iminodiacetic acid scan
(C) MRI of the abdomen
(D) Sestamibi scan
(E) X-ray of the abdomen

43. A 42-year-old man presents for his annual physical examination. His blood pressure is 130/80 mm Hg and pulse is 75/min. His heart rate is regular with no murmurs, rubs, or gallops. Lungs are clear to auscultation bilaterally and abdomen is benign. No subclavicular lymphadenopathy is appreciated, but there is a fixed palpable firm nodule midline that does not shift with swallowing. A fine-needle biopsy is ordered, which is read as "indeterminate for follicular neoplasm." What is the next step in management?

(A) High-resolution ultrasonography
(B) Observation with follow-up every 4 months
(C) Radionucleotide scan
(D) Thyroxine therapy with close follow-up
(E) Total thyroidectomy

44. A 52-year-old man presents for an annual physical examination. He is generally in good health but complains of recent difficulty with urination. He reports that he has a weak, interrupted stream with dribbling. He denies nocturia, urgency, bladder fullness, daytime frequency, hematuria, fevers, chills, or family history of prostate cancer. On examination he is afebrile and has no costovertebral angle tenderness. His abdomen is soft and nontender. What would be the first appropriate screening exam?

(A) Cystoscopy
(B) Digital rectal examination
(C) Prostate biopsy
(D) Prostate-specific antigen level
(E) Urinalysis and urine culture

Questions 45 and 46

For each patient's infection, select the most likely etiologic agent.

(A) *Bacillus cereus*
(B) *Campylobacter jejuni*
(C) *Clostridium difficile*
(D) Enteric adenovirus
(E) *Escherichia coli*
(F) *Giardia lamblia*
(G) *Salmonella enteritidis*
(H) *Shigella*
(I) *Staphylococcus aureus*
(J) *Vibrio cholerae*
(K) *Vibrio parahaemolyticus*

45. A previously healthy 7-year-old girl is brought to the ED for evaluation of prolonged non-bloody watery diarrhea. According to her parents, the episodes began approximately 5 days ago when she simultaneously developed a low-grade fever to 38.2°C (100.8°F). Her travel history is notable for a week-long camping trip that she took with her father to Mexico approximately 1.5 weeks ago, where she went swimming. On physical examination, she is found to have a heart rate of 88/min, blood pressure of 102/65 mm Hg, and respiratory rate of 16/min. She appears tired, but her examination is unremarkable with no abdominal distention, tenderness, or masses. Her stool had a negative fecal occult blood test.

46. The patient seen next in the ED is an otherwise healthy 17-year-old boy who is complaining of recent-onset vomiting and diarrhea. He claims that shortly after eating his home-packed lunch of ham and cheese sandwiches, chips, apple, and cookies, he developed severe nausea and nonbilious, nonbloody emesis. Within 2 hours, he also developed nonbloody diarrhea. Physical examination demonstrates stable vital signs (heart rate 88/min, blood pressure 106/65 mm Hg, respiratory rate 14/min) and an unremarkable abdominal examination with no tenderness, distention, or masses. His stool had a negative fecal occult blood test.

1. **The correct answer is D.** The patient is suffering from primary hyperaldosteronism, and from the effects of elevated aldosterone: hypertension, hypokalemia, and metabolic alkalosis. Symptoms could be alleviated by reversing or blocking the effects of aldosterone. Aldosterone increases sodium reabsorption and increases potassium secretion and hydrogen ion secretion. Spironolactone antagonizes aldosterone at its receptor in the distal convoluted tubule and would be likely be beneficial in this patient.

Answer A is incorrect. Clonidine is a centrally-acting α-adrenergic agonist that might aid in treating the patient's hypertension, but not the electrolyte imbalances caused by the patient's hyperaldosteronism. This class of antihypertensives also could potentially contribute to the patient's complaints of weakness and fatigue.

Answer B is incorrect. Hydrochlorothiazide is a commonly used diuretic that inhibits resorption of sodium and chloride at the distal convoluted tubule. It would be an appropriate choice if this patient were presenting with essential hypertension, but it is inadequate in the context of hypertension secondary to hyperaldosteronism.

Answer C is incorrect. Metoprolol could resolve the patient's hypertension by antagonizing β-adrenergic receptors, but would not address the electrolyte imbalances caused by the patient's hyperaldosteronism. Moreover, fatigue is a common adverse effect of β-blockers, which could potentially exacerbate the patient's complaint of fatigue.

Answer E is incorrect. Selective serotonin agonists such as sumatriptan are first-line agents for treatment of acute migraine headaches. Though this patient does complain of headache, the history is not suggestive of migraines, and this agent would not address the patient's underlying problem of hyperaldosteronism.

2. **The correct answer is E.** The patient described has pyloric stenosis. Pyloric stenosis has a multifaceted etiology, including genetic and environmental factors. It is more common in boys (4–6:1) and is more commonly found in firstborn children. Vomiting after feeding develops 3–6 weeks after birth and is often projectile in nature. Infants with pyloric stenosis are often described as "hungry vomiters," given their desire to feed immediately after episodes of emesis. As a result of the malnourishment and dehydration, infants with pyloric stenosis develop hypochloremic-hypokalemic metabolic alkalosis. This metabolic acid-base disorder is caused by the massive loss of gastric hydrochloric acid (HCl). As HCl is lost, a state of volume depletion is established, and the kidney responds to the metabolic alkalosis by excreting bicarbonate in the urine, which results in obligate potassium and sodium loss. Hypochloremia also induces the renin-angiotensin-aldosterone axis, which induces increased aldosterone production and maintains the hypokalemic alkalosis. In addition, the alkalotic state induces hydrogen ions to move out of the intracellular space, where they are replaced by potassium ions moving into the cells, furthering hypokalemia.

Answer A is incorrect. The loss of gastric hydrochloric acid results in a metabolic alkalosis. Additionally, as the gastric acid is lost, chloride ions are also lost, creating a hypochloremic and not a hyperchloremic state.

Answer B is incorrect. The loss of gastric hydrochloric acid causes a hypochloremic and not a hyperchloremic state.

Answer C is incorrect. Because of the mechanism by which potassium is lost in an obligatory manner secondary to the loss of bicarbonate, the metabolic alkalosis that is produced in pyloric stenosis is of a hypokalemic and not a hyperkalemic nature.

Answer D is incorrect. Loss of hydrochloric acid from the episodes of emesis creates a metabolic alkalosis and not an acidosis disturbance. The hypochloremic and hypokalemic descriptors are correct, however, and describe the electrolyte imbalance that occurs secondary to pyloric stenosis.

3. The correct answer is B. This patient has a pelvic fracture with resultant hemodynamic instability. In such a patient, one must never explore a suspected pelvic or retroperitoneal hematoma. Rather, follow the patient with serial hematocrit and hemoglobin measurements to monitor for sufficient intravenous resuscitation. This patient should not be subjected to major pelvic surgery at this point because these hematomas often are a collection of blood from many vessels, most of which are not amenable to direct surgical control. The best chance to curb the patient's bleeding is external fixation.

Answer A is incorrect. Emergency pelvic angiography with embolization is a treatment option in the hemodynamically unstable patient.

Answer C is incorrect. Prostate examination may demonstrate a high-riding ballotable prostate or lack of a palpable prostate, both of which are suggestive of urethral injury.

Answer D is incorrect. Orthopedic consultation is mandatory in this case.

Answer E is incorrect. Due to the association between pelvic and urethral injury, a retrograde urethrogram must be ordered before Foley catheter placement is considered.

Answer F is incorrect. Rapid volume resuscitation is critical in the hemodynamically unstable patient with a pelvic fracture.

4. The correct answer is B. The differential diagnosis of painless unilateral vision loss can include several possibilities such as central and peripheral vein occlusion, diabetic neuropathy, and hypertensive neuropathy. The patient reports a history of hypertension and diabetes, both of which are risk factors for branch retinal vein occlusion. Additionally, funduscopic examination shows superficial hemorrhages in a sector of the retinal along a retinal vein. The hemorrhages usually do not cross the horizontal raphe (midline).

Answer A is incorrect. In acute ophthalmic artery occlusion, the entire retina typically appears whitened. Such disease occurs in the setting of carotid artery occlusive disease or other ischemic disease such as embolic disease and coagulopathy.

Answer C is incorrect. Central retinal vein occlusion can also present with painless unilateral vision loss. It occurs in patients who are elderly and is often idiopathic. The examination typically shows diffuse retinal hemorrhages in all four quadrants with dilated, tortuous retinal veins. There may also be cotton-wool spots, disc edema, and neovascularization of the disc or retina.

Answer D is incorrect. Diabetic retinopathy usually presents with bilateral visual defects that can lead to blindness because the retina is very sensitive to hyperglycemic effects, leading to loss of retinal pericytes and microvascular endothelial cells and thickening of retinal basement membrane. Funduscopic examination typically shows dot-and-blot hemorrhages and microaneurysms that extend across the horizontal raphe.

Answer E is incorrect. Hypertensive retinopathy usually presents with bilateral visual defects. Hemorrhages are not confined to a sector of the retina and usually cross the horizontal raphe. There are two contributing pathologies to this disease, including arteriolar thickening and acute vascular injury.

5. The correct answer is D. Ophthalmologic complications occur in roughly 20% of patients with sarcoidosis, most commonly in the form of keratoconjunctivitis or chorioconjunctivitis.

Answer A is incorrect. Causes of alopecia include bullous disease, severe folliculitis, and chemical reactions, but it is not a symptom of sarcoidosis.

Answer B is incorrect. Ataxia and dysmetria are not among the neurologic complications of sarcoidosis.

Answer C is incorrect. Although neurologic involvement occurs in a small percentage of patients with sarcoidosis, it typically manifests as cranial nerve palsies, hydrocephalus, or lymphocytic meningitis, and not as extremity weakness.

Answer E is incorrect. Koilonychia, or spooning of the nails, is typically a sign of iron-deficiency anemia, not typically seen in sarcoidosis.

6. The correct answer is E. The sudden onset of this patient's abdominal pain, the presence of guarding and rebound tenderness, and the fact this patient's last menstrual cycle was 2 weeks ago, all suggest the possibility of a ruptured corpus luteum cyst. Normally, a mature follicle transforms into a corpus luteum after ovulation, only to atrophy into a corpus albicans around the time of the next ovulation. Occasionally, a corpus luteum will fail to degenerate and result in the formation of a cyst; when these rupture, the patient experiences acute abdominal pain. It can be difficult to distinguish clinically between this pathology and adnexal torsion, perforated bowel, or ectopic pregnancy.

Answer A is incorrect. Acute appendicitis is a possibility; however, the pain of appendicitis is usually a dull, vague pain originating at the umbilicus and migrating to the right lower quadrant. The rapid onset and sharp nature of this patient's pain is more suggestive of a ruptured cyst.

Answer B is incorrect. Acute gastritis describes an inflammation of the stomach lining. The onset of gastritis is unlikely to occur over half an hour, and would not localize to the right lower quadrant.

Answer C is incorrect. Ectopic pregnancy is effectively ruled out by a negative β-human chorionic gonadotropin test and normal pelvic examination.

Answer D is incorrect. Mesenteric ischemia may be either acute or chronic. The chronic variety leads to pain associated with meals, is linked to vascular comorbidities, and would not likely be a consideration in a patient of this age group. The pain of acute mesenteric ischemia may be sudden in onset, but it is visceral in nature and likely to be poorly localized. Like chronic mesenteric ischemia, it generally affects patients over 60 years of age.

7. The correct answer is C. Given this patient's history, his persistent hypertension is likely to be a withdrawal symptom. Although not ordinarily used as antihypertensives, benzodiazepines are indicated in the supportive treatment of cocaine/amphetamine and alcohol withdrawal, and will treat the underlying cause of this patient's hypertension. In this instance, an ECG should also be ordered to rule out ischemic injury secondary to cocaine use, which may be masked by the abdominal pain.

Answer A is incorrect. Pure β-blockers are contraindicated in the setting of cocaine abuse because unopposed α activity may increase hypertension.

Answer B is incorrect. Pure β-blockers are contraindicated in the setting of cocaine abuse because unopposed α activity may increase hypertension.

Answer D is incorrect. Metoprolol is another pure β-blocker that is contraindicated in the setting of cocaine abuse.

Answer E is incorrect. Verapamil is a calcium channel blocker that may be used as an antiarrhythmic or antihypertensive. Verapamil will not treat the underlying cause of this patient's hypertension and will not prevent additional withdrawal complications.

8. The correct answer is E. This patient is experiencing acute tumor lysis syndrome. This situation occurs when large numbers of rapidly proliferating cells (as are present in acute lymphoid leukemia [ALL]) are exposed to chemotherapeutic agents. Cellular destruction results in release of intracellular contents into the bloodstream, leading to hyperuricemia and hyperkalemia. Uric acid precipitates in the renal tubules, causing oliguric/anuric acute renal failure, and cardiac arrhythmias may occur due to high potassium levels. This syndrome is largely preventable with administration of allopurinol, aggressive hydration, and close monitoring of electrolytes; however, ALL patients with very high WBC values at diagnosis, as well as patients with Burkitt's lymphoma, remain at risk.

Answer A is incorrect. Doxorubicin is a chemotherapeutic agent that is known to cause long-term cardiac damage. This damage does not occur in the acute setting, however.

Answer B is incorrect. Incorrect dosing of anesthesia might cause somnolence or hyperactivity, but would not be expected to cause the reported electrolyte and urinary abnormalities.

Answer C is incorrect. Leukemic infiltrate of the kidneys is extremely rare, and would not be expected to cause such acute renal failure.

Answer D is incorrect. Overhydration would not be expected to cause these symptoms in a patient with well-functioning kidneys.

9. **The correct answer is E.** The treatment algorithm for variceal hemorrhage includes somatostatin therapy or an analog and endoscopic therapy, including band ligation and sclerotherapy. If this is unsuccessful or bleeding recurs continually, then balloon tamponade or portosystemic shunt placement should be considered. Although portosystemic shunt placement is an excellent means to decompress the portal circulation, the main negative consequence is due to the diversion of blood away from the hepatic filtering mechanism. In other words, toxin-filled blood circumvents the liver and goes directly to the systemic circulation, thus putting the patient at risk for hepatic encephalopathy. This patient, a recurrent bleeder, likely underwent shunt placement and is now suffering from encephalopathy.

Answer A is incorrect. Balloon tamponade would be an appropriate measure for bleeding varices that have not been controlled with other measures. However, this would not push the patient into hepatic encephalopathy.

Answer B is incorrect. β-Blocker therapy is used to medically treat portal hypertension due to its effect on the systemic and splanchnic circulations. This therapy is a commonly used as a preventative measure, but not in the case of acute bleeding, and it does not lead to hepatic encephalopathy.

Answer C is incorrect. Endoscopic band ligation is commonly performed simultaneously with sclerotherapy.

Answer D is incorrect. Endoscopic sclerotherapy is an excellent intervention both to treat ongoing variceal bleeding and as a secondary preventative measure for individuals with varices at risk of rebleeding. However, sclerotherapy does not put patients at risk for

hepatic encephalopathy and therefore is likely not the intervention used in this case.

10. **The correct answer is A.** Although this patient suffers from a terminal condition and has indicated through his DNR that resuscitation should not be performed if he suffers from cardiac or respiratory arrest, the advance directive does not apply to action against treatable conditions. A living will in the form of a DNR is an advance directive provided by the patient that indicates the desire to prevent life-sustaining treatment in the event of a terminal disease or a persistent vegetative state. However, feeding, intravenous fluids, treatment of infections or other treatable conditions, and pain management are not restricted under a DNR.

Answer B is incorrect. A durable power of attorney is a legally designated health care proxy who serves as a decision maker if the patient lacks decision-making capacity. Although the health care proxy can make decisions for a patient if his or her wishes are unclear, any advance directive created by the patient when he or she had capacity would supersede the decisions made by the surrogate.

Answer C is incorrect. A DNR does not address adverse effects of appropriate treatment measures, only resuscitation efforts in the case of cardiac or respiratory arrest.

Answer D is incorrect. Although the health care proxy can make decisions for a patient if the his or her wishes are unclear, any advance directive created by the patient when he or she had capacity would supersede the decisions made by the surrogate.

Answer E is incorrect. Although this patient suffers from a terminal condition, his DNR only indicates that resuscitation should not be performed. The advance directive does not apply to action against treatable conditions.

11. **The correct answer is C.** In any child presenting with recurrent pneumonia and poor growth, cystic fibrosis should be considered. Since the pathophysiology results in decreased bacterial clearance from the lungs secondary to impaired ciliary function, these patients are susceptible to a range of pulmonary infections

including *Staphylococcus aureus*, *Burkholderia cepacia*, *Stenotrophomonas maltophilia*, and *Haemophilus influenzae*. However, *Pseudomonas* infection in patients with typical histories for cystic fibrosis virtually assures the diagnosis in the absence of confirmatory sweat chloride or genetic testing.

Answer A is incorrect. *Klebsiella* pneumonia occurs in the elderly, the hospitalized, and in the setting of chronic alcoholism, usually secondary to aspiration.

Answer B is incorrect. *Listeria monocytogenes* is a gram-positive rod which causes pneumonia in the very young and the elderly due to their relatively immunocompromised state, but would not contribute to recurrent pneumonia or poor growth.

Answer D is incorrect. Staphylococcal infections occur commonly in cystic fibrosis patients, but can also be seen in other immunocompromised states. *Staphylococcus aureus* appears as clustered gram-positive cocci.

12. **The correct answer is A.** An aortic dissection occurs when there is a tear in the aortic intima that forms a false lumen for blood to flow through. Patients typically present with acute onset chest pain and/or back pain that is characteristically "tearing" in nature. The pain may radiate as the dissection enlarges. Risk factors for aortic dissection include hypertension, as seen in this patient who may not be compliant with his medications. Although the gold standard for diagnosis of aortic dissection is an angiogram, CT with intravenous contrast, MRI, or transesophageal echocardiography may show a pseudolumen that aids in the diagnosis.

Answer B is incorrect. Lumbar disc herniation involves extrusion of the intervertebral disc and compression of the nerve roots with resultant lower back and lower extremity pain. These patients may have decreased lower extremity reflexes and weakness of their lower extremities. A diagnosis of lumbar disc herniation is not likely in this patient, however, because lumbar disc herniation would not explain the diminished pulses in the lower extremities. A diagnosis of aortic dissection is more likely than a diagnosis of lumbar disc herniation.

Answer C is incorrect. Pancreatic cancer is a chronic process that does not typically present with acute-onset "tearing" back pain and normal laboratory values. Pancreatic cancer in the head of the pancreas is often associated with painless jaundice, weight loss, pruritus, acholic stools, dark urine, and abdominal pain. This patient's history, physical examination, laboratory findings, and radiographic findings are more suggestive of an aortic dissection than pancreatic cancer.

Answer D is incorrect. Perforated peptic ulcer typically presents with sudden-onset abdominal pain; however, it is not associated with decreased pulses in the lower extremities bilaterally. Although patients with perforated peptic ulcers may present with back pain, the history, laboratory findings, physical examination, and radiographic findings are more supportive of a diagnosis of aortic dissection than of perforated peptic ulcer.

Answer E is incorrect. Abdominal aortic aneurysms (AAAs) may be asymptomatic or may present with back or abdominal pain. Risk factors for AAA include hypertension, atherosclerosis, male gender, advanced age, and smoking. A ruptured AAA typically presents with a triad of abdominal pain, hypotension, and a pulsatile abdominal mass. Because this patient is hypertensive and does not show any indication of an AAA or rupture (retroperitoneal hematoma), this diagnosis is less likely than a diagnosis of aortic dissection.

13. **The correct answer is B.** Decreased ceruloplasmin, along with Kayser-Fleischer rings and neurologic abnormalities, is characteristic of Wilson's disease. Patients may also present with jaundice, hematemesis, depression, dysphagia, speech impairment, and abdominal distention with hepatomegaly and/or splenomegaly.

Answer A is incorrect. Elevated serum iron, elevated percentage saturation of iron, and elevated ferritin with decreased serum transferrin are characteristic of hemochromatosis. Symptoms usually do not appear until patients are 40 years old and may include joint pain (the most common complaint), bronze skin, fatigue, loss of sex drive, diabetes, heart problems, abdominal pain, and jaundice. Corneal deposits are unlikely as is rigidity with a tremor.

Answer C is incorrect. Abdominal CT would be appropriate for diagnosing structural liver abnormalities such as hepatocellular carcinoma and sclerosing cholangitis. Both of these entities are unlikely to present with corneal deposits, but may present with corneal injection and jaundice. Both may also present with hepatomegaly. Tremor and rigid extremities are uncharacteristic.

Answer D is incorrect. Hepatitis screening panel will determine whether the patient has been infected with any of the hepatitis viruses, but will not determine any metabolic abnormalities in the liver. Hepatitis may present with jaundice and hepatomegaly, but not corneal deposits and a tremor.

Answer E is incorrect. The patient does not have evidence of ascites, and a paracentesis is inappropriate.

14. **The correct answer is C.** This man is suffering from a major depressive episode, characterized by weight loss, anhedonia, tearfulness, and psychomotor retardation. Feelings of inadequacy and excessive guilt pervade his thoughts. Antidepressant medication is indicated. In addition, his extensive suicidal ideation put him at increased for suicide. Citalopram is a selective serotonin reuptake inhibitor (SSRI); SSRIs have minimal adverse effects in comparison to other antidepressants, such as tricyclic antidepressants and monoamine oxidase inhibitors, both of which can be lethal in overdose or with certain foods or other medications. Other examples of commonly used SSRIs include fluoxetine, sertraline, and escitalopram.

Answer A is incorrect. Amitriptyline is a tricyclic antidepressant (TCA) that can cause significant anticholinergic adverse effects, orthostatic hypertension, and third-degree heart block, especially in patients with second-degree heart block. TCAs can be lethal in overdose.

Answer B is incorrect. Benztropine is an anticholinergic that is used in psychiatry as prophylaxis for extrapyramidal symptoms (EPS) to

antipsychotic medications. As this patient is not currently on any antipsychotics, EPS prophylaxis is not indicated.

Answer D is incorrect. Phenelzine is a monoamine oxidase inhibitor (MAOI) that can cause a hypertensive crisis in combination with sympathomimetic amines (found in some decongestants) and in tyramine-containing foods (e.g., aged wines and cheese). Hypertensive crises can be fatal; therefore the potential for lethal interactions is reason enough to avoid MAOIs in this patient.

Answer E is incorrect. Risperidone is an atypical antipsychotic used to treat impulsivity, lability, agitation, and both the positive and negative symptoms of schizophrenia. This patient does not have any of these, nor does he have any impairment in his reality testing; thus an antipsychotic is not indicated.

15. **The correct answer is C.** *Ehrlichia chaffeensis* is an intracellular bacteria that causes human monocytic ehrlichiosis, carried by the *Ixodes* tick. The disease can present with fever, in addition to nonspecific symptoms such as malaise, myalgias, headache, and chills, in addition to nausea and vomiting. Mental status changes, such as the confusion exhibited by this patient, are common. Laboratory abnormalities include leukopenia, thrombocytopenia, and mildly elevated transaminases. Examination of the buffy coat of a peripheral blood smear can sometimes demonstrate morulae in leukocytes but is rarely seen. Diagnosis can definitively be made on serologies; detection of a four-fold increase in *E. chaffeensis* antibody titer (to 1:64) by indirect immunofluorescence in paired serum samples obtained approximately 3 weeks apart are sufficient for diagnosis. Treatment is with doxycycline.

Answer A is incorrect. Babesiosis is a protozoan disease that is transmitted by ticks, with most cases found in the same geographic distribution as Lyme disease. The clinical presentation can be similar to that of ehrlichiosis, but *Babesia microti* is an intraerythrocytic, not intraneutrophilic, parasite. It is usually treated with a combination of quinine sulfate and clindamycin.

Answer B is incorrect. *Borrelia burgdorferi* is the spirochete that causes Lyme disease, and like *Ehrlichia*, is carried in the *Ixodes* tick. It can present with many of the same symptoms as ehrlichiosis; however, in this case, the presence of intraleukocyte morulae is much more indicative of ehrlichiosis. Note, however, that both *Ehrlichia chaffeensis* and *Borrelia burgdorferi* can be present in the same *Ixodes* tick and therefore co-infect.

Answer D is incorrect. Acute HIV infection can be associated with a flu-like syndrome during which the antibody test is negative but the viral load is extremely high. HIV can also cause leukopenia due to decreases in CD4+ T lymphocytes, but no intracellular bodies are visible on peripheral blood smear.

Answer E is incorrect. *Leishmania donovani*, a parasite found in Bangladesh, northeastern India, Nepal, Sudan, and Brazil, that typically causes visceral leishmaniasis (also known as kala-azar), and has a wide range of symptoms that may include splenomegaly, peripheral lymphadenopathy, pancytopenia, hypergammaglobulinemia, and hypoalbuminemia. The infection can be diagnosed with demonstration of the parasite in slides or in cultures of tissue aspirate or biopsy. This patient's presentation is not consistent with that of leishmaniasis.

Answer F is incorrect. *Rickettsia rickettsii* is the pathogen that causes Rocky Mountain spotted fever. It would not present with neurologic symptoms.

Answer G is incorrect. *Trypanosoma brucei* is the agent of African sleeping sickness, which is transmitted to humans by the tsetse fly. Its diagnosis requires detection of the parasite in blood or lymph node aspirate.

16. **The correct answer is B.** This patient most likely has systemic lupus erythematosus because she fits 5 of the 11 lupus criteria: photosensitivity, malar rash, arthralgias, renal involvement, and oral lesions. Although several of the antibodies listed might be seen in this patient, only anti–double-stranded DNA correlates with glomerulonephritis in lupus.

Answer A is incorrect. Anticentromere antibodies are seen in limited scleroderma, also known as **CREST** syndrome, which is characterized by **C**alcinosis, **R**aynaud's phenomenon, **E**sophageal dysmotility, **S**clerodactyly, and **T**elangiectasias. This woman's presentation is not consistent with CREST syndrome, so she would not be expected to have anticentromere antibodies.

Answer C is incorrect. Anti-Jo-1 is an antibody to the tRNA synthetase that is seen in polymyositis and dermatomyositis. These patients tend to have interstitial lung disease, "mechanic's hands" (dry, cracked skin), Raynaud's phenomenon, and arthritis, and they tend to have treatment-refractory disease.

Answer D is incorrect. Anti-Scl-70 is an antibody to DNA topoisomerase I that is seen in diffuse scleroderma. This patient's presentation is not consistent with scleroderma, which is characterized by thickening and tightening of the skin of the fingers and the skin proximal to the wrists and ankles. Other minor criteria for the diagnosis of scleroderma include sclerodactyly (skin tightening limited only to the fingers), digital pitting scars resulting from ischemia, and bibasilar pulmonary fibrosis.

Answer E is incorrect. La (anti-SSB) antibodies are seen in approximately 10–15% of patients with systemic lupus erythematosus, but their levels do not correlate with disease activity.

Answer F is incorrect. Ro (anti-SSA) antibodies are seen in approximately 30–45% of patients with systemic lupus erythematosus, but their levels do not correlate with disease activity. The presence of Ro antibodies is associated with dry eyes and mouth, subacute cutaneous lupus erythematosus, neonatal lupus, and photosensitivity.

17. **The correct answer is C.** In patients suspected of perforated appendix, percutaneous drainage with interval appendectomy may be an appropriate alternative if the perforation has led to a well-loculated abscess and the patient is not septic. Given the complex history of this patient, if the appendix is indeed perforated and an abscess has formed, then percutaneous drainage can be a viable alternative to performing emergency appendectomy.

Answer A is incorrect. While hypotension and fever can be the presenting symptoms for sepsis, this patient has symptoms of an acute abdomen, which can only be diagnosed via radiologic evaluation.

Answer B is incorrect. MRI is appropriate for patients with contraindications for CT scan, such as metal implants or allergy to intravenous contrast. The patient in this question does not have such contraindications and a CT scan with contrast provides the most informative evaluation of the abdominal symptoms.

Answer D is incorrect. Abdominal ultrasound is the standard diagnostic tool for acute cholecystitis, not for appendicitis.

Answer E is incorrect. This patient has no urinary symptoms such as dysuria or hematuria, and her symptoms are more indicative of a gastrointestinal ailment.

18. **The correct answer is A.** Postinfectious idiopathic thrombocytopenic purpura (ITP) is a self-limited disease process that will resolve on its own; in fact, 70–80% of cases will resolve within 6 months. Because this patient has no clinical evidence of spontaneous bleeding or symptoms due to her low platelets, no additional medical procedures are warranted. If the patient developed spontaneous bleeding as a result of the ITP, further measures to control the symptoms would be indicated. Spontaneous bleeding is likely to occur with platelet counts < 20,000/mm3, and major spontaneous bleeding in not likely to occur with platelet counts < 10,000/mm^3.

Answer B is incorrect. Postinfectious ITP is a self-limited disease process that resolves without additional therapy. Steroids may be useful in severe cases of ITP but would not be indicated for this patient because she is asymptomatic.

Answer C is incorrect. Fresh frozen plasma replaces clotting factors but lacks RBCs, WBCs, or platelets. It has no utility in the treatment of idiopathic thrombocytopenic purpura.

Answer D is incorrect. Packed RBCs do not contain platelets or clotting factors. Although postinfectious idiopathic thrombocytopenic

purpura (ITP) is self-limited, symptomatic thrombocytopenia and/or evidence of spontaneous bleeding may warrant transfusion of platelets. Packed RBCs lack platelets and therefore have no use when managing a patient with ITP.

Answer E is incorrect. There is no indication for platelet transfusion. Platelet counts are high enough to inhibit spontaneous hemorrhage. In addition, this patient has no evidence of serious bleeding and therefore would not be a candidate for a platelet transfusion. Finally, transfused platelets are as rapidly destroyed as endogenous platelets.

19. **The correct answer is E.** This case centers on the concept of medical futility. Treatment is futile when there is no pathophysiologic rationale for treatment, when a maximal intervention is currently failing, when a given intervention has already failed, or when a particular treatment would not achieve the goals of care. If these criteria are met, the physician is neither ethically nor legally required to provide treatment, even if requested by a health care proxy or other family member. In this case, the woman has advanced metastatic ovarian cancer and most recently failed the treatment being requested.

Answer A is incorrect. If a treatment has been shown to be medically futile, the physician is neither ethically nor legally required to provide treatment, even if requested by a health care proxy or other family member.

Answer B is incorrect. This woman has recently failed the treatment being requested. It is therefore medically futile to continue, and the physician is neither ethically nor legally required to provide treatment.

Answer C is incorrect. If a treatment has been shown to be medically futile, the physician is neither ethically nor legally required to provide treatment, even if requested by a health care proxy or other family member.

Answer D is incorrect. If a treatment has been shown to be medically futile, the physician is neither ethically nor legally required to provide treatment, even if requested by a health care proxy or other family member.

20. The correct answer is A. The child in question has the classic triad of West's syndrome: infantile spasms, regression of psychomotor development, and hypsarrhythmia on EEG. This disease typically progresses through three stages, beginning with mild and infrequent spasms that become more frequent and severe during the second stage before resolving during the final stage. They are often followed by the appearance of other seizure disorders and/or neurologic impairment.

Answer B is incorrect. Febrile seizures in infants can occur secondary to disseminated or localized infectious agents of virtually any form, some of which are treatable. However, the child in question has infantile spasms, which do not have an infectious etiology.

Answer C is incorrect. Many benign conditions (e.g., exaggerated Moro reflexes) or stereotyped movements can be mistaken for seizures in children and infants. Unfortunately, the child in question has an abnormal EEG and psychomotor delay, which is indicative of more serious pathology.

Answer D is incorrect. Upper respiratory tract infections are the most common pathology in children and can even result in fever and febrile seizures. A very sick 3-month-old child may even appear to have psychomotor delay, since there are so few milestones to observe at this age. However, the EEG changes seen in this child would not be expected for a febrile seizure.

Answer E is incorrect. Certain patterns of pathology associated with child abuse (e.g., retinal hemorrhages and shaken baby syndrome) should prompt immediate notification of child protective services. This child's symptoms to not readily conform to any well-documented pattern of abuse.

21. The correct answer is A. This patient has Crohn's disease (CD). Among the most common symptoms of CD are abdominal pain, often in the RLQ, and diarrhea. Rectal bleeding, weight loss, and fever may also occur. The segmental distribution of the lesions and "cobblestoning" of the mucosa in this patient indicate that this is CD and not ulcerative colitis. An-

tibiotics, including metronidazole and ciprofloxacin, have been shown to benefit patients with CD, especially in conjunction with immunosuppression and the first-line therapy of mesalamine products.

Answer B is incorrect. Although the RLQ pain and fever raise concerns for appendicitis, this patient's history and physical findings suggest inflammatory bowel disease.

Answer C is incorrect. A proctocolectomy would be curative for ulcerative colitis, but it is only indicated for specific complications of Crohn's disease in severe, medically refractory disease, or for cancer prophylaxis in selected high-risk patients.

Answer D is incorrect. Toxic megacolon is sometimes seen in patients with ulcerative colitis but rarely in those with Crohn's disease.

Answer E is incorrect. A gluten-free diet is indicated for patients with celiac sprue. Although patients with celiac disease may present with diarrhea and weight loss, the results of colonoscopy and colonic biopsy in this patient are indicative of Crohn's disease.

22. The correct answer is C. Although the patient has consented to earlier transfusions, she has the right to change her mind at any time. Therefore, the most appropriate next step is to withhold further transfusions and discuss the alternative plans with the care team.

Answer A is incorrect. The patient appears competent and is aware of the consequences of not receiving blood products. Therefore the ethics committee cannot override the patient's decision despite probable poor outcome.

Answer B is incorrect. The patient does not show any signs or symptoms of depression and/or suicidality. While psychiatry consultation may be appropriate as part of the patient's care plan, the patient's condition requires urgent transfusions and health care decisions need to be made immediately. Gynecological consultation takes precedence.

Answer D is incorrect. The patient has the right to change her mind despite earlier informed consent..

Answer E is incorrect. The patient is not deemed incapacitated, and so her husband cannot serve as surrogate and make any health care decisions on her behalf.

23. **The correct answer is A.** Acute myelogenous leukemia (AML) is the clonal proliferation of blasts that are unable to differentiate into mature myeloid cells. The median age at presentation is 65 years and AML accounts for more than 80% of leukemia in adults. Common symptoms at presentation are those resulting from bone marrow failure, including fatigue, dizziness, or dyspnea on exertion. Infection is common due to low levels of mature neutrophils, and there are often signs of organ infiltration by blasts, usually the spleen, liver, and gums. Complete blood cell count reveals a greatly elevated WBC count and thrombocytopenia, while the peripheral smear shows a predominance of immature myeloid cells, which stain positively with myeloperoxidase.

Answer B is incorrect. Anemia of chronic disease is often associated with renal failure and results from decreased erythropoietin production. Anemia develops from the lack of stimulus driving red blood cell maturation. The peripheral smear usually is normocytic with occasional presence of burr cells.

Answer C is incorrect. Chronic myelogenous leukemia (CML) also involves the myeloid lineage of cells, but in CML they retain the ability to differentiate. As a result, peripheral smear should show an abundance of myeloid cells in all stages of differentiation, including blasts. Most patients present in the chronic phase of the disease. Cytology in the vast majority of cases shows the presence of the Philadelphia chromosome.

Answer D is incorrect. Multiple myeloma can produce anemia and recurrent infections due to bone marrow failure. However, renal disease is much more common, and bone pain due to increased osteoclast activity and lytic lesions is seen.

Answer E is incorrect. Thrombotic thrombocytopenic purpura is characterized by microangiopathic hemolytic anemia and thrombocytopenia. Peripheral smear should show schistocytes without increased blasts.

24. **The correct answer is C.** Although uncommon, the HIV-positive patient can initially present with full-blown AIDS, which is defined as a CD4+ count of $< 200/mm^3$ and/or the presence of an AIDS-defining illness. This patient's presentation and symptoms are consistent with progressive multifocal leukoencephalopathy, which is caused by the JC virus. Polymerase chain reaction assays of cerebrospinal fluid (CSF) for the JC virus are 80% sensitive and 95% specific, but no other CSF changes are notable. Median survival is approximately 6 months after diagnosis.

Answer A is incorrect. Demyelination of the central nervous system is the mechanism that underlies multiple sclerosis (MS). The characteristic presentation of MS includes many neurologic complaints separated in space and time that cannot be explained by a single lesion. An MRI demonstrates multiple periventricular lesions in the white matter. Given this patient's immunodeficiency, however, an infectious cause is much more likely.

Answer B is incorrect. Infection with *Candida albicans* can cause esophagitis, oral thrush, and vaginitis but generally does not affect the central nervous system. Treatment is with 1–3 weeks of antifungal therapy.

Answer D is incorrect. Infection with herpes simplex virus type 1 (HSV-1) can cause HSV encephalitis, which typically presents with headache, fever, and nuchal rigidity as well as with mental status changes. Focal neurologic signs and seizures may also be present. Lumbar puncture demonstrates mononuclear cells and RBCs. The suspicion of HSV encephalitis requires prompt therapy with intravenous acyclovir. This patient's presentation is not characteristic of HSV encephalitis.

Answer E is incorrect. Infection with *Toxoplasma gondii* results in encephalitis that can present with focal neurologic deficits. An MRI of the brain will demonstrate ring-enhancing lesions. Treatment consists of pyrimethamine, leucovorin, and sulfadiazine, to which most patients respond within 1 week. More than

90% of patients will test positive for anti–*Toxoplasma gondii* IgG.

25. **The correct answer is B.** Diabetes is an indication for the vaccine given that diabetic patients are considered to be immunocompromised. Diabetics, especially poorly controlled diabetic patients, are vulnerable to infection. The chronic hyperglycemia of diabetes leads to abnormalities in cell-mediated immunity and phagocyte function. Also, the vascular impairment of diabetes prevents the immune system from responding appropriately to an infectious challenge.

Answer A is incorrect. Age over 65 years old is an indication for the pneumococcal vaccine, as the elderly and very young are especially susceptible to developing pneumococcal pneumonia.

Answer C is incorrect. Health care workers are recommended to receive pneumococcal vaccine due to their exposure in the work setting. However, for this patient, his immunocompromised state secondary to diabetes is a more pressing reason to administer the vaccine.

Answer D is incorrect. Hypertension is not itself an indication for the vaccine although significant heart disease would indicate that the patient should receive the vaccine.

Answer E is incorrect. Current respiratory infection is a contraindication for the vaccine, which is the case prior to the administration of any vaccine. The patient also has a history of one episode of community-acquired pneumonia that was treated as an outpatient. For patients with this history but no further immunocompromised state, such as diabetes, the pneumococcal vaccine would not be indicated.

26. **The correct answer is A.** This patient has sarcoidosis. Activated sarcoid macrophages secrete calcitonin, which can lead to hypercalcemia. Evidence of hypercalcemia in this patient includes fatigue, muscle weakness, constipation, and polyuria.

Answer B is incorrect. Although diabetes mellitus can cause polyuria, fatigue, blurry vision,

and weight loss, it should not cause lymphadenopathy.

Answer C is incorrect. Anemia can be associated with fatigue and dyspnea on exertion, but this patient has many other symptoms.

Answer D is incorrect. Diabetes insipidus can cause polyuria, fatigue, and weight loss; it should not cause lymphadenopathy or blurry vision.

Answer E is incorrect. Lymphocytosis can be due to either infection or malignancy. Patients with tuberculosis (TB) can have a variety of presentations; however, the patient does not report risk factors for TB (e.g., international travel, health care profession), making this diagnosis much less likely. Leukemia would not present with interstitial lung disease.

27. **The correct answer is A.** This patient is suffering from gestational diabetes. Infants of mothers with gestational diabetes have an increased incidence of macrosomia (an infant that is heavier than 4.0 kg for diabetic mothers, or 4.5 kg for nondiabetic mothers). In diabetic patients with poor maternal glucose control, preeclampsia, macrosomia, or evidence of fetal lung maturity, early delivery should be considered. Macrosomia may lead to longer labor, shoulder dystocia, and birth trauma. If early delivery is considered, then the lecithin:sphingomyelin (L:S) ratio and phosphatidylglycerol (PG) level should be obtained to assess fetal lung maturity. An L:S ratio > 2 indicates pulmonary maturity, and an L:S ratio < 2 indicates pulmonary immaturity. If, however, the ratio is < 2 and PG is present, then the chance of neonatal respiratory distress syndrome is < 5%. The test performed to assess these levels is amniocentesis.

Answer B is incorrect. Chorionic villus sampling is performed at 10–12 weeks' gestation, for the purpose of early assessment of fetal karyotype. It would not be appropriate in this patient. Amniocentesis is indicated in the clinical situation described above, as well as in mothers over the age of 35, as their risk for congenital abnormalities, such as Down syndrome, increases with advanced maternal age.

Answer C is incorrect. If delivery is necessary, corticosteroids may be given to the mother to hasten fetal lung maturity. However, a cortisol level has no role in prenatal screening.

Answer D is incorrect. Hemoglobin A_{1c} levels should be drawn in patients with known diabetes at the first prenatal visit. If it is > 8.5%, the mother should be counseled regarding congenital abnormalities and an ultrasound done at about 15 weeks; the fetus should also be aggressively assessed for congenital abnormalities.

Answer E is incorrect. A random blood glucose level is not indicated here. This patient has failed the 3-hour glucose tolerance test, indicating a diagnosis of gestational diabetes. Management for her diabetes should begin with regular exercise, an American Diabetes Association diet with at least 1800 calories/day, and frequent fingerstick glucose readings at home.

28. **The correct answer is D.** The patient is suffering from bradycardia and hypotension secondary to an overdose of β-blockers. Glucagon is an appropriate treatment. Glucagon receptor-mediated effects on many tissues are similar to the effects of β-adrenergic stimulation and include increased intracellular levels of cAMP, leading to relaxation of bronchial, vascular, and gastrointestinal smooth muscle, as well as increased calcium levels in cardiac muscle, which increases contractility. Isoproterenol and atropine are first-line agents to treat heart block and bradycardia in β-blocker toxicity but in refractory or severe cases glucagon should be administered.

Answer A is incorrect. Amiodarone is a class III antiarrhythmic agent that acts on the myocardium to increase the time of the action potential. It also acts as a vasodilator. It is used in treatment of severe ventricular arrhythmias, especially supraventricular arrhythmias.

Answer B is incorrect. Although cardiac pacing may be helpful for stimulating contractility in β-blocker–induced bradycardia, this is more commonly used in patients with Torsades de pointes due to sotalol toxicity.

Answer C is incorrect. Diphenhydramine is an effective histamine blocker antihistamine. This may be used prophylactically to avoid potential anaphylaxis, including respiratory distress, in patients known to have risk factors for drug interactions.

Answer E is incorrect. Albuterol is a selective β_2-agonist and is indicated in exacerbations of restrictive airway disease. Although β-blocker overdose could contribute to bronchospasm, this patient is not in apparent respiratory distress. In albuterol toxicity, β-blockers are often used to decrease heart rate.

29. **The correct answer is D.** Fatigue and weight loss are suspicious for metastatic disease or a metabolically active tumor. The workup has led to the diagnosis of metastatic transitional cell carcinoma. The treatment of this terrible disease is systemic chemotherapy. With today's therapies, patients with metastatic TCC have a median survival of about 12 months and a 3-year survival rate of about 15–20%. MVAC (methotrexate, vinblastine, doxorubicin [Adriamycin], and cisplatin) is the standard chemotherapeutic regimen, but other less toxic combination therapies are used. The utility of surgery in patients with metastatic disease is not well defined. There is some suggestion that it would be warranted in some patients, but given the extent of spread, this man would probably not stand to benefit.

Answer A is incorrect. This combination is not regularly used in the management of bladder cancer. Intravesicular bacille Calmette-Guérin is one of the agents used in the treatment of superficial transitional cell carcinoma without the use of systemic chemotherapy.

Answer B is incorrect. Extensive pelvic exenteration (en bloc resection of all pelvic organs) and systemic chemotherapy would not be the standard treatment for a patient with metastatic disease. There is some evidence that a metastectomy and chemotherapy in addition to local bladder and pelvic dissection may improve survival; however, this is not the standard of care, and given the numerous lung lesions, such an aggressive approach is of limited benefit.

Answer C is incorrect. Supportive care is indeed warranted in some cases if the patient is competent, informed about options, and does not desire treatment. At this point the patient has not voiced any objection to treatment. Therefore, the standard of care should be offered first.

Answer E is incorrect. Transurethral resection of bladder tumor, pelvic radiation, and systemic chemotherapy is not warranted for metastatic bladder cancer. The use of radiation and aggressive surgery does have a role in invasive cancer without evidence of metastases, but this patient has metastatic disease and transurethral resection is not aggressive surgery. Transurethral resection with intravesicular chemotherapy is used in superficial cancers.

30. **The correct answer is C.** This patient has euvolemic hyponatremia. Her urine osmolality and Na are low, which indicates that she is appropriately producing dilute urine. The etiology of her disorder is the intake of too much water, probably related to her psychiatric condition. There can be a relationship between chronic schizophrenia and psychogenic polydipsia. This has been treated with clozapine.

Answer A is incorrect. Adrenal insufficiency presents as euvolemic hyponatremia, but serum potassium levels would be high.

Answer B is incorrect. Dehydration presents as hypovolemic hyponatremia. Urine osmolality and urine sodium would be high.

Answer D is incorrect. Renal failure presents as hypervolemic hyponatremia. This patient's blood urea nitrogen and creatinine are normal, which indicates that she is not in renal failure.

Answer E is incorrect. Syndrome of inappropriate ADH presents as euvolemic hyponatremia, but urine osmolality is usually fixed and elevated.

31. **The correct answer is E.** Myasthenia gravis is an autoimmune disease caused by antibodies against postsynaptic acetylcholine receptors. Treatment is typically aimed at downregulating the immune response or increasing the concentration of acetylcholine within the synapse. In emergency situations such as during myasthenia crisis with impending respiratory failure, plasmapheresis and intravenous immu-

noglobulin after intubation provide a means of temporarily relieving symptoms. Indicators of respiratory compromise include loss of upper airway integrity and decreasing vital capacity or negative inspiratory force. The arterial blood gas is not a good indicator of the need for intubation in these patients. The lifetime risk of a myasthenic crisis is 15–20% and is often precipitated by infection, metabolic stress, or nondepolarizing anesthetic agents.

Answer A is incorrect. Albuterol is helpful as a treatment in asthmatic and chronic obstructive pulmonary disease treatments with obstructive defects. This patient has a neuromuscular disorder leading to restrictive defect.

Answer B is incorrect. Edrophonium is useful in diagnosing myasthenia, although it is rarely used as a treatment.

Answer C is incorrect. Inhaled racemic epinephrine can be a useful bronchodilator in pediatric patients with croup. However, it is not indicated in adults with restrictive defects.

Answer D is incorrect. Intravenous (IV) antibiotics would be useful in a patient whose shortness of breath was caused by pneumonia but not a neuromuscular defect. Although the right middle lobe infiltrate is suggestive of pneumonia, the patient's presentation and declining vital capacity is compatible with a myasthenic crisis that has been precipitated by the infection. Clearly, IV antibiotics would be indicated but only after emergent intubation.

32. **The correct answer is D.** Physicians are ethically and legally obligated to override patient confidentiality in the following cases: (1) suicidal patients, (2) gunshot and knife wounds, (3) infectious diseases (health authorities and at-risk third parties must be informed), (4) child and elder abuse, and (5) impaired automobile drivers. The physician should inform the patient that she is obligated to breech usual confidentiality in the case of HIV status. She should encourage the patient to disclose his HIV status to his partner and other sexual contacts, but she must do so if he will not.

Answer A is incorrect. Physicians must maintain confidentiality in cases of abuse between competent adults because this is not included in the list of activities in which confidentiality may be breached.

Answer B is incorrect. Health authorities and at-risk third parties must both be informed of HIV status.

Answer C is incorrect. Health authorities and at-risk third parties must both be informed of HIV status.

Answer E is incorrect. The physician should inform the patient that she is obligated to breech usual confidentiality in the case of HIV status. She should encourage him to disclose his HIV status to his partner and other sexual contacts, but she must do so if he will not.

33. **The correct answer is C.** This infant has seborrheic dermatitis (SD) of the scalp, or "cradle cap." These lesions are erythematous and characterized by greasy, yellow plaque and scale formation. SD is frequently associated with *Malassezia furfur* colonization, although causality has not been proven. Treatment is with selenium sulfide, tar, or zinc pyrithione shampoos.

    Answer A is incorrect. Seborrheic dermatitis elsewhere on the body is often successfully treated with topical corticosteroids or antifungals; however, the scalp can usually be managed easily with shampoos.

    Answer B is incorrect. Oral griseofulvin is used to treat tinea capitis, which is characterized by erythema and scaling of the scalp, accompanied by alopecia. Plaque formation is atypical of tinea capitis.

    Answer D is incorrect. Topical emollients are often effective treatments of scalp eczema (atopic dermatitis). Eczematous lesions are typically erythematous and scaling but can be distinguished from seborrheic dermatitis by the presence of intense itching and dryness.

    Answer E is incorrect. This is also an appropriate treatment for nonscalp seborrheic dermatitis (SD). The antifungal most commonly used for nonscalp SD is ketoconazole.

34. **The correct answer is E.** Carcinoid syndrome is due to metastasis of tumors that secrete an abnormally high amount of serotonin, which

can eventually lead to damage to the lining of the heart. Restrictive cardiomyopathy may result. This condition is commonly associated with infiltrative diseases such as amyloidosis, sarcoidosis, or hemochromatosis. Congestive heart failure symptoms (right greater than left), as described in this question, may result when left ventricle filling is restricted, with resultant decreased output and compliance, and increased filling pressure. The echocardiogram and ECG help pinpoint this as the cause of the patient's problem. Treatment for this condition is to control the underlying cause (e.g., iron chelation for hemochromatosis), diuretics, angiotensin-converting enzyme inhibitors, and nitrates.

    Answer A is incorrect. There is no indication that the patient has undergone neurologic damage and therefore stroke would not be high on the differential.

    Answer B is incorrect. Coarctation of the aorta may lead to hypertension in adults and is characterized by a midsystolic murmur and notching of the ribs.

    Answer C is incorrect. Mitral stenosis is almost always associated with rheumatic heart disease in adults. It can lead to pulmonary congestion due to increased left atrial pressure. Left-sided heart failure may result. An opening snap, diastolic rumble, and echocardiogram visualization of the valve leaflets are helpful in making this diagnosis.

    Answer D is incorrect. Prinzmetal's, or atypical, angina occurs at rest and is associated with ST elevation. It is due to ischemia and would not present with these symptoms.

35. **The correct answer is E.** The correct answer is the size of the tumor. The staging of breast cancer is predicated largely upon the size of the tumor and whether or not there is nodal involvement. Stage is the critical factor in prognosis for breast cancer.

    Answer A is incorrect. Early age of menarche increased the risk of developing breast cancer in this patient, but it does not change the prognosis.

Answer B is incorrect. The histology of the tumor does not contribute as much to the prognosis of breast cancer. The diagnosis of lobular carcinoma in situ does, however, increase the probability of invasive carcinoma of both breasts.

Answer C is incorrect. Presence of fatigue and fever are not involved in the staging of breast carcinoma.

Answer D is incorrect. While irregular masses on mammography are more likely to be malignant, shape does not contribute to formal staging and prognosis.

36. **The correct answer is E.** Odds ratios are used in retrospective case-control studies to analyze the relationship between an exposure and disease or condition of interest. The starting point is the presence or absence of the disease, and among patients in those two categories, an odds ratio describes the likelihood that each had the exposure of interest.

Answer A is incorrect. Although the study demonstrates a correlation between nonsteroidal anti-inflammatory drug (NSAID) use by patients with rheumatoid arthritis and subsequent stroke risk, it does not prove causation. The increase in stroke incidence may be due to a feature of the disease and not a sequela of NSAID use, in which case not using NSAIDs in the treatment of arthritis might not reduce stroke risk.

Answer B is incorrect. This answer describes relative risk (RR), which is used in prospective cohort studies and starts with the absence of disease. RR describes the likelihood of developing a particular disease or condition after a given exposure.

Answer C is incorrect. Attributable risk is the difference in incidence rate between exposed and unexposed patients and is used in prospective studies.

Answer D is incorrect. This answer confuses the putative underlying relationship and assigns the increased risk for stroke to rheumatoid arthritis (RA) as the risk factor, rather than NSAID use in the treatment of RA.

37. **The correct answer is C.** This is a patient with Cushing's syndrome presenting with depression. In addition to hyperglycemia, central obesity, and hypertension, these patients are often depressed due to the effects of elevated cortisol. In this case, the hypercortisolism is due to ectopic ACTH secretion by a bronchial tumor. The most common sites of ectopic ACTH production are the lung, thymus, and pancreas. The first-line treatment for an ectopic ACTH-producing tumor is surgical resection. If resection is not possible, medical therapy is used. Therapy consists of adrenal enzyme inhibitors, such as ketoconazole, metyrapone, and aminoglutethimide.

Answer A is incorrect. Fludrocortisone is a mineralocorticoid, and therefore would not be useful in treating this patient, who has hypercortisolism.

Answer B is incorrect. Fluoxetine is a selective serotonin reuptake inhibitor that is used to treat depression. While this will be useful in treating this patient's depression, it will not treat the hypercortisolism.

Answer D is incorrect. Metformin may be necessary to treat diabetes mellitus in these patients. However, it will not treat their hypercortisolism.

Answer E is incorrect. Mitotane causes adrenal cortical atrophy and is used to treat hypercortisolism from a pituitary or adrenal source. It is equivalent to performing a medical adrenalectomy. It is not, however, an effective treatment for hypercortisolism from ectopic ACTH production.

38. **The correct answer is E.** Amyotrophic lateral sclerosis is a slowly progressive, generalized motor muscle paralysis involving both lower and upper neurons that typically progresses to death in 3–5 years. Drooling is a common symptom and is due to facial muscle weakness and reduced swallowing ability rather than increased secretions. However, anticholinergic drugs such as glycopyrrolate can be useful in decreasing secretions in order to manage these symptoms.

Answer A is incorrect. Baclofen is potentially useful for treating muscle spasticity in amyotrophic lateral sclerosis.

Answer B is incorrect. Carbamazepine is potentially useful for treating muscle spasms and cramps that accompany amyotrophic lateral sclerosis.

Answer C is incorrect. Although depression, pseudobulbar symptoms (outbursts of laughter or tearfulness), and cognitive loss are symptoms in amyotrophic lateral sclerosis, this patient's current problem is medical and does not require psychiatric evaluation.

Answer D is incorrect. Diphenhydramine is a sedative and is potentially a useful treatment for insomnia, which is very common in patients with amyotrophic lateral sclerosis. Sedatives should be used sparingly in these patients.

39. **The correct answer is B.** This patient has uric acid renal calculi, which are nonopaque on plain film but detectable by CT scan. Uric acid stones are common in patients with gout who are not receiving effective treatment for hyperuricemia. There are three mainstays of treatment for this condition: hydration, which reduces the concentration of uric acid in the urine; alkalinization of the urine, which decreases the precipitation of uric acid; and allopurinol, which lowers uric acid production and excretion.

Answer A is incorrect. Alkalinization and hydration alone are highly effective in dissolving uric acid stones, and extracorporeal shock wave lithotripsy is therefore unnecessary in these patients.

Answer C is incorrect. A low-sodium diet is effective in treating calcium stones, but is not part of the management of uric acid stones.

Answer D is incorrect. Penicillamine is an effective treatment for cystine stones, but has not been used in treatment of uric acid stones.

Answer E is incorrect. Thiazide diuretics can be used to treat hypercalciuria in patients with calcium stones, but are not used in patients with uric acid stones.

40. **The correct answer is E.** Rifampin is an inducer of the cytochrome P450 enzymes. That is, it causes the enzymes to metabolize the drugs that they act on at a faster rate, decreasing blood concentrations of these drugs, which are oral contraceptive pills in this case.

Answer A is incorrect. Albuterol would not induce the cytochrome P450 enzymes. Therefore, it would not increase the metabolism of the oral contraceptive pills.

Answer B is incorrect. Competition for binding sites is incorrect because rifampin does not share binding sites with estrogen or progesterone, the components of combined oral contraceptive medications.

Answer C is incorrect. This answer is incorrect because sex hormones are not pumped into or out of cells but rather diffuse across the lipid bilayer.

Answer D is incorrect. Patient error is possible but is not likely in the presence of a known mechanism for drug interaction.

41. **The correct answer is A.** Autosomal dominant polycystic kidney disease (ADPCKD) is the more common type of polycystic kidney disease. Symptoms usually begin in the third to fourth decade of life. Renal cyst formation, chronic interstitial inflammation, and recurrent urinary tract infections (UTIs) lead to chronic kidney disease manifest as hypertension and an elevated creatinine. Other complications of ADPCKD include intracranial berry aneurysms, mitral valve prolapse, and UTIs. Physical examination may reveal palpable and tender kidneys. Rupture of renal cysts can cause flank pain and hematuria.

Answer B is incorrect. Autosomal recessive polycystic kidney disease (ARPCKD), with an incidence of 1:20,000 births, is less common than the autosomal dominant type (1:400–2000 births). This disease affects infants and children, with a majority of cases being diagnosed in the first year of life. The gene responsible for ARPCKD has been located on chromosome 6p21. The cysts are formed from the distal tubules and are typically arranged in a radial fashion. In addition to renal failure and loss of urine-concentrating ability, these patients may develop portal hypertension, likely secondary to hepatic fibrosis.

Answer C is incorrect. Medullary cystic disease is an autosomal dominant disease that leads to small kidneys with medullary cysts, generally sparing the cortex and papillae. Cysts range from 1 to 10 mm in size and can originate from various parts of the nephron including the loop of Henle, distal convoluted tubule, and collecting duct. This disease presents in third or fourth decade of life. The symptoms are polyuria, anemia, and progressive renal insufficiency. There is no cure for this disease.

Answer D is incorrect. Medullary sponge kidney is usually an asymptomatic disease, but can present with hematuria, flank pain, or dysuria. The disease is characterized by renal tubular ectasia and enlargement of medullary collecting ducts, papillae, and calyces. Although patients are at risk for nephrolithiasis, urine-concentrating defects, and urinary tract infections, patients have an excellent renal prognosis and a normal life expectancy.

Answer E is incorrect. Kidney stones can cause flank pain and hematuria. However, acute nephrolithiasis rarely if ever causes palpable kidneys or renal failure. Additionally, this patient's clinical presentation necessitates the provisional diagnosis of simultaneous bilateral stones, which would be unusual.

Answer F is incorrect. Pyelonephritis is an infection of the kidney parenchyma. Bacteria from the lower tract, most commonly *Escherichia coli*, enter the upper tract. The patient has a history of urinary tract infections; however, pyelonephritis would be an unusual cause of hypertension and bilateral palpable kidneys. Furthermore, the urinalysis showed no bacteria, making infection unlikely.

42. **The correct answer is B.** In a hepatic iminodiacetic acid scan, iminodiacetic acid is absorbed from the bloodstream and secreted in the bile ducts. If there is cholecystitis, then the gallbladder will not be visualized. This is the next appropriate test after an equivocal abdominal ultrasound.

Answer A is incorrect. CT is not an appropriate test when evaluating right upper quadrant

pain because it is unable to detect most gallstones.

Answer C is incorrect. MRI is not an appropriate test when evaluating right upper quadrant pain because it is too costly and time consuming.

Answer D is incorrect. A sestamibi scan is useful in the evaluation of parathyroid disease. Radiolabeled sestamibi is injected into the bloodstream and becomes concentrated in overactive parathyroid adenomas, allowing them to be visualized.

Answer E is incorrect. X-ray of the abdomen is not very helpful in the evaluation of biliary colic or cholecystitis because only 10% of stones are radiopaque. X-ray of the abdomen can be useful in the evaluation of gallstone ileus, which will demonstrate air in the gallbladder (pneumobilia) and radiodensity near the ileocecal valve.

43. **The correct answer is C.** If a radionucleotide scan shows a hot nodule, the patient should be evaluated for hyperthyroidism and observed carefully. If the scan indicates a cold nodule, the mass is more likely to be malignant and surgery should be the next option. Most nodules (70–90%) are cold, and most of these are benign. Therefore, if a nodule is scanned as warm the chance of malignancy is significantly reduced.

Answer A is incorrect. High-resolution ultrasonography offers better anatomic definition than scintigraphy but is not a cost-effective initial test. Scintigraphy is also the only test that can elucidate the functional status of a nodule.

Answer B is incorrect. Observation alone is not sufficient in this instance, as the patient's age, gender, and nature of the mass suggest a possible malignancy.

Answer D is incorrect. Thyroxine therapy with close follow-up may be appropriate depending on the results of the radionucleotide scan and thyroid function tests.

Answer E is incorrect. Surgery is not appropriate immediately; further studies should be done to evaluate the nature of the nodule.

44. **The correct answer is B.** An annual digital rectal examination after reaching 50 years of age is the most universally recommended screening tool for prostate cancer, and is a mandatory part of the physical examination for a middle-aged man with recent-onset urinary complaints.

    Answer A is incorrect. Cystoscopy is not recommended for screening or longitudinal benign prostatic hypertrophy monitoring. This would be an appropriate test in a younger male patient with recurrent urinary tract infections.

    Answer C is incorrect. Ultrasound-guided biopsy of the prostate is used to provide the definitive diagnosis of suspected prostate cancer but would not be used as an initial test.

    Answer D is incorrect. A prostate-specific antigen (PSA) level is recommended yearly for screening patients at high risk or over the age of 50, and start at age 40 for African-Americans. With a PSA > 4.1 ng/mL, transrectal ultrasonography with biopsy of suspicious areas is recommended. However, an elevated PSA may be due to benign prostatic hypertrophy, prostatitis, urinary tract infection, pancreatic trauma, or carcinoma.

    Answer E is incorrect. Urinalysis and urine culture would be appropriate to rule out infection and hematuria; however, the patient denies fever, chills, urgency, frequency, costovertebral angle tenderness, or bladder fullness. Urinary tract infection are uncommon in men of this age.

Questions 45 and 46

45. **The correct answer is F.** *Giardia lamblia* is a flagellated protozoan that infects the duodenum and small intestine in affected patients. Infection is often asymptomatic, but in patients with manifesting symptoms, watery diarrhea is the most common presentation. Other symptoms include malaise and weakness, flatulence, abdominal distention, foul-smelling greasy stools, weight loss, and anorexia. The key to this patient's history is found in the timetable of her illness, in addition to her recent travel and exposure. *G. lamblia* has an in-cubation period of approximately 1–2 weeks and diarrhea can be prolonged, lasting in some patients for several weeks. The organism has been associated with waterborne outbreaks, and the child's recent swimming in natural water sources with nearby wildlife is the likely area where she was infected.

46. **The correct answer is I.** *Staphylococcus aureus* is a pathogen implicated in multiple cases of food-borne illness each year. The mechanism of infection is based on preformed toxins that are found in infected foods and are able to illicit the clinical symptoms described. The incubation period for *S. aureus* food poisoning is within hours after ingestion, and emesis is commonly the first and most significant symptom. Precooked, prepackaged meats with high salt contents (i.e., the ham from the patient's sandwiches) are commonly implicated in cases of *S. aureus* food poisoning.

    Answer A is incorrect. *Bacillus cereus* is a gram-positive spore-forming rod that causes food poisoning when the spores land on food and germinate, creating a toxin. Ingestion of the toxin will lead to sudden-onset nausea, vomiting, and diarrhea. Because the reaction is due to preformed toxins, antibiotics are not useful and treatment is supportive.

    Answer B is incorrect. *Campylobacter jejuni* is a gram-negative flagellated rod that, along with rotavirus and enterotoxigenic *Escherichia coli*, is one of the three most common causes of diarrhea in the world. Domestic animals and poultry are a reservoir for these bacteria, which are passed by the fecal-oral route and unpasteurized milk. Infection presents with a prodrome of fever, headaches, and malaise, followed by bloody, loose diarrhea. Treatment is with a fluoroquinolone and fluid resuscitation.

    Answer C is incorrect. *Clostridium difficile* is the pathogen of antibiotic (usually clindamycin or ampicillin)-associated colitis. Symptoms include diarrhea, fever, and abdominal cramping. *C. difficile* toxins can be tested for in stool samples. Treatment is usually with metronidazole and discontinuation of antibiotics.

Answer D is incorrect. Enteric adenovirus is another common viral etiology of diarrhea in infants and children. However, this virus is most prevalent in the spring and summer seasons. Infection is often accompanied by fever, rhinorrhea, cough, and acute respiratory disease. No antivirals or vaccines are appropriate for the treatment of adenovirus, and aggressive hydration is the treatment of choice.

Answer E is incorrect. *Escherichia coli* bacterial colitis is caused by several subtypes of the *E. coli* bacteria. Enterotoxigenic *E. coli* causes a rice water–type stool and is often seen in travelers to third-world countries. Enterohemorrhagic *E. coli* causes a hemorrhagic colitis, and the specific subtype *E. coli* O157:H7 results in hemolytic uremic syndrome (HUS). HUS is characterized by thrombocytopenia and renal failure. Enteroinvasive *E. coli* results in colitis along with fever, and WBCs can be found in the stool. Treatment is aggressive oral hydration without antibiotic therapy.

Answer G is incorrect. *Salmonella enteritidis* causes < 1 week of nausea, abdominal pain, and watery diarrhea. Diarrhea can be trace heme positive, and fever may or may not be present. *Salmonella* infections occur as a result of contamination by animal feces of foods. Common animal carriers are turtles and chickens. Treatment is aggressive hydration without antibiotic therapy.

Answer H is incorrect. *Shigella* is a nonflagellated gram-negative rod. It is found only in humans and passed by the fecal-oral route often in communal living situations or day care. Infection presents with fever and abdominal pain, along with blood and pus-speckled diarrhea. Treatment is with fluoroquinolones and fluid resuscitation.

Answer J is incorrect. *Vibrio cholerae* is a gram-negative flagellated rod that is passed by the fecal-oral route, usually through drinking contaminated water. It presents with sudden onset voluminous "rice water" diarrhea. Treatment is primarily with fluid resuscitation and oral rehydration because patients can lose up to 1 L of fluid in an hour, and death is commonly from dehydration. Definitive treatment is with antibiotics—either doxycycline or a fluoroquinolone.

Answer K is incorrect. *Vibrio parahaemolyticus* is a gram-negative rod that is found in marine water and is a common cause of diarrhea in Japan, where raw seafood is commonly consumed. Infection presents similarly to *Vibrio cholerae* with "rice water" diarrhea; however, *V. parahaemolyticus* typically resolves within 3 days without need for treatment.

Test Block 5

1. A 54-year-old woman with a history of rheumatoid arthritis (RA) presents to the rheumatology clinic complaining of swelling in her ankles and puffy eyes present for the last week. She has had RA for the past 15 years, and is currently being managed with several medications. She has no other significant past medical history, and has had no recent change in her diet. She does not smoke or drink alcohol. She has a temperature of 36.9°C (98.4°F), a heart rate of 110/min, and a blood pressure of 144/92 mm Hg. Her face appears puffy, with significant bilateral periorbital edema. Examination of her heart and lungs is normal. Her abdomen is soft and nondistended with no hepatosplenomegaly. She has 2+ pitting edema in both legs. Urinalysis shows 3+ protein. Renal biopsy is read as "renal disease consistent with membranous nephropathy." Which of the following medications most likely caused her acute presentation?

(A) Aspirin
(B) Corticosteroids
(C) Cyclophosphamide
(D) Methotrexate
(E) Penicillamine

2. A 29-year-old woman presents to the emergency department (ED) concerned that she is having a stroke. Her husband states, "My wife just can't seem to walk right." When the patient is asked about this, she meekly says that for the past month, her legs just won't work, as if she has no strength in them. She denies numbness or tingling, and otherwise feels well. During the interview, the husband repeatedly answers questions for his wife. He notes that the weakness began just after the patient's mother died 1 week ago. Tearfully, the patient states that she did not visit her mother before her death because "my mom and my husband didn't get along." The patient's cranial nerves II–XII are grossly intact; motor activity is 5/5 in the upper extremities and 1/5 in the lower extremities; sensation is intact to pinprick and vibration; the patient is unable to ambulate without significant assistance; and her cerebellar function is intact. Results of an MRI are nor-

mal. Which diagnosis best explains the patient's current presentation?

(A) Conversion disorder
(B) Depression
(C) Hypochondriasis
(D) Multiple sclerosis
(E) Somatization disorder

3. A 62-year-old woman presents to the ED after a sudden syncopal episode. She has no chronic medical conditions and takes no medications. However, during the past 36 hours she has felt acutely ill, with abdominal pain and repeated episodes of diarrhea and vomiting. On examination, blood pressure is 144/85 mm Hg, pulse is 70/min, respiratory rate is 10/min, and temperature is 37.9°C (100.3°F). Laboratory studies are shown as follows:

Na^+	155 mEq/L
K^+	2.1 mEq/L
Cl^-	105 mEq/L
HCO_3^-	36 mEq/L

An ECG demonstrates flattened T waves and prominent U waves that normalize after potassium repletion. Further tests reveal normal 24-hour urine-free cortisol levels and persistently diminished plasma renin activity. Which of the following is the most likely diagnosis?

(A) Addison's disease
(B) Conn's syndrome
(C) Cushing's disease
(D) Cushing's syndrome
(E) 21-Hydroxylase deficiency

4. A 60-year-old man with idiopathic dilated cardiomyopathy presents for a routine visit. Over the past few years his symptoms have been stable. He has significant fatigue and dyspnea upon mild to moderate exertion with marked limitation of daily activity. His past medical history is negative for hypertension, diabetes, smoking, or coronary artery disease. Echocardiogram reveals four-chambered dilatation and global hypokinesis of the myocardium. Which of the following therapies may worsen the patient's condition?

(A) Adult-dose aspirin
(B) Carvedilol
(C) Enalapril
(D) Exercise training
(E) Spironolactone

5. A 37-year-old obese, multiparous woman presents with severe epigastric pain that began several hours ago. Initial laboratory findings are:

Na^+	128 mEq/L
K^+	3.8 mEq/L
Cl^-	97 mEq/L
HCO_3^-	15 mEq/L
Ca^{2+}	7.8 mEq/L
Mg^{2+}	2.0 mEq/L
Phosphate	4.7 mg/dL
Blood urea nitrogen	9 mg/dL
Creatinine	0.5 mg/dL
Glucose	188 mg/dL
WBC count	14,000/mm^3
Hemoglobin	11.9 g/dL
Hematocrit	37%
Platelet count	347,000/mm^3
Aspartate aminotransferase	456 U/L
Alanine aminotransferase	562 U/L
Alkaline phosphatase	201 U/L
Total bilirubin	3.3 mg/dL
Direct bilirubin	2.9 mg/dL
Amylase	432 U/L
Lipase	256 U/L

Which of the following is included in Ranson's criteria?

(A) Alanine aminotransferase > 150 U/L
(B) Blood glucose < 200 mg/dL
(C) Fluid sequestration ≥ 4 L
(D) Fatigue/lack of energy
(E) Serum calcium > 8 mg/dL

6. A hypothetical study is performed that examines the link between breast cancer and red wine consumption. Patients who have been diagnosed with breast cancer are paired with subjects who do not have breast cancer, as shown on mammography. Data are collected about each patient's use of red wine. Which of the following data analyses is most suitable for this study?

(A) Attributable risk
(B) Number needed to treat
(C) Odds ratio
(D) Prevalence
(E) Relative risk

7. A 4-year-old Asian girl is brought to the ED because of a persistent fever. Her father reports she has had a fever to 38.3°C (101°F) for the past 5 days that was difficult to manage with acetaminophen. Additionally, he has noticed her eyes appear to be red, her tongue looks scarlet and "pitted," and she is complaining of neck pain. On physical examination, the child is febrile (38.7°C [101.6°F]) with otherwise stable vital signs. She has bilateral conjunctivitis, a reddened tongue, a scarlatiniform rash on her trunk, and a single palpable 2.5-cm lymph node of her right anterior cervical chain. If left untreated, what condition is this patient at highest risk for developing?

(A) Cardiomyopathy
(B) Coronary artery aneurysms
(C) Encephalitis
(D) Epidermal necrolysis
(E) Retropharyngeal abscess
(F) Stroke

8. A 79-year-old woman with no significant past medical history has become progressively more forgetful in the past 9 months. She has trouble remembering familiar places and people, can no longer balance her checkbook, and has increased trouble verbally expressing her thoughts. These symptoms have progressively worsened in the past several months. She has no history of head trauma or of anxiety disorder. Her neurologic examination is within normal limits except for a mini-mental status examination score of 22 of 30, missing points on calculation, recall, and orientation. A rapid plasma reagin test was negative, and the thyroid-stimulating hormone, vitamin B_{12}, folate, and electrolytes were normal. CT scan of the head is shown below. What is the most likely diagnosis?

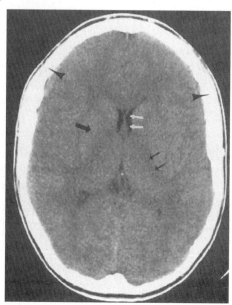

Reproduced, with permission, from Chen MYM, Pope TL, Ott DJ. *Basic Radiology.* New York: McGraw-Hill, 2004: Figure 12-2.

(A) Alzheimer's disease
(B) Creutzfeldt-Jakob disease
(C) Delirium
(D) Depression
(E) Normal pressure hydrocephalus

9. A 26-year-old man with HIV and a history of intravenous drug use presents to the ED with 5 days of low-grade fever, nonproductive cough, and dyspnea on exertion that progressed to dyspnea at rest. His oxygen saturation in the ED is 88% on room air. An arterial blood gas shows an arterial-alveolar gradient of 45 and a partial arterial oxygen pressure of 65 mm Hg. X-ray of the chest reveals diffuse bilateral infiltrates. What is the most appropriate treatment?

(A) Ampicillin + gentamicin
(B) Intravenous clindamycin
(C) Isoniazid + pyrazinamide + rifampin + ethambutol
(D) Third-generation cephalosporin + doxycycline
(E) Trimethoprim-sulfamethoxazole + oral prednisone

10. An 18-year-old man is brought to the ED following a high-speed motor vehicle crash. He is in stable condition and reports no loss of consciousness following the accident. His vital signs are temperature 36.8°C (98.3°F), heart rate 86/min, blood pressure 135/84 mm Hg, and respiratory rate 15/min. The patient describes chest pain that worsens with inhalation and with abduction of his right arm. An x-ray of the chest shows a widened mediastinum, along with loss of the aortic knob. In addition, first and second rib fractures are noted on the x-ray. Which test should be completed next to workup this patient?

(A) Aortogram
(B) MRI scan
(C) Transthoracic echocardiography
(D) Upper endoscopy
(E) Ventilation-perfusion scan

11. A 44-year-old woman presents to her primary care physician for a routine checkup. She states that over the past year, she has become more bowlegged, and that her hats are now too small to fit her comfortably. She denies any focal pain or tenderness, but does admit to occasional dull aching in her lower legs that is exacerbated by exercise. Her temperature is 36.9°C (98.4°F), pulse is 76/min, and blood pressure is 119/83 mm Hg. Physical examination findings include frontal bossing and bilateral bowing of her tibias. Suspecting Paget's disease, the physician orders a set of laboratory tests. Which of the following laboratory abnormalities is most likely to be associated with this disorder?

(A) Decreased alkaline phosphatase levels
(B) Elevated alkaline phosphatase levels
(C) Elevated serum calcium
(D) Elevated serum phosphate
(E) Positive rheumatoid factor

12. The concerned parents of a 3-month-old boy present to the ED because of their son's behavior during feedings. His mother reports that he often chokes and gags during feedings and "spits up" significant amounts of material after such episodes. Additionally, his parents have noticed he is often irritable and has been seen to arch his back when seated. His pediatrician has advised close monitoring of his weight because he has moved from the 60th percentile to the 45th percentile since birth. His birth, family, and social histories are unremarkable. Vital signs are stable and there are no remarkable findings. Relevant laboratory findings are:

Na^+	141 mEq/L
Cl^-	105 mEq/L
Mg^{2+}	1.5 mEq/L
K^+	4.2 mEq/L
Ca^{2+}	9.8 mEq/L
HCO_3^-	23 mEq/L
Phosphate	2.1 mEq/L
Glucose	96 mg/dL
Creatinine	0.5 mg/dL
Blood urea nitrogen	15 mg/dL

What is the best course of action for the pediatrician to take?

(A) Conservative management with parental reassurance
(B) Initiation of daily antacid treatment
(C) Prescription of a histamine$_2$-receptor antagonist
(D) Prescription of a prokinetic agent
(E) Prescription of a proton pump inhibitor

13. A 16-year-old girl comes to see her pediatrician alone, complaining of itchy, greenish vaginal discharge for 4 days. When questioned about her sexual practices, the patient blushes and admits that although she is usually careful about using condoms, she was at a party recently where she drank too much and forgot to insist that her boyfriend use a condom. After disclosing this information, she suddenly looks alarmed and says, "You're not going to tell my parents this, are you? They don't know that my boyfriend and I have sex, and they would kill me." In addition to gently reminding the patient about safe sex, how should the pediatrician respond?

(A) "Although I would encourage you to be open and honest with your parents, your health is most important, and everything you tell me about your sexual practices is completely confidential."
(B) "Although this is not generally my practice, I will make an exception for you because you are a long-standing patient. However, as your physician I do not approve of your refusal to tell your parents about your habits."
(C) "I'm sorry, but because you are under 18 I will have to get your mother's consent before treating you for vaginitis."
(D) "I really will need to tell your parents because now that you have had unprotected sex I need their consent to do an HIV test."
(E) "Unless you agree to tell your parents about your sexual activity, I cannot treat you for your vaginal infection."

14. A 40-year-old white woman presents to the ED with 2 days of constant moderate abdominal pain accompanied by nausea and vomiting. She has not had a bowel movement or passed flatus in 4 days. Her medical history is significant for a chronic pain syndrome for which she takes opiates regularly. Her vital signs are normal. On examination, she is in mild distress, her abdomen is distended with mild diffuse tenderness to palpation, and bowel sounds are absent. She does not have rebound tenderness. Complete blood cell count, urinalysis, and basic metabolic panel with extended tests were unremarkable. Flat and upright abdominal films reveal general distension of the small intestine and colon with air present throughout the bowel. Which of the following is the most likely diagnosis?

(A) Acute appendicitis
(B) Acute cholecystitis
(C) Complete bowel obstruction
(D) Paralytic ileus
(E) Partial small bowel obstruction

15. A 52-year-old high school teacher is seen in the clinic with a chief complaint of reduced exercise tolerance. An avid soccer player, she has had to sit out portions of league games due to shortness of breath and reports having to pause to rest when bringing in groceries. She worked as a welder 20 years ago, prior to earning her degree in education. Medications include combined estrogen and progesterone tablets for menopausal symptoms and occasional ibuprofen for aches and pains. X-ray of the chest reveals honeycombing, and bronchoalveolar lavage is positive for two asbestos bodies per milliliter. Which of the following pulmonary function tests is expected in this patient?

CHOICE	FEV_1	FVC	FEV_1:FVC RATIO
A	↓	↓	normal
B	↓	normal	normal
C	↓	↑	↓
D	normal	normal	normal
E	↑	↑	normal

(A) A
(B) B
(C) C
(D) D
(E) E

16. A 58-year-old man is brought to the trauma bay unresponsive and intubated. He was an unrestrained driver in a high-speed motor vehicle crash. Medical transporters report that the car's windshield was broken. His vital signs on admission are pulse 58/min and regular, blood pressure 80/50 mm Hg, and respiratory rate 15/min. Chest auscultation reveals good air flow bilaterally and no adventitial lung sounds. He opens his eyes to command and his pupils are equally round and reactive to light. He is unable move his extremities or withdraw to pain. His extremities are pink and warm. Which of the following is most likely the diagnosis?

(A) Addisonian crisis
(B) Anaphylaxis
(C) Atrial fibrillation
(D) Bacteremia
(E) Congestive heart failure
(F) Inadequate fluid repletion
(G) Spinal cord injury

17. A 2-year-old girl has had repeated infections with opportunistic pathogens, including *Pneumocystis jiroveci* (formerly *carinii*). She also has had a right-sided aortic arch with congenital ventricular septal defect and an underdeveloped thymus. She has a short philtrum of the upper lip with cleft palate, an antimongoloid slant to her eyes, and a hypoplastic mandible. Relevant laboratory findings are:

Na^+	140 mEq/L
Cl^-	104 mEq/L
Mg^{2+}	1.1 mEq/L
K^+	4.0 mEq/L
Ca^{2+}	7.0 mg/dL
HCO_3^-	24 mEq/L
Phosphate	2.0 mg/dL
Glucose	97 mg/dL
Creatinine	0.6 mg/dL
Blood urea nitrogen	13 mg/dL

What chromosomal segment has been implicated in the constellation of these signs and symptoms?

(A) 7q11
(B) 8q24
(C) 11p13
(D) 15q11
(E) 17p13
(F) 20p12
(G) 22q11

18. A 78-year-old man presents to clinic with fatigue over the past few weeks. He lives in a second-story apartment and has increasing difficulty walking up the stairs. Vital signs are significant for a blood pressure of 165/86 mm Hg. The height of the QRS waves in leads V_1 and V_5 on the 12-lead ECG are greater than 35 mm. Echocardiogram reveals increased wall thickness, left atrial dilatation, E to A reversal, and an ejection fraction of 60%. What is the most likely etiology of this patient's heart failure?

(A) Diastolic dysfunction caused by constrictive pericarditis
(B) Diastolic dysfunction caused by hypertensive cardiomyopathy
(C) Diastolic dysfunction caused by restrictive cardiomyopathy
(D) Systolic dysfunction caused by diastolic cardiomyopathy
(E) Systolic dysfunction caused by hypertrophic cardiomyopathy
(F) Systolic dysfunction caused by ischemic heart disease

19. A G1P1 mother presents with her 5-month-old daughter to her pediatrician's office. The infant was delivered by cesarean section at 37 weeks' gestation because of breech presentation. There were no complications during delivery. The infant has reached all developmental milestones as expected and is up to date with immunizations. However, on physical examination, the pediatrician senses a palpable "click" about the infant's hip joint when the pediatrician gently adducts the hip and directs a posterior force. What is the most appropriate treatment at this time?

(A) A flexion-abduction orthosis
(B) A removable extension splint
(C) Closed reduction and spica cast
(D) No treatment is necessary
(E) Surgical correction

20. After losing his wife to ovarian cancer 5 weeks ago, a 58-year-old man with no psychiatric history presents to his primary care physician with a 2.3-kg (5-lb) weight loss. He complains of not eating or sleeping well since his wife was admitted to inpatient hospice. He reports hearing the voice of his wife as he lies in bed attempting to fall asleep. His physical examination is unremarkable, but he appears tearful throughout the encounter. What is the most appropriate treatment plan?

(A) Administer 10 cycles of electroconvulsive therapy
(B) Offer supportive reassurance
(C) Prescribe olanzapine
(D) Prescribe zolpidem
(E) Refer to an inpatient psychiatric facility

21. The mother of a 7-year-old girl brings her to the pediatrician because she is concerned that her daughter has already begun to develop breasts. She has been an otherwise healthy child with no significant illnesses or surgeries. The mother states that she went through menarche at age 14 years, and her other two daughters began puberty at around age 12 years. On physical examination, the pediatrician notes that the girl has Tanner stage III breasts, but lacks pubic hair. Laboratory evaluation reveals elevated gonadotropin-releasing hormone, luteinizing hormone, and follicle-stimulating hormone. What is the most likely diagnosis?

(A) Adrenal tumor
(B) Central precocious puberty
(C) McCune-Albright syndrome
(D) Ovarian tumor
(E) Primary hypothyroidism

22. A 65-year-old man is brought to the ED in a confused state following a seizure in public. Witnesses report the seizure as occurring suddenly and lasting at least 2 or 3 minutes. A call to his family reveals that he has no major medical problems other than hypertension and high anxiety, and that both are well controlled by his medications. On examination, the patient's tongue is unharmed, although his pants are covered in fresh urine and feces. He is oriented to person, but not place or time, and has no recollection of what occurred. Physical examination is otherwise unremarkable. Withdrawal from which drug might be responsible for this patient's seizure?

(A) Captopril
(B) Cocaine
(C) Diazepam
(D) Lithium
(E) Verapamil

23. A 36-year-old woman presents at the primary care clinic for a routine health check-up. She has no complaints aside from occasional low-back pain and states that she has been generally healthy. She smokes cigarettes on occasion and drinks 4–5 glasses of wine each week. She is currently on no medications. Her family history is significant for type 2 diabetes and endometrial cancer at age 46 years in her paternal grandmother, as well as colon cancer in her father at 50 years of age, and in her half-brother at 44 years. Her physical examination, including digital rectal examination, is normal. What recommendation should be given at this time?

(A) Colonoscopy beginning at age 50, and every 5 years after that
(B) Immediate colonoscopy
(C) Immediate CT scan of the abdomen
(D) Immediate double-contrast barium enema
(E) Yearly digital rectal examinations and sigmoidoscopy every 2–3 years, beginning at age 44 years

24. A 35-year-old homeless woman is brought to the ED after having been found unconscious in the street. Her pupils are 2 mm, her respiratory rate is 6/min, and she has extensive scarring across her forearms. It is assumed that she has taken a drug of some type, and a urine toxicology screen is ordered. Which of the following statements is true of this woman's condition?

(A) Lorazepam is the treatment of choice for this woman's condition
(B) The fatal consequence of this condition is myocardial infarction
(C) The substance that caused her condition only binds effectively to μ receptors
(D) Tolerance to the euphoric effects of this substance develops slowly
(E) Withdrawal from this substance is life-threatening

25. A 5-year-old boy with an "itchy rash" is brought to the pediatrician by his mother. She states that the rash first appeared 3 weeks ago. He had a similar rash on his face when he was about a year old, but that resolved. This rash first appeared on his left arm and is now on the backs of his knees. He has otherwise been well.

She thought he was allergic to their new laundry detergent, but the rash has failed to resolve despite changing back to their previous detergent. He had bronchiolitis as an infant, but has otherwise been healthy. On examination, the lesions shown in the image are present on the flexor surfaces of both proximal upper extremities and the popliteal fossae bilaterally. The diaper area is spared. The plaques are erythematous and dry, with scattered papules and excoriations. Which of the following is the most appropriate diagnosis?

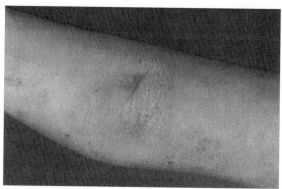

Reproduced, with permission, from Wolff K, Johnson RA, Surmond D. *Fitzpatrick's Color Atlas & Synopsis of Clinical Dermatology*, 5th ed. New York: McGraw-Hill, 2005: Figure 2e-12.

(A) Allergic contact dermatitis
(B) Atopic dermatitis
(C) Pityriasis rosea
(D) Psoriasis
(E) Seborrheic dermatitis

26. A 2-year-old boy is brought in to the ED by his parents. His mother reports that he developed a fever to 38.8°C (101.9°F) today and additionally began to complain of throat pain while eating. Shortly after dinner, he began to drool and had "noisy" breathing. The patient is sitting on the examining table with his neck hyperextended and chin protruding. His lung examination is normal without rales, rhonchi, or wheeze. The advent of what immunization greatly reduced the incidence of this condition?

(A) Diphtheria-tetanus-pertussis
(B) *Haemophilus influenzae* type B (Hib)
(C) Measles-mumps-rubella
(D) Pneumococcus
(E) Varicella

27. An 83-year-old woman with a history of hypertension, emphysema, and a 90 pack-year smoking history presents to a gastroenterologist for a follow up appointment. Six weeks ago, she was seen in the ED presenting with acute severe abdominal pain that began earlier that morning. The patient recalled having had several episodes of painless bright red blood per rectum during the weeks preceding her visit to the ED. The patient complained of fever, chills, nausea, and emesis, which accompanied the pain. CT scans of the abdomen and pelvis were obtained in the ED in which an abscess was noted, and the patient was subsequently begun on oral antibiotics. Which of the following is most likely to have reduced the likelihood of this condition?

(A) Blood pressure control
(B) Exercise
(C) High-fiber diet
(D) Reduction of caffeine intake
(E) Smoking cessation

28. A 58-year-old woman presents to her primary care physician for her annual health maintenance examination. Overall she feels well, but she does complain of pain in her hands that has progressively worsened over the past year. She notes that the pain is worst at the end of the day, and she is experiencing pain and stiffness. She has had some relief with ibuprofen. On physical examination, her fingers are tender to palpation at the proximal and distal interphalangeal joints bilaterally. She also has limited flexion at these joints. What is the most likely diagnosis in this patient?

(A) Calcium pyrophosphate deposition disease
(B) Gout
(C) Osteoarthritis
(D) Psoriatic arthritis
(E) Rheumatoid arthritis

29. A 26-year-old G1P0 woman at 37 weeks' gestation presents to her obstetrician's office for a routine prenatal checkup. The fetal head is palpated by the obstetrician in the upper abdomen with Leopold maneuvers, and a breech presentation is suspected. Cervical examination reveals a cervix that is posterior, moderate in consistency, and 20% effaced. The fetus is not yet engaged in the pelvis, and the amniotic sac is intact. Breech presentation is then confirmed by ultrasound. A biophysical profile of the fetus is performed, with a reactive non-stress test and an overall score of 10/10. Which of the following is the most reasonable next step in management?

(A) Elective cesarean section delivery
(B) Emergent cesarean section delivery
(C) Expectant management for vaginal breech delivery
(D) Induction of labor with intravaginal prostaglandin E_2 for a vaginal delivery
(E) Offer the patient an external cephalic version

30. A 10-month-old boy is brought to the clinic with cough, fever, and wheezing. The parents report that he has had recurrent episodes of pneumonia, otitis media, and sinusitis during the past 4 months. His temperature is 39°C (102.2°F), heart rate is 95/min, respiratory rate is 30/min, and blood pressure is 110/65 mm Hg, and crackles are auscultated on the left chest. On physical examination no tonsillar tissue is seen, and no lymph nodes are palpated. X-ray of the chest shows left lower lobe consolidation. Further work-up yields a normal absolute lymphocyte count and low levels of IgG, IgA, IgM, and IgE, and flow cytometry demonstrates the absence of circulating B lymphocytes. What is the most likely underlying immune deficiency?

(A) Bruton's agammaglobulinemia
(B) Common variable immunodeficiency
(C) DiGeorge's syndrome
(D) IgA deficiency
(E) Severe combined immunodeficiency

31. In a study of predictive factors for failing extubation in the intensive care unit (ICU), patients who failed extubation (and consequently had to be reintubated) were matched with ICU patients who were successfully extubated. For each patient, the physiologic data routinely measured prior to extubation was collected from charts, and was analyzed to see which data differed between the successfully and unsuccessfully extubated patients. What type of study is described?

(A) Case-control
(B) Clinical trial
(C) Correlation
(D) Prospective cohort
(E) Retrospective cohort

32. A 24-year-old man is brought to the ED after suffering from blunt trauma to his chest in a motor vehicle accident. His respiratory rate is 32/min, heart rate is 125/min, and blood pressure is 80/45 mm Hg, with a decrease to 65/40 mm Hg on inspiration. Physical examination demonstrates decreased heart sounds and a pericardial friction rub. Which other symptoms would the physician expect to see as part of the patient's presentation?

(A) Bounding pulse
(B) Bradycardia
(C) Holosystolic murmur
(D) Hypertension
(E) Jugular venous distention

33. A 68-year-old African-American woman presents with palpitations, breathlessness, and fatigue of 2 months' duration. She also reports an unintentional 6.8-kg (15.0-lb) weight loss during this time period, which she ascribes to stress at her workplace. The patient is currently taking captopril for high blood pressure, amiodarone for arrhythmias, and omeprazole for gastroesophageal reflux disease. She is a nonsmoker. On examination, her temperature is 36.8°C (98.2°F), blood pressure is 125/80 mm Hg, and heart rate is 86/min and regular. What is the appropriate next step in management?

(A) Check thyroid-stimulating hormone and thyroid hormone levels
(B) Provide reassurance and follow-up in 6 months
(C) Refer the patient to a psychiatrist for possible anxiety disorder
(D) Substitute nifedipine for captopril
(E) Substitute procainamide for amiodarone

34. A 28-year-old man comes to see an infectious disease specialist after being told he is HIV-positive. Upon testing, his CD4+ count is 400/mm^3 and his HIV viral load is 126,000 copies/mL. He believes he was infected 2 months earlier while sharing a needle to inject drugs. He reports no symptoms, denying lymphadenopathy, fevers, chills, and night sweats; he says he feels "fine." What is the next appropriate step?

(A) Begin highly active antiretroviral therapy immediately because his CD4+ count is falling rapidly and is unlikely to rebound
(B) Begin trimethoprim-sulfamethoxazole as prophylaxis against *Pneumocystis jiroveci* (formerly *carinii*) pneumonia
(C) Retest for HIV; the patient may have cleared the infection
(D) Retest for HIV; the patient may have had a false-positive result
(E) Schedule a follow-up appointment in 1 month to retest CD4+ count and viral load, and instruct the patient to call if he experiences any symptoms

35. A 68-year-old patient presents to his primary care practice complaining of easy fatigue and shortness of breath over the past year. Six months ago, his identical twin died of an intracranial hemorrhage. His history is notable only for recurrent epistaxis. He claims he is eating well, sleeping well, and is at peace with his brother's passing. Physical examination reveals the lesions shown in the image and pale conjunctivae. What is the most likely cause of this man's symptoms?

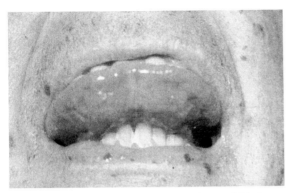

Reproduced, with permission, from Lichtman MA, Beutler E, Kipps TJ, Seligsohn U, Kaushansky K, Prchal JT. *Williams Hematology*, 7th ed. New York: McGraw-Hill, 2006: Figure XXV-41.

(A) Depression
(B) Chronic obstructive pulmonary disease
(C) Gastrointestinal bleed
(D) Intracranial aneurysm
(E) New-onset coronary artery disease

36. The on-call intern in the newborn nursery is paged because a baby girl born at 34 weeks' gestation is experiencing bilious vomiting. The newborn was reportedly doing well since delivery 16 hours ago and had been tolerating oral feeding without complication. The pregnancy was complicated by mild polyhydramnios. There is no parental family history of gastrointestinal abnormalities. The newborn has a heart rate of 117/min, blood pressure of 65/48 mm Hg, respiratory rate of 42/min, and temperature of 37.0°C (98.6°F). Physical examination is unremarkable, except for mild jaundice. The abdomen is not distended. A plain film of the abdomen shows two air-filled structures in the upper abdomen, both showing air and fluid. The first step in management of this patient should involve which of the following treatment strategies?

(A) Radiologic studies of the spine and chest
(B) Gastrostomy tube placement
(C) Immediate surgical correction
(D) Nasogastric decompression
(E) Radiologic studies of the spine and chest

37. A 28-year-old man is brought to the ED by his friend after having a confrontation with his girlfriend. He has a stab wound in the anterior neck just lateral to the left lateral border of the thyroid cartilage. His past medical history is unremarkable. His pulse is 88/min, blood pressure is 138/85 mm Hg, and respiratory rate is 20/min. On examination, it is difficult to assess whether the platysma has been penetrated. Subcutaneous air is palpated. The trachea is midline. What is the most appropriate management for this injury?

(A) Arteriography
(B) Esophagoscopy
(C) Oral and intravenous contrast CT of the neck
(D) Surgical exploration
(E) Tracheobronchoscopy

38. A 55-year-old Asian philosophy professor presents to his primary care physician with months of intermittent watery diarrhea and episodes of wheezing and facial flushing sometimes precipitated by consuming alcohol. He has no past medical history or recent travel history. His vital signs are temperature 37.5°C (99.5°F), blood pressure 130/80 mm Hg, pulse 80/min, and respiratory rate 22/min. Physical examination reveals some facial flushing, moderate elevation in jugular venous pressure, II/VI systolic ejection murmur at the left upper sternal border, wheezes in the lungs, and mild lower extremity edema. Complete blood cell count and basic metabolic panel with extended panel were unremarkable. CT of the abdomen demonstrated a thickened desmoplastic reaction in the mesentery surrounding an area of terminal ileum and three possible lesions in the liver. Which of the following is most likely to confirm the diagnosis?

(A) Serum antigliadin antibody titer
(B) Serum cortisol level
(C) Serum gastrin level
(D) Urine 5-hydroxyindoleacetic acid level
(E) Urine vanillylmandelic acid level

39. A 38-year-old woman presents for a routine health maintenance examination. She has no complaints and physical examination is within normal limits. Relevant laboratory findings include a Ca^{2+} level of 11.8 mg/dL, Mg^{2+} level of 2.9 mg/dL, and parathyroid hormone level of 75 pg/mL (normal: 11–54 pg/mL). On further screening, her mother, brother, and 10-year-old son also have elevated serum calcium levels. The patient has no personal or family history of malignancy. Which of the following is the most likely diagnosis in this patient?

(A) Familial hypocalciuric hypercalcemia
(B) Jansen's disease
(C) Primary hyperparathyroidism
(D) Type I multiple endocrine neoplasia
(E) Type IIB multiple endocrine neoplasia

40. A middle-aged woman drives herself to the ED. When she is seen by the physician, she tells her that her chest pain "has been getting worse" over the past day. Upon questioning, she tells the physician that she is starting to get this chest pain at rest and it is not responding to the sublingual nitroglycerin like it used to. Recognizing that this could be an emergent situation, the physician orders an immediate ECG. What ECG changes would require sending this patient immediately to the revascularization laboratory?

(A) Delta waves
(B) Flipped T waves
(C) Low-voltage ECG
(D) New left bundle-branch block
(E) ST depressions

EXTENDED MATCHING

Questions 41 and 42

For each patient with glomerular disease, select the most likely diagnosis.

(A) Alport's syndrome
(B) Amyloidosis
(C) Cryoglobulinemia
(D) Focal segmental glomerulosclerosis
(E) Goodpasture's syndrome
(F) IgA nephropathy
(G) Lupus nephritis
(H) Membranoproliferative glomerulonephritis
(I) Minimal change disease
(J) Polyarteritis nodosa
(K) Postinfectious glomerulonephritis
(L) Wegener's granulomatosis

41. A 46-year-old man presents to the ED complaining of leg swelling, pink-colored urine, and headache. He was in good health until 3 months ago, when he noticed several days of pink-colored urine following an upper respiratory tract infection. Both the infection and the urine discoloration resolved spontaneously, but after about 6 weeks his urinary symptoms recurred, this time accompanied by flank pain. His symptoms again resolved, and he was asymptomatic until today. His blood pressure is 160/94 mm Hg and he has 2+ edema up to his shins bilaterally. Urinalysis shows 20 RBCs/high-power field and 2+ protein. Antinuclear antibody and antiglomerular basement membrane antibody titers are negative, and serum complement is normal.

42. A 32-year-old man is being evaluated for new-onset hypertension. His only other medical problem is difficulty with hearing, which has been worsening since childhood. Family history is significant for an uncle with kidney problems, but the specifics are not known. His blood pressure is 158/94 mg Hg and heart rate is 64/min. On physical examination the patient is in no acute distress. He has diminished auditory acuity bilaterally. Laboratory studies show a blood urea nitrogen level of 17 mg/dL and creatinine of 1.8 mg/dL. Urinalysis shows 4+ blood and 2+ protein.

Questions 43 and 44

For each patient with nipple discharge, select the most likely diagnosis.

(A) Fibroadenoma
(B) Fibrocystic changes
(C) Galactocele
(D) Intraductal papilloma
(E) Invasive ductal carcinoma
(F) Paget's disease of the breast
(G) Pregnancy

(H) Prolactinoma
(I) Invasive lobular carcinoma
(J) Invasive papillary carcinoma

43. A physician sees a 44-year-old woman in the ED reporting 1 day of serosanguineous discharge from her right nipple. She noticed a discharge this morning, but it was clear at that point and not bloody. When she removed her clothes this evening, however, her underclothing had some blood on it. When she pressed on the right breast, more bloody discharge came out. At that point, she became panicked and rushed to the ED. The patient denies breast pain or tenderness. She reports a past obstetric history of two uncomplicated pregnancies via spontaneous vaginal delivery, and an age of 12 years at menarche. Her last period was 3 months ago and she believes she is experiencing menopause. Family history is negative for neoplasm of any kind. Breast examination reveals a lump in the left upper quadrant of the right breast. When pressed, there is serosanguineous discharge from the nipple.

44. A physician sees a 44-year-old woman in a primary care clinic with the chief complaint of bloody nipple discharge from her right nipple. She says that at first it was clear, but after a couple of weeks it seemed pink, then frankly bloody. The bleeding resolved, but this symptom prompted her to examine her breasts, and at that point she noticed a lump in her breast, close to the axilla. Her family history is significant for a mother and aunt with ovarian cancer. On physical examination, she is in no acute distress. She has a 1-cm lump in the right upper outer quadrant. The lump is hard and immobile, although it is regular in shape. Palpation of the lump elicits no discharge from the nipple.

Questions 45 and 46

For each patient with delirium, select the most likely cause.

(A) Brief psychotic disorder
(B) Creutzfeldt-Jakob disease
(C) Delirium due to a general medical condition
(D) Dementia, Alzheimer's type
(E) Depression
(F) Irritable mania
(G) Normal age-associated cognitive decline
(H) Parkinson's disease
(I) Pseudodementia
(J) Psychotic disorder resulting from a general medical condition
(K) Substance intoxication delirium
(L) Vascular dementia

45. A 72-year-old woman is brought to the ED due to altered mental status and combative behavior. Two weeks ago, the patient had been admitted to a nursing home after sustaining a hip fracture; history also reveals hypertension and recent urinary tract infections. Though normally "calm and loving" per her family's report, the patient has grown restless and combative with staff and residents in past days.

46. A 38-year-old woman with bipolar disorder is brought to the ED for confusion. She appears to be apathetic with a flat affect and highly distractable; she grows lethargic, hypotensive, and unarousable. Her lithium level was found to be > 3.5 mEq/L (normal: 0.4–0.8 mEq/L).

1. The correct answer is E. This patient has had the onset of nephrotic syndrome. Patients with rheumatoid arthritis (RA) are at risk for multiple types of renal disease, due both to their underlying disease as well as the therapies used to manage RA. In this patient with membranous nephropathy, the most likely etiologic agent is penicillamine. Up to 7% of patients treated with penicillamine will develop membranous nephropathy, and proteinuria usually develops within 6–12 months. Cessation of therapy will usually result in resolution of proteinuria. Gold, another disease-modifying antirheumatic drug, can also cause membranous nephropathy.

Answer A is incorrect. Aspirin or nonsteroidal anti-inflammatory drugs (NSAIDs) are very commonly used in the management of patients with RA and may cause renal disease. NSAIDs can cause nephrotic syndrome due to minimal change disease. Another NSAID-induced renal complication is acute interstitial nephritis. Chronic aspirin use may increase the risk of chronic renal failure, causing analgesic nephropathy.

Answer B is incorrect. Corticosteroids are also used in the management of RA, but do not cause nephrotic syndrome. Corticosteroids may actually be used to treat nephrotic syndrome or other renal pathology, including rheumatoid vasculitis.

Answer C is incorrect. Cyclophosphamide is an alkylating agent and a very potent immunosuppressive drug. An important genitourinary complication of cyclophosphamide therapy is acute hemorrhagic cystitis, which presents with hematuria.

Answer D is incorrect. Methotrexate is another disease-modifying antirheumatic drug that is commonly used to treat patients with RA. However, it is not typically associated with renal toxicity. Its primary adverse effects include gastrointestinal upset, oral ulcerations, and dose-dependent liver function abnormalities.

2. The correct answer is A. Although the diagnosis of conversion disorder is a diagnosis of exclusion, it seems to best fit the clinical picture described in the question. The *Diagnostic and Statistical Manual of Mental Disorders*, Fourth Edition, Text Revision criteria for conversion disorder are as follows: (1) neurologic function is lost; (2) psychological factors are associated with the symptom or deficit because the initiation or exacerbation of the symptom or deficit is preceded by conflicts or other stressors. In the question stem, the patient feels conflict because she was unable to visit her mother because of her husband's controlling nature. When her mother died, the patient became unable to walk. This allows the patient to express her resentment of her controlling husband by making herself "unable" to cooperate with him.

Answer B is incorrect. The patient may very well be depressed. One could even argue that her conversion disorder has occurred as a way for her mind to alleviate her depression. However, her current presentation is best explained by conversion disorder.

Answer C is incorrect. Hypochondriasis is defined by a preoccupation with fears of having, or by the idea that one has a serious disease. These feelings are based on the person's misinterpretation of bodily symptoms.

Answer D is incorrect. Multiple sclerosis (MS) is characterized by multiple neurologic events (e.g., blurry vision, bladder incontinence, and neurologic leg pain), which can be linked to white matter tracts in the brain. Moreover, these events must occur in different parts of the body at multiple points in time. MRIs in patients with MS usually show multiple hyperintense white matter lesions. Thus, MS would be an unlikely diagnosis.

Answer E is incorrect. Somatization disorder presents with a history of many physical complaints beginning before age 30, which occur over a period of several years. The patient must have at least four pain symptoms involving multiple sites, at least two unexplained gastrointestinal symptoms such as nausea and indigestion, at least one sexual complaint and/or menstrual complaint, and at least one pseudoneurologic symptom, such as blindness or inability to walk, speak, or move. They must result in the patient seeking frequent medical treatment, or in significant impairment in social, occupational, or other important areas of functioning.

3. **The correct answer is B.** Conn's syndrome, or primary hyperaldosteronism, results from an adrenal adenoma. It is manifested by hypertension, hypokalemia, hypernatremia, low plasma renin, and increased plasma aldosterone. In this case, an episode of viral gastroenteritis likely resulted in gastrointestinal loss of potassium, aggravating the chronic hypokalemia seen with this disorder. The patient's syncopal episode could have been caused by a hypokalemia-induced ventricular arrhythmia.

Answer A is incorrect. Addison's disease is incorrect because this entails adrenal insufficiency and thus the electrolyte disturbances (hyponatremia with hyperkalemia) would be the opposite of those seen here. Hyperpigmentation of the skin, weight loss, weakness, and eosinophilia are often seen in adrenal insufficiency.

Answer C is incorrect. Cushing's disease refers to those cases of Cushing's syndrome caused by a pituitary adenoma. It would be characterized by increased cortisol.

Answer D is incorrect. Twenty-four-hour urine-free cortisol levels would be expected to be elevated in endogenous causes of Cushing's syndrome, and we have no history to suggest that this patient has taken exogenous glucocorticoids (the most common cause of Cushing's syndrome).

Answer E is incorrect. 21-Hydroxylase deficiency is a congenital salt-wasting syndrome. Hypertension and hypernatremia would not be seen.

4. **The correct answer is A.** Based on the patient's symptoms (comfortable at rest but symptoms with less-than-normal activity), he can be classified as having New York Heart Association class III heart failure. Heart failure can be due to restrictive cardiomyopathy (sarcoid and amyloid), hypertrophic (diastolic dysfunction) cardiomyopathy, or dilated cardiomyopathy (systolic dysfunction), as described in this case. Nonsteroidal anti-inflammatory drugs (NSAIDs) have not been proven to improve mortality in patients with heart failure. In contrast, there are several mechanisms by which they may exacerbate the condition and would be contraindicated in this patient. NSAIDs may worsen afterload by inhibiting prostaglandin synthesis (eliminating their effects on vasodilation) and by counteracting the benefits of angiotensin-converting enzyme inhibitors.

Answer B is incorrect. A number of β-blockers, including carvedilol and metoprolol, have been proven to improve survival in patients with heart failure and without other contraindications (including bradycardia, hypotension, atrioventricular conduction abnormalities, and asthma).

Answer C is incorrect. Angiotensin-converting enzyme inhibitors are the most effective drugs for improving survival and slowing the progression of heart failure due to systolic dysfunction regardless of severity.

Answer D is incorrect. Exercise training is associated with both improved morbidity and mortality in patients with heart failure.

Answer E is incorrect. Spironolactone is a competitive inhibitor of aldosterone at the mineralocorticoid receptor that has been shown to improve survival in patients with symptomatic heart failure. The mechanism may be by increased potassium levels or by inhibiting the effects of aldosterone on receptors in the heart.

5. **The correct answer is D.** Acute pancreatitis is a rapid-onset inflammation of the pancreas. Depending on its severity, it can have severe complications and high mortality despite treatment. In addition, in predicting the prognosis, there are several scoring indices that have been used as predictors of survival. One such scoring system is Ranson's criteria. There are a total of 11 Ranson's criteria, which are split into

two groups: On admission criteria include the following: age > 55 years, WBC count > 16,000/mm3, aspartate aminotransferase > 250 U/L, lactate dehydrogenase > 350 U/L, and glucose > 200 mg/dL. Between 24 and 48 hours after admission criteria include the following: hematocrit drop > 10%, blood urea nitrogen rise > 5 mg/dL, calcium < 8 mEq/L, partial pressure of arterial oxygen < 60 mm Hg, fluid sequestration > 6 L, and base deficit > 4. The risk of mortality increases with the number of Ranson's criteria present. If 3–4 are positive, mortality is 20%. If 4–5 are positive, mortality is 40%, and if 7 or more are positive, mortality is 100%.

Answer A is incorrect. Aspartate aminotransferase > 250 U/L is one of Ranson's criteria on admission.

Answer B is incorrect. Glucose > 200 mg/dL is one of Ranson's criteria on admission.

Answer C is incorrect. Fluid sequestration of ≥ 6 L is one of Ranson's criteria between 24 and 48 hours after admission.

Answer E is incorrect. Serum calcium < 8 mg/dL is one of Ranson's criteria between 24 and 48 hours after admission.

6. **The correct answer is C.** The study described is a case-control study in which cases (patients with disease) are paired with controls (without disease) and information is retrospectively collected about past exposure to possible etiologic factors. The odds ratio is determined as the ratio of the odds of exposure in those with disease to the odds of exposure in those without disease in case-control studies. This statistic is mathematically identical to the ratio of odds of disease in exposed persons to the odds of disease in unexposed persons.

Answer A is incorrect. Attributable risk, also called the risk difference, cannot be calculated using a case-control study.

Answer B is incorrect. Number needed to treat, which is the inverse of the absolute risk reduction, cannot be calculated using a case-control study without additional data about the underlying population.

Answer D is incorrect. Prevalence cannot be calculated using a case-control study because it is a property of the underlying population.

Answer E is incorrect. The relative risk, or the risk of developing the disease in those exposed versus those not exposed to a risk factor, cannot be calculated in case-control studies. Because the outcome has occurred with a case-control study, one cannot measure the risk for developing the outcome directly because the prevalence of a risk factor in the underlying population is not known. However, when the incidence of the disease in the underlying population is low, the odds ratio approximates the relative risk.

7. **The correct answer is B.** The patient described in this vignette has a classical presentation of Kawasaki's disease. For a diagnosis of Kawasaki's disease, a patient must have fever for at least 5 days in addition to at least four of the following criteria: bilateral nonexudative conjunctivitis, mucosa changes of the oropharynx, changes of the peripheral extremities such as edema and/or erythema of the hands or feet, rash, and cervical lymphadenopathy (unilateral with at least one node > 1.5 cm). Patients with Kawasaki's disease are treated with intravenous immunoglobulin and aspirin. Before discharge, all patients with Kawasaki's disease should undergo an echocardiogram to examine for the presence of coronary artery aneurysms, a complication affecting up to 40% of untreated patients.

Answer A is incorrect. Although patients with Kawasaki's disease may develop coronary artery aneurysms, pericarditis, myocarditis, or valvular regurgitation, they have not been shown to be at increased risk for the development of any form of cardiomyopathy.

Answer C is incorrect. Aseptic meningitis can be associated with Kawasaki's disease, but encephalitis is not.

Answer D is incorrect. Epidermal necrolysis is a feature of toxic epidermal necrolysis, which is related to Stevens-Johnson syndrome, where a skin rash results from an adverse drug reaction and progresses to skin sloughing. By definition, this involves the mucous membranes. Although Kawasaki's disease also involves the oral mucosa and can be associated with peeling of the fingertips, there is no skin sloughing.

Answer E is incorrect. Although mucous membrane involvement may be severe in patients with Kawasaki's disease, the injected pharynx and strawberry tongue are not linked to an infectious etiology; therefore, patients are not at increased risk for retropharyngeal abscess development.

Answer F is incorrect. Kawasaki's disease represents a multisystem acute vasculitis with potential risk of developing cardiac complications. However, there is no evidence that children with Kawasaki's disease are at an increased risk of stroke or other neurologic complications.

8. **The correct answer is A.** Alzheimer's disease is manifested by a progressive dementia, with memory loss, general cognitive dysfunction, and functional impairments. Statistically, it is the most common cause of dementia. Ten percent of persons over age 70 and 20–40% of individuals over age 85 years have clinically identifiable memory loss. While a head CT can be unremarkable in patients with Alzheimer's disease (as evidenced by this patient's normal CT scan of the head), atrophy can also be seen, especially in the hippocampus. In the image, large arrow points to gray matter in right basal ganglia, small black arrows point to white matter, white arrows point to cerebrospinal fluid, and arrowheads point to the skull.

Answer B is incorrect. Creutzfeldt-Jakob disease is associated with a rapidly progressive dementia with death within a year of onset. There can be other associated neurologic findings such as motor deficits and seizures. These deficits are believed to be caused by prions.

Answer C is incorrect. Delirium has a more acute onset, of days to weeks, not months to years. Patients generally have a more clouded sensorium, with fluctuations in level of consciousness rather than deficits in cognition.

Answer D is incorrect. Patients with depression are more likely to present with more memory loss than the general cognitive deficits seen with dementia. Affect changes are more prominent, as is more psychomotor slowing, while in dementia the intent to perform tasks is present but the cognitive ability is not, which can lead to frustration in these patients, as opposed to the lack of initiative noticed with depression. Depressed patients are aware of their symptoms and tend to present by themselves, while in dementia they are brought to a physician more commonly by a family member. This is also called pseudodementia.

Answer E is incorrect. Although patients with normal pressure hydrocephalus present with cognitive impairment, it is usually accompanied by gait disturbances and urinary incontinence. Further, a CT scan of the head would show dilated ventricles.

9. **The correct answer is E.** This patient has a classic presentation of *Pneumocystis jiroveci* (formerly *carinii*) pneumonia, characterized by low-grade fever, progressive dyspnea, hypoxia, increased arterial-alveolar gradient, and x-ray of the chest with diffuse bilateral infiltrates. First-line therapy is trimethoprim-sulfamethoxazole. If the patient's partial arterial oxygen pressure is < 70 mm Hg, oral prednisone should be added. The other regimens would not be effective against *P. jiroveci* pneumonia.

Answer A is incorrect. Ampicillin + gentamicin is a possible treatment choice for enterococcal septicemia, depending on sensitivity, which would not present with cough, but rather with fever and low blood pressure.

Answer B is incorrect. Intravenous clindamycin has been used in combination with primaquine for treatment of *Pneumocystis jiroveci* pneumonia, but it is not the first-line therapy.

Answer C is incorrect. Isoniazid + pyrazinamide + rifampin + ethambutol is a possible regimen for treatment of *Mycobacterium tuberculosis*, which can also present with a fever and nonproductive cough. However, the most common abnormality on x-ray of the chest is hilar adenopathy.

Answer D is incorrect. A third-generation cephalosporin + doxycycline is a possible treatment for non–*Pneumocystis jiroveci* community-acquired pneumonia, which would most likely present with a productive cough and lobar opacity on x-ray of the chest.

10. **The correct answer is A.** Patients who present after a high-speed motor vehicle crash or rapid deceleration injury must be considered for aortic disruption. The diagnosis of aortic disruption is supported in this case by findings on the x-ray of the chest, including rib fractures, which are often seen along with aortic disruption. Aortography is the gold standard for diagnosis of aortic disruption and is used to confirm a suspected diagnosis. In experienced hands, a sensitivity of 67–100% and a specificity of 98–100% have been achieved using aortography to diagnose an aortic disruption. Although less invasive imaging techniques are currently being studied (including CT scan and transesophageal echocardiography), angiography remains the most reliable means of diagnosis.

Answer B is incorrect. MRI is not indicated for the diagnosis of aortic disruption because of the lengthy time involved in acquiring the image, as well as its limitations in patients with pacemakers and other metallic implants.

Answer C is incorrect. Transthoracic echocardiography (TTE) is a noninvasive method for evaluating cardiac anatomy and function. This imaging modality is limited, however, because thoracic structures such as ribs and lungs do not allow for full evaluation of cardiac anatomy and the aorta. Due to its limitations, TTE would not be the best test to work up a diagnosis of aortic disruption.

Answer D is incorrect. Upper endoscopy is useful for visualizing the upper gastrointestinal (GI) tract; however, it has no utility in the diagnosis of an aortic disruption. This patient shows no clinical signs of acute upper GI injury (i.e., upper GI bleeding and/or mediastinal emphysema) and thus does not require endoscopy.

Answer E is incorrect. A ventilation-perfusion scan would be helpful in the diagnosis of a pulmonary embolism, but it has no utility in diagnosing an aortic disruption. This patient shows no clinical signs of pulmonary embolism (i.e., hypoxia, dyspnea, tachycardia, and/or tachypnea) and thus does not require a ventilation-perfusion scan.

11. **The correct answer is B.** Paget's disease is a disorder of bone remodeling. It is initiated by a pathologic increase in osteoclastic bone resorption, followed by a compensatory increase in osteoblastic bone production. Serum calcium and phosphate levels are generally normal in Paget's disease; however, elevated alkaline phosphatase levels are a common finding in this disorder.

Answer A is incorrect. Alkaline phosphatase should be elevated, reflecting increased bone formation.

Answer C is incorrect. Hypercalcemia is not seen in Paget's disease. Causes of elevated calcium include parathyroid hormone–secreting adenomas, malignancies such as multiple myeloma and lung cancer, granulomatous disease, and vitamin D intoxication.

Answer D is incorrect. Elevated phosphate levels are not seen in Paget's disease. The most frequent cause of hyperphosphatemia is renal failure.

Answer E is incorrect. Positive rheumatoid factor is not commonly associated with Paget's disease. It is found in patients with rheumatoid arthritis.

12. **The correct answer is A.** Gastroesophageal reflux disease (GERD) is a common disorder that generally becomes evident during the first few months of life, peaking at about 4 months of age; most patients will have resolution of symptoms by 12–24 months of age. Common clinical manifestations of GERD include postprandial regurgitation with signs of esophagitis (irritability, arching, gagging, choking) and resultant failure to thrive. Because most cases of GERD will completely resolve by 24 months of age, management is aimed at conservative therapy with parental reassurance. Small, frequent feedings; thickened feedings; and keeping the infant upright, or elevating the head of the bed after feedings, are often sufficient to provide significant improvements in symptoms.

Answer B is incorrect. Although antacids are a commonly employed antireflux medication, they are not routinely recommended for chronic use because of the common adverse effects of diarrhea and constipation.

Answer C is incorrect. Histamine$_2$-receptor antagonists, such as cimetidine, famotidine, nizatidine, and ranitidine, act to selectively inhibit histamine receptors on the gastric parietal cells, thereby reducing acid secretion. They have a favorable safety profile but are not often employed as first-line therapy in infant gastroesophageal reflux disease. They are usually prescribed after conservative measures such as altering feeding techniques and infant positioning have failed.

Answer D is incorrect. Prokinetic agents, such as metoclopramide, bethanechol, and erythromycin, have varying mechanisms of action, but controlled trials have not shown significant efficacy for treating gastroesophageal reflux disease.

Answer E is incorrect. Proton pump inhibitors include omeprazole, lansoprazole, pantoprazole, rabeprazole, and esomeprazole. They act by blocking the hydrogen-potassium ATPase channels involved in gastric acid secretion. Although effective, they are not generally initiated as first-line therapy in childhood gastroesophageal reflux disease.

13. **The correct answer is A.** Minors requesting treatment for sexually transmitted diseases are entitled to complete confidentiality.

    Answer B is incorrect. The physician must respect the confidentiality rights of all minors, and it would be inappropriate to imply that an exception is being made for this particular patient.

    Answer C is incorrect. Minors have the right to confidential treatment and screening for sexually transmitted diseases. Parental consent is not necessary for minors to receive this treatment.

    Answer D is incorrect. Minors have the right to confidential treatment and screening for sexually transmitted diseases. Parental consent is not necessary for minors to receive this screening.

Answer E is incorrect. Minors requesting treatment for sexually transmitted diseases are entitled to complete confidentiality. Physicians are legally and ethically prohibited from withholding treatment.

14. **The correct answer is D.** This patient is presenting with a clinical scenario and radiologic findings consistent with a paralytic ileus. Clinically, she is taking regular doses of a medication that slows bowel motility (opiates), has constant abdominal pain, is obstipated, has absent bowel sounds, and is not focally tender anywhere with no signs of peritoneal irritation. Radiologically, she has air throughout the colon and small intestine, both of which are distended; this is more consistent with an ileus than a small bowel obstruction.

    Answer A is incorrect. Acute appendicitis can begin with diffuse abdominal pain, but will tend to localize to McBurney's point in the lower right quadrant over 4–6 hours, where focal rebound tenderness can develop. It is also associated with a leukocytosis and fever.

    Answer B is incorrect. In acute cholecystitis, the pain would be more localized in the right upper quadrant (positive Murphy's sign), and after 3 hours to 3 days, can develop rebound and guarding. The pain is often related to food intake. Patients often have a low-grade fever. Also, no distension or air-fluid levels would be present on the abdominal films.

    Answer C is incorrect. Complete bowel obstruction would present with crampy intermittent abdominal pain, increased or high-pitched bowel sounds, and obstipation. The abdominal films would show air-fluid levels proximal to the obstruction and the absence of air distal to the obstruction.

    Answer E is incorrect. Partial bowel obstruction would present with crampy intermittent abdominal pain, increased or high-pitched bowel sounds, and passage of flatus without stool. The abdominal films would also likely not show diffuse intestinal distension with air-fluid levels proximal to the obstruction and some air distal to the obstruction.

15. **The correct answer is A.** The patient has asbestosis, as evidenced by the finding of asbestos bodies on bronchoalveolar lavage and suggested by the x-ray of the chest and symptoms in light of a history of possible exposure. A latency period of 20 years or longer between exposure and symptomatic disease in asbestosis is not uncommon. Asbestosis is one of the pneumoconioses and, as a disease of the interstitium, is an example of restrictive lung disease. The pulmonary function test pattern seen in restrictive disease is for FEV_1 and FVC to both decrease preserving a normal FEV_1:FVC.

Answer B is incorrect. In some instances of obstructive lung disease, the FEV_1 decreases, while FVC remains normal. The resultant ratio of FEV_1:FVC still decreases.

Answer C is incorrect. In lung disease with airflow obstruction, pulmonary function tests can reveal decreased FEV_1 and increased FVC, lowering the FEV_1:FVC.

Answer D is incorrect. This patient has a significant fiber burden, is symptomatic, and has evidence of interstitial disease on x-ray of the chest. It is thus very unlikely that her pulmonary function tests would be normal.

Answer E is incorrect. This pattern is the opposite of what is seen in restrictive lung disease and is not noted in obstructive illness either.

16. **The correct answer is G.** The patient likely suffered a cervical spine injury that resulted in neurogenic shock. This spinal cord injury is associated with a sudden loss of sympathetic input to the smooth muscles in vessels. This loss causes a sudden decrease in peripheral vascular resistance and thus a decrease in blood pressure and bradycardia. Unlike other causes of shock, neurogenic shock is associated with warm, dry extremities.

Answer A is incorrect. Addisonian crisis can occur in a patient with adrenal insufficiency who has had an acute stress or with bilateral adrenal hemorrhage or infarction. Patients often complain of nonspecific symptoms, such as anorexia, nausea, vomiting, abdominal pain, weakness, fatigue, and lethargy. Bradycardia is not expected.

Answer B is incorrect. In anaphylactic shock, peripheral vascular resistance is reduced so there is a reflexive tachycardia in an attempt to maintain adequate perfusion. In this case, you would expect hypotension, respiratory distress, urticaria, flushing, and angioedema.

Answer C is incorrect. Atrial fibrillation is a cause of cardiogenic shock. However, the heart rate is typically fast and irregular. In cardiogenic shock, physical examination will reveal hypotension, cool, clammy skin, jugular venous distention, and rapid, weak, and thready pulses.

Answer D is incorrect. Bacteremia is a cause of septic shock. The patient would present with fever, tachycardia, and leukocytosis.

Answer E is incorrect. Congestive heart failure (CHF) is a cause of cardiogenic shock. Cardiac output is reduced and the heart compensates with tachycardia. In cardiogenic shock, physical examination will reveal hypotension, cool and clammy skin, jugular venous distention, and rapid, weak, and thready pulses. Often in cases of CHF the pulmonary examination will reveal congestion.

Answer F is incorrect. Inadequate fluid repletion would cause hypovolemic shock, and reflexive tachycardia to compensate for loss of volume would be expected. In this case, you would expect to see signs of decreased peripheral perfusion such as decreased capillary refill, weakened peripheral pulses, or cool/clammy/cyanotic extremities.

17. **The correct answer is G.** The patient described has DiGeorge syndrome. The translocation responsible and the signs of the disease can best be remembered with the mnemonic "CATCH 22." The Cardiac anomalies, Abnormal facies, Thymic hypoplasia, Cleft palate, and Hypocalcemia are all consistent with a broad spectrum of conditions associated with 22q11.2 deletions, including DiGeorge syndrome, velocardiofacial syndrome, and conotruncal anomaly face syndrome.

Answer A is incorrect. Williams syndrome is associated with a deletion at 7q11.23 and manifests clinically as a round face with full cheeks and lips, strabismus, supravalvular aortic stenosis and other cardiac malformations, variable degrees of mental retardation, and an extremely friendly personality.

Answer B is incorrect. Mild mental retardation with abnormal facies, sparse hair, multiple cone-shaped epiphyses, and multiple cartilaginous exostoses is characteristic of Langer-Giedion (trichorhinophalangeal, type II) syndrome. This disorder is caused by an 8q24 microdeletion.

Answer C is incorrect. WAGR syndrome is caused by microdeletions of 11p13. The syndrome presents with abnormal facies, hypernephroma (**W**ilms' tumor), **A**niridia, and varying degrees of male **G**enital hypoplasia and mental **R**etardation.

Answer D is incorrect. Microdeletions to 15q11 are responsible for Prader-Willi and Angelman syndromes. Both syndromes are characterized by mental retardation and hypotonia. Prader-Willi syndrome also includes obesity with short stature, small hands and feet, and hypogonadism. Angelman syndrome presents with ataxic movements and seizures, uncontrollable episode of laughter, and midface hypoplasia.

Answer E is incorrect. 17p13 Microdeletions result in Miller-Dieker syndrome, presenting clinically as microcephaly with severe mental retardation, seizures, growth failure, hypoplastic male genitalia, and pachygyria (decreased development of brain cortex gyri and sulci).

Answer F is incorrect. Microdeletions affecting chromosome 20p12 give rise to the Alagille syndrome. This syndrome manifests with skeletal defects, including butterfly vertebrae, bile duct paucity with cholestasis, heart defects (especially pulmonary artery stenosis), and ocular abnormalities.

18. **The correct answer is B.** Given the patient's history of hypertension and hypertrophy on ECG, this is the most likely cause of his diastolic dysfunction. Diastolic dysfunction occurs when there is abnormal relaxation of the left ventricle, which impairs filling and results in elevated left ventricular, left atrial, and pulmonary venous pressures. Causes of diastolic dysfunction include acute ischemia, chronic

hypertension, severe aortic stenosis, infiltrative cardiomyopathy (e.g., amyloid), and hypertrophic cardiomyopathy. Systolic dysfunction referrers to the inability for the ventricle to properly squeeze. This results in a decrease in stroke volume and a compensatory rise in preload in order to maintain end-organ perfusion by advancing further to the right on the Frank-Starling curve.

Answer A is incorrect. It is important to diagnose constrictive pericarditis as a cause of diastolic dysfunction, as this is one of the more treatable etiologies. Other findings point to a hypertrophic cause and moreover, echocardiography would likely reveal a constrictive pericarditis if it existed. Symptoms of constrictive pericarditis include leg edema, abdominal fullness, and pain secondary to hepatic congestion, and these may progress to exertional dyspnea, cough, and orthopnea. Signs include Kussmaul's sign, pericardial knock, and others consistent with right-sided heart failure. Echocardiography would show pericardial thickening.

Answer C is incorrect. Restrictive cardiomyopathy (seen in various infiltrative diseases) is a less common cause of diastolic dysfunction. Again, the evidence of hypertrophy makes this even less likely in this patient.

Answer D is incorrect. The patient's imaging results point to diastolic dysfunction, not systolic dysfunction, due to increased wall thickening and normal ejection fraction.

Answer E is incorrect. The patient's imaging results point to diastolic dysfunction, not systolic dysfunction, due to increased wall thickening and normal ejection fraction.

Answer F is incorrect. The patient's imaging results point to diastolic dysfunction, not systolic dysfunction, due to increased wall thickening and normal ejection fraction.

19. **The correct answer is A.** The infant has developmental dysplasia of the hip. If left untreated, the infant is at risk for persistent dysplasia, osteoarthritis, and avascular necrosis of the femoral head. The appropriate treatment for infants younger than 6 months is a flexion-abduction orthosis known as a Pavlik harness,

which is designed to stabilize the affected hip in a reduced position.

Answer B is incorrect. The affected hip in a patient with developmental dysplasia of the hip must be kept in a flexed, abducted position to maintain reduction. Extension does not engage the femoral head in the acetabulum and will not stabilize the dislocatable hip.

Answer C is incorrect. Once the newborn period is complete (after 6 months of age), closed reduction with application of a spica cast is the treatment of choice.

Answer D is incorrect. This infant presented with a dislocatable hip. Without treatment, this may lead to significant deformity from developmental dysplasia of the hip. The long-term complications of developmental dysplasia of the hip include leg-length discrepancy and osteoarthritis.

Answer E is incorrect. The Pavlik harness is the treatment of choice for a newborn with a dislocated or subluxed hip. Once the child is older (15–24 months old), open reduction is indicated when an attempt at closed reduction has failed.

20. **The correct answer is B.** This man is likely suffering from normal bereavement, which is part of the grieving process. Loss of a loved one can have a serious impact on health status. The symptoms of bereavement, including weight loss, decreased appetite, and decreased sleep, can mimic those of major depression. "Searching behaviors," such as auditory or visual hallucinations, can also be seen. If these symptoms resolve within 8 weeks, they are normal. The proper approach with this patient is to listen, support, reassure, and follow up closely to watch for development of a more serious disorder. A diagnosis of major depression would require persistence of these symptoms, in addition to severe feelings of guilt, helplessness, hopelessness, and/or suicidal ideation.

Answer A is incorrect. Electroconvulsive therapy (ECT) induces seizures in an attempt to treat severe psychoses, such as catatonic schizophrenia, major depression with psychotic features, and refractory obsessive-compulsive disorder. This patient does not fit into any of these categories and would hence not achieve any benefit. The adverse effects of headache and retrograde/anterograde memory loss are additional reasons not to use ECT to treat this patient.

Answer C is incorrect. Olanzapine is an atypical antipsychotic that is used to treat depression with psychotic features, schizophrenia, and other psychotic disorders. Although this patient is experiencing some auditory hallucinations, such symptoms are consistent with "searching behaviors" and are related to the grieving process.

Answer D is incorrect. Zolpidem is a sleep aid with a very low addictive potential. Although it would likely enable this patient to get more sleep, it would not combat his other bereavement symptoms.

Answer E is incorrect. This patient is experiencing a normal part of the grieving process and therefore does not require admission to an inpatient psychiatric facility.

21. **The correct answer is B.** This patient is presenting with precocious puberty, which is generally defined as sexual development at age < 8 years for girls and < 9 years for boys. In central, or true, precocious puberty, there is early activation of the normal hypothalamic-pituitary axis. The majority of these cases occur in girls and are idiopathic; however, certain central nervous system lesions, like hamartomas or other tumors, can cause central precocious puberty. Because the disorder is caused by early activation of the normal signaling pathway, the patients tend to have normal sequential pubertal development. However, many patients do not have adrenarche at presentation because the adrenals are under separate control. Laboratory evaluation will reveal elevated levels of gonadotropin-releasing hormone (GnRH) as well as luteinizing hormone (LH), follicle-stimulating hormone (FSH), and estrogen.

Answer A is incorrect. Adrenal tumors can secrete estrogen and cause early sexual development. However, these patients will have decreased GnRH, LH, and FSH due to negative feedback by estrogen on the hypothalamus and pituitary.

Answer C is incorrect. McCune-Albright syndrome is a cause of gonadotropin-independent precocious puberty. In addition to the dysfunctions caused by autonomous activity of other endocrine glands, early sexual development occurs due to autonomous ovarian function, usually from a dominant ovarian cyst that independently produces estrogen. These patients will have decreased LH, FSH, and GnRH due to negative feedback by estrogen on the hypothalamus and pituitary.

Answer D is incorrect. An ovarian tumor that secretes estrogen is another cause of gonadotropin-independent precocious puberty. These patients will have early sexual development, but GnRH, LH, and FSH will be decreased due to negative feedback of estrogen on the hypothalamus and pituitary.

Answer E is incorrect. Patients with chronic hypothyroidism may experience early sexual development. Because thyroid-stimulating hormone (TSH) and FSH are structurally similar, high levels of TSH in primary hypothyroidism can directly activate the FSH receptor. These patients would likely have other signs of hypothyroidism including weight gain, fatigue, dry skin, constipation, and cold intolerance. In addition, GnRH levels would not be expected to be elevated in hypothyroidism.

22. **The correct answer is C.** Benzodiazepines are sedatives that bind at specific receptors and act to enhance the inhibitory tone of γ-aminobutyric acid receptors in the central nervous system. Some common indications include induction of anesthesia, alcohol withdrawal, insomnia, epilepsy, and generalized anxiety. Patients who have developed benzodiazepine dependency are at risk for potentially fatal complications from withdrawal, including seizures. Benzodiazepine withdrawal should be suspected in any patient taking a drug from this class who suffers a seizure.

Answer A is incorrect. Angiotensin-converting enzyme inhibitors would be a logical choice for treating this patient's hypertension, although this class is known to cause severe withdrawal symptoms or seizures.

Answer B is incorrect. Cocaine is among many common illegal drugs known to cause seizures. However, there is no reason to suspect that this man uses cocaine. Furthermore, withdrawal from cocaine is far less likely to cause seizures than its use or abuse.

Answer D is incorrect. Lithium is known to cause seizures; however, there is no evidence of the patient's taking this substance. Furthermore, withdrawal from lithium is far less likely to cause seizures than their use or abuse.

Answer E is incorrect. Calcium channel blockers would be a logical choice for treating this patient's hypertension, although this class is known to cause severe withdrawal symptoms or seizures.

23. **The correct answer is B.** This patient should undergo colonoscopy as soon as possible. Her history is consistent with hereditary nonpolyposis colorectal cancer (HNPCC), the most common hereditary cause of colon cancer. HNPCC is inherited in an autosomal dominant fashion, and patients with this syndrome tend to develop colon cancer at an average age of 44 years. This woman meets the Amsterdam II criteria for HNPCC which includes the following: (1) Three or more relatives with HNPCC-associated cancer (including cancer of the colon, endometrium, small bowel, kidney, and ureter), two of whom are first-degree relatives, (2) At least two successive generations affected, and (3) At least one relative diagnosed before 50 years of age. Patients with a positive family history of HNPCC should undergo colonoscopy every 1–2 years after age 25 (or when 10 years younger than the youngest affected relative), and every year after age 40. This patient is already 36 years old, and should undergo immediate colonoscopy.

Answer A is incorrect. Colonoscopy in a patient with a positive family history for colon cancer should begin before 50 years of age.

Answer C is incorrect. A CT scan of the abdomen is useful in assessing patients with colon cancer that has metastasized to lymph nodes and the liver, as well as in diagnosing recurrence of resected or metastatic colon cancer. A scan at this time would not be the appropriate next step, and would not negate the need for a colonoscopy.

Answer D is incorrect. A double-contrast barium enema (DCBE) can be used to examine the entire rectum and colon and carries less risk than colonoscopy. However, the sensitivity of DCBEs for large polyps and cancers is less than that of colonoscopy, and the procedure does not permit removal of polyps or biopsy of cancers—thus necessitating a follow-up colonoscopy if any abnormalities are found. A DCBE is also more likely than colonoscopy to identify artifacts and other findings (such as stool) as polyps. Although useful in patients with an average risk of developing colorectal cancer, a DCBE would not be appropriate in this high-risk patient.

Answer E is incorrect. While digital rectal examinations (DREs) are useful for detecting rectal or prostate cancer, they are clearly not sufficient in screening for colon cancer, though there is a role for fecal occult blood testing performed three times annually. Flexible sigmoidoscopy can detect lesions 60 cm from the anus, but will not detect lesions in the proximal colon. Yearly DREs and flexible sigmoidoscopy every 2–3 years would not be sufficient in this high-risk patient.

24. **The correct answer is C.** This woman is suffering from a heroin overdose. Heroin is a highly addictive member of the opioid family, which includes morphine and codeine. These drugs activate opioid receptors found in both the central nervous system (CNS) and the gastrointestinal (GI) system. There are three major opioid receptor subtypes: μ (mu), κ (kappa), and δ (delta). Activation of μ receptors in the CNS and GI tract result in heroin's euphoric effects as well as to its adverse effects—constipation (due to decreased bowel motility), sedation, pupillary constriction, and decreased respiration.

Answer A is incorrect. Naloxone is an opioid antagonist that binds strongly to opioid receptors. It acts quickly to reverse the symptoms of opiate overdose, and most patients recover consciousness with intravenous administration. Patients must be closely monitored when naloxone is administered, however, as its half-life is shorter than that of most recreational opiates, and patients can reexperience respiratory compromise once its effects wear off. Lorazepam has no use in the setting of heroin intoxication.

Answer B is incorrect. Patients who overdose on heroin usually present with respiratory compromise and may stop breathing altogether. For this reason, patients who present to the ED with the hallmarks of an opioid overdose—such as pinpoint pupils, needle-track marks, and respiratory compromise—should be closely monitored and an emergency airway secured if necessary. Myocardial infarction due to illicit drug use is usually associated with cocaine overdose.

Answer D is incorrect. Tolerance to the euphoria, sedation, and decreased respiration caused by opiates develops rapidly. Tolerance to the constipation opiates induce is slower to develop.

Answer E is incorrect. Patients in heroin withdrawal have symptoms that are very intense and unpleasant, but such symptoms are not life threatening.

25. **The correct answer is B.** Atopic dermatitis (eczema) typically appears before the age of 7 years and manifests as itchy, often dry, scaling erythematous plaques with excoriations. In infants and very young children, the extensor surfaces, posterior scalp, and face are typically involved, while the diaper region is spared. In older children and adults the flexural areas (though not the groin) are most commonly involved. Chronic atopic dermatitis manifests with thickened skin and excoriated papules.

Answer A is incorrect. The history mentions a possible allergen exposure (detergent), but this is extremely unusual. Furthermore, a dermatitis resulting from detergent exposure would be expected to predominantly manifest in areas in contact with clothing; the initial involvement of the face in this case would be difficult to associate with detergent.

Answer C is incorrect. Pityriasis rosea is typically seen in older children and adults. A "herald patch" is followed by erythematous, oval, scaly papules on the trunk and proximal extremities that spread from the neck down. Involvement of the face is unusual.

Answer D is incorrect. Lesions typical of chronic plaque psoriasis are well-demarcated erythematous papules and plaques with silvery scales with variable pruritus. While lesions are usually found on extensor surfaces (elbows and knees), as in this case, the age of onset is typically much later in childhood. Nail findings (the "oil drop sign," local brownish discoloration of the nail, or pitting) may also be seen in psoriasis, but are not associated with atopic dermatitis.

Answer E is incorrect. Seborrheic dermatitis is an erythematous, scaling rash associated with mild pruritus. In contrast to atopic dermatitis, seborrheic dermatitis is most common in areas rich in sebaceous glands (forehead, scalp, nasolabial folds, nasal bridge, chest, axilla, and groin), and is not usually associated with dry skin.

26. **The correct answer is B.** Epiglottitis is a rapidly progressive infection of the supraglottic structures that can lead to complete airway obstruction. Patients typically present with rapid-onset fever with dysphagia, drooling, muffled voice, inspiratory retractions, cyanosis, and soft stridor. The presentation described is referred to as the "sniffing" position with hyperextension of the neck and protrusion of the chin. The most common cause of this condition was *Haemophilus influenzae* type B before immunizations with the Hib vaccine became available. The primary pathogens of epiglottitis now include *Streptococcus* species, nontypable *H. influenzae*, and viral pathogens.

Answer A is incorrect. The Diphtheria-tetanus-pertussis (DTaP) vaccination is responsible for reducing the occurrence of diphtheria, tetanus, and pertussis. It has not been shown to play a role in reducing the incidence of epiglottitis, since the implicated pathogens are different from those targeted by the DTaP vaccine.

Answer C is incorrect. Measles-mumps-rubella vaccination has significantly reduced the occurrence of measles, mumps, and rubella. However, these viral antigens have not been shown to be implicated in the etiology of epiglottitis.

Answer D is incorrect. The vaccine for pneumococcal species has aided in reducing the incidence of ear infections, meningitis, and pneumonia.

Answer E is incorrect. The introduction of the varicella vaccine has greatly reduced the incidence of chickenpox, but has not impacted the occurrence of epiglottitis.

27. **The correct answer is C.** The patient presented to the ED with an episode of diverticulitis. A diverticulum is a herniation of the colonic mucosa that occurs as a result of increased pressure in the colon. Diverticula are often seen in the sigmoid colon because this area of the colon is subjected to the greatest amount of intraluminal pressure because of its narrow radius (Laplace's law: pressure = wall tension/radius). Diverticulitis is infection of a diverticulum that may result in an abscess or pericolic infection and may present with abdominal pain, peritoneal signs, leukocytosis, fever, chills, nausea, vomiting, change in bowel habits, and/or dysuria. It has been shown that patients who consume low-fiber diets or have chronic constipation may be at increased risk for developing diverticula.

Answer A is incorrect. Increased intraluminal colonic pressure leads to the development of diverticula formation. Although it is a good idea to treat hypertension for the sake of preventing further medical complications, treating hypertension has no impact on preventing diverticula formation.

Answer B is incorrect. There have not been any conclusive studies that show a relationship between exercise and diverticula formation. One study indicated that physical activity may reduce diverticulosis; however, this was not statistically confirmed.

Answer D is incorrect. There have not been any conclusive studies that show a relationship between caffeine and diverticula formation.

Answer E is incorrect. Although smoking cessation should be encouraged in all populations because of the health risks that smoking presents, this would not have had any impact on reducing the likelihood of diverticula formation.

28. **The correct answer is C.** Osteoarthritis (OA) is a common disorder in which articular cartilage is damaged as a result of multiple factors including aging, mechanical trauma, genetics, and biochemistry. Loss of articular cartilage causes narrowing of the joint spaces. Secondary bone remodeling leads to osteophyte development. Pain due to OA is described as dull and aching, which gets worse with activity and may resolve with rest, but as the disease progresses, pain may also be present at rest. Patients may also complain of stiffness and limited mobility of the affected joints. Multiple joints are typically involved, with the hands being a common site of disease. In the hand, the proximal and distal interphalangeal joints are classically affected, while the metacarpophalangeal joints are spared. Enlargement of the distal interphalangeal and proximal interphalangeal joints results in Heberden's and Bouchard's nodes, respectively.

Answer A is incorrect. Calcium pyrophosphate deposition disease (CPPD), a spectrum of disease that includes the clinical entity known as "pseudogout," may resemble osteoarthritis, presenting as progressive joint degeneration. Physical examination findings as well as radiographs may resemble osteoarthritis. However, CPPD most commonly affects the knees.

Answer B is incorrect. Acute gouty arthritis is typically monarticular, and like acute infectious arthritis, presents with redness, swelling, and warmth of the affected joint. Patients with long-standing gout can develop chronic tophaceous gout, in which urate crystals deposit in connective tissue. On x-ray films, chronic tophaceous gout appears as extensive soft tissue swelling with calcifications adjacent to joints, and extensive erosion of the bones.

Answer D is incorrect. Psoriatic arthritis is a disorder associated with psoriasis. It is an inflammatory arthritis, so the pattern of pain resembles that of rheumatoid arthritis, not osteoarthritis. Patients complain of pain and stiffness that is worst in the morning, often in the distal interphalangeal (DIP) joints. Although this patient has DIP joint involvement, by definition, patients with psoriatic arthritis must also have psoriasis. Most patients have evidence of psoriatic skin and/or nail disease prior to presenting with arthritis.

Answer E is incorrect. Rheumatoid arthritis (RA) in the hands typically affects the metacarpophalangeal and proximal interphalangeal joints, with sparing of the distal interphalangeal joints and absence of Heberden's nodes. Patients with RA have pain and stiffness in the hands that is most severe in the morning and after a long period of inactivity. On examination, patients with RA will typically have swollen joints that are warm, red, and tender. Radiographs in RA show erosion of the bone, as opposed to the joint space narrowing, sclerosis, and osteophytes seen in osteoarthritis.

29. **The correct answer is E.** External cephalic version is a series of maneuvers performed via maternal abdomen to convert from breech to cephalic presentation. External cephalic version has been shown to significantly reduce the attendant risks of both vaginal breech delivery and cesarean section. External cephalic version cannot be performed once labor is initiated or the fetus is engaged in the pelvis, without adequate amniotic fluid, or when fetal heart tracings are nonreassuring.

Answer A is incorrect. Cesarean delivery of fetuses in breech presentation has been found in several studies to reduce the rate of perinatal morbidity and mortality, and is associated with higher Apgar scores after delivery. Therefore, planned cesarean delivery of fetuses in persistent breech presentation is recommended.

Answer B is incorrect. Cesarean delivery is the preferred method of delivery of fetuses with persistent breech presentation. However, breech presentation is not an indication for an emergent delivery. Operative delivery may take place on a planned basis to eliminate the risks associated with emergent surgery.

Answer C is incorrect. Cesarean delivery of fetuses in breech presentation has been found in several studies to reduce the rate of perinatal morbidity and mortality, and is associated with higher Apgar scores after delivery. Therefore, planned cesarean delivery of fetuses in persistent breech presentation is recommended.

Answer D is incorrect. External cephalic version followed by vaginal delivery or planned cesarean delivery are the preferred methods of delivering breech presentation infants. Vaginal delivery of a child in breech position is not recommended, and external cephalic version cannot be attempted once labor has begun. Thus, it is inadvisable to induce labor with a fetus in breech presentation.

30. **The correct answer is A.** The patient described has Bruton's (X-linked) agammaglobulinemia. Patients are typically well until 6–9 months of age, at which point maternal IgG antibodies become inactive. Then patients acquire infections with extracellular pyogenic organisms, including *Streptococcus pneumoniae* and *Haemophilus influenzae*, and present with pneumonia, otitis media, and sinusitis. Low levels of IgG, IgA, IgM, and IgE are found on laboratory evaluation, and flow cytometry demonstrates the absence of B lymphocytes. Because the gene that is mutated in this disease, Bruton's tyrosine kinase, is on the X chromosome, the disease is overwhelmingly more common in male patients. B-lymphocyte development can be arrested by mutations in at least four other genes that are inherited in an autosomal recessive manner, resulting in the same clinical phenotype of agammaglobulinemia. Inheritance of two mutant alleles of these genes, however, is extraordinarily rare, and the vast majority of agammaglobulinemic patients has the X-linked variety.

Answer B is incorrect. Common variable immunodeficiency is a syndrome characterized by hypogammaglobulinemia and impaired specific antibody production, with circulating B lymphocytes.

Answer C is incorrect. DiGeorge's syndrome, also know as velocardiofacial syndrome, is largely a disorder of T lymphocytes that results from inappropriate thymic development. In > 80% of cases, it is caused by a microdeletion of chromosome 22. It often presents with hypocalcemia in the first few days of life that can be severe enough to result in tetany or seizures if untreated.

Answer D is incorrect. IgA deficiency is the most common primary immunodeficiency and can be asymptomatic or present with recurrent upper respiratory infections. However, the other immunoglobulins would be found at normal levels.

Answer E is incorrect. Severe combined immunodeficiency is a life-threatening condition affecting T, and in many cases B, lymphocytes. Patients present commonly with failure to thrive, diarrhea, severe bacterial infections, opportunistic infections, and chronic candidiasis. The absolute lymphocyte count is, by definition, decreased.

31. **The correct answer is A.** This study is a case-control study, where those who failed extubation are the cases (disease present) and those who were successfully extubated are the controls (disease not present). Valid matching is facilitated in this case by a well-defined population (intubated ICU patients) from which to draw both cases and controls.

Answer B is incorrect. Clinical trials are prospective studies that examine random use of an intervention and its effect on outcome.

Answer C is incorrect. Correlation studies are used to compare disease frequencies between entire populations (as opposed to individuals).

Answer D is incorrect. Prospective cohort studies take a sample group (a cohort) with a risk factor and match them to a control without the risk factor. The groups are then studied over time to assess development of disease.

Answer E is incorrect. Retrospective cohort studies assemble a cohort based on retrospective identification of risk factors, and then compare current outcome data with that of a matched control group.

32. **The correct answer is E.** Cardiac tamponade classically presents with Beck's triad: hypotension, muffled heart sounds, and jugular venous distention. Cardiac tamponade results from rapid engorgement of the pericardial space with blood, and often results from penetrating trauma to a ventricle or aortic dissection.

Answer A is incorrect. In addition to Beck's triad, cardiac tamponade can present with a narrowed pulse pressure. A bounding pulse is usually associated with aortic insufficiency.

Answer B is incorrect. In cardiac tamponade, impaired diastolic filling leads to a drop in stroke volume, resulting in hypotension. The body attempts to respond by increasing heart rate; thus, tamponade usually presents with tachycardia, not bradycardia.

Answer C is incorrect. Rupture of a papillary muscle may result in mitral regurgitation, which can present with a new-onset holosystolic murmur. This is a common presentation of acute myocardial infarction, not tamponade.

Answer D is incorrect. Cardiac tamponade usually presents with hypotension, not hypertension.

33. **The correct answer is A.** Heart palpitations, breathlessness, and fatigue (the latter often secondary to insomnia) are all signs of hyperthyroidism. This patient's weight loss is also consistent with a hypermetabolic state. Amiodarone has been known to cause both hyper- and hypothyroidism in previously euthyroid individuals. Thyroid hormone levels should be assessed before any medication adjustments are attempted.

Answer B is incorrect. Although providing reassurance is often helpful, this patient's presentation requires further investigation. Instructing her to return in 6 months would not be appropriate.

Answer C is incorrect. Although this patient's symptoms may be linked to an anxiety disorder, there is no strong evidence to suggest this type of disorder to be the cause.

Answer D is incorrect. Captopril is generally well tolerated—a persistent, dry cough is the most common adverse effect—and is unlikely to be contributing to the patient's complaints.

Answer E is incorrect. Substitution of procainamide for amiodarone would not be appropriate before initial laboratory tests have been performed.

34. **The correct answer is E.** The patient appears to be in the acute seroconversion stage of HIV infection. During this stage, the HIV viral load will peak and the CD4+ count will fall before both establish a set point, usually within the first 3–4 months of infection. Treatment is only recommended for this stage of infection if the CD4+ count is < 200/mm^3 or if the patient is experiencing symptoms of "acute viral syndrome," characterized by flulike symptoms, including fever, chills, night sweats, and lymphadenopathy.

Answer A is incorrect. Patients often will experience a transient increase in viral load and dip in CD4+ counts at the time of seroconversion. In the majority of patients, the viral load will fall to a set point, and the CD4+ count will rebound before falling again over several years as the disease progresses.

Answer B is incorrect. The patient's CD4+ count is not yet in the range that requires prophylaxis for *Pneumocystis jiroveci* pneumonia. *P. jiroveci* pneumonia prophylaxis starts when CD4+ counts dip below 200/mm^3. It is expected that his CD4+ count will rebound to near-normal levels, but rechecking within a month is prudent, and if necessary, prophylaxis can be started at that time.

Answer C is incorrect. There are no reported cases of patients "clearing" HIV infection. The HIV viral load shows that the patient has ongoing viral replication.

Answer D is incorrect. The patient's HIV viral load and decreased CD4+ count shows that the patient has ongoing HIV viral replication, and that the test was not falsely positive.

35. **The correct answer is C.** Osler-Weber-Rendu syndrome, also known as hereditary hemorrhagic telangiectasia, is an autosomal dominant condition in which vascular lesions (telangiectasias, arteriovenous malformations, and aneurysms) are found throughout the body, particularly in the lungs, brain, and gastrointestinal (GI) tract. This patient has lesions on his oral mucosa as shown and pale conjunctivae suggesting anemia. The most likely explanation for his symptoms is that he has mucosal telangiectasias in his GI tract that have begun to bleed and are making him anemic.

Answer A is incorrect. Although stressful life events such as the recent death of a loved one can often lead to depression, this patient is complaining of isolated decreased exercise tolerance. The fact that he feels fine and is eating and sleeping well point away from depression and toward a physiologic cause such as anemia.

Answer B is incorrect. Although chronic obstructive pulmonary disease can cause easy fatigue and dyspnea on exertion, this patient has no prior history, and the physical examination findings are more suggestive of anemia.

Answer D is incorrect. Although this patient may have intracranial arteriovenous malformations and/or aneurysms, they are unlikely to be responsible for her chronic fatigue and shortness of breath.

Answer E is incorrect. Although coronary artery disease can cause easy fatigue and dyspnea on exertion, this patient has no prior history, and the physical examination findings are more suggestive of anemia.

36. **The correct answer is D.** This case, in combination with the abdominal film (demonstrating the classic "double-bubble" sign), is characteristic for duodenal atresia. The condition is believed to be caused by failure to recanalize the intestinal lumen after the solid phase of intestinal development during gestation. Most patients present with bilious vomiting within the first day of life and are noted to have nondistended abdomens. Half of patients with duodenal atresia are born prematurely, often following pregnancies complicated by polyhydramnios. Initial treatment of patients with duodenal atresia is aimed at reducing gastric pressure by placement of a nasogastric or orogastric tube, in addition to providing intravenous fluid replacement.

Answer A is incorrect. Congenital heart disease is present in approximately 10% of patients with duodenal atresia. As a result of this high incidence of heart disease, echocardiograms should be performed on patients with duodenal atresia to rule out associated cardiac anomalies. Cardiac studies should be undertaken after fluid replacement and nasogastric decompression in cases of hemodynamically stable patients.

Answer B is incorrect. Gastrostomy tube placement is helpful for draining the stomach and providing protection of the airway. Such management is undertaken after the patient is stabilized and has undergone fluid replacement and gastric decompression.

Answer C is incorrect. In hemodynamically stable patients, surgical intervention is not initially required. The usual surgical repair for duodenal atresia is duodenoduodenostomy, but such repair is performed after nasogastric tube placement and intravenous fluid replacement.

Answer E is incorrect. Radiologic studies of the spine and chest should be performed to evaluate for associated anomalies, but such evaluations are postponed until after initial fluid replacement and gastric decompression.

37. **The correct answer is D.** This is a zone II penetrating neck injury. Zone II is defined as the area between the angle of the mandible and the cricoid cartilage. It contains the internal and external carotid arteries, jugular veins, pharynx, larynx, esophagus, recurrent laryngeal nerve, spinal cord, trachea, esophagus, thoracic duct, and thymus. Surgical exploration is indicated if the platysma is penetrated, if there is subcutaneous air, or if there is an expanding hematoma. Of note, the threshold for intubation should be very low in these patients.

Answer A is incorrect. Arteriography is useful as the initial test for zone I (between the clavicle/suprasternal notch and the cricoid cartilage) and zone III (between the angle of the mandible and the base of the skull) injuries because the clinical examination is less reliable due to the deeper location of the vascular structures.

Answer B is incorrect. Esophagoscopy is useful for zone I and III injuries if there is clinical evidence for esophageal or pharyngeal injury. Signs include dysphagia, bloody saliva, sucking neck wound, blood nasogastric aspirate, crepitus, and bleeding from the mouth. It is important to keep in mind that there is a risk of esophageal perforation during esophagoscopy, so the procedure should only be performed when necessary.

Answer C is incorrect. A CT of the neck should not delay surgical exploration. It is particularly useful in diagnosing laryngeal injury, but it does not replace esophagoscopy if esophageal injury is suspected.

Answer E is incorrect. Tracheobronchoscopy is useful for zone I and III injuries if there is suspicion of larynx or tracheal injury. Signs include hoarseness, stridor, respiratory distress, subcutaneous emphysema, drooling, and hemoptysis. Although this patient's crepitus is suggestive of injury to the aerodigestive tract, surgical exploration is needed because of the large number of vulnerable structures in zone II.

38. **The correct answer is D.** Elevated urine 5-hydroxyindoleacetic acid (a breakdown product of serotonin) levels would confirm the diagnosis of carcinoid syndrome, in this case secondary to a small bowel carcinoid tumor with metastases to the liver. This syndrome can result from carcinoid tumors producing excess serotonin at sites without venous drainage into the portal system (e.g., rectal or bronchial) or from carcinoid metastases to the liver. It manifests as episodic watery diarrhea, cutaneous flushing, vasomotor instability, wheezing and bronchial spasm, and right-sided valvular lesions which can cause right-sided heart failure (peripheral edema). These tumors precipitate a vigorous desmoplastic reaction in the mesentery resulting in small bowel obstruction (the most common presentation of a carcinoid tumor).

Answer A is incorrect. Serum antigliadin antibodies are present in the malabsorption syndrome called celiac disease.

Answer B is incorrect. Serum cortisol levels play no role in the diagnosis of carcinoid tumors, but are used in the diagnosis of Cushing's syndrome.

Answer C is incorrect. Serum gastrin levels are used in the diagnosis of the Zollinger-Ellison syndrome.

Answer E is incorrect. Urine vanillylmandelic acid levels play no role in the diagnosis of carcinoid tumors, but can confirm the elevation of catecholamine levels when a pheochromocytoma is present.

39. **The correct answer is A.** This family has familial hypocalciuric hypercalcemia (FHH), an autosomal dominant inherited disorder causing hypercalcemia, hypocalciuria, and mild hypermagnesemia. Although heterozygotes have a benign hypercalcemia, homozygotes can have severe neonatal hypercalcemia. The disorder is due to inappropriate sensing of serum calcium by receptors in the parathyroid gland and the kidney. This leads to increased secretion of parathyroid hormone (PTH) and increased renal tubular reabsorption of calcium, despite high serum levels. FHH can be differentiated from primary hyperparathyroidism by the following: PTH may be elevated in FHH, but not to the same degree as in patients with primary hyperparathyroidism; the presence of hypercalcemia in multiple family members, especially young children; > 99% of filtered calcium is reabsorbed in FHH, while < 99% is reabsorbed in primary hyperparathyroidism; and absence of abnormal imaging of the parathyroid gland.

Answer B is incorrect. Jansen's disease is another inherited disorder of hypercalcemia. It is due to excessive activity of the parathyroid hormone (PTH) receptor in target tissues. Serum PTH levels will be very low. Patients typically have extensive bone disorders such as short-limbed dwarfism and cystic bone disease. Bone disease is rare in familial hypocalciuric hypercalcemia.

Answer C is incorrect. In most patients with primary hyperparathyroidism, parathyroid hormone (PTH) levels would be expected to be much higher than the mild elevation seen in this patient, although approximately 10% of patients with primary hyperparathyroidism can have normal PTH levels. Primary hyperparathyroidism is rarely genetic (unless inherited as part of a multiple endocrine neoplasia syndrome), so the finding of hypercalcemia in multiple family members, especially in this patient's 10-year-old son, makes this diagnosis less likely.

Answer D is incorrect. Multiple endocrine neoplasia type I is an autosomal dominant disorder causing primary hyperparathyroidism, pituitary tumors, and pancreatic tumors. Primary hyperparathyroidism would usually be expected to have more significantly elevated parathyroid hormone. The absence of malignancy in the patient or the family makes this diagnosis less likely.

Answer E is incorrect. Multiple endocrine neoplasia type IIB consists of medullary thyroid cancer, pheochromocytoma, and mucosal neuromas. Hyperparathyroidism and disorders of calcium homeostasis are not components of this syndrome.

40. **The correct answer is D.** Bundle-branch block occurs when there is abnormal conduction through one of the conductive branches that supplies the left or right ventricle. These blocks occur when the heart is injured, such as during myocardial infarctions. Signs of acute myocardial infarction necessitate immediate revascularization, and include new left bundle-branch block or ST elevations. These signs would distinguish unstable angina (which may have ST depression) from a current myocardial infarction.

Answer A is incorrect. Delta waves are associated with Wolff-Parkinson-White syndrome and are seen on ECG as an initial slowed upstroke of the QRS complex, resulting in its widening. The delta wave occurs because an accessory pathway exists in the heart, exciting the ventricles directly from the atria, as opposed to the normal condition of having the impulse travel solely through the atrioventricular (AV) node. Because this conduction pathway does not have the normal delay at the AV node, the ventricles are excited earlier, resulting in a delta wave. Treatments for Wolff-Parkinson-White syndrome include antiarrhythmics or ablation of the accessory pathway, depending on the patient's symptoms.

Answer B is incorrect. Flipped T waves are nonspecific and are not an indication to bring a patient to the revascularization laboratory unless they occur with other signs that point to current myocardial infarction.

Answer C is incorrect. Myocardial infarction would not cause a low-voltage ECG. Low-voltage ECGs imply that the heart is far from the electrodes and may be seen in conditions like emphysema, pericarditis, and in obese patients.

Answer E is incorrect. ST depressions are consistent with unstable angina or non–ST wave elevation myocardial infarction and it would be left to the discretion of the treating physician to assess the patient's level of risk and to pursue an aggressive/invasive or conservative course.

Questions 41 and 42

41. **The correct answer is F.** IgA nephropathy is the most common cause of glomerulonephritis in adults. Recurrent hematuria with or without flank pain is a common presentation. Occasionally, however, IgA nephropathy can present as acute renal failure with headache, edema, and decreased urine output, in addition to hematuria and flank pain. An immune complex glomerulonephritis, IgA nephropathy, can be differentiated from other immune-mediated nephritides (lupus and postinfectious nephritis) by normal complement levels. Final diagnosis of IgA nephropathy is made by renal biopsy, which shows mesangial IgA deposits on immunofluorescence.

42. **The correct answer is A.** Also known as hereditary nephritis, Alport's syndrome is an X-linked syndrome consisting of progressive glomerular disease (nephritis), sensorineural hearing loss, and ocular findings (anterior lenticonus). It manifests itself in childhood (when detected) as asymptomatic microhematuria and, in most cases progresses to renal failure by 35 years of age. This patient manifests the first overt signs of renal failure with elevated creatinine and hypertension.

Answer B is incorrect. Amyloidosis is a disorder caused by extracellular deposition of insoluble abnormal fibrils that injure tissue. Roughly two dozen different unrelated proteins are known to form amyloid fibrils in vivo. When amyloidosis affects the kidney, bright green fluorescence is observed under polarized light after Congo red staining.

Answer C is incorrect. Cryoglobulins are immunoglobulins that undergo reversible precipitation at low temperatures. Cryoglobulinemia may result in systemic inflammation via cryoglobulin-containing immune complexes.

When the kidney is involved, cryoglobulins are seen in the lumen.

Answer D is incorrect. Focal segmental glomerulosclerosis (FSGS) is the second most common cause of nephrotic syndrome in children. A more aggressive form of FSGS is associated with HIV infection. Light microscopy typically reveals segmental sclerosis or hyalinosis, and electron microscopy can show podocyte effacement. The microscopic findings, however, are inconsistent with this patient's biopsy results.

Answer E is incorrect. Goodpasture's syndrome is a disease characterized by autoantibodies directed against an antigen intrinsic to the glomerular basement membrane, resulting in acute glomerulonephritis and crescent formation. Classically, it may also present with pulmonary hemorrhage and hemoptysis. Goodpasture's syndrome has a predilection for men in their mid-20s. Plasma exchange and pulsed steroids are the treatment of choice. Despite treatment, it may progress to end-stage renal disease.

Answer G is incorrect. Lupus nephritis is a common complication of systemic lupus erythematous (SLE), affecting 40–85% of patients. In fact, the severity of renal disease often determines the overall prognosis for SLE. Renal involvement can range from mild abnormalities to full-blown nephritic or nephrotic syndrome. Lupus nephritis is mediated by immune deposition in the glomerulus. Treatment includes prednisone and cytotoxic therapy.

Answer H is incorrect. Membranoproliferative glomerulonephritis is a hard-to-treat progressive nephritic syndrome often associated with hepatitis C infection. Light microscopy demonstrates the classic "tram track" double-layered basement membrane. Despite treatment with corticosteroids, the disease usually progresses slowly to renal failure.

Answer I is incorrect. Minimal change disease (MCD) is the most common cause of nephrotic syndrome in children and is characterized by minimal histologic change by light microscopy. There is an increased risk of thrombotic events in MCD due to low serum levels of antithrombin III, tissue plasminogen activator, and other derangements in the coagulation cascade secondary to heavy proteinuria. Treatment is with steroids, and prognosis is excellent.

Answer J is incorrect. Polyarteritis nodosa is a form of systemic necrotizing vasculitis that classically affects small to medium-size vessels. It is classically P-ANCA (perinuclear antineutrophilic cytoplasmic autoantibody) positive.

Answer K is incorrect. Postinfectious glomerulonephritis is associated with group A β-hemolytic streptococcal infection within the past 2 weeks. ASO titer is elevated, serum C3 is decreased, and care is supportive because almost all patients have a complete recovery (children more than adults).

Answer L is incorrect. Wegener's granulomatosis is a cause of nephritic syndrome characterized by granulomatous inflammation of the lung and kidney, leading to hemoptysis, sinus symptoms, and nephritis. It is classically C-ANCA (circulating anti-neutrophilic cytoplasmic autoantibody) positive, and patients respond to high-dose steroids, albeit with frequent relapses.

Questions 43 and 44

43. **The correct answer is D.** The most common cause of bloody nipple discharge is intraductal papilloma. It is more common than invasive ductal papillary carcinoma, invasive ductal carcinoma, or invasive lobular carcinoma, all of which may cause nipple discharge. Intraductal papillomas are more likely to develop in menopausal or perimenopausal women. The discharge may be bloody, serous, or turbid. The other answer choices are incorrect due to the fact that intraductal papilloma is the most common cause of this symptom, in addition to the fact that this patient has a very typical presentation of the disease.

44. **The correct answer is E.** This is most likely invasive ductal carcinoma. Although intraductal papilloma is the most common cause of a bloody nipple discharge, bloody nipple discharge is still suspicious for carcinoma. Since 80% of all breast cancers are invasive ductal

carcinomas, this is the most likely diagnosis. Typical clinical features of breast carcinoma are hard, irregular, painless, and immobile masses located in the right outer quadrant.

Answer A is incorrect. Fibroadenoma is a benign, slow-growing breast tumor, and is the most common breast tumor in women who are < 30 years old. It usually presents as a firm but mobile mass.

Answer B is incorrect. Fibrocystic changes are associated with a bloody discharge in about one-third of cases, but usually the discharge is tinged yellow. Fibrocystic changes occur along a spectrum of clinical findings that may include cystic change, nodularity, stromal proliferation, and epithelial hyperplasia. An exaggerated response of breast tissue to hormones and growth factors causes cyclic, premenstrual, bilateral breast pain and tenderness.

Answer C is incorrect. Galactocele is a cystic dilation of a duct that is filled with a thick, milky fluid. It is not associated with a bloody discharge, but there may be a yellow-tinged discharge.

Answer F is incorrect. Paget's disease of the breast is an adenocarcinoma that presents with characteristic eczematous nipple pathology.

Answer G is incorrect. Although pregnancy can cause nipple discharge, it is unlikely to present as seen in either of these cases.

Answer H is incorrect. Prolactinoma does cause nipple discharge; however, it would not account for the breast mass seen in these cases.

Answer I is incorrect. Invasive lobular carcinoma is not as common as invasive ductal carcinoma.

Answer J is incorrect. Invasive papillary carcinoma is not as common as invasive ductal carcinoma. It can then be inferred that in a presentation highly suspicious for any carcinoma, it is not the most likely diagnosis.

Questions 45 and 46

45. **The correct answer is C.** Delirium is defined as an impairment in consciousness, usually accompanied by cognitive deficits, emotional la-

bility, hallucinations, impulsivity, or violent behavior. Delirium is generally considered to be an acute reversible disorder. Delirium is classified according to etiology: delirium due to a medical condition, substance-intoxication delirium, substance-withdrawal delirium, and delirium NOS (not otherwise specified). In this clinical scenario the delirium appears to be brought on by the patient's medical condition (e.g., post-surgery or urinary tract infection).

46. **The correct answer is K.** This patient's acute impairment in consciousness fits the definition of delirium. In this case, the precipitating cause is lithium toxicity.

Answer A is incorrect. Brief psychotic disorder involves inclusion of one of the following: delusions, hallucinations, or disorganized speech. In addition, the symptoms cannot be accounted for by a general medical condition. In this case, both patients have underlying medical conditions.

Answer B is incorrect. Creutzfeldt-Jakob disease is a rare disease of rapid neurodegeneration that is caused by prions. More than 90% of patients experience myoclonus in addition to progressive dementia, and death occurs within 1 year of disease onset.

Answer D is incorrect. Alzheimer's disease is the most common cause of dementia. It typically presents in a person's 50s or 60s, is slowly progressive, and does not affect a person's level of consciousness. Conversely, delirium has an acute onset, typically lasting from days to weeks, and impairs a person's level of consciousness.

Answer E is incorrect. Depression is not generally associated with true delirium, although very depressed patients may appear delirious or demented. The patient in this clinical scenario does not present with signs or symptoms of depression such as sadness, tearfulness, weight change, problems with sleep, or loss of interest in previous activities.

Answer F is incorrect. Mania involves erratic and disinhibited behavior, low frustration tolerance with irritability and violent behavior, and vegetative signs such as excessive energy, insomnia, or weight loss. This patient exhibits an acute onset of irritability coupled with cognitive decline as a result of her medical condition.

Answer G is incorrect. Normal aging is associated with a decreased ability to learn new material and a slowing of cognition; however, it does not show a progressive deteriorating course.

Answer H is incorrect. Parkinson's disease is a movement disorder; in addition, 40–80% of patients become demented.

Answer I is incorrect. Pseudodementia is when depression in the elderly presents as symptoms of cognitive impairment. The patient in this clinical scenario does not present with signs or symptoms of depression such as sadness, tearfulness, weight change, problems with sleep, or loss of interest in previous activities.

Answer J is incorrect. It may be difficult to distinguish the diagnosis of delirium due to a general medical condition from a psychotic disorder resulting from a general medical condition; however, the latter refers to hallucinations or delusions that result from medical illness (e.g., temporal lobe epilepsy or meningitis). In both these cases, the patients do not exhibit psychotic symptoms such as hallucinations or delusions.

Answer L is incorrect. Vascular dementia is the second most common cause of dementia. The disorder progresses in a stepwise fashion due to cerebrovascular disease and intermittent vascular events (i.e., strokes). Neurologic signs are common. Physical findings include carotid bruits and funduscopic abnormalities. Cognitive impairment may be patchy, with cognitive function intact in some areas.

Test Block 6

1. A 76-year-old man returns to his primary care physician for follow-up of a known medical condition. He has no complaints, and his physical examination is unremarkable. Laboratory studies reveal a Ca^{2+} level of 6.1 mEq/L, a phosphate level of 6.2 mg/dL, and a parathyroid hormone level of 150 pg/mL (normal: 11–54 pg/mL). Which of the following is most likely to be the patient's underlying medical condition?

   (A) End-stage renal disease
   (B) Hyperthyroidism
   (C) Lung cancer
   (D) Parathyroid adenoma
   (E) Sarcoidosis

2. A 57-year-old African-American man presents with gradual onset of pain in the right leg over 3 months, and acute onset of back pain. He reports that the pain is right on the bone and becomes worse with walking. He does not recall any inciting trauma to the leg. He has no chronic illnesses but reports two episodes of pyelonephritis over the last 18 months. A review of systems is significant for mild fatigue. Physical examination shows tenderness along the right femur with no pain on straight leg raise. The legs are warm to the touch with good pulses and no sensory or motor deficit. No abdominal bruit is heard. Laboratory results are significant for hypercalcemia, elevated creatinine, and a low hemoglobin level. X-ray of the spine reveals compression fractures. Which of the following additional tests would confirm the diagnosis?

   (A) Abdominal ultrasound showing stenosis of the right iliac artery
   (B) Bone densitometry with diminished T-score
   (C) Bone marrow biopsy showing plasmacytosis
   (D) Decreased serum vitamin D level
   (E) Nerve conduction studies

3. A 65-year-old man with type 2 diabetes mellitus and eczema presents to his physician for a routine office visit. He is currently taking metformin and atorvastatin. On examination, the patient has a blood pressure of 140/86 mm Hg, heart rate of 75/min, and respiratory rate of 26/min. An ECG shows normal sinus rhythm with peaked T waves. Urinalysis shows a urine pH of 5.0; it is negative for ketones, WBC esterase, and nitrite, but is positive for protein. An arterial blood gas is drawn, which shows pH of 7.3, partial pressure of carbon dioxide of 32 mm Hg, HCO_3^- of 14 mEq/L, partial pressure of oxygen of 98 mm Hg, and oxygen saturation of 99% on room air. Relevant laboratory findings are:

Na^+	140 mEq/L
K^+	6.0 mEq/L
Cl^-	120 mEq/L
Blood urea nitrogen	16 mg/dL
Creatinine	1.1 mg/dL

   What is the most likely diagnosis of this acid-base disturbance?

   (A) Hyperkalemia
   (B) Hyperventilation
   (C) Ketoacidosis
   (D) Lactic acidosis
   (E) Renal tubular acidosis

4. A 30-year-old primigravida is in the labor and delivery unit at 7 weeks' gestation. She has had a prolonged active labor and her obstetrician introduces a catheter into the dilated cervix to manually rupture her membranes. With the passage of amniotic fluid into the vaginal canal, the obstetrician notes the fluid to be dark green and thick. Amnioinfusion could help prevent which of the following?

   (A) Brachial plexus injury
   (B) Breech presentation
   (C) Chorioamnionitis
   (D) Early decelerations of fetal heart rate
   (E) Meconium aspiration

5. A 7-month-old boy is brought to the pediatrician by his parents, who are concerned about his recent change in behavior. He was healthy until 3 days prior to this episode, when he presented with severe diarrhea and was diagnosed with gastroenteritis. His parents now describe new-onset vomiting with pallor and lethargy.

Current heart rate is 109/min, blood pressure is 102/68 mm Hg, respiratory rate is 20/min, and temperature is 38.0°C (100.4°F). The infant is pale but hemodynamically stable. He is crying and in significant discomfort, particularly on abdominal palpation. He has bloody mucus in his diaper. Which is the most appropriate next step to both diagnose and potentially treat this condition?

(A) Air contrast or barium enema
(B) Colonoscopy
(C) Endoscopy
(D) Surgery
(E) Watchful waiting

6. A 43-year-old construction worker was renovating a building when he slipped and fell three stories. The patient immediately complained of intense back pain. When paramedics arrived at the scene, the worker's vital signs were temperature 37.1°C (98.8°F), blood pressure 108/62 mm Hg, pulse 92/min, and respiratory rate 16/min. Physical examination was notable for diminished pulses peripherally and a systolic murmur. In the emergency department (ED), an x-ray of the chest was obtained in which a widened mediastinum was noted, along with first through fourth rib fractures on the left side. There was loss of the aortic knob, as well as deviation of the trachea and depression of the left main stem bronchus. Which of the following is indicated to confirm the suspected diagnosis?

(A) Aortogram
(B) MRI of chest
(C) Needle decompression
(D) Transthoracic echocardiography
(E) Upper gastrointestinal endoscopy

7. A 10-year-old boy is brought to the clinic because of a sore throat, rhinorrhea, and rash. His parents report he was well before he developed a severe sore throat 2 days prior to presenting. The child continued to complain of throat pain, and today has been unable to swallow secondary to severe pain. Yesterday, his mother noticed he was developing a diffuse rash (see image) that was nonpainful and nonpruritic. On physical examination his oropharynx is markedly inflamed with tonsillar exudates. A course of antibiotics is prescribed. Which of the following is the most likely diagnosis?

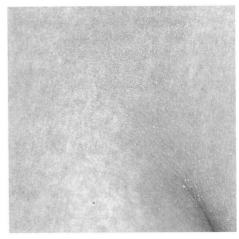

Reproduced, with permission, from Wolff K, Johnson RA, Surmond D. *Fitzpatrick's Color Atlas & Synopsis of Clinical Dermatology*, 5th ed. New York: McGraw-Hill, 2005: Figure 22-35.

(A) Fifth disease
(B) Impetigo
(C) Kawasaki disease
(D) Measles
(E) Mononucleosis
(F) Scarlet fever

8. A 40-year-old African-American woman presents to the ED complaining of confusion, colicky abdominal pain, vomiting, spiking fevers, and chills. She has noted her stools over the past 2 days to be lighter colored than usual. Her temperature is 39.6°C (103.3°F), pulse is 120/min, blood pressure is 85/55 mm Hg, and respiratory rate is 25/min. On examination, she is in obvious distress, sclerae are icteric, bowel sounds are normal, and abdomen is tender to palpation in the right upper quadrant without rebound. Laboratory values reveal a WBC of 18,000, total bilirubin of 4.5, aspartate aminotransferase/alanine aminotransferase of 90/100, and alkaline phosphatase of 250. CT reveals dilated intrahepatic bile ducts with stones in the gallbladder and pneumobilia. Which of the following has first priority in the management of this patient?

(A) Establish vascular access and give intravenous fluids
(B) Further image the biliary system to pinpoint the obstruction
(C) Perform emergent decompression of biliary system
(D) Place nasogastric tube
(E) Prescribe empiric oral antibiotics

9. A 20-year-old white man presents to the ED with a mild cough, weight loss, low-grade fevers, and night sweats. He lives in Tennessee and spends his weekends spelunking (exploring caves). X-ray of the chest shows small apical cavitary lesions bilaterally. The physician diagnosis a cavitary pneumonia. Purified protein derivative test is negative. He denies any history of asthma, allergies, smoking, and immunosuppression. Which of the following is the most appropriate next step in the management of the patient?

(A) Ceftriaxone
(B) Itraconazole and possibly amphotericin B
(C) Nystatin swish and swallow
(D) Pyrazinamide
(E) Trimethoprim-sulfamethoxazole

10. A 24-year-old woman presents to the ED after being involved in a motor vehicle accident. She is moving all extremities and is conversant. She indicates that while driving at 30 mph, she veered off the road to avoid an oncoming car and crashed into a guard fence. Her airbag deployed, and she denies losing consciousness. She was placed in a stabilization collar in the field. In the ED, she complains of some minor cuts on her face and arms as well as neck pain. Her temperature is 37.2°C (99.0°F), blood pressure is 134/80 mm Hg, pulse is 90/min, and respiratory rate is 12/min. On examination she is alert and oriented, and extraocular movements are intact. Her pupils are equally round and reactive to light. She has full strength and sensation in her face and extremities. Neck examination reveals diffuse soreness posteriorly but no midline tenderness. There are no dislocations or step-offs. Breathalyzer test and urine toxicology screen are negative. What is the appropriate next step in management?

(A) Cervical MRI scan
(B) Halo placement
(C) High-dose corticosteroids
(D) Lateral cervical x-rays with flexion and extension
(E) Remove collar and allow patient to slowly flex, extend, and rotate neck

11. A mother and father bring their 7-year-old son to the pediatrician's office because he is developing facial hair. The mother states that he has always been healthy and had been developing normally until his voice began "squeaking" about a month ago. Last week while her son was getting out of the shower, she noticed some chest hair and made an appointment "right away." The father states that he went through puberty very young and was shaving by age 14 years. On physical examination, the boy is a thin, well-appearing 7-year-old. His examination is remarkable only for some hair growth on his upper lip and sparse chest hair. Which of the following hormones would most likely be low in this patient?

(A) Androstenedione
(B) Cortisol
(C) Dihydrotestosterone
(D) 17α-Hydroxyprogesterone
(E) 5α-Reductase

12. A 39-year-old man with a history of hypertension and diabetes presents to the ED with acute-onset painless loss of vision in his left eye. He reports that he has had fleeting episodes of vision loss in the past. Vital signs are blood pressure of 158/88 mm Hg, pulse of 80/min, and respiratory rate of 16/min. Ocular examination shows decreased visual acuity in the left eye and a relative afferent pupillary defect. Funduscopic examination shows a cherry red spot and surrounding retinal edema. Laboratory values reveal a WBC count of 10,600/mm^3, glucose of 120 mg/dL, and erythrocyte sedimentation rate of 10 mm/h. What is the most likely diagnosis?

(A) Acute ophthalmic artery occlusion
(B) Central retinal artery occlusion
(C) Central retinal vein occlusion
(D) Giant cell arteritis
(E) Tay-Sachs disease

13. A 14-month-old boy is playing in the living room with his 3.5-year-old sister. Their mother leaves briefly to answer the phone. On returning to the living room, the mother notices that the children are still playing together with no noticeable change in behavior. Later in the

day, the boy refuses feeding and seems to have excessive salivation. The mother is concerned and decides to have her son evaluated at the local ED. Which of the following is the most logical next step in evaluating this child based solely on the history presented?

(A) Barium contrast radiologic evaluation
(B) Complete blood cell count with differential
(C) Endoscopic evaluation
(D) Parental reassurance that the child is healthy
(E) Radiologic studies of the neck, chest, and abdomen

14. A 14-year-old girl is brought to the ED by paramedics while seizing. Her parents, who report she has a history of seizures, found her in her bedroom and were unsure of how long she had been seizing. On arrival to the ED the patient's vital signs are pulse 125/min, blood pressure 160/100 mm Hg, temperature 38.9°C (102°F), and respiratory rate 22/min. On examination the patient has her arms extended rigidly at her sides and she is arching her back rhythmically and appears to be aspirating. After several failed attempts at nasopharyngeal intubation, rapid sequence induction allowed placement of a nasopharyngeal airway. Several infusions of intravenous benzodiazepines, phenytoin, and phenobarbital produce little effect. Which of the following is true regarding this patient's condition?

(A) Irreversible neuronal injury usually occurs after 10 minutes
(B) Management options are strongly influenced by the cause of the seizure
(C) Mortality following status epilepticus is over 50%
(D) Patients with minimal myoclonic activity are not at risk for serious complications
(E) Rhabdomyolysis is a potential life-threatening complication

15. A 38-year-old G5P4 woman at 37 weeks' gestation has a history of preeclampsia in previous pregnancies. She presented to the obstetric clinic for her initial screening at 10 weeks' gestation but was subsequently lost to follow-up. At her initial visit, the patient had a blood pressure of 140/70 mm Hg and no proteinuria. Since then, the patient reports experiencing headaches, some visual disturbances, and lightheadedness but has not sought health care for any of her symptoms. The patient now presents to the ED complaining of a headache. Vital signs reveal a blood pressure of 162/90 mm Hg. An ultrasound of the uterus is likely to reveal which of the following?

(A) Intrauterine growth retardation
(B) Macrosomia
(C) Placenta previa
(D) Polyhydramnios
(E) Rocker-bottom feet

16. A 22-year-old woman is brought to the hospital by her family for progressive weight loss over the past 4 months, fatigue, depression, and refusal to eat. Vital signs are blood pressure 95/65 mm Hg and pulse 120/min. Her body mass index is 6 kg/m². The patient is hospitalized and undergoes a strict refeeding protocol, in addition to psychotherapy. After 3 weeks of treatment, the patient is started on a pharmacologic agent to treat her persistent symptoms of depression. The following morning, the patient experiences a generalized tonic-clonic seizure. Which medication is the most likely cause of this patient's seizure?

(A) Aripiprazole
(B) Bupropion
(C) Escitalopram
(D) Fluoxetine
(E) Imipramine

17. A 55-year-old otherwise healthy man reports a cough productive of green sputum, fever, chills, and pleuritic chest pain over the past 4 days. His physical examination reveals egophony and increased tactile fremitus in the left lower lobe. A complete blood cell count shows a WBC count of 20,000/mm^3 with 15% bands. X-ray of the chest is shown in the image. What is the most likely pathogen causing this man's illness?

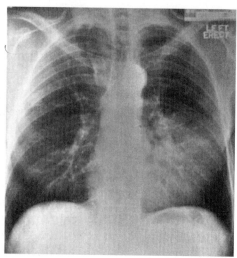

Reproduced, with permission, from Chen MYM, Pope TL, Ott DJ. *Basic Radiology.* New York: McGraw-Hill, 2004: Figure 4-19.

(A) *Escherichia coli*
(B) *Klebsiella*
(C) *Mycoplasma pneumoniae*
(D) *Pseudomonas*
(E) *Staphylococcus aureus*
(F) *Streptococcus pneumoniae*

18. A 47-year-old man presents to his physician with mouth pain for the past 2 weeks. It seems to be getting worse and is making eating uncomfortable. He first noticed a small blister on the inside of his cheek that popped immediately after forming and has been very painful. Two more oral ulcers and four ulcerated lesions on his back have developed since then and are not healing well. He denies fevers, chills, diarrhea, constipation, or abdominal pain, and has no significant past medical history. On examination there are three shallow ulcerations, 5 mm to 1 cm in diameter, located on the buccal mucosa and tongue and four shallow ulcerations, 2–4.5 cm in diameter, on the lumbar and buttock region. Which of the

following is the most likely cause of these symptoms?

(A) Antibodies against basement membrane
(B) Antibodies against desmoglein proteins
(C) Antibodies against hemidesmosome glycoproteins
(D) Aphthous ulcers
(E) Infection with a herpesvirus

19. A 60-year-old with a newly diagnosed focal brain lesion presents with aphasia. His ability to repeat words and his fluency are both impaired, and his language comprehension is also diminished. He has no other symptoms, and the remainder of his neurologic examination is unremarkable. From what kind of aphasia is he suffering?

(A) Broca's aphasia
(B) Conduction aphasia
(C) Global aphasia
(D) Transcortical motor aphasia
(E) Wernicke's aphasia

20. A 40-year-old white woman presents to the ED with 3 hours of cramping abdominal pain and multiple episodes of vomiting after which the pain was temporarily relieved. She says the vomit is greenish. Her last bowel movement was 2 days prior to presentation, but she continues to pass flatus. Her vital signs are normal, except for a pulse of 115/min. On examination, she is in mild distress, and her abdomen is somewhat distended and diffusely tender with high-pitched bowel sounds and multiple old surgical scars. She does not have rebound tenderness. Complete blood cell count, urinalysis, and electrolytes are unremarkable. Flat and upright x-rays of the abdomen reveal multiple air-fluid levels and residual air in the colon. Which of the following is the most appropriate management of this patient?

(A) Admit to hospital, administer intravenous fluids, and perform endoscopic retrograde cholangiopancreatography
(B) Admit to hospital, make "nothing by mouth," place nasogastric tube, and give intravenous fluids
(C) Admit to hospital, place rectal tube, administer enemas, and disimpact bowels

(D) Emergency laparotomy

(E) Make "nothing by mouth" and observe in ED

21. A 68-year-old man presents to his primary care physician with a persistent cough over the past 2 months, with dyspnea on exertion. Physical examination reveals decreased breath sounds in all lung fields and a prolonged expiratory phase. Pulmonary function tests reveal a decreased FEV_1, decreased FEV_1:FVC, and increased residual volume. What would this patient's x-ray of the chest most likely show?

(A) Apical cavitary lesion

(B) Diffuse bilateral infiltrates

(C) Hyperinflation with diaphragmatic flattening and increased anteroposterior diameter

(D) Lobar consolidation

(E) Mass lesion with mediastinal adenopathy

22. A 3000-g (6.6-lb) girl is born at 37 weeks' gestation by spontaneous vaginal delivery to a 26-year-old mother of Chinese origin. Pregnancy and birth were uncomplicated, with Apgar scores of 9 and 10 at 1 and 5 minutes, respectively. Physical examination and newborn laboratory results were normal. The infant is exclusively breast-fed and is latching on and feeding well with adequate urine output. She presents on her fifth day of life because of increasing jaundice and scleral icterus. She is afebrile with stable vital signs. Laboratory results in the ED are notable for the following:

Total bilirubin	22 mg/dL
Unconjugated bilirubin	19.7 mg/dL
Conjugated bilirubin	0.3 mg/dL
WBC count	12,000/mm^3

What is the next step in treatment?

(A) Abdominal ultrasound

(B) Discharge the patient on formula and with a fiberoptic bilirubin blanket

(C) Erythromycin

(D) Exchange transfusion

(E) Phototherapy

23. A 57-year-old man presents to his family physician for routine health maintenance. He has no complaints and takes no medications. Family history is unremarkable. Blood pressure is measured at 158/94 mm Hg at the time of the routine physical, and hypertension is confirmed with a second elevated reading 2 weeks later. After obtaining laboratory studies, the physician diagnoses primary hyperaldosteronism. Which of the following electrolyte panels is likely to be obtained from this patient?

CHOICE	Na$^+$ (mEq/L)	K$^+$ (mEq/L)	Hco$_3^-$ (mEq/L)
A	160	2.8	45
B	124	4.1	27
C	140	4.0	26
D	125	6.0	25
E	141	4.2	15

(A) A

(B) B

(C) C

(D) D

(E) E

24. A 60-year-old man presents to a urologist complaining of difficulty having an erection. The man states that the quality of his erections has been getting worse over the past year. He has a history of hyperlipidemia, for which he is noncompliant with his medications, and has smoked one pack per day for the past 40 years. On review of systems, he notes that his buttocks and lower back hurt when he walks. The patient's heart rate is 70/min and blood pressure is 130/80 mm Hg. His examination is notable for distant breath sounds bilaterally and global atrophy of the lower extremities. Which of the following would the physician expect to find?

Choice	Femoral Pulses	Ankle-Brachial Index (at rest*)	Ankle-Brachial Index (after exercise)
A	absent	0.3	0.3
B	weak	0.3	0.6
C	weak	0.6	0.3
D	increased	0.2	0.2
E	increased	0.6	0.3

* Normal 0.9–1.3.

(A) A
(B) B
(C) C
(D) D
(E) E

25. A 77-year-old woman presents to her primary care physician's office for evaluation. The patient states that other than several episodes of gout in the past 4 years, she has been quite healthy. She currently has no complaints but wants to discuss treatment and/or prophylaxis options to help protect her against recurrent episodes of gout. The patient's musculoskeletal examination is within normal limits, with full range of motion and no focal tenderness in any of her joints. First-line prophylactic therapy for chronic gout involves which treatment or medication?

(A) Allopurinol
(B) Colchicine
(C) Indomethacin
(D) Intra-articular corticosteroid injections
(E) Niacin

26. A 7-year-old boy presents to the local ED in a Maryland hospital after his mother found a tick on him. She states that they have been camping for 2 days in the Appalachians and she noticed a similar tick on their dog. The patient is asymptomatic. The mother is requesting assistance removing the tick. The tick has a hard body and after removal is identified as *Dermacentor variabilis* (American dog tick). Which of the following diseases can be transmitted by *Dermacentor variabilis?*

(A) Aspergilloma
(B) Bubonic plague
(C) Lyme disease
(D) Malaria
(E) Rocky Mountain spotted fever

27. A 22-year-old G0 woman presents to the clinic seeking a refill of her oral contraceptive pills (OCPs). She was started on a combination pill 2 years ago for menorrhagia and has had no complications. She has no other past medical or past surgical history and denies smoking. She is not currently sexually active. Which of the following would constitute an absolute contraindication to administration of OCPs?

(A) Active liver disease
(B) History of atherosclerosis
(C) Lactation
(D) Occasional smoking (three to four cigarettes per week)
(E) Uterine fibroids

28. A 37-year-old woman is admitted to the hospital with hypernatremia. The woman was recently diagnosed with Langerhans cell histiocytosis after a skin biopsy of a raised, pruritic purple lesion in her axilla that was refractory to treatment with topical steroids. The woman

states that she feels fine, and denies any confusion or mental status change. She admits to polyuria, polydipsia, and persistent thirst. On physical examination the patient is awake, alert, and oriented with a blood pressure of 120/80 mm Hg and a heart rate of 70/min. She is afebrile, and has a respiratory rate of 16/min. Cardiac examination reveals a normal S1 and S2 with no murmurs, rubs, or gallops. A pulmonary examination is normal with clear breath sounds throughout. The above-mentioned axillary lesions are noted. Relevant laboratory findings are:

Na^+	155 mEq/L
K^+	4.2 mEq/L
Cl^-	120 mEq/L
CO_2	25 mEq/L
Blood urea nitrogen	22 mg/dL
Creatinine	1.0 mg/dL

The patient's urine osmolality is 100 mOsm/kg (normal: 50–1200 mOsm/kg). The medication used to chronically treat diabetes insipidus in this patient also has what effect?

(A) Binds reversibly to the 30S ribosomal subunit
(B) Decreases plasma factor VIII
(C) Increases von Willebrand factor
(D) Inhibits platelet adhesion
(E) Prevents some adverse cardiovascular outcomes
(F) Stabilizes mood

29. A 47-year-old man involved in a motor vehicle accident is unresponsive and unarousable. On physical examination, he has a respiratory rate of 8/min, heart rate of 120/min, blood pressure of 90/65 mm Hg, and temperature of 37.1°C (98.8°F). He does not open his eyes, nor does he vocalize spontaneously or in response to painful stimuli such as a sternal rub or nail bed stimulation. He makes no spontaneous movements, but his muscles do flex in response to painful stimuli. What is the most appropriate next step?

(A) Administer intravenous mannitol
(B) CT of the head
(C) Intubate
(D) Measure blood glucose
(E) Push tissue plasminogen activator

30. Approximately 8 hours after receiving an injection of haloperidol, an extremely agitated man in the ED begins complaining that his room is "too hot." The nurse subsequently reports a temperature of 40.2°C (104.4°F), a pulse of 114/min, and a blood pressure of 182/115 mm Hg. An hour later, the patient is stiff and sweating profusely. His WBC count is 27,000/mm³ and his creatinine kinase is 52,140 U/L. Over the next 24 hours, he becomes minimally responsive to verbal stimuli. The patient is placed on a cardiac monitor for constant observation of vital signs, and attempts are made to decrease the patient's temperature with cooling blankets and intravenous fluids, but the patient continues to decline. Which of the following should now be used?

(A) Clonidine
(B) Continued use of cooling blankets and intravenous fluids
(C) Dantrolene
(D) Ice packs to the axillae and groin
(E) Lorazepam

31. A 65-year-old man is seen in the doctor's office for a nonproductive cough, 6.8-kg (15-lb) unintentional weight loss, and recurrent pneumonia, all occurring over the past 6 months. The patient's wife, who is currently with the patient, has noticed excessive hair growth and acne over the patient's face, chest, and back. The patient has a 75 pack-year smoking history and continues to smoke one pack per day. He has no significant past medical history and takes no medications. His blood pressure is 155/95 mm Hg, but other vital signs are normal. Physical examination reveals purple striae along the patient's chest and abdomen as well as peripheral muscle wasting. X-ray of the chest shows a focal 3-cm mass lesion in the right lower lobe of the lung that is highly suspicious for bronchogenic carcinoma. A bronchoscopy with brushing is significant for classic small cell carcinoma. A CT scan confirms the presence of the 3-cm mass in the right lower lobe and shows possible involvement of the contralateral mediastinal lymph nodes. Which of the following is the most appropriate management?

(A) Localized irradiation of the involved hemithorax and nodes
(B) Surgical resection
(C) Surgical resection after initial chemotherapy
(D) Surgical resection with radiation
(E) Systemic chemotherapy

32. A 40-year-old Asian mother of two presents to the ED complaining of intermittent epigastric pain. The pain is severe, lasts for a couple of hours, is sometimes accompanied by nausea and vomiting, and often occurs following meals. Her bowel movements have been normal. Her vital signs are temperature 38.2°C (100.8°F), pulse 100/min, blood pressure 135/75 mm Hg, and respiratory rate 22/min. On examination she is in obese, her sclerae are mildly icteric, and her bowel sounds are normal, with an abrupt halt of inspiration with palpation of the right upper quadrant (RUQ), and RUQ tenderness. Laboratory tests reveal a WBC count of 13,000/mm³, total bilirubin of 3.3 mg/dL, and normal liver enzymes and alkaline phosphatase. RUQ ultrasound is performed but is inconclusive. Which of the following is the next diagnostic imaging study that should be performed?

(A) CT scan
(B) Flat and upright abdominal plain films
(C) 5-Hydroxyindoleacetic acid scan
(D) Upper gastrointestinal series with oral contrast

33. A small 5-month-old girl presents to the hospital with signs of severe sepsis and pneumonia. At time of admission, she is hemodynamically unstable with a heart rate of 78/min, blood pressure of 55/38 mm Hg, and respiratory rate of 40/min. She is directly admitted to the pediatric intensive care unit, where she abruptly decompensates and attempts at resuscitation are unsuccessful. Postmortem examination of the child demonstrates a small thymus (0.86 g) that was located within the anterior neck. Pathologic examination of the thymic sample demonstrates few thymocytes and a lack of corticomedullary differentiation. Additional findings at autopsy included absent tonsils, adenoids, and Peyer's patches. What test, if performed, would have diagnosed this patient's condition and possibly saved her life?✱

(A) Blood cultures with antibiotic sensitivities at time of presentation
(B) Echocardiography at time of presentation
(C) Routine neonatal screening at time of birth
(D) Serum uric acid level performed anytime
(E) WBC count with differential at time of birth

34. A 67-year-old woman comes to the ED complaining of a red rash (shown in the image) and fever for more than 3 days. Her past medical history is significant for hypertension, diabetes, obesity, and calcific aortic stenosis. Her temperature is 39.2°C (102.6°F), her blood pressure is 145/86 mm Hg, and her heart rate is 110/min. She has a III/VI systolic murmur at her left sternal border not documented on previous examinations and inspiratory crackles at both lung bases. She has 2+ pitting edema bilaterally in her ankles to the knees. Which of the following treatments is the most appropriate initial pharmacotherapy?

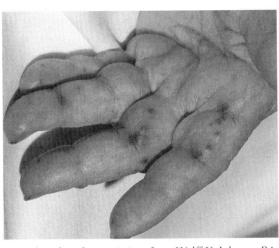

Reproduced, with permission, from Wolff K, Johnson RA, Surmond D. *Fitzpatrick's Color Atlas & Synopsis of Clinical Dermatology*, 5th ed. New York: McGraw-Hill, 2005: Figure 22-38.

(A) Gentamicin
(B) Hydrochlorothiazide
(C) Metoprolol and enalapril
(D) Penicillin
(E) Penicillin and gentamicin

35. Following presentation to his primary care doctor, a 59-year-old man was diagnosed with multiple myeloma. The patient has been participating in a clinical trial for a chemotherapeutic agent and has begun to show early signs of disease remission. The patient has been immobile for 3 weeks due to fatigue and bone tenderness. He now presents to the ED with new-onset erythema, swelling, and tenderness of the right lower extremity. The patient states that he has never had anything like this in the past. At presentation, his temperature is 37.3°C (99.2°F), blood pressure is 136/84 mm Hg, pulse is 74/min, and respiratory rate is 13/min. What is the first step in management of this patient?

(A) Cessation of chemotherapy
(B) Inferior vena cava filter
(C) Intravenous heparin
(D) Ventilation-perfusion scan
(E) Warfarin

36. A 36-year-old white man presents to his primary care physician with a 3-month history of progressive weakness. He complains that it is increasingly difficult to get up from a chair, climb stairs, or lift ordinary household objects. He denies having episodes like this in the past, a family history of neuromuscular disease, or exposure to mycotoxic drugs; however, he does recall a 2-week period 4 months ago where he had "flulike" symptoms. Physical examination reveals no signs of rash and no involvement of the extraocular and facial muscles. He has symmetric 3/5 muscle strength in his upper and lower extremities bilaterally. Muscle biopsy is consistent with polymyositis. Which of the following is the most appropriate initial course of therapy?

(A) Azathioprine
(B) Intravenous immunoglobulin
(C) Methotrexate
(D) Nonsteroidal anti-inflammatory drugs
(E) Oral prednisone

37. An 84-year-old woman suffering from terminal breast cancer is hospitalized and intubated with pneumonia. Her clinical condition worsens, and 1 week later her health care proxy decides to withdraw care and offer comfort measures only. Her family requests that she be given high doses of morphine to ensure that she will not be in pain. Her physicians agree to this, even though they know that opioids may further depress her respirations. The physicians' willingness to treat this patient with potentially fatal drugs for palliative purposes is an example of which principle?

(A) Autonomy
(B) Dereliction
(C) Double effect
(D) Malpractice
(E) Physician-assisted suicide

38. A 65-year-old woman with a history of myocardial infarction, hypertension, and asthma presents with new onset of hallucinations. She can no longer sleep at night because she sees small children and cats in her apartment. She thinks she must be going crazy and is too frightened to explain the symptoms to her husband. She has no prior psychiatric history. Her vital signs are blood pressure supine 115/80 mm Hg and standing 90/60 mm Hg. Physical examination reveals an alert, oriented elderly woman with a slight resting tremor and mild rigidity in her upper and lower extremities, but no cogwheeling. Mini-mental status examination reveals deficits in long-term recall. What abnormal neuronal finding is expected?

    (A) Birefringent crystals
    (B) Dark pigmentation in the substantia nigra
    (C) Eosinophilic cytoplasmic inclusions
    (D) Hypersegmented nuclei
    (E) Neurofibrillary tangles and webs

39. A 6-year-old boy presents with unrelenting fever over 10 days with headache. Acetaminophen has not improved the fever. His mother says that he sounds "stuffed up" and that he has developed a cough over the last 2 days. He had a similar episode 2 months ago and was treated with amoxicillin with resolution of symptoms. On physical examination, the child has a widened nose bridge and nasal polyps, with purulent discharge from the ostiae bilaterally. X-ray of the head is shown in the image, and a sweat chloride test shows a chloride concentration of 70 mEq/L (normal <60 mEq/L). What is the most probable diagnosis?

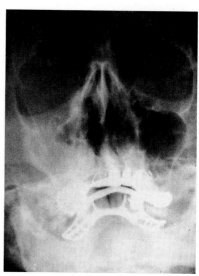

Reproduced, with permission, from Stone CK, Humphries RL. *Current Emergency Diagnosis & Treatment.* New York: McGraw-Hill, 2004: Figure 32-8.

    (A) Allergic rhinitis
    (B) Cystic fibrosis
    (C) Kartagener's syndrome
    (D) Nasal foreign body
    (E) X-linked severe combined immunodeficiency

40. A 75-year-old cognitively intact woman with a history of diabetes, coronary artery disease, hypercholesterolemia, and peripheral vascular disease is diagnosed with glioblastoma multiforme. She is referred to a neurologic oncologist. The treatment for glioblastoma multiforme that has been shown to improve mortality is resection followed by radiation therapy. Given her multiple cardiac risk factors, however, this patient is a poor surgical candidate. The oncologist is concerned that the risks of resection may outweigh the benefits and it is not clear which treatment option would provide the best quality-of-life outcome for the patient. Which of the following is the best way to approach this issue with the patient?

    (A) Asking the patient to take time to digest what has been said and not ask questions
    (B) Detailing the intricate specifics of numerous studies investigating the treatment options so as to completely inform the patient

(C) Discussing the possible treatment modalities while disclosing the relative morbidities and mortality associated with each treatment option

(D) Insist that the patient discuss her medical options with her family members present

(E) Presenting the possible treatment modalities with the highest chance of improving mortality

41. A 72-year-old African-American woman with a long history of gastroesophageal reflux disease and heavy tobacco use presents to her primary care physician complaining of weight loss and difficulty swallowing that has progressed over the past few years such that solids are nearly impossible to get down. She also complains of a constant cough and a "funny sound" when she breathes. Her vital signs are stable. Concerned, the physician orders an endoscopy and finds a sample of columnar epithelium on biopsy. What is the most likely diagnosis?

(A) Achalasia
(B) Adenocarcinoma of the esophagus
(C) Esophageal varices
(D) Gastric cancer
(E) Hiatal hernia

42. A 25-year-old woman is recovering from an uncomplicated open appendectomy for acute appendicitis. She has no significant past medical history and is not taking any medications. Her temperature is 36.7°C (98.1°F), blood pressure is 118/78 mm Hg, pulse is 72/min and regular, respiratory rate is 14/min, and oxygen saturation is 99% on room air. Her physical examination is significant for a 5-cm (2-in) incision in the right lower quadrant, which is clean, dry, and intact. Which of the following should be recommended to prevent the development of a venous thromboembolism?

(A) Early ambulation
(B) Heparin
(C) Intermittent pneumatic compression with or without elastic stockings
(D) Low-molecular-weight heparin
(E) Warfarin plus elastic stockings

43. An 8-year-old boy is brought to the physician because of refusal to walk for 3 days. On questioning, he states that both his legs hurt. His mother states that he has "not been himself" for the past month or so and has been sleeping much more than usual. She has attributed this to her assumption that the boy is about to have a growth spurt. On examination, temperature is 38.4°C (101.1°F), heart rate is 164/min, respiratory rate is 42/min, and blood pressure is 90/54 mm Hg. The child is pale and listless. Severe hepatomegaly is noted. There are no obvious deformities of the lower extremities or hip, knee, or ankle joints. Relevant laboratory findings are:

WBC count	98,000/mm^3
Hemoglobin	8.9 g/dL
Platelet count	75,000/mm^3
Na$^+$	135 mEq/L
K$^+$	4.0 mEq/L
Cl$^-$	104 mEq/L
Blood urea nitrogen	8 mg/dL
Creatinine	0.6 mg/dL

What is the next best step in the patient's management?

(A) Bone marrow biopsy
(B) Delivery of emergent chemotherapy
(C) Platelet transfusion
(D) Typing of his brother's bone marrow to assess the potential for a matched related bone marrow transplant
(E) X-ray of the chest

EXTENDED MATCHING

Questions 44–46

For each of the patients with hematuria, select the most likely diagnosis.

(A) Bladder cancer
(B) Coagulation disorder
(C) Exercise-induced hematuria
(D) Myoglobinuria
(E) Nephrolithiasis
(F) Polycystic kidney disease
(G) Prostate cancer
(H) Pyelonephritis
(I) Renal cell carcinoma
(J) Urinary tract infection

44. A 70-year-old man presents to the physician's office with painless hematuria. He is a heavy smoker and worked in an industrial factory with dyes when he was younger. His temperature is 37.4°C (99.3°F). Examination reveals no abdominal masses and no nodules on prostate examination. Relevant laboratory findings are a WBC count of 5000/mm^3 and creatinine level of 0.9 mg/dL.

45. A 40-year-old man comes to the clinic because of hematuria and occasional flank pain. He has a family history of kidney disease, but he is not sure which type. He knows that his mother and her two sisters had the disease and all three were fine until their 40s. His temperature is 36.9°C (98.4°F) and blood pressure is 130/80 mm Hg. His serum creatinine level is 1.5 mg/dL.

46. A 57-year-old man presents to the physician with hematuria. He denies pain on urination, but reports flank pain that is relatively constant. He has been having the flank pain for the past month. He also notes intermittent fever and weight loss over the past 6 weeks. His temperature is 37.7°C (99.9°F). He has no costovertebral angle tenderness. He has a WBC count of 5200/mm^3 and a hematocrit of 58%.

1. **The correct answer is A.** The patient has hypocalcemia, hyperphosphatemia, and hyperparathyroidism. These findings are consistent with secondary hyperparathyroidism, which is most commonly due to end-stage renal disease. Hyperphosphatemia is due to impaired secretion of phosphate in the proximal tubule. This contributes to hypocalcemia by binding of phosphate to calcium. Hypocalcemia is also due to deficient production of 1,25-dihydroxy-vitamin D in the kidney, which leads to decreased absorption of ingested calcium. Parathyroid hormone levels increase to compensate for the hypocalcemia and hyperphosphatemia.

Answer B is incorrect. Hyperthyroidism can cause **hyper**calcemia, not hypocalcemia. The mechanism is via increased bone turnover, with bone resorption exceeding new bone formation.

Answer C is incorrect. Lung cancer, particularly squamous cell cancer, is a common cause of hypercalcemia due to production of parathyroid hormone (PTH)-related protein. Calcium will be elevated, phosphate will be decreased, and PTH will be low or normal.

Answer D is incorrect. A parathyroid adenoma is the most common cause of primary hyperparathyroidism. Although this condition will present with elevated levels of parathyroid hormone, the patient will have **hyper**calcemia and **hypo**phosphatemia.

Answer E is incorrect. Sarcoidosis is a cause of **hyper**calcemia, not hypocalcemia. The mechanism of hypercalcemia is increased production of 1,25-dihydroxyvitamin D by macrophages in the granulomas. Parathyroid hormone will not be elevated.

2. **The correct answer is C.** Multiple myeloma is a malignant proliferation of plasma cells, which causes them to overproduce monoclonal immunoglobulin. Due to the defective immune system, patients will often have recurrent infections, of which pneumonia and pyelonephritis are the most common. Patients develop bone pain that is worse with movement, lytic bone lesions, compression fractures, and hypercalcemia due to increased osteoclast activity. Renal failure is also common due to deposition of antibody light chains and associated renal amyloidosis. Diagnosis is aided by a bone marrow biopsy showing a clonal plasma cell population of > 10% of the marrow, monoclonal immunoglobulin (M component) in the serum or the urine, and other features like lytic bone lesions, anemia, and elevated serum calcium.

Answer A is incorrect. Abdominal ultrasound that showed stenosis of the iliac artery would be evidence of vascular insufficiency. Peripheral vascular disease would present as claudication (leg pain worse with exertion and relieved by rest). It would not, however, account for the punched-out lesions seen on x-ray.

Answer B is incorrect. A densitometry scan would be useful to rule out osteoporosis, which is unlikely given the patient's age and gender, and is also unlikely given the patient's x-ray findings.

Answer D is incorrect. Decreased serum vitamin D would be seen in osteomalacia, which often presents with pathologic fractures, not lytic lesions on x-ray.

Answer E is incorrect. Nerve entrapment or disease can be diagnosed with nerve conduction studies, and can be the cause of leg pain. This diagnosis, however, is less likely given the lack of pain on the straight leg raise, as well as the radiologic findings.

3. **The correct answer is E.** The clinical scenario represents type IV renal tubular acidosis (RTA), the most common type of RTA. The disturbance can be thought of as relative aldosterone deficiency or resistance, which is most commonly found in diabetic nephropathy. A hypoaldosterone state leads to hyperkalemia, resulting in decreased ammonium production and urine acidification. The patient's arterial blood gas shows a process consistent with a metabolic acidosis with respiratory compensa-

tion, while his electrolyte panel shows that the acidosis is hyperchloremic in nature. The ECG findings reflect the changes found in hyperkalemia. Type IV RTA can also be seen with tubulointerstitial renal diseases, hypertensive nephrosclerosis, and HIV nephropathy. Drugs such as angiotensin-converting enzyme inhibitors, nonsteroidal anti-inflammatory drugs, and trimethoprim can all cause hyperkalemia leading to type IV RTA. Treatment is furosemide and potassium binding agents such as sodium polystyrene sulfonate.

Answer A is incorrect. The hyperkalemia that is present is secondary to relative aldosterone deficiency. Hyperkalemia is not the precipitating event.

Answer B is incorrect. Hyperventilation may cause a primary respiratory alkalosis. This patient has a primary metabolic acidosis with respiratory compensation.

Answer C is incorrect. Ketoacidosis occurs almost exclusively in type 1 diabetes. Furthermore, the urinalysis was negative for ketones, and there is not an anion gap, making overt ketoacidosis unlikely.

Answer D is incorrect. Metformin can cause lactic acidosis, which should cause an anion gap metabolic acidosis. Based on the laboratory values, the anion gap is normal with a value of 6.

4. **The correct answer is E.** Meconium aspiration syndrome results from aspiration of meconium before, during, or after delivery, and results from meconium that is introduced into the tracheobronchial tree below the level of the vocal cords. The thick, dark green amniotic fluid refers to meconium-stained fluid and indicates that the fetus has passed meconium while in the amniotic sac. Amnioinfusion works by diluting the meconium and thereby reducing the risk of aspiration of thick meconium, which can lead to respiratory distress in the newborn.

Answer A is incorrect. Amnioinfusion does not affect the likelihood of injuring the brachial plexus during delivery. Brachial plexus injuries are likely to result during delivery of a large or breech baby.

Answer B is incorrect. Amnioinfusion does not increase the likelihood of breech presentation. Breech presentations can be encountered in women with large fibroids or abnormal uterine shape, history of premature births, oligohydramnios, and multiple gestation pregnancy.

Answer C is incorrect. Amnioinfusion is an indication for prophylaxis against chorioamnionitis in premature rupture of membranes, not in the case being presented.

Answer D is incorrect. Amnioinfusion is indicated for recurrent variable decelerations, which reflect umbilical cord compression and hypoxemic distress to the fetus. Early decelerations are reassuring and do not warrant amnioinfusion.

5. **The correct answer is A.** This case presents a classic picture of intussusception, which is the most common cause of bowel obstruction in the first 2 years of life. Its etiology is unknown, but risk factors include male gender, Meckel's diverticulum, intestinal lymphoma, Henoch-Schönlein purpura, parasites, polyps, adenovirus infection and other upper respiratory infections, celiac disease, and cystic fibrosis. In a hemodynamically stable patient without signs of bowel perforation, air contrast or barium enema is the appropriate first step to both diagnose the intussusception and potentially reduce it. Barium enemas will demonstrate a filling defect or cupping in the head of barium, where the advancement is impeded by the intussusception. An alternative to barium is an air enema under fluoroscopic guidance, reducing the risk of barium spillage. Additionally, such interventions are often therapeutic by way of pressure reduction of the intussusception.

Answer B is incorrect. Colonoscopy has been used to diagnose and treat intussusception in older children and adults. However, in this infant, a barium or air contrast enema should be first-line treatment, followed by surgery if such an intervention fails.

Answer C is incorrect. The most common site of intussusception is at the ileocecal junction, far too distal to be visualized in an upper gastrointestinal endoscopy.

Answer D is incorrect. Surgical reduction, the definitive treatment of this disorder, should only be done as first-line treatment in patients with signs of bowel perforation or bleeding, or after the more conservative approach of air contrast or barium enema fails. Surgery has the additional advantage of allowing the surgeon to remove the lead point of the intussusception, such as a Meckel's diverticulum, reducing the chances of recurrence.

Answer E is incorrect. Intussusception must be diagnosed and treated at the first clinical suspicion. Although the child is currently hemodynamically stable, the presence of bloody mucus ("currant jelly stools") should alert the physician to the need for further workup. Prolonged intussusception can lead to bowel ischemia, perforation, and peritonitis. Prognosis is directly related to the duration of the intussusception before reduction.

6. **The correct answer is A.** All patients who undergo deceleration injuries (falls from heights or high-speed motor vehicle collisions) should be worked up for aortic disruption because this is a highly lethal diagnosis if not managed emergently. This diagnosis must also be considered in patients with sternal fractures or rib fractures. The disruption typically occurs distal to the ligamentum arteriosum because the aorta distal to this is mobile, while the aorta proximal to this is fixed, thereby permitting shearing stress to occur during rapid deceleration. The thoracic aortic adventitia of patients who survive this diagnosis (about 15%) remains intact, therefore preventing fatal hemorrhage. Although this patient's x-ray of the chest demonstrates characteristic findings for aortic disruption, it is not specific. Arteriography remains the gold standard for making the diagnosis.

Answer B is incorrect. MRI is not indicated for the diagnosis of aortic disruption because of the lengthy time involved in acquiring the image, as well as its limitations in patients with pacemakers and other metallic implants.

Answer C is incorrect. Needle decompression is both diagnostic and therapeutic for a tension pneumothorax. Although a pneumothorax may occur during a traumatic injury (espe-

cially one in which there are rib fractures), this patient's history, physical examination, and radiographic findings are more consistent with a diagnosis of aortic disruption than a pneumothorax.

Answer D is incorrect. Transthoracic echocardiography (TTE) is a noninvasive method for evaluating cardiac anatomy and function. This imaging modality is limited, however, because thoracic structures such as ribs and lungs do not allow for full evaluation of cardiac anatomy and the aorta. Due to its limitations, TTE would not be the best test for use in working up a diagnosis of aortic disruption.

Answer E is incorrect. Upper endoscopy is useful for visualizing the upper gastrointestinal (GI) tract; however, it has no utility in the diagnosis of an aortic disruption. This patient shows no clinical signs of acute GI injury (ie, upper GI bleeding and/or mediastinal emphysema) and does not require endoscopy at this time.

7. **The correct answer is F.** Scarlet fever consists of an upper respiratory tract infection that is associated with a characteristic rash. It is caused by group A *Streptococcus*. The rash often appears within 24–48 hours after symptom onset. It usually spares the face, instead affecting the neck, trunk, and extremities. The rash is a diffuse, erythematous, papular eruption (sandpaper rash) that is often bright red in color and blanches on pressure. Antibiotics, such as penicillin, are commonly used in treatment to shorten the clinical course of disease and to prevent rheumatic fever.

Answer A is incorrect. This presentation is not consistent with fifth disease (parvovirus B19), which typically presents without a prodrome and whose major manifestation is a erythematous "slapped cheek" rash that is pruritic and maculopapular in nature, and spreads from the arms to the trunk and legs. Parvovirus B19 may precipitate an anaplastic crisis in susceptible patient populations.

Answer B is incorrect. This presentation is not consistent with impetigo (*Staphylococcus aureus* or group A *Streptococcus*), which typically presents without any constitutional symptoms and is manifest by superficial bacterial infection of the skin. The lesions are vesiculopustular in nature and often rupture ("weepy" lesions), leaking exudate that forms a characteristic golden crust.

Answer C is incorrect. This presentation is not consistent with Kawasaki disease, which is a vasculitic disease that has strict diagnostic criteria, including high-grade fever (> 5 days) plus four of the following: bilateral conjunctivitis, polymorphous rash, cervical lymphadenopathy, diffuse mucous membrane erythema, and/or erythema of the palms/soles or indurative edema of the hands/feet.

Answer D is incorrect. This presentation is not consistent with classic measles (a paramyxovirus), which typically presents with a prodrome of the "3 C's" (Cough, Conjunctivitis, and Coryza), with the appearance of Koplik's spots on the buccal mucosa. The viral exanthem (beginning 1–2 days after the prodrome) is characterized by an erythematous, maculopapular rash spreading from the head toward the feet.

Answer E is incorrect. This presentation is not consistent with mononucleosis (Epstein-Barr virus), which typically presents with pharyngitis, fever, lymphadenopathy, and fatigue, but without a characteristic rash. When patients with mononucleosis are treated with ampicillin, they may develop a diffuse rash resembling that of measles; however, this child had no history of recent antibiotic use.

8. **The correct answer is A.** This patient is presenting with characteristic signs and symptoms of acute suppurative cholangitis with developing sepsis known as Reynolds' pentad (fever, jaundice, right upper quadrant pain, hypotension, and altered mental status). However, more important for management than her high WBC count and dilated intrahepatic ducts with pneumobilia (indicative of suppurative ascending cholangitis) is her hemodynamic instability and evidence of hypoperfusion to vital organs (i.e., brain), in other words, her developing sepsis. Stabilizing her requires large-bore vascular access and fluid resuscitation to bolster her blood pressure. This takes precedence over the decompression of her biliary tree; she would not be able to tolerate

anesthesia (most of which would cause further hypotension) without it.

Answer B is incorrect. Adequate imaging has already been performed, and there are more pressing issues to manage initially.

Answer C is incorrect. Emergent decompression of the biliary tree is the appropriate management for acute cholangitis that does not respond to intravenous (IV) fluid resuscitation, nothing-by-mouth status, and appropriate broad-spectrum empiric IV antibiotics. The development of sepsis and hemodynamic instability takes precedence over the decompression of the biliary tree. Additionally, more than 70% of patients with acute cholangitis will respond to this regimen and will not require decompression. If decompression is eventually required, endoscopic sphincterotomy with stone extraction and/or stent insertion is the treatment of choice for establishing biliary drainage in acute cholangitis. Open surgery or a direct percutaneous interventional radiology procedure is an acceptable consideration, although there are increased rates of morbidity and mortality with open surgery.

Answer D is incorrect. Nasogastric suction may be required if the patient is vomiting and has severely impaired mental status, putting her at high risk for aspiration. This may be necessary; however, intravascular resuscitation in this case is more important due to the developing sepsis.

Answer E is incorrect. Oral antibiotics are not appropriate as a treatment for acute cholangitis, nor does the administration of antibiotic therapy take priority over fluid resuscitation in a septic patient.

9. **The correct answer is B.** The patient is most likely infected with *Histoplasma capsulatum,* a fungus endemic to the Ohio and Mississippi river valleys. The infection causes a mild febrile syndrome in most and a self-limited pneumonia in some. Patients complain of chest pain or cough. Physical examination is generally unremarkable despite radiographic findings of infiltrates and mediastinal and hilar lymphadenopathy. A complement fixation titer of at least 1:32 or a fourfold increase in titer is suggestive of acute histoplasmosis. Dissemi-

nated disease with chronic pneumonia reflects uncontained or poorly contained primary disease, or reactivation of a primary disease in the context of HIV infection. Chronic disseminated disease in a young healthy patient may not always require amphotericin B, but this answer option describes the best drug regimen. Treatment with amphotericin B, or with itraconazole in patients without meningeal disease, is generally curative.

Answer A is incorrect. *Histoplasma capsulatum* is a fungus and antibiotics are less effective than antifungals in treating this class of pathogens.

Answer C is incorrect. Nystatin swish and swallow is predominantly used for oral candidal infections. *Candida* is a fungus characteristically infecting the oral mucosa and tongue of those on broad-spectrum antibiotics, corticosteroids, or those with impaired cell-mediated immunity (i.e., AIDS patients). Without mention of antibiotic course, steroids, or compromised immunity, in the context of signs and symptoms inconsistent with oral candidiasis, nystatin is a poor choice for treatment.

Answer D is incorrect. Pyrazinamide is used to treat tuberculosis in combination with isoniazid and rifampin. Tuberculosis is caused by *Mycobacterium tuberculosis* and is characterized by the formation of tubercles on the lungs and other tissues of the body. Patients tend to present coughing up sputum and blood, with fever, weight loss, and chest pain. Infectious particles are spread via respiratory droplets. Risk factors for acquisition of the disease include close contact with infected individuals generally in the context of military barracks, prisons, and endemic areas of the world. Immunocompromise increases the likelihood for symptomatic, disseminated disease. His purified protein derivative test is negative, and in the absence of severe immunocompromise, it makes tuberculosis less likely.

Answer E is incorrect. Trimethoprim-sulfamethoxazole is useful as an antibiotic and in the treatment of parasitic diseases, notably pneumonia due to *Pneumocystis jiroveci* (formerly *carinii*), a fungus causing pneumonia in those with weakened immune systems, including the young, elderly, and malnourished, and

those with AIDS; and toxoplasmosis, a parasitic disease caused by the protozoan *Toxoplasma gondii*. The most common method of acquisition by humans is consumption or handling of raw or undercooked meat, though handling of cat feces is also a classic risk factor. In healthy adults infection is generally asymptomatic, but in the immunodeficient the disease may prove fatal, with encephalitis, chorioretinitis, and other cardiac and hepatic manifestations. It is not effective in the treatment of histoplasmosis.

10. **The correct answer is E.** This patient presents with neck soreness in the setting of a moderate-speed motor vehicle accident. There are no focal neurologic signs, no other distracting injuries (painful injuries that can mask other concerning injuries), and no signs of intoxication. Neither has there been a loss of consciousness. It is therefore reasonable to trust the patient's symptoms and signs as an indication of the severity of her neck injury. In this case, because midline tenderness, obvious deformities, and focal neurologic findings are absent, radiographic studies are not warranted. A supervised trial without the collar is appropriate.

Answer A is incorrect. Cervical MRI scan is an appropriate intervention to demonstrate the extent of soft tissue injury in the event of neck trauma. It should be used only when there is reason to suspect spinal cord injury or vertebral fracture.

Answer B is incorrect. Halo placement is used to stabilize and immobilize cervical fractures.

Answer C is incorrect. Steroids are used to reduce edema and the possibility of permanent damage when frank spinal cord damage is suspected either clinically or radiographically.

Answer D is incorrect. Flexion/extension films are often employed to clear a patient of possible neck cervical spinal injuries when the criteria for collar removal have not been met. If the patient has focal neurologic symptoms, painful distracting injuries, posterior midline tenderness, any evidence of intoxication, or an altered level of alertness, these studies should be obtained before clearing a patient's neck injuries.

11. **The correct answer is B.** This boy has premature virilization secondary to increased androgens. Of the answers listed here, all should be increased in the case of premature virilization except cortisol. Given that his father also went through puberty at a very young age, this boy's premature virilization is more likely to be caused by an inherited condition than an androgen-secreting tumor. A deficiency in 21-hydroxylase would lead to shunting of the 17α-hydroxyprogesterone from the glucocorticoid pathway into the androgen pathway. This is a benign condition in children, and the parents should be reassured. The child should be followed when he goes through true puberty in the event that his premature virilization is a precursor to other conditions, such as type 2 diabetes.

Answer A is incorrect. Androstenedione is a precursor to testosterone, and therefore would not be expected to be decreased in a case of virilization.

Answer C is incorrect. Dihydrotestosterone is the active form of testosterone. To develop male-pattern hair, testosterone must be converted to dihydrotestosterone by 5α-reductase found in the skin. Levels of dihydrotestosterone would not be decreased in a patient with virilization.

Answer D is incorrect. 17α-Hydroxyprogesterone is the branch point for the glucocorticoid and androgen pathways (using 21-hydroxylase and 17α-hydroxylase, respectively), and is increased in cases of 21-hydroxylase deficiency. Levels of 17α-hydroxyprogesterone would not be expected to be low in a patient with virilization.

Answer E is incorrect. 5α-Reductase is an enzyme found in the skin that converts testosterone to the active dihydrotestosterone, which is responsible for male-pattern hair growth. Levels of 5α-reductase would not be decreased in a patient with virilization.

12. **The correct answer is B.** The differential diagnosis of painless unilateral vision loss can include several possibilities. The patient reports a history of transient ischemic attacks and has a history of hypertension and diabetes, all of which are risk factors for central retinal artery occlusion. Additionally, funduscopic examination shows a cherry red spot and surrounding retinal edema (yellow). Results of treatment remain unsatisfactory; however, the goal is to restore blood flow as soon as possible. This is accomplished by decreasing intraocular pressure to promote retinal perfusion and to potentially dislodge emboli (intravenous acetazolamide, topical β-blockers, and ocular massage).

Answer A is incorrect. In acute ophthalmic artery occlusion, there is usually no cherry red spot in the foveola. The entire retina typically appears whitened.

Answer C is incorrect. Central retinal vein occlusion can also present with painless unilateral vision loss. It occurs in patients who are elderly and is often idiopathic. The examination typically shows diffuse retinal hemorrhages in all four quadrants, with dilated, tortuous retinal veins. There may also be cotton-wool spots, disc edema, and neovascularization of the disc or retina.

Answer D is incorrect. Giant cell arteritis typically occurs in patients older than 50 years with a history of temporal headaches, scalp tenderness, jaw claudication, muscle pains, weakness, or weight loss. Erythrocyte sedimentation rate is also typically elevated.

Answer E is incorrect. A cherry red spot is seen in Tay-Sachs disease, but it typically presents early in life, occurs bilaterally, and is accompanied by other systemic manifestations.

13. **The correct answer is E.** The story described is classic for a foreign body ingestion. Eighty percent of foreign body ingestions occur in children. Most such episodes occur in children 6 months to 3 years old. Older children are often the culprits for the introduction of the foreign body to the younger patient. Initially, an episode of choking, gagging, and coughing may be followed by dysphagia, increased salivation, food refusal, emesis, or pain in the neck, throat, or sternal notch region. The first step in evaluation of suspected foreign body ingestion involves plain anteroposterior radiographs of the neck, chest, and abdomen, with lateral views of the neck and chest.

Answer A is incorrect. Barium contrast radiologic evaluation may be helpful in asymptomatic patients with negative plain films, but this study is discouraged because of the risk of aspiration. Additionally, the use of contrast can make subsequent visualization of the object and removal of it more difficult.

Answer B is incorrect. There is no evidence in the history that this patient has an infectious etiology to his symptoms and presentation. A complete blood cell count with differential would not aid in the diagnosis of foreign body ingestion.

Answer C is incorrect. Endoscopic evaluation is the management strategy for symptomatic patients with negative plain films or patients with respiratory distress or other evidence of a life-threatening condition. Endoscopic evaluation in a stable patient without prior radiologic studies would not be recommended.

Answer D is incorrect. Although this patient is not experiencing respiratory distress or showing evidence of impending distress, a full work-up for suspected foreign body ingestion should be initiated. Given the history, foreign body ingestion is a likely cause for this patient's presentation, so parental reassurance and discharge from the emergency department without a work-up is not a good option. The potential sequelae of foreign body ingestion include impaction, mucosal erosion, abrasion, local scarring, migration, peritonitis, mediastinitis, pneumomediastinum, pneumonia, or even aortoenteric fistula.

14. **The correct answer is E.** Status epilepticus (SE) refers to a continuous state of seizure activity or a series of seizures during which there is no return to consciousness in the inter-ictal period. The minimal duration of seizure activity in SE has traditionally been cited as 15–30 minutes. Practically speaking, anyone who is brought to an emergency department who has been seizing for more than 5 minutes will be treated as having SE. SE is a medical emergency with a wide range of potentially lethal complications. Prolonged intractable muscle contraction secondary to seizures can lead to respiratory compromise, rhabdomyolysis, hyperthermia, and lactic acidosis.

Answer A is incorrect. Irreversible neuronal injury (seen as cortical laminar necrosis) is thought to occur after as few as 30–60 minutes of continuous seizure activity.

Answer B is incorrect. The initial management of patients in status epilepticus is aimed at securing the patient's airway and administering agents to cause cessation of seizure activity and is the same regardless of the underlying cause.

Answer C is incorrect. The mortality of patients in status epilepticus is approximately 20%.

Answer D is incorrect. After 45 minutes of continuous seizure activity, symptoms may become subtle as myoclonic activity decreases. Such patients are often still seizing within the central nervous system and remain at risk for serious neuronal damage.

15. **The correct answer is A.** Tight blood pressure control during pregnancy is important to prevent complications, such as preeclampsia or eclampsia, placental abruption, intrauterine growth retardation (IUGR) with oligohydramnios, or preterm birth. IUGR is presumed secondary to uteroplacental insufficiency due to partial placental abruption or vasoconstriction of the placental vessels.

Answer B is incorrect. Macrosomia, or fetal growth in excess of 5000 grams, is a frequent complication of poorly controlled gestational diabetes, not hypertension.

Answer C is incorrect. Placenta previa is not associated with hypertension during pregnancy. Placental abruption is a frequent complication of hypertension.

Answer D is incorrect. Oligohydramnios, not polyhydramnios, is associated with hypertension during pregnancy.

Answer E is incorrect. Rocker-bottom feet are associated with trisomy 13 and 18.

16. **The correct answer is B.** Bupropion is an atypical antidepressant (blocking norepinephrine and dopamine reuptake) that was found, for unclear reasons, to increase the risk of seizures in patients suffering from anorexia by

decreasing the seizure threshold. Bupropion is also contraindicated in patients undergoing an abrupt withdrawal from alcohol or benzodiazepines and should be used with caution in patients with seizure disorders. Clinicians should use this medication cautiously in patients with eating disorders and only if no other options are available.

Answer A is incorrect. Aripiprazole is an atypical antipsychotic agent and is not a first-line agent in the treatment of depression. Adverse effects include dry mouth, constipation, and anxiety.

Answer C is incorrect. Escitalopram is a selective serotonin reuptake inhibitor used for the treatment of depression. Its adverse effects include restlessness, nausea, blurred vision, difficulty sleeping, and dry mouth.

Answer D is incorrect. Fluoxetine is a first-line agent used in treating depression in patients with eating disorders. It is a selective serotonin reuptake inhibitor, and common adverse effects include nausea, irritability, and sexual dysfunction.

Answer E is incorrect. Imipramine is a tricyclic antidepressant used in the treatment of depression. It has not been shown to be associated with a decreased seizure threshold.

17. **The correct answer is F.** In an outpatient population of otherwise healthy individuals under the age of 60 years, one of the most likely pathogens is *Streptococcus pneumoniae*. The consolidated lobar pneumonia seen in the radiograph is typical of pneumococcal disease.

Answer A is incorrect. *Escherichia coli* most commonly causes pneumonia in patients > 60 years old or with comorbidities, including chronic obstructive pulmonary disease, heart failure, diabetes, liver disease, and alcohol abuse. *E. coli* is a rare cause of pneumonia, and when it is isolated it is typically in a hospital-acquired, not community-acquired, pneumonia.

Answer B is incorrect. *Klebsiella* most commonly causes pneumonia in patients > 60 years old or with comorbidities, including chronic obstructive pulmonary disease, heart failure, diabetes, liver disease, and alcohol

abuse. Classically, *Klebsiella pneumoniae* presents with currant-jelly sputum, and is often due to aspiration (as in an alcoholic).

Answer C is incorrect. *Mycoplasma* is a common cause of community-acquired pneumonia in healthy persons. However, the radiographic appearance of mycoplasmal pneumonia is usually the "atypical" pattern of diffuse infiltrate throughout the lungs, without lobar consolidation.

Answer D is incorrect. *Pseudomonas* should be considered in patients with cystic fibrosis and in those with nosocomial pneumonia, neutropenia, or late-stage HIV infection. It rarely causes community-acquired pneumonia in healthy patients.

Answer E is incorrect. *Staphylococcus aureus* most commonly causes pneumonia in patients > 60 years old or with comorbidities, including chronic obstructive pulmonary disease, heart failure, diabetes, liver disease, and alcohol abuse. It is the most common cause of ventilator-associated pneumonia.

18. **The correct answer is B.** The lesions in pemphigus vulgaris (PV) are a result of antibodies against the intraepidermal desmogleins 1 and 3. When mucosal lesions predominate, anti-desmoglein 3 antibodies can be found in isolation. The appearance of oropharyngeal flaccid bullae that rupture easily to leave ulcerated lesions is an early presentation of PV. The lesions are painful and may cause difficulty eating. Other common areas of skin involvement are the scalp, groin, axillae, and face. The diagnosis of PV requires skin biopsy showing intraepithelial acantholysis with intact basement membrane.

Answer A is incorrect. Anti–basement membrane antibodies are typically found in Goodpasture's syndrome, a pulmonary-renal disorder that does not involve the skin.

Answer C is incorrect. Bullous pemphigoid (BP) is caused by antihemidesmosomal antibodies, resulting in disruption subepidermally, at the basement membrane. Oral mucosa is involved in one-third of all cases, but the predominant areas affected are flexural surfaces, including the groin and axillae. Blisters are tenser, with thicker rims than in pemphigus vulgaris (PV), but may leave erosions and crusting when unroofed. BP typically occurs in adults > 60 years versus middle-age prevalence in PV. Biopsy is required for the diagnosis of BP, showing subepithelial blister formation.

Answer D is incorrect. Multiple painful oral ulcers are often the earliest manifestation of Behçet's disease and may also be seen in Crohn's disease. However, these ulcers are not preceded by vesicles or bullae and do not occur outside the oral mucosa. Instead, they are frequently associated with manifestations of the underlying disease process.

Answer E is incorrect. The oral lesions in herpes simplex virus (HSV) infection can be very painful but are more typically vesicular with evolution to a crusting stage. Recurrent HSV lesions primarily occur on nonkeratinized mucosa such as the lips or gums.

19. **The correct answer is C.** The patient suffers from a global aphasia, characterized by a global impairment in language comprehension, fluency, and word repetition. This occurs when there are both anterior and posterior lesions.

Answer A is incorrect. Broca's aphasia is characterized by problems with language production, but preserved comprehension. The lesion that causes Broca's aphasia affects the third frontal convolution of the left frontal lobe. It corresponds to Brodmann's areas 44 and 45.

Answer B is incorrect. Conduction aphasia is characterized by problems with repeating what is said, but preserved fluency and comprehension. It results from damage to the arcuate fasciculus, a band of nerve fibers that connects Broca's and Wernicke's areas.

Answer D is incorrect. This type of aphasia is characterized by impaired fluency, but preserved repetition and comprehension. Lesions that cause transcortical motor aphasia are typically smaller than those that cause Broca's aphasia and are superior to and often anterior to Broca's area (Broca's area is not affected).

Answer E is incorrect. Wernicke's aphasia represents a problem with language comprehension, which affects both language output and input. Wernicke's area is the posterior region of the left superior temporal gyrus or the first gyrus of the temporal lobe. This area corresponds to Brodmann's areas 21 and 42.

20. **The correct answer is B.** This patient is presenting with clinical and radiologic evidence of a partial small bowel obstruction. She does not appear to have a complete obstruction because she is still passing flatus and has air in her colon on films. Additionally, she has no evidence of necrotic bowel or peritoneal signs on examination, so she is not likely to require emergent surgical intervention. The appropriate management of a partial small bowel obstruction is to admit to the hospital for observation, decompress the bowel proximal to the obstruction with nasogastric (NG) suction, place "nothing by mouth," and replace ongoing fluid losses from vomiting/NG suction to avoid electrolyte abnormalities.

Answer A is incorrect. Although intravenous fluids are important to rehydrate a patient who has been vomiting, the bilious color of her vomitus suggests bowel obstruction, not pancreatitis, making endoscopic retrograde cholangiopancreatography unnecessary. It is important to make the patient "nothing by mouth" and place an nasogastric tube to eliminate bilious fluid from the stomach.

Answer C is incorrect. A rectal tube can be a therapeutic intervention for a large bowel obstruction but plays no role in small bowel obstruction.

Answer D is incorrect. Emergency laparotomy is not necessary in cases of partial bowel obstruction. However, peritonitis due to bowel obstruction is a surgical emergency. In such cases, the clinical, radiologic, and electrolyte picture would have to point toward peritonitis, ischemic bowel, and no air distal to the obstruction.

Answer E is incorrect. Observation in the emergency department is not appropriate, especially if one has not taken steps to manage the obstruction indicated by the films and clinical picture (i.e., nasogastric tube and intravenous fluid replacement).

21. **The correct answer is C.** This patient most likely suffers from chronic obstructive pulmonary disease, as evidenced by his physical examination and pulmonary function tests indicative of obstructive disease. Destruction of lung parenchyma leads to abnormally enlarged airspaces, as suggested by the increased residual volume and hyperinflation on x-ray of the chest.

Answer A is incorrect. An apical cavitary lesion is characteristic of tuberculosis, which would not typically result in prolonged expiration or decreased FEV_1:FVC.

Answer B is incorrect. Diffuse bilateral infiltrates often occur in infectious processes, which would not likely present as insidiously as this patient or cause increased residual volume on pulmonary function tests. Congestive heart failure, another possible cause of this picture, would not produce major abnormalities on pulmonary function testing.

Answer D is incorrect. Lobar consolidation most commonly occurs in infectious processes, which would not likely present as insidiously as this patient or cause increased residual volume on pulmonary function tests.

Answer E is incorrect. Mass lesion with mediastinal adenopathy may be seen in lung carcinoma, which would not likely cause increased residual volume (although changes associated with emphysema, the correct answer, are not uncommon in patients with lung cancer for obvious reasons).

22. **The correct answer is E.** This infant is at risk of developing hyperbilirubinemia because of several factors: she is breast-fed, was carried nearly to full term, and is of east Asian descent. Maternal age > 35 years is also a risk factor. It is physiologic for bilirubin to increase after birth, peaking between postpartum days 5 and 7. However, levels this high are abnormal. Bilirubin can be neurotoxic, so it is important to reduce bilirubin levels in the neonate to prevent kernicterus (also known as bilirubin encephalopathy). Phototherapy is the principal treatment for unconjugated hyperbilirubinemia, as it converts unconjugated bilirubin into water-soluble compounds that can be excreted in the urine.

Answer A is incorrect. In conjugated hyperbilirubinemia, abdominal ultrasound is usually the initial test to evaluate for structural abnormalities of the biliary tree.

Answer B is incorrect. Fiberoptic bilirubin blankets are only appropriate for term infants with nonhemolytic disease and mild hyperbilirubinemia. This neonate's bilirubin level is significantly elevated and requires close observation rather than discharge. Breast milk and poor hydrational status can lead to an increased bilirubin level, so supplementing breast milk with formula or temporarily switching to formula might be advisable.

Answer C is incorrect. Jaundice can occur in the setting of sepsis, in which case it is important to treat both the jaundice and the underlying cause (the infection). Sepsis is less likely in this infant because of her normal WBC count and lack of risk factors. If she were to be treated for sepsis, ampicillin and gentamicin are the most common empiric treatment.

Answer D is incorrect. Exchange transfusions are rarely performed. This is reserved for neonates with signs of bilirubin neurotoxicity (seizures, high-pitched cry, lethargy, poor feeding, and hypertonicity) or when bilirubin levels are exceptionally high. The specific bilirubin level that requires a transfusion is based on an algorithm that takes into account the infant's age, gestational age, failure of prior attempts at phototherapy, presence of isoimmune hemolytic disease, sepsis, glucose-6-phosphate dehydrogenase deficiency, asphyxia, temperature instability, and acidosis.

23. **The correct answer is A.** These values indicate a hypokalemic, alkalotic patient, as expected in primary hyperaldosteronism. In primary hyperaldosteronism, there is autonomous, unregulated production of aldosterone. Aldosterone causes potassium wasting by acting on the cortical collecting ducts to stimulate potassium secretion into the tubular fluid and by enhancing sodium retention, thereby encouraging potassium loss through the Na^+-K^+ countertransport. Hypokalemia results in an increased hydrogen ion loss that causes the associated metabolic alkalosis.

Answer B is incorrect. These findings indicate isolated hyponatremia. Aldosterone hypersecretion results in sodium retention.

Answer C is incorrect. These values represent normal serum electrolytes.

Answer D is incorrect. P Hyponatremia with hyperkalemia is seen in acute adrenal insufficiency. Low levels of aldosterone result in sodium loss and thus potassium retention through the Na⁺-K⁺ transporter.

Answer E is incorrect. A decrease in bicarbonate results in metabolic acidosis, rather than the alkalosis seen in hyperaldosteronism.

24. **The correct answer is C.** The man has aortoiliac occlusive disease which is causing his constellation of symptoms including impotence, claudication of the buttocks, and global lower extremity atrophy. This classic presentation is called Leriche's syndrome. Vascular disease must be considered when patients complain of impotence. Thirty to fifty percent of men with aortoiliac occlusive disease have impotence. In aortoiliac occlusive disease, you should expect to see a weak or absent femoral pulse, an ankle-brachial index (ABI) which is slightly sub-normal to normal at rest (this patient has no rest pain), and an ABI that is decreased with exercise. ABI = ratio of blood pressure (BP) in the ankle to BP in the arm. Normal is > 1.0, with claudication (pain with exercise) < 0.7, and with rest pain < 0.4.

Answer A is incorrect. An ankle-brachial index at rest of 0.3 would likely cause rest pain

Answer B is incorrect. This answer is incorrect because an ankle-brachial index (ABI) at rest of 0.3 would likely be causing pain at rest, which this patient does not have. Also, if occlusive disease is suspected, the ABI should not increase with exercise.

Answer D is incorrect. One would not expect the femoral pulse to be increased in the setting of aortoiliac occlusive disease. The ankle-brachial index is also too low not to be associated with rest pain.

Answer E is incorrect. This answer is incorrect because the femoral pulse should not be increased in this patient. The ankle-brachial

indices at rest and with exercise are what would be expected.

25. **The correct answer is A.** Allopurinol, a xanthine oxidase inhibitor, assists in lowering plasma urate and urinary uric acid concentrations. This effect aids in tophus mobilization and is the first-line therapy for prophylaxis of recurrent gout. Allopurinol will transiently raise uric acid levels.

Answer B is incorrect. Colchicine can be used for treatment of chronic gout (as well as acute gout flares) but is less preferred due to its adverse effect profile. Up to 80% of colchicine users suffer gastrointestinal adverse effects, including cramping, nausea, and diarrhea.

Answer C is incorrect. In cases of acute gout, the pharmacologic treatment of choice is a nonsteroidal anti-inflammatory drug, often indomethacin.

Answer D is incorrect. Use of corticosteroids is mainly reserved for treatment of acute gout in patients who cannot tolerate nonsteroidal anti-inflammatory drugs.

Answer E is incorrect. Niacin use can be associated with acquired hyperuricemia and would potentiate, not prevent, recurrent episodes of gout.

26. **The correct answer is E.** Rocky Mountain spotted fever is caused by infection with *Rickettsia rickettsii*. It may be transmitted by either *Dermacentor andersoni* or *D. variabilis*. Symptoms include fever, conjunctival redness, severe headache, and a rash that initially appears on the wrists, ankles, soles, and palms, and later spreads to the trunk. Infection is endemic in the southeast United States. Treatment is with doxycycline and chloramphenicol, and is considered curative.

Answer A is incorrect. Aspergillomas are formed when the fungus *Aspergillus* grows in a clump in a preexisting pulmonary cavity, or when the organism invades previously healthy tissue, causing an abscess. Risk factors for the development of this infection include conditions that create pulmonary cavities, including histoplasmosis, tuberculosis, lung abscess, cystic fibrosis, sarcoidosis, or previous lung cancer. Presenting symptoms include hemoptysis (in up to 75% of patients) chest pain, shortness of breath, weight loss, and fever. Diagnosis is confirmed with x-ray or CT of the chest, sputum culture, bronchoalveolar lavage, and/or serum precipitins for *Aspergillus*. Treatment is often not needed, but if bleeding is a concern it may be dealt with surgically. Infection in an immunocompromised patient warrants treatment with itraconazole, voriconazole, or amphotericin B. Patients generally recover fully. The primary route of *Aspergillus* transmission is inhalation.

Answer B is incorrect. Bubonic plague is caused by *Yersinia pestis*, a gram-negative bacterium with a bipolar staining pattern. Patients present with grossly swollen lymph nodes, fever, headache, and a blackish discoloration of the skin. The disease resides in rodents and is transmitted to humans by the bite of the flea. It is most common in the southwestern United States. Treatment is with gentamicin, which is considered curative. Untreated *Yersinia pestis* infection carries a 75% mortality rate.

Answer C is incorrect. Lyme disease is caused by an infection with *Borrelia burgdorferi* and typically presents with fever, headache, fatigue, and a characteristic skin rash called erythema chronicum migrans. Treatment is generally curative and is accomplished with oral doxycycline, amoxicillin, or cefuroxime axetil. Patients with certain neurologic or cardiac forms of illness may require intravenous treatment with drugs such as ceftriaxone or penicillin. The infection is transmitted by the deer tick or white-footed mouse tick. Endemic areas include New York, New Jersey, Connecticut, Rhode Island, Massachusetts, Wisconsin, and Minnesota, though infections are becoming more common in nonendemic areas.

Answer D is incorrect. Malaria is not endemic to Maryland and is not transmitted by ticks, but rather by the *Anopheles* mosquito. It may be caused by one of four protozoa: *Plasmodium falciparum*, *P. vivax*, *P. ovale*, and *P. malariae*. The disease presents with episodic severe chills and high fevers along with profuse sweating. Treatment is with chloroquine with the addition of primaquine for *P. vivax* and *P. ovale* infections. Infection is endemic to the tropics.

27. **The correct answer is A.** Active liver disease is an absolute contraindication to oral contraceptive administration for two reasons. First, orally administered steroid hormones are metabolized in the liver and thus will not be appropriately cleared in patients with liver disease. Second, studies have suggested a theoretical increase in the risk of liver disease in users of high-dose oral contraceptives.

Answer B is incorrect. Oral contraceptive administration is absolutely contraindicated in a patient with a history of thromboembolic disease. A history of arterial disease such as atherosclerosis, however, is not a contraindication.

Answer C is incorrect. Pregnancy, not lactation, is a contraindication to oral contraceptive use. Although oral contraceptive use in early pregnancy has not generally been associated with an increased risk of congenital abnormalities, studies suggest that there may be an increased risk of congenital urinary tract defects.

Answer D is incorrect. Active heavy smoking (> 15 cigarettes a day) in women older than age 35 years is an absolute contraindication to oral contraceptive administration. Occasional smoking, particularly in a woman younger than 35 years of age, is a relative risk but not an absolute contraindication.

Answer E is incorrect. OCPs are commonly prescribed to treat hemorrhage associated with uterine fibroids. The presence of fibroids is thus not a contraindication to oral contraceptive administration. However, undiagnosed abnormal uterine bleeding is a contraindication, and the source must be identified before oral contraception can be used.

28. **The correct answer is C.** The patient described has diabetes insipidus (DI), as evidenced by her polyuria, polydipsia, and persistent thirst. Though the laboratory tests do not distinguish between central and nephrogenic DI, given her diagnosis of Langerhans cell histiocytosis (LCH), central DI is more likely, with histiocytic infiltration of the posterior pituitary. In fact, when patients with "isolated" central DI were tested, approximately 15% were diagnosed with LCH. The medication that is used to treat central DI is DDAVP or

desmopressin. This antidiuretic analog is also used in treating patients with von Willebrand's disease, the most common inherited disorder of bleeding. Such patients have a defect in the synthesis or action of von Willebrand factor and DDAVP raises serum levels of von Willebrand factor.

Answer A is incorrect. Symptoms of liver disease will usually be present (e.g., jaundice, pruritus, abdominal pain). Tetracyclines reversibly bind to the 30S ribosomal subunit; this is the mechanism by which they exert their antimicrobial action. However, demeclocycline, a tetracycline, can actually cause nephrogenic diabetes insipidus (DI), and thus using it to treat DI would be counterproductive.

Answer B is incorrect. Desmopressin (DDAVP) indirectly causes an **increase** in plasma factor VIII since von Willebrand factor is also a protein carrier for factor VIII. DDAVP is therefore used in the treatment of some patients with hemophilia type A, in whom factor VIII is deficient.

Answer D is incorrect. Desmopressin is not known to inhibit platelet function.

Answer E is incorrect. Desmopressin has no known effect on cardiovascular outcomes. A drug class that this answer choice could be referring to is thiazide diuretics, which some evidence suggests may prevent adverse cardiovascular outcomes in patients with mild hypertension. Thiazides can also be used in nephrogenic diabetes insipidus to cause volume depletion and increase proximal salt and water absorption.

Answer F is incorrect. Desmopressin has no effect on mood. Lithium is a drug that can cause nephrogenic diabetes insipidus and it is used to stabilize mood.

29. **The correct answer is C.** The patient is comatose, characterized by unresponsiveness to painful stimuli, including a sternal rub or nail bed stimulation. He has a Glasgow Coma Scale (GCS) score of 5 (no eye or verbal response, and decorticate posturing to pain). Furthermore, the toxicology screen and glucose test rule out intoxication or hyperglycemic coma. Anyone with a GCS score < 8 requires immediate intubation due to the likelihood of increased intracranial pressure and consequent respiratory depression.

Answer A is incorrect. Mannitol can be used to temporarily reduce brain swelling secondary to trauma, and it may be useful in this patient if signs of increased intracranial pressure (ICP) appear. However, to stabilize the patient's airway and breathing in the event of increased ICP, intubation is a higher priority.

Answer B is incorrect. A head CT is an important step in this patient's workup because a brain injury is likely, but the patient's breathing must be secured first.

Answer D is incorrect. P An important cause of coma that must be ruled out is hyperglycemia. However, a Glasgow Coma Scale of < 8 in this trauma patient indicates severe brain damage, and measuring blood glucose is secondary to stabilizing the patient's respiration.

Answer E is incorrect. It is possible that this patient has had a severe embolic stroke. However, given that the internal bleeding of this trauma patient has not yet been assessed, tissue plasminogen activator is not appropriate at this time. After stabilizing the patient and imaging studies, this option may be reconsidered.

30. **The correct answer is C.** Neuroleptic malignant syndrome (NMS) is a life-threatening reaction to antipsychotic medications. Symptoms of NMS include sudden altered mental status, stiffness or tremor, and hyperthermia. Autonomic instability (in this case, tachycardia and hypertension) is often associated. Mortality can be as high as 10%, and rhabdomyolysis, myoglobinuria, and acute renal failure can occur, in addition to myocardial infarction, respiratory failure, and seizures. Rapid cooling (with blankets and ice) plus intravenous access for fluid administration are necessary. Dantrolene (a direct acting muscle relaxant) and bromocriptine (a dopamine agonist) are two agents that can be used in cases of neuroleptic malignant syndrome.

Answer A is incorrect. Clonidine is a centrally acting adrenergic agonist that inhibits the sympathetic nervous system via central α_2-adrenergic receptors. While clonidine might work to lower this patient's hypertension, it will not combat the central disease process (neuroleptic malignant syndrome [NMS]). It is not indicated in treatment of NMS.

Answer B is incorrect. The use of cooling blankets and intravenous fluids are methods of rapid cooling that may be beneficial to the patient, but they will not reverse the effects of central dopaminergic blockade from the neuroleptics. Dantrolene will directly relax muscles and bromocriptine will serve as a dopamine agonist.

Answer D is incorrect. Ice packs placed on the patient's axillae and groin are another effective method of rapid cooling. So too is evaporative cooling using water spray with fans. However, these methods do not reverse the effects of central dopaminergic blockade from the neuroleptics. Dantrolene will directly relax muscle and bromocriptine will serve as a dopamine agonist.

Answer E is incorrect. Lorazepam is a benzodiazepine anxiolytic that is relatively quickly absorbed. The drug is used in panic attack for treatment of anxiety and agitation, and for prevention of alcohol and other sedative withdrawal. It would not be effective in the treatment of neuroleptic malignant syndrome.

31. **The correct answer is E.** This patient has signs and symptoms consistent with bronchogenic lung cancer, specifically small cell lung cancer (SCLC). SCLC can be associated with a variety of syndromes, such as syndrome of inappropriate antidiuretic hormone and ACTH production, which are related to the ectopic production of hormones. The patient's combination of hirsutism, purple striae, acne, and hypertension are signs and symptoms consistent with ectopic ACTH production. Staging of SCLC is divided into two categories: limited and extensive. Limited disease is defined as that limited to the ipsilateral hemithorax, while extensive disease is defined as that which has metastasized outside the ipsilateral hemithorax. The use of staging in SCLC is to guide the use of chest radiotherapy, which is indicated in limited, but not extensive, disease. This patient has nodal involvement of the contralateral hemithorax (extensive disease) and

would instead be managed with systemic chemotherapy because of SCLC predilection for metastasis.

Answer A is incorrect. Localized forms of treatment, including radiation and surgical resection, are not the preferred treatment modality in small cell lung cancer because the disease is usually disseminated at time of diagnosis.

Answer B is incorrect. Patients with stage I non-small-cell lung cancer are best managed by surgical resection alone. Surgical resection does not have a role in small cell lung cancer because it is disseminated at time of diagnosis.

Answer C is incorrect. Surgical resection after initial chemotherapy is a therapeutic option for patients with stage IIIa non-small-cell lung cancer. These patients are not suitable for primary resection alone and are often managed via a combined protocol such as surgical resection after initial chemotherapy. In contrast, surgical resection is not commonly performed in small cell lung cancer because the disease is usually metastatic at time of diagnosis, and resection has not been shown to increase long-term survival.

Answer D is incorrect. Surgical resection with radiation (or chemotherapy) is the therapeutic modality employed for patients with stage II non-small-cell lung cancer. In contrast, surgical resection is not commonly performed in small cell lung cancer because the disease is usually metastatic at time of diagnosis, and resection has not been shown to increase long-term survival.

32. **The correct answer is C.** This patient is presenting with signs and symptoms that are highly suspicious for acute cholecystitis. She has all of the "four F's" for typical cholelithiasis patients (**Fat, Forty, Female,** and **Fertile**); in addition, her pain as described is suspicious for biliary colic. On physical examination, mild icterus, low fever, positive Murphy's sign, and tenderness/guarding in the right upper quadrant should prompt evaluation for acute cholecystitis. Since the first-line imaging study was inconclusive, a 5-hydroxyindoleacetic acid (HIDA) (radionuclide biliary scanning) study is the appropriate choice. HIDA is very sensi-

tive and specific for obstruction of the cystic duct.

Answer A is incorrect. CT scanning is not the second-line choice for imaging in suspected cholecystitis due to its lower sensitivity (versus 5-hydroxyindoleacetic acid scan). CT is very useful in the evaluation of neoplasms in the pancreas and hepatobiliary tree.

Answer B is incorrect. Plain abdominal films are rarely diagnostic for stones, because only 10–15% are radiopaque. This imaging modality is useful in the evaluation of acute emphysematous cholecystitis, pneumobilia secondary to a gastrointestinal-biliary fistula, and small bowel obstruction. However, in this case these diagnoses are not likely.

Answer D is incorrect. MRI is not commonly used in the evaluation of acute cholecystitis, due to its high cost and the availability of other highly effective imaging modes for this purpose.

33. **The correct answer is E.** Severe combined immunodeficiency (SCID) is a group of genetic syndromes marked by absent adaptive immune function caused by a failure of lymphocytes to proliferate. All cases have T lymphocyte defects, although some will also have B-lymphocyte and/or natural killer cell problems. Patients affected with SCID generally present within the first few months of life with failure to thrive, diarrhea, recurrent infections, and opportunistic infections caused by *Candida albicans, Pneumocystis jiroveci* (formerly *carinii*), measles, varicella, cytomegalovirus, Epstein-Barr virus, adenovirus, and other such organisms. Patients will have small thymuses that are often < 1 g and can fail to descend from the neck, as well as absence or underdevelopment of other lymphoid tissues (tonsils, adenoids, lymph nodes, and Peyer's patches). Infants with SCID are, by definition, lymphopenic (< 3000/mm^3) at birth, and, therefore, all cases could be identified with a complete blood cell count with differential at the time of birth, a simple screening that can save these children's lives.

Answer A is incorrect. Blood cultures with sensitivities performed at time of presentation would have aided in identifying the etiology of sepsis in this patient but would not have helped in diagnosing severe combined immunodeficiency. Given the acuity of her presentation, blood culture results would not have been available in time to be definitive in identifying the opportunistic pathogens likely implicated in her infections.

Answer B is incorrect. Although cardiac failure eventually developed in this patient as a result of her overwhelming infections, cardiac function is not affected in patients with severe combined immunodeficiency. Therefore, an echocardiogram would not have provided significant information for diagnosing this patient's condition.

Answer C is incorrect. Routine neonatal screening at time of birth is performed for all infants born in hospital settings and was therefore most likely performed for this child. Screening tests are done for a variety of conditions, including congenital hypothyroidism, cystic fibrosis, sickle cell disease, and multiple metabolic disorders, such as phenylketonuria, galactosemia, and homocystinuria, to name a few. Presently, severe combined immunodeficiency is not a routine neonatal screen.

Answer D is incorrect. Serum uric acid can be used as a screening test for deficiency of purine nucleoside phosphorylase (PNP), which results in a mild form of severe combined immunodeficiency (SCID). In PNP deficiency, the level of uric acid will be extremely low. This variant almost never causes immunodeficiency at this young age. Furthermore, PNP deficiency is extremely rare, and only about 50 cases have been described in the medical literature. For these reasons, a WBC count is a much more appropriate general screening test for SCID.

34. **The correct answer is E.** Endocarditis is diagnosed by persistently positive blood cultures (for viridans streptococci, *Streptococcus bovis, Staphylococcus aureus,* enterococci, or **HACEK** group organisms [*Haemophilus* spp., *Actinobacillus actinomycetemcomitans, Cardiobacterium hominis, Eikenella corrodens,* and *Kingella kingae*]), new murmur or cardiac vegetation seen on echocardiography, fever,

petechiae, splinter hemorrhages (linear red-brown lesions in the nail beds), Janeway lesions (painless lesions on palms/soles, as shown in the image), Osler's nodes (painful nodules in pulp of fingers and toes), and Roth spots (retinal hemorrhages). Diagnosis is based on Duke criteria. Endocarditis occurs most commonly in patients with valvular heart disease, congenital heart disease, prosthetic valves, or intravenous drug abusers. Other risk factors include diabetes, advanced age, and the use of anticoagulants or steroids. The patient's presentation with fever, new murmur, and petechiae are highly suggestive of infective endocarditis, and immediate medical management should be started with a α-lactam and an aminoglycoside, pending blood cultures.

Answer A is incorrect. Gentamicin alone is not indicated. It should be combined with a β-lactam to cover resistant streptococci and enterococci.

Answer B is incorrect. A diuretic may be indicated to treat the patient's systolic dysfunction, but antibiotic therapy should be initiated first for treatment of infective endocarditis.

Answer C is incorrect. Metoprolol and enalapril are indicated in the treatment of congestive heart failure. The patient's basilar crackles and edema could be indicative of systolic dysfunction, but this is presumably due to endocarditis, which should be treated first. Congestive heart failure in the absence of infective endocarditis rarely manifests with fever and petechiae. The new-onset murmur also suggests an acute process.

Answer D is incorrect. Penicillin alone is not indicated when the causative organism is unknown, or when there could be an extracardiac source of infection. Penicillin (α-lactam) and gentamicin (aminoglycoside) together cover for the most common microorganisms in infective endocarditis (streptococci and enterococci). Penicillin will cover *Streptococcus bovis* and viridans streptococci. Penicillin alone will not cover enterococci and certain streptococcal strains (C and G).

35. **The correct answer is C.** This patient has a diagnosis of multiple myeloma, a malignancy

of the plasma cells which is associated with hypercoagulability. It is not uncommon for these patients to develop deep venous thrombosis (DVT). This patient also has an increased risk of DVTs because he has been immobile for several weeks. Full anticoagulation must be initiated in order to prevent the development of additional thrombi and progression of the DVT. Since 50% of patients with symptomatic DVTs will develop pulmonary emboli if left untreated, it is recommended that anticoagulation therapy be started in this patient. Anticoagulation in patients with an existing DVT is achieved by either intravenous heparin or low-molecular-weight heparin.

Answer A is incorrect. Patients with malignancy (including multiple myeloma) may have an acquired hypercoagulable state. The treatment in these patients includes traditional treatment for the DVT as well as treatment of the underlying disorder. Since this patient has begun to show signs of disease remission, chemotherapy should be continued at this time.

Answer B is incorrect. Inferior vena cava (IVC) filters are indicated in the treatment of DVTs for patients with contraindications to medical anticoagulants, a history of a recurrent thromboembolism with adequate anticoagulation, pulmonary hypertension with recurrent emboli, or for those patients undergoing surgical pulmonary embolectomy or thromboendarterectomy. IVC filter placement is not considered a first-line treatment in a patient with a DVT. This patient should be started on heparin immediately. Placement of an IVC filter may be considered at a later time if this patient does not respond to medical management.

Answer D is incorrect. The patient is not presenting with any of the signs of pulmonary embolism (dyspnea, pleuritic chest pain, cough, tachypnea, and tachycardia) and does not have physical exam findings or ECG findings suggestive of a pulmonary embolism. Although DVTs in the lower extremities account for about 95% of pulmonary emboli, there is no indication to work-up the diagnosis of a pulmonary embolism in this patient at this time.

Answer E is incorrect. Patients with a history of a DVT are maintained on warfarin as outpatients in order to prevent the development of additional thromboses. Warfarin, however, is not begun immediately in these patients because it is associated with a transient hypercoagulable state due to inhibition of protein C and protein S.

36. **The correct answer is E.** Polymyositis is an inflammatory myopathy. Although rare, this group of disorders (which also includes dermatomyositis and inclusion body myositis) usually presents with symmetric and progressive muscle weakness. Oral prednisone is the preferred agent for initial treatment of polymyositis. The treatment should be started as a high-dose (1 mg/kg daily) regimen for 3–4 weeks, and then slowly tapered over a period of 10 weeks to 1 mg/kg every other day. Following this, the dosage should be reduced by 5–10 mg every 3–4 weeks until the lowest possible dosage with control of symptoms can be determined.

Answer A is incorrect. Immunosuppressive drugs such as azathioprine or methotrexate are second-line agents that are used if initial prednisone therapy is unsuccessful.

Answer B is incorrect. Intravenous immunoglobulin is generally considered a third-line agent to be used when both prednisone therapy and second-line immunosuppressive therapy have failed.

Answer C is incorrect. Methotrexate is not used for initial treatment of polymyositis but is reserved as a second-line agent if prednisone fails.

Answer D is incorrect. Nonsteroidal anti-inflammatory drugs do not have much efficacy in treating polymyositis.

37. **The correct answer is C.** "Double effect" is the ethical principle that states that a palliating treatment is acceptable even if it may hasten death because the intended effect is to relieve the patient's suffering. In this case, opioids may cause respiratory depression and hasten the patient's death after extubation; however, this is ethically acceptable because of the importance of providing palliative comfort measures for the patient.

Answer A is incorrect. Autonomy is the principle stating that physicians must respect the individual rights and opinions of their patients. Although this applies in all cases, this case is not specifically a case of autonomy.

Answer B is incorrect. Dereliction is one of the four elements of a malpractice suit. The physicians in this case are not committing malpractice. After discussion with the patient's family and consideration of the patient's rights and wishes, the physicians are acting in accordance with sound ethical principles.

Answer D is incorrect. The physicians in this case are not committing malpractice; after discussion with the patient's family and consideration of the patient's rights and wishes, the physicians are acting in accordance with sound ethical principles.

Answer E is incorrect. The physicians in this case are offering opioids as a palliative measure, not a treatment intended to hasten the patient's death. This case, in which the patient lacks capacity and her family and physicians decide to withdraw care, is not an example of suicide.

38. **The correct answer is C.** Eosinophilic cytoplasmic inclusions are also known as Lewy bodies and are prevalent neuronal findings in patients with this form of dementia. Lewy body dementia is characterized by new-onset hallucinations, delusions, extrapyramidal signs, and/or repeated loss of balance. Patients may experience periods of lucidity and may undergo extensive delirium evaluations.

Answer A is incorrect. Birefringent crystals are found in joint aspirate of patients with gout.

Answer B is incorrect. Lewy body disease causes neuronal loss in the frontal lobes, locus ceruleus, and substantia nigra. However, darkly pigmented neurons are normal neuronal findings in the substantia nigra, so this answer does not reflect expected abnormal findings.

Answer D is incorrect. Hypersegmented nuclei are features of polymorphonuclear neutrophils, not neurons in Lewy body disease.

Answer E is incorrect. Neurofibrillary tangles and webs can be seen in other forms of dementia but are not specific for Lewy body disease. Neurofibrillary tangles may also be found in Alzheimer's disease and Lewy bodies of Parkinson's disease.

39. **The correct answer is B.** Cystic fibrosis (CF) commonly presents as sinonasal disease in children, often as recurrent sinusitis. Typical symptoms of sinusitis include headache, fever, and cough due to postnasal drip. However, any child with recurrent sinusitis should be evaluated for other structural or immunologic contributors. In cystic fibrosis, the frequency of nasal polyposis is quite variable, but it is rare in individuals without cystic fibrosis. CF is confirmed by a chloride sweat test > 60 mEq/L.

Answer A is incorrect. Allergic rhinitis can cause nasal polyps due to chronic inflammation of the nasal mucosa. However, the disease shows definite seasonal variability, and while it may cause headache and congestion, it also would not cause fever or purulent discharge from the nose unless severe enough to cause acute sinusitis.

Answer C is incorrect. Patients with ciliary dyskinesias, of which Kartagener's is one cause, have structural defects in ciliary function, as opposed to cystic fibrosis, in which there is a mechanical obstruction. The symptoms can appear similar, in that patients with Kartagener's syndrome can present with recurrent sinusitis as well as bronchopulmonary infections. Sterility and situs inversus are classically present. However, the positive sweat chloride test rules out ciliary dyskinesia.

Answer D is incorrect. Nasal foreign bodies, which are common in young children, can cause recurrent sinusitis due to obstruction of the nasal ostiae. However, sinusitis is usually unilateral unless both nostrils are involved.

Answer E is incorrect. Immunodeficiency should be a concern in patients with recurrent sinopulmonary or cutaneous infections. X-linked severe combined immunodeficiency involves mutations in the common γ chain of interleukin receptors, which leads to severe T- and B-lymphocyte dysfunction. Clinically, the patients have recurrent infections and failure to thrive, generally presenting early in life. A sweat chloride test should be negative.

40. **The correct answer is C.** The patient has a right to know and understand the risks and benefits associated with each treatment option. Although the physician should help guide the patient's decision, he should have a frank discussion of the morbidity and mortality, including the life expectancy and possibility of decreased quality of life, associated with each treatment.

Answer A is incorrect. Requesting that the patient not ask questions will not help ensure that the patient understands her options. Asking the patient to summarize what has been said is a good way for the physician to ensure that the patient understands each option. This ensures that the patient is making a truly informed decision about her care.

Answer B is incorrect. Although the physician should discuss treatment options and their relative risks and benefits, it would be too confusing for the patient to discuss the details of all relevant clinical trials. The physician should not simply act as an information repository; he or she must synthesize the clinical knowledge about the subject and present it in a format that the lay person can understand.

Answer D is incorrect. By omitting family members from such discussions, the physician is protecting the patient from potentially coercive influences and ensuring that the patient is making her own decision. The patient can also decide which information to disclose to family members. However, such decisions are not under the discretion of the physician, and if the patient does want her family present, the physician should support the decision.

Answer E is incorrect. The physician is obligated to disclose to the patient all treatment options for her condition, not just those that the physician thinks will work best.

41. **The correct answer is B.** Most adenocarcinomas arise from Barrett's esophagus, which is characterized by columnar epithelium replacing normal squamous tissue. This change is

largely precipitated by constant inflammation due to reflux from the stomach and is strongly associated with malignancy, increasing the risk nearly 40 times. Due to the malignancy, patients often complain of a slow history of dysphagia, especially of solids, and resulting weight loss. Stridor and nocturnal cough are also prominent features. Endoscopy is the diagnostic procedure of choice.

Answer A is incorrect. Achalasia is due to an unknown etiology that affects the neuronal control of the esophagus and affects solids and liquids. It is characterized by a "bird's beak" appearance on barium swallow.

Answer C is incorrect. Esophageal varices are nearly always due to an increase in portal pressure and may present with upper gastrointestinal bleeding. Symptoms of liver disease will usually be present (e.g., jaundice, pruritus, abdominal pain).

Answer D is incorrect. Gastric cancer in the United States continues to decrease. Family history, tobacco, vitamin C deficiency, and preserved foods are risk factors (there has been a rise of gastric cancer in Japan and Eastern Europe possibly for this reason). It is characterized by weight loss and gastric pain.

Answer E is incorrect. Hiatal hernias are asymptomatic but may lead to reflux. Unless they become entangled, they would not present as in this question.

42. **The correct answer is A.** Thromboprophylaxis is an important part of postsurgical care. The risk of deep vein thrombosis (DVT)/pulmonary embolism (PE) after surgery can be classified as low, moderate, and high. Patients who are < 40 years of age and undergo an uncomplicated surgery, such as the one referred to here, have only a 0.4% risk of DVT/PE. In this patient population, early ambulation is the prophylaxis of choice. Although not an answer choice, pulmonary toilet should also be recommended because it decreases the incidence of postoperative pneumonia and atelectasis.

Answer B is incorrect. Patients with a moderate risk of deep vein thrombosis (DVT)/pulmonary embolism (PE) are typically > 40 years and have a history of recent general surgery, myocardial infarct, cerebrovascular accident, bed rest, or chronic illnesses such as cancer, inhibitor deficiency states, or antiphospholipid syndrome. These patients have a 2–4% risk of DVT/PE and should have prophylaxis consisting of heparin 5000 units subcutaneously twice a day or intermittent pneumatic compression with or without elastic stockings.

Answer C is incorrect. Treatment with pneumatic compression and elastic stockings is generally reserved for patients with a moderate risk of deep vein thrombosis/pulmonary embolism, patients > 40 years old, and those with a history of recent general surgery, myocardial infarct, cerebrovascular accident, bed rest, or chronic illnesses such as cancer, inhibitor deficiency states, or antiphospholipid syndrome.

Answer D is incorrect. Patients with a high risk of deep vein thrombosis (DVT)/pulmonary embolism (PE) have a history of recent orthopedic surgery, trauma, or DVT. These patients have a 10–20% risk of DVT/PE and should have prophylaxis consisting of low-molecular-weight heparin using either enoxaparin 30 mg subcutaneously twice a day or dalteparin 2500 IU subcutaneously once daily **or** warfarin plus elastic stockings.

Answer E is incorrect. Patients with a high risk of deep vein thrombosis (DVT)/pulmonary embolism (PE) have a history of recent orthopedic surgery, trauma, or DVT. These patients have a 10–20% risk of DVT/PE and should have prophylaxis consisting of low-molecular-weight heparin using either enoxaparin 30 mg subcutaneously twice a day, or dalteparin 2500 IU subcutaneously once daily **or** warfarin plus elastic stockings.

43. **The correct answer is A.** This patient is presenting with a classic case of acute lymphoid leukemia (ALL). Although ALL may be difficult to differentiate from acute myelogenous leukemia, the next step in treatment is the same for both illnesses. Patient evaluation prior to beginning therapy requires a complete blood cell count, chemistry studies assessing major organ function, a bone marrow biopsy, and a lumbar puncture to rule out occult central nervous system involvement. The latter

two procedures are generally performed together so that conscious sedation is necessary only once.

Answer B is incorrect. Although chemotherapy should be initiated without delay in a patient such as this, lumbar puncture should be performed first if possible.

Answer C is incorrect. A patient with a platelet count of 75,000/mm^3 is not considered at risk for spontaneous bleeding. An emergent platelet transfusion would be considered for a patient with a platelet count of 25,000/mm^3 and would be indicated in one with 10,000/mm^3.

Answer D is incorrect. For the most part, bone marrow transplant is not employed as a first approach to curing childhood acute leukemia. The one exception to this is the acute myelogenous leukemia patient with a matched sibling donor, for whom bone marrow transplant would be considered first-line therapy. This is never the case for an acute lymphoid leukemia patient. Even when sibling typing is required, it can be carried out after initial chemotherapy has been initiated. Lumbar puncture should be done beforehand.

Answer E is incorrect. In the absence of evidence of chest pathology on history or physical examination, x-ray of the chest is generally not required as part of the initial workup of pediatric patients with acute leukemia.

Questions 44–46

44. **The correct answer is A.** In an older man, painless hematuria is classic for bladder cancer. The case also lists two risk factors for transitional-cell carcinoma: smoking and exposure to industrial dyes.

45. **The correct answer is F.** Patients with polycystic kidney disease often present in their 40s with some degree of renal failure. This disease is inherited in an autosomal dominant fashion, as the case suggests. The hematuria and flank pain may be caused by the cysts and cyst rupture, which can cause bleeding.

46. **The correct answer is I.** Renal cell carcinoma (RCC) is the most likely diagnosis here. The disease can cause hematuria without dysuria. The pain described here is not an acute process, but rather a deep, subacute pain. Furthermore, the man has experienced weight loss and fevers, both evidence of a neoplastic process. The final piece of data that should clinch the diagnosis is the elevated hematocrit. Polycythemia is often seen in RCC tumors that secrete erythropoietin.

Answer B is incorrect. While hematuria is a rare symptom of some coagulation disorders, none of these patients have other stigmata of coagulopathy such as bruising, epistaxis, or other mucosal bleeding. In addition, flank pain is not associated with coagulation disorders.

Answer C is incorrect. Exercise-induced hematuria may be gross or microscopic, begins after strenuous exercise, and remits within several days of the exercise. Exercise-induced hematuria is a diagnosis of exclusion and more serious causes must be ruled out.

Answer D is incorrect. Myoglobinuria causes a red discoloration of urine similar to hemoglobinuria. The presence of urine myoglobin can be determined by a urine dipstick positive for blood, but an absence of RBCs on microscopic evaluation. Approximately 200 grams of muscle must be destroyed before urine is colored. None of these patients has a history suggestive of muscle destruction.

Answer E is incorrect. Nephrolithiasis may present with hematuria and flank pain and is also known to run in families. The flank pain is generally severe and persistent until a stone is passed. Treatment is supportive, as stones will pass spontaneously. Nephrolithiasis does not cause systemic symptoms.

Answer G is incorrect. Hematuria is rarely the presenting symptom of prostate cancer, unless the tumor has invaded the bladder. At this locally advanced stage, symptoms such as urinary frequency, retention, or dysuria would be expected.

Answer H is incorrect. Patients with pyelonephritis present with dysuria, urinary frequency, fevers, costovertebral angle tenderness, and increased WBC count. Hematuria is a rare finding in pyelonephritis.

Answer J is incorrect. Hematuria may be a presenting symptom of urinary tract infection (UTI), and one would also expect dysuria, frequency, increased WBC count, and positive urine culture. UTI is more common in women and is rarely a cause of increased creatinine.

Test Block 7

1. A 45-year-old white mother of three presents to the emergency department (ED) complaining of intermittent epigastric pain that awakens her from sleep. The pain is severe, lasts for a couple of hours, and is sometimes accompanied by vomiting. The pain sometimes occurs after large meals. Her bowel movements have been normal. Her vitals are temperature 38.0°C (100.4°F), pulse 100/min, blood pressure 125/60 mm Hg, and respiratory rate 20/min. On examination, she is obese, her sclerae are anicteric, and her bowel sounds are normal with a positive Murphy's sign. Laboratory tests reveal no abnormalities on presentation. Which of the following is most likely responsible for the patient's signs and symptoms?

(A) Adhesions in her abdominal cavity
(B) Cancer in the head of her pancreas
(C) Gallstones in her common bile duct
(D) Gallstones intermittently obstructing her cystic duct
(E) Inflammation of her appendix

2. A 36-year-old woman with a history of systemic lupus erythematosus presents to her gynecologist because of recurrent spontaneous abortions. She has been pregnant three times in the past. However, two of the pregnancies ended in miscarriages prior to the tenth week of gestation, and the most recent pregnancy resulted in unexplained death of the normal fetus at 13 weeks' gestation. No chromosomal abnormalities were detected on karyotypes of both parents and the 13-week-old fetus. The patient then underwent a hysterosalpingogram and vaginal ultrasound which revealed normal maternal anatomy. The patient denies any history of sexually transmitted infections or a change in vaginal discharge, though both rapid plasma reagin and Venereal Disease Research Laboratory tests are found to be positive. She denies any abnormalities in her menstrual cycle and states that she gets her period every 28 days during which time she uses three to four pads per day. The patient is a thin, pale woman who avoids the sun because of a facial rash that develops with sun exposure. Physical examination is notable for arthritis in the hands and a rash on the lower extremities bilaterally. Which of the following tests would have predicted the increased risk of recurrent spontaneous abortions?

(A) CT scan of the pelvis
(B) Lupus anticoagulant
(C) Pituitary function
(D) Potassium hydroxide whiff test
(E) Prothrombin time

3. A homeless 57-year-old African-American veteran, well known to the ED, is brought in by police. He became combative when the police tried to arrest him for harassing a Vietnamese restaurant owner. The police state that the patient insists he has been seeing "those Viet Cong bastards again." He is a known abuser of alcohol and opioids. On mental status examination, the patient continues to insist that anyone with a gun is "one of the enemy." The patient, when asked about the incident with the store owner, states that he usually tries to avoid anything that reminds him of the Vietnamese. When he is faced with such reminders, he becomes extremely agitated and behaves in ways he "wishes he didn't." A toxicology screen in the ED is negative. His temperature is 32.3°C (99.1°F), blood pressure is 140/82 mm Hg, heart rate is 71/min, and respiratory rate is 18/min. What is the best first treatment for this patient?

(A) Chlordiazepoxide with later cognitive behavioral psychotherapy
(B) Chlorpromazine
(C) Cognitive behavioral psychotherapy alone
(D) Methadone maintenance
(E) Sertraline with later cognitive behavioral psychotherapy

4. A 23-year-old man presents to the ED with a chief complaint of fever, facial pain, and epistaxis developing over the last 36 hours. His past medical history is significant for focal segmental glomerulosclerosis that required renal transplant 4 months ago. He had previously been relatively stable on his immunosuppressive regimen. His temperature is 39.1°C

(102.4°F) and his other vital signs are within normal limits. On examination, the physician notices that there is blood-tinged purulent nasal discharge, and there are necrotic areas in the nasal septum. He was brought to the hospital by his parents, who were concerned that he wasn't "acting normally." Which of the following is the most appropriate therapy?

(A) Intravenous amphotericin B
(B) Intravenous vancomycin
(C) Oral azithromycin
(D) Oral ketoconazole
(E) Topical corticosteroid

5. One evening, a nurse gives medication to a 62-year-old man who is 1 day status post-hemicolectomy. The nurse hands the patient two pills, and the patient notices that one does not look familiar to him. He asks the nurse what it is called and what it is for. She explains that it is propranolol prescribed for high blood pressure. The patient insists that he has never had high blood pressure and refuses to take the medication. The nurse contacts the night float intern, who reviews the man's chart and concludes that the propranolol was ordered by mistake. The order should have been written for the patient in the next room. What should the intern do next?

(A) Ask the nurse to remind the patient to always be alert to the medications he receives
(B) Do not dwell on it because the error was discovered before any harm was done
(C) Reprimand the nurse for not double-checking the patient's medications before bringing them to the bedside
(D) Sign out to the team in the morning the details of the medication error
(E) Visit the patient's bedside and explain that an error was made in writing the medication order, but thankfully the patient was alert and noticed the error before taking the wrong medication

6. A 7-year-old boy diagnosed last year with sickle cell disease after a pain crisis comes to the office for a routine checkup. He has been well on hydroxyurea with no pain crises or acute chest episodes since starting the medication a year ago. He has had no infections over the last year and today has no fevers or evidence of increasing splenomegaly. Which of the following is an appropriate preventive measure for this patient?

(A) Monthly RBC transfusion
(B) Pneumococcal vaccine
(C) Splenectomy
(D) Treatment with deferoxamine
(E) Weekly intramuscular benzathine penicillin

7. A 5-year-old girl with no significant past medical history is brought to the ED because of a change in mental status. For the past 4 days she has had rhinorrhea, a dry cough, and a low-grade fever. One hour prior to presentation, she had a 3-minute episode during which her extremities shook rhythmically, and she did not respond to her name. Following the event she is sleepy but arousable. She denies having a headache. There is no history of head trauma or family history of seizures. Her temperature is 39°C (102.2°F), but other vitals are normal. Physical examination reveals a drowsy but otherwise well-appearing girl. Her neural examination is nonfocal. Serum electrolytes, leukocyte count, and hemoglobin are all within normal limits. What is the most likely cause of this seizure?

(A) Arteriovenous malformation
(B) Elevated core temperature
(C) Intracerebral tumor
(D) Meningitis
(E) Subdural hematoma

8. An 87-year-old woman with a history of hypertension and osteoporosis trips and falls over her sleeping poodle. She does not lose consciousness, and head and neck imaging rules out cervical fracture and intracranial bleed. Pelvic films demonstrate a nondisplaced fracture of the pubic ramus and rule out concomitant fractures of the femur or acetabulum. What is the appropriate management of this patient?

(A) Avoid weight bearing prior to follow-up radiography in 1 week; further recommendations are dependent on radiographic evidence of healing
(B) Mandatory 2 weeks of bed rest, followed by weight bearing as tolerated
(C) Pain management and weight bearing as tolerated
(D) Pelvic stabilization with an external fixation device
(E) Surgical reduction of the fracture

9. A 65-year-old man with a history of uncontrolled hypertension presents to the ED with altered mental status. His blood pressure is 210/130 mm Hg and his pulse is 110/min. His oxygen saturation on room air is 99%. A CT scan of the head reveals a posterior fossa bleed. One hour later, the patient goes into respiratory failure. Which of the following is the most likely etiology?

(A) Central herniation
(B) Cerebellar tonsillar herniation into the foramen magnum
(C) Cingulate herniation under the falx cerebri
(D) Epidural hemorrhage
(E) Uncal herniation

10. A 66-year-old man with a past medical history significant for hypertension, peptic ulcer disease, and melanoma presents to the ED with sudden onset of severe (9 of 10) abdominal pain in the left upper quadrant. The patient denies nausea or vomiting, although he explains that he has no appetite despite his last meal being more than 6 hours ago. The pain radiates to the left shoulder and back, and has been getting worse with time. He is lying still on the bed with his knees drawn up to his chest and is taking shallow breaths. His temperature is 37.9°C (100.2°F), blood pressure is 152/88 mm Hg, pulse is 94/min, and respiratory rate is 18/min. On physical examination, the abdomen is very tender, rigid, and distended, with increased tympany. Bowel sounds could not be appreciated. The remainder of the physical examination is noncontributory. Relevant laboratory findings are:

WBC	14,000/mm³
Hemoglobin	13.2 g/dL
Platelets	303,000/mm³
Direct bilirubin	0.2 mg/dL
Total bilirubin	0.9 mg/dL
Amylase	210 U/L
Lipase	20 U/L (normal 0–160 U/L [laboratory-specific])
Aspartate transaminase	33 U/L
Alanine transaminase	30 U/L

Which of the following is the most likely diagnosis?

(A) Cholecystitis
(B) Hepatitis
(C) Pancreatitis
(D) Perforated peptic ulcer
(E) Small bowel obstruction

11. A 2-week-old child who has developed respiratory distress has higher blood pressure in his upper extremities than in his lower extremities. On radiologic examination, there is constriction of his aorta just proximal to where the ductus arteriosus is in communication with the aorta. Given this child's condition, which of the following is the appropriate initial management?

(A) Antibiotics
(B) Coil embolization of the patent ductus arteriosus
(C) Indomethacin administration
(D) Open surgical closure of the patent ductus arteriosus
(E) Prostaglandin E_1 administration

12. A 2-year-old white girl presents with cough beginning 1 month ago, which was initially dry but is now productive of purulent sputum. She has a history of two previous episodes of pneu-

monia, the first at age 1 month, and one episode of sinusitis. The brother of a maternal grandmother died at age 13 of "recurrent pneumonia." Physical examination shows mild tachypnea, diffuse wheezing with retractions, nasal polyps, and digital clubbing. What is the most likely etiology of this presentation?

(A) Foreign body aspiration
(B) Impaired chloride conduction across secretory epithelial cells
(C) Infection with gram-positive bacteria
(D) Infection with respiratory syncytial virus
(E) Reversible bronchoconstriction and acute airway inflammation

13. An 84-year-old woman with chronic obstructive pulmonary disease has been on a ventilator for 3 weeks in the intensive care unit, despite multiple spontaneous breathing trials. When she was admitted to the hospital 4 weeks ago for pneumonia, she signed a "Do Not Resuscitate" (DNR) form and gave her niece durable power of attorney in writing. One day the patient's temperature spikes to 40°C (104°F), and the team tells the family that intravenous antibiotics would be a necessary step to keep the patient alive. The niece instructs the medical team to withhold any additional life-sustaining treatment. How should the medical team proceed?

(A) According to the DNR, all treatments should be given until the patient goes into cardiac or respiratory arrest
(B) The team should call the hospital ethics committee before further decisions are made
(C) The team should discuss the matter with the patient's daughter because she is the closest family member and therefore should be the surrogate decision maker
(D) The team should give the dose of antibiotics necessary to cure the current infection
(E) The team should withhold any additional treatment

14. An HIV-positive 33-year-old man who refuses antiretroviral therapy presents to the ED complaining of a 6-week history of fever, cough, and night sweats. His current CD4+ count is 46/mm^3 and his viral load is 54,000/mL. X-ray of the chest reveals hilar lymphadenopathy and bilateral infiltrates. A complement fixation test reveals a titer of 1:128. His physician suspects coccidioidomycosis. Which of the following would be an appropriate treatment regimen?

(A) Intravenous amphotericin B followed by 2 months of oral itraconazole
(B) Intravenous vancomycin for 2 months
(C) Intravenous vancomycin for 14 days
(D) Oral itraconazole for 2 weeks
(E) Supportive care only; the disease is self-limited

15. A 22-year-old woman presents to the ED with a chief complaint of sharp chest pain for the past day. The pain radiates to her shoulders and worsens when she lies down. In addition, she complains of being short of breath and having a mild cough. She has no significant past medical history and takes no medications except for oral contraceptive pills. On physical examination, the patient is crying and leaning forward. Her lungs are clear to auscultation bilaterally. Her cardiac examination reveals a regular rate and rhythm, normal S1 and S2, and a soft friction rub. Her temperature is 38.8°C (101.8°F), pulse is 100/min, blood pressure is 102/73 mm Hg, and respiratory rate is 23/min. Her O$_2$ saturation is 100%. An ECG is performed and showed diffuse ST-segment elevation. X-ray of her chest shows an enlarged, flask-shaped cardiac silhouette. Which of the following is the most likely etiology of this patient's condition?

(A) Aortic dissection
(B) Myocardial ischemia
(C) Thromboembolism
(D) Thyroid storm
(E) Viral infection

16. A 19-year-old woman undergoes a bone marrow transplant from her human leukocyte antigen-matched sister for refractory acute lymphoid leukemia. In addition to antibiotic prophylaxis, her oncologist recognizes the need for vaccination against likely pathogens. What is the appropriate vaccination schedule for protection against the infectious organisms *Streptococcus pneumoniae, Haemophilus influenzae,* and *Neisseria meningitidis?*

(A) Advise the patient and all close contacts to avoid vaccination to avoid the risk of live viral reactivation

(B) Forgo vaccination of the patient because of the risk of pathogen reactivation in the immunosuppressed host, but vaccinate all household members

(C) Vaccinate immediately after giving donor bone marrow to condition the marrow as it engrafts

(D) Vaccinate 12 months and 24 months after transplantation and confirm that all household members have been vaccinated

(E) Vaccinate the patient prior to beginning the immunosuppressive transplant protocol

17. A 70-year-old man with a history of well-controlled hypertension has an asymptomatic carotid bruit during a routine physical examination. An ultrasound of the patient's neck reveals 80% stenosis of the right carotid artery. The current recommended management in this situation includes which of the following?

(A) Carotid angioplasty

(B) Carotid endarterectomy

(C) Medical management with aspirin 325 mg every day

(D) Medical management with warfarin titrated to International Normalized Ratio 2–3

(E) Medical risk factor management followed by carotid endarterectomy with the onset of neurologic symptoms

18. A 17-year-old girl presents to a family practice clinic with her mother. Her mother states that she has noticed that her daughter's hair is thinning. The patient states that sometimes she pulls her hair out "because it calms me down when I am alone." After pulling it out, she sometimes places the hair in her mouth. The patient states that she has impulses to do this which she cannot control, but that these impulses are "okay with me, they don't really bother me." The patient does note, however, that because she has become self-conscious about her hair, she has stopped socializing with her friends. The patient further states that she occasionally feels sad, but denies guilt, anhedonia, or decreased energy. On physical examination, the patient appears to have patchy hair loss, but no rashes or scalp lesions. What is the patient's most likely diagnosis?

(A) Alopecia areata

(B) Major depression

(C) Obsessive-compulsive disorder

(D) Schizophrenia

(E) Trichotillomania

19. A 13-year-old white girl has had a recurrent cough that is productive of white sputum for the past 6 months. She is the product of a normal pregnancy, delivered at 37 weeks' gestation. She also had recurrent upper respiratory infections as a child. She is at the 10th percentile for weight and height, even though her parents and brother are at the 50th percentile for weight and height. She is unhappy with her weight and stature and reports minimal weight gain despite having a large appetite and eating large meals. She also reports chronic large, foul-smelling, floating stools. She had her first period 2 years ago but has not had her period in the past 6 months. Examination reveals blood pressure of 117/81 mm Hg, pulse of 60/min, respiratory rate of 20/min, and temperature of 38.3°C (101°F). She appears small for her stated age and has digital clubbing. The rest of the physical examination is unremarkable. X-ray of the chest shows hyperinflated lungs. Which of the following is the most appropriate next step in management of the nutritional status of this patient?

(A) Administer laxatives

(B) Dietary supplements alone

(C) Encourage a lower caloric intake

(D) Pancreatic enzyme replacement and dietary supplements

(E) Withhold fat from her diet

20. A 58-year-old man presents to his primary care physician for follow-up. Five years ago, he was diagnosed with diabetes mellitus type 2, and 9 years ago, he was diagnosed with hypertension. At present, his medications include metformin and hydrochlorothiazide. There is a family history of cerebrovascular accident. On examination, there is no evidence of retinopathy or neuropathy, and his blood pressure is 126/72 mm Hg. Laboratory studies indicate hemoglobin A_{1c} of 6.8% and trace albumin in the urine. Which of the following additions to the patient's medication regimen is most appropriate at this time?

(A) Furosemide
(B) Gemfibrozil
(C) Labetalol
(D) Lisinopril
(E) Lispro insulin

21. A 31-year-old G1P1 woman returns to the ED complaining of worsening lower abdominal pain and vaginal bleeding. She presented to the ED 3 days ago with the same complaints. Serum β-human chorionic gonadotropin (βhCG) at that time was 1250 mIU/mL, and transvaginal ultrasound was negative for an intrauterine or extrauterine gestational sac, and did not show an adnexal mass or echogenic or large volume cul-de-sac fluid. She is sexually active with her husband, and she uses a diaphragm for contraception. She had a chlamydial infection 7 years ago, but otherwise her past medical history is unremarkable. Her last menstrual period was 6 weeks ago. She is afebrile with normal vital signs. Laboratory studies show:

WBC count   5.4/mm³
Hemoglobin   13.9 g/dL
Platelet count   200,000/mm³
Quantitative serum β-hCG   1100 mIU/mL

What is the next step in diagnosis?

(A) CT scan with contrast
(B) Dilation and curettage
(C) Follow weekly β-hCG
(D) Laparoscopy
(E) Repeat transvaginal ultrasound

22. A 64-year-old woman with a history of Graves' disease presents to the ED with several hours of vomiting and diarrhea. She is accompanied by her husband who says that she has been very agitated and does not remember her name or where she is. One week ago she was diagnosed with viral pneumonia. On physical examination she has a temperature of 40°C (104°F), a heart rate of 145/min, and a blood pressure of 145/92 mm Hg. Her skin is jaundiced. On cardiac examination, she is tachycardic but has a regular rhythm with a normal S1 and S2; no murmurs are heard. Pulmonary examination is significant for diffusely coarse breath sounds. Her abdomen is soft and nondistended with no masses. On neurologic examination, she has a coarse tremor in both hands and 3+ reflexes bilaterally in the biceps, knees, and ankles. Which of the following is the best agent for initial management of this patient?

(A) Dobutamine
(B) Enalapril
(C) Levothyroxine
(D) Methimazole
(E) Propranolol

23. A 16-year-old female immigrant from Vietnam has a positive purified protein derivative (PPD) test and was never immunized against tuberculosis (TB). Why are PPDs used throughout the United States as a screening test for TB?

(A) It has a low negative predictive value
(B) It has a low positive predictive value
(C) The test is dependent on disease incidence
(D) The test is dependent on disease prevalence
(E) The test is highly sensitive

24. A 27-year-old heroin addict presents to the ED with mental status changes and severe headache. Physical examination reveals substantial meningismus, a positive Brudzinski sign, and track marks on both arms. There are no focal neurologic signs, so a lumbar puncture is performed, which shows:

WBC count	257,000/mm^3, 62% lymphocytes
RBC count	4/mm^3
Glucose	81 mg/dL
Total protein	40 mg/dL
Gram stain	No organisms seen

Blood cultures are negative. Given the patient's known risk factor of intravenous drug use, a rapid HIV antibody test is also performed, and the results are indeterminate. Titers for herpes simplex virus type 1 are sent as well, along with other viral tests; acyclovir is started prophylactically. Which of the following measures is most immediately appropriate?

(A) Determine the HIV viral load
(B) Obtain an echocardiogram
(C) Repeat the lumbar puncture
(D) Start highly active antiretroviral therapy
(E) Start intravenous ceftriaxone and vancomycin

25. A 45-year-old obese white man comes to his physician for a routine visit. He complains of burning chest pain for the past month that occurs with meals and sometimes awakens him from sleep. He smokes one pack of cigarettes and drinks two beers daily. His temperature is 36.5°C (97.7°F), his heart rate is 65/min, his blood pressure is 137/78 mm Hg, and his respiratory rate is 9/min. Which of the following would be appropriate initial treatment for his symptoms?

(A) Avoiding spicy foods
(B) Histamine$_2$-receptor blockers
(C) Lifestyle modification including weight loss, cessation of smoking, and avoiding alcohol
(D) Nissen fundoplication
(E) Proton pump inhibitors

26. A 43-year-old woman who works as a nurse has a 10-year-old son who was diagnosed with in-sulin-dependent diabetes at age 7. It is later discovered that she has been injecting her son with glucagon to simulate her child's illness. What is most likely true about the mother?

(A) She has a history of investigation by child protective services
(B) She has an abnormal psychological profile
(C) She has used one doctor for most of her life
(D) She will appear to those who know her to be a poor mother in the past
(E) She will not stop her behavior even after being found out

27. A 72-year-old woman presents to the ED with a chief complaint of headache. She says that the pain, that has been present for the last week, is constant, 7/10 in severity, and localized to the left side of her forehead and above her left ear. She also notes pain in her jaw when she chews. She also complained of blurry vision. On review of systems, she notes a 4.5-kg (10-lb) weight loss over the past month. She denies chest pain, shortness of breath, abdominal pain, change in bowel movements, or weakness or numbness in her extremities. She has a temperature of 37.2°C (99.0°F), a heart rate of 86/min, and a blood pressure of 116/78 mm Hg. She has tenderness to palpation of the left temporal area. On neurologic examination, cranial nerves II through XII are intact, she has normal sensation to light touch and vibration bilaterally, and strength is 5/5 in all four extremities. Laboratory tests show:

WBC count	98,000/mm^3
Hemoglobin	10.1 g/dL
Platelet count	560,000/mm^3
Erythrocyte sedimentation rate	110 mm/h
C-reactive protein	3.2 ng/mL (normal 0.7– 1.89 ng/mL)
Alanine aminotransferase	38 U/L
Aspartate aminotransferase	62 U/L
Alkaline phosphatase	410 U/L

Which of the following should be the first step in the management of this patient?

(A) Antineutrophil cytoplasmic antibody titer
(B) Initiation of glucocorticoid therapy

(C) Initiation of therapy with nonsteroidal anti-inflammatory drugs

(D) Magnetic resonance angiography of the brain

(E) Temporal artery biopsy

28. A nurse in the newborn care nursery is concerned because a white newborn boy has had one episode of emesis and has failed to pass meconium. His heart rate is 125/min, blood pressure is 75/50 mm Hg, respiratory rate is 40/min, and temperature is 37.1°C (98.7°F). Physical examination is unremarkable, except for a noticeably distended abdomen. A radiograph after water-soluble air contrast enema is shown in the image below. What is the most likely underlying cause of this condition?

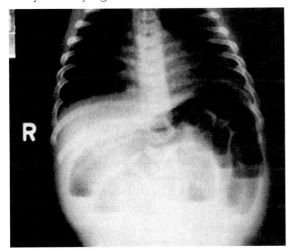

Reproduced, with permission, from Tintinalli JE, Kelen GD, Stapczynski S, Ma OJ, Cline DM. *Tintinalli's Emergency Medicine: A Comprehensive Study Guide*, 6th ed. New York: McGraw-Hill, 2004: Figure 127-1.

(A) Cystic fibrosis

(B) Edwards syndrome

(C) Meckel's diverticulum

(D) Trisomy 21

(E) Williams syndrome

29. A 42-year-old homeless man is brought to the ED. He is obtunded, and there is vomit on his clothing. His breathing is rapid and deep. He has a glucose of 430 mg/dL and a blood urea nitrogen:creatinine ratio of 28. The presence of which of the following is important in distinguishing nonketotic hyperglycemia from diabetic ketoacidosis?

(A) Dehydration

(B) Hyperglycemia

(C) Kussmaul breathing

(D) Mental status change

(E) Vomiting

30. A 35-year-old homosexual man presents to the office expressing concern that he might have contracted a sexually transmitted disease (STD) through several instances of unprotected sex with anonymous partners over the past several years. He requests STD testing. His HIV Western blot test is read as positive. He asks what the chances are that the result is wrong. What is the correct reply?

(A) This is possible, as the test has low positive predictive value in this circumstance

(B) This is unlikely, as the HIV test is highly sensitive

(C) This is unlikely, as the HIV test is highly specific

(D) This is unlikely, as the test has 100% validity

31. A 36-year-old, G1P0 woman presents for her first prenatal visit late in her first trimester of pregnancy complaining of persistent vaginal bleeding, nausea, and pelvic pain. Physical examination is notable for a gravid uterus larger than expected for gestational age. Fetal heart tones are absent. Which of the following is most likely to be true?

(A) Hematocrit will be increased

(B) β-hCG level will be higher than normal

(C) Laboratory evaluation will reveal an increase in thyroid-stimulating hormone

(D) No theca lutein cysts will be visualized on pelvic ultrasound

(E) Pelvic sonogram will show a normal-sized uterus

32. A 60-year-old man visits a health clinic for the third time since moving to the United States from Ireland about a year ago. On the first two visits, his blood pressure was 140/90 mm Hg and 142/86 mm Hg. As recommended by the clinic physician, he eats a healthful, low-salt diet including plenty of fruits and vegetables, and exercises regularly. Today, he notes that for about the past 6 months he has had difficulty urinating. He states that it often takes him a while to start his stream, and the stream is not as forceful as it used to be. He has a blood pressure of 142/88 mm Hg and a heart rate of 70/min. Physical examination shows that his prostate is firm and large without nodularity. Urinalysis is normal, and his serum creatinine is 0.8 g/dL. An ECG is done and is read as normal sinus rhythm. What medication should be started in this patient?

(A) Finasteride
(B) Lisinopril
(C) No medication is needed
(D) Terazosin
(E) Thiazide diuretic

33. A 46-year-old man notices that over the past several years his shoe size has increased and his wedding ring feels tighter. On physical examination, he has an unusually prominent forehead (frontal bossing), a widened space between the lower incisors, and increased heel pad thickness. Laboratory evaluation reveals elevated serum levels of insulin-like growth factor-1. Appropriate initial therapy for this patient might include which of these?

(A) Cortisol
(B) Growth hormone
(C) Metyrapone
(D) Octreotide
(E) Thyroid hormone

34. A 64-year-old woman presents with difficulty breathing and mild chest pain. The chest pain is not exertional or positional and is not relieved by rest. She has no cough or fever, and no other symptoms. Review of systems is significant for morning stiffness of the knees and hands. Physical examination shows some decreased breath sounds and dullness to percussion in both lung bases. There are normal heart sounds and no evidence of cardiomegaly or jugular venous distention. A decubitus x-ray of the chest is shown in the image. Which of the following is now indicated?

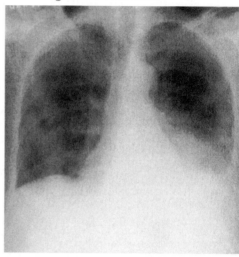

Reproduced, with permission, from Chen MYM, Pope TL, Ott DJ. *Basic Radiology*. New York: McGraw-Hill, 2004: Figure 4-52.

(A) Furosemide
(B) Ibuprofen
(C) Intravenous ceftriaxone
(D) No treatment is indicated
(E) Thoracentesis

35. A 47-year-old man with hypertension is prescribed hydrochlorothiazide by his primary care physician. Which of the following is a potential effect of this medication?

(A) Hyperkalemia
(B) Hyperlipidemia
(C) Hypernatremia
(D) Hypocalcemia
(E) Hypouricemia

36. A 35-year-old woman returns to her primary care physician for follow-up 2 weeks after passing a kidney stone. This is the third stone that the patient has passed in the past year. The stones were evaluated, and all three were composed of calcium phosphate. She has no other past medical history. She mentions that she has not been taking any medications but just started using over-the-counter eye drops for her dry eyes. The patient has a temperature of 37.1°C (98.8°F), heart rate of 80/min, blood pressure of 120/80 mm Hg, and respiratory rate of 18/min. On examination, her mucous mem-

branes appear dry. Her lungs are clear to auscultation, and her abdomen is soft and nontender. A chart review reveals that her urine pH since she passed the first stone has been consistently > 7.0. The physician decides to give her oral challenge with 1.9 mmol/kg of ammonium chloride and repeats a measurement of her urine pH. The pH after this challenge is 6.8. The physician desires to continue the work-up after this finding. What antibodies test(s) would most likely yield the diagnosis?

(A) Antiglomerular basement membrane
(B) Antihistone
(C) Anti-Ro/SSA and anti-La/SSB
(D) Circulating anti-neutrophilic cytoplasmic autoantibody
(E) Perinuclear anti-neutrophilic cytoplasmic autoantibody

37. An 85-year-old white man with a history of hypertension and cerebrovascular disease presents to his physician's office for a routine check-up. Review of systems is positive only for periodic "ringing in the ears." On examination, the physician notes left facial paralysis and poor hearing on the left side. Based on the physician's findings, a stroke in which vascular territory is suspected?

(A) Anterior cerebral artery
(B) Anterior inferior cerebellar artery
(C) Middle cerebral artery
(D) Posterior cerebral artery
(E) Posterior inferior cerebellar artery

38. A 23-year-old man with a history of major depression with psychotic features fails to refill his medication prescriptions for several months. He calls his psychiatrist and states that he is very upset because a fellow student who is clearly in love with him has not returned his calls. While speaking to the psychiatrist, he sounds agitated, displays flight of ideas and clanging speech patterns, and begins making threats against the fellow student. What is the most appropriate next step for the physician to take?

(A) Call the patient's roommate and ask him to "keep an eye on" the patient until he can safely be brought to the hospital
(B) Call the police and ask them to help emergency medical services apprehend the

patient, and inform them of the patient's specific threats against the young woman
(C) Contact the student who is threatened directly and inform her of the situation, allowing her to contact the police herself; the physician's obligation is fulfilled at this point
(D) Do nothing because it is a violation of patient confidentiality to disclose the details of his conversation with the patient to the authorities
(E) Do nothing because the patient has made similar threats during previous manic episodes and has not carried them out

39. A 56-year-old man with hypertension presents with progressive confusion over 2 days. He was also noted to have a rash on his hands. He has no history of trauma to the head, no preceding headache or neck stiffness, and does not drink alcohol or use any illicit drugs. His only medication is a thiazide diuretic. On examination, he is afebrile with intact pupillary reflexes and negative Brudzinski sign. Laboratory studies show:

Na^+	138 mEq/L
K^+	4.3 mEq/L
Blood urea nitrogen	17 mg/dL
Creatinine	1.1 mg/dL
Glucose	93 mg/dL
Total bilirubin	3.2 mg/dL
Direct bilirubin	0.6 mg/dL
Albumin	3.6 g/dL (normal 3.4–4.7 g/dL)
Aspartate aminotransferase	15 U/L
Alanine aminotransferase	12 U/L
WBC count	8600/mm^3
Hemoglobin	8.5 g/dL
Platelet count	90,000/mm^3
Reticulocytes	3.2%
Salicylate level	Undetectable

Results of a urine toxicity screen are negative, and a CT of the head is negative for intracranial hemorrhage and mass lesions. What is the most likely diagnosis?

(A) Diuretic overdose
(B) Drug-induced hemolytic anemia
(C) Liver failure
(D) Thrombotic thrombocytopenic purpura
(E) Viral meningoencephalitis

40. A 32-year-old diabetic woman is postoperative day 4 after an elective cesarean delivery of a 4-kg (9-lb) baby boy at 43 weeks' gestation. On postoperative day 1, she developed a fever of 38.7°C (101.7°F) in the setting of vague uterine tenderness. She was treated with intravenous clindamycin and gentamicin for endometritis. The patient continued to spike fevers over the next few days and complained of worsening abdominal pain, with extension to the right flank and lower back. On the morning of postoperative day 4, the patient's fever spiked to 39.9°C (103.8°F). Pelvic examination was unremarkable, and an MRI demonstrated a thrombosed left ovarian vein. What is the most appropriate treatment strategy?

(A) Add additional β-lactamase coverage to the current antibiotic regimen, without heparin administration
(B) Change the antibiotic regimen without heparin administration
(C) Continue the current antibiotic regimen and add heparin
(D) Discontinue the antibiotic treatment and administer heparin alone
(E) Surgically remove the clot

41. A 70-year-old man is brought to the ED after his family found him to be extremely pale and acting weak and confused. On arrival at the ED the patient is noncommunicative but arousable and is found to have a fever of 38.6°C (101.5°F), a blood pressure of 85/50 mm Hg, and a pulse of 95/min. Physical examination demonstrates clear lung fields and normal cardiac and abdominal examinations, but the patient is clearly pallid. Laboratory studies reveal a WBC count of 17,000/mm³ with 94% neutrophils, and urinalysis reveals > 100,000 bacteria/mL with increased leukocyte esterase, elevated nitrites, and > 5 leukocytes per high-power field. The patient is given aggressive fluid resuscitation and central venous access is established. Although his central venous pressure has risen to above an appropriate level of 8 mm Hg, his mean arterial pressure remains below 65 mm Hg. What is the most appropriate subsequent medication?

(A) Dobutamine
(B) Epinephrine
(C) Isoproterenol
(D) Labetalol
(E) Norepinephrine

42. A 63-year-old woman presents to psychiatry clinic for an initial visit. She states that her husband has recently fallen ill, and that he may die in the next month. She spends most of her time at the local church, praying that her husband will be cured. Even though her husband is currently in a coma, she hears him talk to her at the church. She also sees his image at times when she walks along the street. The patient's preoccupation with her husband's illness has kept her from spending any time with her other family or friends, and it has also kept her from paying her bills. The patient denies any psychiatric history previous to her husband falling ill. She further denies changes in energy, sleep, or appetite. What is the most appropriate diagnosis at this point?

(A) Adjustment disorder
(B) Major depressive disorder
(C) Major depressive episode
(D) Normal grief
(E) Psychotic disorder not otherwise specified

43. A 60-year-old man with a history of congestive heart failure presents to his physician with an 8-month history of exertional fatigue and excessive daytime sleepiness. His wife has told him that he also has episodes of choking in his sleep. He has been taking enalapril, metoprolol, and hydrochlorothiazide for congestive heart failure and is compliant. He denies chest pain, palpitations, or swelling in his legs. He is afebrile and vital signs are normal. His oxygen saturation is 99% on room air and his body mass index is 30.2 kg/m². On cardiac examination his apical impulse is diffuse and shifted 2 cm to the left of the midclavicular line. Heart sounds are normal. Jugular venous distention and peripheral edema are absent. X-ray of the chest shows no active disease and ECG is significant for left ventricular hypertrophy. Which of the following is the most likely cause of the patient's exertional fatigue?

(A) Decreased left ventricular afterload
(B) Decreased right ventricular afterload
(C) Hypertension

(D) Increased negative intrathoracic pressure

(E) Pulmonary vasodilation

44. A 40-year-old man was playing basketball at his company's annual executive picnic when he fell directly onto his left elbow. He had instant pain and was unable to straighten his elbow. In obvious distress, he was taken immediately to the ED by his wife. He had a bag of ice on his left elbow, which was very swollen. On examination, he is unable to sense light touch and two-point discrimination in his left fifth digit and the medial aspect of his left hand. All other areas are neurologically intact. What motor test will be most useful to assess the integrity of the nerve most likely to be damaged?

(A) Abduction of the second and third digits

(B) Extension of the fifth digit

(C) Extension of the wrist

(D) Flexion of the thumb

(E) Flexion of the wrist

EXTENDED MATCHING

Questions 45 and 46

For each patient with urinary frequency, select the most likely diagnosis.

(A) Acute cystitis

(B) Asymptomatic bacteriuria

(C) Benign prostatic hypertrophy

(D) Central diabetes insipidus

(E) Detrusor instability

(F) Diabetes mellitus

(G) Gonorrhea

(H) Interstitial cystitis

(I) Nephrogenic diabetes insipidus

(J) Prostatitis

(K) Psychogenic polydipsia

(L) Urethral stricture

45. A 70-year-old man presents to the physician with urinary frequency for several weeks. He states that he was urinating well after a transurethral resection of the prostate 5 months ago, but his urinary stream decreased again over the past 3 weeks. He denies pain or blood in his urine. He is afebrile and has a palpable bladder dome above the pubic symphysis. On digital rectal examination, the prostatic fossa is empty. Relevant laboratory findings are a WBC count of 4000/mm^3, a creatinine of 1.0 mg/dL, and a serum potassium of 5.0 mEq/L.

46. A 40-year-old woman with a history of multiple sclerosis presents to her physician for routine follow-up. She has been utilizing clean intermittent self-catheterization for the past 3 months. She denies any abdominal or flank pain. She has a temperature of 37°C (98.6°F) and a blood pressure of 120/80 mm Hg. She has a WBC count of 4000/mm^3. A urine culture is positive for *Escherichia coli*.

ANSWERS

1. **The correct answer is D.** This patient is presenting with characteristic signs and symptoms of cholelithiasis with intermittent obstruction of the cystic duct. This accounts for the duration of her pain, association with large meals, vomiting, and the presence of a Murphy's sign (pain upon deep inspiration during palpation of the right upper quadrant). Her personal characteristics should have also pointed towards cholelithiasis. The four **F**'s put a person at higher risk for stones: Fat, Forty, Female, and Fertile. Cholecystectomy is recommended if patients have recurrent symptoms or signs of complications such as acute cholecystitis (fever, right upper quadrant pain, and leukocytosis).

Answer A is incorrect. Adhesions in the abdomen would likely be the cause of a partial or complete small bowel obstruction (SBO), not biliary colic. SBO would present with crampy abdominal pain, possibly with changes in stools, and would not have pain localizing to the right upper quadrant with a positive Murphy's sign. Surgical laparotomy would be necessary if SBO was suspected.

Answer B is incorrect. Cancer in the head of the pancreas commonly presents with painless jaundice and is not often accompanied by intermittent postprandial epigastric pain. Findings on palpation of the right upper quadrant would likely not be tenderness and a Murphy's sign, but could include a painless palpable gallbladder (Courvoisier's sign). If localized, pancreatic cancer may be amenable to surgical resection.

Answer C is incorrect. Stones in the common bile duct (choledocholithiasis) could present with similar epigastric pain, but would most likely be more constant. As well, one would expect signs of an increased bilirubin level on laboratory tests, and physical examination findings (jaundice and scleral icterus). Treatment is via endoscopic retrograde cholangiopancreatography and endoscopic sphincterotomy.

Answer E is incorrect. Appendicitis would present with diffuse abdominal pain which later localizes to the right lower quadrant. It is associated with an elevation in WBC count and temperature, along with nausea, vomiting, and anorexia. On physical examination, one would see pain at McBurney's point, and sometimes a Rovsing's, psoas, or obturator sign. It also is much more likely to occur in young people rather than middle-aged women. The treatment of appendicitis entails surgical removal of the appendix.

2. **The correct answer is B.** Antiphospholipid antibody syndrome (APS) is characterized by a hypercoagulable state with circulating antibodies that leads to recurrent fetal loss and/or arterial or venous thrombosis as well thrombocytopenia. Thrombus formation and infarction may account for the pregnancy morbidity observed in APS. APS may occur as a primary disorder or in association with an underlying disorder, most commonly systemic lupus erythematosus, as in the case described, but also with infection, neurologic disease, or the use of specific drugs (procainamide, chlorpromazine, phenytoin, and quinidine, among others). False-positive syphilis serology may occur in patients with APS because the anticardiolipin antibodies in the patient's serum cross-react with the syphilis antigen used in the test. It should be noted that although rapid plasma reagin and/or Venereal Disease Research Laboratory tests may be falsely positive, antitreponemal antigen assays and fluorescent treponemal antibody assay will remain specific for syphilis. APS should be considered when at least one clinical criterion (vascular thrombosis or pregnancy morbidity) and one laboratory criterion (positive anticardiolipin antibody or lupus anticoagulant assay) are met.

Answer A is incorrect. Anatomic abnormalities may contribute to recurrent spontaneous abortions. Although hysterosalpingograms have a diagnostic accuracy of only 55% when used alone, this imaging modality used in combination with ultrasound examination improves the diagnostic accuracy to 90%. CT scan, on the other hand, has limited utility in diagnosing uterine anatomic abnormalities and would be less likely to show an underlying abnormality that could contribute to recurrent spontaneous abortions. Evidence of systemic lupus erythematosus in the context of recurrent spontaneous abortions is more likely due to antiphospholipid antibody syndrome than to an anatomic abnormality.

Answer C is incorrect. Pituitary disorders may cause alterations in hormone levels that lead to infertility and absence of ovulation with oligo- or amenorrhea. One study showed that women with hypopituitarism have a miscarriage rate of 28% and a mid-trimester fetal death rate of 11%. Although the patient may have a pituitary disorder leading to the recurrent spontaneous abortions, this diagnosis is less likely, as she has been able to conceive and has had normal menstrual cycles without amenorrhea or oligomenorrhea. Evidence of systemic lupus erythematosus in the context of recurrent spontaneous abortions with normal menstrual history is more likely to be due to antiphospholipid antibody syndrome than to a deficiency in pituitary function.

Answer D is incorrect. Cervical cultures are useful for diagnosing sexually transmitted infections as well as bacterial, trichomonal, and fungal infections of the female reproductive tract. The potassium hydroxide whiff test is useful to support a diagnosis of bacterial vaginosis. Bacterial vaginosis is the most common cause of vaginitis in women. Although this diagnosis may be associated with increased incidence of preterm delivery, postpartum fever, and cervical intraepithelial neoplasia, it has not been shown to be associated with recurrent spontaneous abortions.

Answer E is incorrect. Prothrombin time (PT) is used to assess coagulation factors involved in the extrinsic pathway of the clotting cascade. Although lupus anticoagulants may cause prolongation of the activated partial thromboplastin time because the prothrombinase complex cannot assemble properly, lupus anticoagulants have no direct effect on the PT. An abnormal PT therefore would not have predicted a diagnosis of antiphospholipid antibody syndrome as the underlying cause of recurrent spontaneous abortions.

3. **The correct answer is E.** Patients with posttraumatic stress disorder (PTSD) are often misdiagnosed with schizophrenia, especially African-American combat veterans. Core deficits in PTSD include symptoms of constant reexperiencing of traumatic events, avoidance of stimuli associated with the traumatic event, and persistent symptoms of increased arousal. The reexperiencing of traumatic events can often be misinterpreted as hallucinations. Moreover, efforts to avoid reminders of the traumatic events can make the patient appear delusional. Patients who are suffering from PTSD benefit from cognitive psychotherapy oriented toward PTSD and selective serotonin reuptake inhibitors.

Answer A is incorrect. Chlordiazepoxide may be used to treat alcohol withdrawal or mild anxiety. However, both diagnoses are unlikely given the patient's normal vital signs and extremely agitated behavior on certain cues.

Answer B is incorrect. It is possible that the patient has schizophrenia and needs antipsychotics. However, his hypervigilance, as well as the content of his hallucinations and thoughts, make it more likely that the disorder is the result of trauma and stress.

Answer C is incorrect. The patient's symptoms go far beyond a specific fear of guns or of Vietnamese people. Phobias should not, for example, cause persistent re-experiencing of traumatic situations. Thus, behavioral treatment, the option of choice for a simple phobia, would not be recommended. Cognitive behavioral therapy for a phobia would focus on examining the automatic thoughts that occur when a person is faced with the phobia. Then, time would be taken to decatastrophize the experience with the phobic object or situation (e.g., "Now, what would happen if people did really laugh at you while you were speaking?"). Finally, graded exposure to the phobic situation would be used.

Answer D is incorrect. The patient is displaying agitation, which would not typically be seen in someone suffering from opiate intoxication. Thus, posttraumatic stress disorder is more likely than opiate withdrawal.

4. **The correct answer is A.** In the setting of an immunocompromised host with sinus symptoms, a high degree of suspicion should be maintained for invasive fungal sinusitis. This patient's symptoms developed over a short time frame, and he presented with systemic symptoms, indicative of acute fungal sinusitis. Diagnosis depends on pathologic demonstration of the organism from a biopsy specimen, but the usual fungi causing acute sinusitis are Zygomycetes and *Aspergillus*. While these infections are difficult to treat, especially in the presence of central nervous system invasion, intravenous amphotericin B would be the antimicrobial of choice. Emergent surgical biopsy and d,bridement would also be indicated.

Answer B is incorrect. The clinical picture of rapid-onset nasal septum necrosis and systemic symptoms is more suggestive of an invasive fungal infection, rather than a bacterial etiology. While a bacterial source is possible, this patient's immunocompromised state significantly raises the possibility of fungal infection. Furthermore, if this patient had bacterial sinusitis, the most common bacterial agents would be *Streptococcus pneumoniae* and *Haemophilus influenzae*, and vancomycin would be an inappropriate antibiotic choice for these bacteria.

Answer C is incorrect. While antibacterials may play a role in this patient's care, the likelihood of fungal disease makes an intravenous antifungal a more appropriate therapy.

Answer D is incorrect. The fungi typically responsible for invasive fungal sinusitis (*Aspergillus*, *Fusarium*, and the Zygomycetes) are typically unresponsive to ketoconazole.

Answer E is incorrect. Topical corticosteroids would not play a role in the treatment of invasive fungal sinusitis.

5. **The correct answer is E.** Physicians are obligated to disclose to patients errors made in their medical care. In this case, the error was harmless because the patient discovered the mistake before taking the wrong medication, but he nonetheless has a right to know about the error. Furthermore, knowing about the error could encourage him to continue being an active and conscientious participant in his own medical care.

Answer A is incorrect. Although this is generally a good practice, and it is worthwhile to remind patients to be alert and active participants in their own medical care, the intern's first priority should be disclosure of the error.

Answer B is incorrect. Physicians are obligated to disclose to patients errors that are made in their medical care.

Answer C is incorrect. This error was not the fault of the nurse, who followed orders as written and distributed medication she believed was correct for the patient. Blaming the situation on the nurse is an inappropriate response and ignores the physician's true responsibilities.

Answer D is incorrect. Having discovered the error himself, the intern should do his best to fully disclose the error to the patient. Even though the error was not his fault, it is his responsibility to discuss the situation with the patient and not to wait for the next team to make a decision about disclosure. Although the person who wrote the order should be made aware of his or her mistake, this answer does not go far enough. The patient must also be informed.

6. **The correct answer is B.** Sickle cell patients generally have splenic dysfunction due to red blood cell sickling within splenic microvasculature. The subsequent repeated splenic infarctions lead to functional asplenism or "autosplenectomy" by adulthood. This places them at increased risk for infection by encapsulated organisms, which include *Streptococcus pneumoniae* and *Haemophilus influenzae*. Recommended vaccinations include those against pneumococcus, *H. influenzae*, hepatitis B, and influenza virus.

Answer A is incorrect. Chronic red cell transfusion can decrease the percentage of hemoglobin S by three mechanisms: (1) dilution, (2) suppression of endogenous erythropoietin production due to increased hematocrit, and (3) longer half-life of normal hemoglobin as compared to hemoglobin S. However, transfusion is only indicated during aplastic crises and splenic sequestration, to prevent worsening of acute chest syndrome, and to prevent initial or recurrent stroke due to intracerebral thrombosis

Answer C is incorrect. Splenectomy is indicated after the first episode of a splenic sequestration crisis.

Answer D is incorrect. Deferoxamine is an iron chelating agent, and is used with chronic transfusion to prevent iron overload syndrome. This is particularly useful in beta-thalassemia.

Answer E is incorrect. Intramuscular benzathine penicillin injections are the treatment of choice for syphilis infection and have no place in preventive measures for sickle cell patients. However, daily oral penicillin is a good prophylactic measure against pneumococcal infections, and is recommended for all children with sickle cell disease up to the age of 5. However, children older than age 5 who have never had a severe pneumococcal infection or splenectomy may discontinue penicillin prophylaxis without increase in infection rate.

7. **The correct answer is B.** A seizure in a febrile child that occurs without another precipitating cause can be attributed to the fever. Febrile seizures are the most common cause of seizure activity in children from the ages of 6 months to 5 years, and approximately 1 in every 25 children will have a febrile seizure during childhood. This is a benign condition, and > 95% of children who experience a febrile seizure will not develop epilepsy later in life. The workup of a suspected febrile seizure should consist of ruling out most serious conditions that can present with seizure activity, such as meningitis, electrolyte imbalance, or trauma. Treatment is supportive: the fever should be controlled and the child protected from injury should the seizure recur.

Answer A is incorrect. Arteriovenous malformations are abnormal connections of arteries and veins. They can bleed and cause seizures, usually generalized tonic-clonic seizures. They are not associated with fever or upper respiratory infections.

Answer C is incorrect. Brain tumors can present with seizures, but they usually present with other symptoms such as headache, nausea, vomiting, low-grade fever, lethargy, and weight loss. They are not associated with high-grade fever or upper respiratory infections.

Answer D is incorrect. Meningitis can cause seizures, and fever is a sign of meningitis. However, the patient does not have nuchal rigidity or an elevated WBC count, which are classically seen in patients with meningitis. Although nuchal rigidity is typically not seen in very young patients, this child is old enough to demonstrate this cardinal sign of meningitis.

Answer E is incorrect. Subdural hematomas result from rupture of the cerebral bridging veins and can cause seizures, headache, changes in mental status, and contralateral hemiparesis. This usually happens after trauma, and is more unlikely if headache and history of trauma are absent.

8. **The correct answer is C.** This patient has suffered a low-energy pelvic fracture, which is the most common type of fracture in the elderly, and is more common in women than men. Most patients with this injury have sustained a low-energy fall. After a diagnosis of a low-energy pubic ramus fracture is confirmed, and additional fractures of the pelvis and femur are ruled out, treatment is generally nonsurgical and aimed at pain reduction and regaining function, with an emphasis on mobilization as soon as tolerated.

Answer A is incorrect. Repeat radiographic examination is important, and should be done 1–2 weeks following mobilization of the patient. However, weight bearing should not be delayed.

Answer B is incorrect. No clearly defined amount of bed rest is indicated for this injury. The goal in this patient's treatment should be pain management and a return to her previous level of functioning.

Answer D is incorrect. An operative approach is indicated for acetabular and pelvic fractures, but would not be necessary in this patient.

Answer E is incorrect. An operative approach is indicated for acetabular and some other pelvic fractures, but is not necessary for a low-energy fracture of the pubic ramus.

9. **The correct answer is B.** Herniation of the cerebellar tonsils downward can cause respiratory depression and death by compressing the brainstem/medulla. In fact, posterior fossa lesions, as in this case, can also cause upward herniation of the cerebellum. The most likely etiology of this respiratory failure is compression of the respiratory center in the brainstem by herniation through the foramen magnum.

Answer A is incorrect. The history and location of the bleed is more consistent with a tonsillar herniation. Central herniation is also known as transtentorial herniation, in which the diencephalon and parts of the temporal lobes are forced through a notch in the tentorial membrane. Decreased consciousness occurs early in this type of herniation. Central diabetes insipidus may also result from compression of the pituitary stalk.

Answer C is incorrect. Cingulate gyrus herniation typically presents by compressing the anterior cerebral artery, and can cause infarction. This may manifest as a stroke of the frontal lobe.

Answer D is incorrect. Epidural hemorrhage was not present on the CT. However, if the bleed was large enough it could cause a herniation.

Answer E is incorrect. Uncal herniation can compress the third cranial nerve and classically results in increased intracranial pressure causing hypertension, bradycardia, and altered respiratory pattern.

10. **The correct answer is D.** This patient has a history of peptic ulcer disease and now presents to the emergency department with a perforated peptic ulcer. The anterior gastric or duodenal walls are the most common site of such perforation. Patients with an anterior wall perforation do not present with acute bleeding because of the lack of major blood vessels on the anterior gastric surface. Instead, patients may present with acute upper abdominal pain that may radiate to the shoulder or back and a mildly elevated WBC count and amylase level. Peptic ulcer perforation frequently occurs several hours after a meal. In addition, patients will have free air in the abdomen that may

lead to increased tympany and abdominal distention. An upright x-ray of the abdomen will show free intraperitoneal air. Physical examination often reveals abdominal rigidity and inaudible bowel sounds.

Answer A is incorrect. The patient in this case presents with left upper abdominal pain that began 6 hours after his last meal. Patients with cholecystitis characteristically present with right upper quadrant pain that is accompanied by nausea and vomiting. In addition, cholecystitis is associated with increased bilirubin, alkaline phosphatase, and possibly amylase. Cholecystitis is often diagnosed with ultrasound and is not associated with the presence of free intraperitoneal air.

Answer B is incorrect. Hepatitis is not associated with free intraperitoneal air but is associated with abnormal liver function tests, including elevated aspartate transaminase and alkaline phosphatase and right upper quadrant pain. The history, physical, laboratory, and radiographic findings are more supportive of a diagnosis of perforated peptic ulcer than hepatitis.

Answer C is incorrect. Pancreatitis is not associated with free intraperitoneal air as seen in the x-ray of the chest. In addition, patients with pancreatitis often present with elevated amylase and lipase, as well as epigastric pain, nausea, and vomiting. The history, physical, laboratory, and radiographic findings are more supportive of a diagnosis of perforated peptic ulcer than pancreatitis.

Answer E is incorrect. Small bowel obstruction inhibits the passage of intestinal contents and is therefore often seen with nausea and emesis. In addition, these patients present with crampy abdominal discomfort, distention, and high-pitched bowel sounds. It is common to see distended loops of small bowel and air-fluid levels radiographically; however, free intraperitoneal air is not seen in small bowel obstruction. The history, physical, and laboratory findings are more supportive of a diagnosis of perforated peptic ulcer than small bowel obstruction.

11. **The correct answer is E.** This child has a preductal aortic coarctation. The obstruction of the aorta has increased the afterload on the left

ventricle and resulted in congestive heart failure, manifested as respiratory distress. Because the obstruction is proximal to the entry of the ductus arteriosus, blood flow to the abdomen and lower extremities has been supplied primarily by the ductus arteriosus and collateral flow through the intercostal arteries. As the ductus arteriosus begins to close, however, a significant fraction of the blood supply to the lower body is impaired. Although definitive surgical repair of the coarctation is necessary for long-term survival, administration of prostaglandin E_1 will help maintain the patency of the ductus arteriosus, a temporizing measure until definitive repair.

Answer A is incorrect. Endocarditis, or more appropriately, endarteritis, can occur at the site of coarctation. Therefore, endocarditis prophylaxis with antibiotics is appropriate in these patients. Because the child is in respiratory distress and at imminent risk for hypoperfusion of his abdomen and lower extremities, maintaining patency of the ductus arteriosus is of primary importance over reducing the risk of endocarditis/endoarteritis.

Answer B is incorrect. Along with surgical closure and indomethacin administration, coil embolization is a third, minimally invasive way to close the ductus arteriosus. However, continued patency, not closure of the ductus arteriosus, is the desired effect.

Answer C is incorrect. Patency of the ductus arteriosus is important for survival in this child. Although prostaglandins help maintain patency, indomethacin (a prostaglandin inhibitor) promotes the closure of the ductus arteriosus, the opposite of what is needed.

Answer D is incorrect. Surgical closure of the patent ductus arteriosus is analogous to indomethacin administration; both will lead to rapid decompensation in this patient because perfusion to the lower half of the body is reliant in part on the patency of the ductus arteriosus.

12. **The correct answer is B.** Cystic fibrosis is a genetic autosomal recessive disorder of chloride transport across secretory epithelium. The patient typically presents with recurrent pulmonary infections, particularly with *Pseudomonas*, sinusitis, and signs of chronic hypoxia. Family history may be significant for children who died early with recurrent infections. Physical examination often shows nasal polyps, tachypnea, retractions, and wheezing or crackles.

Answer A is incorrect. Foreign body aspiration, if unnoticed, can cause chronic cough with sputum production and is common in this age group. However, the report of multiple infections and family history is not consistent with this diagnosis.

Answer C is incorrect. Most consolidated lobar pneumonia are caused by gram-positive bacteria and would present in this fashion, but the child's history of recurrent infections makes cystic fibrosis more likely.

Answer D is incorrect. Respiratory syncytial virus can cause coughing and respiratory distress but is often a self-limiting infection and does not cause purulent secretions.

Answer E is incorrect. Asthma would cause wheezing and retractions but would not result in purulent sputum or recurrent infections.

13. **The correct answer is E.** On admission, this patient took all necessary steps to make sure that resuscitation did not take place and that a surrogate decision maker was chosen to act if the patient no longer had decision-making capacity. The niece, the chosen health care proxy, requests that life-sustaining care be withheld. This is ethically the same as a withdrawal of care, a right that all patients and their decision makers can exercise. Examples of life-sustaining interventions that can be withheld or withdrawn include ventilation, fluids, nutrition, and medications, such as antibiotics.

Answer A is incorrect. Although the "Do Not Resuscitate" is a form of living will created by the patient and should be abided by if cardiac or respiratory arrest occurs, withdrawal or withholding of care is another right that patients or elected decision makers can exercise in situations such as the one presented.

Answer B is incorrect. In this case, the hospital ethics committee does not need to be involved because a clear surrogate decision maker was chosen when the patient had capacity.

Answer C is incorrect. Decisions should be made by close family members (e.g., the daughter), friends, or a personal physician if a living will or durable power of attorney is not on file. However, the patient chose the niece as her legal health care proxy, and this supersedes the requests of another family member not designated by the patient.

Answer D is incorrect. Because the patient's chosen surrogate health care decision maker has requested that additional life-sustaining treatment, such as antibiotics, be withheld, the team should act in accordance to the niece's wishes.

14. **The correct answer is A.** In immunocompetent patients, isolated pulmonary infection with coccidioidomycosis does not require treatment beyond supportive care. In immunocompromised patients or patients with disseminated disease, the recommended first-line therapy is intravenous (IV) amphotericin B, with or without several months of oral itraconazole following the initial IV therapy. Sometimes itraconazole is given for many years for long-term suppression of the infection in immunocompromised hosts.

Answer B is incorrect. Vancomycin is not an antifungal.

Answer C is incorrect. Intravenous vancomycin for 14 days.

Answer D is incorrect. In this severely immunocompromised patient, oral itraconazole for only 2 weeks is not effective to prevent recurrence.

Answer E is incorrect. In this severely immunocompromised patient, the coccidioidomycosis infection must be treated. His immune system is not capable of clearing the infection without antifungal therapy.

15. **The correct answer is E.** This patient has acute pericarditis, an inflammatory process of the pericardial space. Pericarditis often presents with pleuritic chest pain radiating to the back, dyspnea, pericardial friction rub, and occasionally fever. Common causes of pericarditis include infectious, autoimmune, traumatic, and neoplastic processes. Nine of 10 cases of pericarditis are believed to be viral or idiopathic, so it is quite likely that this patient has a viral etiology. Diagnostic tests included ECG, echocardiography, and x-ray of the chest. An enlarged, flask-shaped cardiac silhouette, as seen in the image, is often apparent on x-ray of the chest. Treatment is through nonsteroidal anti-inflammatory drugs and, if symptoms of tamponade appear, pericardiocentesis.

Answer A is incorrect. Although aortic dissection can cause chest pain, this pain typically presents as a sudden, intense, tearing chest pain that may radiate to the neck and jaw. Imaging is typically used to make the diagnosis and usually involves either CT or transesophageal echocardiography.

Answer B is incorrect. Myocardial ischemia can cause chest pain, but classically presents as a dull pain radiating from the patient's chest to the left arm. It can also be associated with dyspnea and palpitations. Diagnostic tests include ECG, cardiac enzyme levels, and, ultimately, angiography.

Answer C is incorrect. This patient has pericarditis, not a pulmonary embolism (PE). Although this patient has risk factors (family history, smoking, and oral contraceptives) and symptoms (dyspnea, chest pain, and cough) that could be consistent with PE, the positional nature of her pain, her friction rub, her slight cardiomegaly on x-ray of the chest, and her ECG findings suggest that she has pericarditis. Thromboembolism is not a possible etiology of pericarditis, so it is not the correct answer.

Answer D is incorrect. Symptoms consistent with thyroid storm include tachycardia, systolic hypertension, delirium, and fever. This patient's clinical picture does not suggest this diagnosis.

16. **The correct answer is D.** This is the current protocol for posttransplant vaccination. In bone marrow transplant patients, optimal responses to vaccines cannot be reached until

the immune system is reconstituted, a process that may take up to 2 years. In the case of an allogeneic transplant, memory cells are eliminated during the pretransplant conditioning protocol, and so the recipient requires a new primary and booster series against common pathogens. Immunization of close contacts is given to prevent local spread via direct contact and secretion.

Answer A is incorrect. The vaccines in question do not confer risk of reactivation infection to the patient. The risk of reactivation of the live polio vaccine is high enough that patients and their family members should avoid receipt of the vaccine for 24 months posttransplant. The measles-mumps-rubella vaccine confers a lower risk to transplant patients when given to family members, but should still be given with caution.

Answer B is incorrect. Reactivation concerns may be appropriate when the live polio and measles-mumps-rubella vaccines are considered. For this reason, these vaccines should not be given to bone marrow transplant patients for 24 months posttransplant. The vaccines in question, however, are all killed or partial organisms, so reactivation is not a concern.

Answer C is incorrect. Vaccinating the patient immediately after transplant will not offer protection, as her immune system will not be able to mount an appropriate response to the vaccine.

Answer E is incorrect. Because the pretransplant protocol consists of eliminating the patient's own marrow, including memory T and B lymphocytes, vaccinating prior to the transplant will likely not confer protection posttransplant. Additionally, cancer patients undergoing chemotherapy do not respond adequately to vaccinations.

17. **The correct answer is B.** Recent double-blind, randomized controlled clinical trials have demonstrated that patients with asymptomatic carotid stenosis measuring ≥ 60% who were healthy enough to undergo surgery were at a reduced risk of ipsilateral cerebrovascular accident if they underwent carotid endarterectomy versus medical management with aspirin

alone. Therefore, given the patient's stable condition and the finding of an asymptomatic 80% carotid stenosis, this patient would most likely benefit the most from surgery.

Answer A is incorrect. Recent studies indicate that carotid angioplasty with stenting may play a role similar to carotid endarterectomy (CEA), but with fewer adverse effects and lower morbidity. However, angioplasty on its own has not yet been shown to be superior to CEA.

Answer C is incorrect. Medical management with aspirin has been shown to be inferior to surgery in treating asymptomatic carotid stenosis measuring ≥ 60%.

Answer D is incorrect. Warfarin has not been shown to have therapeutic value in carotid disease. In fact, it actually may be of some detriment due the profound anticoagulation, vigilant monitoring, and possible adverse effects that accompany treatment.

Answer E is incorrect. Surgery is indicated in this patient due to the extent of the stenosis despite being asymptomatic. Medical risk factor management followed by surgery may be a rational therapeutic plan in a patient with high surgical risk and is therefore deemed unsafe for elective surgery. However, in a patient with minor comorbidities, such as this patient, surgical risk would be low.

18. **The correct answer is E.** The *Diagnostic and Statistical Manual of Mental Disorders*, Fourth Edition, Text Revision criteria for trichotillomania are recurrent pulling out of one's hair resulting in noticeable hair loss, along with an increasing sense of tension immediately before pulling out the hair or when attempting to resist the behavior. There is also pleasure, gratification, or relief when pulling out the hair. Finally, the disturbance causes clinically significant distress or impairment in social, occupational, or other important areas of functioning. A biologic theory of etiology has been postulated. Researchers have proposed a serotonergic abnormality in trichotillomania and have suggested that this disorder may be a pathologic variant of species-specific grooming behaviors. Supporting a theoretical serotonergic

mechanism in the disorder is the fact that selective serotonin reuptake inhibitors are used to treat trichotillomania, along with cognitive-behavioral therapy.

Answer A is incorrect. Alopecia areata is an autoimmune disease involving the hair follicles. In most cases, hair falls out in small, round patches about the size of a quarter. In many cases, the disease does not extend beyond a few bare patches. In some people, hair loss is more extensive. Although uncommon, the disease can progress to cause total loss of hair on the head (referred to as alopecia areata totalis) or complete loss of hair on the head, face, and body (alopecia areata universalis).

Answer B is incorrect. The patient does not meet the diagnostic criteria for depression (must have five depressive symptoms such as suicidal ideation, decreased interest, guilt, decreased energy, decreased concentration, and decreased appetite, among others). Furthermore, pulling out hair is not a feature typically associated with depression.

Answer C is incorrect. Although patients with trichotillomania often have comorbid obsessive-compulsive disorder (OCD), they are not the same disorder. Those with OCD have specific recurrent thoughts which are ego dystonic. These thoughts cause anxiety, which is then alleviated by compulsive behavior.

Answer D is incorrect. The patient has no thought disorganization, delusions, or hallucinations causing her to pull out her hair. Thus, schizophrenia would be an unlikely diagnosis.

19. **The correct answer is D.** Cystic fibrosis (CF) is an autosomal recessive disease that is more common in the white population. Life expectancy for patients with CF is 30 years, although patients are now living longer due to recent advances in treatment. The hallmark of CF is an abnormal exocrine gland function that involves multiple organ systems and leads to chronic respiratory infections, pancreatic insufficiency, and musculoskeletal manifestations. A defect in the *CFTR* (cystic fibrosis transmembrane regulator) gene results in decreased secretion of chloride, resulting in thicker, viscid secretions, making them hard to

clear and a more favorable environment for bacterial growth. X-ray of the chest reveals hyperinflated lungs, increased interstitial markings, and cysts. Pulmonary function tests reveal obstructive airway disease. Pancreatic insufficiency leads to poor weight gain in association with frequent stools that are malodorous, greasy, and associated with flatulence and colicky pain after feeding. Poor weight gain and failure to thrive results from the combination of increased energy intake at baseline, added energy intake demand of chronic disease, anorexia associated with ongoing lung inflammation, and malabsorption. Treatment of pancreatic insufficiency involves the replacement of pancreatic enzymes and eating a high-calorie diet. Dietary supplements, including fat-soluble vitamins, should also be administered to replace lost nutrients.

Answer A is incorrect. Laxatives may be administered to treat intestinal obstruction in older patients, and would be inappropriate in this case, as the patient is not obstructed.

Answer B is incorrect. Because pancreatic insufficiency results in poor absorption of fat-soluble vitamins A, D, E, and K, they must be replaced with dietary supplements. However, pancreatic enzyme replacement is also necessary to aid in.

Answer C is incorrect. Patients with pancreatic insufficiency are encouraged to maintain a higher-than-normal-calorie diet, not lower, with unrestricted fat intake due to their propensity for malabsorption and failure to thrive.

Answer E is incorrect. Even when a patient has significant steatorrhea, fat is not withheld from the diet. They are actually encouraged to have an unrestricted fat intake once pancreatic enzyme supplementation has been instituted.

20. **The correct answer is D.** Lisinopril is an appropriate addition at this time given the patient's microalbuminuria and history of both hypertension and diabetes mellitus type 2. Angiotensin-converting enzyme inhibitors have been demonstrated to delay nephropathic progression in patients with diabetes and microalbuminuria.

Answer A is incorrect. Furosemide is incorrect because adding an additional diuretic is not necessary given the degree of hypertensive control his current regimen has achieved.

Answer B is incorrect. Gemfibrozil is not indicated because there is no information given regarding the patient's lipid status.

Answer C is incorrect. Adding a β-blocker is incorrect because no further antihypertensive therapy is needed at this time.

Answer E is incorrect. Adding insulin is incorrect because the patient's hemoglobin A_{1c} indicates good glycemic control on metformin alone.

21. **The correct answer is C.** β-hCG can be detected in the serum 8 days after the luteinizing hormone surge, assuming a pregnancy has occurred. The β-hCG concentration in a normal intrauterine pregnancy rises steadily until 41 days of gestation, at which time it plateaus at approximately 100,000 mIU/mL. The average doubling time for β-hCG levels is 2 days. A β-hCG level that does not double within 2 days suggests an at-risk pregnancy, and a decrease in β-hCG levels indicates a failed pregnancy, whether intrauterine or extrauterine. In such an event, patients should be monitored weekly until the pregnancy has passed.

Answer A is incorrect. A CT scan with or without contrast is not an appropriate diagnostic tool in assessing the presence of an intrauterine or extrauterine pregnancy.

Answer B is incorrect. Dilation and curettage is not used to investigate the presence of an ectopic pregnancy, due to the potential for disruption of a viable intrauterine pregnancy. In this patient with a failed pregnancy, dilation and curettage may be indicated in the future if she fails to pass the products of conception. At this point, however, it is inappropriate.

Answer D is incorrect. Laparoscopy or laparotomy is not indicated in this patient, as there is evidence that her pregnancy is failing. Surgical interventions are indicated in a patient with a rising β-hCG and a documented adnexal mass on transvaginal ultrasound.

Answer E is incorrect. The gestational sac is generally evident on transvaginal ultrasound in a viable pregnancy when the serum β-hCG level is > 1500 mIU/mL (4.5–5 weeks of gestation). A negative transvaginal ultrasound in a patient with a β-hCG level < 1500 mIU/mL is nondiagnostic and should be repeated after 72 hours as long as the serum β-hCG level continues to rise. A repeat transvaginal ultrasound, however, is not indicated when the serum β-hCG level is falling, as this is a sign of a failed pregnancy.

22. **The correct answer is E.** The patient is presenting with thyrotoxic shock, or thyroid storm. This is a complication of thyrotoxicosis that is usually preceded by infection, trauma, surgery, or diabetic ketoacidosis. Patients typically present with jaundice, nausea and vomiting, diarrhea, seizure, delirium, fever, tachycardia, and hypertension. If untreated, thyrotoxic shock can be rapidly fatal, and even with treatment, mortality is as high as 30%. Mortality is usually due to cardiac failure, arrhythmias, and hyperthermia. β-Blockers such as propranolol are mainstays in the initial management of patients with thyrotoxic shock.

Answer A is incorrect. Dobutamine is a β-agonist that would worsen this patient's condition. It would further increase her heart rate and increase her risk of developing high-output cardiac failure. β-*Antagonists* are the preferred therapy.

Answer B is incorrect. Enalapril is an angiotensin-converting enzyme inhibitor that is used in the management of hypertension, renal disease, and congestive heart failure. It is not used in acutely managing thyroid storm.

Answer C is incorrect. Levothyroxine would worsen this patient's condition significantly. All attempts should be made to **reduce** levels of circulating thyroid hormone.

Answer D is incorrect. Methimazole is a thionamide that decreases synthesis of thyroid hormone. Although methimazole helps to decrease production of new thyroid hormone, it has no effect on the release of already synthesized hormone or the level of circulating hormone. A better choice is propylthiouracil, another thionamide that in addition to the actions of methimazole, also blocks the peripheral conversion of thyroxine to triiodothyronine.

23. **The correct answer is E.** Highly sensitive tests are used to rule out disease and have a low false-negative rate, so if the patient has a negative result one can rule out disease in the patient.

Answer A is incorrect. A low negative predictive value would indicate that a negative result did not often indicate that the disease could be ruled out in the patient and would suggest the test was not as useful.

Answer B is incorrect. A low positive predictive value would indicate that a positive result did not necessarily indicate that the patient had the disease and would suggest the test was not as useful.

Answer C is incorrect. The test is independent of disease incidence, which is the occurrence of new cases in a defined interval of time. For screening purposes, a highly sensitive test is preferred for the purpose of ruling out disease.

Answer D is incorrect. The test is independent of disease prevalence, which is the occurrence of a disorder or trait in a given population. For screening purposes, a highly sensitive test is preferred for the purpose of ruling out disease.

24. **The correct answer is A.** This patient's symptoms are consistent with aseptic meningitis, which can be caused by any number of viruses. However, given this patient's HIV risk factor (intravenous drug use), the diagnosis of acute HIV syndrome should be high on the differential. Acute HIV syndrome usually occurs 2–3 weeks after the initial exposure. Given the "indeterminate" antibody test (which is possible because it takes many weeks to mount an antibody response to the virus), a viral load would be diagnostic. In acute HIV infection, the viral load is extremely high (up to 100,000 RNA copies per milliliter).

Answer B is incorrect. An echocardiogram would be helpful in diagnosing valvular dis-

ease, wall motion abnormalities, endocarditis, or thrombi in one of the chambers of the heart. However, because there are no focal neurologic signs in this patient, stroke is not high on the differential. Therefore, there is no need to look for a source of emboli.

Answer C is incorrect. Given the low RBC count in the cerebrospinal fluid from the original lumbar puncture, this was not a traumatic tap; there is no reason to believe that the first lumbar puncture was inaccurate.

Answer D is incorrect. Starting an HIV-positive patient on antiretroviral therapy is decided based on the CD4+ count, viral load, and positive symptoms of the disease. Patients should begin a regimen if they have a CD4+ count $< 200/mm^3$, high viral load ($> 100,000/mL$), fall in CD4+ count $> 100/y$, or symptoms such as thrush, wasting, or an AIDS diagnosis.

Answer E is incorrect. Intravenous ceftriaxone and vancomycin are the prophylactic treatments of choice for bacterial meningitis. Since there was a lymphocytic predominance and no organisms were seen on Gram stain, a bacterial meningitis is unlikely. Therefore, empiric antibiotics are not indicated in this case.

25. **The correct answer is C.** The patient likely has gastroesophageal reflux disease (GERD), which often presents with heartburn, regurgitation, and dysphagia that is typically worse with meals and when lying supine. Mild symptomatic GERD can usually be managed empirically; lifestyle and dietary modifications along with antacids and nonprescription histamine$_2$-receptor antagonists are usually sufficient. Lifestyle modifications include cessation of smoking, sleeping with the head of bed elevated, avoiding excessive alcohol, and avoidance of late meals. Patients with debilitating symptoms usually require more pharmacologic acid-suppressive therapy or antireflux surgery.

Answer A is incorrect. Avoiding spicy foods has not been shown to be effective to treat gastroesophageal reflux disease.

Answer B is incorrect. Histamine$_2$-receptor blockers, while providing symptomatic relief, may be unnecessary given the probable improvement in symptoms with lifestyle modifications. However, they can be effective as supplementary therapy to lifestyle modification.

Answer D is incorrect. This surgical procedure has been shown to prevent active reflux and further damage to the esophagus; however, it is reserved for cases that have been refractory to maximal medical management, which this patient has not attempted yet.

Answer E is incorrect. Proton pump inhibitors, as with histamine$_2$-blockers, should be used in cases that are refractory to lifestyle modifications.

26. **The correct answer is E.** This case is an example of factitious disorder by proxy, more commonly known as Munchausen syndrome by proxy. In this disorder, caregivers deliberately exaggerate, fabricate, and/or induce physical and psychological problems in others. In most cases, the perpetrators of Munchausen by proxy will continue their behavior even after they have been discovered. Factitious disorder must be differentiated from malingering because factitious disorder has a goal of primary, or psychological, gain. Malingering means the perpetrator has a secondary goal (e.g., food, shelter, and money).

Answer A is incorrect. In many cases, there is no history of investigation by child protective services.

Answer B is incorrect. Unfortunately, many perpetrators of Munchausen syndrome by proxy appear psychologically healthy.

Answer C is incorrect. Many perpetrators "doctor shop," or move from doctor to doctor, when physicians become suspicious.

Answer D is incorrect. Mothers who are later diagnosed with Munchausen syndrome by proxy often give the semblance of being the "ideal mother." It often appears that they are taking excellent, dutiful care of their sick child, when it is they who are inducing the illness.

27. **The correct answer is B.** This patient presents with signs and symptoms suggestive of temporal, or giant cell, arteritis. Patients are usually aged 50 years or older. Clinical presentation includes headache that is unilateral and localized to the temporal or frontal regions. The temporal artery may appear enlarged and tender to palpation. A bruit may be auscultated over the temporal or carotid artery. Patients may complain of jaw or arm claudication and visual changes. Without appropriate therapy, temporal arteritis can lead to ischemic optic neuropathy and blindness. Patients can also have systemic symptoms including fever, weight loss, and fatigue. A key laboratory finding is elevated erythrocyte sedimentation rate (ESR), often > 100 mm/h. The diagnosis of temporal arteritis should be considered in patients over age 50 presenting with fever, anemia, and elevated ESR. The diagnosis is confirmed by biopsy of the temporal artery as soon as possible. However, initiation of therapy with glucocorticoids should not be delayed while the biopsy is pending, as the risk of permanent vision loss is high.

Answer A is incorrect. Antineutrophil cytoplasmic antibody is found in patients with Wegener's granulomatosis, another type of vasculitis that affects medium- and small-sized vessels, among other disorders. Wegener's classically affects the lungs and kidneys. Pulmonary symptoms include cough, dyspnea, and hemoptysis. Renal involvement is usually a pauci-immune glomerulonephritis.

Answer C is incorrect. Nonsteroidal anti-inflammatory drugs may be used to abort migraine or tension headaches. Migraines may be unilateral and cause visual disturbances. However, in a patient over age 50 presenting with temporal tenderness, jaw claudication, constitutional symptoms, and a significantly elevated erythrocyte sedimentation rate, temporal arteritis should be highest on the differential.

Answer D is incorrect. Magnetic resonance angiography may show large-artery involvement, but temporal artery biopsy is considered the gold standard for diagnosing temporal arteritis.

Answer E is incorrect. Temporal artery biopsy is the gold standard for diagnosing temporal arteritis. However, sight-preserving management should not be delayed in patients who present with the clinical signs and symptoms of temporal arteritis. Following steroid induction, temporal artery biopsy would be the next step in management.

28. **The correct answer is A.** Meconium ileus, as described in this vignette, often presents in the first 24–48 hours of life as abdominal distention, emesis, and failure to pass meconium (the first stool after birth). Abdominal radiographs typically show loops of dilated bowel with air-fluid levels and frequently demonstrate a granular "ground-glass" material in the lower central abdomen. Meconium ileus occurs primarily in newborn infants with cystic fibrosis, occurring in approximately 10% of infants with the condition. Eighty percent to 90% of infants presenting with meconium ileus have cystic fibrosis (CF), and it is considered pathognomonic of CF unless proven otherwise.

Answer B is incorrect. Edwards syndrome is a chromosomal trisomy caused by meiotic nondisjunction of chromosome 18. The characteristic clinical findings in Edwards syndrome include low birth weight, short sternum, rocker-bottom feet, microcephaly with prominent occiput, micrognathia, mental retardation, cardiac and renal anomalies, and a distinguishing hand positioning of closed fists with the index finger overlapping the third digit and the fifth digit overlapping the fourth. Gastrointestinal abnormalities, specifically meconium ileus, are not commonly associated with Edwards syndrome.

Answer C is incorrect. A Meckel's diverticulum is a remnant of the embryonic yolk sac and is the most frequent congenital gastrointestinal anomaly. Symptoms usually present during the first 2 years of life, but primary symptoms generally manifest within the first decade. Most symptomatic patients have diverticula that are lined by an ectopic mucosa that is acid secreting and can cause intermittent painless rectal bleeding by way of ulceration of the adjacent normal ileal mucosa. Episodes of bowel obstruction with Meckel's diverticula have been described but are relatively rare. Meconium ileus is not associated with Meckel's diverticula.

Answer D is incorrect. Trisomy 21 (Down's syndrome) is caused by meiotic nondisjunction or a translocation of chromosome 21. It most commonly presents clinically with hypotonia, flat face, upward and slanted palpebral fissures and epicanthic folds, mental retardation, growth failure of varying degrees, pelvic dysplasia, cardiac malformations, speckled irises (Brushfield spots), and simian crease of the palms. Intestinal atresia can be seen in Down's syndrome patients, but meconium ileus is uncommon.

Answer E is incorrect. Williams syndrome is caused by a microdeletion of 7q11.23 with clinical manifestations, including round face with full lips and cheeks; iris with stellate pattern; strabismus; variable degrees of mental retardation; cardiac malformations, especially supravalvular aortic stenosis; and an extremely friendly personality. Gastrointestinal complaints, specifically meconium ileus, are not associated with Williams syndrome.

29. **The correct answer is C.** Kussmaul breathing is the term for the deep, rapid breathing often seen in diabetic ketoacidosis (DKA). It is the physiologic response to extreme acidosis as the body tries to eliminate excess acid in the form of expired carbon dioxide. Because nonketotic hyperglycemia (NKH) does not result in the formation of ketones or the onset of acidosis, Kussmaul breathing is not normally seen in patients suffering from NKH. Fruity, acetone breath is the result of the acidosis and is another distinguishing characteristic of DKA.

Answer A is incorrect. Dehydration often precipitates both diabetic ketoacidosis and nonketotic hyperglycemia. Because glucose is an osmotic diuretic, patients with extreme hyperglycemia will be dehydrated regardless of the cause.

Answer B is incorrect. Hyperglycemia is a hallmark of both diabetic ketoacidosis (DKA) and nonketotic hyperglycemia (NKH), although DKA has a concomitant acidosis, whereas NKH does not.

Answer D is incorrect. Mental status changes, to varying degrees, are commonly seen in both diabetic ketoacidosis and nonketotic hyperglycemia.

Answer E is incorrect. Vomiting is a common symptom seen in both diabetic ketoacidosis and nonketotic hyperglycemia.

30. **The correct answer is C.** Specificity allows one to rule in a disease with confidence. Specificity is defined as [true negatives/(true negatives + false positives)]. The confirmatory step of the HIV test, a Western blot test for viral proteins, is known to have high specificity, and thus a low chance of being incorrect.

Answer A is incorrect. Positive predictive value is dependent on the sensitivity and specificity of the test, as well as the prevalence of the disease in the population being tested. The pair of tests used for HIV testing collectively have very high sensitivity and specificity. Because this patient falls into a high-risk population for HIV infection, the positive predictive value of the test in this circumstance is higher than it would be for a lower-risk subject.

Answer B is incorrect. High sensitivity increases the negative predictive value of a test, allowing one to rule out a disease if the result is negative. This would be relevant if the patient was asking about a negative test result and whether he might still have the disease. The HIV screening test (enzyme-linked immunosorbent assay) has high sensitivity for infection of more than a month's duration.

Answer D is incorrect. Other diseases can cause false-positive HIV tests, decreasing the validity of the test.

31. **The correct answer is B.** This patient is presenting with the classic signs of a gestational trophoblastic tumor from either a complete or partial hydatidiform mole. Gestational trophoblastic disease is a rare, highly treatable condition in which cancer cells grow in the trophoblast (tissue formed immediately after fertilization that eventually forms the placenta). Typically, this disease affects primigravid patients at the extremes of maternal age and presents with vaginal bleeding as the tumor separates from the underlying decidua. With continued growth of the tumor, pressure on the uterus results in pelvic pain. In addition, the uterus will be larger than expected due to the growth of the tumor. Regardless of

whether this mole is partial or complete, β-human chorionic gonadotropin (hCG) will be higher than normal, resulting in extreme nausea. Serial β-hCG measurements must be monitored after treatment to ensure all parts of the hydatidiform mole have been removed.

Answer A is incorrect. Secondary to continuous vaginal bleeding, patients presenting with molar pregnancies are typically anemic.

Answer C is incorrect. The β-subunit of human chorionic gonadotropin (hCG) is the same as the β-subunit for thyroid-stimulating hormone (TSH). As a result, the elevated hCG stimulates the thyroid gland to produce a hyperthyroid state. Therefore, TSH levels will be decreased.

Answer D is incorrect. Ovarian cysts arising in the normal process of ovulation are called functional or theca lutein cysts. These cysts can be stimulated by gonadotropins, including follicle-stimulating hormone and β-hCG. Because of higher-than-normal β-hCG levels, multilocular theca lutein cysts are classically seen in patients with gestational trophoblastic disease.

Answer E is incorrect. Because the tumor is located within the uterus, a pelvic ultrasound will show an enlarged uterus. An ultrasound will also show a lack of fetal tissue and amniotic fluid.

32. **The correct answer is D.** Terazosin, an α-blocker, should be the first-line treatment in this patient. Based on his symptoms and physical exam, he has benign prostatic hypertrophy (BPH). He also has hypertension that has been noted on three separate occasions despite a healthy low-salt diet and exercise. At this point, terazosin monotherapy, which can address both his hypertension and BPH, is indicated. The prostate and base of the bladder contain α_1 adrenoreceptors. The prostate contracts when these receptors are stimulated by an agonist. Terazosin blocks effects of the α_{1a} subtype in the prostate, improving the symptoms and signs of BPH. These receptors are the same as those found in the vascular system, where the postsynaptic α_1-adrenergic receptors cause peripheral constriction when stimulated. Thus,

pharmacologic blockade causes a decrease in systemic blood pressure. Because terazosin is a selective α-blocker and does not have any effect on presynaptic α_2-receptors, it will not cause reflex tachycardia.

Answer A is incorrect. Finasteride is a medication that has a role in treating benign prostatic hypertrophy. However, it has no role in the treatment of hypertension; terazosin is a better choice.

Answer B is incorrect. Lisinopril is an angiotensin converting enzyme (ACE) inhibitor that is used in treatment of hypertension. This class of drug is thought to prevent progression of microalbuminuria to proteinuria in diabetics. However, an ACE inhibitor would not help the man's urinary symptoms.

Answer C is incorrect. The man has hypertension and benign prostatic hypertrophy, and he needs treatment, as long as there are no contraindications to starting therapy.

Answer E is incorrect. Thiazides are popular as first-line agents in treating hypertension, but in this case terazosin is preferred because it can simultaneously treat the patient's benign prostatic hypertrophy.

33. **The correct answer is D.** Acromegaly is caused by excessive release of growth hormone (GH), most commonly due to an adenoma in the anterior pituitary. Because GH is secreted in a pulsatile fashion, measuring serum GH levels is not a reliable method of diagnosing acromegaly. Instead, serum insulin-like growth factor-1, a growth factor secreted by the liver under GH stimulation, is measured to confirm the diagnosis. Octreotide is a somatostatin analogue that counteracts GH hypersecretion. It is often used for immediate relief of symptoms or for preoperatively shrinking large macroadenomas.

Answer A is incorrect. Cortisol is used to treat patients with glucocorticoid deficiency due to adrenal insufficiency or pituitary deficiency of ACTH. Although a pituitary adenoma can decrease secretion of ACTH, the patient is not currently presenting with findings consistent with low cortisol. Therefore, cortisol would not be the primary therapy.

Answer B is incorrect. Acromegaly is due to excessive secretion of growth hormone (GH), not GH deficiency. Therefore, administration of growth hormone would worsen his signs and symptoms.

Answer C is incorrect. Metyrapone is an antagonist of cortisol production that is used to treat patients with Cushing's disease due to an ACTH-producing pituitary adenoma.

Answer E is incorrect. Thyroid hormone is used to treat patients with hypothyroidism due to intrinsic thyroid disorders or hypopituitarism. Although a pituitary adenoma can suppress secretion of other hormones in the anterior pituitary, including thyroid-stimulating hormone, the patient is not currently presenting with signs of hypothyroidism. His immediate problem is the excessive level of GH, so thyroid hormone would not be considered primary therapy. Thyroid levels should be checked, however.

34. **The correct answer is E.** Patients with long-standing rheumatoid arthritis can develop lung manifestations of the disease, including pleural diseases such as effusions, empyemas, necrosis, or cavitations. This x-ray of the chest shows a pleural effusion with layering of the fluid. Effusions greater than 1 cm in the decubitus view are usually large enough to be safely sampled. While it is not necessarily an indication to absolutely do a thoracentesis, in this case thoracentesis is both diagnostic and therapeutic. To aid in determining the cause of the effusion, one can use the Light's criteria to distinguish between a transudate and an exudate.

Answer A is incorrect. Furosemide would be indicated for congestive heart failure (CHF) contributing to pleural effusion. However, the patient's symptoms are not consistent with CHF.

Answer B is incorrect. A likely cause of this patient's effusion is rheumatoid arthritis, which is suggested by her morning stiffness. However, further workup is indicated before that diagnosis can be confirmed and treatment started.

Answer C is incorrect. Parapneumonic effusions occur with bacterial pneumonias; however, these often do not resolve with antibiotics alone and require drainage via a chest tube. Additionally, this patient has no evidence of infection to make her a candidate for antibiotics.

Answer D is incorrect. Any new effusion with no clear etiology (e.g., congestive heart failure or pneumonia) should be tapped and analyzed for possible oncologic or rheumatologic etiologies.

35. **The correct answer is B.** Thiazides can cause hyperlipidemia with an increase in both total and LDL cholesterol.

Answer A is incorrect. Hypokalemia (not hyperkalemia) with thiazide diuretics is a common early complication of treatment. Increased sodium and water delivery to the aldosterone-sensitive potassium secretory site in the collecting tubules, as well as increased aldosterone secretion in response to volume depletion, leads to increased potassium loss.

Answer C is incorrect. Hyponatremia (not hypernatremia) is a rare but potentially fatal complication of several types of diuretic therapy, but most severe cases are secondary to thiazide diuretic use.

Answer D is incorrect. Thiazide diuretics sometimes result in hypercalcemia secondary to active calcium resorption in the distal tubule.

Answer E is incorrect. Hyperuricemia (not hypouricemia) is a relatively common complication of thiazide diuretics, which cause decreased excretion by increasing net reabsorption of urate.

36. **The correct answer is C.** The patient has a type I renal tubular acidosis (RTA) that was confirmed by challenging her with ammonium chloride. Patients with a distal RTA cannot make the urine pH < 5.5. As a result, they are at risk for calcium phosphate stones. The antibodies that would reveal a cause of this distal RTA would be anti-Ro/SSA and anti-La/SSB. These antibodies are found in high frequency in patients with Sjögren's syndrome. The patient's dry mucous membranes and use of eye drops could also suggest this as a diagnosis and cause of the RTA. Patients with Sjögren's may present with a distal RTA and no other clinical findings.

Answer A is incorrect. Antiglomerular basement membrane antibody is associated with Goodpasture's syndrome. The effect on the kidney is a rapidly progressive glomerulonephritis, which can cause renal failure. The patient is not described as having renal failure, nor does this disease classically present with kidney stones.

Answer B is incorrect. Antihistone antibody is seen in drug-induced systemic lupus erythematosus. Because the patient is not taking any medication, this diagnosis is unlikely. The drugs that are commonly implicated include procainamide, hydralazine, phenytoin, sulfonamides, and isoniazid.

Answer D is incorrect. Circulating antineutrophilic cytoplasmic autoantibody is found in patients with Wegner's granulomatosis. This disorder is more common in men. These patients may present with fever, fatigue, and malaise. The upper airway is also involved, including nasal and sinus discomfort and upper respiratory infections.

Answer E is incorrect. Perinuclear antineutrophilic cytoplasmic autoantibody is found in patients with microscopic polyangiitis. This condition is not associated with distal renal tubular acidosis.

37. **The correct answer is B.** Although there are other possible causes for this man's symptoms, an ischemic stroke of the anterior inferior cerebellar artery (AICA) is most likely. Strokes in this distribution typically present with gaze palsy, deafness, tinnitus, and ipsilateral facial weakness. Unlike strokes in the posterior inferior cerebellar artery, there is no Horner's syndrome, dysphagia, or dysarthria. The AICA is a branch of the basilar artery.

Answer A is incorrect. Anterior cerebral artery strokes present with leg paresis, amnesia, personality changes, foot drop, gait dysfunction, or cognitive changes.

Answer C is incorrect. Middle cerebral artery strokes typically present with aphasia (dominant hemisphere), neglect (nondominant hemisphere) contralateral hemiparesis, gaze preference, or homonymous hemianopsia.

Answer D is incorrect. Posterior cerebral artery strokes present with homonymous hemianopsia, memory deficits, or dyslexia/alexia.

Answer E is incorrect. Posterior inferior cerebellar artery strokes present with sudden-onset nausea/vomiting, vertigo, hoarseness, ataxia, ipsilateral palate and tongue weakness, contralateral disturbance of pain/temperature, dysphagia/dysarthria/hiccup, and ipsilateral Horner's syndrome.

38. **The correct answer is B.** This patient is manic and has a history of psychosis. The Tarasoff decision states that if a patient presents a serious, credible danger to another person, physicians have an obligation to protect the threatened party. In this case it would be reasonable to disclose to police that the patient is psychotic and has made specific threats to harm the young woman. Until the patient is hospitalized and treated for mania, he may pose a serious threat to her.

Answer A is incorrect. The physician must take reasonable steps to protect the threatened party; asking the patient's roommate to control a potentially manic and psychotic person is not a reasonable measure under these circumstances.

Answer C is incorrect. The physician must take a more active role than that described in this answer choice. He may contact the threatened party to inform them of the patient's statements, but he must also contact emergency medical services to take the patient into custody. As a physician, his opinion would expedite the apprehension of the patient.

Answer D is incorrect. The Tarasoff decision states that it is ethically sound and appropriate to override patient confidentiality in cases of potential harm to third parties.

Answer E is incorrect. The physician cannot rely on previous behavior or actions of the patient; he must act on the current information and take steps to protect the threatened party.

39. **The correct answer is D.** For the patient with mental status changes, it is important to rule out life-threatening causes such as intracranial hemorrhage and meningoencephalitis. In this

case, there is a low suspicion of both due to the history negative for trauma, the negative CT, and a lack of signs of infection. Mass lesions causing herniation are also ruled out by CT. Metabolic causes of mental status change should always be considered. Besides a low platelet count and hemolytic anemia, thrombotic thrombocytopenic purpura (TTP) can also present with change in mental status, which can range from mild confusion to coma. The etiology of the mental status change is thrombotic microvascular occlusion within the brain parenchyma. Although TTP can be associated with medications (e.g., cyclosporine and antiplatelet drugs), most cases are idiopathic.

Answer A is incorrect. Diuretics are not associated with mental status changes. Even if the patient had taken enough to cause volume depletion and hypotension, there would be other electrolyte disturbances.

Answer B is incorrect. Hemolytic anemia can be precipitated by medications such as penicillin or quinidine but would not be associated with mental status changes.

Answer C is incorrect. Liver failure may lead to uremia and encephalopathy (the hepatorenal syndrome). However, in the absence of elevated aspartate aminotransferase and alanine aminotransferase and with a normal albumin level, liver failure is unlikely.

Answer E is incorrect. Viral meningoencephalitis is unlikely due to the absence of a fever, normal WBC count, and absence of meningeal signs.

40. **The correct answer is C.** Septic ovarian vein thrombosis (OVT) is a rare complication of delivery, occurring in < 1 in 500 deliveries. OVT generally occurs as a consequence of a pelvic infection and is the result of intimal injury in the setting of a hypercoagulable state. Treatment includes antibiotics and heparin. The current antibiotic regimen is appropriate and does not need to be changed. Typically, patients retain normal function in the affected ovary. Patients should be counseled that the recurrence of septic OVT is rare.

Answer A is incorrect. No further β-lactamase coverage is needed. The combination of clindamycin and gentamicin provide adequate coverage.

Answer B is incorrect. The current antibiotic regimen provides appropriate aerobic and anaerobic coverage of organisms that typically colonize the pelvis and genital tract and should not be changed. The patient's persistent fever spikes are not a sign of antibiotic failure, but rather are due to the production of clot, which necessitates heparin administration.

Answer D is incorrect. Heparin alone will not adequately treat ovarian vein thrombosis because the ovarian vein and clot are generally infected.

Answer E is incorrect. Surgery is not needed at this time. Initial therapy is broad-spectrum antibiotics and heparin. A rapid response to treatment is not expected and may take up to 7 days. Thromboses generally resolve with antibiotics and heparin. Surgery is only rarely indicated in cases of inadequate response to therapy.

41. **The correct answer is E.** This patient is in shock due to urosepsis. As aggressive fluid resuscitation has failed to bring the mean arterial pressure up to acceptable levels, and because the administration of further fluid infusions would render the patient vulnerable to pulmonary edema, a pressor would be the next treatment. Of the medications noted, norepinephrine is the appropriate choice because it specifically targets the cause of the low pressure, namely the relaxation of peripheral blood vessels due to sepsis. It is a predominantly α-adrenergic agonist, and as such will constrict peripheral blood vessels.

Answer A is incorrect. Dobutamine, which is predominantly a positive inotropic agent, would not be as useful as norepinephrine, as it does not address the major cause of the hypotension. However, if the patient achieves an appropriate mean arterial pressure but cannot maintain an appropriate cardiac output, dobutamine is the subsequent medication of choice.

Answer B is incorrect. Epinephrine, which has predominantly either α- or β-adrenergic effects, typically has no role as a pressor in septic shock, although it may be used in patients unresponsive to other agents. Its use in septic shock may cause the patient to experience myocardial ischemia, arrhythmias, and decreased splanchnic blood flow.

Answer C is incorrect. Isoproterenol, a nonselective β-agonist, could actually worsen the relaxation of the peripheral vasculature due to its β-adrenergic effects.

Answer D is incorrect. Labetalol is a combined α and β sympatholytic and is used in the treatment of hypertensive urgency.

42. **The correct answer is A.** Adjustment disorder is the development of emotional or behavioral symptoms in response to an identifiable stressor(s) occurring within 3 months of the onset of the stressor(s), and disappearing within 6 months of the resolution of the stressor. These symptoms or behaviors are clinically significant as evidenced by marked distress that is in excess of what would be expected from exposure to the stressor or significant impairment in social or occupational functioning. The patient meets this description.

Answer B is incorrect. Major depressive disorder requires that a patient has two major depressive episodes, separated by at least 2 months' time, within a 1-year period. The patient described in the stem does not meet criteria for major depressive episodes.

Answer C is incorrect. A major depressive episode requires five of the following: insomnia, decreased interest in pleasurable activities, increased guilt, decreased energy, decreased concentration, decreased appetite, psychomotor retardation, and suicidal ideation. Also, these symptoms must last for 2 weeks. The patient in the stem does not have five of these criteria. Moreover, her symptoms are better accounted for by an inability to adjust to her husband's illness.

Answer D is incorrect. Normal grief does not include being preoccupied to the point that one withdraws from all contact with loved ones and friends, and that one is unable to tend to issues such as bills. These characteristics are what separates adjustment disorder from grief.

Answer E is incorrect. During an adjustment disorder or grief, it is common for patients to see and talk to deceased or sick loved ones. Without a further history of psychotic symptoms, this diagnosis would be difficult to support.

43. **The correct answer is D.** The patient's presentation is consistent with obstructive sleep apnea (OSA) superimposed on a known diagnosis of congestive heart failure (CHF). While polysomnography is necessary for definitive diagnosis of OSA, the findings in this case are still typical of OSA: male aged 30–60 years, history of nocturnal choking, daytime sleepiness, witnessed apneic episodes, mild hypertension, and moderate obesity. Obstructive sleep apnea can adversely affect left ventricular function in patients with congestive heart failure. A compromised left ventricle decreases cardiac output and results in exertional fatigue and weakness. This complication results from a number of causes. During each obstructive apneic event, negative intrathoracic pressure increases, thereby increasing left ventricular (LV) afterload and adversely affecting LV function. In addition, recurrent hypoxia and chronically elevated sympathoadrenal activity in patients with OSA can also precipitate LV dysfunction in patients with CHF. Treatment of OSA in patients with CHF often results in improvement of LV function.

Answer A is incorrect. Left ventricular afterload (the load against which the left ventricle ejects after the opening of the aortic valve) increases, not decreases, during apneic events. The increase in afterload is a result of an increase in negative intrathoracic pressure, which provides further resistance against which the heart must pump.

Answer B is incorrect. Right ventricular afterload increases, not decreases, during apneic events. The increase in afterload is a result of an increase in negative intrathoracic pressure and pulmonary vasoconstriction.

Answer C is incorrect. While hypertension is a cause of systolic dysfunction, it is not the most likely cause in this patient. A blood pressure of 132/82 mm Hg while on medication reflects hypertension that is under control.

Answer E is incorrect. During apneic events, there is a decrease in the amount of oxygen reaching the lungs. Physiologically, pulmonary vasoconstriction, not vasodilation, occurs. Clinically, pulmonary hypertension and right heart failure are consequences of prolonged pulmonary vasoconstriction. At that point, the patient might display symptoms and signs such as shortness of breath (nonexertional), jugular venous distention, and peripheral edema.

44. **The correct answer is A.** The medial aspect of the forth and fifth digits, as well as medial aspect of the hand (both the volar and dorsal surface), is supplied by the ulnar nerve. This nerve can be injured in a fracture of the medial condyle of the humerus. These patients can present with weakness of the hand intrinsic muscles because the ulnar nerve supplies many of these muscles. For example, testing abduction of the second and third digits against resistance tests the dorsal interossei, which are supplied by the ulnar nerve.

Answer B is incorrect. Extension of the fifth digit is supplied by the radial nerve and one of its terminal branches, the posterior interosseus nerve. These nerves do not supply the area involved in this case.

Answer C is incorrect. Wrist extension is supplied by the radial nerve, which can be damaged in a humeral shaft fracture. These patients would have decreased sensation on the dorsal surface of their hand.

Answer D is incorrect. The thumb is mostly supplied by the median nerve, which can be injured in a supracondylar humerus fracture. One would also expect sensation changes over the palmar aspect of the first, second, and third digits, and the lateral palm.

Answer E is incorrect. Wrist flexion is also supplied by the median nerve. An injury to the median nerve would produce sensory deficits over the palmar aspect of the first three digits and the lateral palm, none of which are present in this patient.

Questions 45 and 46

45. **The correct answer is L.** Given the history of instrumentation and the timing of the new symptoms, a urethral stricture is the likely

cause of the man's symptoms. It is likely that his transurethral resection of the prostate was successful, but during the procedure, he sustained an injury to his urethra. A stricture developed, causing the man to have difficulty voiding completely. This residual urine makes the man feel like he has to urinate shortly after the last urination.

46. **The correct answer is B.** Patients that practice clean intermittent self-catheterization can become colonized with bacteria. The bacteria in this case are not causing any symptoms. This scenario does not warrant any treatment, as the significance of the bacterial colonization is unclear.

Answer A is incorrect. Acute cystitis would present with symptoms of pain or burning on urination in addition to urinary frequency. Patients are likely to be febrile and have an elevated WBC count.

Answer C is incorrect. Benign prostatic hypertrophy (BPH) occurs in 90% of men over 80. Symptoms include urinary frequency, hesitancy, urgency, straining, decreased force of urinary stream, and incomplete bladder emptying with a large postvoid residual volume. This man has likely had transurethral resection of the prostate performed to treat BPH. Pharmacologic interventions that would have prevented the development of a urethral stricture include α-adrenergic blockers (such as terazosin) and 5α-reductase inhibitors (such as finasteride). Complications of untreated BPH include urinary retention, bladder calculi, recurrent infections, and renal insufficiency.

Answer D is incorrect. Central diabetes insipidus presents with extreme thirst and urinary frequency due to decreased secretion of antidiuretic hormone (ADH or vasopressin) by the posterior pituitary gland or hypothalamus. Decreased ADH results in an inability to effectively concentrate urine. It may be idiopathic, or patients may report recent head trauma, cranial surgery, or symptoms consistent with a brain neoplasm. Serum levels of ADH are low and water deprivation (Miller-Moses) test fails to produce more concentrated urine.

Answer E is incorrect. Detrusor instability causes uninhibited bladder contractions and leads to symptoms of urge incontinence (inability to hold urination until the appropriate facilities can be reached, once an urge is felt). In addition to urgency, patients complain of frequency and nocturia. Elderly patients may not perceive an urge and may simply experience large-volume urinary loss; however, the mechanism is the same. A causative urinary tract infection should be ruled out before detrusor instability itself is treated with anticholinergic agents (such as tolterodine) or tricyclic antidepressants.

Answer F is incorrect. Patients with undiagnosed or poorly controlled diabetes mellitus (DM) may present with polydipsia and polyuria, caused by osmotic diuresis secondary to hyperglycemia. Urinalysis will show glycosuria. Patients with type 1 DM are typically < 30 years old and may report fatigue, malaise, and weight loss in spite of adequate food consumption. Patients with type 2 DM tend to be older and obese, and may also suffer from hypertension, hyperlipidemia, cardiovascular disease, or polycystic ovary syndrome.

Answer G is incorrect. Infection with *Neisseria gonorrhoeae* most commonly causes cervicitis in women and urethritis in men. Women typically complain of purulent, yellow-green vaginal discharge and occasionally have dysuria if urethritis is also present; however, they may be completely asymptomatic. More severe symptoms, such as fever, pelvic pain, nausea, and vomiting, indicate disease due to other disorders such as pelvic inflammatory disease, salpingitis, endometritis, and/or tubo-ovarian abscesses. Men with gonococcal urethritis complain of urethral discomfort, dysuria, and purulent discharge. Unilateral scrotal pain and swelling suggests epididymitis. In a patient < 35 years old, epididymitis is most likely due to *N. gonorrhoeae* or *Chlamydia trachomatis*. Patients should be treated with a single dose of intramuscular ceftriaxone and oral azithromycin for gonorrhea and chlamydia, respectively, as the two infections often coexist. More intensive antibiotic regimens are required for more extensive infection. Disseminated disease (including a migratory polyarthritis, petechial rash, endocarditis, or meningitis) occurs in 1% of patients.

Answer H is incorrect. Interstitial cystitis is characterized by urgency and chronic pelvic pain in addition to urinary frequency. Approximately 90% of patients are female, 94% are white, and the median age of diagnosis is 40 years. The etiology is poorly understood and thought to involve bladder hypersensitivity, although there appears to be an association with autoimmune diseases, irritable bowel syndrome, fibromyalgia, and atopy. Cystoscopy may be normal or reveal ulceration, especially on overdistension. Potassium sensitivity testing (infusion of KCl solution via Foley catheter) is sometimes used in diagnosis. No definitive treatment exists, though analgesics, anti-inflammatory drugs, antidepressants, sodium pentosan polysulfate (Elmiron, thought to increase production of the protective glycosaminoglycan layer in the bladder wall), electrical stimulation, and acupuncture may provide some relief.

Answer I is incorrect. Nephrogenic diabetes insipidus (DI) presents with similar symptoms to central DI; however, it is due to renal resistance to the effects of ADH. Patients do not concentrate their urine in response to exogenous ADH. Causes include chronic renal insufficiency and drugs such as lithium.

Answer J is incorrect. Patients with prostatitis suffer from obstructive urinary symptoms similar to those associated with benign prostatic hypertrophy or urethral strictures; however, these patients also report fever, chills (in acute bacterial cases, more common in men < 35 years old), malaise, urethral discharge, and pain in the lower back, abdomen, pelvis, and scrotum. On rectal examination the prostate is tender and boggy. Evidence of infection may be found on complete blood cell count, urinalysis, and urine culture.

Answer K is incorrect. Patients with psychogenic polydipsia drink excessively and thus urinate excessively. They may develop symptoms of hyponatremia secondary to water intoxication. A water deprivation test will exclude diabetes insipidus and lead to the diagnosis.

Test Block 8

1. A 5-year-old boy is brought to the pediatrician for persistent hypercalciuria discovered on routine urinalysis. The boy has a past history of renal stones and Ehlers-Danlos syndrome. His family history is notable for a sister, age 22 years, who was diagnosed with EDS as a child. The child is examined and is in no distress. He is in the 5th percentile for height and the 10th percentile for weight. He has a respiratory rate of 30/min, a heart rate of 100/min, and a blood pressure of 110/70 mm Hg. The boy has a soft late-systolic murmur that is heard best at the apex. His lungs are clear and abdomen is soft. His lower extremities are notable for laxity of his knee joint. Relevant laboratory findings are:

Na^+	140 mEq/L
K^+	2.6 mEq/L
Cl^-	119 mEq/L
HCO_3^-	9 mEq/L
Blood urea nitrogen	8 mg/L
Creatinine	0.5 mg/L

Arterial blood gas analysis reveals a pH of 7.2. What is the most appropriate treatment for this boy's renal disorder?

(A) Acetazolamide
(B) Ammonium chloride
(C) Potassium citrate
(D) Sodium polystyrene sulfonate
(E) Vitamin D

2. A 57-year-old woman is referred for colposcopy following an abnormal Pap smear finding of high-grade squamous intraepithelial lesion. Her last Pap smear 3 years ago was normal and she has never had an abnormal Pap smear. She denies weight loss, abdominal pain, vaginal bleeding, or dyspareunia. On colposcopy, two lesions are identified near the squamocolumnar junction. What is the next best step in management?

(A) Endocervical curettage and directed biopsy of the lesions
(B) Observe with Pap smears every 4 months for 1 year
(C) Radiation and/or chemotherapy
(D) Radical hysterectomy
(E) Repeat colposcopy in 3 months

3. A 2-year-old boy is brought to the clinic for evaluation after 2 days of low-grade tactile fever, irritability, and decreased activity. His mother reports that on waking him this morning, his pillow was stained with a small amount of yellow fluid. His heart rate is 92/min, blood pressure is 104/70 mm Hg, respiratory rate is 22/min, and temperature is 38.8°C (101.8°F). His external ear canal is normal, but otoscopic examination shows the tympanic membrane appears dull, erythematous or injected, and bulging. What is the most likely bacterial pathogen implicated in this condition?

(A) *Haemophilus influenzae* (type B)
(B) *Neisseria meningitidis*
(C) *Pseudomonas aeruginosa*
(D) *Staphylococcus aureus*
(E) *Streptococcus pneumoniae*

4. A physician gets paged to the emergency department (ED) to evaluate a young, well-muscled man weighing 102 kg (225 lb) who came to the ED complaining of weakness. While his history is taken, the physician notices that he is using accessory neck muscles to breathe. In the course of a complete history it is revealed that he is a nurse who recently received the influenza vaccine. The doctor places him on oxygen by nasal cannula and orders pulmonary function tests that show a vital capacity of 1.5 L. The physician decides to intubate due to impending respiratory failure. Subsequent electromyographic and cerebrospinal fluid studies are pending. First-line treatment of this disorder consists of which of the following?

(A) Antithymic immunoglobulin
(B) Corticosteroids
(C) Cyclosporine and tacrolimus
(D) Plasmapheresis and intravenous immune globulin
(E) Tumor necrosis factor-1α receptor blockers

5. A 46-year-old African-American mother of three presents to the ED complaining of colicky abdominal pain, vomiting, fevers, and

chills. She has noted her stools over the past 2 days to be lighter colored than usual. She has had similar pain before, but it resolved with time and was never this bad. Her temperature is 39.6°C (103.3°F), pulse is 115/min, blood pressure is 95/60 mm Hg, and respiratory rate is 22/min. On examination she is in obvious distress and the sclerae are icteric. Bowel sounds are normal and the abdomen is tender to palpation in the right upper quadrant (RUQ) without rebound. Laboratory studies show a WBC count of 15,000/mm³, total bilirubin of 4.0 mg/dL, and elevated levels of alanine aminotransferase, aspartate aminotransferase, and alkaline phosphatase. RUQ ultrasound revealed dilated intrahepatic bile ducts with a few stones in the gallbladder. Which of the following is the most likely diagnosis?

(A) Acute cholangitis
(B) Acute cholecystitis
(C) Complete small bowel obstruction
(D) Hepatitis
(E) Pancreatic cancer

6. A problem-based learning case being discussed in class regards an immunodeficiency disorder involving a 12-year-old boy. Shortly after he began walking, he developed worsening instability and imbalance until he was eventually confined to a wheelchair at 9 years of age. Additionally, he developed oculocutaneous telangiectasias beginning at approximately 3 years of age. During the discussion of this patient's case, it is added that such patients commonly have chronic sinopulmonary disease and also have a high incidence of malignancy, particularly lymphoreticular malignancies. What is the mechanism of action responsible for this patient's condition?

(A) Absent respiratory burst
(B) Blocked lysosomal trafficking
(C) Defective DNA repair
(D) Defects in peroxisome function
(E) Impaired toll-like receptor signaling

7. A 46-year-old African-American diabetic woman visits her primary care physician with an ulcer on her toe. The ulceration has a dark-

ened keratinous base with central necrosis involving skin, fat, muscle, and bone. There is also a thick purulent discharge present. She denies any pain, tenderness, or discomfort, and states that sensation in her feet is diminished. X-ray of the foot shows erosion of the phalanges. Her temperature is mildly elevated at 38°C (100°F). Which of the following will be the most appropriate initial pharmacology?

(A) Clindamycin
(B) Doxycycline
(C) Metronidazole
(D) Penicillin G
(E) Piperacillin and gentamicin

8. A 34-year-old woman presents to her gynecologist complaining of incontinence. She states that for the past year, ever since the birth of her third child, she has been leaking small amounts of urine such that she needs to wear liners in her underwear to prevent her clothes from being soiled. She states that it occurs all the time but is worse when she drinks a lot of coffee or water. Which of the following procedures or tests is most likely to indicate the correct diagnosis?

(A) A voiding cystourethrogram
(B) Bladder capacity measurement
(C) Catheterization
(D) Cystometry with bethanechol chloride
(E) Sphincteric function analysis

9. In a nationwide study, 10% of the screening tests performed on patients with disease X resulted in false-negative outcomes, while 25% of the tests falsely identified healthy patients as having the disease. To determine the probability that a patient who tests positive for disease X actually does have the disease, what additional information is necessary?

(A) No additional information is necessary
(B) The incidence of the disease must be known
(C) The prevalence of the disease must be known
(D) The sensitivity of the test must be known
(E) The specificity of the test must be known

10. A 23-year-old Asian woman, G2P1, delivers a 3100-g (6.8-lb) boy at term by spontaneous vaginal delivery after a pregnancy without complication. Her prenatal laboratory results are notable for a positive group B *Streptococcus* screen and an A negative blood type. The infant's Apgar scores were 8 and 9 at 1 and 5 minutes, respectively, and his blood type is AB positive. He is being exclusively breast-fed, but the mother notes that he is not feeding well. On his discharge at 48 hours of life, he is in no distress but is jaundiced with a bilirubin level of 15 mg/dL. His unconjugated bilirubin is 13.2 mg/dL, and his conjugated bilirubin is 1.8 mg/dL. His hematocrit is 50%. Coombs' test is negative. What is the most likely etiology of the child's jaundice?

(A) Bile duct obstruction
(B) Breast-feeding
(C) Hemolytic disease
(D) Physiologic
(E) Sepsis

11. A 15-year-old boy presents to his family physician after noticing a small, hard nodule on testicular self-examination. The patient denies pain in his testicles or scrotum, or any difficulty or pain associated with urination. He denies any testicular trauma. Genital examination shows a 2-cm fixed, firm nodule on the lateral aspect of the right testicle. The patient also has mild bilateral gynecomastia. An ultrasound confirms a solid testicular lesion, and a CT scan shows no apparent metastatic disease. The testicle is removed, and the tumor is revealed to be a choriocarcinoma. What tumor marker is elevated in all patients with this lesion?

(A) Carcinoembryonic antigen
(B) α-Fetoprotein
(C) β-Human chorionic gonadotropin
(D) Protein-specific antigen
(E) The expression of tumor markers in this lesion is variable

12. Which of the laboratory findings in the table below are characteristic of immune thrombocytopenic purpura? PT refers to prothrombin time, and aPTT refers to activated partial thromboplastin time.

(A) A
(B) B
(C) C
(D) D
(E) E
(F) F

13. An 18-year-old girl comes to her pediatrician for a precollege medical evaluation. She got straight As throughout high school, and she recently performed in her dance troupe's spring ballet. She has no physical complaints but mentions in passing that she wants to lose more weight so she can be "skinny like the rest of the girls." On physical examination, her

CHOICE	BLEEDING TIME (MIN)	PT (S)	aPTT (S)	PLATELET COUNT (/MM³)	FACTOR IX	FACTOR VIII
A	3	17	27	202,000	abnormal	normal
B	4	12	42	190,000	abnormal	normal
C	4	12	45	230,000	normal	abnormal
D	8	13	27	58,000	normal	normal
E	9	20	28	143,000	normal	abnormal
F	9	20	29	67,000	normal	normal

height is 168 cm (66 in), her weight is 45.9 kg (101 lb), and her body mass index is 16.3 kg/m². Her pulse is 55/min, and her blood pressure is 95/50 mm Hg. The physician notes dry, yellow-tinged skin, and soft, fine hair on her arms and trunk. She is not currently sexually active and denies drinking alcohol and doing drugs, but she does smoke two to three cigarettes a day. Her chart indicates that she reached menarche at age 13. Which of the following is most likely to be diagnosed in this patient?

(A) Hirsutism
(B) Hypothyroidism
(C) Pituitary adenoma
(D) Secondary amenorrhea
(E) Small bowel obstruction

14. An otherwise healthy 27-year-old woman presents to the ED with lower abdominal pain, nausea, vomiting, anorexia, and fever that began yesterday morning. The patient states that the pain is present bilaterally; however, it is more severe in the right lower quadrant of the abdomen than the left. The patient has had five sexual partners in the past year with whom she sometimes used condoms and sometimes had unprotected intercourse. Her menstrual cycles have been regular with a moderate amount of bleeding. At presentation, her vital signs are temperature 38.2°C (100.8°F), blood pressure 112/72 mm Hg, pulse 72/min, and respiratory rate 13/min. On physical examination, there is bilateral lower quadrant abdominal pain, along with cervical discharge and cervical motion tenderness. A urine β-human chorionic gonadotropin was negative, and a complete blood count revealed WBCs 13,500/mm³, hemoglobin 13.8 g/dL, and platelets 315,000/ mm³. What is the next step in the management of this patient?

(A) Abdominal plain films
(B) Begin oral contraceptives

(C) Laparotomy
(D) Potassium hydroxide whiff test
(E) Ultrasound

15. A 56-year-old woman with congestive heart failure, managed with diuretics and an angiotensin-converting enzyme inhibitor, presents with progressive difficulty breathing over the past week. She states that it is difficult for her to take a full breath, and occasionally she will develop pain over the right lateral chest that becomes worse with inspiration. The patient quit alcohol use after her heart attack but has continued to smoke two packs of cigarettes a day, which she has done for more than 25 years. A review of systems is significant for brief episodes of fever and occasional blood-tinged sputum over the past 5 months. On examination, she is afebrile, with 99% oxygenation on room air. Her respiratory rate is 17/min. She has decreased breath sounds at the right base with dullness to percussion; the left lung field is clear. There is no jugular venous distention. An ECG shows no acute changes. An x-ray of the chest shows a fluid collection in the right base and a spiculated mass at the right hilum with a normal cardiac silhouette. The results of the thoracentesis are given below.

Appearance	Turbid
WBCs	43,000/mm³; lymphocyte predominant
RBCs	11,000/mm³
pH	7.32
Glucose	87 mg/dL

What is the likely etiology of the patient's effusion?

(A) Alcoholic cirrhosis
(B) Collagen vascular disease
(C) Exacerbation of congestive heart failure
(D) Malignancy
(E) Pneumococcal pneumonia

16. A 55-year-old man recently diagnosed with colon cancer and familial adenomatous polyposis sees his doctor with regard to the care of his 5-year-old son. If the son is genetically tested and found to have a mutated *APC* gene, what should the physician recommend to the father as colon cancer screening for his son?

    (A) Colonoscopy every 2–3 years with yearly sigmoidoscopy starting at the age of 10
    (B) Colonoscopy every 2–3 years with yearly sigmoidoscopy starting at the age of 30
    (C) Colonoscopy every 2–3 years with yearly sigmoidoscopy starting at the age of 40
    (D) Digital rectal examinations only starting at the age of 10
    (E) Digital rectal examinations only starting at the age of 40

17. A 53-year-old white woman presents to her primary physician complaining of flu-like symptoms, including muscle and joint pains, which have developed gradually over the course of a month. The woman also reports a low-grade fever during this time period. Her past medical history is significant for hypertension, for which she takes clonidine and captopril. She also takes procainamide for arrhythmia, methimazole for hyperthyroidism, and amitriptyline for depression. The patient's temperature is 37.7°C (99.8°F), blood pressure is 132/86 mm Hg, pulse is 82/min and regular, and respiratory rate is 18/min. Physical examination is normal. Laboratory studies reveal anti-histone antibodies and the presence of anti-ss DNA. C3 and C4 complement levels are within normal limits. Resolution of this patient's symptoms will most likely occur following discontinuation of which of the following drugs?

    (A) Amitriptyline
    (B) Captopril
    (C) Clonidine
    (D) Methimazole
    (E) Procainamide

18. A 19-year-old college sophomore presents to the university health clinic with a 2-day history of burning upon urination. Her vital signs are within normal limits and physical examination reveals moderate suprapubic pain. Physical examination is also negative for vaginal discharge and cervical motion tenderness. She has been sexually active for the past 15 months with four different partners. She admits to infrequent condom use but has been taking oral contraceptives. Which of the following organisms is most likely to be causing her symptoms?

    (A) *Chlamydia trachomatis*
    (B) *Enterococcus faecalis*
    (C) *Klebsiella pneumoniae*
    (D) *Neisseria gonorrhoeae*
    (E) *Pseudomonas aeruginosa*
    (F) *Staphylococcus saprophyticus*

19. A 28-year-old woman presents to her primary care physician with complaints of vaginal itching and discomfort for the past day, as well as white "cottage cheese" discharge for the past 3 days. The patient's medical history is significant for epilepsy well controlled on phenytoin. Genital erythema and excoriation is noted on pelvic examination, and potassium hydroxide preparation reveals pseudohyphae. Which of the following is the most appropriate definitive treatment?

    (A) Clindamycin
    (B) Doxycycline
    (C) Metronidazole
    (D) Oral fluconazole
    (E) Topical miconazole

20. Which of the following is associated with the development of primary central nervous system lymphoma?

    (A) Epstein-Barr virus
    (B) JC virus
    (C) *Mycobacterium avium* complex
    (D) Previous radiation exposure
    (E) *Toxoplasma gondii*

21. An 11-day-old is diagnosed with tuberous sclerosis following the discovery of a heart rhabdomyoma and an intraventricular hamartoma in the region of the foramen of Monroe. In addition, the baby is also discovered to have bilateral kidney masses, but as of yet, no obvious skin lesions. The parents of the child soon meet with a developmental pediatrician, who warns that which of the following is a known major complication of tuberous sclerosis?

(A) Glioblastoma multiforme
(B) Liver adenocarcinoma
(C) Pancreatic adenocarcinoma
(D) Seizures

22. A 24-year-old man with a history of type 1 diabetes mellitus is brought to the ED after he was found unconscious by a family member. His brother reports that there have been financial problems, and he does not think that the patient has been taking his insulin. Urine dipsticks are markedly positive for ketones, and there is a smell of acetone on his breath. Among other initial measures, a STAT blood chemistry is sent. Which set of values represents this patient's anion gap?

Choice	Na$^+$ (mEq/L)	Cl$^-$ (mEq/L)	HCO$_3^-$ (mEq/L)
A	135	99	16
B	135	100	21
C	138	105	29
D	140	107	25
E	142	99	31

(A) A
(B) B
(C) C
(D) D
(E) E

23. A 16-month-old, full-term boy is brought to the ED with burns on his chest and left arm. His mother states that she was boiling water and accidentally splashed some onto him when he startled her. She applied ice at home and immediately brought him to the ED for evaluation. His temperature is 37.0°C (98.6°F), pulse is 150/min, and respiratory rate is 22/min. He cries during the examination, but touching the lesions lightly does not cause increased distress. The burns are brightly erythematous in some areas, with patchy whitish, waxy spots. Several large, thin blisters have unroofed. The burns do not blanch with pressure, although this maneuver does elicit pain. What is the depth of the described burns?

(A) Deep partial-thickness burn
(B) Full-thickness/third-degree burn
(C) Superficial/first-degree burn
(D) Superficial partial-thickness burn

24. An obese 75-year-old man with a history of coronary artery disease and prior three-vessel bypass graft is brought to the ED with the complaint of chest pain. Upon entering the ED the patient becomes unresponsive and stops breathing. He is pulseless and found to be in ventricular tachycardia, and is subsequently shocked with no response. The patient is then intubated, epinephrine is administered, and the patient is again shocked without response. Which of the following antiarrhythmic medications would be the best choice for the patient's present state?

(A) Amiodarone
(B) Digoxin
(C) Diltiazem
(D) Metoprolol
(E) Procainamide
(F) Tocainide

25. A 24-year-old man presents with a chief complaint of neck pain that has become more severe over the past several months. He describes the pain as dull and says he feels very stiff in the morning, but this improves with activity. He also notes that the pain often awakens him during the night. On physical examination his lungs are clear to auscultation bilaterally, but he seems to have diminished air entry due to impaired chest wall expansion. Palpation of the cervical spine causes pain, and an x-ray of this area is shown in the image. Which of the following is the patient at risk for developing?

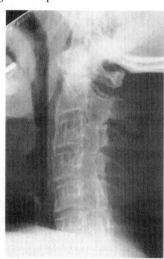

Reproduced, with permission, from Chen MYM, Pope TL, Ott DJ. *Basic Radiology.* New York: McGraw-Hill, 2004: Figure 7-38.

(A) Anterior uveitis
(B) Gastroesophageal reflux disease
(C) Malar rash
(D) Mitral stenosis
(E) Pleuritis

26. A patient presents to the clinic with complaints of difficulty swallowing and says that "the food seems to get stuck in my throat when I try to swallow." A barium swallow shows smooth narrowing at the lower esophageal sphincter (LES). What is most commonly seen in this condition on manometry?

Choice	LES Tone	LES Relaxation	Peristalsis
A	↓	normal	aperistalsis
B	↓	normal	hyperperistalsis
C	↑	normal	aperistalsis
D	↑	impaired	aperistalsis
E	↑	impaired	hyperperistalsis

(A) A
(B) B
(C) C
(D) D
(E) E

27. A young man with no history of neurologic disorder is playing basketball when he falls on the court and hits the side of his head. Although he reports a headache immediately after the injury, he is otherwise neurologically intact. Three hours later, his friends notice that he has slumped over in his chair and does not respond to their questions. On evaluation in the ED, he is observed to have a fixed, dilated pupil. What is likely to be found on a CT scan of this patient?

(A) Blood in the subarachnoid space
(B) Crescent-shaped, concave hyperdensity that does not cross the midline
(C) Irregularly shaped hyperdensity within the parenchyma
(D) Lens-shaped, convex hyperdensity limited by the sutures
(E) Normal CT scan

28. A 27-year-old woman presents to her psychiatrist with a 6-week history of 6.8-kg (15-lb) weight gain, increased sleep, generalized "moodiness," and generalized fatigue. She notes that she has been eating much more than usual, especially sugary and carbohydrate-rich foods. Approximately 2 months ago, her fiancé ended their engagement. She had several episodes of this same feeling while in college, during which time she initially sought psychiatric help. She denies any suicidal or homicidal ideation. Which of the following might be an appropriate pharmacologic option?

(A) Desipramine
(B) Lithium
(C) Olanzapine
(D) Sertraline
(E) Zolpidem

29. A 30-year-old man with type 2 diabetes mellitus presents to the office complaining of nocturnal sweating and headaches. He states that since his insulin regimen was changed 1 month ago, he has been waking up at night with these symptoms. He also notes that his morning glucose levels via fingersticks have been 250–300 mg/dL. Last night when this occurred, he checked his blood sugar and it was 50 mg/dL. He currently takes 30 U of neutral protamine Hagedorn (NPH) every morning and 15 U of NPH every night. Which of the following is the most appropriate next step in patient care?

(A) Decrease the evening dose of insulin
(B) Decrease the morning dose of insulin
(C) Increase the evening dose of insulin
(D) Increase the morning dose of insulin
(E) Monitor plasma glucose levels in the morning more closely

30. A 45-year-old man with no known past medical history underwent a total knee replacement 3 days ago. Postoperatively, the man had nausea that necessitated the placement of a nasogastric tube. On postoperative day 2, the patient's nasogastric tube was discontinued. On postoperative day 3, relevant laboratory findings are:

Na⁺	145 mEq/L
K⁺	7.2 mEq/L
Cl⁻	110 mEq/L
HCO₃⁻	24 mEq/L
Blood urea nitrogen	9 mg/dL
Creatinine	0.8 mg/dL

ECG is within normal limits. The house officer examines the man, who has a heart rate of 89/min, blood pressure of 136/86 mm Hg, respiratory rate of 12/min, and temperature of 36.9°C (98.4°F). The man states that he feels fine except for 4/10 incisional pain and mild nasal congestion. What is the most likely cause of the man's hyperkalemia?

(A) Accidental insulin injection
(B) Addison's disease
(C) Hemolysis (in collected blood sample)

(D) Nasogastric suction
(E) Renal failure
(F) Rhabdomyolysis

31. A 67-year-old woman with a family history of heart disease is seen in the clinic for follow-up of elevated total cholesterol. Dietary modification and initiation of an exercise program have not yielded change in her lipid profile, so she began taking atorvastatin. Which complaint from the patient regarding her new medication would be most concerning?

(A) Aching limbs
(B) Cognitive decline
(C) Headache
(D) Malar rash
(E) Shortness of breath

32. A 66-year-old man presents to the ED with epigastric pain after being discharged 1 week ago for an episode of acute pancreatitis. A CT scan of the abdomen is performed (see image). Which of the following statements about this diagnosis is true?

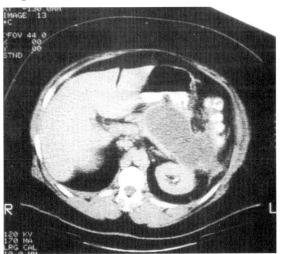

Reproduced, with permission, from Chen MYM, Pope TL, Ott DJ. *Basic Radiology.* New York: McGraw-Hill, 2004: Figure 26-3.

(A) The mature form of this structure will contain blood, necrotic debris, and WBCs
(B) This structure cannot be caused by pancreatic trauma
(C) This structure communicates with the exocrine ductal system
(D) This structure is at risk for rupture and bacterial superinfection
(E) This structure is best diagnosed with MRI

33. A 16-year-old boy is brought to the ED by paramedics while seizing. The patient's parents are known drug addicts and are nowhere to be found. The neighbors who called 911 claim they saw the boy seizing in the backyard and were not sure how long he had been there, but state that it took the ambulance at least 10 minutes to arrive. They are aware that the child has a long-standing seizure disorder of some kind and add that they believe he often abuses cocaine. On arrival to the ED the patient's pulse is 125/min, blood pressure is 160/100 mm Hg, temperature is 38.9°C (102°F), and respiratory rate is 22/min. On examination the patient has his arms extended rigidly at his side and is arching his back rhythmically and appears to be aspirating blood. The patient is covered in his own urine and blood is coming from his mouth. Nasopharyngeal intubation is unsuccessful after several attempts. Which of the following is the most appropriate next step in management?

   (A) Intravenous glucose, thiamine, and naloxone
   (B) Intravenous lorazepam and phenytoin
   (C) Intravenous phenobarbital
   (D) Placement of an electroencephalography monitor
   (E) Rapid sequence intubation

34. A 68-year-old man with a past medical history significant for hypertension, coronary artery disease, and previous inferior myocardial infarction presents to the ED with sudden onset of severe "tearing" chest pain that radiates to the back. The pain is accompanied by diaphoresis, nausea, and lightheadedness. The patient denies loss of consciousness or evidence of syncope. Administration of sublingual nitroglycerin has not provided any relief. On physical examination, the right arm blood pressure is 80/40 mm Hg, while that in the left arm is 190/110 mm Hg. A diastolic murmur is heard at the left sternal border, which is consistent with aortic insufficiency. An ECG was obtained that showed no acute ischemic ST segment changes. On x-ray of the chest, there was evidence of a widened mediastinum. Which of the following is the most appropriate next step in diagnosis?

   (A) Transesophageal echocardiogram
   (B) Transthoracic echocardiogram
   (C) Upper endoscopy
   (D) Ventilation-perfusion scan
   (E) X-ray of the abdomen

35. A 15-year-old boy presents to the physician's office complaining of fatigue, headache, myalgias, and sore throat that have been continuous for 1.5 weeks. The patient has generalized lymphadenopathy of the cervical, submandibular, and epitrochlear nodes, in addition to splenomegaly. His tonsils are significantly enlarged with exudates. Peripheral blood smear shows 65% lymphocytes, with 15% atypical lymphocytes. Heterophile antibody test is positive. Which is the most likely cause of his syndrome?

   (A) Cytomegalovirus
   (B) Epstein-Barr virus
   (C) HIV-1
   (D) Human herpes virus-6
   (E) Infection with *Toxoplasma*

36. Dr. Goodheart is a cardiologist and researcher who, after years of hard work, creates a new, more flexible coronary artery stent that is easier to manipulate during cardiac catheterization. The initial response to this invention is so positive that he decides to take a business partner. He begins a small company that manufactures and sells these stents. Dr. Goodheart knows that the interventional cardiologists at Hospital A purchase and use his stents, while those at the hospital downtown, Hospital B, do not use his stents. He also knows that outcomes at the two hospitals are similar, although no data have yet emerged about which stent is better. What is the most appropriate way for Dr. Goodheart to approach cardiac catheterization for his private patients?

   (A) Dr. Goodheart should not be involved in commercial interests as long as he is involved in patient care in the same medical field
   (B) He may refer patients to either hospital and does not need to disclose his economic interests in Hospital A; the patients can ultimately decide to which hospital they want to go

(C) He may refer patients to either hospital but must inform them of his economic interests in Hospital A

(D) He should only refer patients to Hospital A so they may benefit from his superior technology

(E) He should only refer patients to Hospital B so as not to take advantage of patients for his own economic benefit

37. A patient presents to her primary care physician with vague complaints of epigastric pain. X-ray of the abdomen is suggestive of a type II (paraesophageal) hiatal hernia, and this is later confirmed on barium swallow. The patient is recommended to undergo surgical repair. The goal of surgery is to prevent which complication?

(A) Barrett's esophagus
(B) Gastric cancer
(C) Gastric ulcer
(D) Gastric volvulus/incarceration
(E) Gastroesophageal reflux disease

38. A 68-year-old woman presents to the ED with acute onset of a frontal headache, blurry vision with halos around lights, and pain in the right eye. Her past medical history is notable for hypertension and tobacco use. She was recently seen by her ophthalmologist for treatment of anterior uveitis. Ocular examination shows mid-dilated pupils, corneal edema, and conjunctival hyperemia. Tonometry reveals intraocular pressure of her right eye to be 55 mm Hg. What is the most appropriate initial option in the management of this patient?

(A) Laser iridotomy
(B) Oral pilocarpine
(C) Topical acetazolamide (eyedrops)
(D) Topical atropine (eyedrops)
(E) Topical prednisone (eyedrops)

39. An 18-year-old unconscious teenager is brought by his school's athletic trainer to the ED after he passed out during practice. The trainer indicates that the patient experienced shortness of breath, said that he was having "weird heartbeats," and then fell to the ground. He drove the patient to the ED because the school is located next door to the hospital, and he figured that he should get him checked out. However, he believes that the teenager's condition is just due to the heat. While he is relating the story, the patient awakens and is confused. On questioning, he denies using drugs or any medical problems. His father died when he was young, but he does not know the cause of death. His vital signs are stable, except for a pulse of 104/min. Laboratory values are:

Na$^+$	141 mEq/L
K$^+$	4.2 mEq/L
Cl$^-$	103 mEq/L
CO$_2$	21 mEq/L
Blood urea nitrogen	14 mg/dL
Creatinine	1 mg/dL
Glucose	90 mg/dL
Hemoglobin	16 g/dL
Hematocrit	45%
WBC count	6000/mm^3
Platelet count	250,000/mm^3
RBC count	5/mm^3
Iron	120 µg/dL
Iron saturation	40%
Prothrombin time	12 s
Partial thromboplastin time	30 s

Urinalysis shows no hematuria and no evidence of alcohol or narcotics. Physical examination reveals a systolic crescendo-decrescendo murmur that increases when he squats and a split-second heart sound. What is the most likely diagnosis?

(A) Cocaine toxicity
(B) Hypertrophic cardiomyopathy
(C) Iron-deficiency anemia
(D) Mitral valve prolapse
(E) Pericarditis

EXTENDED MATCHING

Questions 40 and 41

For each patient with rash, select the most likely diagnosis.

   (A) Drug reaction
   (B) Erythema migrans
   (C) Guttate psoriasis
   (D) HIV seroconversion
   (E) Nummular eczema
   (F) Pityriasis rosea
   (G) Secondary syphilis
   (H) Tinea corporis

40. A 45-year-old woman presents to the clinic with a lesion on her posterior right thigh, just above the knee. The lesion is erythematous with an area of central clearing. It appeared 2 days ago and has grown larger since then. She also complains of fever, occasional chills, headache, and achy muscles.

41. A 32-year-old man visits his doctor because of an extremely itchy rash on his left arm for the past week. The lesion is oval, papular, and erythematous, with central clearing and a dry scale at the periphery. He recently spent time with his 7-year-old nephew who is being treated by the pediatrician for a scaly, red, pruritic rash on his chest.

Questions 42–44

For each of the patients with vaginal bleeding during pregnancy, select the most likely diagnosis.

   (A) Abruptio placentae
   (B) Bacterial vaginitis
   (C) Candidal vaginitis
   (D) Cervical carcinoma
   (E) Ectopic pregnancy
   (F) Endometrial cancer
   (G) Foreign body
   (H) Gonococcal cervicitis
   (I) Molar pregnancy
   (J) Normal labor
   (K) Normal menses
   (L) Placenta previa
   (M) Threatened abortion
   (N) Trichomoniasis
   (O) Vesicovaginal fistula
   (P) Vulvar carcinoma

42. A 36-year-old G2P1 presents to the ED at 35 weeks' gestation complaining of abdominal pain. She has had an uneventful pregnancy until this point with regular prenatal care. Her temperature is 36.9°C (98.4°F), blood pressure is 168/102 mm Hg, pulse is 74/min, and respiratory rate is 14/min. Pelvic examination reveals blood pooled in the posterior fornix and pain on palpation of the uterus. Tocometry reveals irregular contractions, and fetal heart tones are in the 180s.

43. A 27-year-old G1P0 presents to her obstetrician's office at 29 weeks' gestation with bright red vaginal bleeding which began 2 hours ago. Tocometry reveals a quiescent uterus; fetal heart tones are in the 150s and reactive.

44. A 29-year-old G2P1 presents at 37 weeks' gestation with a singleton fetus who is moving regularly. The mother noted abdominal pain and a small amount of vaginal bleeding mixed with mucous vaginal discharge. Tocometry demonstrates regular contractions, and fetal heart tones are in the 140s and reactive.

Questions 45 and 46

For each of the following patients, choose the most likely diagnosis.

   (A) Acute lymphoid leukemia
   (B) Acute myelogenous leukemia
   (C) Burkitt's lymphoma
   (D) Chronic lymphocytic leukemia
   (E) Chronic myelogenous leukemia
   (F) Common variable immunodeficiency
   (G) Hodgkin's lymphoma
   (H) Hyper-IgE syndrome
   (I) Hyper-IgM syndrome
   (J) Multiple myeloma
   (K) Nodular sclerosing lymphoma
   (L) Osteomyelitis
   (M) Posttransplant lymphoproliferative disease

45. A 10-year-old boy presents with pallor, fatigue, and hepatosplenomegaly. Bone marrow aspirate reveals eosinophilic needle-like inclusions.

46. A 55-year-old woman presents with fatigue and frequent infections. Radiographic imaging of the bone marrow reveals lytic lesions.

1. **The correct answer is C.** This patient has type I renal tubular acidosis (RTA). His laboratory tests show a nongap acidosis. This renal disorder is also known to cause nephrolithiasis, and is associated with collagen vascular diseases (i.e., Ehlers-Danlos syndrome). The defect in type I RTA is a defect in H$^+$ excretion. Treatment of both type I and type II RTA involves potassium citrate. Potassium citrate is preferred over bicarbonate salts in this case because it will help with the boy's hypokalemia and requires less frequent dosing. Treating this boy's acidemia will reduce his chances of forming stones.

Answer A is incorrect. Acetazolamide is not used in the treatment of type I renal tubular acidosis (RTA). The drug can actually be a cause of type II RTA. The drug inhibits carbonic anhydrase activity, and thus causes an acidosis because of decreased HCO$_3^-$ production.

Answer B is incorrect. Ammonium chloride is not used in the treatment of renal tubular acidosis (RTA). This is an acid that can be used to help diagnose defects in urine acidification. It is given to cause acidemia, after which the urine pH is followed. If the patient cannot adequately acidify the urine, the diagnosis of RTA is made.

Answer D is incorrect. Sodium polystyrene sulfonate (Kayexalate) would not be recommended for treatment of type I or type II renal tubular acidosis (RTA). This medication helps lower serum potassium, and the boy has a serum potassium that is already below normal. Sodium polystyrene sulfonate is useful in treating patients with type IV RTA that frequently have an elevated serum potassium secondary to decreased aldosterone levels or decreased aldosterone effectiveness.

Answer E is incorrect. Vitamin D is not used to treat type I renal tubular acidosis. Chronic acidosis does lower tubular reabsorption of calcium, but correcting the acidosis should result in less loss of calcium.

2. **The correct answer is A.** The majority of cervical dysplasia and cancers arise adjacent to the squamocolumnar junction of the cervix. Thus, endocervical curettage and directed biopsy to search for carcinoma is the appropriate evaluation following a finding of high-grade squamous intraepithelial lesion, because of the much higher risk of finding precancerous lesions such as cervical intraepithelial neoplasia 2 or 3, or invasive cancer. Biopsy specimens will be considered satisfactory if the entire lesion and the boundaries of the transformation zone (squamocolumnar junction) are included.

Answer B is incorrect. Observation with Pap smears, a screening test, is not acceptable for an initial Pap smear that shows a high-grade intraepithelial lesion. According to the Bethesda 2001 guidelines, observation is acceptable only for low-grade intraepithelial lesions and only in certain circumstances (e.g., reliable patients that are also immunocompetent).

Answer C is incorrect. Radiation and chemotherapy are modalities reserved for invasive carcinoma.

Answer D is incorrect. Radical hysterectomy is part of the treatment for biopsy-proven invasive carcinoma.

Answer E is incorrect. Repeat colposcopy is not part of the acceptable management of a patient with a high-grade intraepithelial lesion. The lesions observed via colposcopy following the abnormal Pap smear must be addressed with biopsy to evaluate for carcinoma.

3. **The correct answer is E.** The patient described is typical for a young child with acute otitis media (AOM). Although patients with AOM can be asymptomatic, many present with myriad symptoms, including ear pulling, ear pain, ear drainage, fever, lethargy, irritability, decreased activity, and decreased appetite, to name a few. Combining the history and the physical examination, this patient is most likely to have a bacterial AOM. The most common pathogen causing about 40% of AOM episodes is *Streptococcus pneumoniae*.

Answer A is incorrect. Nontypeable *Haemophilus influenzae*, not the type B form, may cause 25–30% of episodes of acute otitis media (AOM) and is the second most common cause of this frequent pediatric ailment. *H. influenzae* type B does not usually cause AOM. Although it was once a major cause of meningitis and epiglottitis, it has almost completely disappeared due to widespread inoculation with the Hib vaccine in infancy.

Answer B is incorrect. *Neisseria meningitidis* is not an important cause of otitis media or otitis externa.

Answer C is incorrect. *Pseudomonas aeruginosa* is the most common cause of otitis externa but is not a major cause of otitis media and is therefore not the correct answer for this question.

Answer D is incorrect. Studies have implicated *Staphylococcus aureus* in about 5% of episodes of acute otitis media, making it a relatively rare pathogen for inner ear infections.

4. **The correct answer is D.** The diagnosis is Guillain-Barré syndrome, suggested by the patient's weakness and recent vaccination. It is an inflammatory demyelinating polyneuropathy characterized by the acute onset of muscle weakness, areflexia, and eventually flaccid paralysis, commonly occurring after a viral infection of the upper respiratory or gastrointestinal tract. The ascending paralysis of Guillain-Barré is somewhat unpredictable and can progress rapidly (over hours) to compromise respiratory function. First-line treatment consists of plasmapheresis and intravenous immune globulin. The presumed mechanism of action of both is inhibition of antibody-mediated autoimmune demyelination, although the details remain obscure.

Answer A is incorrect. Antithymic immunoglobulin has not been found to be beneficial in Guillain-Barré syndrome.

Answer B is incorrect. Corticosteroids have not been found to be beneficial in Guillain-Barré syndrome.

Answer C is incorrect. Cyclosporine and tacrolimus have not been found to be beneficial in Guillain-Barré syndrome.

Answer E is incorrect. Tumor necrosis factor-1α receptor blockers have not been found to be beneficial in Guillain-Barré syndrome.

5. **The correct answer is A.** This patient is presenting with characteristic signs and symptoms of acute cholangitis known as Charcot's triad (fever, jaundice, and right upper quadrant [RUQ] pain). She also has hypotension, one of the two additional indicators of poor prognosis in Reynolds' pentad (the other being altered mental status). Moreover, she is in a high-risk group for gallstones, and likely has had episodes of undiagnosed biliary colic in the past. Her laboratory values are also consistent with an infectious process involving the biliary system and causing some mild inflammation of the liver. RUQ ultrasound indicated stones in the gallbladder and, more importantly, dilated intrahepatic ducts from a biliary obstruction.

Answer B is incorrect. Acute cholecystitis would present with colicky abdominal pain and tenderness to palpation in the RUQ, but the patient would not likely present with such overt signs of a serious infection (hypotension, high-grade fevers, and tachycardia/tachypnea). Acute cholecystitis can cause mild jaundice, but the magnitude of this patient's problem is too great for that diagnosis. Although the ultrasound indicated stones in the gallbladder, the major problem is biliary obstruction (most likely from choledocholithiasis) and the resulting infection (shown by dilation of intrahepatic ducts).

Answer C is incorrect. The patient is still passing stool, although it is light colored. The patient has normal bowel sounds and no distention of the abdomen and has focal rather than diffuse tenderness. Also, jaundice or elevated liver enzyme levels would not be seen.

Answer D is incorrect. Hepatitis has a more subacute onset and does not have many of the signs of acute bacterial infection on its way to septic shock, which are presented in this case. The jaundice and RUQ tenderness often follow a viral prodrome that includes fever, nausea, vomiting, and upper respiratory tract symptoms. Laboratory tests would reveal a normal WBC count and markedly elevated aspartate aminotransferase and alanine aminotransferase levels, as well as abnormalities in liver synthetic function.

Answer E is incorrect. Cancer in the head of the pancreas commonly presents with painless jaundice and is not often accompanied by such obvious signs of infection as spiking fevers and elevated WBC count. The right upper quadrant would likely not be tender, but a painless palpable gallbladder (Courvoisier's sign) could be present. Evidence of impending sepsis (hypotension, tachycardia, and tachypnea) is not often a presenting feature.

6. **The correct answer is C.** Ataxia-telangiectasia is a syndrome with cutaneous, immunologic, neurologic, and endocrinologic abnormalities. Patients have oculocutaneous telangiectasias with progressive cerebellar ataxia that eventually leads to confinement to a wheelchair, often by the age of 10–12 years. Additional findings often include a selective IgA absence with low concentrations of IgE; IgM is often present in the low-molecular-weight form. Ataxia-telangiectasia is an autosomal recessive disorder that is due to defective DNA repair and results from a mutation in the *ATM* gene.

Answer A is incorrect. Absent respiratory burst is the biochemical hallmark of chronic granulomatous disease. These patients present in childhood with recurrent bacterial and fungal infections and granuloma formation in the skin, gastrointestinal, and genitourinary tracts. Movement function is unaffected in these patients.

Answer B is incorrect. Blocked lysosomal trafficking is seen in mucolipidosis III, a rare lysosomal storage disease leading to accumulated glycoproteins and glycolipids. In this autosomal recessive disorder (also called pseudo-Hurler's syndrome), symptoms develop at 3–5 years of age, and include skeletal and joint abnormalities, coarse facial features, and corneal clouding. Ataxia is not a feature of this disease.

Answer D is incorrect. Defects in peroxisome function are seen in many rare disorders of inborn errors of metabolism, the most common of which is adrenoleukodystrophy (ALD). In this disease, very long-chain fatty acids accumulate in cells and lead to dysfunctional myelination. Usually, ALD presents in childhood with seizures, ataxia, adrenal insufficiency, and loss of sight and hearing. Telangiectasias are not seen with this disorder.

Answer E is incorrect. Although genetic defects in toll-like receptor signaling have been identified, they are very uncommon and do not cause clinically significant immunodeficiency.

7. **The correct answer is E.** Patients with diabetes are at increased risk of developing non-healing ulcers secondary to distal symmetric polyneuropathy, peripheral arterial insufficiency, limited joint mobility and bony deformities, obesity, and chronic hyperglycemia. Patients may present with lesions ranging from a small blister or cellulitis to a ulcer involving the bone as in the case described in the stem. The best treatment is tight glucose control combined with patient education about daily foot inspection, appropriate footwear, drying and nail trimming, and referral to a podiatrist when necessary. Treatment of ulcers may include debridement, growth-stimulating factors, reduction of weight bearing, and improvement in arterial supply. Penetrating infections are due to secondary infection with anaerobes and or other bacilli. The correct answer includes a broad-spectrum penicillin and an aminoglycoside that are able to combat such organisms.

Answer A is incorrect. Clindamycin, a lincosamide antibiotic, treats anaerobic infections including those caused by gram-negative bacilli. This medication may be used as second-line treatment of such an infection when paired with ciprofloxacin, but it is considered less suitable than piperacillin and gentamicin, secondary to increased side effects (including eradication of commensals) and higher cost.

Answer B is incorrect. Doxycycline is a tetracycline. It is commonly used to treat *Haemophilus influenzae*, *Streptococcus pneumoniae*, *Mycoplasma pneumoniae*, *Chlamydia psittaci*, *Chlamydia trachomatis*, and *Neisseria gonorrhoeae*. It will not combat *Pseudomonas aeruginosa* and other anaerobes that inhabit diabetic ulcers.

FULL-LENGTH EXAM

Test Block 8

Answer C is incorrect. Metronidazole is commonly used against flagellated protozoa, and works well against anaerobic bacteria, among others; however, it is not very effective against *Pseudomonas aeruginosa*, a gram-negative bacillus commonly found in invasive diabetic ulcers.

Answer D is incorrect. Penicillin G is primarily used to treat staphylococcal and streptococcal infections. It is not very effective against *Pseudomonas aeruginosa*, a gram-negative bacillus commonly found in penetrating diabetic ulcers. Broad-spectrum penicillins like piperacillin are more effective.

8. **The correct answer is A.** Given the fact that the urine leakage is constant, worse when urine production is increased (by caffeine or volume), and began after childbirth, the most likely cause of this woman's incontinence is a vesicovaginal fistula. Fistulas can develop following trauma (as during childbirth) and require surgical correction. A fistula can sometimes be directly visualized on physical examination, but a voiding cystourethrogram has more sensitivity.

Answer B is incorrect. Increased bladder capacity can be seen in cases of bladder outlet obstruction (prostatic hypertrophy or stricture) but is usually associated with overflow incontinence (which is seen when the bladder is full). In this patient, her bladder capacity should be normal or even low, based on the fact that urine continuously leaks out and does not allow the bladder to reach full capacity.

Answer C is incorrect. Catheterization is both therapeutic and diagnostic for overflow incontinence (secondary to outflow inhibition). In this scenario, catheterization would likely demonstrate a normal or low-normal bladder volume.

Answer D is incorrect. Bethanechol chloride is a parasympathomimetic drug that can be used to test whether incontinence is due to a lower motor neuron lesion or a muscle lesion. Lack of a detrusor contraction to bethanechol chloride administration suggests muscle damage, and an increased response suggests lower motor neuron involvement. In this woman's case, her response should be normal.

Answer E is incorrect. A common cause of incontinence in multiparous women is pelvic floor laxity resulting in sphincteric insufficiency. However, this usually presents as stress incontinence, which is urine leakage in conditions of increased abdominal pressure (e.g., sneezing or coughing). This woman's description of total incontinence is more consistent with a vesicovaginal fistula.

9. **The correct answer is C.** To determine the probability that a patient who tests positive for disease X actually does have the disease (the positive predictive value [PPV] of the test), one must know both the sensitivity of the test and the test specificity. Both values can be derived from information provided. However, to determine the PPV, one must also know the prevalence of the disease so the absolute number of true and false positives can be calculated: PPV = (true positives)/(true + false positives). Lower disease prevalence results in a lower PPV, and results in a less reliable positive test.

Answer A is incorrect. The positive predictive value of a test depends on the prevalence of the disease within a specific population, but no population-specific information is given.

Answer B is incorrect. The incidence of a disease is the number of new disease cases per population at risk over a specified time interval. This information is not necessary in determining the positive predictive value of a test.

Answer D is incorrect. The false-positive ratio, listed as 10%, is equal to 1 − sensitivity. Therefore, we know the test has 90% sensitivity.

Answer E is incorrect. Specificity can be calculated as 1 − false-positive ratio. From the information given, we know that the specificity is 75%.

10. **The correct answer is B.** Breast-feeding jaundice is the most common cause of nonphysiologic jaundice. It occurs in neonates who are being exclusively breast-fed, usually because of poor intake. Decreased milk intake leads to increased enterohepatic circulation and abnormally high reabsorption of bilirubin that is normally excreted in the feces. Jaundice is usually apparent on the third day of life and peaks

at > 12 mg/dL between days 3 and 6. In contrast with physiologic jaundice, total and conjugated bilirubin levels are higher.

Answer A is incorrect. Obstructive jaundice in a newborn is most often caused by biliary atresia. It is usually diagnosed when jaundice persists for more than 2 weeks and is accompanied by acholic stools and/or dark urine. However, at this age (2 days old) breast-feeding jaundice is much more likely.

Answer C is incorrect. Rh isoimmune hemolytic disease of the newborn causes immediate severe unconjugated hyperbilirubinemia, anemia, and eventually increased hematopoiesis (including frontal bossing). This diagnosis is supported by a positive Coombs' test. This occurs when Rh-negative women have previously been exposed to Rh factor and subsequently make Rh antibodies that cross the placenta and destroy fetal RBCs. Giving Rh-negative women $Rh_O(D)$ immune globulin when they are exposed to Rh-positive blood can prevent Rh isoimmune hemolytic disease of the newborn.

Answer D is incorrect. Physiologic jaundice results in a mild unconjugated hyperbilirubinemia after the third day of life, and resolves by 1 week in full-term neonates and 2 weeks in preterm neonates. Notably, the conjugated bilirubin is always normal, and total bilirubin is always less than 14 g/dL in physiologic jaundice.

Answer E is incorrect. Sepsis causes a conjugated hyperbilirubinemia. The mother's group B *Streptococcus* status puts this boy at increased risk for neonatal sepsis. However, aside from his jaundice, this child is otherwise well appearing, which would not be the case if he was septic.

11. **The correct answer is C.** A pure choriocarcinoma is uncommon (< 1%). The lesions are usually small but tend to hematogenously metastasize early. In recent studies, 100% of these lesions exhibit elevation of β-human chorionic gonadotropin (β-hCG). The gynecomastia that the patient is exhibiting is likely secondary to this tumor and its β-hCG secretion.

Answer A is incorrect. Carcinoembryonic antigen is a tumor marker that is often associated with colorectal cancer.

Answer B is incorrect. α-Fetoprotein (AFP) is a tumor marker that is elevated in various testicular tumor types, including teratomas, teratocarcinomas, and embryonal cell tumors, but it is not elevated in choriocarcinomas. AFP is most commonly elevated in embryonal testicular tumor types.

Answer D is incorrect. Protein-specific antigen is a marker that is used in following disease of the prostate. It is frequently employed as a screening test for prostate cancer.

Answer E is incorrect. It is true that tumor marker expression is variable for other types of testicular tumors (e.g., embryonal, teratoma, and teratocarcinoma), but this is not the case for choriocarcinoma. All of these tumors express β-hCG.

12. **The correct answer is D.** Idiopathic thrombocytopenic purpura (ITP) is associated with isolated thrombocytopenia that results from primary immune-mediated platelet destruction. This may cause prolonged bleeding time, but it would have no impact on the prothrombin time or activated partial thromboplastin time and is not associated with abnormalities of coagulation factors.

Answer A is incorrect. Idiopathic thrombocytopenic purpura is not associated with abnormalities of coagulation factor IX and is associated with decreased platelet levels not seen in these laboratory values. These laboratory values also display an increased prothrombin time (PT) and activated partial thromboplastin time (aPTT). A deficiency in factor IX would only lead to a prolonged aPTT, not PT.

Answer B is incorrect. ITP is not associated with abnormalities of coagulation factor IX. Due to thrombocytopenia seen in ITP, there will be a prolonged bleeding time and decreased platelet count. Factor IX is part of the intrinsic coagulation pathway and would indeed lead to increased PTT and a diagnosis of hemophilia B. Hemophilia B is associated with normal platelet counts but abnormal activated partial thromboplastin time.

Answer C is incorrect. These laboratory values are significant for a prolonged activated partial thromboplastin time and abnormal levels of factor VII. Factor VII is a coagulation factor in the extrinsic pathway. Therefore, abnormal levels of factor VII should lead to increased prothrombin time, not aPTT. A deficiency of coagulation factors is not seen in idiopathic thrombocytopenic purpura.

Answer E is incorrect. ITP is not associated with abnormalities of coagulation factor VII. These values show a prolonged PT and abnormal levels of factor VII. Factor VII is part of the extrinsic pathway, and decreased levels should lead to prolonged PT. However, ITP is associated with decreased platelets and is not associated with abnormal coagulation factors.

Answer F is incorrect. These laboratory values are significant for thrombocytopenia and prolonged bleeding time and PT. ITP causes only a prolonged bleeding time because of the decrease in platelet number. Thrombocytopenia has no effect on the coagulation cascade and therefore should not prolong PT or aPTT.

13. **The correct answer is D.** Anorexia nervosa is a serious psychiatric disorder characterized by refusal to maintain a normal body weight, distorted body image, and amenorrhea (≥ 3 months). Secondary amenorrhea is seen in > 90% of women with anorexia nervosa.

Answer A is incorrect. The patient's fine hairs are most consistent with lanugo, often seen in patients with anorexia nervosa and other conditions of starvation. Lanugo is the body's attempt to insulate itself as the percentage of body fat decreases. Hirsutism is the abnormal growth of dark thick hair in women in areas where hair growth is usually absent or minimal.

Answer B is incorrect. Patients with anorexia nervosa can present with abnormal thyroid tests. However, these laboratory values are most consistent with "sick euthyroid syndrome," or low triiodothyronine (T_3) and thyroxine concentrations accompanied by low thyroid-stimulating hormone levels and high reverse T_3 levels.

Answer C is incorrect. A pituitary adenoma can present with a variety of symptoms, including eye problems (bitemporal hemianopsia), acromegaly, and hyperprolactinemia. Although high levels of prolactin can lead to amenorrhea, this case is much more suggestive of amenorrhea secondary to anorexia nervosa.

Answer E is incorrect. Small bowel obstruction is usually associated with severe cramping, abdominal pain, nausea, and vomiting. The patient has no abdominal pain, cramping, nausea, or vomiting, and because this patient has no history of previous surgeries, small bowel obstruction is highly unlikely.

14. **The correct answer is E.** This patient's history, physical examination findings, and laboratory findings are suggestive of pelvic inflammatory disease (PID). This sexually active woman has a history of multiple sexual partners and does not use condoms consistently. In addition, abnormal vaginal discharge may indicate a history of gonorrhea, chlamydia, or other sexually transmitted infections. Minimal criteria for a diagnosis of PID include abdominal pain, cervical motion tenderness, and/or purulent cervical discharge. Because the differential diagnosis also includes appendicitis, ectopic pregnancy, adnexal torsion, diverticulitis, ileitis, and ulcerative colitis, further tests should be conducted to work up this patient. An ultrasound may be used to rule out an abscess resulting from this patient's PID and can also be used to rule out many of the other differential diagnoses.

Answer A is incorrect. X-rays of the abdomen have limited utility in diagnosing PID. Although an x-ray of the abdomen may be useful for ruling out some of the potential diagnoses, an ultrasound has greater utility in this case because the history, physical examination, and laboratory findings suggest PID.

Answer B is incorrect. This patient has a presentation that is consistent with a diagnosis of PID. Although she may be interested in starting oral contraceptives because she is sexually active, this would not be an appropriate next step in a patient with gynecologic pathology. This patient must be diagnosed and treated appropriately for her condition to reduce the risk of long-term complications.

Answer C is incorrect. Laparoscopy provides a definitive diagnosis in the case of PID. However, laparotomy is not indicated in the diagnostic workup of a patient with suspected PID. Because the patient is otherwise healthy, non-invasive diagnostic studies such as ultrasound and subsequent treatment with antibiotics are indicated before considering invasive procedures.

Answer D is incorrect. A potassium hydroxide (KOH) whiff test is useful in making a diagnosis of bacterial vaginosis. These patients usually present with vaginal discharge and vulvovaginal pruritus. The presentation and history in this case is not consistent with a diagnosis of bacterial vaginosis and, therefore, the KOH whiff test has limited utility.

15. **The correct answer is D.** Pleural effusion secondary to malignancy is most commonly due to primary lung cancer, although other sources such as breast and lymphoma are seen. The fever and blood tinged sputum are some manifestations of the likely endobronchial location of the mass, and her long history of smoking is the major risk factor. The development of pleural effusion represents regional spread of the malignancy. Thoracentesis often reveals a turbid or bloody fluid with a lymphocytic predominance and a normal pH and glucose concentration. However, it is important to remember that up to 30% of patients can have a low pH and up to 20% a low glucose because low pH and low glucose correlate with a higher burden of tumor cells in the fluid. Therefore, if an exudate has a low pH or glucose, malignancy is still on the differential, although it is less likely.

Answer A is incorrect. Although the patient has a history of alcohol use, she does not have any other symptoms or signs associated with cirrhosis, such as jaundice, hepatomegaly, or caput medusa. Effusions secondary to cirrhosis are similar in character to those produced by congestive heart failure, and clinically they are usually unilateral and on the right side.

Answer B is incorrect. Collagen vascular disease such as rheumatoid arthritis and lupus can cause exudative effusions, often with low pH and decreased glucose concentration. In

this patient, however, there are none of the classic symptoms of rheumatic disease.

Answer C is incorrect. Although the patient has a history of congestive heart failure, the presentation of this effusion is atypical for those caused by heart failure. When pulmonary vascular pressures rise secondary to left ventricular dysfunction, fluid shifts across the vascular endothelium into both lung fields in 80% of cases. The effusion is commonly clear or straw colored with few WBCs. X-ray of the chest often shows evidence of cardiomegaly.

Answer E is incorrect. Parapneumonic effusions are caused by local disruption of pulmonary vasculature, often secondary to a bacterial pneumonia. The effusion is commonly purulent with a predominance of polymorphonuclear cells.

16. **The correct answer is A.** The 5-year-old son should start undergoing screening and colonoscopy starting at the age of 10 according to recent guidelines. Familial adenomatous polyposis (FAP), caused by mutation of the APC gene, can lead to the development of hundreds to thousands of colonic polyps capable of malignant transformation (risk approaches 100% by age 45). These polyps tend to develop in the second and third decades of life with a mean age of 16, but they can appear in those as young as 8. All patients with FAP will require colectomy because of the extremely high risk of cancer, but often this is delayed as long as possible due to the psychological consequences. Colonoscopy is needed for surveillance prior to the surgical removal to monitor for multiple large (> 1 cm) adenomas or adenomas with villous histology, and/or high-grade dysplasia, any of which would necessitate the removal of the colon earlier than planned.

Answer B is incorrect. Age 30 is too late to start screening in someone with a family history of familiar adenomatous polyposis.

Answer C is incorrect. Age 40 is when a person with a first-degree relative with colorectal cancer should begin sigmoidoscopic screening (or 10 years before the earliest age of onset of colorectal cancer in the family). Again, this age would be too late to screen somebody with a positive family history of familial adenomatous polyposis.

Answer D is incorrect. A digital rectal examination would be insufficient to detect early polyps that may be in the colon.

Answer E is incorrect. Age 40 is too late to start looking for signs of colorectal cancer in someone with a first-degree relative with familial adenomatous polyposis. Also, a digital rectal examination would be insufficient to detect early polyps that may be in the colon.

17. **The correct answer is E.** This patient exhibits signs of drug-induced lupus erythematosus (DILE), a milder version of systemic lupus erythematosus (SLE) that generally resolves within weeks to months after discontinuation of the offending medication. Severe but noninflammatory joint pain is common in patients with DILE, as is myalgia. Patients may also experience a low-grade fever. The usual absence of central nervous system and renal involvement in DILE helps to distinguish it from SLE. While DILE may be induced by a number of medications, the two most common culprits are procainamide and hydralazine.

Answer A is incorrect. Use of amitriptyline is not a known risk factor for drug-induced lupus erythematosus. Amitriptyline most commonly causes anticholinergic adverse effects (blurred vision, constipation, dry mouth, lightheadedness, confusion, and loss of urinary control).

Answer B is incorrect. While captopril has been reported to cause drug-induced lupus erythematosus, the risk is very low as compared to procainamide. Four to seven percent of patients report an urticarial or maculopapular rash on captopril, and < 2% report a cough or dysgeusia (diminished sense of taste).

Answer C is incorrect. While clonidine has been reported to cause drug-induced lupus erythematosus, the risk is very low as compared to procainamide. The most common adverse effects of clonidine are drowsiness or dizziness.

Answer D is incorrect. This patient is taking methimazole for hyperthyroidism, but it is not a drug reported to cause drug-induced lupus

erythematosus (DILE). However, propylthiouracil (another antithyroidal) has been associated with a low risk of causing DILE. Methimazole infrequently causes a number of nonspecific adverse effects, such as gastrointestinal complaints and a rash.

18. **The correct answer is F.** The most likely pathogen for urinary tract infections in this age group is *Escherichia coli*. Of the choices available, you should be aware that *Staphylococcus saprophyticus* is the cause of approximately 10% of uncomplicated urinary tract infections in sexually active college-age women.

Answer A is incorrect. Although the patient may be at risk for sexually transmitted disease, the symptoms are more consistent with a lower urinary tract infection.

Answer B is incorrect. While most urinary tract infections are caused by gram-negative bacteria, *Enterococcus faecalis* is one of the gram-positive organisms that can be involved, often in the setting of nosocomial infections.

Answer C is incorrect. *Klebsiella* is a common cause of urinary tract infections but is not the most likely pathogen listed.

Answer D is incorrect. Gonococcal urethritis/cervicitis would likely have a different clinical presentation. Nevertheless, urinary symptoms in sexually active young adults should never be assumed to be due to a urinary tract infections unless cervicitis/pelvic inflammatory disease have been considered.

Answer E is incorrect. *Pseudomonas* is commonly associated with nosocomial infections of the bladder and would be unlikely given the clinical scenario.

19. **The correct answer is E.** The patient's complaints, as well as the potassium hydroxide preparation, are suggestive of vaginal candidiasis. Miconazole and fluconazole both treat candidiasis; however, fluconazole is an inhibitor of the cytochrome P450 enzyme system and would lead to increased serum concentrations of phenytoin, possibly leading to toxicity. Topical miconazole avoids this risk.

Answer A is incorrect. Clindamycin could be used to treat bacterial vaginosis. Bacterial vaginosis is caused by *Gardnerella vaginalis*. It is associated with an increased amount of a thin, gray, liquid, homogenous vaginal discharge and an often fishy odor that is especially recognizable after sexual intercourse.

Answer B is incorrect. Doxycycline is appropriate treatment for chlamydia infection and may lead to candidal vulvovaginitis. In acute vulvovaginal candidiasis, vulvar pruritus and burning are the main symptoms with erythema and edema of the vestibule and labia majora and minora. Chronic candidiasis includes edema and lichenification of the vulva, often with a grayish sheen. This patient is typically older, obese, and often has long-standing diabetes mellitus.

Answer C is incorrect. Metronidazole would not treat *Candida* but could be used to treat *Trichomonas*. *Trichomonas* presents with a yellow discharge, dyspareunia, and vulvar itching.

Answer D is incorrect. Oral fluconazole is incorrect because it would increase serum levels of phenytoin through cytochrome P450 metabolism interaction. Topical miconazole is the safer choice in a patient on phenytoin.

20. **The correct answer is A.** Virtually all cases of primary central nervous system (CNS) lymphoma in HIV patients are associated with Epstein-Barr virus. Before the use of highly active antiretroviral therapy, the frequency of central nervous system (CNS) lymphoma was 1000 times higher among HIV-positive patients than in the general population. Symptoms of CNS lymphoma can be focal or nonfocal, and the development of the disease is usually associated with a very low CD4+ count (i.e., < 50/mm^3).

Answer B is incorrect. The JC virus is not associated with central nervous system lymphoma. The disease caused by the JC virus is known as progressive multifocal leukoencephalopathy, which can present with focal or nonfocal neurologic symptoms over a short period of time. An MRI of the brain shows nonenhancing white matter lesions. Polymerase chain reaction assays for the JC virus

are 80% sensitive and 95% specific. The median duration of survival is approximately 1–6 months after diagnosis; there is no specific treatment.

Answer C is incorrect. *Mycobacterium avium* complex can infect the lung and the gastrointestinal tract and can become disseminated, but it is not associated with primary central nervous system lymphoma.

Answer D is incorrect. Previous radiation exposure is associated with the development of many other types of cancers, including leukemia (e.g., chronic myelogenous leukemia), thyroid cancer, and multiple myeloma, but it is not specifically linked to the development of central nervous system lymphoma.

Answer E is incorrect. Infection with *Toxoplasma gondii* leads to encephalitis that can present with focal neurologic deficits. An MRI of the brain will demonstrate ring-enhancing lesions. More than 90% of patients will test positive for anti–*Toxoplasma gondii* IgG. Treatment is with pyrimethamine, leucovorin, and sulfadiazine, and most patients respond within 1 week. *T. gondii* is not associated with the development of CNS lymphoma, but if such a response does not occur, an alternative diagnosis (e.g., CNS lymphoma) should be considered.

21. **The correct answer is D.** The classic triad of tuberous sclerosis is mental retardation, seizure activity, and facial hamartoma, in addition to the aforementioned heart rhabdomyoma, intraventricular hamartoma, and angiomyolipoma of the kidney. Other dermatologic lesions include: ash leaf spots (hypopigmented macules), and shagreen spots (leathery cutaneous thickening). Tuberous sclerosis may occur sporadically or with familiar autosomal dominant inheritance. Most children present with seizures.

Answer A is incorrect. There is no known association between glioblastoma and tuberous sclerosis. Glioblastoma multiforme is a brain tumor which commonly presents with nonspecific complaints and increased intracranial pressure. It is a rapidly progressive cancer, and the most common primary brain cancer.

Answer B is incorrect. There is no known association between liver adenocarcinoma and tuberous sclerosis. Hepatocellular carcinoma is the most common primary liver malignancy. It is associated with cirrhosis, hepatitis B virus, hepatitis C virus, alcoholism, hemochromatosis, Wilson's disease, and α_1-antitrypsin deficiency.

Answer C is incorrect. There is no known association between pancreatic adenocarcinoma and tuberous sclerosis. Most pancreatic cancers are adenocarcinoma located in the head of the pancreas. Pancreatic cancer is more often seen in African-Americans, cigarette smokers, males, and people with diabetes or chronic pancreatitis. Pancreatitis presents with abdominal pain, weight loss, jaundice, and occasionally migratory thrombophlebitis (Trousseau's sign).

22. **The correct answer is A.** The anion gap is the measured difference between the serum sodium (cation) and the sum of the serum chloride and bicarbonate (anions). A normal value is between 8 and 14 mEq/L. The anion gap is commonly elevated in patients in diabetic ketoacidosis, which is the most likely diagnosis for this patient, given the history of type 1 diabetes, and the constellation of possibly not taking the insulin, acetone breath, and ketones in the urine. Other conditions that lead to an increased anion gap are summarized in the mnemonic "**MUD PILES**," which is short for **M**ethanol intoxication, **U**remia, **D**iabetic ketoacidosis, **P**araldehyde ingestion, **I**ron ingestion (or isoniazid treatment), **L**actic acidosis, **E**thylene glycol ingestion, and **S**alicylate ingestion.

Answer B is incorrect. The normal range for the anion gap is 8–14 mEq/L, and patients in diabetic ketoacidosis have an increased anion gap.

Answer C is incorrect. This answer is an anion gap that is below the normal range. This can occur in hypoalbuminemia, hypergammaglobulinemia, and when there is an increase in unmeasured cations, such as magnesium, calcium, or lithium.

Answer D is incorrect. The normal range for the anion gap is 8–14 mEq/L, and patients in diabetic ketoacidosis have an increased anion gap.

Answer E is incorrect. The normal range for the anion gap is 8–14 mEq/L, and patients in diabetic ketoacidosis have an increased anion gap.

23. **The correct answer is A.** This is a classic description of a deep partial-thickness or deep second-degree burn. The epidermis and most of the dermis are involved. There is some loss of pain sensation, but pain with deep pressure is still experienced. The capillary supply is somewhat compromised in these deeper burns, and blanching may not occur when pressure is applied. These burns can be difficult to distinguish from full-thickness burns, and careful observation may lead to reclassification as the lesions evolve.

Answer B is incorrect. Full-thickness, or third-degree, burns involve both the epidermis and the entire dermis. The area is typically painless and white-gray to black, dry, and does not blanch.

Answer C is incorrect. Superficial, or first-degree, burns are quite painful, erythematous, and blanch with pressure. Because only the epidermis is involved, these burns are dry and do not blister.

Answer D is incorrect. Superficial partial-thickness or superficial second-degree burns are typically quite painful and involve blistering. Blanching occurs when pressure is applied because the capillary supply is intact. The epidermis and less than half of the dermis are involved in superficial second-degree burns.

24. **The correct answer is A.** At this point in the advanced cardiac life support algorithm for pulseless ventricular tachycardia, amiodarone should be administered. If amiodarone is unavailable, lidocaine or magnesium sulfate are acceptable alternatives.

Answer B is incorrect. Digoxin is not indicated for ventricular tachycardia. It is primarily used for supraventricular arrhythmias.

Answer C is incorrect. Diltiazem is not indicated for ventricular tachycardia. It is useful for supraventricular arrhythmias.

Answer D is incorrect. Metoprolol is not indicated in pulseless ventricular tachycardia, but it is useful for polymorphic stable ventricular tachycardia.

Answer E is incorrect. Procainamide would be indicated for a stable ventricular tachycardia, but not pulseless ventricular tachycardia.

Answer F is incorrect. Tocainide is often used for long-term management of ventricular arrhythmias, as it is available in an oral formulation.

25. **The correct answer is A.** This patient is presenting with signs and symptoms consistent with ankylosing spondylitis (AS), a chronic inflammatory disease of the axial skeleton. AS is most common in white males, with onset of symptoms at age 20–30. There is an association between AS and the human leukocyte antigen HLA-B27. The criteria for diagnosing AS include a history of inflammatory back pain, limitation of both flexion/extension and lateral flexion of the spine, impaired chest wall expansion, and radiographic findings of sacroiliitis, including blurring of the cortical margins of subchondral bone followed by erosions and sclerosis. Inflammatory back pain is further defined as insidious in onset and lasting longer than 3 months, with morning stiffness and improvement of pain with activity. Patients with AS are at risk for a variety of extra-articular manifestations, one of the most common of which is acute anterior uveitis. This complication occurs in 25–40% of patients with AS, and presents with unilateral eye pain, blurred vision, and photophobia. The disorder is treated with local steroids and atropine, and often recurs. AS is also associated with fracture of the spine, aortic regurgitation, IgA nephropathy, and bowel ulcerations.

Answer B is incorrect. AS is not associated with an increased risk of gastroesophageal reflux disease. Patients with AS are at increased risk of developing ulcerations in the ileum and colon, which are typically asymptomatic. However, some patients with AS have endoscopic and clinical findings of inflammatory bowel disease.

Answer C is incorrect. Malar rash is a cutaneous finding in patients with systemic lupus erythematosus, and is not typically found in patients with ankylosing spondylitis.

Answer D is incorrect. Patients with AS are at risk for cardiac complications, including aortic insufficiency, mitral valve prolapse, and third-degree heart block. AS is not associated with an increased risk of developing mitral stenosis.

Answer E is incorrect. Pleuritis is an extra-articular finding in patients with rheumatoid arthritis, and may also be seen in patients with systemic lupus erythematosus. It is not typically found in patients with AS. Patients with AS may have abnormal pulmonary function due to impaired chest wall expansion, and some patients are found to have pulmonary apical fibrosis.

26. **The correct answer is D.** Achalasia is a condition that commonly leads to dysphagia, or difficulty swallowing. Manometry is an excellent test to assess for achalasia, and classically shows increased lower esophageal sphincter (LES) tone, impaired LES relaxation, and aperistalsis. Besides the "bird's beak" appearance on barium swallow, the esophagus itself will commonly be dilated.

Answer A is incorrect. Decreased lower esophageal sphincter tone would be expected to lead to symptoms of gastroesophageal reflux, the opposite result from the dysphagia that is associated with achalasia.

Answer B is incorrect. In addition to demonstrating on manometry increased LES tone and impaired LES relaxation, achalasia is marked by aperistalsis.

Answer C is incorrect. One of the fundamental elements of achalasia is impaired LES relaxation that does not allow for substances to easily pass the LES. Therefore, normal LES relaxation would not be expected to create symptoms of dysphagia.

Answer E is incorrect. One of the hallmarks of achalasia is aperistalsis, not hyperperistalsis.

27. **The correct answer is D.** This patient has the classic presentation of an epidural hematoma (EDH). Trauma to the side of the skull (most commonly affecting the middle meningeal

artery) is immediately followed by a lucid interval. As blood accumulates in the hematoma and compresses the brain, progressive obtundation is seen, often accompanied by a fixed, dilated, "blown pupil" (60% of patients with EDH present with a blown pupil, 85% of which are ipsilateral). Because the blood is in the epidural space, it is bound by the sutures, and therefore the classic finding is a lens-shaped, convex hyperdensity.

Answer A is incorrect. In a subarachnoid hemorrhage (SAH), blood is seen in the subarachnoid space. The common presentation of a SAH is acute onset headache ("the worst headache of my life"), often accompanied by neck stiffness. Although SAH can occur secondary to trauma, the onset is much more likely to be immediate and acute in onset, instead of delayed and more progressive, as is the case in epidural hematomas.

Answer B is incorrect. A crescent-shaped, concave hyperdensity that does not cross the midline is seen in a subdural hematoma. This is caused by tearing of the bridging veins that penetrate the dura and perfuse the brain parenchyma. Although this is a possibility in this patient, it is much more likely in persons who are elderly and/or alcoholics. Therefore, this patient's demographics, as well as the lucid interval between injury and onset of symptoms, make it much more likely to be an epidural hematoma.

Answer C is incorrect. An irregularly shaped hyperdensity within the parenchyma is the most likely radiologic finding in a parenchymal hemorrhage. This scenario is less likely than an epidural hematoma in this patient because parenchymal hemorrhage is more commonly associated with hypertension, tumors, vascular malformations, and amyloid angiopathy. Although a parenchymal bleed may occur in severe head trauma, the "lucid interval" would not have been observed.

Answer E is incorrect. Given that this patient does not have a history of neurologic disorder and given the temporal relationship between his injury and the onset of symptoms, it is highly unlikely that he would have a normal CT scan. The blood of intracranial hemor-

rhage is resorbed, so it is possible that days after the injury there is no radiologic evidence of the hemorrhage. However, this would not be the case because of the relatively short period between injury and treatment in the emergency department.

28. **The correct answer is D.** This patient's symptoms of hyperphagia, weight gain, and hypersomnolence, are consistent with atypical depression. Sertraline is a selective serotonin reuptake inhibitor (SSRI), which, like the monoamine oxidase inhibitors (MAOIs) has a 55–75% success rate in the treatment of atypical depression. Because adverse effects and drug interactions are drawbacks to treatment with MAOIs, most patients with atypical depression are treated first with an SSRI. Adverse effects of MAOIs include weight gain, dry mouth, and hypertensive crisis if the patient does not avoid tyramine-rich foods, such as cheese. Other examples of commonly used SSRIs include fluoxetine, citalopram, and escitalopram.

Answer A is incorrect. Desipramine is a tricyclic antidepressant. Although tricyclics have been shown to be effective in the treatment of major depression, atypical depression responds more preferentially to SSRIs and MAOIs.

Answer B is incorrect. Lithium is a mood stabilizer often used in the treatment of bipolar disorder. As this woman has no history of mania, a diagnosis of bipolar disorder is unlikely; therefore, lithium would not be helpful.

Answer C is incorrect. Olanzapine is an atypical antipsychotic medication used for treatment of agitation and the positive and negative symptoms of schizophrenia. Two major adverse effects include somnolence and weight gain.

Answer E is incorrect. Zolpidem is a nonbenzodiazepine used in treating insomnia. This patient has no symptoms consistent with insomnia; therefore, zolpidem is not indicated.

29. **The correct answer is A.** This patient is experiencing the Somogyi effect, which is episodic nocturnal hypoglycemia followed by morning rebound hyperglycemia. Hypoglycemia is

caused by an excess of insulin at night, often as a result of a change in the insulin regimen. This leads to a hyperadrenergic state that consists of increased gluconeogenesis and glycogenolysis and decreased peripheral glucose uptake, all of which contribute to rebound hyperglycemia. The appropriate management is to decrease the nighttime dose of insulin to avoid hypoglycemia. This is in contrast to the dawn phenomenon, which is morning hyperglycemia that occurs in diabetes mellitus (DM) type 1, in DM type 2, and in nondiabetics. Growth hormone, an insulin antagonist, as well as cortisol, glucagons, and adrenaline, rise between 2 and 4 A.M. until between 10 and 11 A.M. Thus, as the sun rises (dawn phenomenon), so does the blood glucose.

Answer B is incorrect. Decreasing the morning insulin dose would exacerbate morning hyperglycemia.

Answer C is incorrect. Increasing the evening dose of insulin would exacerbate nocturnal hypoglycemia and would therefore worsen rebound hyperglycemia.

Answer D is incorrect. Increasing the morning dose of insulin treats the patient's symptoms but not the cause of the problem. Although it would decrease morning hyperglycemia, it would do nothing to affect nocturnal hypoglycemia.

Answer E is incorrect. This patient's symptoms are due to his insulin regimen, which must be adjusted to prevent continued morbidity.

30. **The correct answer is C.** Pseudohyperkalemia should always be considered when evaluating hyperkalemia. Poor phlebotomy technique can cause RBCs to hemolyze, which allows intracellular potassium to leak into the sample being tested. The house officer, however, was correct in checking the patient. If the clinical picture were suspicious, emergent measures to protect the cardiac membrane from depolarizing and to lower serum potassium would be necessary.

Answer A is incorrect. Insulin causes potassium to shift intracellularly. Administration of insulin in an otherwise healthy person would cause hypokalemia.

Answer B is incorrect. Addison's disease refers to primary adrenal insufficiency. This can cause hyperkalemia. Addison's disease also causes hyponatremia, hypotension, fatigue, anorexia, nausea, and vomiting. The patient's blood pressure and sodium are normal, and his nausea is easily attributable to other causes (e.g., recent anesthetics or narcotics).

Answer D is incorrect. Gastric contents are acidic. Their removal, either by nasogastric tube or vomiting, causes alkalemia and volume depletion. Volume depletion results in increased aldosterone levels, and alkalemia causes forced natriuresis due to spilling bicarbonate into the urine (Na^+ delivery to the distal nephron is enhanced due to obligatory HCO_3^- loss in the urine). The combination of distal Na^+ delivery and high aldosterone levels leads to urine K^+ excretion at the collecting duct. As a result, nasogastric suction is a cause of hypokalemia, not hyperkalemia.

Answer E is incorrect. Renal failure may also cause hyperkalemia. However, this patient has a normal creatinine, making renal failure unlikely.

Answer F is incorrect. Though orthopedic surgery is the most common iatrogenic cause of rhabdomyolysis, the clinical presentation is not suggestive of rhabdomyolysis, which is a cause of hyperkalemia. If the laboratory draw were repeated and confirmed the diagnosis of hyperkalemia, an elevated creatine phosphokinase would help diagnose muscle breakdown.

31. **The correct answer is A.** Patients who are new to taking statin medications, as well as those whose doses have recently been changed, are at risk for rhabdomyolysis and renal damage from accumulation of creatinine. Serum creatine kinase levels can be measured in patients suffering from muscle pain to determine whether tissue breakdown is occurring. Patients on statins can experience muscle pain without creatine kinase elevation; one study suggested that this may be due to reversible mitochondrial myopathy. Because of the potential for progression to renal failure, a complaint that might herald the onset of rhabdomyolysis, such as limb aches or other

musculoskeletal pain, should be taken seriously.

Answer B is incorrect. Randomized trials have shown decline in memory and cognitive function with statin use, and it appears that the elderly are at increased risk for these adverse effects. Although troublesome and especially concerning from a quality-of-life standpoint, this would not be an urgent issue.

Answer C is incorrect. Headache is a nonspecific adverse effect of many types of medications, as well as being a common complaint in patients not on medications. Unless it has unusual features, it is not of particular concern.

Answer D is incorrect. A lupus-like syndrome has been reported as a potential adverse effect of statin therapy but would not require immediate evaluation.

Answer E is incorrect. Myopathy from statin initiation can sometimes be accompanied by shortness of breath without identifiable etiology on cardiopulmonary workup. This symptom is reversible with statin discontinuation, unlike the potential for kidney damage with widespread rhabdomyolysis.

32. **The correct answer is D.** This is a pancreatic pseudocyst, which is so named because the wall does not have an epithelial lining. Instead, the wall is a fibrous capsule, formed by the body to wall off the hemorrhage and fat necrosis from pancreatitis or pancreatic trauma. This structure is not a true cyst and therefore does not communicate with the exocrine ductal system. They form as a result of pancreatic trauma or pancreatitis, and are best visualized with CT or ultrasound. If the cysts are small, they may be reabsorbed by the body and can therefore be managed medically. Larger cysts will need either internal (pancreaticogastrostomy) or external (percutaneous) drainage. Internal drainage is favored if possible, with possible fistula formation if an external drainage procedure is used. Bacterial superinfection and rupture (leading to peritonitis) are two of the complications of pancreatic pseudocysts.

Answer A is incorrect. New pancreatic pseudocysts contain blood, necrotic debris (fat

necrosis and pancreatic autodigestion), and WBCs. After a period of time the contents degenerate into a straw-colored, serous fluid.

Answer B is incorrect. This patient had a previous episode of pancreatitis, which can lead to pseudocyst formation. Pancreatic trauma, such as impact of the steering wheel on the abdomen, can also lead to pseudocysts.

Answer C is incorrect. This structure is not a true cyst and therefore does not communicate with the exocrine ductal system.

Answer E is incorrect. Pancreatic pseudocysts are best visualized with abdominal ultrasound or CT.

33. **The correct answer is E.** Status epilepticus (SE) refers to a continuous state of seizure activity or a series of seizures during which there is no return to consciousness in the interictal period. The minimal duration of seizure activity in SE has traditionally been cited as 15–30 minutes. Practically speaking, anyone who is brought to an emergency department who has been seizing for > 5 minutes will be treated as having SE. SE is a medical emergency with a wide range of potentially lethal complications and 20% mortality. The most important initial step in management, however, is simply to attend to basic **ABC**s, or **A**irway, **B**reathing, and **C**irculation. Due to the inaccessibility of the oropharynx in such patients, this is often best accomplished with nasopharyngeal airway placement or even intubation. If intubation is unsuccessful in a patient who is in danger of aspirating, rapid sequence induction must be employed to secure the patient's airway.

Answer A is incorrect. At many centers intravenous glucose, thiamine, and naloxone, and oxygen by facemask are given presumptively to all unconscious patients that arrive in the emergency department. While these therapies have little risk and may be appropriate in this patient, the next logical step in a patient with presumed status epilepticus would be securing an airway via intubation and the administration of medication capable of ending seizure activity.

Answer B is incorrect. Following a basic primary survey (airway, breathing, and circulation), the next step in management is the administration of a benzodiazepine and a loading dose. If intravenous benzodiazepines and phenytoin are ineffective, phenobarbital may be given intravenously. However, the patient's airway is the more pressing issue.

Answer C is incorrect. The primary objective in this clinical scenario is to address airway, breathing, and circulation. Since this patient is unable to protect his airway, it is imperative to intubate him prior to any other medical intervention.

Answer D is incorrect. Complex studies such as EEG and brain imaging, although they may be useful in establishing diagnosis, are best deferred until the patient has been stabilized.

34. **The correct answer is A.** The patient presents with a very high suspicion for a thoracic aortic dissection. This diagnosis is supported by a presentation of severe, tearing chest pain that radiates to the back, pressure differences between the right and left upper extremities, and a widened mediastinum on x-ray of the chest. The transesophageal echocardiogram (TEE) is becoming the gold standard for diagnosing aortic dissection. The information obtained from TEE is frequently used to guide patient management. TEE is a portable procedure that can be performed at the bedside and can yield diagnostic information in just a few minutes. It allows for direct visualization of the thoracic aorta and determination of disease extent. TEE can assess the ascending arch, aortic insufficiency, and proximal coronary arteries. With a sensitivity of 97–99% and a specificity of almost 100% with the addition of M-mode imaging, TEE is the best test for further workup of an aortic dissection and for guiding management.

Answer B is incorrect. A transthoracic echocardiogram (TTE) has limited use in the evaluation of a thoracic aortic dissection. This imaging modality has a lower sensitivity and specificity when compared to transesophageal echocardiogram, CT scan, or MRI. In addition, TTE is most frequently used to assess the proximal aortic root and to confirm aortic insufficiency, but it is limited in that it is difficult to visualize the distal ascending, transverse,

and descending aorta. Because patient management often depends on the site of dissection entry and the extent of the aortic dissection, TTE would not be the first-line diagnostic test ordered.

Answer C is incorrect. Upper endoscopy is not indicated in diagnosing an aortic dissection or in determining specifics about the dissection such as its extent. Although upper endoscopy may be useful when visualizing the esophagus and stomach in the case of peptic ulcer disease or other upper gastrointestinal abnormality, this patient most likely presents with an aortic dissection and would benefit little from an upper endoscopy.

Answer D is incorrect. A ventilation-perfusion scan is used to diagnose or rule out a pulmonary embolism and has no potential for diagnosis in cases of aortic dissection.

Answer E is incorrect. X-ray of the abdomen is not indicated in the workup of a thoracic aortic dissection. Although further workup may be indicated if the dissection is believed to extend to the abdominal aorta, this would not be the most appropriate next step in diagnosis. In addition, transesophageal echocardiogram and CT scan are more sensitive and specific for determining the extent of a dissection than an x-ray of the abdomen.

35. **The correct answer is B.** The patient described has infectious mononucleosis, the most common cause (90% of cases) of which is Epstein-Barr virus (EBV). Symptoms typically consist of malaise, fatigue, fever, headache, sore throat, nausea, abdominal pain, and myalgias. Generalized lymphadenopathy is common (90% of cases), and epitrochlear lymph node enlargement is particularly suggestive of infectious mononucleosis. Splenomegaly is found in 50% of cases. The diagnosis of infectious mononucleosis is made by the characteristic peripheral blood smear, with 60–70% lymphocytes and > 10% atypical forms. The heterophile antibody test is a sensitive, specific test that confirms EBV as the infectious agent.

Answer A is incorrect. Cytomegalovirus (CMV) is a herpesvirus that generally causes latent, asymptomatic infection in immunocompetent hosts. It is the second most common cause of infectious mononucleosis. Patients with CMV mononucleosis will have a negative heterophile antibody test. Although the clinical presentation can be similar, there are some differences: CMV mononucleosis rarely causes the lymphadenopathy, splenomegaly, and tonsillar exudates so often seen in EBV infection.

Answer C is incorrect. Primary HIV infection can cause a generalized viral syndrome similar to EBV mononucleosis. However, the heterophile antibody test would be negative. Symptoms seen in acute HIV infection but not in EBV include mucocutaneous ulceration, rash, and diarrhea.

Answer D is incorrect. Human herpes virus rarely causes a heterophile antibody–negative infectious mononucleosis. The syndrome is usually quite mild.

Answer E is incorrect. Toxoplasmosis is usually asymptomatic, although it is estimated to cause 1% of acute mononucleosis syndromes. Heterophile antibody test would be negative. It rarely causes pharyngitis, and rarely would a peripheral blood smear show more than 10% atypical lymphocytes.

36. **The correct answer is C.** This case is one of a conflict of interest; that is, the physician has both a financial interest and a patient care interest. Patients have a right to full disclosure of these interests and of the financial gain for Dr. Goodheart if they choose Hospital A.

Answer A is incorrect. Although there is a conflict of interest inherent in Dr. Goodheart's business and medical practice, he is allowed to do both as long as he fully discloses his interests to his patients.

Answer B is incorrect. This answer would be appropriate if Dr. Goodheart had evidence that his stent is better; however, given the current lack of evidence and his own knowledge that outcomes at the two hospitals are similar, this is not a justification to refer solely to one hospital.

Answer D is incorrect. This answer would be appropriate if Dr. Goodheart had evidence

that his stent is better; however, given the current lack of evidence and his own knowledge that outcomes at the two hospitals are similar, this is not a justification to refer solely to one hospital.

Answer E is incorrect. Because outcomes at the two hospitals are similar, Dr. Goodheart is justified in referring patients to either hospital. They will receive good care at either one, and he will have fulfilled his obligation in patient care.

37. **The correct answer is D.** Gastric volvulus or incarceration is the feared complication of type II (paraesophageal) hiatal hernia, and while surgical repair of the asymptomatic patient is still the standard of care, there are increasing data to suggest that nonoperative management might be preferable, as the incidence of gastric volvulus is lower than historically believed.

Answer A is incorrect. Barrett's esophagus, or columnar metaplasia of the distal esophagus, is a complication of long-standing gastroesophageal reflux disease (GERD), and can potentially lead to esophageal adenocarcinoma. As GERD is not commonly seen in type II hiatal hernia, Barrett's esophagus is not a common complication of this type of hernia. It is, however, commonly seen as a complication of type I hiatal hernia.

Answer B is incorrect. Gastric cancer has two forms: intestinal type and diffuse type. Intestinal type is associated with diet, *Helicobacter pylori* colonization, and chronic gastritis. The risk factors for diffuse type are unknown. There is no known association between gastric cancer and type II (paraesophageal) hiatal hernia.

Answer C is incorrect. While there is a slightly increased risk of gastric ulcer in patients suffering from type II (paraesophageal) hiatal hernia, the greatest risk is of gastric volvulus.

Answer E is incorrect. Gastroesophageal reflux disease is a common complication of type I (sliding) hiatal hernia, but not of type II hernia.

38. **The correct answer is C.** Immediate reduction of intraocular pressure in acute (also

called angle-closure or narrow-angle) glaucoma is a medical emergency in order to prevent blindness. Reduction can be achieved by using a carbonic anhydrase inhibitor such as acetazolamide, which acts to decrease the production of aqueous humor. In the past these agents were given by mouth as pills, but now they are available as eyedrops. Other agents that also decrease aqueous humor inflow are β-adrenergic blockers (timolol, betaxolol, and levobunolol) and α-agonists (apraclonidine and brimonidine).

Answer A is incorrect. This treatment is indicated only after medical reduction of intraocular pressure. An iridotomy is a procedure that uses lasers to open a new channel in the iris. This new channel then relieves pressure and prevents another attack.

Answer B is incorrect. Oral pilocarpine is used for the treatment of xerostomia caused by salivary gland hypofunction resulting from radiotherapy for cancer of the head and neck, or for Sjögren's syndrome. Topical pilocarpine eyedrops, however, would be effective in lowering the intraocular pressure, as it facilitates fluid drainage through the canal of Schlemm.

Answer D is incorrect. Atropine is helpful in treating iritis and uveitis, not glaucoma. Atropine is an antimuscarinic agent that results in mydriasis, which will further exacerbate her symptoms of closed-angle glaucoma (which typically presents as this patient did) because of its effects on the closure of the trabecular meshwork around Schlemm's canal, which acts to drain the aqueous humor from the anterior chamber. Prevention of attacks with eyedrops is essential for the treatment of closed-angle glaucoma. This drug should not be used in patients with open-angle glaucoma either. Patients with open-angle glaucoma tend to have few symptoms, but may begin to notice blind spots in their field of vision, especially in the periphery. Although open-angle glaucoma cannot be cured, patients can generally prevent the progression of symptoms with eyedrops.

Answer E is incorrect. While steroids are indicated for treatment of her anterior uveitis, it also elevates intraocular pressure and will exacerbate her symptoms. She requires emergent

treatment for closed-angle glaucoma to prevent permanent vision loss.

39. **The correct answer is B.** Mostly affecting young, athletic men after exercise, hypertrophic cardiomyopathy (HCM) can be fatal and is believed to be due to a sarcomere protein mutation. Common symptoms are dyspnea, angina, and syncope. It is most often inherited in an autosomal dominant fashion, as in this case, with the patient's father most likely suffering from it as well. The murmur is classic for HCM. Other findings can include left ventricular hypertrophy on ECG, left ventricular outflow tract obstruction on echocardiography, and cardiomegaly on x-ray of the chest. Treatment is with β-blockers or calcium channel blockers to decrease the heart rate and increase diastolic filling time.

Answer A is incorrect. The patient denies drug use, and his urine test is negative.

Answer C is incorrect. Not only are the patient's iron levels normal, but it would also be very unlikely for a young man to be suffering from this condition.

Answer D is incorrect. Mitral valve prolapse might present with chest pain and palpitations. Heart sounds are usually normal (maybe an elevated S1).

Answer E is incorrect. Pericarditis patients often report a viral infection 1–2 weeks preceding onset of symptoms, which classically includes a pericardial knock or rub and a prominent S4 heart sound.

Questions 40 and 41

40. **The correct answer is B.** Erythema migrans is usually due to Lyme disease. It is classically described as an erythematous oval lesion with central clearing, which may be confused with the herald patch of pityriasis rosea. The classic "bull's-eye" occurs in only a minority of cases. Erythema migrans may be pruritic. The lesion typically occurs near the tick bite in a warm area of the body. Systemic symptoms may include fever and chills in approximately two-thirds of patients, as well as headache, arthralgias, myalgias, diffuse lymphadenopathy, and meningitis.

41. **The correct answer is H.** Tinea corporis, or "ringworm," is a dermatophyte infection commonly seen in children or their close contacts. The lesion is erythematous, scaled, and papular. As it expands there is central clearing. Tinea corporis is often very pruritic.

Answer A is incorrect. Cutaneous drug reactions vary in appearance but most often manifest as a diffuse morbilliform or urticarial rash. The rash remits when the offending drug is discontinued.

Answer C is incorrect. Guttate psoriasis causes a scaling rash with multiple small well-defined papules with a tendency to coalesce.

Answer D is incorrect. Approximately 50–70% of HIV-infected patients experience acute HIV syndrome, which is associated with a rapid increase in plasma viremia. Acute HIV syndrome varies but may include fevers, lymphadenopathy, arthralgias, nausea, vomiting, encephalitis, and an erythematous maculopapular rash.

Answer E is incorrect. The rash of nummular eczema appears as closely-grouped vesicles and papules that coalesce into large plaques. The plaques are often crusted and excoriated secondary to scratching. Nummular eczema is a chronic inflammatory dermatitis often seen on the lower legs during cold, dry seasons.

Answer F is incorrect. The rash of pityriasis rosea is erythematous and pruritic with central clearing and peripheral scaling. The distribution is typically on the trunk and begins with a herald patch and then spreads downward and peripherally but rarely spreads as far as the distal extremities.

Answer G is incorrect. Secondary syphilis affects the palms and soles and is associated with systemic symptoms.

Questions 42–44

42. **The correct answer is A.** Placental abruption classically presents with bright red vaginal bleeding and uterine pain. If the abruption is significant there may also be fetal distress as indicated by the fetal tachycardia in this scenario.

43. **The correct answer is L.** In contrast to abruption, placenta previa presents with painless vaginal bleeding without notable uterine contractions or irritability.

44. **The correct answer is J.** Normal labor can occur spontaneously between 37 and 42 weeks' gestational age and has as its hallmark regular uterine contractions with progressive cervical effacement and dilatation. The loss of the cervical mucous plug may be accompanied by a small amount of vaginal bleeding.

Answer B is incorrect. Bacterial vaginitis presents with thin white or gray vaginal discharge which may have an unpleasant odor. Vaginal pain or vulvar irritation is atypical.

Answer C is incorrect. Thick, odorless, clumpy white ("cottage cheese") discharge along with pruritus that may be intense are commonly seen with vaginal candidiasis.

Answer D is incorrect. With routine screening, cervical cancer is commonly found in its asymptomatic stages via an abnormal Pap smear result. If advanced, disease may present with abnormal vaginal bleeding, vaginal pain, and dyspareunia, and abnormal vaginal discharge.

Answer E is incorrect. Unilateral pelvic pain, vaginal bleeding, and low rate of increase in β-human chorionic gonadotropin (β-hCG) for stage of pregnancy are seen in ectopic pregnancy.

Answer F is incorrect. Most patients with endometrial carcinoma are postmenopausal, and postmenopausal bleeding is the heralding symptom. In perimenopausal patients, irregular or abnormally heavy bleeding patterns should raise suspicion for endometrial carcinoma.

Answer G is incorrect. The most common symptoms of a vaginal foreign body are malodorous discharge and vaginal bleeding. Vaginal pain or dysuria may also be present.

Answer H is incorrect. Many women with gonococcal infection are asymptomatic. Patients with symptoms may present with vaginal discharge, dyspareunia, and pelvic pain.

Answer I is incorrect. Symptoms of molar pregnancy may include size greater than dates, vaginal bleeding, and unusually high β-hCG concentration for stage of pregnancy. "Snow-storm" on ultrasound and the vaginal passage of small bits of hydatidiform tissue may also be seen.

Answer K is incorrect. In addition to regular bleeding, normal menses may present with mild to moderate lower abdominal pain, mild nausea, loss of appetite, bloating, and mood symptoms.

Answer M is incorrect. Vaginal bleeding or spotting in the presence of pregnancy and a closed cervix is seen with threatened abortion.

Answer N is incorrect. *Trichomonas* infection can be asymptomatic, or patients may present with yellow or green vaginal discharge that is usually profuse.

Answer O is incorrect. Patients with vesico-vaginal fistula present with leakage of urine from the vagina that may be continuous or in-termittent. The patient may complain of in-creased vaginal discharge following pelvic radi-ation or pelvic surgery.

Answer P is incorrect. Vulvar carcinoma may present as a mass, or more commonly as vulvar pruritus. Advanced vulvar cancer may be ac-companied by bleeding, pain, and discharge.

Questions 45 and 46

45. **The correct answer is B.** The bone marrow aspirate is pathognomonic for acute myeloge-nous leukemia (AML) due to the presence of Auer rods. Auer rods, seen in the cytoplasm of leukemic cells, are eosinophilic needle-like in-clusions that are not always seen in AML but that are pathognomonic for myeloid disease. Other characteristics of AML cells include a high nuclear-to-cytoplasmic ratio and open nu-clear chromatin, as seen in the bone marrow aspirate. AML accounts for approximately 20% of childhood leukemias. The presentation can be similar to that of acute lymphoid leukemia, and bone marrow aspirate may be required for diagnosis. When a diagnosis of AML is sus-pected, histochemical stains demonstrating

myeloid enzymes (e.g., peroxidase) may be helpful for diagnosis.

46. **The correct answer is J.** Multiple myeloma is a malignancy of plasma cells. As the atypical malignant cells fill the bone marrow, normal plasma cells and other cell lines are not pro-duced adequately. The result is an increased susceptibility to infection, anemia, and easy bruising. Most patients with newly diagnosed multiple myeloma are older than 50 years but may be as young as 25.

Answer A is incorrect. Acute lymphoid leukemia is characterized by proliferation of immature lymphocytes and is common in chil-dren.

Answer C is incorrect. Burkitt's lymphoma is caused by an 8:14 translocation and is a B-lymphocyte lymphoproliferative disorder.

Answer D is incorrect. Chronic lymphocytic leukemia is characterized by proliferation of nearly mature lymphocytes and is common in persons who are elderly.

Answer E is incorrect. Chronic myelogenous leukemia is characterized by proliferation of nearly mature myeloid cells without eosino-philic inclusions and is common in persons who are elderly.

Answer F is incorrect. Common variable im-munodeficiency is an immunodeficiency of humoral immunity that presents insidiously in persons who are elderly.

Answer G is incorrect. Hodgkin's lymphoma is characterized by Reed-Sternberg cells and mediastinal lymphadenopathy.

Answer H is incorrect. Hyper-IgE syndrome is an immunodeficiency characterized by aller-gies and increased susceptibility to staphylo-coccal infection.

Answer I is incorrect. Hyper-IgM syndrome is caused by a deficiency in B-lymphocyte class switching due to the loss of CD40/CD40L in-teractions.

Answer K is incorrect. Nodular sclerosing lymphoma is a fibrosing form of Hodgkin's lymphoma.

Answer L is incorrect. Osteomyelitis is caused by bacteremia seeding to the bones and may cause lytic lesions.

Answer M is incorrect. Posttransplant lymphoproliferative disease occurs in transplant recipients, likely secondary to immunosuppression.

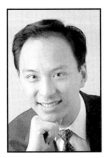

Tao Le, MD, MHS

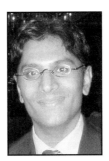

Anil Shivaram, MD

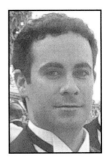

Joshua Klein, MD, PhD

Tao Le, MD, MHS

Tao has been having fun with medical education for the past 15 years. As senior editor, he led the expansion of *First Aid* into a global educational series. In addition, he is the founder and editor-in-chief of the *USMLERx* online test bank series as well as a cofounder of the *Underground Clinical Vignettes* series. As a medical student, he was editor-in-chief of the University of California, San Francisco *Synapse,* a university newspaper with a weekly circulation of 9000. Tao earned his medical degree from the University of California, San Francisco, in 1996 and completed his residency training in internal medicine at Yale University and fellowship training at Johns Hopkins University in allergy and immunology. In addition, he completed an MHS at the Johns Hopkins Bloomberg School of Public Health. At Yale, he was a regular guest lecturer on the USMLE review courses and an adviser to the Yale University School of Medicine curriculum committee. He is currently chief of allergy and immunology in the Department of Medicine at the University of Louisville.

Anil Shivaram, MD

Anil is currently a second-year resident in ophthalmology at Boston Medical Center. He was born and raised in Chicago, Illinois, and attended college at Columbia University, where he majored in Sanskrit. After undergraduate, he went on to pursue graduate studies at Oxford University and then completed a fellowship in medical ethics at the American Medical Association. During medical school at Yale, his thesis research focused on the migration of retinal microglia in inherited retinal degenerative disorders. When he is not in pursuit of things optical, he spends time pampering his wife Lisa, a pediatrician. This is Anil's sixth year working on the *First Aid* series. He can be reached via e-mail at shivaram@aya.yale.edu.

Joshua Klein, MD, PhD

Josh is a graduate of the Medical Scientist Training Program at Yale University School of Medicine. He is originally from Roslyn, New York, and attended the University of Pennsylvania, where he studied biology and music theory. He completed his PhD dissertation in Dr. Stephen Waxman's neurology lab, where he studied activity-dependent modulation of neuronal sodium channel expression. He has authored more than ten journal articles based on his work, and has presented at numerous research conferences. His current research interests are focused on the pathogenesis and neurobiology of epilepsy. Last year, he was selected as an International Student Delegate of the Academy of Achievement. Following a year of internal medicine at Beth Israel Deaconess Medical Center, he is now a resident in neurology at Massachusetts General Hospital and Brigham and Women's Hospital. Josh has been an author and editor on multiple *First Aid* projects over the past six years. He can be contacted at joshua.p.klein@aya.yale.edu.

ABOUT THE EDITORS

Pourya M. Ghazi, MD

Pourya is currently an intern in internal medicine at the San Joaquin General Hospital, University of California in French Camp. He was a senior fellow at the Department of Laboratory Medicine at University of Washington in Seattle. He is planning a career in endocrinology. Pourya earned his medical degree at Beheshti Medical School in Tehran, Iran. He has authored three books and contributed to five books in the *Underground Clinical Vignettes* series. He also contributed to *First Aid Q&A for the USMLE Step 1.* Other interests include history, independent artistic cinema, and traveling.

Jessica Merlin, MD, MBA

Jessica is a resident in internal medicine at the Hospital of the University of Pennsylvania. She is originally from Pittsburgh, Pennsylvania. She is a Phi Beta Kappa graduate of Carnegie Mellon University, where she received a Bachelor of Science degree in biological sciences with an additional major in history and policy. While in medical school at the University of Pennsylvania, she developed an interest in academic medical administration, and as a result, pursued a Masters in Business Administration at the Wharton School. While at Wharton, she co-founded www.md-mba.org <http://www.md-mba.org/>, a website for students interested in the intersection of business and medicine. She also traveled to Botswana, where she both cared for patients and helped design a tuberculosis isolation facility at the country's tertiary care hospital. As a resident, Jesse serves as vice-president of the hospital's housestaff committee. She plans to pursue a career in infectious disease and residency administration. Her research interests include end-of-life care in HIV patients and the financing of hospice programs. She may be reached at jessica.merlin.wg05@wharton.upenn.edu.

Russell J. H. Ryan, MD

Russell is a resident in anatomic and clinical pathology at the Massachusetts General Hospital, and a graduate of the Yale University School of Medicine. He previously contributed to the 2005 edition of *First Aid for the USMLE Step 1*. Russell grew up in Marblehead, Mass. and studied neuroscience as an undergraduate at Amherst College, where he also competed interscholastically in cross-country and track. Following his third year of medical studies, Russell pursued a one-year research fellowship in the laboratory of Dr. Bhuvanesh Singh at the Memorial Sloan-Kettering Cancer Center, where he studied the role of the novel oncoprotein SCCRO in the activation of ubiquitin ligase complexes. He ran his first New York City Marathon in a time he now describes only as "two minutes faster than Lance Armstrong." He is thankful for the support of his family, especially his lovely and talented wife, Honor. He can be reached at Rustavo@gmail.com.

Esteban Schabelman, MD, MBA

Esti is currently an emergency medicine resident at the University of Maryland. In addition to attending medical school at the University of Pennsylvania, he received a Masters of Business Administration degree with dual concentrations in public policy and healthcare management from the Wharton School of Business. During medical school Esti served as the coordinator of Language Link, a program that provides free interpreting services to patients; he was also the founder of a political advocacy class that taught medical students and other health professionals how to identify and campaign for a political goal. In his free time he enjoys traveling, soccer, and brewing his own beer. He hopes to pursue a career that keeps him busy and juggles his interests in emergency medicine and health policy. Esti can be contacted at escha003@umaryland.edu.

Flora Waples, MD

Flora is currently an intern in the University of Chicago emergency medicine program. She began working on First Aid and USMLERx.com projects while she was a second-year medical student at Weill Medical College of Cornell University. Over the last two years she has had the opportunity to be a part of several different projects for both Step 1 and Step 2 as an author, editor, and now as a senior editor. During the generous amount of free time that emergency medicine residents enjoy, Flora runs a small construction/rehab business for distressed real estate, dives, snowboards, works on the family ranch in Montana, and generally attempts to live up to the ER physician ideal of being a shiftless dilettante.

Omeed Zardkoohi, MD

Omeed currently is a resident in internal medicine at Massachusetts General Hospital with an interest in cardiac electrophysiology. In his spare time he enjoys cooking, weight training, and playing classical guitar.

ABOUT THE AUTHORS

J. Geoff Allen, MD
Geoff grew up in Santa Cruz, Calif. with his parents and two younger brothers. After high school, he attended Saint Mary's College of California, graduating summa cum laude with a double major in biology and chemistry. Geoff completed medical school at the Johns Hopkins University School of Medicine, where he was a member of Alpha Omega Alpha and Phi Beta Kappa honor societies. He then stayed on as a general surgery resident. Currently Geoff is undecided as to the subspecialty of general surgery he will choose. Geoff is married to Erin Hamer Allen, who works as a speech pathologist.

Neeti Bathia, MD
As an avid runner and Duke basketball fan (go Blue Devils!), Neeti is pursuing a career in physical medicine and rehabilitation and eventually wants to specialize in sports medicine. She also enjoy reading fiction and living in New York City.

Donald Lee Boyer, MD
Don is a pediatrics resident at The Children's Hospital of Philadelphia and clinical instructor at the University of Pennsylvania. He will complete his training in 2008. Don is originally from Bradford, Pa., and graduated Phi Beta Kappa from Case Western Reserve University with a Bachelor of Arts degree in chemistry. Following college, he attended the University of Pennsylvania College of Medicine, where he was actively involved with admissions interviewing and the campus Christian fellowship. Don plans to pursue a pediatric critical care fellowship and Masters Degree in education and would like to focus on pediatric critical care in an international setting, combining academic medicine with his faith. Don is actively

involved in his local church, where he works with the high school ministry. In his spare time, he enjoys running, biking, rollerblading, downhill skiing, camping, hiking, and just about anything outdoors. Don is a recipient of the Penn Pearls Award for Clinical Teaching.

Arianne Boylan
Arianne is currently a fourth-year medical student at Yale School of Medicine in New Haven. She spent the past year in Dr. Murat Gunel's neurovascular lab looking at molecular mechanisms of cerebral cavernous malformations. She recently contributed to the *First Aid Cases for the USMLE Step 1*. Arianne graduated from Wellesley College in 2002 with Bachelor of Arts degrees in biology and English.

Benjamin Brucker, MD
Benjamin graduated from the University of Pennsylvania School of Medicine in 2005. He is currently a resident at the Hospital of the University of Pennsylvania in the urology department. Prior to his urology residency, he completed a 1-year surgical internship at the Hospital of the University of Pennsylvania. Benjamin is originally from Scarsdale, N.Y., and graduated from Cornell University in 2001 with Bachelor of Science degrees in ecology and evolutionary biology. Though an avid scuba diver and PADI Dive Instructor, Benjamin has given up the warm waters of the Caribbean for the cold waters of cystoscopy. Benjamin would like to thank his wife Elizabeth and his family for all of their support.

Jessica Buckley, MD
Jessica attended the University of California, San Diego, during which time she studied abroad at the Institute for American Universities in Aix-en-Provence, France and at the University of Otago in Dunedin, New Zealand. She graduated summa cum laude with Bachelor of Science degrees in biochemistry and cell biology. After graduation, Jessica spent a year as a staff research associate in the UCSD Department of Biology, which resulted in three publications in peer-reviewed journals. She completed her Medical Doctorate degree as a 21st Century Scholar at the University of Pennsylvania in Philadelphia. Currently she is a licensed pediatrics resident at the University of California, San Francisco.

Kerry Case, MD
Kerry's interest in medical education began as a senior undergraduate student at the University of Wisconsin when she led MCAT preparation classes. After graduating with a Bachelor of Science degree in Zoology in 2000, she attended the Rosalind Franklin University of Medicine and Science, from which she received her Master of Science degree in applied physiology in 2001 and her Medical Doctorate degree in 2005. Currently a family medicine resident in her hometown, Kerry enjoys blogging, biographies, and spending time with her husband and daughter. She plans a broad-based primary care career with an emphasis on mentoring and education, and thanks her family and friends for their support.

Connie Youhua Chang, MD
Connie was born in Boston, where she fell in love with rollerblading. After college, she took a year off to spend some time with the Christian organization Youth With a Mission (YWAM), and she went to Mongolia with them. Later in the year she explored the hospital system in Taiwan through Massachusetts Institute of Technology's International Science and Technology Initiative program while volunteer teaching English with YWAM and learning Chinese calligraphy. She has grown to love New York City in the past 5 years, and enjoys going to musicals, visiting the Met, and biking. However, she also looks forward to joining her family in Boston next year for the rest of her residency.

Kimberly S. Chhor, MD
Kimberly graduated from medical school in 2005 from Johns Hopkins University School of Medicine. She is now in her second year as a resident in orthopedic surgery in the New York University-Hospital for Joint Diseases program.

Alana Cohen, MD
Alana grew up in New York with her parents and older sister. After attending Benjamin N. Cardozo High School, she attended the University of Pennsylvania, graduating magna cum laude with Bachelor of Arts degrees in the biological basis of behavior as well as Spanish. She then completed medical school, also at the University of Pennsylvania. She is currently a second-year resident in internal medicine at Columbia Presbyterian Hospital, and has recently been published in the *American Journal of Medicine* for research within the subspecialty of infectious diseases.

Melinda Costa, MD
Melinda is a graduate of the University of Pennsylvania. Currently she is a resident in plastic and reconstructive surgery at the University of Southern California.

Monya De, MD
Monya graduated from Stanford University with honors in human biology and from the University of California, Irvine School of Medicine with special distinction in the arts and humanities. She is currently pursuing graduate study in public health at the University of California, Berkeley. She has written for *Virtual Mentor*, *The Economist*, *The Stanford Daily*, and the *New Physician*, and has had a column in the Stanford alumni magazine since 2000.

Steven Dong, MD
Steven graduated from Weill Medical College of Cornell University in 2006, and he is currently a urology resident at Thomas Jefferson University Hospital in Philadelphia.

Daniel J. Durand, MD
Dan grew up on Long Island and attended Wake Forest University prior to earning his doctorate degree from Johns Hopkins. After completing the Osler internship at Hopkins, he will stay on as a resident within the department of radiology. Some of his interests include molecular imaging, cell therapy, and medical informatics.

Trevor Ellison, MD
Trevor is currently a general surgery resident at Johns Hopkins Hospital with interests ranging from pediatric surgery to cardiac surgery. He plans on being involved in medical instrument development during the research years of his residency. His other interests include international medical work, learning foreign languages, and medical education. Trevor attended Brigham Young University, where he earned his Bachelor of Science degree before moving to Baltimore to attend the Johns Hopkins School of Medicine. Trevor is from a family of five siblings, and his parents and two sisters currently reside in Maine.

Douglas Elwood, MD, MBA
Douglas completed his undergraduate training at Amherst College, where he majored in English and wrote his thesis on James Joyce. He then attended Jefferson Medical College, earning a combined MD/MBA degree and publishing research on physician-owned practices. An active writer, he co-founded a literary magazine at Jefferson and has short stories appearing in the *American Medical Student Association* journal. He continues to stay involved in the business side of medicine while completing his residency at New York University Medical Center, publishing on major policy issues affecting his field of physical medicine and rehabilitation and interning at a healthcare financial firm.

Victor Ikechukwu Esenwa, MD
Victor grew up in Nigeria and moved to the United States at the age of 15. He went to Stony Brook University and received a Bachelor of Science degree in biochemistry. In 2002, Victor was accepted to Weill Medical College of Cornell University and received his Medical Doctorate degree in 2006. He is now working as an intern resident at New York Hospital in Queens. Victor plans to continue his training in the radiology program at New York Presbyterian Hospital.

Payam Farjoodi, MD
Payam is originally from Los Angeles and was raised in the San Fernando Valley. He attended the University of California-Los Angeles, where he received his Bachelor of Science degree in biochemistry. Payam left California to study medicine at the Johns Hopkins University School of Medicine, from which he graduated in 2005. Currently Payam is a second-year resident in orthopedic surgery at the Johns Hopkins Hospital in Baltimore. He enjoys travel and sports.

Jorge Galvez, MD
Jorge is a 2006 graduate of the Yale University School of Medicine. He is currently completing a preliminary internship in the Yale primary care program, after which he will continue to the Yale anesthesiology residency program. He completed his undergraduate education at the University of Miami in Coral Gables, Fla.

Jesse A. Goldstein, MD
Jesse graduated from the University of Pennsylvania in 2000 with a degree in English and attended the School of Medicine. During his time at Penn Med, he was granted a Doris Duke Clinical Research Fellowship to spend a year studying health policy and economics. His current research interests include surgical outcomes research and quality of life.

Renu Gupta, MD
Renu is currently a resident in psychiatry at the University of Illinois-Chicago. Prior to medical school she had been a doctoral student in psychology at Loyola University of Chicago. Her interests include women's mental health and international psychiatry/public health. She has also completed a certificate in medical writing and editing from the University of Chicago. Her hobbies include writing, travel, cooking, and spending time with her family.

Alia Hbeib, MD
Alia was born and grew up in Bucharest, Romania. In 1992, Alia moved to the United States to join her parents who had moved here three years prior. Alia attended high school and college in Beckley, West Va. In 2001, Alia started medical school at Johns Hopkins in Baltimore. From a very early age Alia became interested in neurosurgery. During medical school, she decided to further pursue that interest by spending a year conducting research, concentrating on studying brain and spinal cord tumors in a neurosurgical laboratory at

Johns Hopkins. In 2006 Alia earned her medical degree and started neurosurgery residency at the Case Western School of Medicine/University Hospitals of Cleveland program in Cleveland, Ohio. Aside from medicine, Alia enjoys art and sports.

Peter W. Henderson, MD
Peter is a native of Seattle, and after graduating from Harvard University in 2002, he attended Weill Medical College of Cornell University until graduation in 2006. He is currently in residency in the general surgery program at the Cornell campus of New York Presbyterian Hospital in New York City.

Daniel Jamieson, MD
Daniel received his Bachelor of Arts degree in psychology from Wesleyan University in 1999. He graduated from Weill Medical College of Cornell University in 2006. He is currently a resident in internal medicine at the University of Colorado in Denver, and plans to pursue a career in pulmonary and critical care medicine.

Phoebe Este Koch, MD
Phoebe is a 1998 graduate of Brown University. She recently received her Medical Doctorate degree from Yale University School of Medicine, and began a residency in dermatology here in June 2007. In addition to studying medicine, Phoebe likes to spend time in the outdoors with her partner Timmy and 1-year-old son Oak.

Cindy Man-Yan Ku, MD
Cindy is currently an intern at New York Hospital Medical Center of Queens and will begin her training in anesthesiology at Beth Israel Deaconess Medical Center in Boston in July 2007. A native of Hong Kong, Cindy received a Bachelor of Science degree from the Massachusetts Institute of Technology and earned her medical degree from Weill Medical College of Cornell University. During her free time Cindy can be seen cooking for friends, enjoying the city's offerings such as theater and museums, and catching up with friends and family across the globe.

Erica Lee, MD
Erica was born in Ann Arbor, Mich. She completed her undergraduate studies at the Massachusetts Institute of Technology and graduated with a major in biology and minor in anthropology. She is currently a transitional intern at Albert Einstein College of Medicine.

Jason David Lee, MD
Jason received his undergraduate degree in molecular, cellular, and developmental biology from Yale University, and a Doctor of Medicine degree from Weill Medical College of Cornell University. He is currently serving his residency in pediatrics at the Harbor-UCLA Medical Center in Torrance.

David M. Lieberman, MD
David recently completed his medical school training at the Weill Medical College of Cornell University in New York City. He completed his undergraduate education at Stanford University, receiving a Bachelor of Science degree in human biology with a focus in neuroscience. He has returned to Stanford as a resident in otolaryngology-head and neck surgery. Additional interests include international medicine, hiking, running, and movies.

Emily Nelson Maher, MD
Emily is a Virginia native. She received her Bachelor of Science degree in biology with a minor in creative writing at the University of North Carolina at Chapel Hill, where she was a Morehead scholar. She then attended medical school at Johns Hopkins University, completed an internal medicine internship at Brigham and Women's Hospital, and is now an anesthesiology resident at Brigham and Women's Hospital. She currently resides in Brookline, Mass., with her husband Todd.

Nicholas Mahoney, MD
Nick graduated from the University of Pennsylvania School of Medicine and is training in ophthalmology at the Scheie Eye Institute.

Tzivia Moreen, MD
Originally from New Jersey, Tzivia went to medical school at Weill Medical College of Cornell University and stayed for her residency in internal medicine. Tzivia now lives in New York with her husband and daughter, where she is hoping to pursue a career in primary care/geriatrics.

Ikechi John Nwankwo MD
Ikechi is American born, but Nigerian raised. He attended college at the University of San Francisco and also completed research at Merck Pharmaceuticals. He studied abroad in Keble College in Oxford, England. Ikechi attended medical school at Johns Hopkins and he completed an internship at Sinai Hospital in Baltimore. He is in residency at St. Vincent's Hospital in New York. Ikechi's interests include the advancement of radiology as a field through research, all competitive team sports (especially soccer and basketball), paintball, rock climbing, and drawing with charcoal.

Eleanor Pitt, MD
Eleanor grew up in Louisville, Kentucky, but much to her chagrin she doesn't have even the slightest bit of a southern accent. She spent some time in Pennsylvania for college, lived in Washington, D.C. for a year, and then moved north to take up residency in the quirky city of Baltimore. In addition to work on this study guide while in medical school at Johns Hopkins, she did some research in HIV, put up with some interesting roommates, and played in a bar trivia league for beer money. She's currently back in the south, working as a lowly intern in internal medicine residency at Vanderbilt University in Nashville.

Hindi E. Stohl Posy, MD
Hindi graduated cum laude from Columbia College, where she earned a double concentration in economics and pre-medical studies. She completed her medical school training at the University of Pennsylvania School of Medicine, where she graduated with honors in obstetrics and gynecology. She has led numerous community service initiatives in the United States and abroad and is currently a resident at Johns Hopkins University in the department of obstetrics and gynecology.

Siva P. Raman, MD
After graduating from the University of Southern California with a degree in psychobiology, Siva graduated from the Johns Hopkins School of Medicine. Siva is currently a resident in radiology at the University of Washington. In his spare time he enjoys traveling abroad, reading fiction, and spending time with his family.

Sarah Schellhorn, MD
Sarah is a resident at Beth Israel Deaconess Medical Center. She graduated in May 2006 from Weill Medical College of Cornell University. She graduated magna cum laude from Harvard University in 2000 with a Bachelor of Arts degree in biochemical sciences. In her spare time, you can find her knitting, playing poker, or rooting for her beloved Boston Red Sox—sometimes all at the same time.

Lindsey Sukay, MD
Lindsey is currently a pediatric resident at The Children's Hospital in Denver and has special research interests in neonatology and pain management. To relieve the stress of studying for the boards, she loves to run, hike, play Frisbee with her dog, and spend time with her family and friends.

Mathew A. Thomas, MD
Mathew was born and raised in Bradenton, Fla., with three brothers (George, Joe, and Jacob). His father is a practicing cardiologist and founder of the Bradenton Cardiology group. Currently Mathew is in the second year of the plastic surgery training program at Harvard with a preliminary interest in reconstructive microsurgery.

ABOUT THE ASSOCIATE AUTHORS

Anna Awdankiewicz, MD

Anna grew up in Warsaw, Poland, and came to the United States at the age of 18. She completed her undergraduate education at the State University of New York at Stony Brook, where she earned a Bachelor of Science degree in biochemistry. In 2006 she graduated from Weill Medical College of Cornell University. She is currently a resident at Vanderbilt Medical Center, where she pursues interests in pulmonary and critical care medicine.

Ravi Kant Bashyal, MD

Ravi grew up just outside Chicago in the town of Oak Park. As an undergraduate, he attended the University of Illinois at Urbana-Champaign, and conducted life science research during the summers with the National Aeronautics and Space Administration at the Kennedy Space Center in Cape Canaveral, Fla. Soon after graduation, he earned his private pilots license and continues to pursue his interest in aviation. Ravi attended medical school at the University of Pennsylvania, where he was the recipient of the Ernest Scholarship awarded to an outstanding student entering the field of orthopedic surgery. He is currently a resident in orthopedic surgery at Barnes-Jewish Hospital, Washington University School of Medicine in Saint Louis. Ravi would like to thank his parents for all the support and assistance they have given him throughout his academic career.

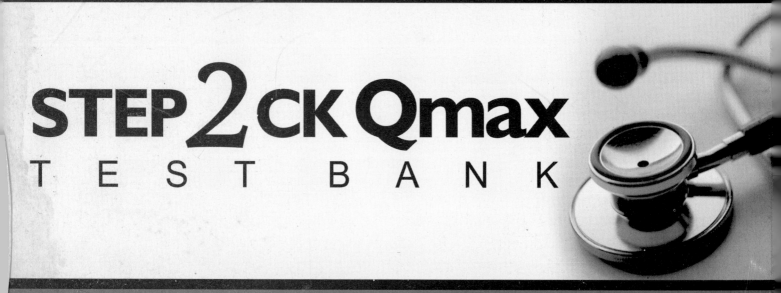